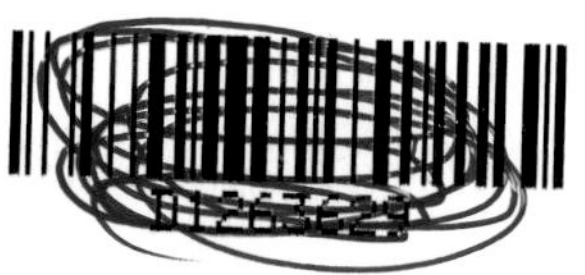

The Malalignment Syndrome

Diagnosing and treating a common cause of acute and chronic pelvic, limb and back pain

DEDICATION

Dedicated to the memory of Jan Boyd (1950–2008)

A physiotherapist, renowned as a manual therapist, who believed in teaching professionals and patients how to recognize and treat malalignment.

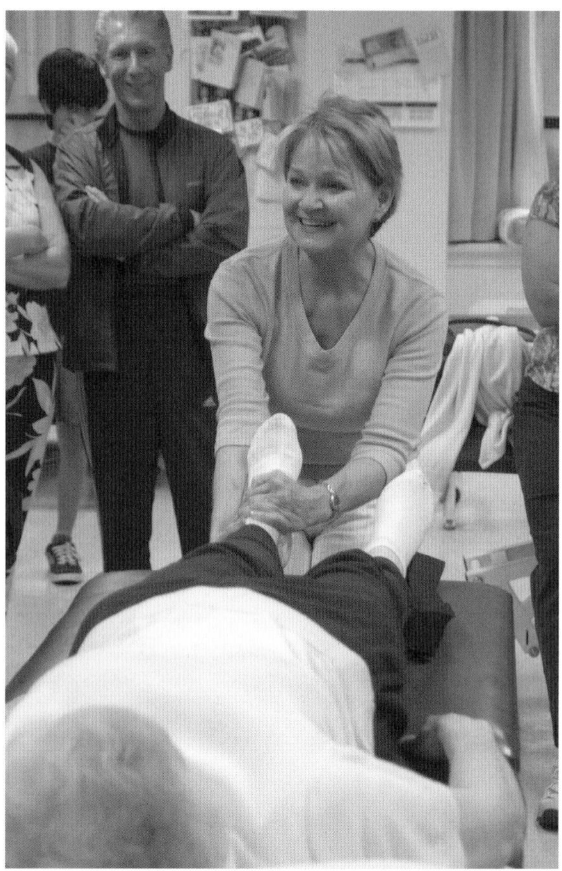

Content Strategist: Rita Demetriou-Swanick
Content Development Specialist: Carole McMurray
Senior Project Manager: Beula Christopher
Designer: Kirsteen Wright/Alan Studholme
Illustration Manager: Merlyn Harvey/Jennifer Rose

The Malalignment Syndrome

Diagnosing and treating a common cause of acute and chronic pelvic, limb and back pain

Wolf Schamberger MD FRCP (C) Dip Sports Med
Clinical Associate Professor, Department of Medicine, Division of Physical Medicine and Rehabilitation, and The Allan McGavin Sports Medicine Centre, University of British Columbia, Vancouver, Canada

With contributions by
David Lane DVM **and Lauren Fraser** (riding instructor)
Chapter 6: Horses, Saddles and Riders

Sarah Stevens BScPT, CAFCI, RCAMT (hons) **and**
Karina Steinberg BScPT, FCAMT, CAFCI, CGIMS
Chapter 8: Treatment: the Manual Therapy Modes

Foreword by
Dr. Jack Taunton BSc, MSc, MD, Dip Sports Med
Professor, Deptartment of Family Practice/Human Kinetics; Director, The Allan McGavin Sports Medicine Centre; Faculty of Medicine and School of Human Kinetics, University of British Columbia, Vancouver, Canada

CHURCHILL LIVINGSTONE

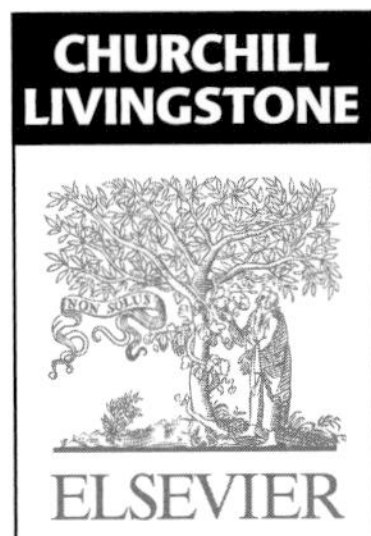

Edinburgh London New York Oxford Philadelphia St Louis Sydney Toronto 2013

CHURCHILL
LIVINGSTONE
ELSEVIER

First edition 2002
Second edition 2013

ISBN 9780443069291

British Library Cataloguing in Publication Data
A catalogue record for this book is available from the British Library

Library of Congress Cataloging in Publication Data
A catalog record for this book is available from the Library of Congress

Notices
Knowledge and best practice in this field are constantly changing. As new research and experience broaden our understanding, changes in research methods, professional practices, or medical treatment may become necessary.

Practitioners and researchers must always rely on their own experience and knowledge in evaluating and using any information, methods, compounds, or experiments described herein. In using such information or methods they should be mindful of their own safety and the safety of others, including parties for whom they have a professional responsibility.

With respect to any drug or pharmaceutical products identified, readers are advised to check the most current information provided (i) on procedures featured or (ii) by the manufacturer of each product to be administered, to verify the recommended dose or formula, the method and duration of administration, and contraindications. It is the responsibility of practitioners, relying on their own experience and knowledge of their patients, to make diagnoses, to determine dosages and the best treatment for each individual patient, and to take all appropriate safety precautions.

To the fullest extent of the law, neither the Publisher nor the authors, contributors, or editors, assume any liability for any injury and/or damage to persons or property as a matter of products liability, negligence or otherwise, or from any use or operation of any methods, products, instructions, or ideas contained in the material herein.

Printed in China

Contents

Foreword

It is an honour to write this Foreword for Dr. Wolf Schamberger's 2nd edition of 'The Malalignment Syndrome'.

I have known Dr. Schamberger for a long time, as an excellent marathon runner and sport and physical medicine/rehabilitation physician. He has always had a passion to educate the clinicians and therapists on the diagnosis and management of the malalignment syndrome. The 1st edition was an attempt to make medical doctors aware that being out of alignment does occur and is the cause of local/referred symptoms in over 60% of the people they see 'out of alignment'.

Dr. Schamberger has added over 90 new illustrations and has redrawn a number of the previous illustrations to make the clinical examination and management easier. He has updated this new edition with the developments of the last 10 years. His new approaches to the one- or two-person assessment and treatment are excellent. With his rewriting, the three most common presentations can be very easily recognized and treated. The one-person assessment more easily allows the individual to maintain day-to-day alignment.

Dr. Schamberger felt the title of the 1st edition - 'The Malalignment Syndrome: Implications for Medicine and Sport' - may have misled physicians, physiotherapists and manual therapists. This new edition speaks about 'persons' and 'patients', not just 'athletes', as the syndrome is so common. Hence, the new title - 'The Malalignment Syndrome: Diagnosing and treating a common cause of acute and chronic pelvic, limb and back pain'. He emphasizes that 50-60% of low back pain is associated with malalignment.

This edition has gone a long way in giving physicians and therapists the tools to be able to treat common presentations and typical symptom patterns. It offers new updated material in two excellent chapters with new authors. 'Horses, saddles and riders' (Ch. 6) is written by Dr. David Lane, veterinarian and chiropractor, and Lauren Fraser, riding instructor, on malalignment of the rider and of the horse, including assessment of horse anatomy and gait. Chapter 8 is a very useful review by physiotherapists Sarah Stevens and Karina Steinberg of manual therapy models and complementary techniques, including intramuscular stimulation, trigger point injection, active release, yoga, Pilates and Rolfing.

This new edition is a must for those in the medical field who deal with musculoskeletal problems, particularly sports physicians, physiatrists, rheumatologists, orthopaedic surgeons and neurologists. It should prove an asset for those already practicing or going through training involving manual medicine, chiropractors, osteopaths, physiotherapists, manual therapists, kinesiologists and athletic trainers. It has taken a lot of the mystique out of the malalignment terminology, presentation and treatment which will hopefully make it more readily understood and accepted as another approach available for helping people, both in the clinic and on the field.

Dr. Jack Taunton
Vancouver 2012

Acknowledgements

My thanks go out to those in my life who made it possible to commit myself to writing the 2nd edition. Foremost, to Alison, for always being there to answer 'those questions' about grammar, spelling and other vagaries of the English language to allow me to best express a thought, for respecting my endless hours 'away' in the study, but assuring there was 'time out' by regularly taking my 'little gray cells' to the theatre and other venues to allow them to 'rest and recover'. Also, to Eva, for all those hours spent lying at my feet, tolerating repeats of Beethoven, Chopin, Mozart and a host of other musicians unknown to dogs, while waiting patiently to take me for a walk, with similar beneficial effects for both of us. My colleague and friend, Jan Boyd, helped me complete a video on the topic, produced her own on how to do 'Alignment' exercises correctly in 2005 and was set to rewrite Chapter 8 when she passed away unexpectedly in 2008. Her cheerful personality, her ability to engage patients in their specific treatment protocol (both in the clinic and at home) and her contributions to the clinical and teaching scene have been sadly missed. Thankfully, Sarah Stevens and Karina Steinberg together were able to provide the new version of that chapter. Similarly, Dr. David Lane and Lauren Fraser were able to pool their extensive resources, working with horses and riders both from the clinical and practical side, to provide a welcome revision of the original Chapter 6 written by Cynthia Webster PT. The excellent additional drawings by Jeff MacDonald-Bain and photographs by Michael Noon should help clarify points made in the text. Alison, Alastair McKenzie, Jerred Friday and Kerrie Elchuk (at that time still very obviously carrying my soon-to-be grandson, Mateo) were kind enough to serve as models. During the past year, my friend Terry Treasure has suffered through hours of hearing about malalignment, the ups and downs of getting the book ready, and deadlines slipping by as we hiked the local trails; it is largely thanks to his encouragement, computer savvy and willingness to help me out through many a crisis (that might have otherwise ended with me for once carrying out my repeated threats to throw the laptop out of the window) that I was able to forge ahead with the proofs over this past year. Again, I am indebted to the staff of the Allan McGavin Sports Medicine Centre (University of BC) - in particular, Drs. Jack Taunton, Douglas Clement, Rob Lloyd-Smith and Don McKenzie - for their ongoing support dating back to the early years of my endeavours to define the abnormal biomechanics of malalignment and their clinical importance. My thanks also to Drs. Charles Cass, David Evans, Peter Golpin, Danika Olenick, Richard Sweeting, Andrew Travlos and Heather Underwood, who provided feedback from a medical perspective, and my friends Maureen Baker, Lora Finan, Colleen Shook, son Anton and daughter Iona for their critical reviews of the text. Finally, I am grateful to the staff at Elsevier who were involved in helping bring about the publication of the 2nd edition. In particular, to Sarena Wolfaard, senior commissioning editor (who in 1997 encouraged me to proceed with writing the 1st and, subsequently, this edition) and to Carole McMurray, Content Development Specialist (who so efficiently supervised this project over the past three years).

Introduction 2012

In my introduction to the 1st edition, I indicated that my aim in writing the book was to create an awareness of malalignment, the 'malalignment syndrome' and the problems that these can cause (see 'Introduction – 2002'). The book was intended particularly for those practising medicine, whose education even to date rarely includes the recognition of common presentations of malalignment and appropriate treatment techniques. In that regard, the book has been successful to some extent. In my own referral practice, I have become increasingly aware of the number of physicians who have attended workshops and who, subsequently, on the basis of their modified examination approach, came to:

1. realize that malalignment was actually evident, or
2. suspect an underlying alignment problem was at the root of their patient's problem, especially when all standard examinations and investigations were negative and other treatment attempts had failed.

Teaching continues to make the greatest impact on medical students, interns and residents, who are not yet set in their ways of looking at the patient. Also, there have been more requests to present on the topic and conduct workshops at medical meetings.

However, it was also a pleasant surprise to see from the reviews and subsequent feedback how well the book had been received by professional groups that already deal, to varying extent, with alignment-related problems. For some - particularly those physiotherapists, massage therapists, kinesiologists and athletic trainers who had not yet had any formal training in the area - it was a matter of learning more about something they knew they could readily apply to benefit their clients. For others - particularly osteopaths, chiropractors and physiotherapists trained in manipulation and/or manual therapy - the book appeared to bring together some of the basics taught during their initial training. Subsequently, most of these groups seem to have undergone a 'division within', so to speak, as members began to ascribe to different theoretical and treatment approaches: NUCCA, high- or low-velocity manipulation, acupressure, IMS, Mackenzie technique, to name a few. Unfortunately, these divisions have, in some settings, let to outright separation from, and often intolerance of, others within the original group. It appears that the book had managed to present a number of basic ideas that at one time unified them but that seemed to have been forgotten as these 'specialized' sub-groups evolved.

Unfortunately, the title of the 1st edition and the fact that I referred to 'athletes' throughout the text, misled some into thinking that the book was aimed primarily at those practising sports medicine. Hence the change to the present title and reference in the text to a 'person', 'patient' or 'athlete', as appropriate.

The years since the 1st edition appeared have seen publications and ongoing research that have led to some changes in our perception of how the lumbo-pelvic-hip complex functions to cope with its challenging tasks, the prime ones being load transfer in standing or allowing movement of the trunk and the lower limbs while maintaining stability. There has been further confirmation of many of the original ideas (e.g. concepts of 'form' and 'force' closure), while some more recent thoughts have become increasingly evident from studies (e.g. the hypo- or hypermobile SI joints are more likely to be symptomatic if the 'abnormal' mobility is asymmetrical). The research in this area is carried out more and more by interdisciplinary teams and results of their studies have frequently been published in *Spine, BMJ* and other reputable medical journals. In addition to the increasing number of books published on the topic in recent years, education both for professionals and laymen has also been improved the provision of DVDs (e.g.: DG Lee 1998, 2011, L-J Lee 2004b, W Schamberger 2003, J Boyd 2005) and the publication of new journals, including 'International Musculoskeletal Medicine' and the 'Journal of Prolotherapy'.

Writing this second edition was initially discussed in 2006. In retrospect, the delay has been of benefit in terms of:

1. providing further confirmation of the value of applying the basics of diagnosis and treatment of malalignment to clinical practice
2. finding ways to simplify teaching as regards recognition of the common presentations of malalignment and the 'malalignment syndrome'
3. incorporating recent advances in research looking particularly at the lumbo-pelvic-hip complex.

Clinical experience, practice, publications and courses continue to emphasize that:

1. malalignment is present in some 80% of the population and is the prime cause and/or an aggravating factor in 50-60% of those presenting with back pain
2. recognition of sacral and vertebral rotational displacement, the 3 common presentations of pelvic malalignment and the manifestations of the 'malalignment syndrome' can make a major difference in helping establish the diagnosis and deciding on the appropriate course of treatment in the case of a person suffering from problems related to these
3. treatment measures capable of decreasing or temporarily abolishing pain and tension (e.g. acupuncture, massage, medication) but which fail to eliminate the root cause of the problem (in this case, the malalignment) are inadequate. However, compensatory treatment measures such as these must always be considered as adjuncts to manual therapy as they may be able to resolve any residual pain, increase in tension or muscle spasm to help the person finally achieve and maintain alignment
4. realignment is an essential step in the initial treatment of someone presenting with symptoms that can be attributed to malalignment. However, while realignment can sometimes have a dramatic effect in terms of relieving symptoms, the key to achieving a lasting cure is a supervised, progressive course of treatment based on strengthening of the core muscles to re-establish stability of the pelvis and spine, maintaining alignment from one day to the next, regaining cardiovascular fitness and concentrating on ease and symmetry of movement. The person's success in using this approach is improved by education and involvement in a self-assessment, self-treatment and home exercise programme to help them achieve and maintain the alignment between scheduled treatment sessions, improve their day-to-day comfort, speed up their recovery or simply prevent them from becoming symptomatic or suffering a needless injury in the first place. Maintaining symmetry as much as possible while carrying out daily activities is another key to preventing recurrences of malalignment.

Those physicians who still ignore the fact that there is such a problem as 'malalignment', or feel there are 'not enough evidence-based' research findings to confirm its presentations, are merely indicating that they are not informed about the subject. Possibly they are caught in a world that did not prepare them to accept changes they should be incorporating into their clinical practice and need to be reminded that a false diagnosis is likely to lead to inappropriate, prolonged and sometimes outright harmful treatment. At the same time, those doing research that involves the biomechanics of the pelvis and lower extremities, but who fail to determine whether or not malalignment is present, are publishing results that should be suspect because they have ignored the fact that the results may have been affected by the asymmetrical biomechanical changes attributable to malalignment. DonTigny (2007: 277) could not have stated it more bluntly:

> *Research of low back pain that does not include the appropriate biomechanics or uses inappropriate biomechanical models will result in inappropriate*

findings, the inappropriate interpretation of evidence, inappropriate treatment and will delay recovery.

Misconceptions concerning malalignment still persist; ones commonly encountered include: 'the SI joint does not move', 'with the bone scan negative, the SI joint is unlikely to be the cause of the pain', 'asymmetry of the pelvis is common and hence not likely to be responsible for the problem at hand'. The solution may be simply to let go of these misconceptions and finally allow the practitioner to get on with learning more about this condition. Practice is so much more enjoyable if one has an understanding of malalignment and, therefore, of one more medical entitity and its manifestations that may help explain a person's presenting complaint(s).

Extensive rewriting and editing, the complete revision of two chapters by new contributing authors and the addition of new sections and over 90 new illustrations should make it easier for the reader to understand the concepts discussed and apply this knowledge to the diagnosis and treatment of those presenting with malalignment. I am able to present some new ways to simplify recognition and treatment approaches for an 'upslip', 'rotational malalignment' and 'outflare/inflare' that have proven invaluable in practice and the workshops. There are also now available 2 DVDs which complement each other and this 2nd edition; they are intended for teaching both professionals and anyone having to deal with the consequences of malalignment:

1. 'The malalignment syndrome: treating a common cause of pelvic, back and leg pain', on the recognition of malalignment, aspects of treatment and modification of specific activities to best avoid recurrences (Schamberger 2003), and
2. 'Alignment: the missing piece of the pelvic puzzle', covering the appropriate way to carry out core strengthening and other exercise programmes aimed at maintaining alignment once achieved (Boyd 2005).

This 2nd edition updates the basics of malalignment and manual therapy treatment using primarily the muscle energy technique. I can only hope that it will be successful in reaching more of those in professions that every day have to deal with the problems typically seen with malalignment and the 'malalignment syndrome': in particular, pelvic, limb and back pain.

Introduction 2002 (1st edition)

At one time, I was a national caliber, 2 hour 20 minute marathon runner. My running career from high school in the 1960s through 39 marathons in the 1970s had been relatively injury free. It was in 1980, following a run on narrow, winding trails, that I first became aware of right heel pain. There had been no obvious injury, no twisting or unexpected jarring. The pain fluctuated in intensity and could be present both on weight-bearing and at rest. Sometimes there was no pain at all; the pain was most likely to recur with running. There was not even temporary improvement with standard physiotherapy, anti-inflammatory medication, acupuncture and a lift for a right leg supposedly shorter than the left.

The tendency to pronation was so pronounced on the right side that the heel cup of a racing flat or lighter running shoe would start to collapse noticeably inward on the right within 3 or 4 weeks (Fig. I.1). Orthotics with a 4 degree medial raise on the right failed to control this marked pronation. An injection of local anaesthetic around the heel did not provide even short-term relief. The pain impaired heel-strike and push-off and with time resulted in a noticeable wasting of the entire right leg. With runs of 10 miles or more, the right thigh muscles - particularly the quadriceps - would ache as with overuse, similar to how the leg muscles usually felt just after having completed a marathon.

In 1987, 7 years after the onset of the pain, I attended the annual meeting of the American Association of Orthopedic Medicine in Montreal. One speaker projected a drawing of patterns of pain and/or paraesthesias referred from the sacrotuberous and sacrospinous ligaments, as delineated by Hackett (1958) with hypertonic saline injections (Fig. I.2). It was the circle around the heel that caught my eye - I wondered whether my pain could be on the basis of referral from these more proximal structures. That would explain why the injection around the right heel had failed to affect the pain.

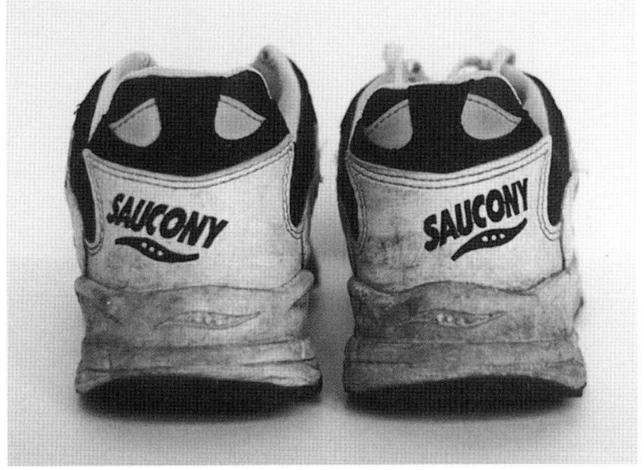

Fig. I.1 Heel cup collapse, inward on the right and outward on the left running shoe, reflecting a malalignment-related tendency to right pronation and left supination, respectively.

My suspicions were confirmed at a workshop that afternoon. One of the instructors, an osteopath, noted that I was out of alignment: my right innominate bone was rotated anteriorly relative to the sacrum. He proceeded with correction using a gentle muscle energy technique (MET), described in detail in Chapter 7 (Figs 7.8–7.15). Basically, I lay supine and he offered resistance to my attempts to extend my flexed right thigh. This MET in effect reversed the origin and insertion of the right gluteus

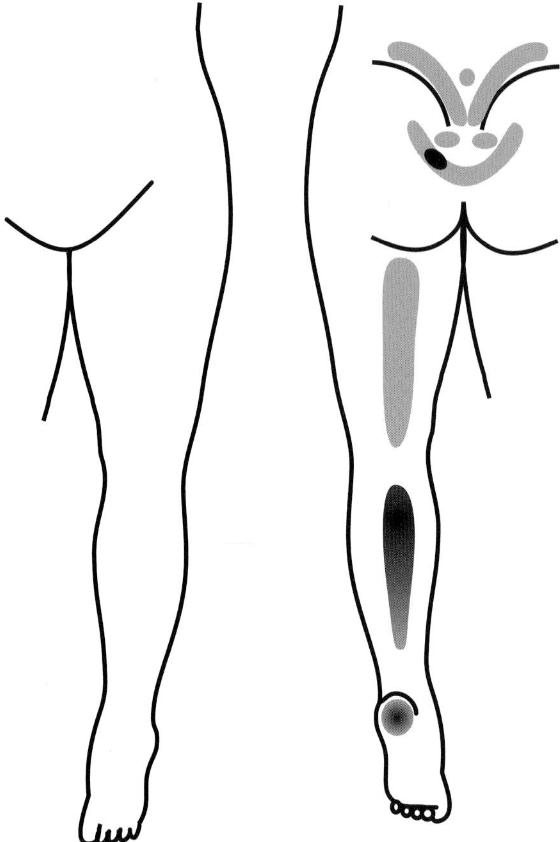
Fig. I.2 Referred pain - sacrospinous and sacrotuberous ligaments (sacroiliac joint instability). *(After Hackett 1958.)*

maximus, resulting in posterior traction and rotation of the right innominate.

The manoeuvre, simple as it may seem, was successful; better still, my heel pain disappeared immediately on realignment. However, on stepping back into my shoes I felt awkward: the right side of my pelvis now seemed higher than the left. Then I remembered the lift incorporated into the right orthotic for the 'shorter' right leg. After removing the orthotics, the pelvis felt level again. The best part was yet to come. I went for a 12 mile run later that day and, for the first time in years, came back without the ache in my right thigh muscles. Within 3 months, the muscle bulk on the right leg had increased to match that on the left. I continued to do the MET daily. Over the next 4 years, I occasionally went out of alignment, usually as a result of some asymmetrical activity such as hiking or climbing. Eventually, I came to recognize these recurrences just from the fact that my gait pattern felt different, with my right foot not only pronating excessively but also pointing outward from midline more than the left. If I delayed correction, the right heel pain would come back within 24 hours. Much less often, I would switch sides: the left innominate rotating forward and the right backward, with associated pain from the left posterior pelvic ligaments.

In addition, although recurrence of this 'rotational malalignment' decreased gradually over the years, and correction was usually fairly immediate, my shoes continued to collapse in the same pattern: right inward, left outward. It was not until more recently that I realized this problem was attributable to a recurrent left 'outflare' and right 'inflare' (see Figs 2.13, 7.21), causing the pelvis and the legs to rotate. Barring the occasional recurrence, which I can usually correct easily on my own, I am now staying in alignment more or less continuously.

The months following the meeting in Montreal stand out as the most exciting in my years of medical practice as I gradually became aware of the other changes that occurred with malalignment. I began to piece together the biomechanics, symptoms and signs that constitute what I now call the 'malalignment syndrome'. Probably foremost was the awareness that my right leg was no longer rotated outward and that I was no longer pronating with my right foot; in fact, I have turned out to be a supinator.

People presenting with malalignment were noted to show consistent patterns of asymmetry involving muscle function, weight–bearing and ranges of motion in particular. Eventually, knowledge of a certain presentation of malalignment allowed for the prediction of the associated pattern of asymmetry and vice versa. In addition, the specific changes could be related to specific problems with which the person presented. Even more important was the recognition that simply correcting the malalignment was often adequate treatment for problems that had evaded cure for months, sometimes years, using standard therapy approaches. This aspect has now been corroborated by my clinical experience and the studies presented here.

The concept of malalignment often evokes feelings of anxiety in those not familiar with the terminology and the examination techniques. The reader has to realize that, like anything else practiced by any one group to the exclusion of all else, the subject can appear more difficult than it really need be to someone looking in from the outside. I myself had arrived at the scene by accident and from the feet up, so to speak, rather than through one of the traditional approaches (e.g. chiropractic or osteopathic) that teaches a detailed examination of the alignment of the various parts of the pelvis and spine. In the intervening period, I have learned some of these more detailed assessments and have obtained more training in manual therapy techniques. This additional knowledge has repeatedly emphasized the fact that the initial assessment should always establish whether or not malalignment is one of the problems one may be dealing with and, as I will try to show in this book, that is usually not a complicated matter.

I recognize that the majority of the readers are, like myself, primarily interested in being able to establish whether malalignment is present, and whether it might be the cause of the person's complaints, in which case they can then refer him or her to someone who has the skill to correct it. I have tried to provide an easy method for determining the presence of malalignment. To this end, I have limited discussion to the four most common, and usually treatable, presentations: vertebral rotational displacement, 'rotational malalignment', sacroiliac joint 'upslip' and 'outflare/inflare'.

I am also a strong believer that the more people can do for themselves, the better their chances of recovery. I look at the therapist as doing the 'fine tuning'; whereas those afflicted need to get involved in their day-to-day treatment to help maintain alignment between visits. It is important that they learn to recognize any recurrence of malalignment; the sooner they do, the sooner they can get on with self-correction manoeuvres and/or seek help. A spouse or friend can easily be taught how to help with the assessment, although most people will quickly learn how to do this on their own - they themselves can usually carry out some of the techniques that may correct the malalignment or, failing that, at least achieve partial correction and decrease their discomfort until they can reach their therapist for further treatment. By these means, they can often speed up their recovery and, at the same time, decrease their dependence on the therapist.

Most of them will eventually come to recognize the changes that occur at the time of a recurrence, such as a shift in gait pattern. An earlier recognition of recurrence allows for an earlier initiation of treatment, usually easier correction and often an avoidance of the pain and other problems that are likely to bother the person the longer the malalignment persists.

My intent here is to create an awareness of the 'malalignment syndrome' and the problems it can create in anyone afflicted with it, particularly athletes, who may be more at risk of becoming symptomatic because of the very nature of their sport. If I can get others to start looking at those presenting for help in what may at first seem a completely different way, and hopefully stimulate some research along new lines, then I will have succeeded.

Chapter 1

The malalignment syndrome: A synopsis

CHAPTER CONTENTS

Malalignment of the pelvis and/or spine is present in 80-90% of the adult population and has been held responsible for being the prime cause and/or an aggravating factor in anywhere from 50-60% of those suffering from back pain. While medicine in general continues to be relatively unaware of malalignment, how it presents and what problems it can cause, it is encouraging that over the past decade those involved in sports medicine, rheumatology and some other specialties have become increasingly aware that malalignment:

1. is one of the major causes of back pain and other musculoskeletal complaints, also the fact that it
2. can seemingly mimic or actually cause problems in every organ system (Ch. 4).

Those engaged in physically-demanding work or athletic activities, in particular, are at increased risk of injury to a musculoskeletal system already subjected to abnormal biomechanical forces by the malalignment (Chs 2, 3). These abnormal forces not only predispose to injury but, if they persist, may also impair recovery and return to a work setting or sport; at worse and, in athletes particularly, they may interfere with the person's ability to realize their full potential (Chs 5, 6). In addition, there continues to be a major problem in that much of the research dealing with matters relating to weightbearing, ground reaction forces and muscle strength fails to take into account the biomechanical effects of malalignment. Reports of side-to-side differences in joint ranges of motion or weight-bearing, for example, lack meaning when we do not know whether the person enrolled in a particular study was in alignment or not. Asymmetries in muscle tension and strength may be simply secondary to the presence of malalignment

DOI: 10.1016/B978-0-443-06929-1.00001-6

that, to date, had not been diagnosed and any attempts at stretching and strengthening may prove futile until realignment has been achieved. Similarly, orthotics made while someone is out of alignment will just perpetuate the shift in weight-bearing subsequently, regardless of whether the subject is in or out of alignment, as well as increasing the risk of injury (Ch. 7).

The present chapter will outline:

1. the common presentations of malalignment of the pelvis and spine seen in clinical practice
2. the basic implications of malalignment in terms of altered biomechanics
3. the two presentations - an 'upslip' and 'rotational malalignment' - with which the 'malalignment syndrome' is associated
4. diagnostic features and appropriate treatment measures

While the author does come from an athletic background, and while athletes who are out of alignment admittedly are more at risk of suffering complications with any further increase in activity because of the increased asymmetrical stresses already imposed on the musculoskeletal system, symptoms attributable to malalignment are similar in 'athletes' and 'non-athletes' alike. Also, please note that:

1. those with malalignment evident on examination are not necessarily symptomatic (Ch. 2), and
2. any symptoms reported may not necessarily be linked to the malalignment

There are, therefore, 12 possible combinations relating to alignment that one may encounter in clinical practice, namely:

1. the 'athlete' or 'non-athlete' who presents in alignment and is:
   a. asymptomatic
   b. symptomatic for some other reason (e.g. low back pain attributable to disc degeneration)
2. the 'athlete' or 'non-athlete' who presents with malalignment and is:
   a. asymptomatic
   b. symptomatic as a result of the malalignment
   c. symptomatic as a result of causes other than the malalignment
   d. symptomatic as a result of a combination of problems, not all of which are attributable to the malalignment (see Ch. 4: 'Implications for cardiology')

Reference, therefore, will henceforth be to a symptomatic or asymptomatic person presenting with malalignment, with the understanding that most of the material discussed applies to the 'athletic', 'non-athletic' and patient populations, unless specifically indicated otherwise; whereas:

1. Chapter 4 addresses particular pain phenomena caused by malalignment, also malalignment-related symptoms and signs that may confuse physicians dealing with patients in certain medical and surgical specialties
2. Chapters 5 and 6 address aspects of malalignment that can cause problems for athletes in specific sports

MALALIGNMENT AND TRADITIONAL THINKING

Malalignment has traditionally been thought of in terms of involvement of the pelvis and spine.

1. One or more vertebrae may show excessive rotation, or rotational displacement, relative to the vertebra(e) immediately above and/or below (or the sacrum, in the case of L5). Barring a traumatic cause, this asynchrony of vertebrae:
   a. may have been caused by the pelvic malalignment, or
   b. may actually have been responsible for occurrence of the pelvic malalignment (Fig. 2.52).
2. While there are numerous presentations of pelvic malalignment, three are particularly prevalent and together account for somewhere from 80-90% of those presenting with malalignment in a practice dealing primarily with neuromusculoskeletal problems, also defined as 'orthopaedic medicine' (Box 1.1). Their specific axes and planes of movement are noted in Figure 2.9.

BOX 1.1 Three common presentations of pelvic malalignment

'Rotational malalignment'
'Anterior' or 'posterior' rotation of an innominate relative to the sacrum, referring to the direction of movement around the coronal axis, in the sagittal plane (Figs 2.9, 2.10A, 2.42, 2.76)

An 'upslip' of the sacroiliac joint
Direct upward translation of an innominate relative to the sacrum, in the vertical plane (Fig. 2.61)

'Outflare/inflare'
Movement of an innominate outward or inward, respectively, in the transverse (horizontal) plane (Fig. 2.13)

All three result in some form of asymmetry.

1. *pelvic 'outflare/inflare'*
   a. pelvic ring distortion in the transverse plane (leg length, therefore, remains normal)
   b. asymmetrical tension in some ligaments, muscles and tendons
   c. some predictable asymmetry affecting weight-bearing and particular hip joint ranges of motion
2. *an 'upslip' and 'rotational malalignment'*

These two presentations both cause:

   a. distortion of the pelvic ring and the joints that are part of that ring: the symphysis pubis and the two sacroiliac joints (Fig. 2.42)
   b. pelvic obliquity and a functional leg length difference (Fig. 2.73)
   c. compensatory curves of the spine, to keep the head level and in midline (Figs 2.90, 3.7, 3.8)

In addition, both the 'upslip' and 'rotational malalignment' are part of a well-defined clinical entity, designated as the 'malalignment syndrome'.

MALALIGNMENT SYNDROME

The malalignment syndrome is characterized by the features listed in Box 1.2. Recognition of the syndrome rests on the findings of:

1. asymmetrical alignment of the bones of the pelvis, trunk and extremities
2. compensatory curvatures of the spine, with or without associated rotational displacement of one or more vertebrae
3. asymmetrical ranges of motion of the head and neck, trunk, pelvis and joints of the upper and lower extremities
4. asymmetrical tension in the muscles, tendons and ligaments
5. asymmetrical muscle bulk and strength
6. an apparent (functional) leg length difference
7. an asymmetrical weight-bearing pattern

BOX 1.2 Features of the 'malalignment syndrome'

1. distortion of the pelvic ring
2. associated changes in the alignment of the axial and appendicular skeleton, so that there appears to be a reorientation of the body from head to foot
3. asymmetries of weight-bearing, tension, strength, joint ranges of motion and leg length
4. compensatory changes in the soft tissue structures
5. possible involvement of the viscera and the genitourinary, gastrointestinal and reproductive systems

ADDITIONAL CLINICAL ASPECTS

Associated with these three presentations of malalignment, there may be:

1. tenderness to palpation in soft tissues and joints that are put under increased tension, compressed or otherwise stressed as a result of the asymmetries
2. pain localizing to these structures, which can also be the cause of typical patterns of referred pain and/or paraesthesias, and
3. possibly visceral symptoms and dysfunction of bowel, bladder and/or the pelvic floor

INVESTIGATIONS

Investigations may be required to rule out underlying pathological conditions that can:

1. present with symptoms overlapping with those related to malalignment (e.g. underlying disc degeneration or protrusion, nerve root compression, sciatica, sacroiliitis)
2. predispose to the recurrence of malalignment following correction (e.g. ovarian cyst, uterine fibroids, central disc protrusions).

TREATMENT

Treatment consists primarily of:

1. correction of the malalignment using manual therapy techniques
2. 'inner' and 'outer' core muscle strengthening to increase the stability of the pelvis and spine, with simultaneous or subsequent postural and balance retraining and a graduated cardiovascular program

The chance of recovery is improved by teaching the person:

1. self-assessment techniques
   - to determine whether or not malalignment is present and what type

2. some self-treatment methods
   - these include muscle energy techniques and traction, which can be helpful for achieving and/or maintaining alignment on a day-to-day basis

Depending on the person's presentation and response to treatment, other measures to consider include:

1. addition of foot orthotics, a sacroiliac belt or compression shorts
   - to help increase the stability of the pelvis
2. acupuncture and/or massage
   - to decrease pain, relax muscles and help achieve/maintain alignment
3. prolotherapy injections
   - to incite a soft tissue reaction which triggers a natural sequence of events leading to formation of new collagen fibres and strengthening of connective tissue, particularly when there is evidence of laxity in specific ligaments, capsules and/or tendons that allows malalignment to recur
4. other types of injection, including:
   a. cortisone, particularly when there is persisting inflammation and ligament tenderness even though alignment is being maintained
   b. prolotherapy, with the intent of decreasing ongoing pain from connective tissue structures while at the same time inciting collagen formation for strengthening
   c. neural therapy and nerve desensitization (Chs 7, 8)
5. emphasis on symmetrical exercise (especially as long as malalignment keeps recurring), unless the therapist specifically recommends an asymmetrical stretching or strengthening routine

The response to this treatment protocol has been excellent in people who often have failed to benefit, or have done so only temporarily, from a variety of therapeutic approaches including acupuncture, massage and standard physiotherapy. Prior treatment attempts have usually been aimed at the localized problems (e.g. pain, muscle tension or spasm), while completely ignoring the underlying malalignment that aggravated these symptoms or may actually have precipitated them in the first place.

One of the more common complaints of persons presenting with malalignment is that of back pain and abnormal sensations or pain that subsequently turn out to be paraesthesias/dysaesthesias referred primarily to the hips, groin and lower extremities. A failure to recognize these symptoms as one of the manifestations of malalignment sets the stage for misdiagnosis and mistreatment. Minor changes seen with imaging techniques receive more attention than is their due. Neurological and/or orthopaedic lesions are considered and may be extensively investigated, to no avail. Sometimes whatever seemingly 'abnormal' findings there are end up being misinterpreted in the search for an explanation of the symptoms, leading to unwarranted surgery that, not surprisingly, fails to bring relief and, predictably, sets the stage for accelerated disc and facet joint degeneration and secondary complications.

MALALIGNMENT, WORK AND SPORT

Further confusion can arise from a tendency to attribute asymmetries in style and recurrence of injuries, especially unilateral injuries, to preferences acquired over a lifetime, the repetition of certain patterns of movement and right or left handedness and footedness. Factors of style, sidedness, or repetition have little to do with the pain or an actual injury that turns out to be yet another predictable manifestation of the presentations of malalignment being discussed. Consider the following examples:

1. a left ankle inversion sprain which responds to routine physiotherapy treatment but keeps recurring because the underlying malalignment responsible for the asymmetrical ankle weakness and shift in weight-bearing has not been corrected (Fig. 3.37)
2. the downhill skier who finds it easier to execute a turn to the left than to the right (Fig. 5.23)
3. the carpenter or plumber who has an obvious restriction to turning to the left and always finds it easier to get into a crawl-space with the pelvis and trunk rotated clockwise (Figs 3.5. 3.49)
4. the horseback rider whose horse keeps veering off to the left and is chagrined to find that switching to another horse does not solve the problem that is actually attributable to the rider (Ch. 6)

Side-to-side differences of this type may be simply attributable to the biomechanical changes that occur with malalignment, as will become apparent throughout the following chapters.

ETIOLOGY AND RECURRENCE OF MALALIGNMENT

Where and when does the problem of malalignment start? Perhaps we can take some comfort from the fact that most of us go out of alignment somewhere between the ages of 8 and 12 years (Ch. 2). The initiating factor may be as basic as a fall or a collision while playing in the school yard or at home. More likely, however, it is a developmental problem related to subtle asymmetries in muscle tension that is determined at the level of the spinal tract, brain stem or cortex. Possibly it may relate to something as simple as the fact that most of us are either right or left motor dominant (Ch. 2). However, the picture is probably more complicated, perhaps involving a disturbance of the craniosacral rhythm, a facilitation of the reticular activating system or pressure on central nervous system structures as they exit from the cranial foramina (see Ch. 8).

One might think of malalignment as being one of the prices that we have to pay for walking upright, were it not for the fact that quadrupeds such as horses and other animals can also be afflicted by this condition (see Ch. 6). In addition, we now know that pelvic malalignment may result from a problem elsewhere, such as:

1. rotational displacement of a vertebra, protrusion of a disc, temporomandibular joint dysfunction, leg length difference or favouring one leg (e.g. antalgic weight-bearing pattern)
2. malalignment of any particular bone or joint, which is known to result in an increase ('facilitation') or contralateral decrease ('inhibition') of tension in specific pairs of muscles (e.g. facilitate the left, inhibit the right TFL/ITB complex)

The important thing is to keep an open mind, to be aware that malalignment can be triggered by various mechanisms and to search for these if the person fails to respond to initial attempts at realignment. Correction of the malalignment, and maintenance of realignment, can be achieved in the majority. It may well be what finally allows them to get back on the road to recovery and, in the case of athletes, allows them to return to and, perhaps, to finally progress in their chosen sport.

Chapter 2

Common presentations and diagnostic techniques

CHAPTER CONTENTS

DOI: 10.1016/B978-0-443-06929-1.00002-8

An understanding of the 'malalignment syndrome' requires a knowledge of the common presentations of malalignment and the techniques used to diagnose and treat these. Key to this is an understanding of the sacroiliac (SI) joint and the role it plays in the normal and abnormal functioning of the unit formed by the lumbosacral spine, pelvic ring and hip joints (henceforth referred to as the 'lumbo-pelvic-hip complex'). Interestingly, in the early 20th century, the SI joint was thought to be the main source of low back pain and was the focus of many scientific investigations. The publication, in 1934, of a paper by Mixter and Barr on rupture of the intervertebral disc quickly changed the direction of these investigations; over the next four decades, the SI joint was more or less ignored in favour of the disc as a primary cause of back pain.

The resurgence of interest in the SI joint since the 1970s can be attributed in large part to the following:

1. a failure of disc resection and subsequent desperation measures, such as disc-to-disc or lumbo-pelvic fusions, to relieve the persisting low back pain
2. the recognition of the short-and long-term complications of chymopapaine 'discectomy'
3. the evolution of the computed tomography (CAT) scan and, subsequently, magnetic resonance imaging (MRI), with gradual recognition of the fact that disc protrusions were common but did not necessarily cause back pain.

A CAT scan study of fetuses in utero by Magora & Schwarz (1976) was the first to report the coincidental finding that disc degeneration was evident in about 25% and disc protrusion in 1-2% of the pregnant women. The findings were confirmed by further CAT scan and eventually MRI studies, such as the one by Boos et al. (1995) who, in a study of asymptomatic subjects, found that as many as 75% had evidence of disc degeneration and some an actual disc protrusion.

From the late 1930s into the 1990s, research focused largely on SI joint anatomy and biomechanics (Bernard & Kirkaldy-Willis 1987; Bowen & Cassidy 1981; DonTigny 1985; Vleeming et al. 1989a, 1989b, 1990a, 1990b, 1992a, 1992b). More recent interest in rehabilitation involving the SI joint may be attributable in large part to the following two factors:

1. Publications of studies in the mid-1990s suggesting initially that approximately 20–30% of low back and referred pain came from the SI joint itself and/or the surrounding ligaments, muscles and other soft tissues involved in the functioning of the joint (Maigne et al. 1996, Schwarzer et al. 1995).
2. Presentation of the first International World Congress on 'Low Back Pain and its Relationship to the Sacroiliac Joint', hosted by San Diego in 1992 and, subsequently, by other major cities on a tri-annual basis. The congress has become a forum for the presentation of clinical experience and ongoing research on the SI joint and the lumbo-pelvic hip complex and has led to the publication of a number of books and articles in this field (e.g. Vleeming et al. 2007; Lee 2011).

Over the past decade, ongoing integration of clinical experience and research (e.g. Willard 2007, DeRosa & Porterfield 2007; Barker & Briggs 1998, 1999, 2004, 2007) has led us to recognize that:

1. The 'inner core' muscles help stabilize the pelvis and lumbar spine and, in tandem with the 'outer core' muscles, ligaments and myofascia form a system of well-defined 'slings' or 'cylinders' that can:
   a. absorb shock
   b. help support the bony structure of the spine, pelvis and hip joints and allows for weight transfer through the acetabular, sacroiliac and lumbosacral regions
   c. provide stability in preparation for carrying out activities with other parts of our body
   d. ensure balance and facilitate motion of the pelvis, spine/trunk and the limbs to carry out a specific action, such as throwing a ball
2. As a result of the functional kinetic interlinkage of the skeleton with these core muscles and myofascial 'slings', pathology affecting any of these structures can stress other proximal and even distal sites, sometimes to the point of interfering with their proper function and causing them to become another 'pain generator' (Vleeming & Stoeckart 2007; see also Ch. 8). Rotation of a vertebra, pelvic malalignment, excessive tension in a particular ligament or muscle are all interlinked and affect the function of the rest of the musculoskeletal system. Treatment needs to address that fact; it cannot be restricted to one site and will often require use of more than one treatment modality in order to be successful.
3. Malalignment of the pelvis and spine initially may not be painful. However, with time the stress on an increasing number of structures is more and more likely to result in:
   a. irritation and eventual hypersensitivity of the nociceptive nerve fibres supplying these structures (Willard 2007)
   b. chronic reactive contraction of specific muscles that are attempting to decrease movement of a painful structure and/or to stabilize a lax joint, with eventual complicating compromise of their own blood supply to the point where the muscles become symptomatic as well
   c. adaptive changes in gait as a result of the biomechanical changes and/or in reaction to pain.
4. All these factors combined are now felt to be the primary cause and/or an aggravating factor in as many as 50-60% of those presenting with low back pain and referred pain symptoms from this site, or 'pain generator' (Vleeming & Stoeckart 2007). Pain may localize to the structure initially involved (i.e. vertebra, lumbosacral junction, SI joint or other) but even at the onset can present as referred pain felt only nearby or at a distant site on the same or opposite side (see 'Introduction 2002'; Fig. 3.63). Eventually, the abnormal stress pelvic malalignment exerts on soft tissues and joints throughout the body may cause them to become painful and a source of referred pain, so that the actual site or sites where the pain is felt may be misleading to the person reporting the pain and to those trying to determine and treat the underlying problem that precipitated this chain of events. An example is the common complaint of pain 'from the hip joint' on one side, when the pain is actually:
   a. originating from the nearby SI joint or trigger points in piriformis (Fig. 3.45), or
   b. referred from the iliolumbar or sacroiliac ligaments to the hip joint, groin or greater trochanter regions (Figs 3.46, 3.62, 3.63).
5. Recognition of malalignment and the typical problems it can cause is, therefore, a key factor in helping determine whether the symptoms and signs on clinical examination are attributable to the malalignment *per se*, or whether the malalignment is covering up an underlying clinical problem.

This chapter will examine some old and new concepts regarding the SI joint and lumbo-pelvic-hip complex, then proceed to look at what will be the focus of this book: the common presentations of malalignment - 'rotational malalignment', 'upslip' and 'downslip', 'outflare/inflare', sacral torsion and 'vertebral rotational displacement' - before discussing some of the tests that have, over the past decade, gained acceptance as being the more reliable ones for examining the pelvis and spine in order to diagnose an alignment problem.

THE SACROILIAC JOINT

The SI joints are planar joints that function to:

1. transfer the loads generated by gravity and the weight of the trunk and upper body to the ilia and onto the ischial tuberosities in sitting and through the hip joints to the lower extremities in standing (Fig. 2.1A)

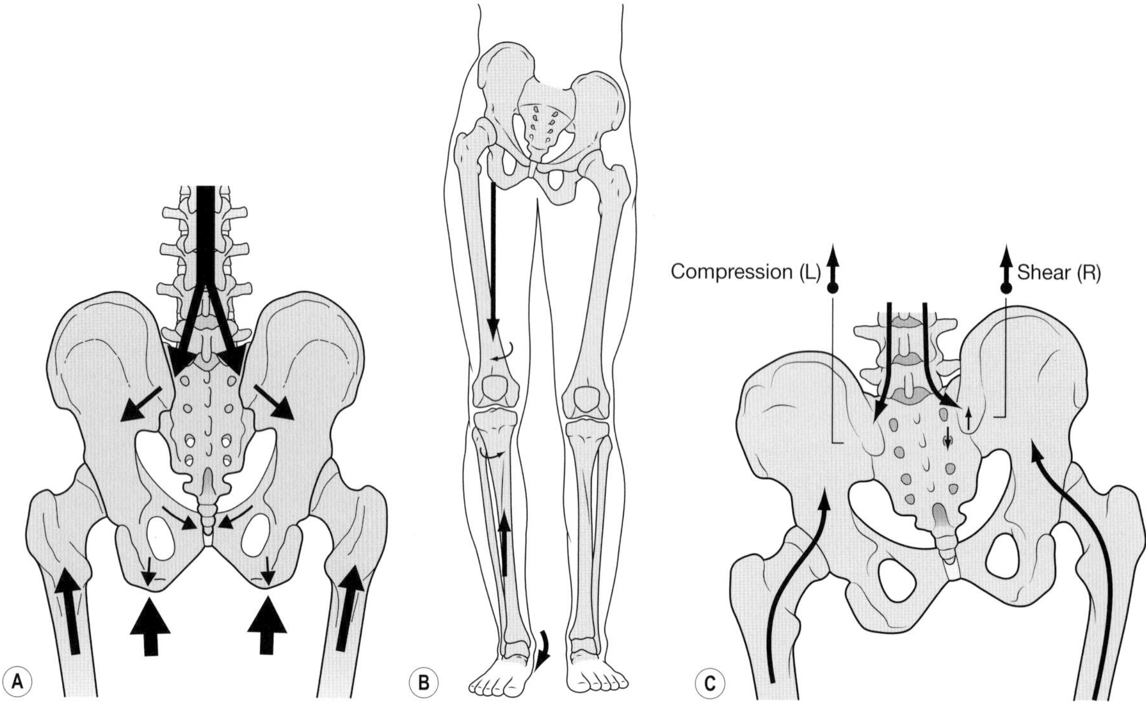

Fig. 2.1 Weight transfer forces through the lumbo-pelvic-hip complex from above and below. (A) In standing and sitting (pelvis in alignment, leg length equal). (B) On right one leg stance. (C) Changes in loads and forces imparted to the sacroiliac joint with a left frontal plane asymmetry. The right joint is more vertical, creating greater shear. *(Courtesy of DeRosa & Porterfield 2007.)*

2. transfer weight in the opposite direction, in sitting, standing, walking or falling onto one or both ischial tuberosities or the knees or feet – through the ilia onto the sacrum and upward by way of the lumbosacral junction (Fig. 2.1,B,C)
3. act as a shock absorber, particularly at heel-strike and
4. diminish any iliac-on-sacral surface translation or actual shear, when properly positioned (Fig. 2.1A).

Some SI joint motion does occur and seems to:

1. decrease the energy cost of:
   a. ambulation (DonTigny 1985, 1990, 2007)
   b. lifting (Masi et al. 2007)
2. aid delivery

   The comparatively flat joint surfaces allow movement in a way that makes it possible for women to deliver what are, in evolutionary respects, rather large babies.
3. help decrease stress on the pelvic ring of bones

   Combined with movement at the symphysis pubis, they are felt to decrease the risk of the pelvic ring 'cracking' that a solid ring would be subjected to (Vleeming & Stoeckart 2007; Adams et al. 2006).
4. absorb stresses and store energy

   Stresses are absorbed in large part by the complex of ligaments and myofascial slings (see below; Figs 2.35-2.39) that act on each SI joint, helping to absorb shock, to stabilize the joint for load transfer and to store or provide energy at select points when walking and lifting

A basic knowledge of SI joint development, configuration and biomechanics is crucial to the understanding and diagnosis of asymmetries of the pelvis and spine. At the same time, it must be emphasized that the SI joints are but two of the joints inherent to the lumbo-pelvic-hip complex and comprise but one aspect of what has here been designated the 'malalignment syndrome'. It is unfortunate that, in the past, discussion so often centred on the SI joints, and it is really only since the 1990s that there has been more recognition of the other structures that are part and parcel of the lumbo-pelvic-hip complex and how they all interact. The discussion that follows in this and subsequent chapters should help put the role of the SI joints into proper perspective.

For a more detailed discussion of the most recent thinking and scientific studies on pelvic and SI joint embryology, development and ageing, and on the kinetic interaction of the pelvis with the spine and the hip joints, the reader is referred to the excellent presentations on these topics in 'Muscle Energy Techniques' (Chaitow 2006), 'The Pelvic Girdle' (Lee 2004a), 'Diagnosis and Treatment of Movement Impaired Syndromes' (Sahrmann 2002), 'Movement, Stability and Pelvic Pain' (Vleeming, Mooney, Stoeckart et al. 2007) and other publications in text and as individual papers.

ANATOMY, DEVELOPMENT AND AGING

The exquisite work by Bowen and Cassidy (1981), Bernard and Cassidy (1991) and others revealed the following:

First, at birth, one finds the well-defined cartilaginous surfaces, synovial fluid and capsular enclosure typical of a synovial joint (Bernard & Cassidy 1991; Bowen & Cassidy 1981; Cassidy 1992; Dihlmann 1967; Sashin 1930; Solonen 1957; Willard 2007; Williams & Warwick 1980).

A thin fibrocartilagenous cover then develops over the iliac surface, in contrast to the thick layer of hyaline cartilage evident on the sacral surface.

Second, as growth continues:

1. the articular surfaces of the SI joint eventually assume an L-shape, with a shorter, almost vertical, upper arm and a longer, lower arm directed posteriorly and inferiorly (Figs 2.2, 2.3C)
2. these arms can be oriented in a different plane relative to the vertical axis, creating a propeller-like appearance (Fig. 2.3B).
3. with time, the 'propeller' aspect of this 'L-shape' is accentuated by the development of complementary convexities and concavities, variously described as follows:
   a. by Resnick et al. (1975)
      - in the upper (cephalad) arm, a sacral convexity complementing an innominate concavity
      - in the lower (caudad) arm, an innominate convexity that fits into a sacral concavity
   b. by Masi et al. (2007)
      - upper and lower 'ileal convexities that match sacral concavities' (Fig. 2.2)
4. in addition, the sacrum widens anteriorly, creating an anterior-to-posterior wedging effect (Figs 2.2, 2.3, 2.4B, 2.10A, 2.11A, 2.46BD).

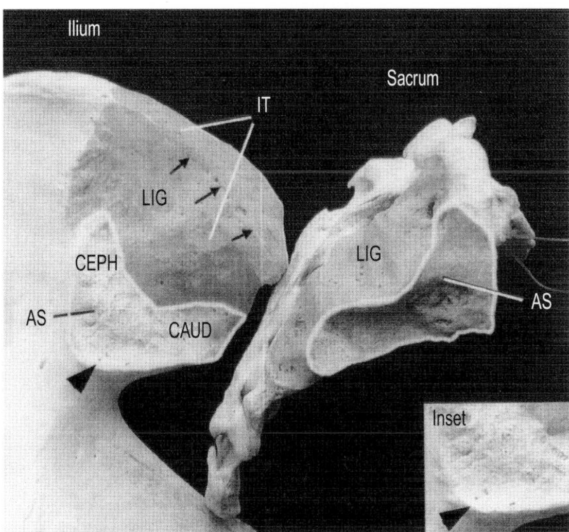

Fig. 2.2 The right sacroiliac joint is opened so that the opposing surfaces can be viewed simultaneously. . .The topography of the articular surfaces (AS) is irregular but congruent, with slight convexity on the ilial side, and complementary concavity on the sacral side. Both articular surfaces have numerous pits and surface roughenings and these are clearly visible in the inset [which] is an enlargement of the iliac auricular surface. Corresponding pits on the two photographs are indicated by arrowheads. The more posterior part of the joint is shaded and is a syndesmosis. It provides extensive areas of ligamentous attachment (LIG), particularly the strong interosseous ligament. . .at the centre of an 'axial joint', the pivotal point around which the sacrum rotates in nutational and counternutational movements. The erector spinae muscle is attached to the most posterior part of the iliac tuberosity (IT). . .Note the wedge shape of the sacrum, with the superior part of the bone, nearer the sacral promontory, being wider anteroposteriorly than the inferior part. *(Courtesy of Masi et al. 2007.)*

Third, the joint capsule thickens anteriorly to form the anterior or ventral sacroiliac ligament; this is a weak ligament that has been shown to be continuous with the anterior fibres of the iliolumbar ligament (Fig. 2.4A). The interosseous ligament forms the posterior border of the joint; it constitutes the

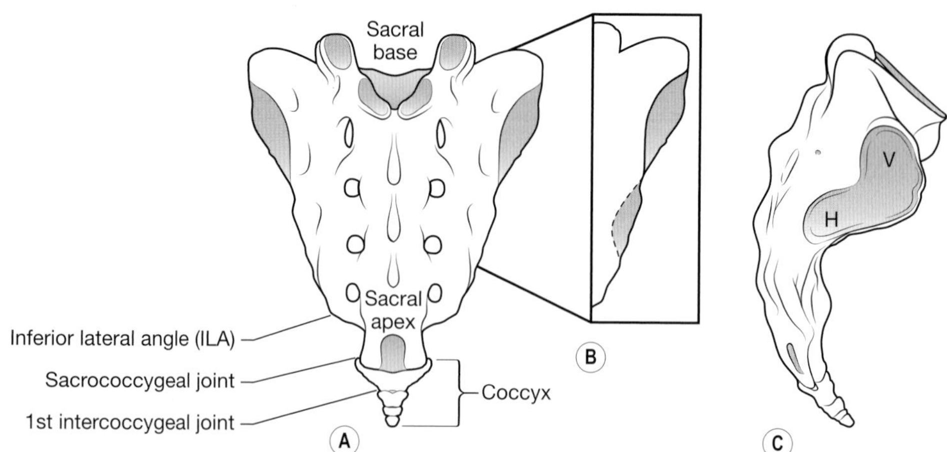

Fig. 2.3 Posterior aspect of the sacrum and coccyx, and configuration of the adult sacroiliac joint. (A) Anteroposterior view: major bony landmarks. (B) Angulated inset showing orientation of the two main arms of the sacral articular surface along different planes relative to the vertical axis, which creates a propeller-like shape. (C) Lateral view: L-shape of the sacroiliac joint (H = horizontal arm; V = vertical arm). *(Redrawn courtesy of Vleeming et al. 1997.)*

strongest ligament supporting the SI joint and makes up for what is usually a rudimentary or even absent posterior joint capsule (Figs 2.4B, 2.13Aiii). Additional support comes from the short posterior (dorsal) sacroiliac ligaments, the long posterior (dorsal) sacroiliac ligament, also the iliolumbar, sacrotuberous and sacrospinous ligaments (Figs 2.5A, 2.45). The sacrum literally ends up suspended between the ilia by these ligaments.

Fourth, Bellamy et al. (1983) observed that the SI joint is surrounded by the largest and most powerful muscle groups in the body but that none of these directly influenced the movement of this joint. However, as Lee pointed out (1992a), very few articulations in the body are actually capable of independent motion, and although the muscles crossing the SI joint are not typically described as prime movers of that joint, motion can occur at the SI joint as a result of their contraction. Lee went on to list 22 muscles that do affect SI joint movement, ranging from latissimus dorsi proximally to sartorius distally. Richard (1986) observed that 36 muscles have their insertion on each ilium but that only 8 of these are also attached to the sacrum; some of the others just cross the joint but provide a key function in establishing and maintaining the axes of movement (e.g. gluteus maximus posteriorly; see Figs 2.5B, 2.37) or stabilizing the joint (e.g. iliacus anteriorly; see Figs 2.46B, 4.2).

The work of Vleeming et al. (1989a) is of particular interest in this respect. From their initial dissections on 12 cadavers, these authors reported that gluteus maximus was attached to the sacrotuberous ligament in all cases. In 50% of dissections, there was also a 'fusion' of the sacrotuberous ligament, unilateral or bilaterally, with the tendon of the long head of biceps femoris at its origin (Figs 2.6, 2.37). In some specimens, 'fusion' to the ligament was complete so that there was actually no connection of this muscle to the ischial tuberosity itself.

Vleeming et al. (1989b) showed how load application to the sacrotuberous ligament, either directly to the ligament or by way of its continuations with the long head of biceps femoris or the attachments of gluteus maximus, significantly diminished the ventral (forward) rotation of the base of the sacrum (Figs 2.6, 2.59). They went on to demonstrate that these forces resulted in a compression of the sacral and iliac surface, increasing the coefficient of friction and thereby decreasing movement at the SI joint by what they termed 'force

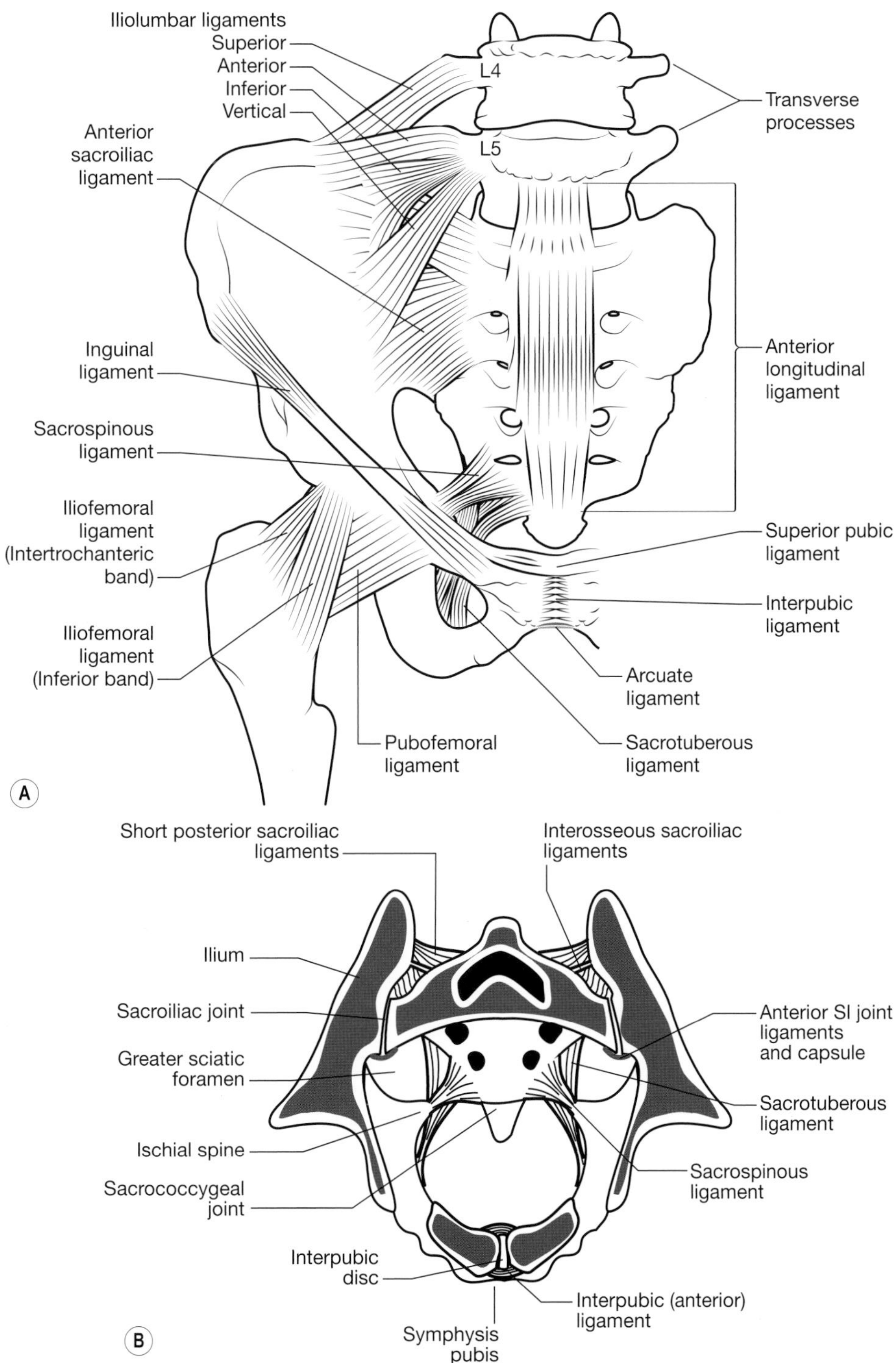

Fig. 2.4 Pelvic ring: articulations and ligaments. (A) Anterior view. (B) Superior view (note the anterior widening of the sacrum).

Posterior superior iliac spine
Short dorsal sacroiliac ligaments
Long dorsal sacroiliac ligament
Greater sciatic foramen
Lesser sciatic foramen
Falciform edge
Sacrotuberous ligament
Ischial tuberosity
Biceps femoris
A
Long dorsal sacrotuberous ligament
Piriformis
Capsule and ligaments of hip joint:
Iliofemoral
Ischiofemoral
Greater trochanter
Sacrospinous ligament
Sciatic nerve
B

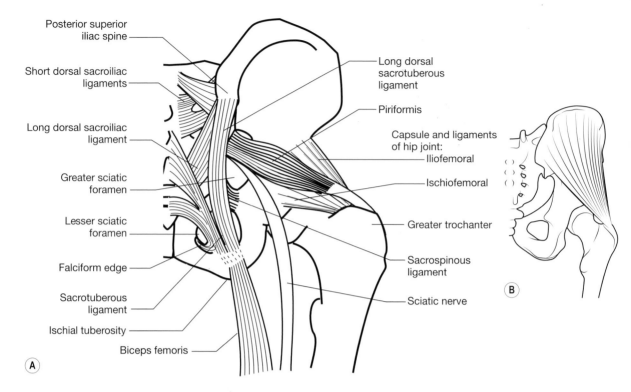

Fig. 2.5 (A) Posterior pelvic ligaments and muscles that act on the sacroiliac joint (see also Figs 2.37, 2.45). (B) Gluteus maximus.

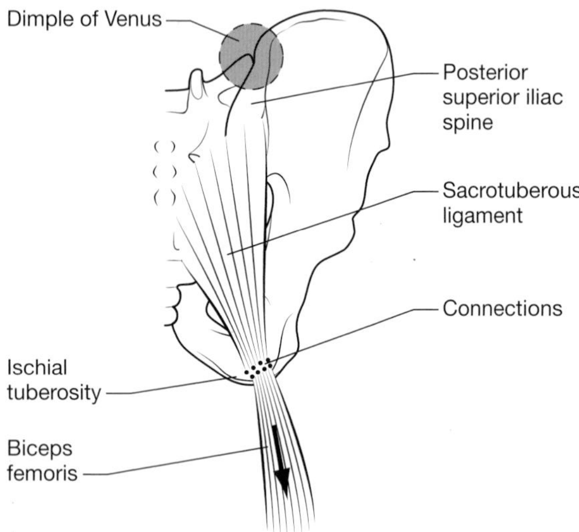

Fig. 2.6 Tension in the sacrotuberous ligament can be augmented by increasing tension in the biceps femoris, and vice versa, when there are fibrous connections between the ligament and the muscle (see also Figs 2.37, 2.59). Note the left 'dimple of Venus', overlying the depression formed at the underlying junction of the sacral base with the left ilium. *(Redrawn courtesy of Vleeming et al. 1997.)*

closure', which will be discussed further under 'self-locking mechanisms' and 'form and force closure' below (Vleeming et al. 1990a, 1990b). The link of the sacrotuberous (ST) ligament to rectus femoris has been repeatedly verified subsequently and also, more recently, evidence that this ligament is usually connected to semimembranosus as well (Barker & Briggs 2004).

These findings are but one illustration of how specific muscles may indirectly affect the sacrum, the innominate bones and hence the function of the joints of the pelvic girdle by causing joint motion, compression or both. Recent work by these and other authors (e.g. Pool-Goodzwaard et al. 2003; DeRosa & Porterfield 2007) has more clearly defined the role of these so-called 'inner' and 'outer' pelvic 'core' muscles as dynamic stabilizers of the SI joints in particular and of the lumbo-pelvic-hip girdle and trunk in general (see 'Kinetic function and stability' below; Figs 2.29-2.40).

Fifth, the pre-pubertal SI joint surface is described as planar – flat opposing sacral and iliac surfaces that allow for small gliding movements in all directions (Fig. 2.7A). After puberty, most

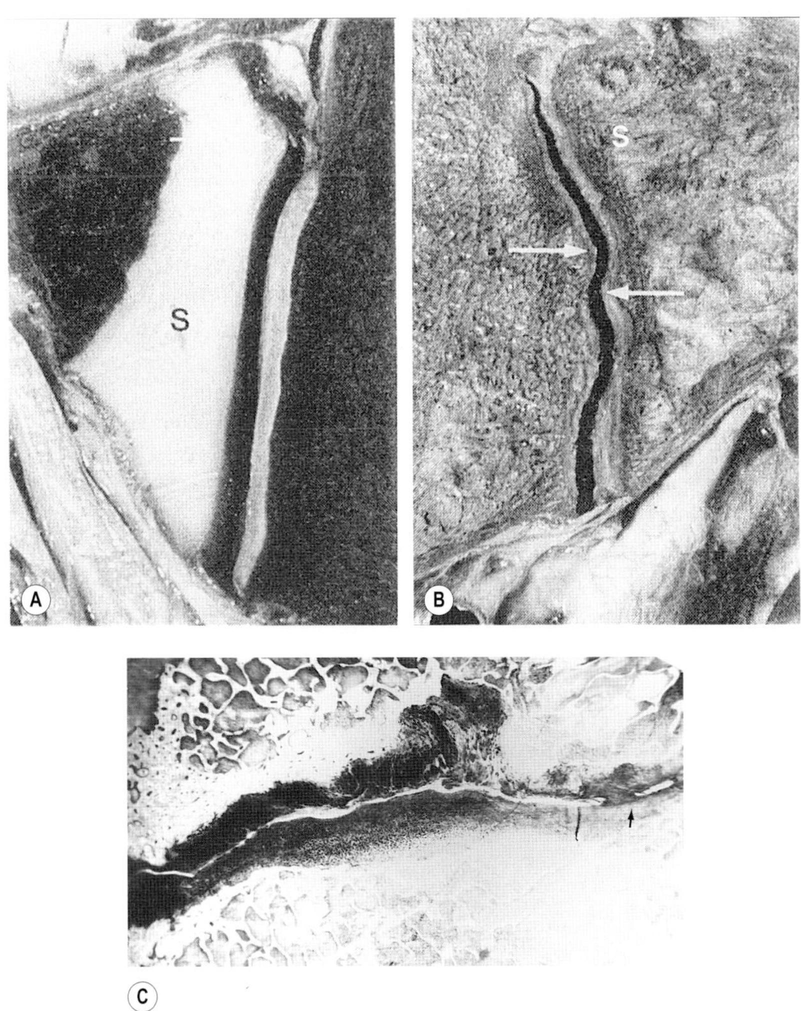

Fig. 2.7 (A,B) Coronal section through two embalmed male specimens: (A) Age 12 - the planar appearance of the sacroiliac joint (S denotes the sacrum). (B) Over age 60 - the presence of ridges and grooves is denoted by arrows. *(Courtesy of Vleeming et al. 1990a.)* (C) Sacroiliac joint of a female, 81 years of age. Note the erosion of the articular cartilage [but the sacroiliac joint is still visible except for] . . . the intra-articular fibrous connection (arrow). *(From Lee 2004a, reproduced courtesy of Walker 1986.)*

individuals develop 'a crescent-shaped ridge running the entire length of the iliac surface with a corresponding depression on the sacral side' (Fig. 2.7B); this complimentary ridge and groove are now felt to lock the surfaces together and increase stability of the SI joint (Vleeming et al. 1990a; Gracovetsky 2007). Also, 'with increasing age the surfaces become more irregular and prominent' (Cassidy 1992, 41). The apparent 'roughening' of these surfaces may be an adaptation to adolescent weight gain; certainly, work by Vleeming et al. (1990a, 1990b) supported the conjecture that these macroscopic changes represent functional, rather than pathological, adaptations. These authors presented evidence that articular surfaces with both a coarse texture and ridges and depressions have high friction coefficients, consistent with their view that the roughening represents a 'non-pathological adaptation to the forces exerted at the SI joints, leading to increased stability' (Vleeming et al. 1990a). The same authors raised two points of particular interest:

1. These physiologically normal intra-articular ridges and depressions could easily be misinterpreted as osteophytes on radiological studies. They pointed out that:

   'it might well be that a textbook statement like 'The sacroiliac synovial joint rather regularly shows pathologic changes in adults, and in many males more than 30 years of age, and in most males after the age of 50, the joint becomes ankylosed ...' (Hollinshead 1962) is based on an incorrect interpretation of anatomical data'

   and that:

   'with standard radiological techniques, the [cartilage-covered] ridges and depressions easily can be misinterpreted as pathologic, because of the well known overprojection in SI joints'

   (Vleeming et al. 1990a)

   The angle of projection and whether or not the subject is weight-bearing asymmetrically, as he or she would do when out of alignment, are other factors to consider (see Ch. 4 – 'Implications for Radiology and Medical Imaging'; Figs 4.24, 4.30, 4.31, 4.33)
2. SI joints with intact cartilage showed the friction coefficient to be particularly high 'in preparations with complementary ridges and depressions'. This led them to conjecture that:

   'Under abnormal loading conditions ... it is theoretically possible that an SI joint is forced into a new position where ridge and depression are no longer complementary. Such an abnormal joint position could be regarded as a blocked joint'

   (Vleeming et al. 1990b: 135)

This 'blocked joint' may refer to the frequent finding of a decrease or even absence of movement, also referred to as 'locking', in one or other SI joint on clinical examination of those presenting with 'malalignment' (discussed in detail under 'Functional or dynamic tests' below, and in Ch. 3). Note that this decrease or loss of mobility occurs 'under abnormal loading conditions'. Normal interlocking of the surfaces contributes to joint stability and limitation of range of motion of the SI joint when this is functionally required; for example, to enhance the force-closure mechanism occurring on the weight-bearing side during the gait cycle (Snijders et al. 1993a, Vleeming et al. 1997, Hungerford & Gilleard 2007).

Sixth, the joint may retain its synovial features well into the patient's 40s or 50s. The fibrocartilage covering the iliac side consistently starts to degenerate early in life, usually by the third decade in males and the fourth or fifth decade in females. By this time, narrowing of the joint space, sclerosis, osteophyte formation, cysts and erosions of the articular surfaces may be evident on X-Rays (Figs 2.8A, 4.38) and on CAT scan/computed tomography (Shibata et al. 2002). Given that these changes could be evident so early on yet were usually asymptomatic, Vleeming et al. (1990a) remarked that they most likely represented a functional adaptive change to an increase in weight. Shibata et al. (2002) and others (Schunke 1938; Bowen & Cassidy 1981; Walker 1986, 1992; Faflia et al. 1998) felt these were 'degenerative changes'. Iliac osteoarthrosis is indicated by an initial fibrillation of the cartilage, plaque formation and eventual peripheral erosions and subchondral sclerotic changes.

In contrast, osteoarthritic changes are rarely evident on the sacral side by the fifth decade. With advancing age, the typical changes of worsening osteoarthritis (deep erosions, areas of exposed subchondral bone, enlarging osteophytes and increasing fibrous connections) result in both articular surfaces becoming totally irregular. In some individuals, this change may progress to a complete replacement of the joint space with fibrous tissue, eventual calcification and a complete loss of movement. However, 'in most cases, the joint remains patent throughout life. Fusion can occur by synostosis or by fibrosis' (Cassidy 1992: 41).

Fibrous adhesions, although more common in older specimens, have been seen in younger males, but 'to a lesser degree'. Faflia et al. (1998) reported a higher prevalence of advanced, asymmetric non-uniform SI joint degenerative changes in obese, multiparous females compared to age-matched normal-weight, non-multiparous women and to men (Lee 2004a). Whereas bony ankylosis is rare, para-articular synostosis has been reported to be a common finding in both males and females over the age of 50 (Valojerdy et al. 1989). Most will continue to show some SI joint movement well into their 70s and 80s (Bowen & Cassidy 1981, Cassidy 1992, Colachis et al. 1963). Some studies have actually refuted the existence of absolute intra-articular ankylosis in the elderly, suggesting that at these age levels they show primarily intra-articular fibrous connections and osteophytes, cartilagenous erosions, plaque formation (Resnick et al. 1975; Walker 1986) – all

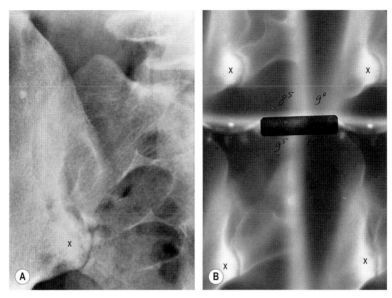

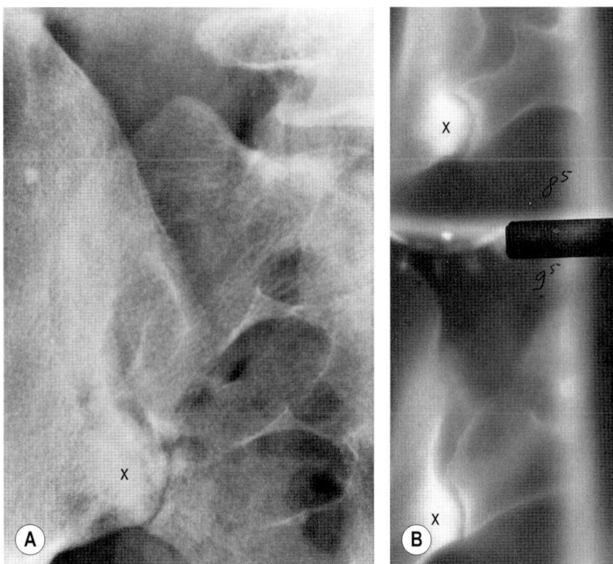

Fig. 2.8 Iliitis condensans. (A) Plain X-ray of the right sacroiliac joint (SIJ) with irregular and sclerosing changes in S3 (X). This type of sclerosis of the ilium can cause confusing plain X-rays. (B) Tomography of the posterior parts of the same SIJ. There is sclerosis of the same ilium (X) with subchondral cysts and slight sclerosis of the sacrum, but normal joint width. The numbers 8.5 to 10 denote the distance from the table top. *(Courtesy of Dijkstra 2007.)*

these resulting in narrowing of the SI joint space (Fig. 2.8B). Schunke back in 1938 reported that actual SI joint fusion attributable to ankylosing spondylitis was more likely to be found in younger subjects; if such a fusion was found in an older person, it was more likely attributable to them having suffered ankylosing spondylitis somewhere in their younger years.

Finally, the clinical significance of the premature osteoarthrosis on the iliac side is not known. However, similarly to other sites in the body, osteoarthrosis does not necessarily cause symptoms. As Magora & Schwartz already reported in 1976, and others have since confirmed, osteoarthrosis of the spine correlates more with increasing age than with back pain. The same is probably true for the SI joint.

SI JOINT MOBILITY

There has been much debate over whether movement can occur at the SI joint, despite a wealth of studies dating back as far as the turn of the 19th century indicating that small measures of movement around specific axes were indeed possible (Albee 1909; Ashmore 1915; Beal 1982; Bowen & Cassidy 1981; Colachis et al. 1963; Dihlman 1967; Egund et al. 1978; Frigerio et al. 1974; Meyer 1878; Miller et al. 1987; Pitkin & Pheasant 1936; Sashin 1930; Solonen 1957; Strachan 1939; Weisl 1955).

Methods of assessment have included:

1. analysis of the SI joint in various positions of the trunk and lower extremities by:
   a. X-rays (Albee 1909; Brooke 1924)
   b. inclinometer measurements of surface markers on the innominate, sacrum and femur (Hungerford et al. 2001; Hungerford 2002)
2. computerized analysis using a metronome skeletal analysis system (Smidt 1995)
3. Doppler imaging of vibrations across the SI joint (Buyruk et al. 1995a, 1995b, 1997, 1999; Damen et al. 2002a)

The question was settled more definitively by *in vivo* sudies using:

1. roentgen stereophotogrammetric analysis - a computerized dual-radiographic technique for assessing the relative movement of implanted titanium balls serving as reference points on the ilium and sacrum (Sturesson et al. 1989, 2000a, 2000b).

2. Kirschner rods implanted in both ilia and the sacrum in healthy volunteers (Jacob & Kissling 1995; Kissling & Jacob 1997).

Fig. 2.9 shows how the pelvis as a unit can:

1. rotate around the 3 basic axes
   a. the coronal axis, to tilt anterior and posterior in the sagittal plane
   b. the vertical axis, to rotate right (clockwise) and left (counter-clockwise) in the transverse (horizontal) plane
   c. the sagittal axis, to side-flex right and left in the coronal (frontal) plane
2. move, or 'translate', along the 3 planes indicated
   a. to right or left (medial, lateral) along the coronal axis
   b. up or down (cephalad or caudad, respectively) along the vertebral axis
   c. forward or backward (anterior or posterior, respectively) along the sagittal axis

Movement of the SI joint is also triplanar and amounts to approximately 2–4 degrees of rotation and translation at best (Egund et al. 1978, Sturesson et al. 1989, 2000a, 2000b). Stevens and Vyncke reported 3.3 degrees mean axial rotation of the sacrum in the 'transverse plane' on side-bending in 1986. Previous reports suggested that asymmetry, both of the configuration and the amount of mobility possible on one side compared with the other, appears to be the rule (Bowen & Cassidy 1981; Vleeming et al. 1992a, 1992b). However, the studies using Doppler imaging of vibrations across the SI joint, mentioned above, have consistently shown that:

1. stiffness is variable between individuals, which is probably a key factor why range of motion is also likely to be variable
2. subjects with symmetrical side-to-side stiffness are more likely to be asymptomatic (no pelvic pain); whereas those with asymmetric stiffness are more likely to be symptomatic.

Most studies to date have, however, used a static approach to investigating a dynamic phenomenon. Even though studies have become increasingly refined, there is still some truth even now to the observation by Cassidy (1992) that 'a valid and reliable method for measuring this motion in patients has not yet been developed'. Also, none of the authors cited have indicated whether or not there was malalignment of the pelvis at the time of the study, nor mentioned any particular presentation. Malalignment results in asymmetrical opposition of the SI joint surfaces and can cause unilateral SI joint hypermobility, hypomobility or even 'locking', all factors that would result in an asymmetry of configuration and/or mobility (see Chs 3, 4).

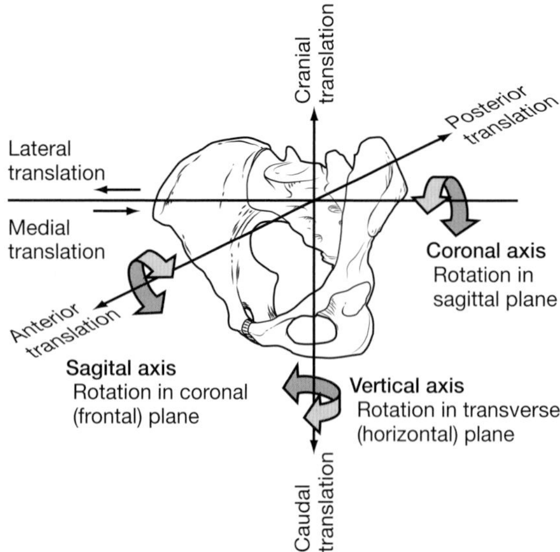

Fig. 2.9 Axes and planes around which sacroiliac joint movement occurs.

AXES OF MOTION

Motion at the SI joint is complex, probably not occurring around just one fixed axis but being a movement combining rotation and translation (Beal 1982; Bernard & Cassidy 1991; Egund et al. 1978; Frigerio et al. 1974; Kissling & Jacob 1997; Walker 1992). A good description of the directions and degrees of freedom of movement at the SI joints was already found in Gray's Anatomy in 1980 (Williams & Warwick). At risk of oversimplification, the primary motions that can occur are outlined in Box 2.1 and Figure 2.9.

Rotation and/or translation of the sacrum or an innominate results in a relative displacement of the SI joint surfaces (Figs 2.10, 2.11). Excessive rotation and/or translation in any direction can have a shearing effect. These surfaces may also become pathologically 'stuck' in any one position, Panjabi's so-called 'compressed' joint (see 'Kinetic function and stability' below; Figs 2.23, 2.24). SI joint nutation makes for stability, and counternutation for instability; the amount of nutation, or counternutation, can be of a normal or pathological degree.

BOX 2.1 Axes of motion of the sacroiliac joint

Rotational movement, 'anterior' or 'posterior' around the coronal axis in the sagittal plane

1. of one or both ilia relative to the sacrum; if both rotate, this may be:
   a. in the same direction simultaneously; e.g. as occurs usually on flexion or extension of the trunk (Fig. 2.116), or tilting of the pelvis when sitting (Fig. 2.80)
   b. in opposite directions (e.g. as occurs in the course of the normal gait cycle; Figs 2.10A, 2.21, 2.22, 2.41)
2. of the sacrum relative to both ilia; forward movement of the base has been designated as *nutation* and backward movement as *counternutation* (Figs 2.11, 2.17, 2.18, 2.19)

Upward or downward translation along the vertical or Y-axis

- also described as 'cranial and caudal translation', respectively; this may involve one or both ilia relative to the sacrum, or the sacrum relative to the ilia (Fig. 2.9)

Axial rotation of sacrum and ilia in the transverse plane

1. sacrum and ilia rotating as one unit around the vertical axis
   - normally occurs with clockwise or counterclockwise rotation of the pelvis when standing or walking (Figs 2.12, 2.13A)
2. an ilium relative to the sacrum
   a. the anterior part of the ilium moving either outward from or inward to the midline in the transverse plane (i.e. an outflaring and inflaring, respectively (Figs 2.13A, 2.17)
   b. some outflaring occurs in association with anterior, and inflaring with posterior, innominate rotation during normal gait (Fig. 2.13A) and flexion/ extension manoeuvres (Fig. 2.17)
3. the sacrum relative to the innominates around the vertical axis, in the transverse plane (Fig. 2.89):
   - this normally occurs with trunk rotation in sitting (when the innominates are fixed by bearing weight on the ischial tuberosities) and during gait (Fig. 2.41)

Torsion of the sacrum around an oblique axis

1. torsion around the right or left oblique or 'diagonal' axis is one form, and usually happens in conjunction with some rotation around the vertical axis (Figs 2.14, 2.21 and Point 3 above)
2. the mean transverse axes (MTA) run from the sacral base down and over to the opposite innominate, crossing where the two parts of the L-shaped SI joint meet, at about the level of S2 (Richards 1986; Figs 2.3A, 2.10B, 2.14, 2.21, 2.42, 2.50)
3. these axes are named according to the side of origin from the sacral base (e.g. the right oblique axis starts from the right corner of the sacral base and runs downward and across to the left apex; Fig. 2.14)

Muscles that can effect nutation, and increase stability, include those that can:

1. rotate the innominates posteriorly relative to the base of the sacrum (Figs 2.10, 2.21); e.g. rectus abdominis (Fig. 2.31B) and biceps femoris (Fig. 2.59)
2. rotate the sacral base anteriorly (Fig. 2.11A); e.g. semispinalis or erector spinae muscles (Figs 2.37, 2.38) and multifidi (Fig. 2.29)

Muscles that effect counternutation, and decrease stability, include those that can:

1. rotate the innominates anteriorly (Figs 2.10, 2.21); e.g. iliacus, rectus femoris and the tensor fascia lata/iliotibial band complex (Figs 2.46B,C, 2.59)
2. rotate the sacral base posteriorly (Fig. 2.11B); e.g. pubococcygeus, ischiococcygeus and iliococcygeus, all levator ani muscles originating from the pubic rami and pulling forward on the apex of the sacrum by way of their insertions into the coccyx (Fig. 2.53B)

BIOMECHANICS

Movement around the various axes of the SI joints occurs as part of normal movement patterns involving the spine, pelvis and lower extremities throughout our day-to-day activities (DonTigny 1985, Greenman 1992, 1997; Figs 2.12-2.16). The sacrum influences the relative movement of the innominates, and vice versa, as tension is increased in the connecting soft tissues - primarily ligaments and

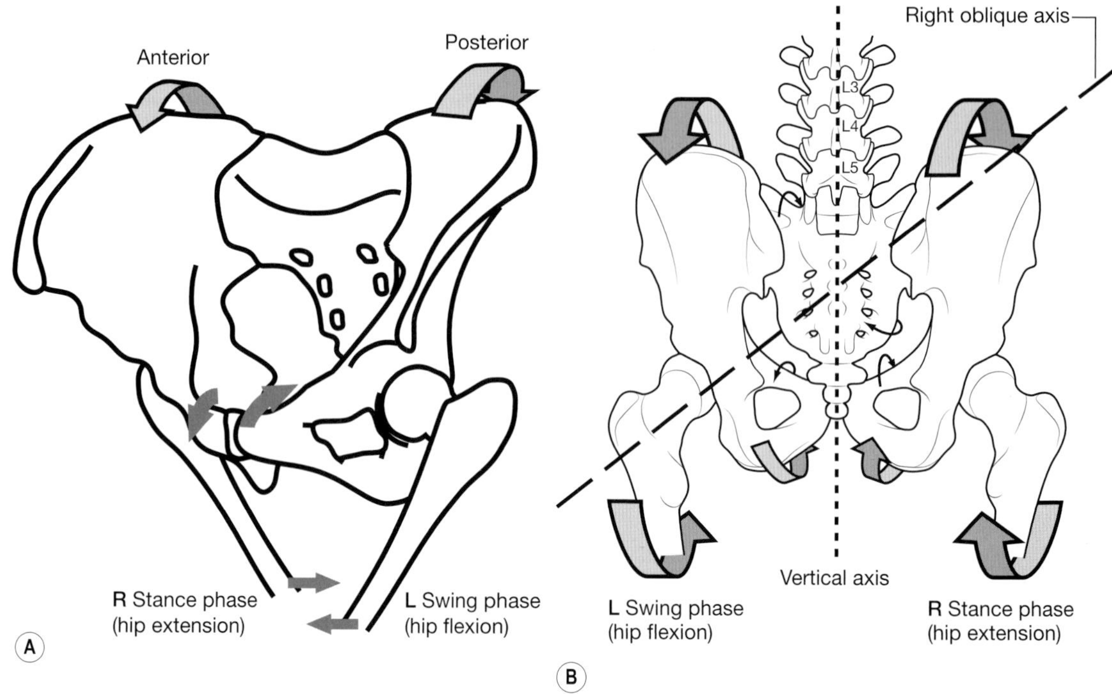

Fig. 2.10 Movement of the pelvic ring with normal gait. (A) Contrary rotation of the innominates relative to the sacrum. (B) Sacral torsion around the right oblique axis associated with 'right anterior, left posterior' innominate rotation (posterior view.)

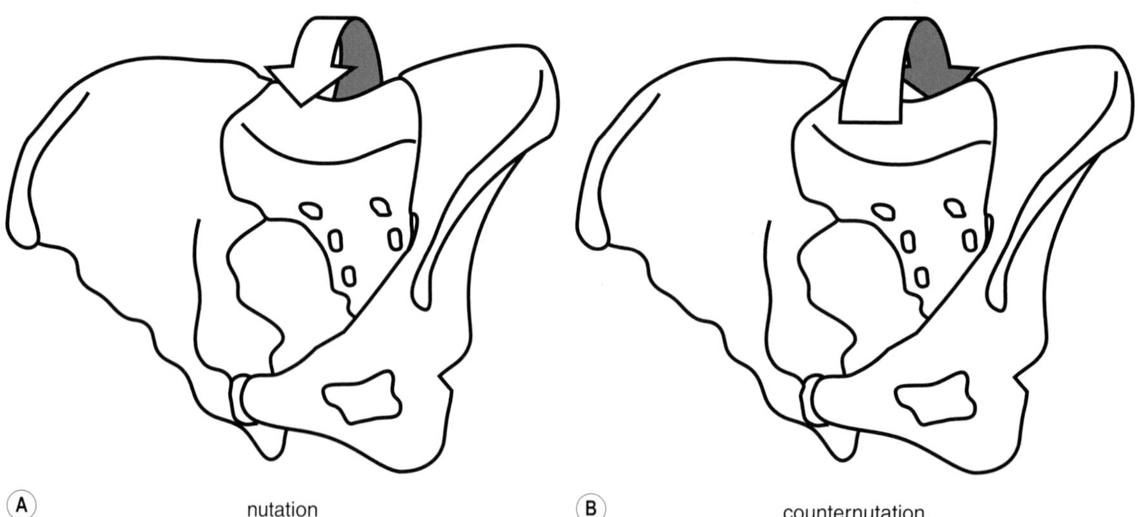

Fig. 2.11 Movement of the sacral base relative to the ilia. (A) Nutation (B) Counternutation

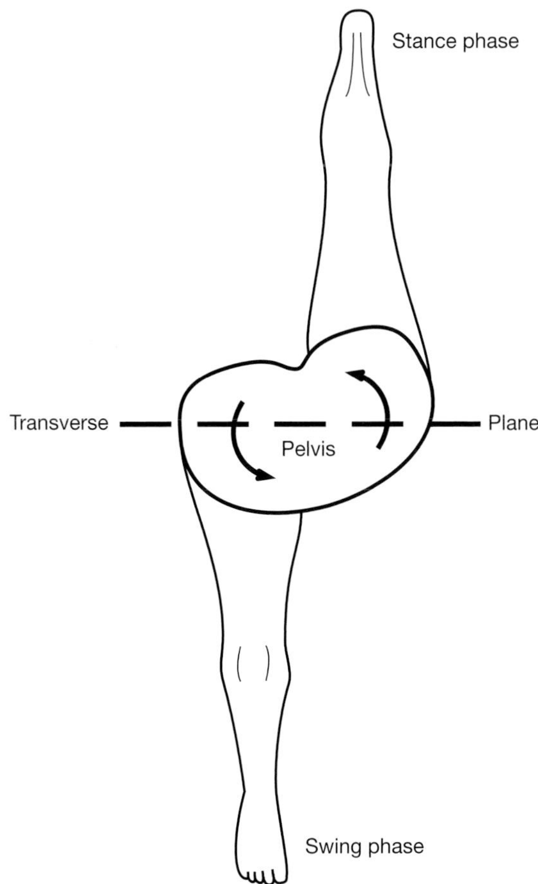

Fig. 2.12 Pelvic rotation in the transverse (horizontal) plane with normal gait: counterclockwise during the right swing, left stance phase (shown); clockwise with left swing, right stance.

muscles - that act on the SI joint(s). This is a normal phenomenon, as described, but will be affected by the presence of tight structures; for example, a tight biceps femoris acting on an SI joint by way of its connections to the sacrotuberous ligament (Fig. 2.6). In addition, the movement is likely to be asymmetrical when such tightness is worse on one side compared to the other. When sitting, this tightness is less of a problem as the innominates are relatively 'fixed' and less mobile than when standing.

Trunk flexion

In standing

Flexion initially results in a simultaneous forward rotation of the sacrum and innominates around the coronal axis in the sagittal plane which may continue through full flexion (Kapandji 1974; Figs 2.17, 2.116A, 2.117). The right and left innominate should move an equal amount. Flexion somewhere past 50–60 degrees sees the innominates and sacrum continuing to rotate forward symmetrically in most people. In some, however, the sacrum now starts to counternutate, the base moving posteriorly and the apex (coccyx) anteriorly, decreasing the lumbosacral angle and, therefore, the lumbar lordosis (Fig. 2.18A). Counternutation from this point on may occur on account of:

1. a posteriorly directed force applied to the sacral base by the flexing lumbar spine
2. a maximal tightening of the ligaments (interosseous, sacrotuberous and sacrospinous) effected by the initial nutation (Fig. 2.19A)
3. the presence of any other factor capable of opposing the progressive nutation of the sacrum; for example, tightness of:
   a. pubo-, ilio- and/or ischio-coccygeus (Fig. 2.53)
   b. the sacrotuberous ligament if continuous, in part or completely, with a tight rectus femoris (Fig. 2.6)

In sitting

The initial movement on trunk flexion is one of sacral counternutation as the innominates rotate anteriorly relative to the sacrum. Counternutation increases the tension in the long dorsal sacroiliac ligament in particular, eventually resulting in posterior rotation of the innominates and sacral nutation on further trunk flexion (Figs 2.19B, 2.80B).

Trunk extension

In standing

On extension, the innominates should rotate posteriorly to an equal extent and the sacrum nutates, increasing the lumbosacral angle and hence the lumbar lordosis (Figs 2.16, 2.18C).

In sitting

Initially, the innominates do not move as the spine extends and the sacrum nutates. Once nutation has taken up all the slack in the interosseous, sacrospinous

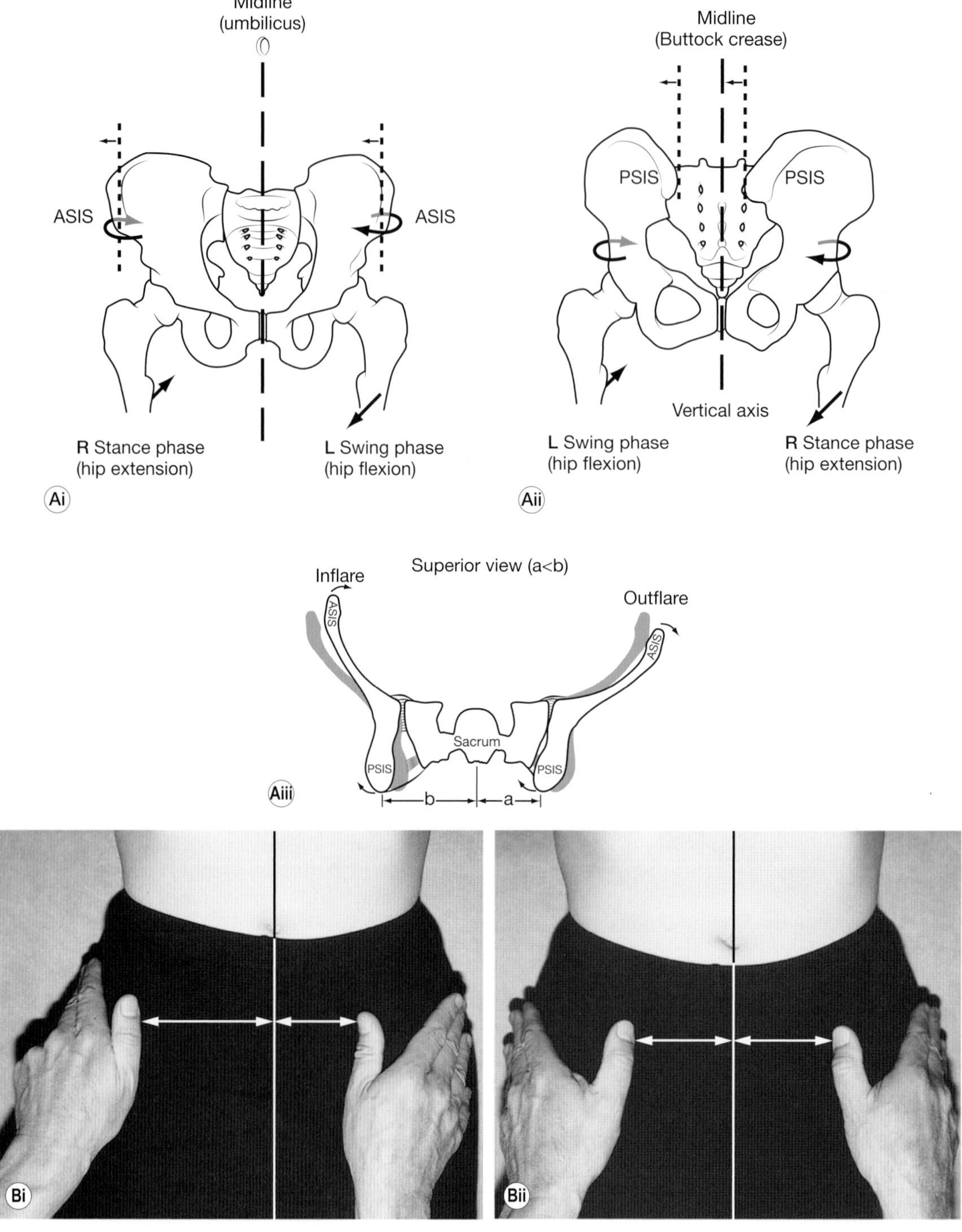

Fig. 2.13 'Inflare' and 'outflare' of the innominates in the transverse plane. (A) During normal gait cycle (right stance, left swing phase = the left inflares, the right outflares): (i) anterior view; (ii) posterior view; (iii) superior view. ASIS = anterior superior iliac spine; PSIS = posterior superior iliac spine. (B) With an actual 'outflare/inflare' presentation: relative to umbilicus (assuming that it is central in location), the thumbs resting against inside of the ASIS show: (i) initial asymmetry with a 'right outflare' (thumb away from the midline) and 'left inflare' (closer to the midline); (ii) symmetry following correction (equidistant from the midline).

(Continued)

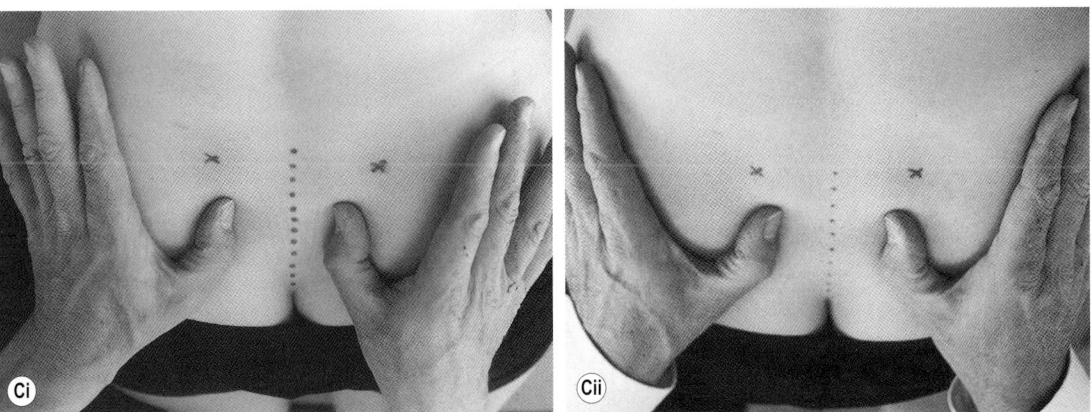

Fig. 2.13—cont'd (C) Relative to the buttock (gluteal) crease, thumbs against the inner aspect of the PSIS show: (i) initial asymmetry with 'right outflare' (thumb closer to the midline) and 'left inflare' (thumb away from the midline); (ii) right and left equidistant after correction of the 'outflare/inflare'.

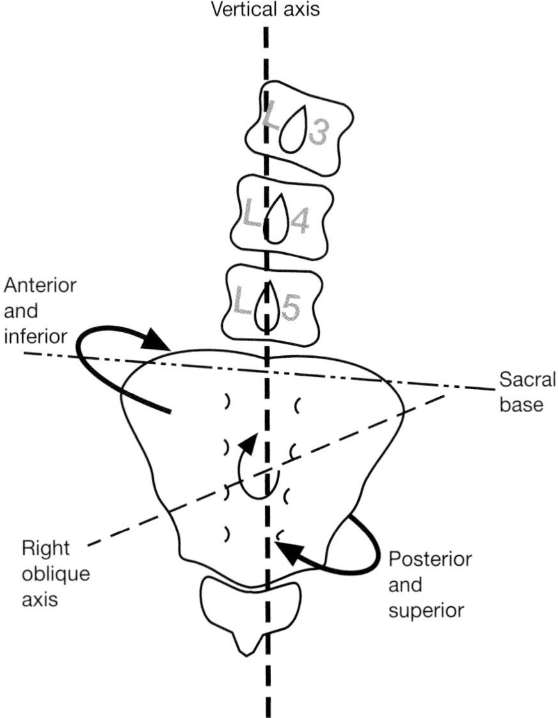

Fig. 2.14 Sacral torsion around the right oblique axis; also known as 'right-on-right' or R/R torsion pattern (see also Fig. 2.50)

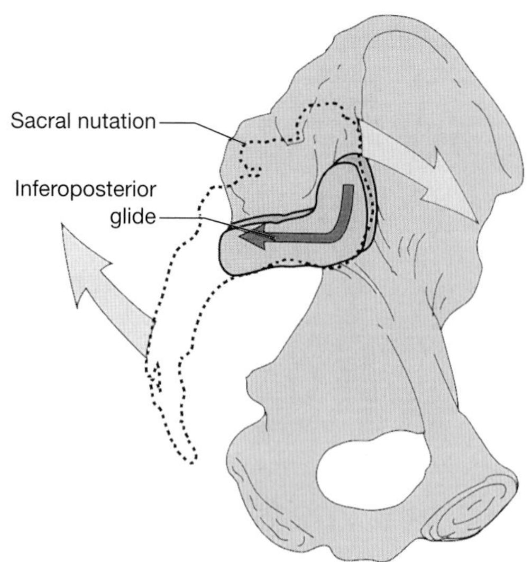

Fig. 2.15 When the sacrum nutates, its articular surface glides inferoposteriorly relative to the innominate (anterosuperiorly on counternutation). *(Courtesy of Lee 1999.)*

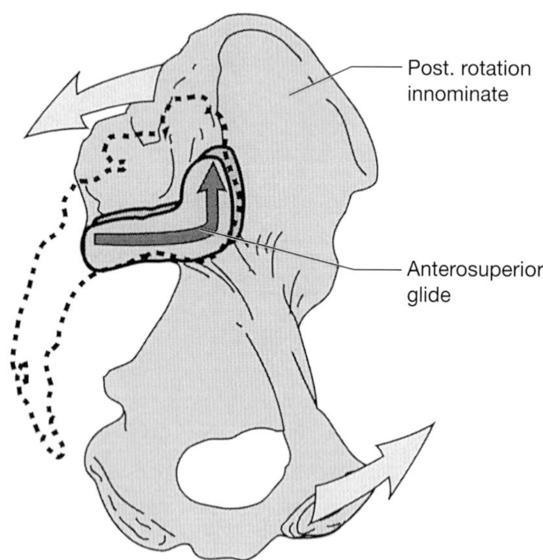

Fig. 2.16 When the innominate rotates posteriorly, its articular surface glides anterosuperiorly relative to the sacrum (inferoposteriorly on anterior rotation). *(Courtesy of Lee 1999.)*

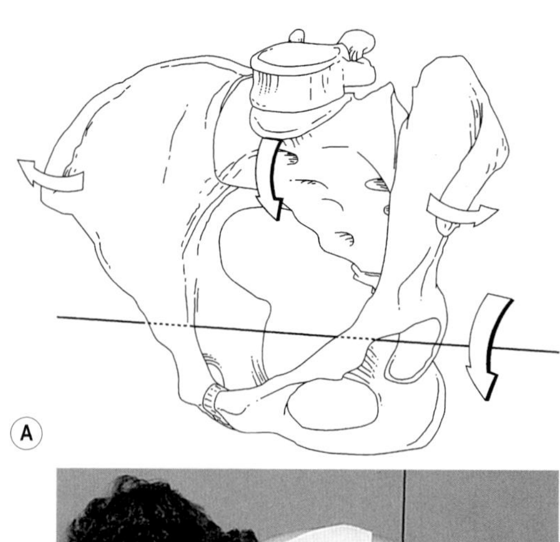

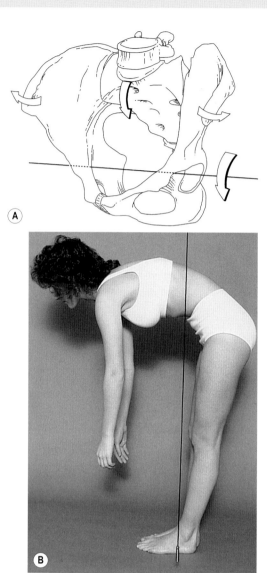

Fig. 2.17 Forward flexion of the trunk from the erect standing position normally results in initial sacral nutation, anterior rotation of the innominates and a concomitant outflare of both innominates. *(Courtesy of Lee 1999.)*

and sacrotuberous ligaments (Fig. 2.19A) and in the pelvic floor muscles and ligaments that attach to the coccyx, further extension will result in anterior rotation of the innominates (e.g. by increasing the traction force of the tight sacrotuberous ligament on the ischial tuberosity, pulling the innominate anteriorly).

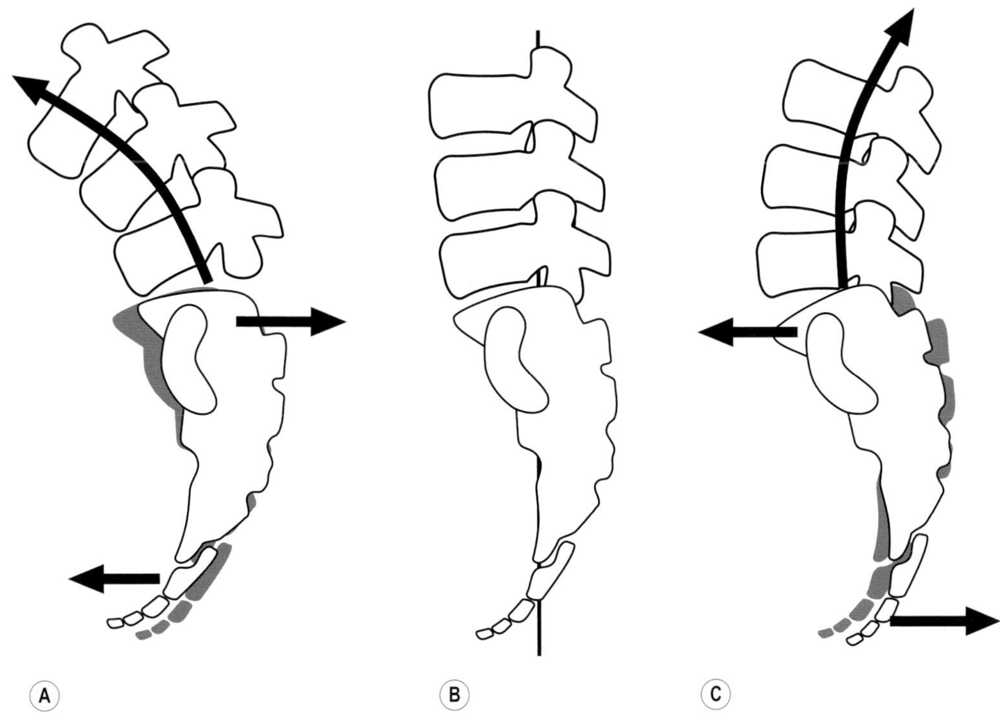

Fig. 2.18 Normal movement of the sacrum relative to the ilia. (A) Flexion past 45 degrees: sacral counternutation. (B) Neutral (standing). (C) Extension: sacral nutation.

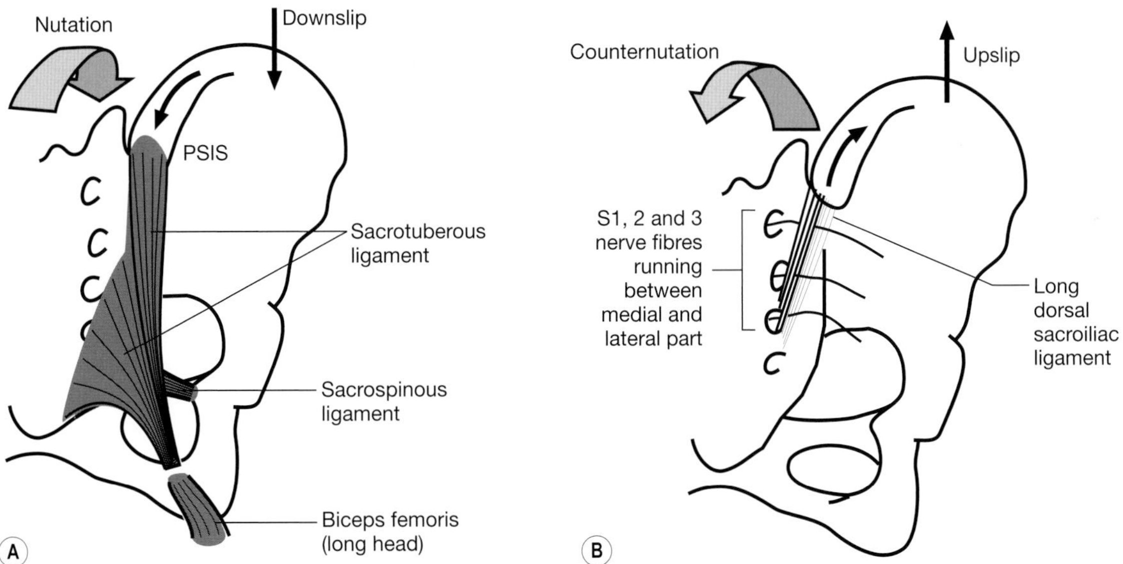

Fig. 2.19 Ligaments put under tension by the movement of an innominate or the sacrum relative to each other. (A) 'Posterior' rotation (= sacral nutation) and 'downslip' of an innominate: sacrotuberous, sacrospinous; also interosseous ligaments (not shown; see Figs 2.4B, 2.13Aiii). (B) 'Anterior' rotation (= sacral counternutation) and 'upslip' of an innominate: long dorsal sacroiliac ligament.

Landing on one leg

When jumping or missing a step and landing with the straight leg vertical and the foot directly underneath, the forces transmitted upward result in an ipsilateral SI joint movement consisting primarily of an upward translation of the innominate in the vertical plane relative to the sacrum (Fig. 2.20A). If there is a degree of angulation of the leg relative to the vertical axis at the moment of impact, there may be an element of anterior or posterior rotation in the sagittal plane. For example, missing the step(s) and landing with the straight leg angulated forward creates a force that can rotate the innominate anteriorly on that side, resulting in sacral counternutation and SI joint instability (Fig. 2.20B). Landing with the leg angulated backward can rotate the innominate posteriorly, resulting in sacral nutation and increasing SI joint stability. These changes are of particular importance when we come to consider the abnormal forces that can result in an 'upslip' and 'rotational malalignment' (Ch. 3). The biomechanics of standing on one leg are discussed in detail below (see 'Functional or dynamic tests'; Figs 2.121-125)

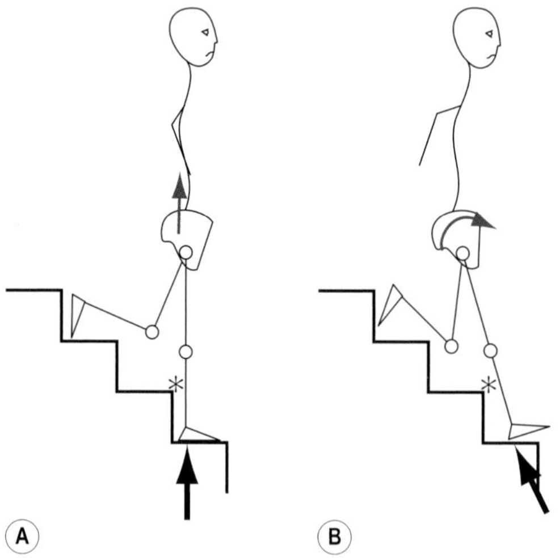

Fig. 2.20 Missing a step and landing with increased force on one extremity can cause malalignment of the pelvis.
A) With the leg vertical on impact, the force transmitted through the hip joint can result in upward displacement of the innominate relative to the sacrum (a so-called 'upslip').
B) Landing with the leg at a hip-flexion angle on impact results in an 'anterior rotational' force on the innominate, as illustrated.

Vertical forces on the sacrum

In standing, the sacrum is literally suspended between the innominate by the ligaments and may be in a slightly nutated or counternutated position (Fig. 2.4A,B). As proposed by Strachan in 1939, a force transmitted vertically downward from the lumbar region causes the sacrum to glide downward and flex (Fig. 2.15); traction applied from above causes the sacrum to move upward and extend (Fig. 2.16).

Ambulation

During ambulation, there is:

1. rotation of each innominate around the coronal axis in the sagittal plane - anteriorly on the side of hip extension, posteriorly on the side of hip flexion (Figs 2.10, 2.21, 2.41-1,3,5,7)
2. rotation of the pelvic unit as a whole around the vertical axis in the transverse plane - the ASIS moves forward with the leg during swing phase, backward on the side of the extending leg during stance phase (Fig. 2.12)
3. rotation of the pelvic unit as a whole around the sagittal axis in the coronal plane - the iliac crest is initially higher on the side of heel-strike and drops progressively on going past mid-stance to toe-off while the reverse is happening on the opposite side from toe-off to heel-strike (Fig. 2.41-4,8)
4. torquing of the sacrum, alternately to the right and left around the vertical and oblique axes with each gait cycle, concomitant with displacement of the pelvis as described (Figs 2.10B, 2.21).

For example, as the right leg swings forward, there is posterior rotation of the right innominate which results in a left rotation of the sacrum (around the left oblique axis), increase in sacral nutation and with this an increase in tension in the right sacrotuberous (ST), sacrospinous and interosseous ligaments. Contraction of biceps femoris to further increase ST ligament tension (Fig. 2.22), combined with contraction of specific muscles that cross the right SI joint (e.g. piriformis, gluteus maximus and iliacus), has the overall effect of stabilizing the right SI joint in preparation for heel-strike and weight-bearing on that side (Figs 2.32, 2.46, 2.62).

KINETIC FUNCTION AND STABILITY

The ability of the SI joints to transfer weight and to absorb shock is closely linked to the proper functioning of the hip joints and the spine, in particular

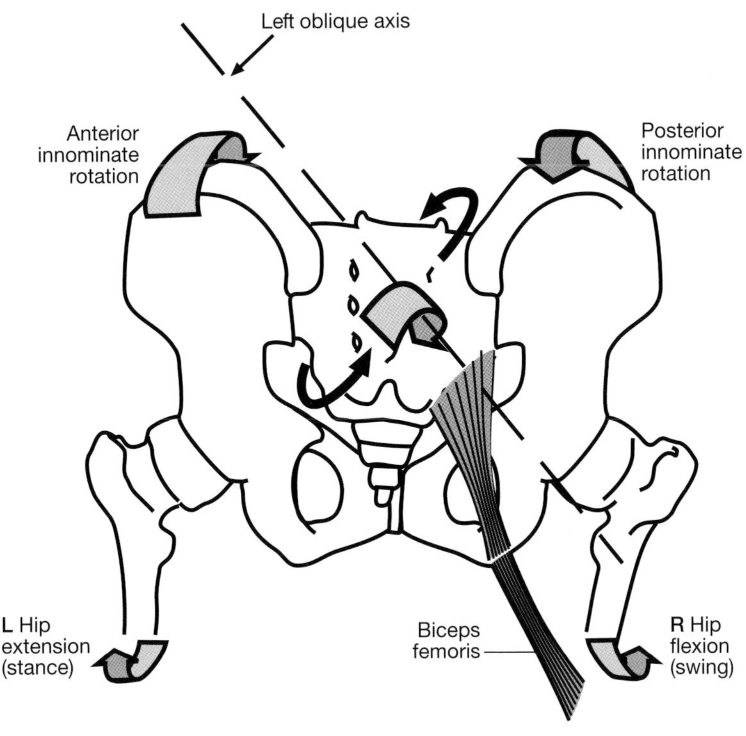

Fig. 2.21 Gait: right swing, left stance phase with 'right posterior, left anterior' innominate rotation, and sacral torsion around the left oblique axis. This results in increasing right SI joint stabilization, partly owing to increasing sacral nutation and a tightening of the right sacrotuberous, sacrospinous and interosseous ligaments, in preparation for heel-strike.

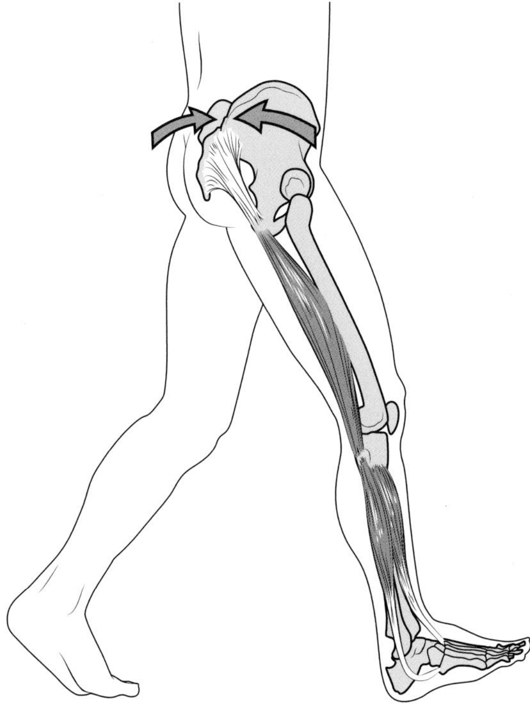

Fig. 2.22 At heel-strike, posterior rotation of the right innominate increases the tension in the right sacrotuberous ligament. Contraction of the biceps femoris further increases tension in this ligament, preparing the sacroiliac joint for impact. *(From Lee 2004a, redrawn courtesy of Vleeming et al. 1997.)*

the lumbar segment. Normal kinetic function involves all three regions simultaneously and depends on the availability of normal ranges of motion, appropriate muscle function and the ability to stabilize the various components adequately and in a coordinated manner. The following concepts are helpful in understanding the interaction between the pelvis, spine and lower extremities, in particular with regard to stability.

Panjabi: active, passive and neural control systems

Panjabi's conceptual model (1992a,b), originally intended to explain the stabilizing system of the spine, finds application 'to the entire musculoskeletal system' (Lee 1999), including the pelvic floor (Fig. 2.53) and is particularly helpful when trying to understand the factors that have a bearing on SI joint stability. Panjabi proposed the following interacting systems (Fig. 2.23):

1. the *'passive system'*: the 'osteoarticular ligamentous' structures; that is, the support derived from the actual shape of the joint and from its capsule and ligaments
2. the *'active system'*: the 'myofascial' or contractile tissues acting on the joint

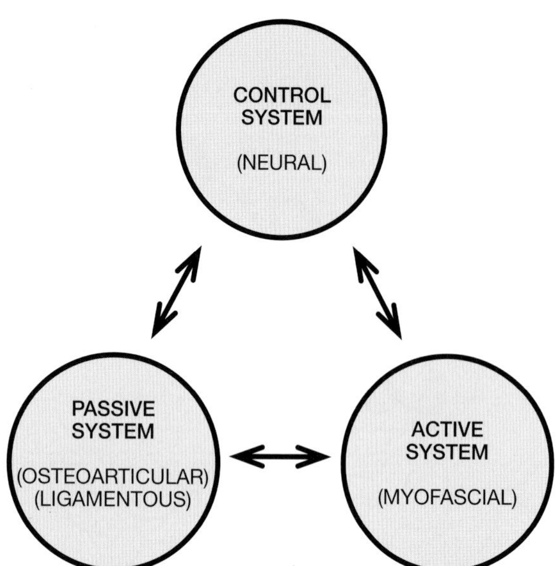

Fig. 2.23 Conceptual model by Panjabi illustrating the systems that interact to provide stability (see also Fig. 2.27). *(Redrawn courtesy of Panjabi 1992.)*

3. the '*control system*': the central and peripheral nervous systems that coordinate the interaction between the passive and active systems.

Normal interplay of these systems results in a small amount of displacement of the joint surfaces with minimal resistance, the so-called '*neutral zone*', and makes for stability (Fig. 2.24A). The neutral zone needs to be evaluated both quantitatively (the actual range of motion available - smaller or larger) and qualitatively (e.g. amount of resistance encountered on increasing or decreasing compression of the joint; Lee & Vleeming 1998, 2003); also, one must always do a side-to-side comparison of both factors. Injury to or degeneration of articulations and/or supporting ligaments (passive system), muscle weakness (active system) and incoordination or failure of muscle function (control system) can all result in instability, with abnormal displacement of the joint surfaces around an enlarged neutral zone (Fig. 2.24B).

Restriction of the 'neutral zone' may occur with:

1. contracture of the capsule and ligaments, with restriction of movement and stiffness of the joint (Fig. 2.24C)
2. active forces bringing the joint surfaces too close together, resulting in a so-called 'compressed' joint; for example, excessive tension in muscles acting on the joint (Fig. 2.24D)
3. excessive movement of the joint surfaces relative to each other to the point that they literally end up

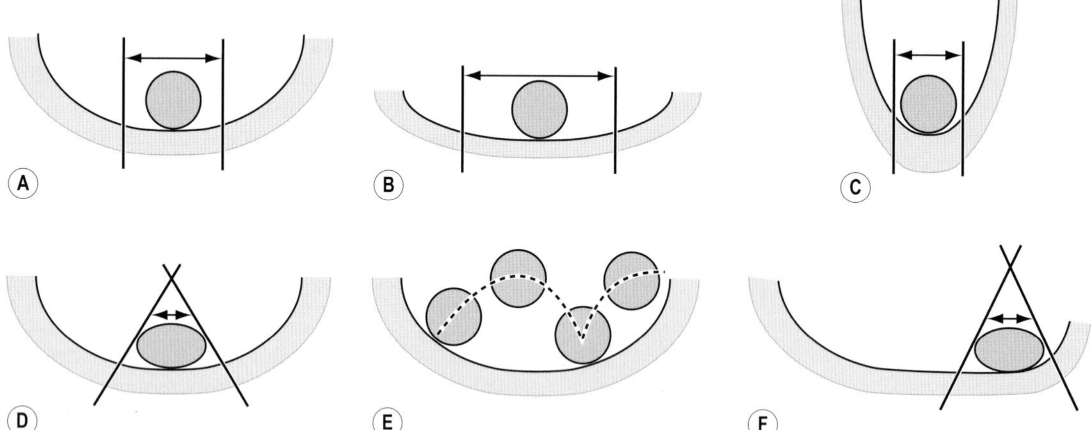

Fig. 2.24 The neutral zone can be affected by altering compression forces across the joint. (A) A graphic illustration of the neutral zone of motion in a hypothetically normal joint. (B) A joint which is insufficiently compressed due to the loss of either form or force closure will have a relative increase in the neutral zone of motion. (C) A joint which is excessively compressed due to fibrosis will have a relative decrease in the neutral zone of motion. (D) A joint which is excessively compressed due to overactivation of the global system will also have a relative decrease in the neutral zone of motion. (E) When there is an intermittent motor control deficit, *passive* motion within the neutral zone can be normal since the dysfunction is *dynamic*. The bouncing ball reflects the intermittent loss of compression during functional activities (dynamic instability). (F) A joint which is fixed (subluxed) is excessively compressed and no neutral zone of motion can be palpated (complete joint block). *(Courtesy of Lee 2004a.)*

getting 'stuck' in an abnormal position with the joint again 'compressed'; for example, subluxation of a joint, or excessive 'anterior' rotation of an innominate relative to the sacrum in the sagittal plane may actually result in 'joint compression' to the point of creating a so-called 'blocked' or 'locked' SI joint (Fig. 2.24F).

However, when a seemingly 'locked' joint is 'decompressed' by relaxing the muscles and/or manually moving the surfaces back into proper alignment, the neutral zone may now turn out to be enlarged because the capsule and ligaments were stretched initially when the excessive forward rotation occurred (e.g. a shear-force injury; Fig. 2.51B) or, subsequently, from being under increased tension as a result of the joint having been in this abnormal position for some time.

Failure of the control system can result in an aberrant movement of the surfaces relative to each other. A problem with control will become obvious with activity, when the muscles need to be activated or relaxed in proper sequence to carry out specific patterns of movement. On examination, passive movement within the neutral zone may be normal. However, active stabilization of the joint varies so that joint mobility is at times excessive, at other times normal, and sometimes inadequate as the appropriate distance between the joint surfaces is repeatedly lost and regained (Fig. 2.24E). In addition to the dynamic instability, chronic failure of the control system can eventually also result in passive instability as the joint surfaces deteriorate and the supporting capsule and ligaments are repeatedly stretched. The instability that results, for whatever reason, may present as a sudden 'giving way' of what is often mistakenly localized to the 'hip joint' but may actually be a manifestation of the 'slipping clutch' phenomenon which is discussed below and in Ch. 3 (Dorman 1994, 2001; Dorman et al. 1998; Vleeming et al. 1995a; Fig. 3.94).

'Self-locking' mechanism and 'form' and 'force' closure

The strong ligamentous support system that allows for proper SI joint function is, nevertheless, felt to be inadequate to prevent dislocation of the joints under postural load unless supplemented by other forces. This has led to the concept of a 'self-bracing' or 'self-locking' mechanism based on the fact that:

> *'In combination with load transfer through fascia, muscle forces that cross the SI-joints can produce joint compression. This [compression] counteracts mobility by friction and interlocking ridges and grooves'*
>
> (Snijders et al. 1993)

The terms 'form' and 'force' closure delineate the passive and active components of this self-locking mechanism, respectively (Snijders et al. 1993a,b, 1995a,b); Vleeming et al. 1990a, 1990b, 1997):

> *Shear in the SI-joints is prevented by the combination of specific anatomical features (form closure) and the compression generated by muscles and ligaments that can be accommodated to the specific loading situation (force closure) . . . If the sacrum would fit the pelvis with perfect form closure, no lateral forces would be needed. However, such a construction would make mobility practically impossible.*
>
> (Vleeming et al. 1995a)

In other words, 'form closure' refers to the stability provided by the joint structure itself and the capsular and ligamentous support; whereas 'force closure' refers to the any additional forces provided by muscles and myofascial structures on demand to ensure the stability of that joint for particular activities carried out under variable conditions (Figs 2.25, 2.26).

Because 'joint mechanics can be influenced by multiple factors...and that management requires attention to all', Lee & Vleeming (2003) proposed the 'dynamic' 'integrated model of function' that one should always consider on assessment and treatment in any attempt to achieve and maintain joint stability that is adequate for load transfer (Fig. 2.27). The model has the following four components:

1. form closure (structure, joint congruency)
   - depends on 'optimal function of the bones, joints and ligaments' (Vleeming et al. 1990a,b; Vleeming & Stoeckart 2007)
2. force closure
   - forces produced by myofascial action and, therefore, dependent on optimal function of the muscles and fascia (Vleeming et al. 1995b, Vleeming & Stoeckart 2007; Richardson et al. 1999, 2002; O'Sullivan et al. 2002; Hungerford 2002; van Wingerden et al. 2004)
3. motor control
   - specific timing of muscle action and inaction during loading (Hodges 1997, 2003; Hodges & Richardson 1997; Hodges & Gandevia 2000a; Hungerford et al. 2003)

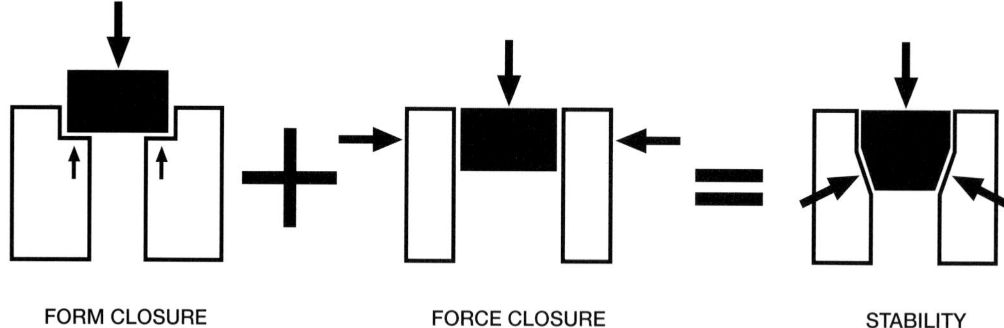

Fig. 2.25 Model of the self-locking mechanism: the combination of form and force closure establishes stability in the sacroiliac joint. *(Redrawn courtesy of Vleeming et al. 1997.)*

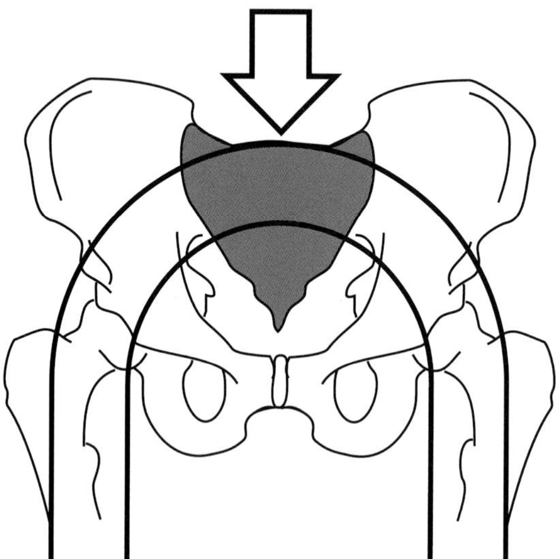

Fig. 2.26 'Form' closure: minimizing sacroiliac joint shear through the 'keystone in a Roman arch' effect, with the sacrum being 'trapped' vertically. *(Redrawn courtesy of Dorman & Ravin 1991.)*

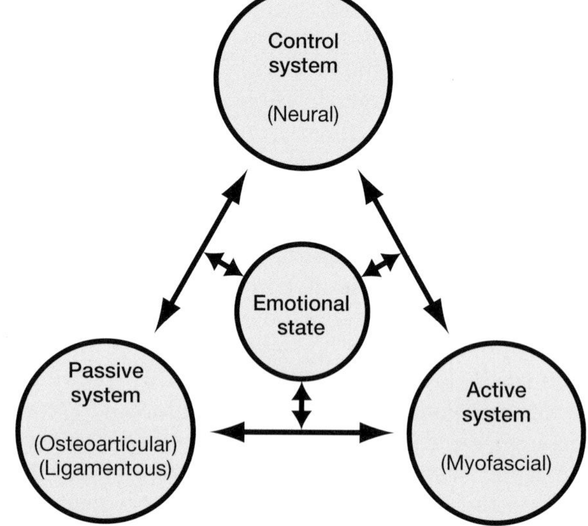

Fig. 2.27 Redrawing of Panjabi's model (see Fig. 2.23), to emphasize current acknowledgement of the interaction of psychological factors with the passive, active and control systems.

4. emotion

Psychological factors can affect form, force and neuromotor control unfavourably (Vlaeyen et al. 2000, 2007). The problem is discussed further in Ch. 4 under 'Psychiatry and psychology', to improve awareness of how emotional factors:

a. can play a role in causing musculoskeletal problems like the 'malalignment syndrome', or
b. may actually be a complication of such musculoskeletal problems.

Typical features in regards to emotional factors, cited by Lee and Vleeming (2007), include:

1. 'chronic pelvic or back pain', a history of 'traumatized life experiences', adopting motor patterns 'indicative of defensive posturing which suggests a negative past experience, [sustained] fight and flight reactions influencing basic muscle tone and patterning'
2. persistent increase in muscle tension resulting in increased levels of adrenaline (epinephrine) and cortisole which help perpetuate this vicious cycle (Holstege et al. 1996)
3. hypertonicity of pelvic muscles which can cause compression of the SI joints (Richardson et al. 2002; van Wingerden et al. 2001, 2004)

Treatment should include:

1. explaining the problem, time factors; restoring hope through education and awareness of the

underlying mechanical problem (Butler & Moseley 2003; Hodges & Moseley 2003)
2. 'professional cognitive-behavioural therapy...to retrain more positive thought patterns'
3. teaching individuals to become 'mindful' or aware of what is happening in their body whenever it is subjected to the effect(s) of physical and/or emotional loading, so as to reduce 'sustained, unnecessary muscle tone and therefore joint compression' (Murphy 1992)

Sacroiliac joint 'form' and 'force' closure

As concerns the lumbo-pelvic-hip region, 'a primary function is to transfer the loads generated by body weight and gravity during standing, walking and sitting' (Snijders et al. 1993a). In turn, how well this load is managed dictates how efficient function will be. Just the right amount of stability required for any effective load transfer is achieved when the passive, active and control systems work together (Panjabi 1992a,b). These systems produce approximation of the joint surfaces - the amount required is variable and depends on the individual's structure (form closure) and the forces needed for control (force closure). The term 'adequate' has been used, 'just enough to suit the existing situation' (Lee & Vleeming 1998, 2007). Too much force would result in 'stiffness' of the joint, impaired movement, or even inability to move at all; too little, in instability of the joint which, in turn, may result in a 'loose', unstable, or even totally uncontrolled motion.

'Local' and 'global' motor systems

Force closure and motor control depend on the adequate functioning of the muscles and the neural control. Increasingly sophisticated research has shown that any physical action can be divided into two phases: a preparatory phase which helps stabilize a particular part of the body and, in turn, allows the proposed action itself to be carried out safely and efficiently. Bergmark in 1989 suggested classifying muscles into two categories: a 'local' and a 'global' system. These are now commonly referred to as the 'inner' and 'outer' core muscles. When throwing a ball, for example, there are actually three phases to the muscle action:

1st Phase: the 'local system' or 'inner core' muscle contraction, to achieve segmental stabilization (Figs 2.28, 2.29)

1. involves the thoracic diaphragm, transversus abdominis, the pelvic floor muscles and deep fibres of [the lumbosacral] multifidi

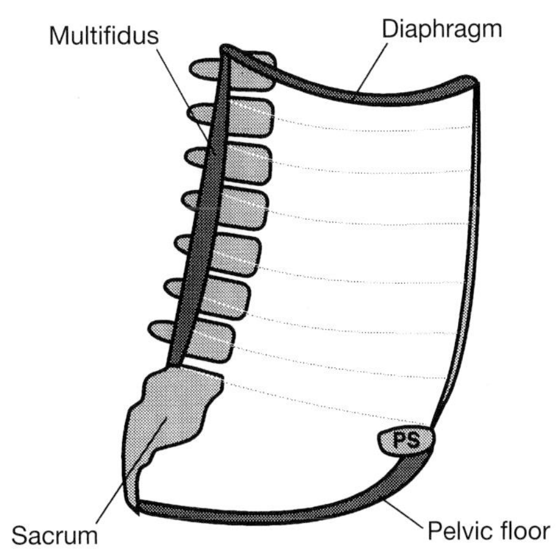

Fig. 2.28 The muscles of the 'inner core' unit include the multifidus, transversus abdominis (light lines), thoracic diaphragm and pelvic floor muscles. PS, pubic symphysis. *(Courtesy of Lee 1999.)*

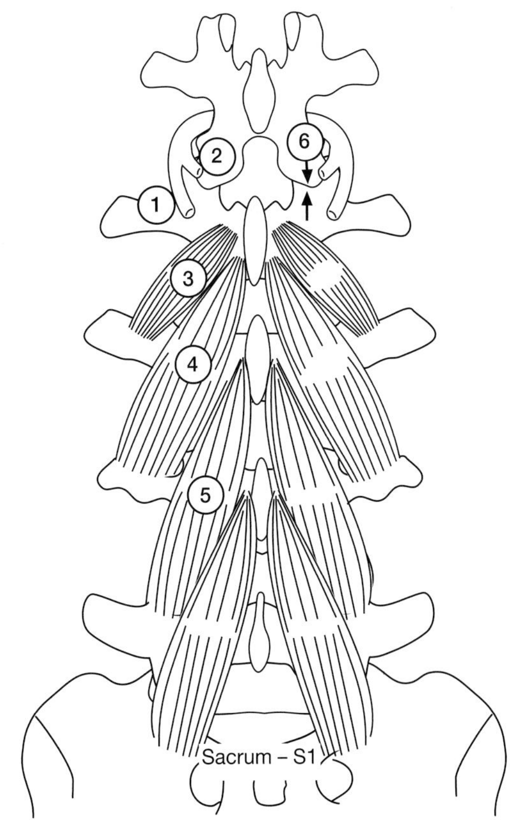

Fig. 2.29 Posterior elements of the lumbosacral spine.

2. ongoing research continues to identify other muscles that probably belong to this 'inner core' group (Lee 2004a): deep (medial) psoas (Gibbons et al. 2002), medial quadratus lumborum (Bergmark 1989; McGill 2002), lumbar part of iliocostalis and longissimus (Bergmark 1989), posterior part of internal oblique
3. achieves primarily 'intrapelvic', also segmental, stabilization (particularly with the multifidi acting on the lumbar spine) in preparation for carrying out this action
4. apparently is not direction dependent (Hodges 1997, 2003; Hodges & Richardson 1997; Hodges et al. 1999; Moseley et al. 2002, 2003)

2nd Phase: the 'global system' or 'outer core' muscle contraction to achieve regional stabilization (Figs 2.30–2.40)

1. involves contraction of muscles running from thorax to pelvis and pelvis to a lower extremity
2. achieves stabilization of thorax, pelvis and hip girdle and may be involved in initiating the actual motion (Lee 2004a; Lee et al. 2009, 2010)
3. contraction starts after that of the 'inner core' has been initiated; it is direction-dependent (Radebold et al. 2000, 2001; Hodges 2003)

3rd Phase: contraction of the peripheral muscles to carry out the action of throwing the ball

1. involves muscles in the upper and lower extremities, trunk and pelvis
2. given adequate stabilization has been achieved by the 1st and 2nd phase, this is the final phase of an action that involves considerable side-flexion to alternate sides, trunk rotation, torquing while transferring weight from one leg to the other (e.g. right-to-left with a right hand throw) as well as co-ordinated contraction of peripheral muscle and timing of release.

The end-result of this three-phase sequence is an action that:

1. can be carried out safely and efficiently on a stable base, given that stability of the pelvis and trunk has been established by contraction of 'inner' and then 'outer' core muscles in anticipation of the action
2. results in throwing the ball the distance required by correctly matching speed and the angle of release.

Throwing events will be discussed further in Chapters 3 and 5 (Figs 3.51, 5.30, 5.31).

Sacroiliac joint 'form' closure

In the case of the SI joint, form closure is derived from the following:

1. The triangular shape of the sacrum makes it fit between the innominates 'like a keystone in a Roman arch' (Dorman and Ravin 1991). The two ends of the arch are firmly connected by the sacrotuberous and sacrospinalis ligaments, so that the relatively flat SI joint surfaces are loaded only with compression and shear is minimized (Fig. 2.26).
2. The interlocking of the complementary articular surfaces of the sacrum and innominates helps to counter vertical and anteroposterior translation (Figs 2.2, 2.3).
3. The anterior widening of the sacrum restricts movement between the innominates by causing wedging in an anterior-to-posterior direction, thereby restricting counternutation (Figs 2.4B, 2.10A, 2.11A, 2.46B,D).
4. The increasing joint friction coefficient detected with advancing age as a result of:
   a. the formation of the interlocking ridges and grooves (Fig. 2.7B)
   b. roughening of the joint surfaces, which usually starts with the deterioration of the fibrocartilagenous cover of the iliac surface.
5. The ligaments that influence the SI joint and literally 'suspend' the sacrum between the innominates when a person is standing: the SI joint ligaments (anterior and posterior, interosseus and long dorsal) and the pelvic floor ligaments (Figs 2.4, 2.5, 2.13Aiii, 2.19, 2.52A, 2.53, 2.59, 3.64-3.66, 3.68).

Sacroiliac joint 'force' closure

SI joint force closure is achieved by two means.

First, there may be an active force that results in nutation of the sacrum (Figs 2.11A, 2.18C, 2.19A, 2.22, 2.31, 2.59). Nutation comes about either by anterior rotation of the sacral base (e.g. contraction of multifidi, extensor spinae or sacrospinalis) or posterior rotation of the innominates (e.g. contraction of rectus abdominis, biceps femoris or gluteal muscles). Nutation results in a tightening of the interosseous, sacrotuberous and sacrospinous ligaments (Fig. 2.19A). This tightening appears to facilitate the force closure mechanism, thereby increasing the compression of the SI joint articular surfaces which, in turn, increases the stability of the joint in preparation for load transfer (Vleeming et al.

1997). Conversely, counternutation, by decreasing tension in these same ligaments, decreases SI joint stability (Fig. 2.19B).

Second, force closure arises from the contraction of the 'inner' and 'outer' myofascial units, or 'core' muscles (see above). These units help to stabilize not only the pelvis but also the lumbar spine and hip joints, or 'lumbo-pelvic-hip complex'.

The 'inner core' or unit

The 'inner core' (Fig. 2.28) consists primarily of the deep fibres of multifidi, thoracic diaphragm, transversus abdominis and pelvic floor muscles.

1. Work by Sanford et al. (1997), using fine-wire electromyography, suggested that the contraction of specific abdominal muscles was coupled with the contraction of specific pelvic floor muscles (e.g. the co-contraction of transversus abdominis with pubococcygeus, the oblique abdominals with ilio/ischiococcygeus, and rectus abdominis with puborectalis).
2. This 'inner core' may be able to set up a force couple capable of affecting the stability of the SI joint and lumbosacral junction. For example, the multifidi originating from the lower lumbar vertebrae insert into the upper sacrum (Fig. 2.29), and ilio- and ischiococcygeus insert into the coccyx (Fig. 2.53). Contraction of the multifidi causes sacral nutation; contraction of ilio- and ischiococcygeus, counternutation. A change in these two forces that favours one group compared to the other could move the sacrum into a stable or unstable position, repectively.
3. Transversus abdominis contraction appears to occur in preparation for carrying out an action (Richardson et al. 1999) by:
    a. the co-activation of pubococcygeus; that is, part of the pelvic floor
    b. the force closure of the anterior aspect of the SI joints (Fig. 2.30); simultaneous compression of that part of the joint caused by inward movement of the innominates is resisted by the strong ligaments running across the back of the SI joint on that side (Snijders et al. 1995b)
    c. lateral traction forces by way of insertions into the thoracolumbar fascia posteriorly and abdominal fascia anteriorly (Porterfield & DeRosa 1998; Fig. 2.31A,B) and forces that act on the ilia anteriorly (Richardson et al. 2002), including the external and internal oblique (Figs 2.32 and 2.33, respectively); these forces, in turn:

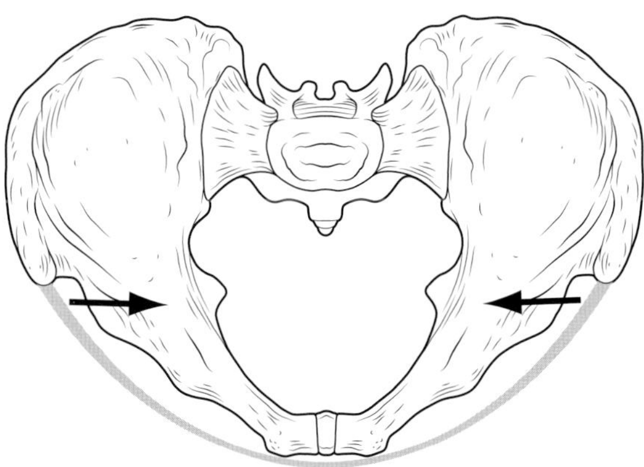

Fig. 2.30 Contraction of the transversus abdominis is proposed to produce a force which acts on the ilia perpendicular to the sagittal plane (i.e. approximates the ilia anteriorly: arrows). *(Courtesy of © Diane G. Lee Physiotherapy Corp.)*

    i. increase the intra-abdominal pressure, believed to contribute to lumbar spine stability (Aspden 1987; Barker & Briggs 1999)
    ii. increase tension within the thoracolumbar fascia, stabilizing the fascia and thereby making it more effective in its role as part of the 'outer unit'; in particular, as part of the posterior oblique and deep longitudinal systems, discussed below.

4. Contraction of superficial lumbar multifidi extends the lumbar spine as they create a lever arm by way of their attachments to the spinous processes. In contrast, contraction of the deep fibres of the lumbar multifidi, which lie next to the body of the lumbar vertebrae, actually compress these vertebrae. Also, contraction makes the deep muscle broaden and swell between the sacrum and overlying thoracodorsal fascia (Fig. 2.34); this has been likened to 'pumping up' the fascia, increasing tension in the fascia particularly in the thoracolumbar region 'by virtue of... broadening effect of the muscle as it contracts' (Gracovetsky 1990; Vleeming et al. 1995a; Lee 2004a; DeRosa & Porterfield 2007). Using Doppler imaging, Richardson et al. (2002) were able to show that simultaneous contraction of deep multifidi and transversus abdominis now anchored to a tighter thoracodorsal fascia, increased 'stiffness' of the SI joints. Clinically, the effect would appear to be a stabilization of the pelvic ring of bones, similar to that achieved with a sacroiliac belt. Also, contraction of the deep

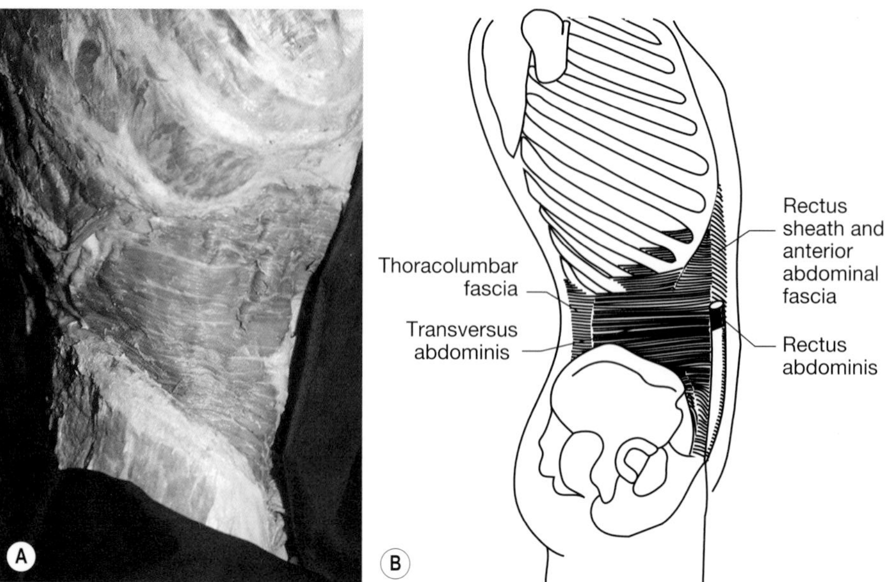

Fig. 2.31 (A) The transversus abdominis is attached posteriorly to the thoracolumbar fascia and anteriorly to the abdominal fascia. Note that it has an optimal muscle fibre orientation to pull posteriorly on the abdominal fascia, complementing the more angled forces on the fascia exerted by the external and internal abdominal oblique muscles. *(Courtesy of Porterfield & DeRosa 1998: 92.)* (B) Muscles that are part of the 'inner' (transversus abdominis) and 'outer' core (rectus abdominis).

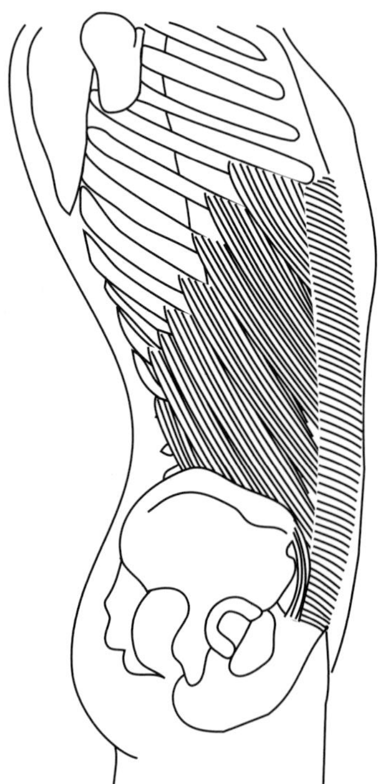

Fig. 2.32 Muscles that are part of the 'outer core' unit: External oblique.

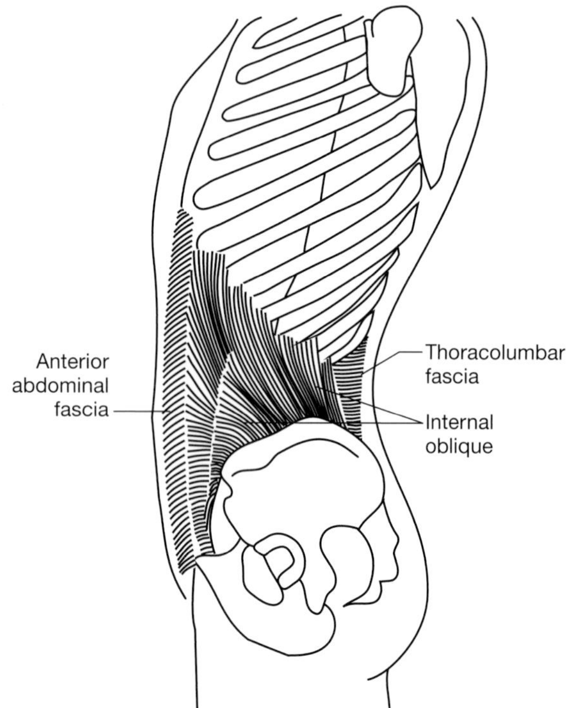

Figure 2.33 Muscles that are part of the 'outer core' unit. Internal oblique.

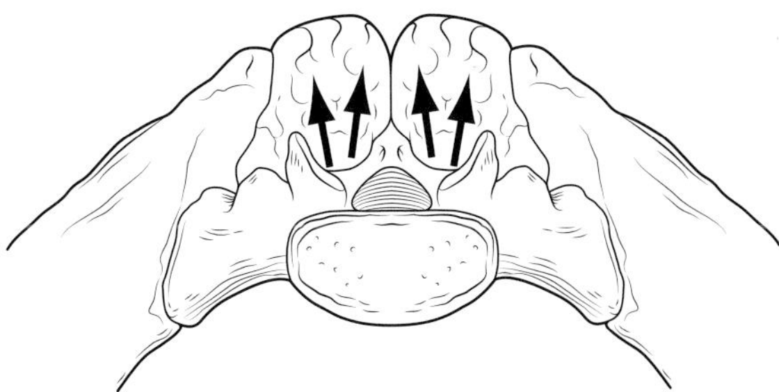

Fig. 2.34 When the deep fibres of the multifidi contract, the muscle can be felt to broaden or swell (represented by the arrows in the deep layers of the muscle). This hydraulic amplifying mechanism (proposed by Gracovetsky 1990) 'pumps up' the thoracolumbar fascia much like a balloon (Vleeming et al. 1995a) *(Courtesy of the © Diane G Lee Physiotherapy Corp.)*

multifidi has been observed to occur just prior to use of the upper extremities 'when the load is predictable' (e.g. throwing a ball) in order to stabilize the lumbar spine in anticipation of carrying out that action (Moseley et al. 2002; Hodges & Cholewicki 2007).

Uni- or bilateral segmental atrophy of multifidi visualized using Real-Time ultrasound (RTUS) and other dynamic techniques has been described in association with chronic back pain, failure to activate multifidi in proper sequence or not at all. RTUS is helpful in that it allows for instant feedback with selective muscle strengthening and activation (see Chs 4, 7).

The 'outer core' or unit

The 'outer core' is made up of the *oblique, longitudinal and lateral systems* of 'slings' of interconnecting muscles, tendons, ligaments and fascia. While contraction of an individual muscle may exert a force on a specific joint, if that muscle is part of one or more of these slings it can also:

1. exert a force on a distant site
2. increase stiffness of the SI joint by compressing the surfaces, even though the muscle does not itself cross the joint (van Wingerden et al. 2001; Lee 2004a; DeRosa & Porterfield 2007).

The four basic sling systems of the 'outer' unit

1. *the posterior (dorsal) oblique sling*

   The continuum of latissimus dorsi connected, by way of the thoracolumbar fascia, to the contralateral gluteus maximus constitutes the upper part of this system (Fig. 2.35) which will, on contraction:

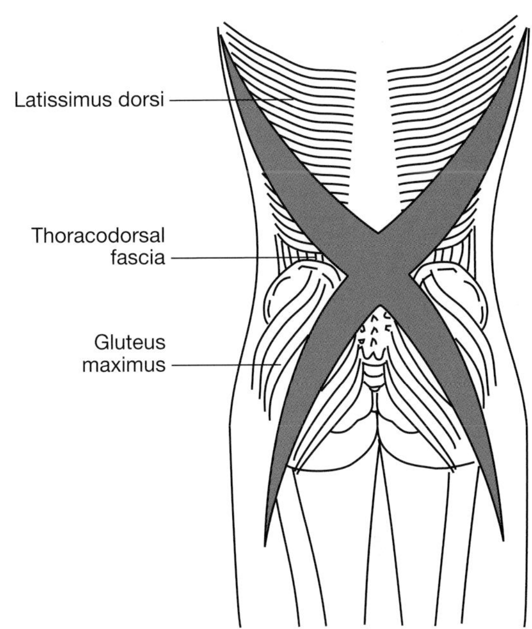

Fig. 2.35 The oblique systems of the 'outer unit'. Posterior oblique system. *(From Lee 1999, as redrawn courtesy of Snijders et al. 1995.)*

   a. compress the SI joint on the side of gluteus maximus, improving SI joint ability to attenuate shear loads (Porterfield and DeRosa 1998; Vleeming et al. 1990a,b)
   b. stiffen the lumbar spine 'over multiple spinal segments. . .minimizing translatory motion between the lumbar vertebrae' (DeRosa and Porterfield 2007)
   c. contribute to load transfer through the pelvic region with rotational activities (Mooney et al. 1997) and during gait (Gracovetsky 1997; Greenman 1997; Fig. 2.41)

   The lower part of this system is comprised of the continuations of gluteus maximus that act to tense the ITB. Concomitant contraction of TFL and vastus lateralis further increase tension in ITB which helps stabilize the knee during the 'single support' or stance phase (Fig. 2.36A)

2. *the deep longitudinal sling*

   This sling was initially described as the continuum of the ipsilateral erector spinae muscle and contralateral iliocostalis connected, by way of the deep lamina of the thoracodorsal fascia, to the contralateral sacrotuberous ligament and biceps femoris (Gracovetsky 1997; Vleeming et al. 1997; Lee 2004a; Figs 2.37, 2.38A).

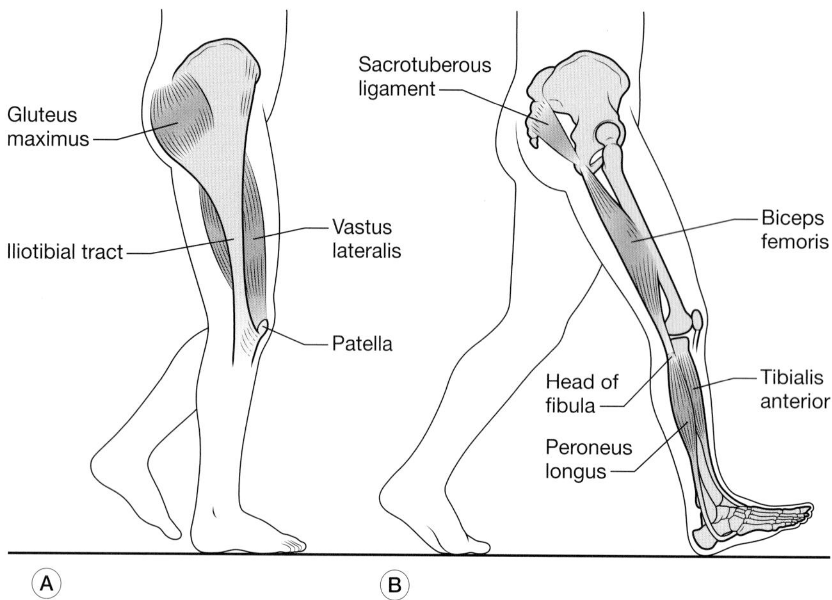

Fig. 2.36 (A) Lower part of the oblique dorsal muscle-fascia-tendon sling. Relationship between gluteus maximus muscle, iliotibial tract, vastus lateralis muscle and knee in the single support phase. The iliotibial tract can be tensed by action of the dorsally located gluteus maximus and ventrolaterally located tensor fascia lata muscle. The tract can also be tensed by contraction of the vastus lateralis muscle. (B) The longitudinal-tendon-fascia sling. Relations at the end of the swing phase. *(Courtesy of Vleeming & Stoeckart 2007.)*

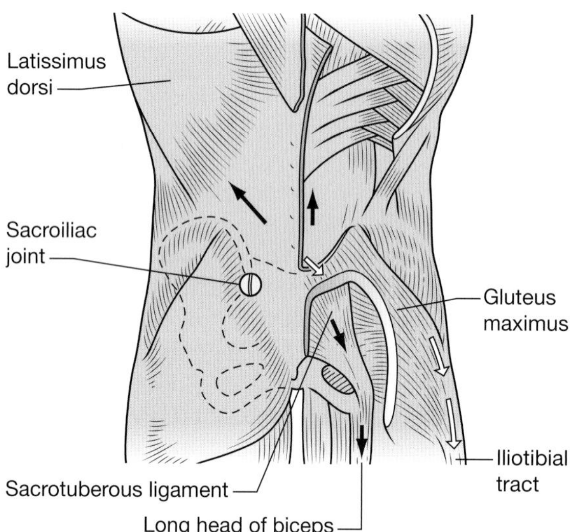

Fig. 2.37 Schematic dorsal view of the low back. The right side shows a part of the longitudinal muscle-tendon-fascia sling. Below this is the continuation between biceps femoris tendon and sacrotuberous ligament, above this is the continuation of the erector spinae. To show the right erector spinae, a part of the thoracolumbar fascia has been removed. The left side shows the sacroiliac joint and the cranial part of the oblique dorsal muscle-fascia-tendon sling, latissimus dorsi muscle and thoracolumbar fascia. In this drawing the left side of the thoracolumbar fascia is tensed by the left latissimus dorsi and the right gluteus maximus muscle. *(Courtesy of Vleeming & Stoeckart 2007.)*

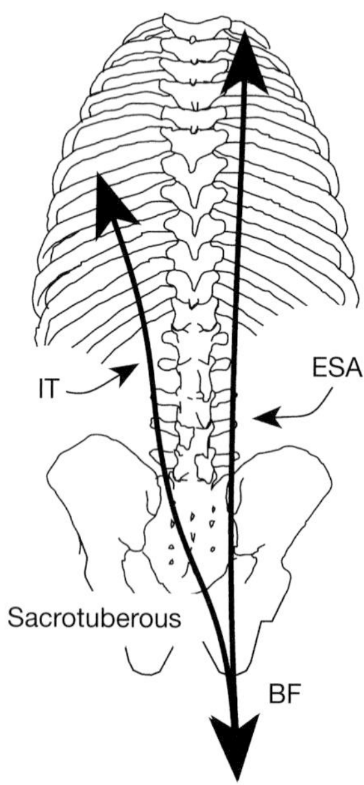

Figure 2.38 Deep longitudinal system of the 'outer' unit: the biceps femoris (BF) is directly connected to the upper trunk via the sacrotuberous ligament, the erectores spinae aponeurosis (ESA) and iliocostalis thoracis (IT). *(Courtesy of Gracovetsky 1997.)*

It is now felt to include peroneus longus and probably also tibialis anterior, both of which have been shown to contract in preparation for heel-strike (Fig. 2.36B). The effect of activating this 'deep longitudinal system' is to:

a. compress the SI joint because of biceps femoris connections and the increase in tension on the sacrotuberous ligament (van Wingerden et al. 1993)
b. increase tension in the thoracodorsal fascia and, thereby, enhance the ability of the fascia to contribute to any SI joint force closure mechanisms acting across it
c. decrease downward movement of the fibula by way of contraction of biceps femoris which inserts into the head of the fibula
d. probably help support the longitudinal arch of the foot by tightening the sling formed by peroneus longus and tibialis anterior (both of which insert into the medial cuneiform and the base of the 1st metatarsal.

3. *the anterior oblique sling*

The external obliques on one side are connected, by way of the anterior abdominal fascia, to the contralateral internal abdominal obliques and adductors of the thigh (Fig. 2.39A). The lower horizontal fibres of the internal abdominal oblique may augment transversus abdominis in its role of supporting the SI joint (Richardson et al. 1999). Posteriorly, the internal oblique attaches to the upper and the external oblique to the lower part of the thoracolumber fascia, allowing them to exert a stabilizing effect on the upper and lower part of the lumbar spine, respectively; whereas the more extensive transversus abdominis attachments can affect the length of the lumbar segment (Barker & Briggs 2004). Interaction of the anterior shoulder girdle muscle groups has been well delineated by DeRosa and Porterfield (Fig. 2.39B).

4. *the lateral sling*

This sling is comprised of the lateral stabilizers of the thoracopelvic region (e.g. quadratus lumborum) and the primary stabilizers of the hip, namely gluteus medius and minimus (G. med/min), tensor fascia lata and the contralateral adductors of the thigh (Fig. 2.40). The gluteus medius and minimus are more involved with stabilizing the pelvic girdle at the hip joint rather than with SI joint force closure,

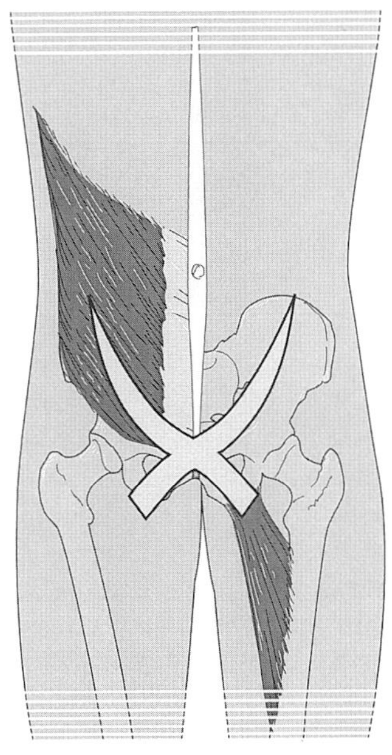

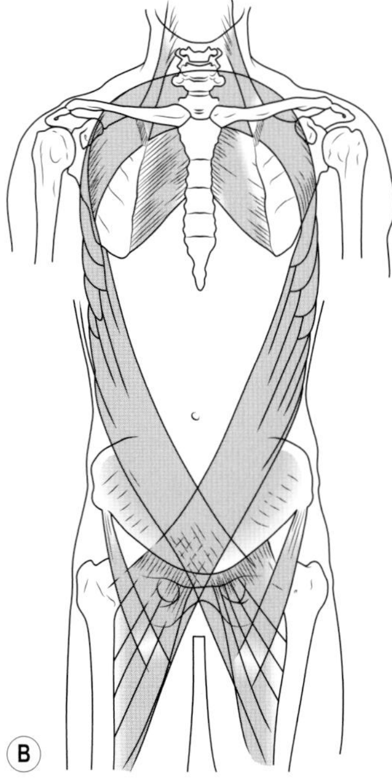

Fig. 2.39 (A) Anterior oblique system. *(Courtesy of Lee 1999.)* (B) Muscle sling of the shoulder girdle and the abdominal mechanism. The muscle fibre line of the rhomboids is continuous with the line of pull of the serratus anterior. The serratus anterior interdigitates and is often fused with the external abdominal oblique, which has a muscle fibre line of force in parallel with the internal abdominal oblique on the opposite side of the body. *(Courtesy of Porterfield & DeRosa 2004.)*

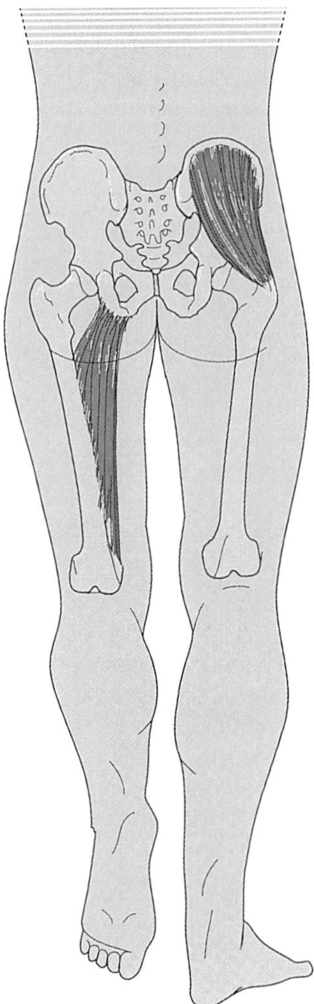

Fig. 2.40 The lateral system of the outer unit includes: lateral stabilizers of the hip (gluteus medius and minimus) and the tensor fascia lata (not shown), the contralateral adductors of the thigh, and the lateral stabilizers of the thoracopelvic region (e.g. quadratus lumborum). *(Courtesy of Lee 1999.)*

acting in particular to stabilize the femoral head in the acetabulum just prior to heel strike and throughout single-leg stance (Gottschalk et al. 1989). SI joint instability, however, is thought to possibly result in a reflex inhibition of these muscles which could be one mechanism to account for the feeling of the hip 'giving away', or 'slipping clutch syndrome' (Dorman 1994, 1995, 2001; Dorman et al. 1998; Vleeming et al. 1995a; Fig. 3.94)

The four basic 'sling systems' described are also interlinked and part of larger systems that allow for controlled load transfer and mobility, ensure balance and stability and also help to absorb shock. Contraction of the obliques may actually initiate movement, provided that the trunk has been stabilized by prior contraction of transversus abdominis (Richardson & Jull 1995; Hodges & Richardson 1996).

Force closure of the SI joints will suffer as a result of problems within the active system and/or the control system:

1. actual muscle weakness; atrophy
2. the inadequate recruitment of muscles in one or several interacting slings, which can also result in weakness affecting a whole system
3. uncoordinated contraction and relaxation of these local and global systems, resulting in failure to provide adequate stability and consistent control of motion (Hodges & Gandevia 2000b; Hodges 2003; Hodges & Cholewicki 2007)

The movement patterns that a patient starts to use in order to compensate for these insufficiencies - weakness, impaired muscle tension and control - results in abnormal stresses on the musculoskeletal system and may lead to an 'eventual decompensation of the low back, pelvis, hip and knee joints' (Lee 1997), including earlier, more rapidly progressing and more marked degenerative changes, ligament laxity and joint instability (see Fig. 3.82).

Given that the problem involves not isolated muscles but these well-defined interacting slings, Lee (2004a) has provided an excellent summary of the overall role of the core muscles and the slings:

> *'In conclusion, when the local system is functioning optimally, it provides anticipatory intersegmental stiffness of the joints of the lumbar spine (Hodges et al. 2003) and pelvis (Richardson et al. 2002). This external force (force closure) augments the form closure (shape of the joint) and helps prevent excessive shearing at the time of loading. This stiffness/compression occurs prior to the onset of any movement and prepares the low back and pelvis for additional loading from the global system. Simultaneously, the diaphragm maintains respiration while the pelvic floor assists in maintaining the position of the pelvic organs (continence) as load is transferred through the pelvis'.*

Treatment now emphasizes working on the 'local' and 'global' system as a whole in trying to re-establish strength, coordinated activation of contraction, and neural control (Richardson et al. 1999, Lee 2004a, 2007, Lee & Vleeming 2003).

Functional evaluation of 'form' and 'force' closure

There are a number of functional tests for the evaluation of form and force closure that are coming into common usage in clinical practice, both to help one arrive at a proper diagnosis and to determine the appropriate treatment. These are discussed under 'Functional or dynamic tests' below.

Sacroiliac joint function during the gait cycle

Right swing phase

The right SI joint becomes progressively more stable in preparation for weight-bearing, as a result of:

1. rotation of the sacrum around the left oblique axis, so that the right sacral base drops forward and down into nutation, while the apex rotates backward and to the left (Fig. 2.21); the rotation is initiated by the contraction of left piriformis and gluteus maximus, key stabilizers of the oblique axes, during the left stance phase
2. rotation of the right innominate posteriorly relative to the sacrum (Fig. 2.22)

Both of these actions result in increasing nutation of the right SI joint, with a passive increase in tension in the sacrotuberous, sacrospinous and interosseous ligaments (form closure). At the same time, tension in the 'posterior oblique' sling is increased both:

1. actively, with contraction of the right gluteus maximus, and
2. passively, with the simultaneously swinging forward of the left arm and clockwise rotation of the trunk, stretching left latissimus dorsi and, through the thoracodorsal fascia connections, involving gluteus maximus and distal muscles of this sling (Figs 2.35, 2.36).

The right iliopsoas is already contracting to help swing the leg forward, at the same time acting across the right SI and hip joint (force closure). The onset of right hamstring contraction just before heel-strike further increases the tension in the sacrotuberous ligament, augmenting form closure. The combined effect is a compression of the right SI joint, increasing its stability and, hence, ability to deal with load transfer at heel-strike.

Right stance phase

During the late stance phase, gradual destabilization of the now weight-bearing right SI joint (in preparation for the next swing phase) is accomplished by:

1. the onset of counternutation of the right sacral base, as the sacrum begins to rotate around the right oblique axis with the left leg swinging forward (Figs 2.10B, 2.41)
2. anterior rotation of the right innominate bone relative to the sacrum, passively with hip extension and actively with contraction of the ipsilateral iliacus and rectus femoris (Fig. 2.59)
3. contraction of piriformis (one of the prime hip extensors).

Tension in the right sacrotuberous ligament decreases even further as the hamstrings gradually start to relax. Form closure of the right SI joint is, therefore, gradually lost during late stance phase, so that stability during this phase is provided primarily by force closure. Active contraction of the left latissimus dorsi and right gluteus increases tension in the thoracolumbar fascia that connects them (Fig. 2.35) and compresses the right SI joint; this contraction also starts to reverse the forward swing of the left arm and clockwise rotation of the trunk that had occurred during the right swing phase. Iliacus and rectus femoris act across the joint while helping the anterior rotation of the innominate. Once hip extension has been completed at the end of right stance, gluteus maximus and piriformis begin to relax, at which point sacral torsion around the right oblique axis can proceed unhindered to its maximum range in preparation for left heel-strike.

As the right leg begins to swing forward following toe-off, the sacrum again begins to rotate around the left oblique axis, and the cycle repeats itself. During a complete cycle, therefore:

1. the SI joints move reciprocally in a figure-of-8 pattern
2. there is need to control vertebral and pelvic unit motion in all six degrees of freedom, as well as translation/rotation of any segments of the pelvis relative to each other (Fig. 2.9)

The interaction between the spine, pelvic unit and hips during the gait cycle is further deliniated in Figure 2.41.

Ongoing research and clinical presentations continue to clarify SI joint anatomy, the forces normally acting on the joint especially during weight transfer and its role in the normal and abnormal function of the lumbo-pelvic-hip complex as a whole. The part that the joint plays in the pathological presentations of malalignment will be discussed throughout the following sections. However, granted that the SI joint is in a key position to influence the function of the spine, pelvis and legs, it cannot be stressed enough that it is but one part of a system of muscles and bones that are interconnected and can affect each other detrimentally especially when malalignment is present.

COMMON PRESENTATIONS OF PELVIC MALALIGNMENT

Studies have repeatedly shown malalignment of the pelvis to be present in 80 to 90% of high school graduates (see 'aetiology' below; Klein 1973). About one-third are asymptomatic, two-thirds symptomatic

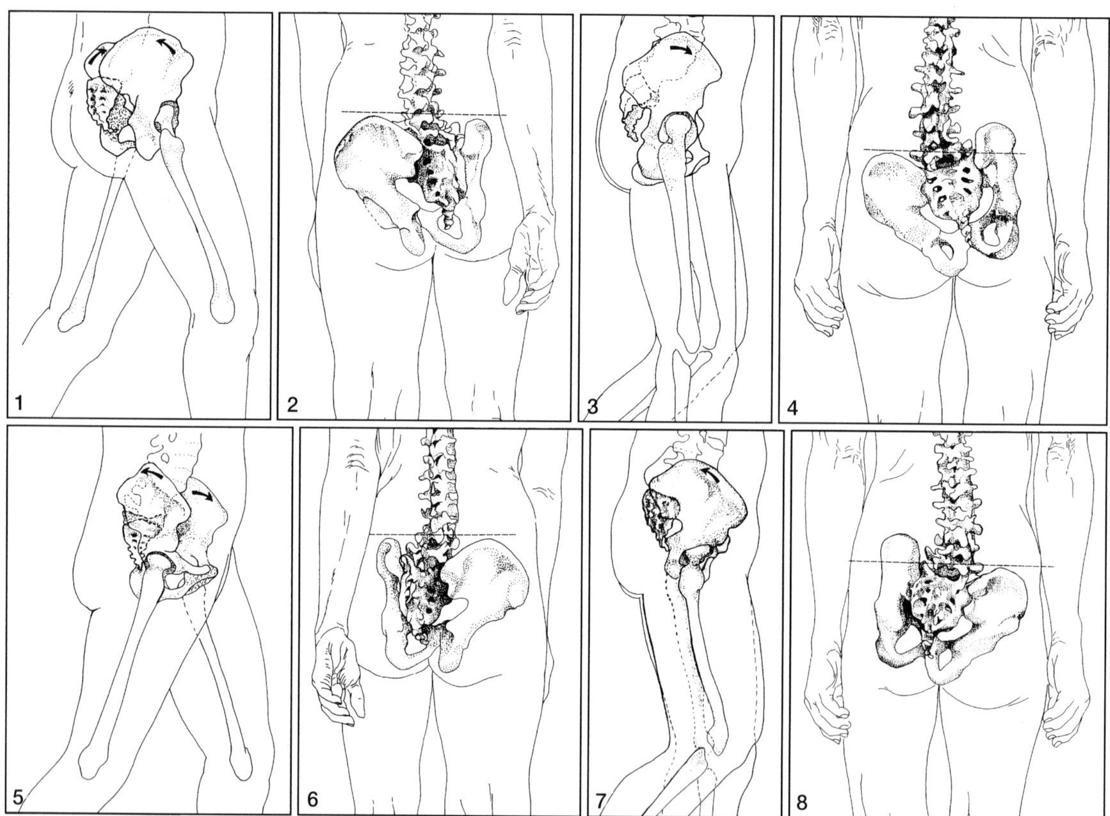

Fig. 2.41 Combined activities of right and left innominates, sacrum and spine during walking. ***At right heel strike***: 1. the right innominate has rotated in a posterior and the left innominate in an anterior direction; 2. the anterior surface of sacrum is rotated to left and superior surface is level, while the spine is straight but rotated to the left. ***At right midstance***: 3. the right leg is straight and the innominate is rotating anteriorly; 4. the sacrum has rotated to the right and side-bent left; whereas the lumbar spine has side-bent right and rotated left. ***At left heel strike***: 5. the left innominate begins rotation anteriorly; after toe-off, the right innominate begins rotation posteriorly; 6. Initially the sacrum is level but with the anterior surface rotated to right. The spine, although straight, is also rotated to right, as is the lower trunk. ***At left leg stance***: 7. the left innominate is high and the left leg straight; 8. the sacrum has rotated to the left and side-bent right, while the lumbar spine has side-bent left and rotated right. *(Courtesy of Greenman 1997.)*

(e.g. low back, leg or groin pain) with or without evidence of coincident facet or disc degeneration, root irritation or radiculopathy on investigation. Three common presentations account for some 90-95% of those found to be out of alignment. These presentations (with frequency noted in studies quoted in the text) are:

1. 'rotational malalignment' (80-85%)
2. pelvic 'flare' - innominate 'outflare'/'inflare' (40-50%), and the
3. 'upslip' (15-20%)

A presentation may appear in isolation or in combination with one or both of the others. For example, an 'upslip' appears on its own in about 10%, in combination with either 'rotational malalignment' or 'flare' or both in another 10%, for a total of 20% overall.

The following remarks should clarify some of the upcoming discussion:

1. ***'malalignment'***

   This refers to the abnormal biomechanical changes seen in conjunction with each of these three presentations; whereas
2. ***the 'malalignment syndrome'***

   The 'syndrome' refers to the clinical symptoms and signs that are typically associated with two of these presentations, namely: 'rotational malalignment' and an 'upslip'. It will be discussed in Ch. 3 and thereon.
3. ***'flare' presentations ('outflare'/'inflare')***

   These have their own distinct clinical features when seen in isolation but not those of a 'malalignment syndrome'. However, when seen in association with an 'upslip' and/or 'rotational malalignment', all the features of the 'malalignment syndrome' will also be present.

Discussion of the gait cycle above indicated how the innominates and sacrum normally move through a figure-of-8 pattern, from swing to stance phase and back again. The three presentations of malalignment suggest that the pelvic ring has seemingly become 'stuck' in one or a combination of the three patterns that the innominates normally move through relative to each other and to the sacrum with each gait cycle.

Looking at someone walking, with the right leg moving forward through 'swing', left leg through 'stance' phase (Fig. 2.41), these patterns are:

1. counterclockwise rotation of the pelvic unit around the vertical axis in the transverse plane (Fig. 2.12), so that the innominate (ASIS/PSIS)
   - moves relatively forward on the side of the right leg and backward on the side of the weight-bearing left leg
   - may arrest, or get 'stuck', in this particular 'flare' combination, which would present as a 'right inflare, left outflare'.
2. 'posterior' rotation of the right, 'anterior' rotation of the left innominate around the coronal axis in the sagittal plane
   - arrest of movement would result in a 'rotational malalignment' presentation; in this case, in the 'right posterior, left anterior' pattern
3. clockwise rotation around the sagittal axis in the coronal (frontal) plane, so that the innominate (iliac crest) rises on the left (weight-bearing) side, falls on the right (non-weight-bearing) side
4. sacral rotation around an oblique axis, in this case the 'left-on-left' axis (Figs 2.21, 2.50)
   - 'fixation' in this pattern would see the sacrum 'frozen' in a position where the right sacral base has moved forward and down, the left inferior angle backward and up.

'ROTATIONAL MALALIGNMENT'

'Rotational malalignment' refers to fixation of an innominate bone relative to the sacrum in excessive anterior or posterior rotation in the sagittal plane. Such rotation can affect an innominate on one side only but is more likely to be seen in association with:

1. compensatory rotation of the contralateral innominate, with arrest in the opposite direction and failure to move on through the figure-of-8 pattern as it should during a normal walking cycle (Figs 2.10, 2.21, 2.41)
2. displacement of the pubic bones relative to each other (Figs 2.42, 2.76C,D, 3.86)

The overall effect is a completely asymmetrical distortion of the pelvic ring (Fig. 2.76). There may also be:

1. movement dysfunction, involving one or both SI joints
2. torsion of the sacrum, most often around one of the oblique axes

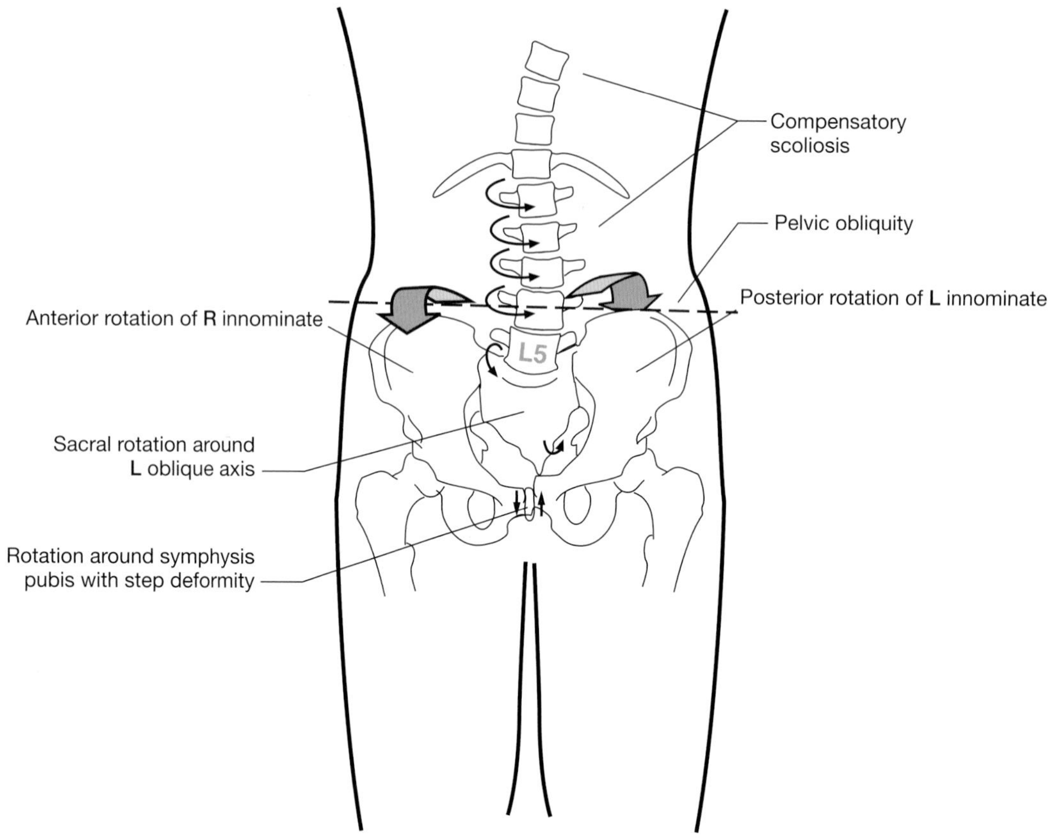

Fig. 2.42 Typical pelvic ring distortion associated with 'rotational malalignment': 'right anterior', compensatory 'left posterior' innominate rotation, as shown. Pubic bones are rotated and displaced at the symphysis; sacrum in torsion around the left oblique axis. Pelvic obliquity (here inclined to right) and compensatory scoliosis (lumbar segment here convex to left; L1-L4 rotated into convexity).

On passive examination, SI joint movement dysfunction may occur in the form of:

1. hypermobility, hypomobility, or actual 'locking', of one of the SI joints
2. compensatory hypermobility of the the SI joint contralateral to the one known to be hypomobile or 'locked' (Fig. 2.125)
3. instability of one or both SI joints attributable to muscle weakness or fatigue, ligament laxity, joint degeneration, impaired neural control or a combination of these

> The most common pattern of 'rotational malalignment' is that of 'right anterior, left posterior' innominate rotation with 'locking' of the right SI joint

Examination findings typical of the 'most common' rotational patterns are detailed in Appendix 1.

Aetiology of 'rotational malalignment'

Individuals are sometimes able to recall a specific incident that seemed to have triggered their problem. They may blame a fall, a collision or a lifting, twisting or reaching incident. Females may date onset around the time of a pregnancy (see Ch. 4, 'Implications for . . . obstetrics') when they are especially vulnerable because of the increase in weight, ligament laxity attributed to increased relaxin hormone levels pre-partum and while breastfeeding, the mechanical and emotional stress of delivery and asymmetrical stresses incurred in caring for the infant (e.g. an unexpected torsional force lifting the baby from the crib or change-table at an angle).

There is, however, often no obvious history of trauma, raising the question whether 'rotational malalignment' is really the result of some forgotten traumatic incident or is more likely a developmental phenomenon. The following are some of these other mechanisms that may have resulted in 'rotational malalignment'.

Developmental

Several studies have found a high percentage of children already presenting with asymmetries before reaching their teens. Pearson (1951, 1954), undertaking progressive standing radiological studies on 830 children from 8 to 13 years of age, found some degree of pelvic obliquity in 93%. Longitudinal studies by Klein and Buckley (1968) and Klein (1973) showed an increasing prevalence of asymmetry on going from elementary (75%) to junior (86%) to senior high school (92%). One might think that the an innominate fixed in 'anterior' or 'posterior' rotation may be the result of an accumulation of minor traumas and insults. However, as Fowler had already suggested in 1986 (810), the rotation is thought to be 'primarily the result of muscular imbalances which secondarily restrict sacroiliac joint motion', a clearly identified traumatic or mechanical stress being a less frequent cause. Perhaps the 'muscular imbalance' relates to a craniosacral problem (see Ch. 8), a C1–C2 instability or a prevalent one-sidedness in motor dominance. For example:

1. 70% of us are left, 15% right motor dominant. In other words, the combined total of some 85% showing 'asymmetric motor dominance' might correspond to that of the approximately 85% found to be out of alignment with one or more of the three most common presentations: 'rotational malalignment', 'flare' and/or an 'upslip'
2. 80-85% of these individuals whose pelvis is found to be out of alignment present with a 'rotational malalignment': approximately 75-80% of them with a 'right anterior, left posterior' innominate rotation and the remaining 5-10% with a 'left anterior, right posterior' rotation
3. the 70% who are left and 15% right motor dominant also matches the approximately 70% who are right, 15% who are left hand dominant.

One might speculate that:

1. the approximately 70% with left and 15% right motor dominance and/or the 70% with right and 15% left-sidedness correspond to the split of those with 'rotational malalignment' into 80-85% with 'right anterior/left posterior' and 5-10% with 'left anterior, right posterior' pattern, respectively
2. any one, or combination of two or all three presentations, can result in an asymmetry in muscle tension that predisposes to the occurrence and subsequent recurrence(s) of malalignment
3. this would leave approximately 10-15% with symmetrical motor dominance and symmetrical muscle tension, who are ambidextrous and present in alignment on examination.

However, studies on alignment, handedness and patterns of muscle tension to date have failed to bear out these speculations.

Combinations of bending, lifting, twisting and reaching

A particular traumatic incident or mechanical stress later in life may have made a pre-existing 'rotational malalignment' symptomatic rather than actually having caused that malalignment. A common mechanism involves bending forward and twisting the trunk to reach to either the right or left side. The intent may be simply to pick up a piece of paper from the floor (Fig. 2.43), or reaching above horizontal to a high shelf (Fig. 2.44). These movements often constitute an action of either extension or forward flexion combined with side-flexion and axial rotation of both the sacrum and the vertebrae. The onset of pain is usually acute, often felt on trying to get back to the upright position. Sometimes the pain comes on more gradually, over the next few hours or even days, which is more suggestive of injury to ligaments or tendons and the prolonged time required for inflammation to develop because of the relatively poor blood supply to these structures.

Stevens (1992) postulated how a strong activation of gluteus maximus and biceps femoris on the side opposite to the lateral bending, in conjunction with the asymmetrical loading of the spine and pelvis inherent to side-flexion while standing, may result in a side-to-side difference in the amount of anterior rotation that is possible in the SI joints on attempting this manoeuvre (Fig. 2.43). For example, on simultaneous reaching forward and bending to the right, anterior rotation in the SI joints is:

1. restricted on the contralateral (left) side with the increase in tension in the left sacrotuberous ligament, in part due to contraction of muscles that can be interlinked with this ligament; e.g. gluteus maximus, piriformis, biceps femoris and deep multifidi (Figs 2.6, 2.45)

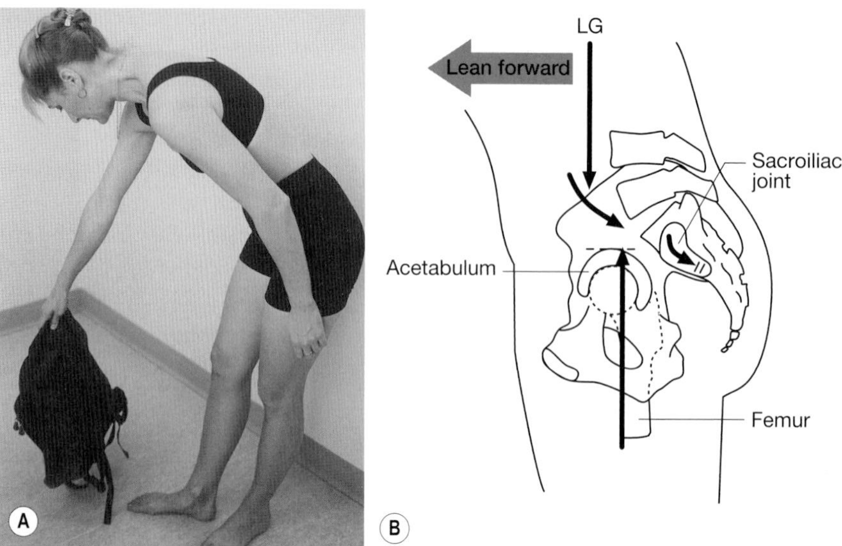

Fig. 2.43 A common way of causing a pre-existing asymptomatic 'rotational malalignment' to become symptomatic. (A) Simultaneously bending forward and twisting to the right or left (or returning back to neutral from that position), especially when attempting to lift or just hang on to a weight. (B) When the trunk leans forward, the line of gravity (LG) moves anteriorly, causing an anterior rotation of the pelvis around the acetabula; caudal gliding of the sacroiliac joint is impaired, relaxing the posterior pelvic ligaments and making the joint vulnerable. *(Redrawn courtesy of DonTigny 1990.)*

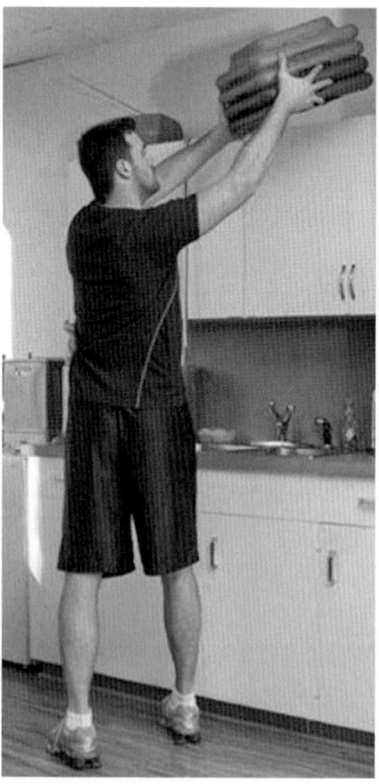

Fig. 2.44 Stocking shelves often requires simultaneous reaching and twisting which predisposes to recurrence of malalignment of the pelvis and spine and precipitation or aggravation of symptoms.

2. normal or possibly even increased on the ipsilateral side (Willard 1997)

DonTigny (1990, 2005) described how, on bending forward in standing, the weight of the trunk shifts the line of gravity anterior to the acetabula and 'the innominates tend to rotate anterior and downward around the acetabula and appear to limit caudal gliding [of the sacrum]' (1990: 483). In this position, the SI joints become vulnerable: the sacrum is counternutated, the posterior SI joint ligaments – with the exception of the long dorsal sacroiliac ligament - are now in a relaxed position, and the anterior ligaments never do offer much support at the best of times (Figs 2.4A, 2.5, 2.19):

> *Because the sacrum is placed within the innominates and is wider anteriorly, when the innominates move anteriorly and downward on the sacrum the innominates tend to spread on the sacrum. On reaching their limit of motion, they may wedge and become fixed in the anterior position. There is no problem when the spine and the innominates flex anteriorly at the same rate, or if the spine flexes prior to the innominates. Dysfunction occurs*

> *when the innominate bones rotate anteriorly prior to flexion of the spine, or if the innominates lag and the spine extends prior to posterior rotation of the innominates.*
> (DonTigny 1990: 485)

In both situations, the innominates rotate anteriorly and the sacrum into relative counternutation, making the SI joint unstable and vulnerable to displacement.

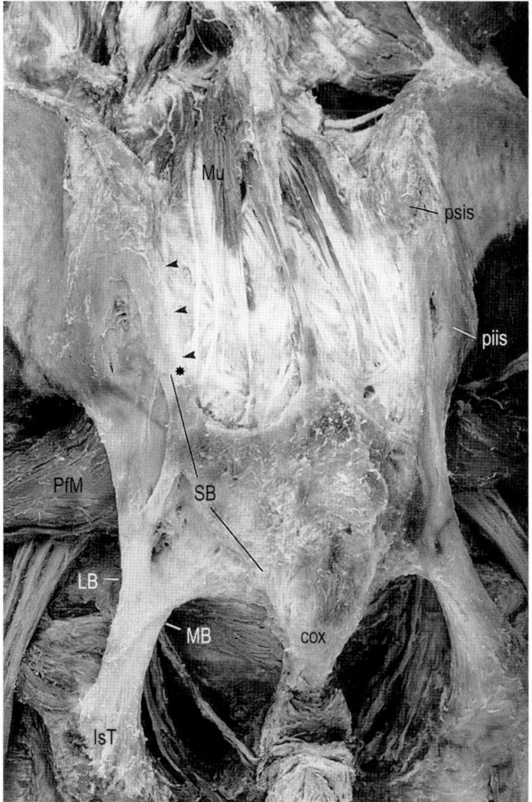

Fig. 2.45 Dorsal view of the male sacroiliac joint (SIJ) and sacrotuberous ligament. All but the deepest laminae of the multifidus muscle (Mu) have been removed. The sacrotuberous ligaments [are] seen stretching from the ischial tuberosity (IsT) to the coccyx (cox) medially and the posterior iliac spines superolaterally. . . . The arrowheads mark the course of the long posterior interosseous ligament under the lateral band of the sacrotuberous ligament. Three major bands of the ligament are seen: lateral (LB), medial (MB) and superior (SB). The lateral band spans the piriformis (PfM) to reach the ilium inferior to the (piis). As the lateral band climbs toward the (psis), it blends with the raphe. The medial band attaches to the coccyx and the superior band. . .[connects] the coccyx with the posterior ilial spines. Tendons of the multifidus pass between the superior band and the long dorsal SI ligament to insert into the body of the sacrotuberous ligament. *(Courtesy of Willard 2007.)*

Spasm occurring in specific muscles can also result in wedging of the bones of the pelvis in an abnormal position. For example, iliacus normally contracts to stabilize the SI joint in preparation for heel-strike and early weight-bearing phase; if it goes into spasm, it can cause the innominate on that side to become stuck in an 'anterior' rotated position relative to the sacrum (Figs 2.46B,C, 3.42). Iliacus would have the effect of rotating the innominate anteriorly and wedging it against the widening sacrum. Piriformis contraction actually rotates the sacrum posteriorly on that side, in effect pulling it against the innominate as the latter is attempting to rotate forward (Fig. 2.46A,C). However, as Grieve pointed out in 1988, and as indicated in the discussion in Chapter 3:

> *Sacroiliac sprain and pelvic torsion are so often associated with spasm or tightness of the piriformis that it is difficult to decide whether sacroiliac dysfunction is primary or secondary to piriformis overactivity.*
> (Grieve 1988:177)

Certainly, increased tone or outright 'spasm' is commonly detected in iliacus, piriformis and also gluteus maximus in someone presenting with malalignment; the tension sometimes decreases or resolves immediately on realignment. This phenomenon suggests that the increase in tone was in reaction to the malalignment rather than the cause of it, very likely indicative of facilitation and/or reflex contraction of these muscles as they attempt to counter the SI joint instability and decrease any discomfort caused by the malalignment (see Chs 3, 4: 'orthopedics' and 'piriformis syndrome').

Rotational forces acting on an innominate

Forces can act directly on the innominates to cause excessive anterior or posterior rotation relative to the sacrum which may result in a partial-to-complete impairment of movement between the sacrum and ilium. Unilateral rotational forces can result in three ways:

Leverage effect of a lower extremity

Excessive leverage forces can be exerted on one or other innominate with passive movements of the femur, either deliberately or such as may occur unintentionally in sports and during surgical, obstetric and gynaecological procedures (Grieve 1976; Figs 2.47, 7.16). There comes a point on passive right hip extension, for example, at which

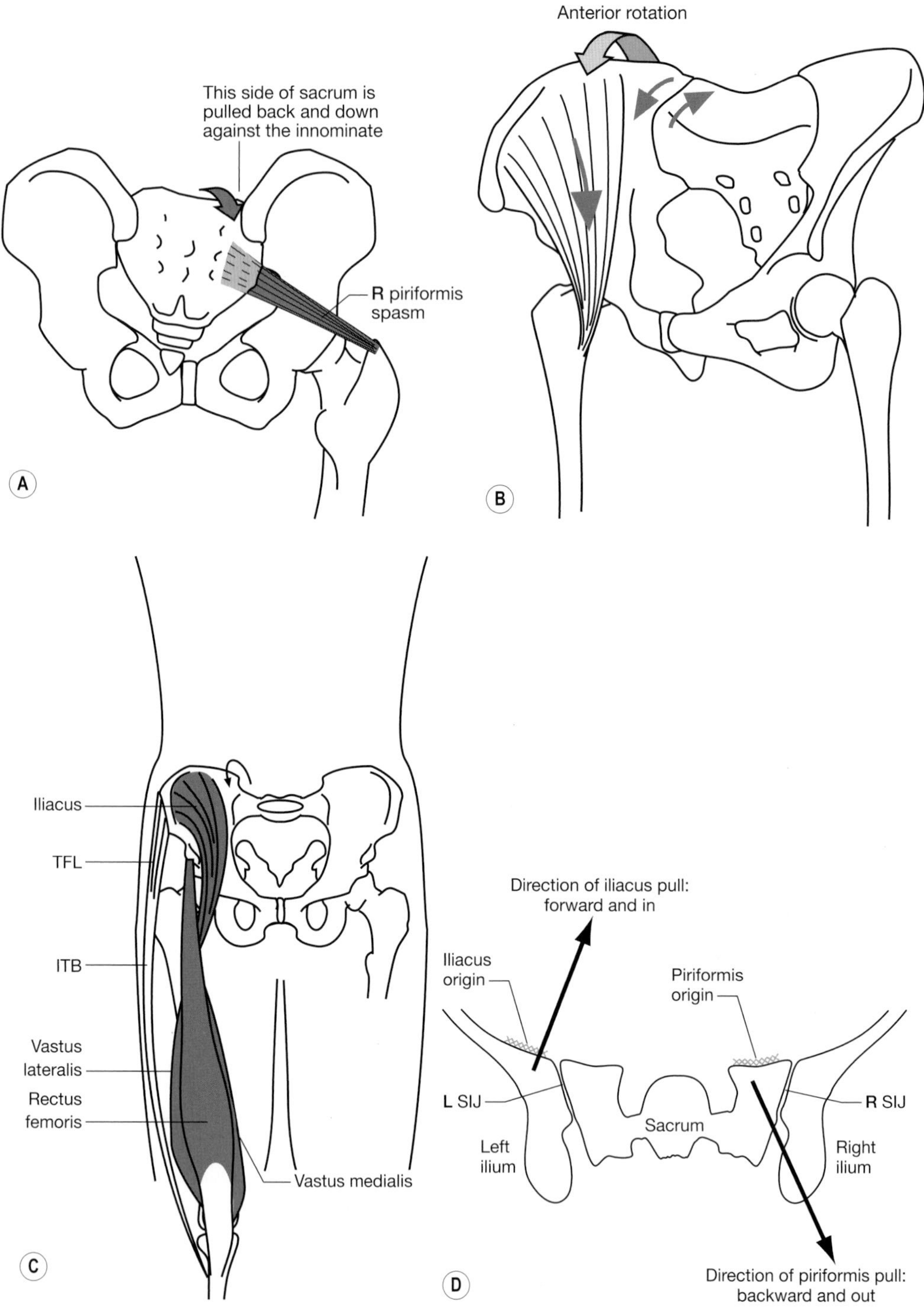

Fig. 2.46 Stabilization of the sacroiliac joint (SIJ) through wedging of the anteriorly widening sacrum (see also Figs 2.2B, 2.3, 2.4B, 2.10A, 2.11A). (A) Piriformis pulling the sacrum backward against the innominate. (B) Iliacus pulling the innominate forward against the sacrum. (C) Anterior innominate rotation through the action of iliacus, rectus femoris and the tensor fascia lata/iliotibial band complex. (D) Wedging effect viewed from the top of the joint.

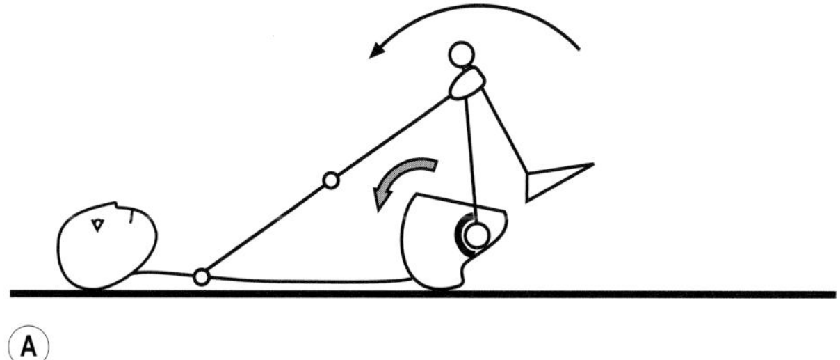

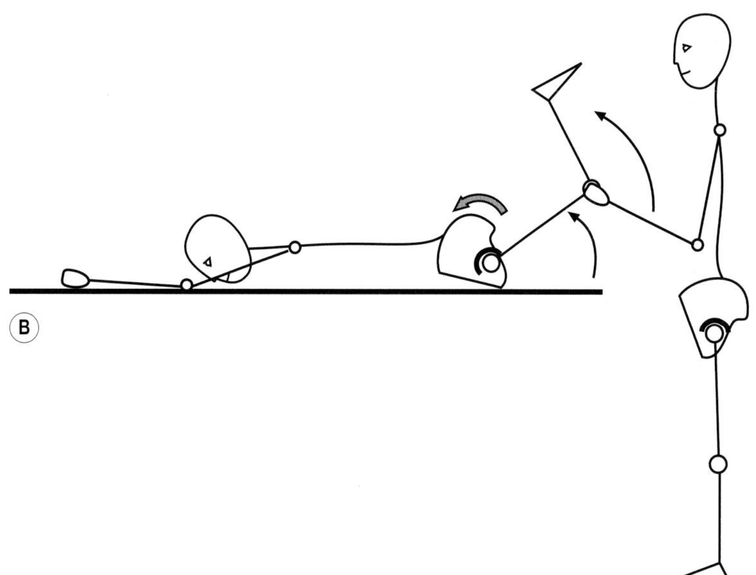

Fig. 2.47 Leverage effect of the femur on the innominate, by impingement against the acetabular rim (see also Figs 7.16-7.18). (A) Against anterior rim: results in posterior rotation. (B) Against posterior rim: results in anterior rotation.

movement of the femur independent of the ipsilateral innominate reaches its:

1. *physiological limit*

   This refers to the end point attained because of limitation by increasing tightness in the anterior muscles (e.g. iliacus, rectus femoris; Fig. 2.46C), ligaments (ilio- and pubofemoral; Figs 2.4A, 4.3) and anterior capsule (Fig. 2.48), without causing any damage.
2. *the anatomical limit*

   Once the femoral head engages the posterior acetabular rim (Fig. 2.48), the right femur and innominate move together on further active or passive hip extension, the femur now acting as a lever, the anterior muscles and ligaments as a traction force. Similarly, when flexing the hip by pulling or pushing the thigh onto the chest, the femur eventually turns into a lever as it engages

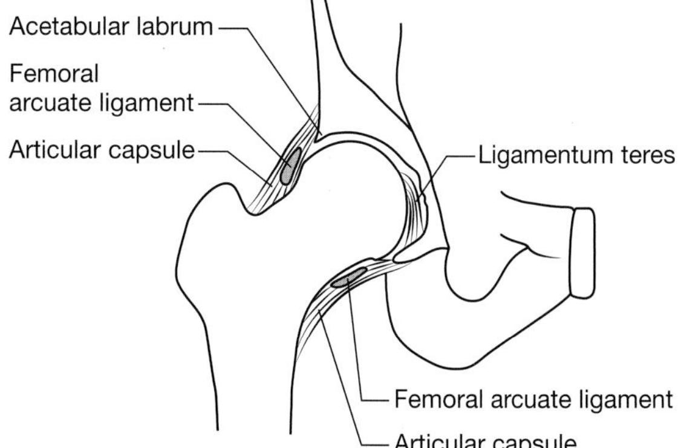

Fig. 2.48 Acetabular rim/labrum, joint capsule, and ligaments that can limit hip extension or flexion and can be injured when using the femur as a lever.

the anterior acetabular rim and any tight posterior muscles and ligaments (e.g. gluteus maximus, hamstrings, sacrotuberous ligament) to act as a posterior rotational torsion force (Fig. 2.47A).

It is for this reason that stretches involving unilateral hip flexion are best avoided on the side of a previously corrected 'posterior' innominate rotation during the initial period of treatment of a 'rotational malalignment' disorder, for fear of precipitating a recurrence of that 'posterior' rotation (Figs 3.74B, C, 7.22A,C). Conversely, the same manoeuvre may be useful to effect the correction of an 'anterior' rotation (Figs 7.16A,C, 7.17, 7.18).

Direct rotational force applied to an innominate

The application of specific forces, either actively (e.g. with walking or running or as part of a treatment regimen) or passively as the result of a fall or collision, can result in innominate rotation. There is some ongoing debate regarding the axes of rotation. DonTigny (2007) felt that there is a force-dependent transverse axis established 'through the sacrum, but not necessarily through the joints.... at the most posterion aspect of the S3 segment...this axis should probably be considered as being the axis for sacral rotation rather than an axis for the sacroiliac joint *per se*' (Fig. 2.49). Richards (1986) described the axis of rotation of the sacrum around the mean transverse axis (MTA), passing through the point at which the two parts of the L-shaped sacral articulating surfaces meet, at about the level of S2; whereas the axis of rotation of the wings of the ilia was observed to be around the inferior transverse axis, passing though the inferior pole of the sacral articulating surfaces at the S3 level (Fig. 2.50). There is also the previously mentioned element of the sacral and innominate joint surfaces 'gliding' relative to each other on sacral nutation/counternutation (Fig. 2.15) and innominate anterior/posterior rotation (Fig. 2.16).

'Anterior' rotational forces on the innominate result when:

1. an anterior force is applied to its posterior aspect above the level of the inferior transverse axis or ITA (e.g. against the posterior iliac crest)
2. a posterior force is applied to its anterior aspect below the level of the inferior transverse axis (e.g. the anterior or superior aspect of the pubic bone).

'Posterior' rotational forces on the innominate result when:

1. a posterior force is applied to its anterior aspect above the level of the inferior transverse axis (e.g. against the anterior iliac crest)

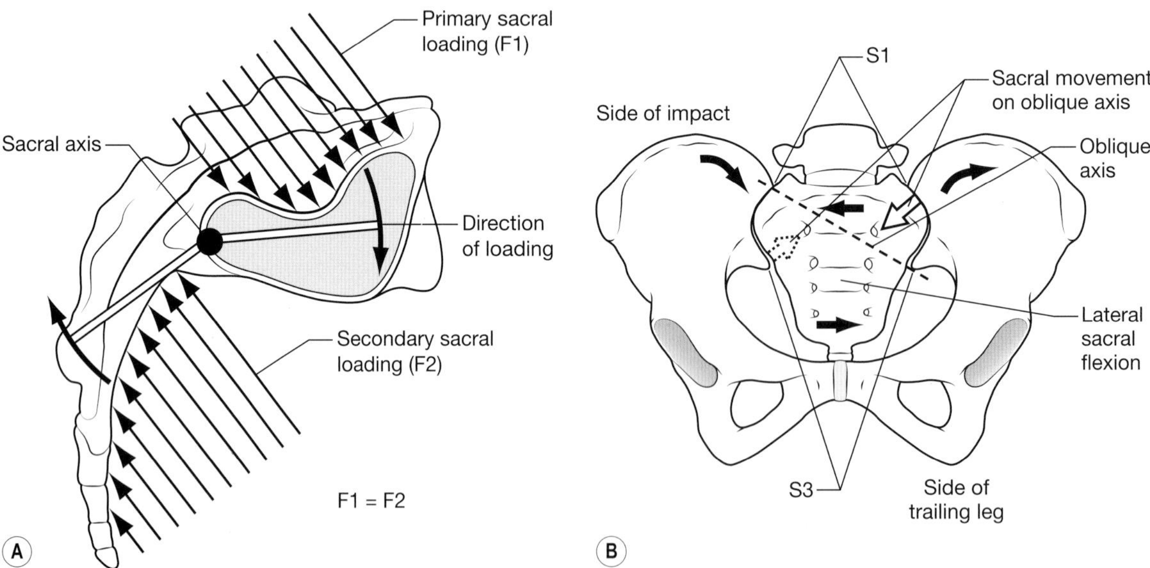

Fig. 2.49 (A) Two equal and parallel forces acting in opposite directions define the sacral axis. If the forces are spread, the force-dependent axis is more narrowly defined. (B) Posterior rotation (right) and anterior rotation (left) demonstrating joint closure at S1(right) and S3 (left) to create an oblique axis (OA). A functional destabilization occurs at S1 (left) and S3 (right), allowing the joint to open and move on that oblique axis. *(Reproduced from DonTigny 2004, courtesy of DonTigny 2007.)*

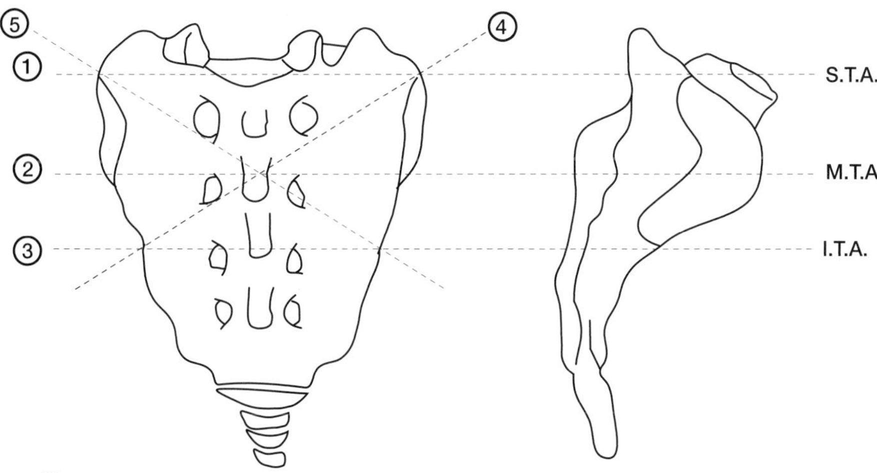

(1) S.T.A. = Superior Transverse Axis – primary respiratory axis of Sutherland

(2) M.T.A. = Mean Transverse Axis – axis of rotation of the sacrum in respect to the ilia

(3) I.T.A. = Inferior Transverse Axis – axis of rotation of the ilia in respect to the sacrum, at the inferior aspect of the SI joint

(4) Right Oblique Axis

(5) Left Oblique Axis

Fig. 2.50 Axes of rotation around the sacroiliac joint.

2. an anterior force is exerted on its posterior aspect below the level of the inferior transverse axis (e.g. ischial tuberosity or inferior pubic bone).

Forces acting on a lower extremity

An impact to a lower extremity can affect the innominate if the force is transmitted upward through the hip joint when:

1. there is already some 'anterior' or 'posterior' rotation of the innominates, which results in the centre of the acetabulum being placed increasingly forward or backward of the vertical force-line, respectively
2. the femur is at an angle relative to the innominate at the time of impact.

Typical examples include:

1. at heel-strike (Figs 2.36A,B; 2.41-1,5)
2. falling forward and landing on one knee
3. coming down hard on one extremity while the trunk is lurched either forward or backward, (e.g. an uneven dismount in gymnastics, an asymmetrical landing following a jump, misjudging a change in floor level or simply missing a step when going down a staircase (Fig. 2.20)
4. the impact transmitted through an extended lower extremity on hitting against the wall in a luge event, or while jammed against the floorboards of a crashing bobsled or toboggan
5. the impact of a collision, absorbed by the knee hitting the dashboard or transmitted upward through the extended knee from the foot pushing on the clutch or brake, when the hip joint is partially flexed (Fig. 2.51).

Asymmetrical impact forces like these can sometimes work in the person's favour. The author is reminded of a woman who initially presented with 'right anterior, left posterior' innominate rotation, and the right ASIS prominent because of counterclockwise rotation of the innominates around the vertical axis ('right inflare, left outflare'). Two weeks later she was found to be in perfect alignment without having had any form of treatment in the interval. She recalled having tripped recently, landing initially on both knees, her trunk then being flung forward. In the process, she had seemingly effected a correction, either by exerting a 'left anterior' or a 'right posterior' rotational force through a femur on hitting the ground, or perhaps by way of reflex muscle contraction(s). Trauma can obviously work both ways!

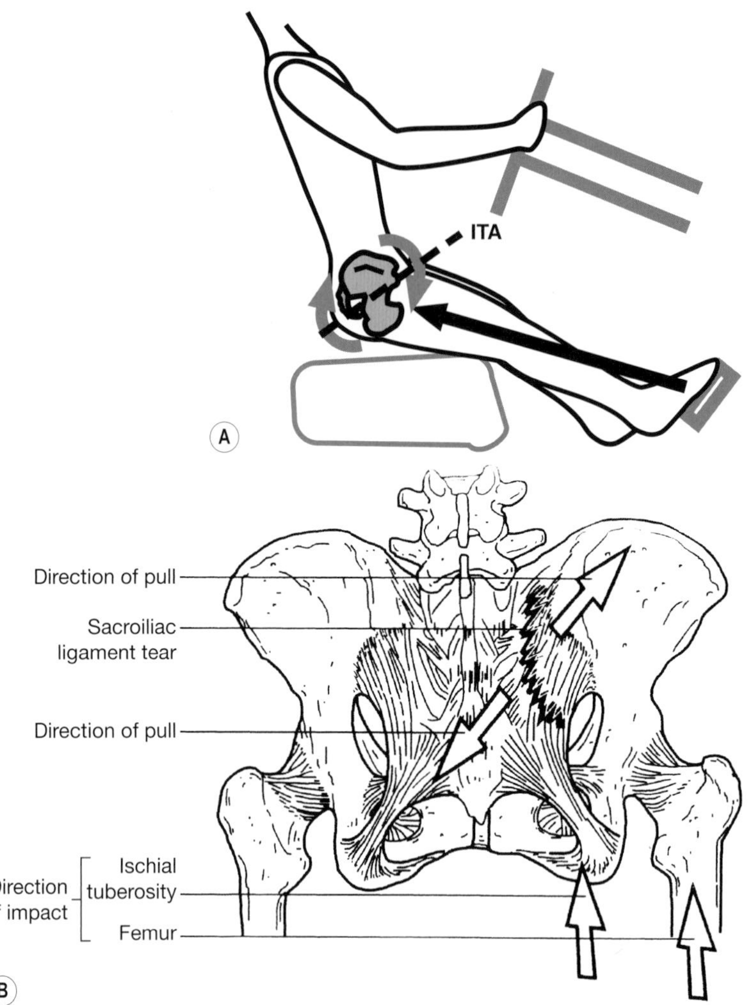

Fig. 2.51 Common mechanisms of injury. (A) In an automobile accident: the force, impacting on the acetabulum at an angle below the inferior transverse axis (ITA; see Figs 2.20, 2.50) results in anterior rotation of the right innominate. (B) In a fall: forcing the leg upward or landing on the ischial tuberosity can shear the ligaments between the sacrum and ilium.

Asymmetrical forces exerted by the spine, pelvis or legs

Torsion of the sacrum and rotation of the innominates can result from abnormal forces being transmitted to these bones from the spine, pelvic floor or lower extremities.

Spine

Excessive rotation of vertebrae from C1 down to L5 can result in forces capable of causing malalignment of the pelvis. These forces include a reactive asymmetrical increase in muscle tension and/or direct torsion and traction forces. A rotation of L4 or L5, for example, exerts a rotational or torquing force on each other and the sacrum by their interlinkage through the facet joints (Beal 1982; Kirkaldy-Willis & Cassidy 1985; Richard 1986; Gracovetsky & Farfan 1986; Lee 2004a). Rotational or torquing forces at the lumbosacral junction are recognized as one cause for recurrent malalignment of the pelvis (Fig. 2.52).

A right (clockwise) rotation of the body of L4 or L5 results in a posterior movement of the right transverse processes, and with it the origins of the attaching iliolumbar ligaments (Fig. 2.4A). The increase tension in these ligaments creates a posterior rotational force on the right ilium by way of the superior insertions into the posterior iliac crest and deep ones to the anterior ilium (Fig. 2.52A). The simultaneous anterior movement of the left transverse processes increases tension in the left iliolumbar ligaments

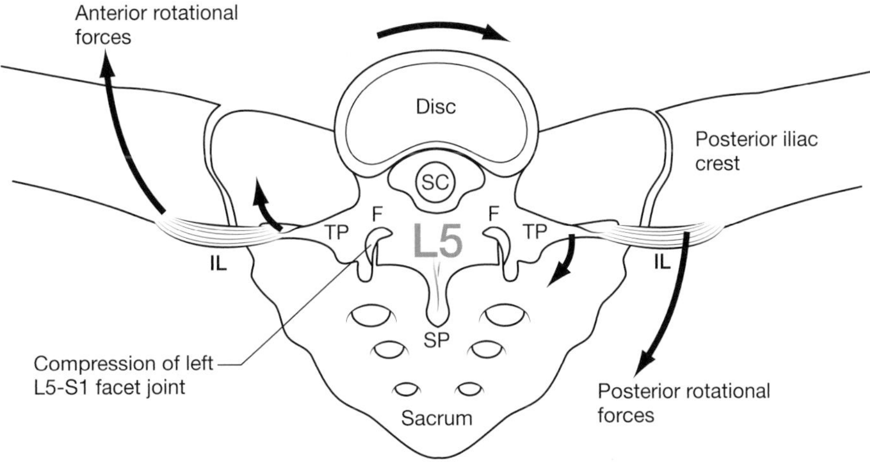

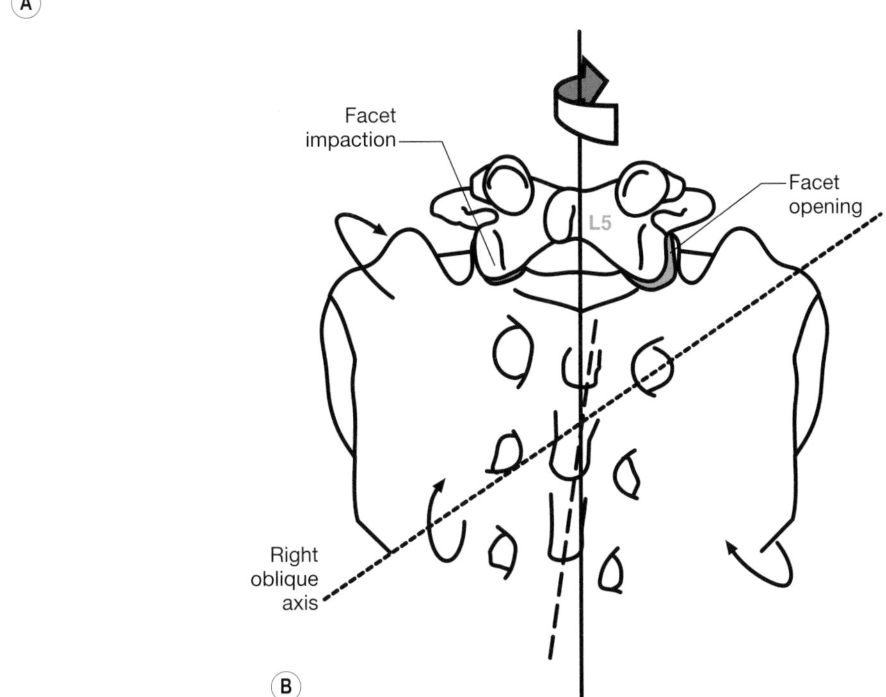

Fig. 2.52 Rotational effect on the innominates caused by right axial (clockwise) rotation of the L5 vertebral complex. (A) 'Right posterior' and 'left anterior' innominate rotation as a result of increased tension in the iliolumbar ligaments as these are being pulled backward on the right and forward on the left. (B) Rotation of the sacrum around the right oblique axis as a result of compression (impaction) of the left L5–S1 facet joint. IL=iliolumbar ligament; TP=transverse process; F=facet joint surface; SC=spinal cord.

and creates an anterior rotational force on the left innominate. The shorter the transverse process, the longer the iliolumbar ligament and the greater the torsional force (Farfan 1973). Vertebral rotation is coupled with side-flexion and some movement either into extension or forward flexion:

1. the L1-L3 vertebral right rotation around the vertical axis is accompanied by left side-flexion and some extension or forward-flexion
2. the pattern for L4 has been found to be variable; whereas L5 rotates and side-flexes to the same side (Pearcy & Tibrewal 1984;

Bogduk 1997) - Fig. 2.52B illustrates this 'motion coupling' effect (Lee 2004a)

Torsional forces with right rotation are, therefore, compounded if there is simultaneous:

1. upward movement of the left transverse process as L5 right side-flexes
2. L5 forward flexion

With L5 right-rotation, the right L5 inferior process separates from the superior process of S1, opening the space and increasing tension on the facet joint ligaments, capsule and nerves. The L5 right-rotation simultaneously exerts a left anterior torsional force through the left inferior L5-S1 facet joint as the inferior articular process of L5 impacts increasingly against the superior process of S1. Once these surfaces have been maximally compressed, the left L5 facet joint starts to act as a fulcrum so that any further rotation of L5 will now cause torsion of the sacrum around the right oblique axis (Fig. 2.52B). Excessive L4 right-rotation can have a similar effect, with initial compression of the left L4-5 facet surfaces eventually working as a fulcrum to rotate L5 vertebral body, then left L5-S1 facet and the sacrum in succession. The innominates, being attached to the sacrum, simply follow. In other words, excessive rotation of L4 or L5, by acting on the sacrum, can cause rotation of the whole pelvic ring as a unit, regardless of whether pelvic malalignment – 'rotational', 'flare' or an 'upslip' – is already present or not. However, assuming that malalignment is also present:

1. treatment that corrects the excessively rotated lumbar vertebra(e) and helps decrease reactive muscle spasm may simultaneously achieve realignment by allowing the bones of the pelvic ring to rotate back into place
2. initial treatment aimed at achieving pelvic realignment may actually allow L4 and/or L5 to rotate back into place by helping decrease pain and settle down any reactive muscle spasm that may have been pulling asymmetrically on one or both vertebrae

With both approaches, resolution of pain and muscle spasm are key factors that allow for pelvic realignment and/or rotation of any displaced vertebra(e) back into place (e.g. pelvic realignment allowing resolution of spasm in deep multifidi, extensor spinae so that L4 and/or L5 can rotate back into normal position or vice versa).

Pelvic floor

The components of the levator ani muscle constitute a major part of the pelvic floor. The location of these muscles and other structures can be defined on external (Fig. 2.53A) and on rectal (or vaginal) examination (Fig. 2.53B):

1. *puborectalis and pubococcygeus*, originating from the pubic bone and anterior obturator fascia
   a. puborectalis, running posteriorly to form a muscular sling by way of connections at the anorectal flexure with its partner on the opposite side
   b. pubococcygeus, attaching posteriorly to the midline raphe (fascial junction) or anococcygeal body, running from the rectum to the coccyx
2. *ilio- and ischiococcygeus*, arising from the ischial spine, posterior obturator fascia and sacrospinous ligament, and inserting posteriorly into the lowest part of the sacrum.

These various attachments of the levator ani muscles directly to parts of the pelvis, or indirectly by way of their ligamentous or fascial connections, puts them in a strategic position to influence alignment. For example, any asymmetry of tension in these structures caused by irritation of the pelvic floor muscles on one side by a unilateral ovarian cyst, uterine fibroid or other mass can result in recurrent malalignment of the sacrococcygeal joint, the innominates and/or the sacrum and, secondarily, the spine (Fig. 2.53C).

Diagnostic techniques such as Real-time ultrasound (RTUS), colour and duplex Doppler analysis (O'Neill & Jurriaan 2007) have been instrumental in assessing particularly the function of the 'inner core' muscles - the deep multifidi, transversus abdominis, diaphragm and pelvic floor muscles - and also of the bladder and organs as they inter-relate with these muscles (see also Chs 4, 7; Fig. 4.43). Examples include assessment of:

1. appearance and function of specific muscles, such as the multifidi (Figs 2.54, 2.55A,B):
   a. appearance is normal or there is evidence of hypertrophy or atrophy; e.g. confirming uni- or bilateral wasting of deep multifidi which, on paravertebral palpation, may have been felt as a dip on one or both sides at the level(s) involved
   b. function of superficial and deep fibre is normal or there is evidence of malfunction, such as failure to contract at all or hyperactivity of individual muscle layers
2. sequence of muscle activation; e.g. hamstring contraction inadvertently precede that of gluteus maximus when initiating hip extension

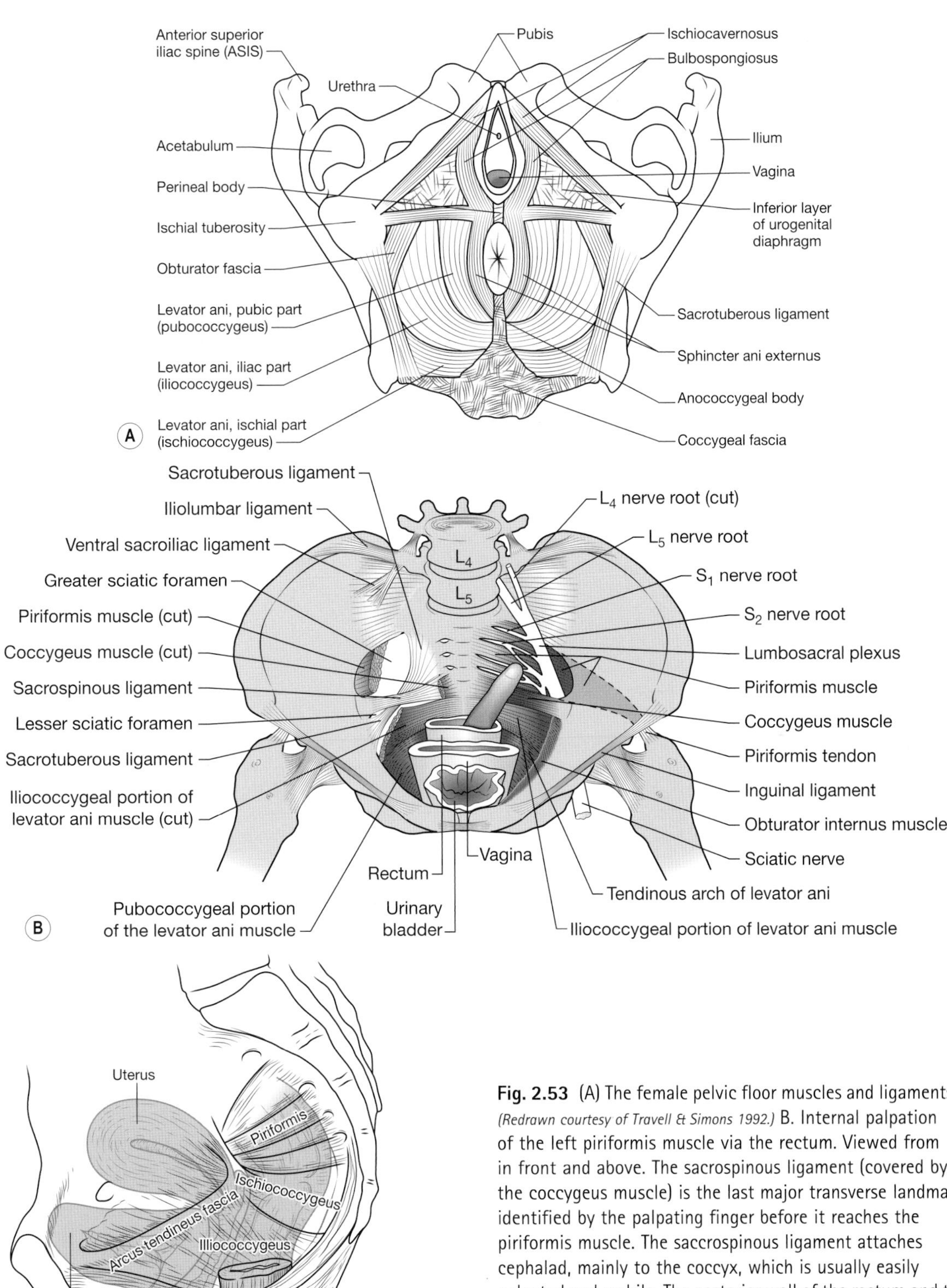

Fig. 2.53 (A) The female pelvic floor muscles and ligaments. *(Redrawn courtesy of Travell & Simons 1992.)* B. Internal palpation of the left piriformis muscle via the rectum. Viewed from in front and above. The sacrospinous ligament (covered by the coccygeus muscle) is the last major transverse landmark identified by the palpating finger before it reaches the piriformis muscle. The saccrospinous ligament attaches cephalad, mainly to the coccyx, which is usually easily palpated and mobile. The posterior wall of the rectum and the S3 and S4 nerve roots lie between the palpating finger and the piriformis muscle *(Redrawn courtesy of Travell & Simons 1992.)* (C) The relationship between the muscles, fascia, and organs (transparent) of the pelvic floor. *(Courtesy of Lee 2004a.)*

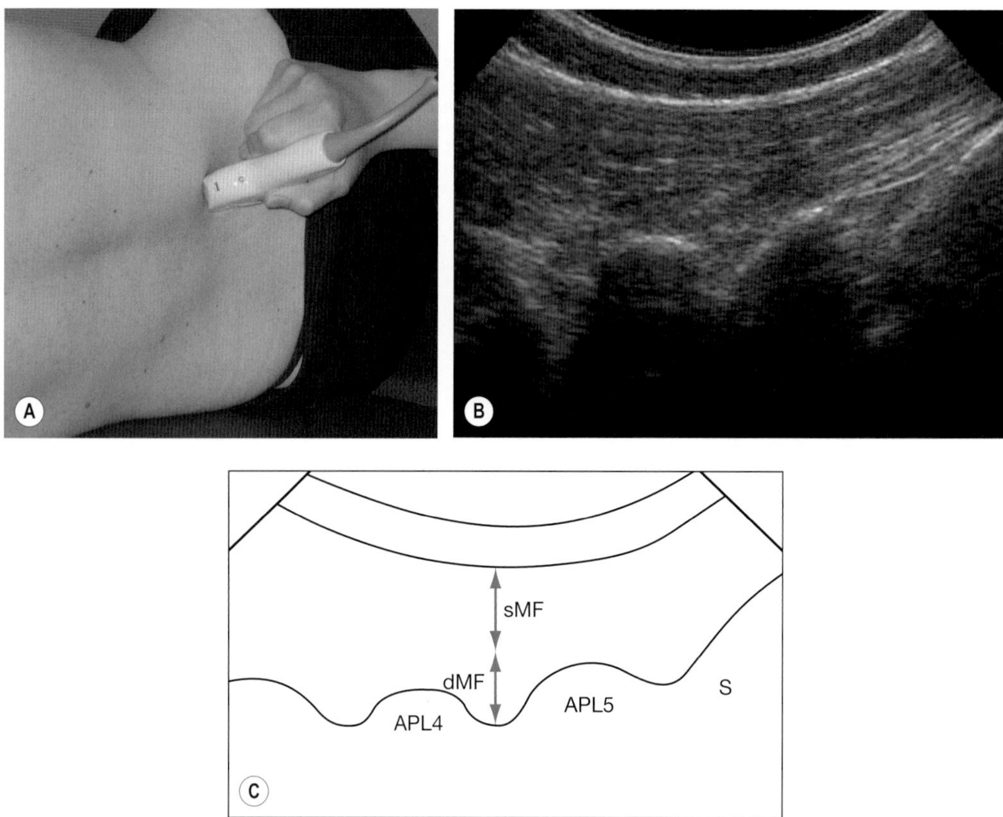

Fig. 2.54 (A) Ultrasound transducer placement for longitudinal imaging of the lumbar multifidus. (B) Longitudinal resting image of lumbar multifidus just lateral to the spinous processes and over the L3-S1 articular column. (C) Outline of the same image. APL4, articular process L4; APL5, articular process L5; S, sacrum; dMF, deep multifidus; sMF, superficial multifidus. *(Courtesy of Lee 2004a.)*

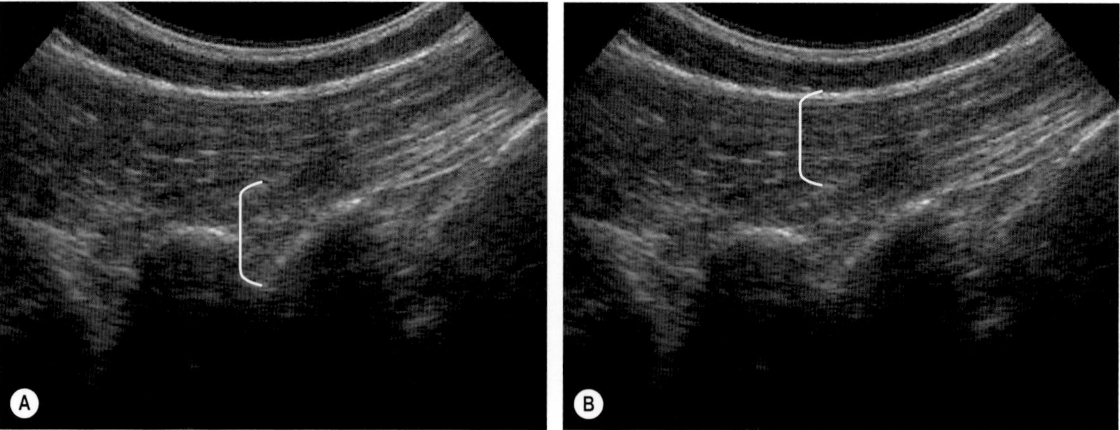

Fig. 2.55 (A) Ultrasound image indicating the location for an isolated response of the deep fibres of lumbar multifidus. (B) Ultrasound image indication the location for a hyperactive response from the superficial fibres of lumbar multifidus. *(Courtesy of Lee 2004a.)*

3. interaction of 'inner' and 'outer' core muscles
4. pelvic floor
   a. delineation of the bladder (Fig. 2.56A,B)
   b. functioning of the levator ani mucles and their effect (Bo et al. 2001, Whittaker 2004, 2007, 2010), including encroachment on the bladder with voluntary normal and abnormal pelvic floor contraction and the Valsalva manoeuvre (Fig. 2.57A,B)
   c. muscle tone; specifically, evidence of unilateral hypertonicity or hypotonicity (looking for evidence of encroachment or seeming 'widening' of the bladder, respectively, on the side affected)
   d. pathology such as organomegaly, ovarian cysts, fibroids, masses which can encroach on the 'inner core' muscles or the bladder itself and result in either a reactive increase in tension or an inhibition of core muscle contraction, very likely asymmetrically and, therefore, predispose to malalignment (Fig. 2.53C).

Assessment with the patient's awareness enhances treatment protocols as it allows for feedback that helps the person understand the problem at hand, learn how to activate or relax some muscles and in proper sequence, also to initiate progressive stretching and strengthening routines for specific muscles.

Lower extremities

Any condition that results in a lower extremity exerting an asymmetrical torquing force on a hip

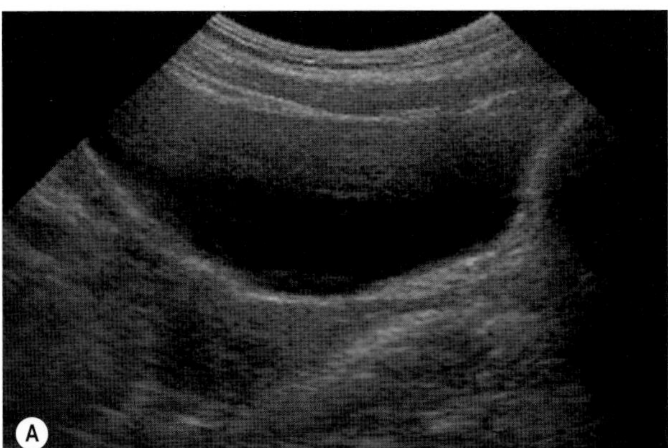

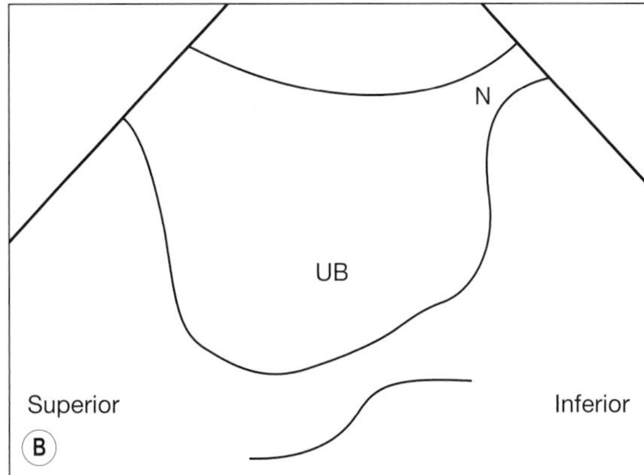

Fig. 2.56 Parasagittal abdominal ultrasound imaging. (A) Resting parasagittal abdominal image of the urinary bladder. (B) Labelled outline of the same image. UB, urinary bladder; N, neck of the bladder. *(Courtesy of Lee 2004a.)*

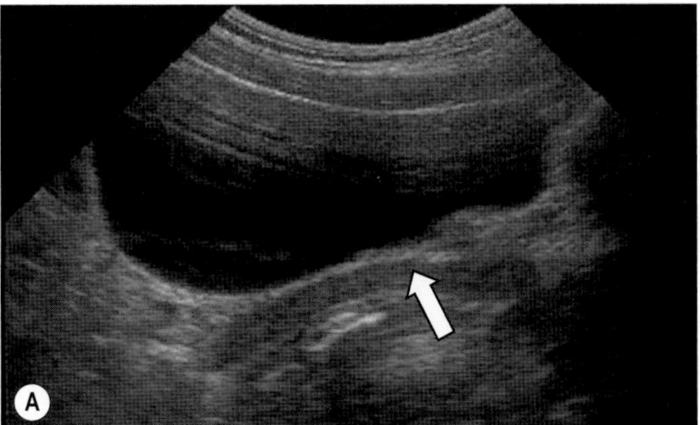

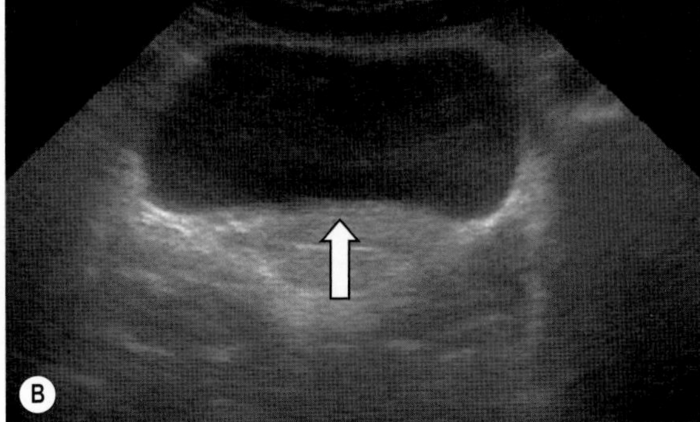

Fig. 2.57 Ultrasound image showing an isolated response of the pelvic floor muscles. The arrow notes where the bladder can be seen to indent with a proper pelvic floor contraction. (A) parasagittal abdominal view; (B) transverse abdominal view. *(Courtesy of Lee 2004a.)*

joint can, in turn, cause a 'rotational malalignment' as the force is transmitted, in succession, to the innominate, the SI joint, the sacrum and, finally, the lumbosacral junction. Torquing forces of this kind can result from:

1. asymmetrical weight-bearing on account of an anatomical (true) or a functional leg length difference
2. attempts by the pelvic girdle to compensate for problems to transfer load through the lumbo-pelvic-hip complex in order to reduce vertical shear forces through the SI joint:
   a. *compensated Trendelenburg gait for insufficient 'force' closure*
      Weakness in the left hip abductors makes them less effective (= decreased force closure) for stabilizing the left hip and SI joint for proper load transfer through the hip, SI joint and up through the lumbosacral junction. When walking, the person can compensate by leaning the trunk into the impaired left side during mid-stance, moving the centre of gravity outward from midline and more directly over top of the hip joint, thereby
      i. decreasing the need for left abductor muscle action to achieve stability of the left hip joint
      ii. decreasing vertical shear forces through the left SI joint (Figs 2.58A, 2.1C)
   b. *true Trendelenburg gait for insufficient 'form' closure*
      Left hip instability can be caused by degeneration (osteoarthritis) of the joint and/or ligament laxity and the joint may be inflamed and painful. The person may compensate for the impaired ability to transfer loads through the left hip by leaning away from that side (adducting the pelvis, abducting the left femur) in mid-stance, thereby
      i. bringing the centre of gravity closer to midline (away from the left hip joint and toward the SI joint
      ii. decreasing stress on the painful left hip joint
      iii. depending more on the strong left hip abductors to ensure stability of the left hip joint and also of the pelvic unit in the coronal plane (Fig. 2.58B)

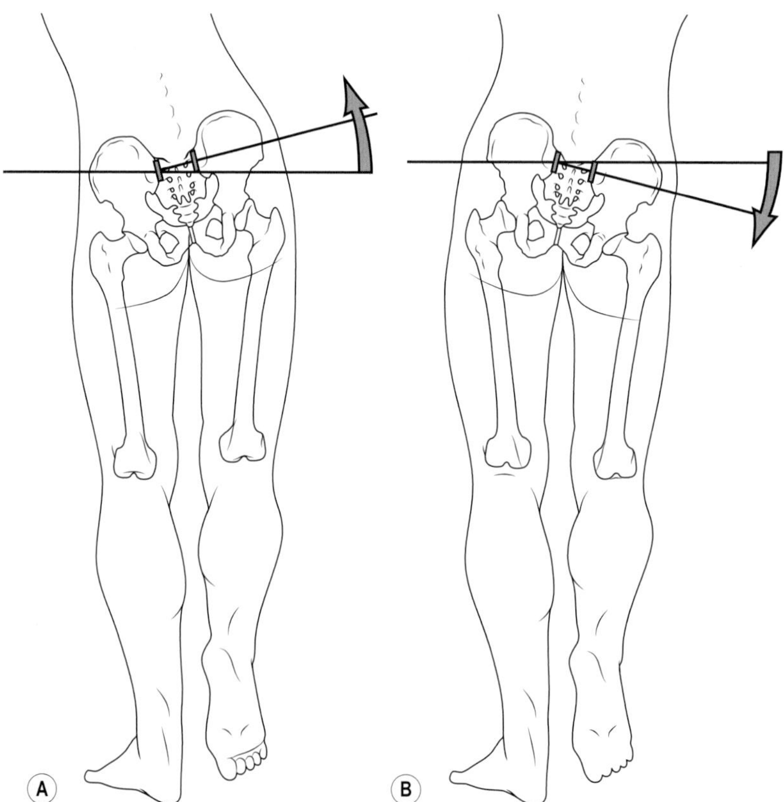

Fig. 2.58 A. Compensated Trendelenburg; B. True Trendelenburg (see also Fig. 3.93). *(Courtesy of Lee 2004a.)*

3. a change in weight-bearing caused by trying to avoid a painful condition involving a lower extremity; e.g. excessive supination of the foot and external rotation of the leg to avoid a painful osteoarthritic 1st and/or 2nd MTP joint
4. unilateral or asymmetrical muscle tightness or contracture acting on an innominate; for example:
   a. an 'anterior' rotational force exerted by a tight
      i. rectus femoris by way of its origin from the anterior inferior iliac spine (AIIS)
      ii. iliacus, TFL or the inferior band of the iliofemoral ligament pulling on the ilium when the hip joint is stabilized and cannot flex (Figs 2.4A, 2.46B,C, 2.59)
   b. a 'posterior' rotational force exerted by a tight biceps femoris, either directly, by way of its attachments to the ischial tuberosity, or indirectly, when continuations with the sacrotuberous (ST) ligament allow it to exert a pull all the way up to the ST origins from the sacrum and ilium (Figs 2.6, 2.59)
   c. asymmetrical forces created by contracture or scarring of the fascia that envelops the muscles of the trunk, hip girdle and thigh, with its extensive connections to the hip joint capsule and ligaments, the pelvis itself and proximally to the thoracolumbar and anterior abdominal fascia (Figs 2.31, 2.33)

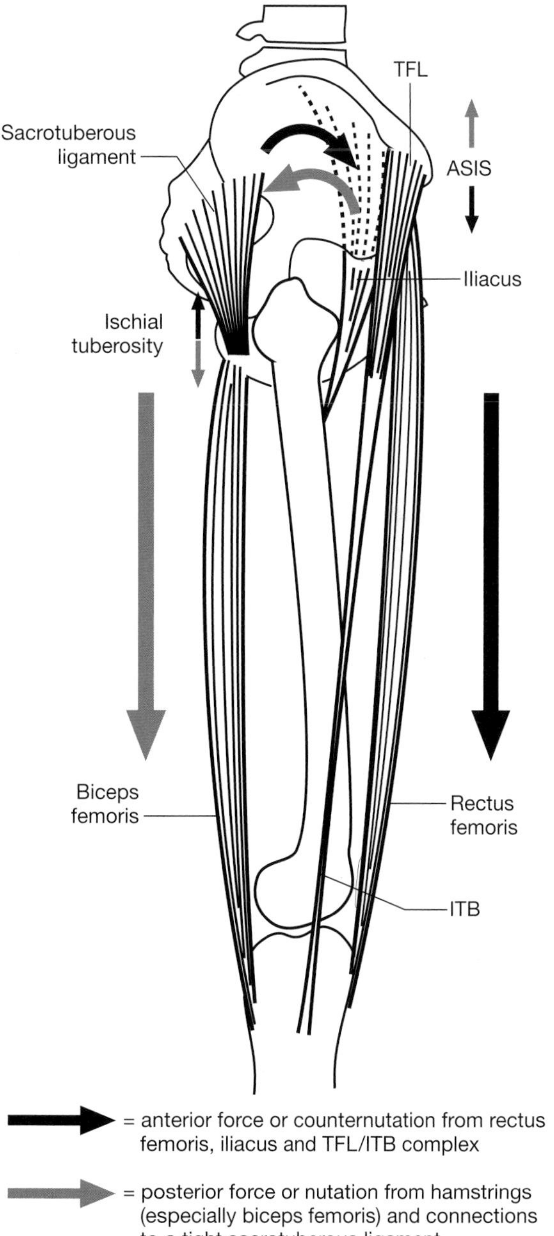

Fig. 2.59 Torquing/rotational forces on the innominate caused by tightness in the attaching muscles or ligaments (see Figs 2.46B,C for an anterior view). ASIS, anterior superior iliac spine.

Myofascial contracture and lengthening

Myofascial problems and treatment are discussed at length in Ch. 8. At this point, suffice it to say that contracture or lengthening of the fascia, musculotendinous units, ligaments and capsules are one of the major long-term complications of malalignment and a frequent cause of its recurrence. It is the nature of soft tissues to contract when placed in a shortened position and to lengthen when put under increased tension for prolonged periods of time.

Contracture can occur:

1. actively (e.g. as a result of chronic shortening of a muscle as it contracts continuously in reaction to joint instability or pain) or
2. passively (e.g. wherever the origin and insertion are moved closer together, as would happen to right rectus femoris when the right innominate is 'stuck' in an 'anterior' rotated position)

Alternatively, these tissues can undergo lengthening when subjected actively or passively to forces that increase tension by stretching on the muscle or by moving its origin and insertion further apart. Someone with 'rotational malalignment' usually presents with a pelvic obliquity and compensatory scoliosis (Fig. 2.60). The myofascial tissue:

1. on the relatively shortened concave side
   - may eventually shorten and augment any compressive force on the ipsilateral facet joints and aspects of the vertebrae and discs
2. on the relatively lengthened convex side
   - may elongate with time and decrease its ability to help counter joint instability on that side

There may also be contracture of muscles that have been in a chronic state of contraction in reaction to joint instability and/or pain. Myofascial tissue that is constantly placed in a shortened position will eventually undergo some reorganization. The gradual replacement of the muscle element with an increasing amount of fascial tissue between the muscle fibres and muscle fibre atrophy may eventually lead to end stage contracture (see Ch. 8).

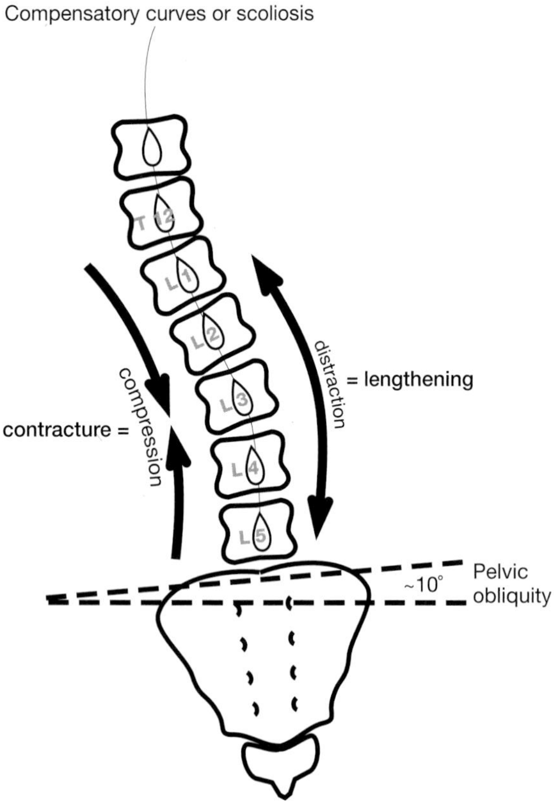

Fig. 2.60 Typical pelvic obliquity and compensatory scoliosis seen with an 'upslip' and 'rotational malalignment'. With time, myofascial lengthening occurs on the lumbar convex side and contracture on the concave side.

Failure to treat myofascial contractures has been identified as one of the factors responsible for the recurrence of malalignment following realignment of the bony elements of the pelvis and spine (Shaw 1992). Recurrence may also be attributable to connective tissue lengthening that has resulted in joint instability.

Contractures must be considered as a possible cause of some of the new aches and pains, often in areas which were not previously a problem, that people frequently report during the first 2-4 weeks following initial realignment. On achieving realignment, tension is increased in the structures that have shortened with long-standing malalignment; they may now unexpectedly become a cause of localized and/or referred discomfort and outright pain. These new symptoms gradually abate and eventually disappear altogether as normal length is regained and alignment finally maintained.

SACROILIAC JOINT 'UPSLIP' AND 'DOWNSLIP'

The degrees of freedom of the SI joint normally allow for approximately 2 degrees of upward and downward (craniocaudal) translation of an innominate relative to the sacrum (Fig. 2.9; William & Warwick 1980, 2004). Excessive upward or downward movement can result in the 'fixation' of an innominate - getting 'stuck', so to speak - in what are referred to as an SI joint 'upslip' and 'downslip' position, respectively.

Sacroiliac joint: unilateral 'upslip'

An 'upslip':

1. may co-exist with a 'rotational malalignment' and/or an 'outflare/inflare'
2. occurs considerably less often than 'rotational malalignment' (about 10-20% versus 80%, respectively, of all those noted to have one or more of the three common presentations)

The more obvious causes of a right or left 'upslip' include:

1. *traumatic upward forces*

   These would have to be transmitted straight upward:

a. through the innominate itself, such as on falling and landing directly on the ischial tuberosity on one side
b. through the leg to the acetabulum, with the knee straight and the hip joint in a relatively neutral position, so that the leg does not exert a rotational force on the innominate; such a situation might occur, for example, when:
   i. landing hard on the extended extremity in a fall, on a dismount or just missing a step (Figs 2.20A, 2.61A)
   ii. the foot is jammed against the floorboards of a crashing car, bobsled or other vehicle (Fig. 2.51A)

A traumatic 'upslip' like this can cause or aggravate a shear injury involving the ipsilateral SI joint and/or symphysis pubis that may increase joint instability and predispose to recurrence of the 'upslip' (Fig. 2.51B).

2. *injury to a muscle that can pull upward on the innominate*

For example, left quadratus lumborum can be sprained or strained on leaning forward and side-flexing to the right to pick an item up from the floor, especially if this proves heavier than expected (Figs 2.43A, 2.62). An ongoing increase in tension in that muscle subsequently, pulling upward by way of its origin from the posterior iliac crest, can eventually result in a 'left upslip' which may persist until tension in that muscle is finally released to allow the left innominate to slide down to the point where the SI joint surfaces are once again aligned.

However, in the absence of a history of trauma, more subtle forces that could cause an 'upslip' to

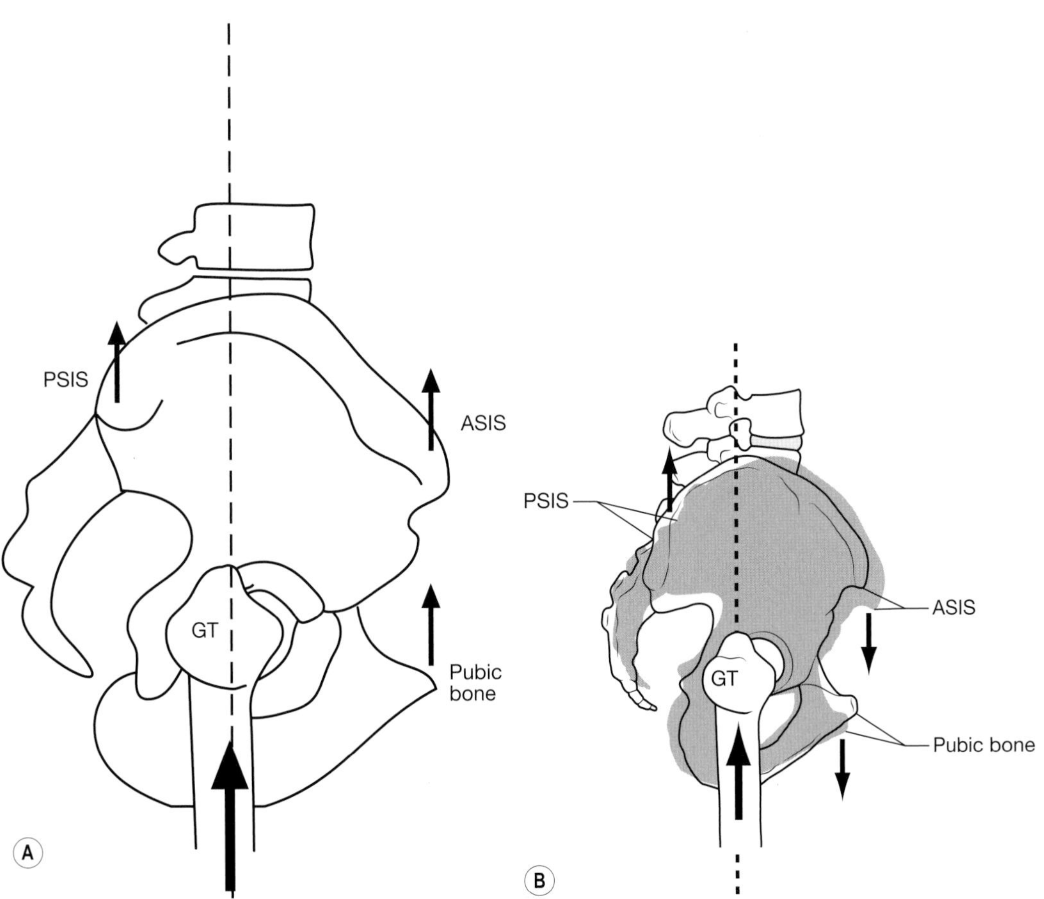

Fig. 2.61 (A) 'Right upslip' caused by a unilateral femoral upward force transmitted through the hip joint to the innominate. (B) The 'upslip' is hidden by the shift of all the pelvic landmarks with a coexistent 'right anterior rotational malalignment'. ASIS, anterior superior iliac spine; GT, greater trochanter; PSIS, posterior superior iliac spine.

occur initially and are probably to blame for its persistance/recurrence include:

1. *an imbalance of tension in right compared to left hip girdle muscles*

   This involves in particularly those that show 'facilitation' as part of the 'malalignment syndrome' (see Ch. 3); typical of these is:
   - a unilateral increase in the resting tone involving quadratus lumborum, latissimus dorsi, psoas major/minor (Figs 2.62, 3.43), external and/or internal abdominal obliques, in isolation or in combination (Figs 2.32, 2.33).
2. *coronal (frontal) plane asymmetry*

   Rotation of the pelvic unit around the sagittal axis in the coronal plane for whatever reason results in a secondary pelvic obliquity; e.g. as caused by an anatomical (true) LLD or a functional LLD seen with 'rotational malalignment'. Counterclockwise rotation of the pelvis, for example, results in the sacrum now 'tilting' to the left and would change the direction of the SI joints so that:

   a. the left is now at a greater angle, increasing surface compression forces and stability of the joint on this side

   b. the right SI joint is now more vertical and the surfaces subjected to greater shear stresses on loading (Fig. 2.1C), increasing the possibility of an 'upslip' occuring on this side as the right innominate is at increased risk of moving craniad relative to the sacrum on right weight-bearing or with an upward force applied to the right iliac crest (e.g. tense quadratus lumborum), femur or ischial tuberosity (e.g. fall onto the right knee or buttock, respectively)

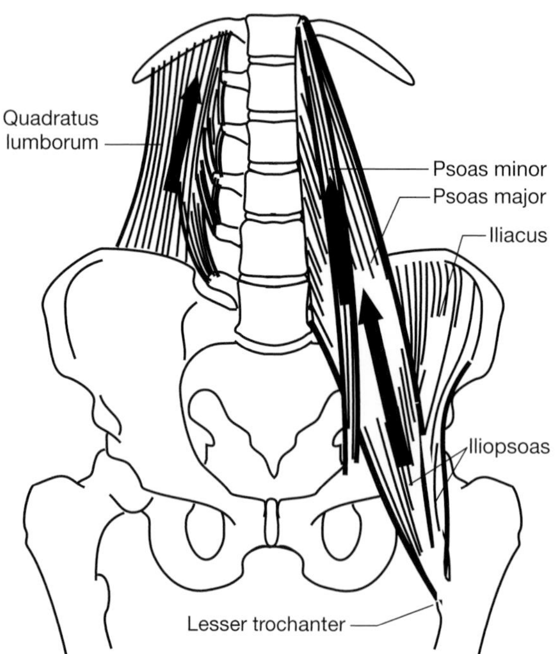

Fig. 2.62 Muscles capable of generating forces (arrows) that can result in an 'upslip'.

As with 'rotational malalignment', a unilateral 'upslip' is associated with the findings typical of the 'malalignment syndrome' (Ch. 3). In addition, on the side of the 'upslip':

1. the leg will be shorter to an equal extent both in long-sitting and lying (see 'sitting-lying' test below)
2. there results a specific pattern of pelvic ring distortion in that all ipsilateral landmarks, anterior and posterior, have moved upward relative to the sacrum itself and to the innominate on the opposite side.

Appendix 2 gives the examination findings typically seen with a right 'upslip' and these findings are detailed below in the discussion on 'Establishing the diagnosis of malalignment'.

Sacroiliac joint: 'bilateral upslip'

A 'bilateral upslip' is present when both innominates have moved upward an equal amount and 'jammed', something that may occur with a straight upward force when landing fairly symmetrically on:

1. both ischial tuberosities (e.g. falling backward onto ice or other hard surface)
2. both feet, with the knees in exension, provided the hip joint is in 'neutral' alignment so that forces end up being transmitted straight up through the acetabulum bilaterally
3. the distal femur or the patella bilaterally, with the knees in flexion and hip joints in 'neutral'

Sacroiliac joint: 'downslip'

A unilateral 'downslip' occurs rarely and the diagnosis is frequently delayed or missed altogether. Typically, there is a history of excessive traction on an extremity; examples of this include:

1. incidents where the person is hurled forward while one leg remains tethered, such as can occur with the failure of one ski binding to release, or

with entrapment of one foot in the toe straps of a crashing bicycle or the stirrup while riding horseback

2. trying to rapidly extract an extremity that has sunk into a hole; for example, a foot suddenly stuck in mud on a boggy running trail or in quicksand

A 'downslip' is frequently misdiagnosed and the person treated initially for an 'upslip' of the opposite SI joint. It is often only when measures aimed at correction of the so-called 'upslip' repeatedly fail that the therapist begins to suspect that the problem is actually a 'downslip' on the opposite side and appropriate treatment is finally started. Sometimes, a person who has been instructed in how to use traction ends up with a 'downslip' on account of having overcorrected for an 'upslip' by applying traction: too much, too often or when it was not even indicated because the 'upslip' had already been corrected.

'Bilateral downslips' can occur but will not be discussed further other than to say they should be considered in the differential diagnosis whenever there is a history of the body having been catapulted forward or downward while both legs/feet were entrapped or secured (e.g. failure of bindings to release when both skies suddenly get stuck in a mogul/snow bank and the skier is thrown forward; inadvertent excessive traction on lower extremities of a bunji jumper as a result of retraining bindings having been applied incorrectly).

PELVIC 'OUTFLARE' AND 'INFLARE'

'Outflare' and 'inflare' refer to movement of the innominates outward and inward, respectively, around the vertical axis in the transverse plane (Figs 2.13, 2.17). A normal bilateral 'outflaring' and 'inflaring' have invariably been linked to simultaneous 'anterior' or 'posterior' rotation of the innominates around the coronal axis. The following are some of the descriptions offered as to how and why this should happen.

'Outflare' linked to 'anterior innominate rotation'

As previously described (DonTigny 1990), the anterior widening of the sacrum causes the innominates to 'spread on the sacrum'; i.e. flare out whenever the innominates rotate anteriorly and downward relative to the sacrum (Fig. 2.17). More recently, he suggested that 'SIJD [SI joint dysfunction] is essentially always caused by an anterior rotation of the innominate bones cephalad and laterally [= 'outflare'] on the sacrum' (DonTigny 2007). 'Inflare' supposedly occurs with a 'posterior' rotation of the innominates relative to the sacrum and with sacral nutation.

'Outflare' linked to trunk flexion in standing

During the initial 50-60 degrees forward flexion in standing the sacrum nutates; the ilia rotate anteriorly 'in the sagittal plane' (Kapandji 1974) and flare outward (see 'Biomechanics' above; Fig. 2.17).

'Outflare' or 'inflare' linked to innominate rotation?

1. the posterior aspect of innominates that are rotating posteriorly have been described as gliding medially because of the posterior narrowing of the sacrum, causing the pelvis to open anteriorly; the same would occur with sacral nutation (Lee 1999)
2. 'inflare' has also been seen in conjunction with 'anterior' rotation and sacral counternutation (JS Gerhardt, pers. comm. 1999).

Other factors that may determine whether an 'outflare' or 'inflare' occurs, and the extent of it, include:

1. tightening or actual contracture of posterior and anterior SI joint ligaments, respectively
3. contraction of transversus abdominis, producing a force that would tend to pull the right and left ASIS together - predisposing to inflare of the innominates (Fig. 2.30)
4. tight muscles; e.g. adductors and gracilis, predisposing to 'outflare'; abductors and piriformis, predisposing to 'inflare'.

'Outflare'/'inflare' in the normal gait cycle

During the normal gait cycle (Figs 2.12, 2.13A, 2.41), the pelvic unit rotates around the vertical axis and there occurs:

1. an inflaring on the swing-side, as the innominate moves forward in the transverse plane; simultaneous posterior rotation of the innominate places the sacrum into relative nutation on this side, which helps stabilize/'lock' the SI joint in preparation for heel-strike and weight-bearing
2. an outflaring on the weight-bearing side, as the innominate moves backward in the transverse plane; simultaneous anterior rotation of the innominate results in relative sacral counternutation, SI joint laxity and increased ability to absorb shock

The malalignment presentations of 'outflare' and 'inflare'

When there is malalignment in the form of a 'flare' presentation, the person typically seems to have become 'stuck' in either a:

1. 'right outflare, left inflare' pattern, with the innominates rotated clockwise around the vertical axis, or
2. 'right inflare, left outflare' pattern, with the innominates rotated counterclockwise around the vertical axis

When considering pathological 'outflare' and 'inflare', other facts to appreciate include the following:

First, a unilateral 'outflare' or 'inflare' can be seen in isolation; for example, a 'right outflare' only (with the left innominate and sacrum still in alignment) could occur as the result of:

1. lax anterior, tight posterior right SI joint ligaments
2. chronic increase in tension or spasm in right hip adductors and/or gracilis, pulling outward and up on their origin from the pubic bone, just lateral to the symphysis pubis (Fig. 2.63)

Second, the more common clinical presentation is with the innominate fixed in a position of an 'outflare' on one, 'inflare' on the opposite side, as if one is compensating for the other. Aside from some of the possible contributing causes cited above, other factors to consider include:

1. Reversal of the convex-concave relationship of the SI joint surfaces in the long and short arms (Figs 2.2, 2.3B) allows for innominate rotation medially or laterally around a vertical axis which could result in inflare or outflare dysfunction, respectively (Greenman 1990).
2. Normally, in the course of each gait cycle, the innominate passing through the swing phase is observed to rotate from outflare-to-inflare, while that on the opposite side passing through the stance phase rotates from inflare-to-outflare. The abnormal presentation shows the pelvic ring seemingly 'fixed' in the transverse plane in sitting, standing and during the gait cycle, with the innominates either in:
   a. the 'right outflare, left inflare' pattern
      - in this case, the landmarks of the pelvic unit (e.g. ASIS, PSIS - Fig. 2.13Ai-iii) consistently end up forward on the left side relative to the right and the left ASIS ends up higher when lying supine (Fig. 2.64)
   b. the 'right inflare, left outflare' pattern
      - all the pelvic landmarks are forward on the right side and the right ASIS is higher when lying supine.

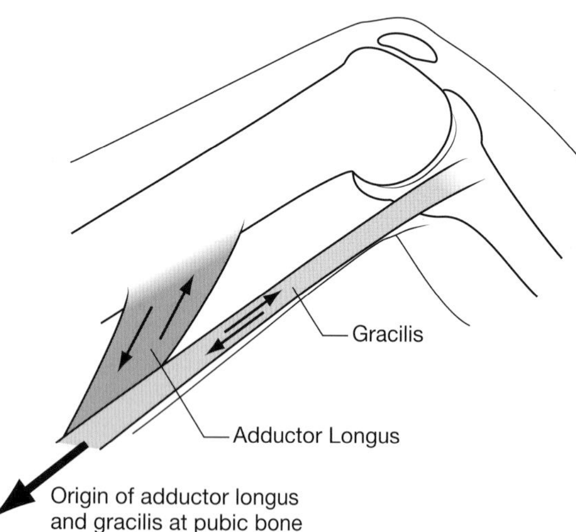

Fig. 2.63 Forces generated by adductor longus and gracilis: 1) adduction of leg; 2) traction forces on inner pubic bone origin, which (a) can result in an innominate 'outflare', (b) can be harnessed to correct an innominate 'inflare' using muscle energy technique (MET; see Ch. 3).

On realignment, right and left pelvic landmarks will again be symmetrical and the previous side-to-side difference detected when using a level for comparison of the height of the ASIS in supine-lying no longer apparent (Fig. 2.65).

Third, a pelvic 'outflare/inflare' presentation may possibly be the result of the changes caused by one of the other presentations when seen in conjunction with:

1. a 'rotational malalignment' - the 'outflare' can be seen on the side of the 'anterior' rotation and the 'inflare' on that of the 'posterior' rotation, or vice versa; commonly noted patterns are:
   a. 'right anterior and outflare, left posterior and inflare'
   b. 'left anterior and outflare, right posterior and inflare'
2. an 'upslip' - either the 'outflare' or 'inflare' can appear on the side of the 'upslip'.
3. both of these presentations at the same time.

Finally, tightness or adhesions in the surrounding tissues may determine whether an 'outflare' or

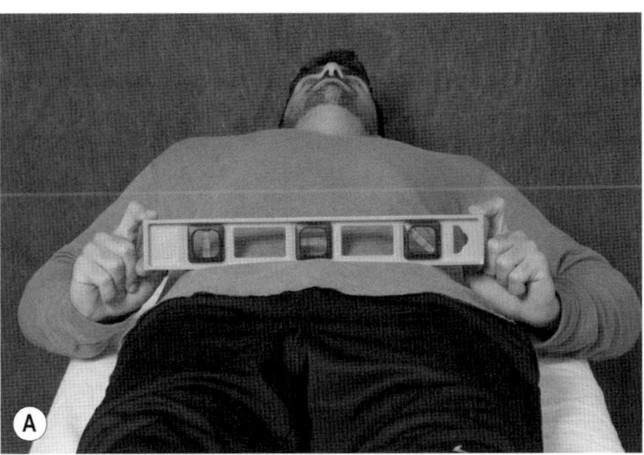

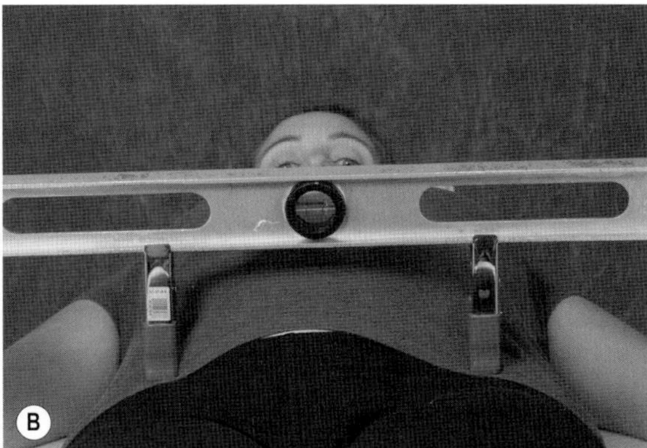

Fig. 2.64 'Right outflare, left inflare': (A/B) a level resting on top of the right and left ASIS shows elevation of left side; (B) 'feet' (clamps) attached to the level rest on right and left ASIS; they raise the level to help bring the bubble into view (e.g. for someone who is obese, pregnant)

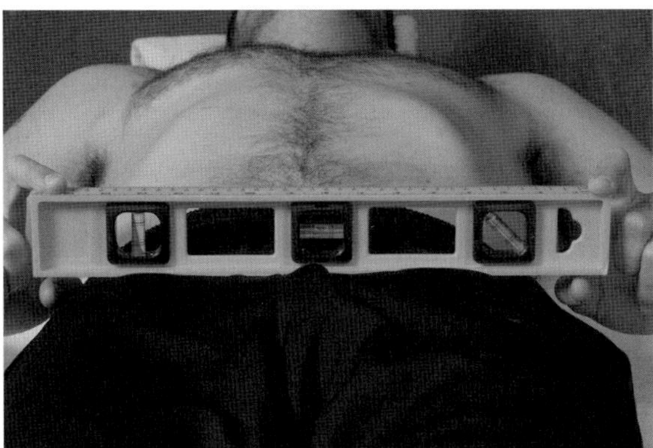

Fig. 2.65 ASIS now level, bubble in centre, following correction of the 'outflare/inflare' (same subject as in Fig. 2.64A).

'inflare' occurs together with innominate rotation in the sagittal plane. Factors to consider include:

1. adhesions and/or scar tissue formation involving the lower posterior pelvic ligaments (considering a sacral axis of rotation around the S3 level; Fig. 2.49) and the long (dorsal) sacroiliac ligament would tend to hold the posterior aspect of the innominate medially and predispose to persistence of an 'outflare' as well as 'posterior' innominate rotation (Figs 2.5A, 2.19B)
2. contracture or scarring of the inguinal ligament would predispose to an 'inflare' and 'anterior' rotation because of its interconnections with ligaments and fascia crossing the symphysis pubis and anchoring to the opposite pubic bone (Fig. 2.4A)

The umbilicus and the gluteal cleft conveniently demarcate the anterior and posterior midline, respectively. If a 'right outflare/left inflare' are present:

1. the right ASIS will have moved outward and the left inward relative to the umbilicus; with the thumbs resting against the inside of the ASIS:
   a. the thumb on the 'inflare' side will appear closer to centre; whereas that on the 'outflare' side ends up further away (Figs 2.13Bi; 2.66)
   b. the index fingers meet off-centre, on the 'outflare' side, when the palms are swung inward (pivoting on the thumbs; Fig. 2.67)
2. the right PSIS will have moved inward and the left outward relative to the gluteal cleft (Fig. 2.13Aii,iii and Ci).

On realignment, the thumbs are again equidistant from midline (Figs 2.13Bii,Cii; 2.71Ei) and the index fingers meet in centre (Fig. 2.69).

Correlation of the PSIS to the gluteal cleft is more likely to be accurate, as it allows for an easier comparison with the landmarks lying closer together. Also, the umbilicus is frequently off-centre pre- and post-partum or as a result of previous surgery (e.g. appendectomy, unilateral hernia repair) and visceral adhesions (e.g. traumatic, surgical or post-partum). In addition, the umbilicus may appear in centre when an 'outflare/inflare' is actually present; for example, it may appear equidistant from the right and left ASIS as a result of having been pulled

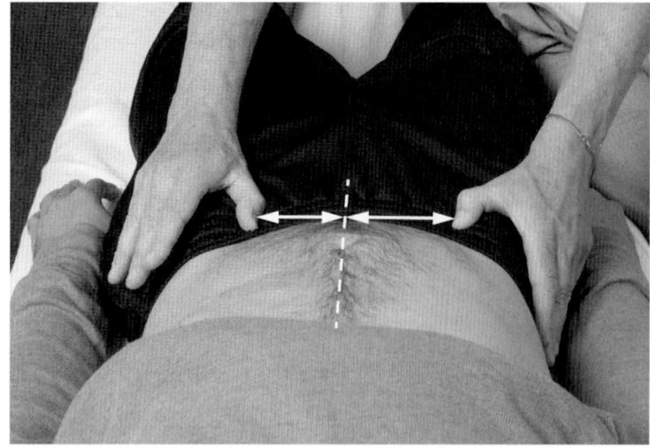

Fig. 2.66 'Right outflare, left inflare' present: thumbs anchored to inside of ipsilateral ASIS are not equidistant from umbilicus and central hairline marker (left ASIS is closer, right further away); left finger tips end up off the bed, right touching.

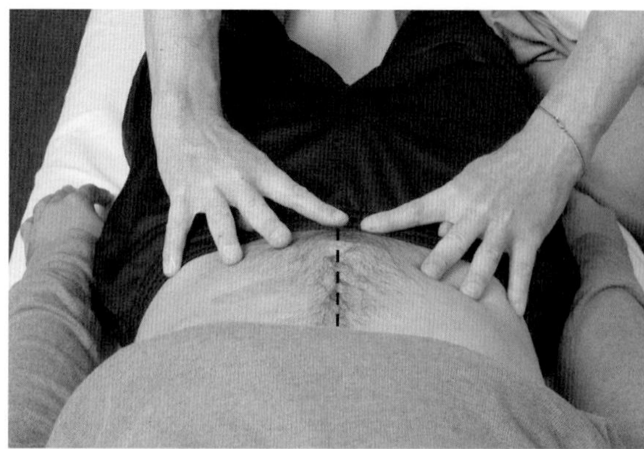

Fig. 2.67 Index fingers pivoted inward fail to meet in centre; index on subject's right ends up outward from, left inward (actually across) the centre line, in keeping with the right 'outflare' and left 'inflare', respectively.

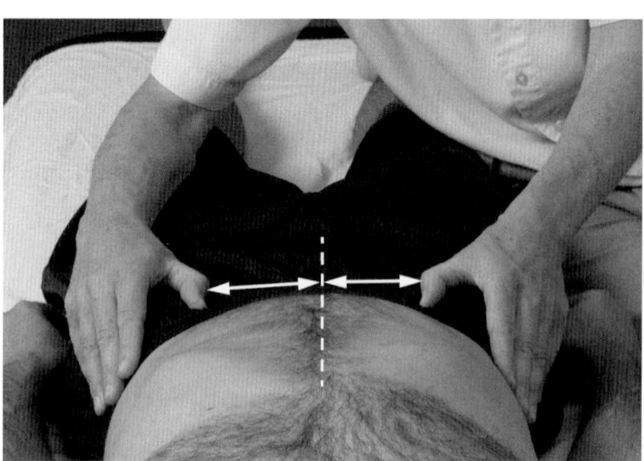

Fig. 2.68 With correction of the 'outflare/inflare', thumbs anchored to inside of ipsilateral ASIS are now equidistant from midline; right/left finger tips now equal distance off the bed.

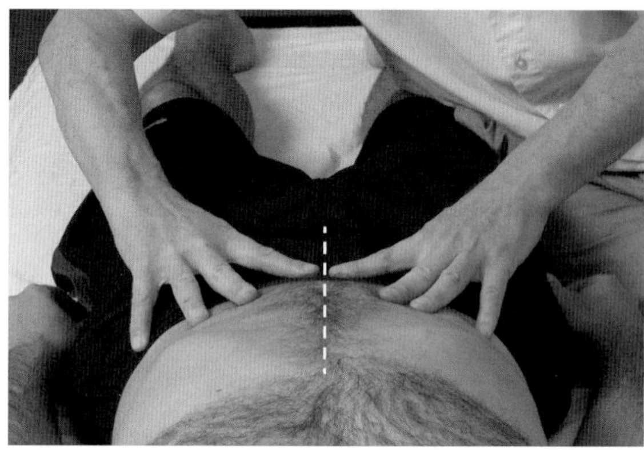

Fig. 2.69 Following realignment, index fingers again meet in midline.

toward the side of the 'outflare' by a unilateral tightness caused by scar tissue or adhesions or an increase in tension in muscles such as transversus abdominis, rectus abdominis or external/internal obliques. An even easier, and probably more accurate way of determining 'outflare' and 'inflare' that depends on determining ASIS/PSIS displacement, both relative to the centre and forward/backward position in the transverse plane, is outlined in Box 2.2 and will be discussed at length in Ch. 7.

The recognition of an 'outflare' and 'inflare' is important from a treatment perspective in that:

1. they can result in specific clinical problems relating to altered biomechanics, stress being placed particularly on the hip and SI joints, lumbosacral region and specific muscles, ligaments and other soft tissues (see Ch. 3)
2. 'rotational malalignment' and 'upslip' may resist treatment efforts using the muscle energy technique of manual therapy until a coexistent 'outflare' or 'inflare' has been corrected first (see Ch. 7)
3. attempts aimed at first correcting the 'outflare' and 'inflare' are successful in simultaneously correcting a coexistent 'rotational malalignment' in 70 to 80% of cases but are unlikely to correct a coexistent 'upslip'

BOX 2.2 Determining 'outflare' and 'inflare'

Look for a change in the relative position of:

1. the ASIS when lying supine
   a. relative to the umbilicus: outward with an 'outflare', inward with an 'inflare' (Figs 2.13A,Bi, 2.66, 2.67)
   b. relative to the table: low on the 'outflare', high on the 'inflare' side (Figs 2.13Aiii, 2.64)
2. the PSIS when lying prone
   a. relative to the sacral spinous processes or gluteal crease:
      -inward on the 'outflare', outward on the 'inflare' side (Fig. 2.13 Ci)
   b. relative to the plinth or table top: relatively high on the 'outflare', low on the 'inflare' side

Always remember that:

1. the height will also be affected by a 'sacral torsion' around the vertical or an oblique axis; to lesser extent, by 'rotational malalignment' (e.g. the ASIS displacement forward and down to the table with 'anterior' and backward and up from the table with 'posterior' rotation of an innominate)
2. assessment in prone-lying is usually a more accurate way of determining 'outflare/inflare', even when there is a coexistent 'rotational malalignment'.

ESTABLISHING THE DIAGNOSIS OF MALALIGNMENT

The initial step in the diagnosis of malalignment is to establish whether asymmetry is present and, if so, whether it is caused by one (or a combination) of the following:

1. an anatomical (true) leg length difference (LLD),
2. one of the 3 common presentations of pelvic malalignment, with a functional LLD (seen with an 'upslip' and 'rotational malalignment')
3. vertebral rotational displacement
4. sacral torsion

Examination is preferably carried out on a firm, even surface. Sitting or lying on a soft or sagging support, or across a break in the surface (a feature common to medical plinths; Fig. 3.20A), may affect the assessment and lead to incorrect conclusions and possibly misdiagnosis. If the reader is interested in carrying out mobilization procedures other than the simple manual therapy techniques presented in this text, a more thorough determination of the type of pelvic and spine malalignment present is of the utmost importance. Such a detailed assessment is, however, not usually necessary in order to apply the material presented here to the clinical setting. Advanced assessment and treatment techniques are best learned in a formal teaching setting, hands-on workshops and from selected papers, books and educational videos/DVDs (see DVD information provided and listings under 'References' and 'Useful addresses and web sites').

Box 2.3 outlines the basic questions to be answered by the examination.

PELVIC OBLIQUITY

The presence of a pelvic obliquity may become obvious from noting that the pants, a belt or underwear are up on one side as the person walks, stands or sits (Figs 2.70, 2.76B, 2.90, 6.4, 6.5). A more accurate examination to determine whether the pelvic landmarks are lying level or obliquely relies on side-to-side comparison with:

1. visualization or palpation of the sometimes very easily apparent 'dimples of Venus' on the buttocks, about 1 cm above the PSIS and overlying the hollows - or sacral 'sulci' - formed

BOX 2.3 Examination for pelvic malalignment

1. Is the pelvis level or oblique?
2. Are the bony landmarks of the pelvis symmetrical or asymmetrical?
3. What happens on the 'sitting-lying' test (described in detail below)?
4. Is there any sacral torsion or excessive nutation or counternutation of the sacrum?
5. Is there an obvious curvature of the spine (e.g., a scoliosis, increased lumbar lordosis, thoracic kyphosis) and/or any rotational displacement of isolated vertebrae?
6. Is there excessive gapping and/or displacement of the symphysis pubis at rest or on stressing the joint?
7. Is there an abnormal increase in tension and/or tenderness localizing to specific muscles and ligaments?
8. What are the findings on sacroiliac joint and pelvic girdle testing for:
   a. function, motion/mobility and stability
   b. 'form' and 'force' closure?
9. Is the basic musculoskeletal, neurological and vascular examination normal?

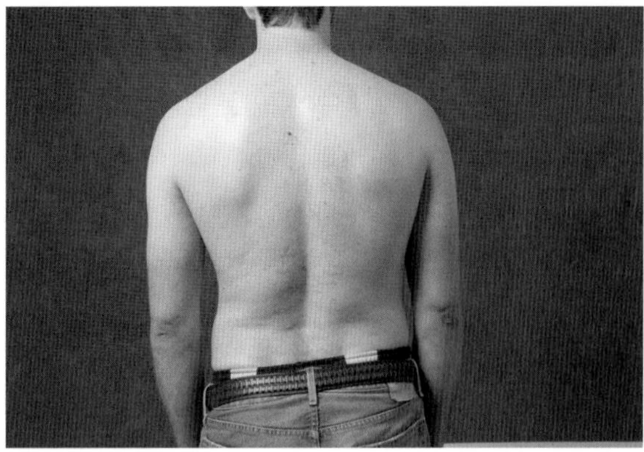

Fig. 2.70 Belt angled up on right in standing, indicating pelvic obliquity (inclined to right).

by the junction of the base of the sacrum with the posterior iliac crest on either side (Figs 2.6, 2.71A, 2.87B)

2. the index and/or middle fingers lying on the lateral iliac crests (Fig. 2.71B)
3. the thumbs or index fingers resting on the superior rim of the pubic bones (Fig. 2.71C)
4. thumbs pressed upward against the inferior aspect of the ASIS (Fig. 2.71D), PSIS ('X' on Fig. 2.71Eii), ischial tuberosities (Fig. 2.71F), ILA (Figs 2.3A 2.71 G, 2.87B) or inside of PSIS (Fig. 2.71Ei)

Assessment of the sacral base/sulci and ILA prove helpful in determining sacral alignment, torsion and rotation around the vertical axis (Box 2.1; Figs 2.21, 2.71Gi,ii, 2.87-2.89).

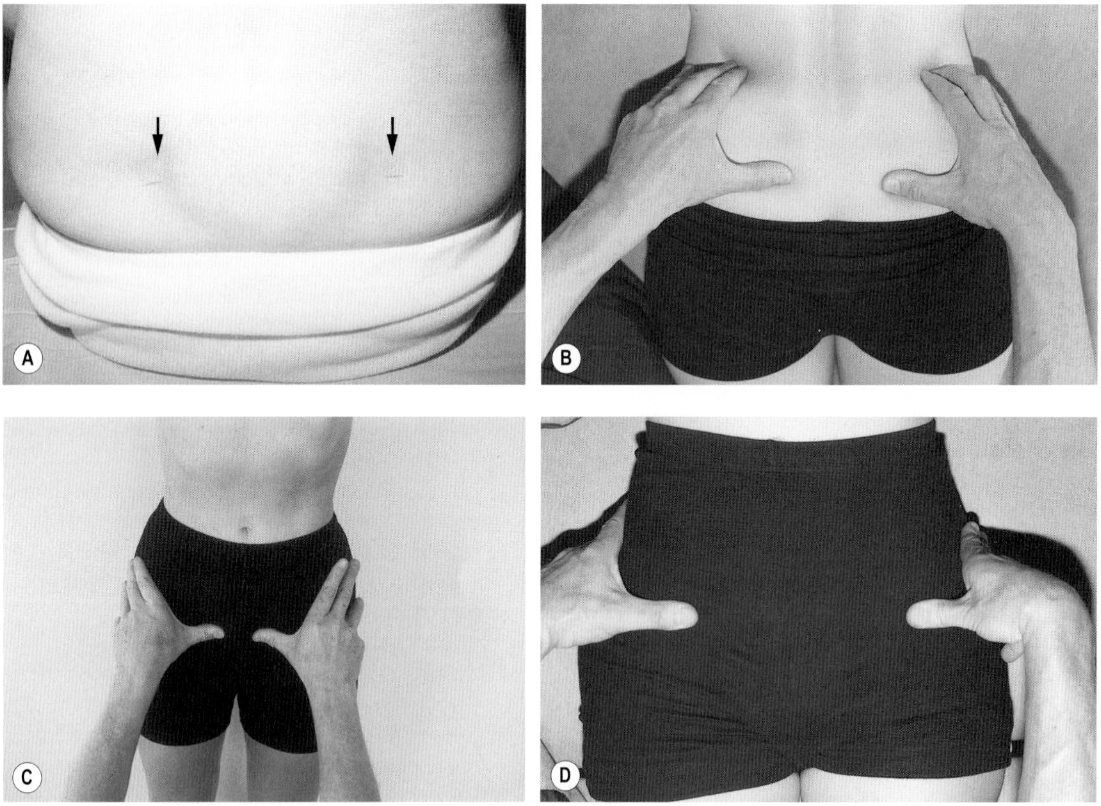

Fig. 2.71 Landmarks when the pelvis is aligned and the leg length equal. (A) 'Dimples of Venus', about 1 cm above the inner margin of the posterior superior iliac spine (PSIS) - see also Fig. 2.6A. (B) Fingers on the iliac crests, thumbs against the inferior aspect of the PSIS. (C) Superior pubic bones (thumbs resting on the superior aspect). (D) Anterior superior iliac spine (thumbs resting against the inferior aspect).

(Continued)

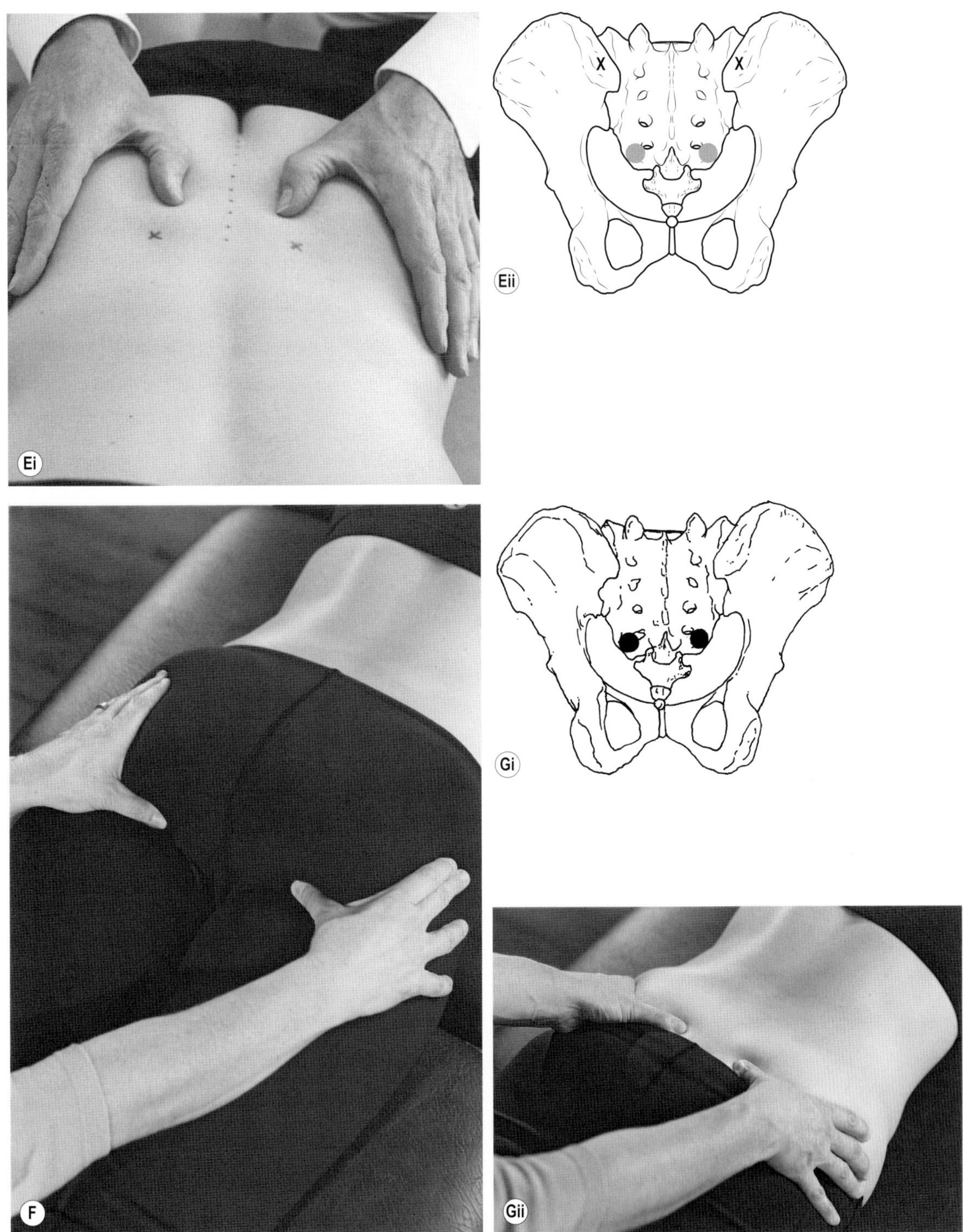

Fig. 2.71—cont'd (E) PSIS: i) thumbs resting against the inner aspect are equidistant from midline (broken line running upward from gluteal cleft) ii) 'X' marks the right/left PSIS. (F) Ischial tuberosities. (Gi,ii) Inferior lateral angle, at the S5 level. (Figs 2.71Eii, F,G: *Courtesy of © Diane G. Lee Physiotherapist Corp.)*

In standing

1. If the pelvis appears level, this suggests (but does not confirm) that the person has equal leg length and that there is no indication of 'rotational malalignment' and/or an 'upslip'; it does not rule out an underlying 'outflare/inflare' (Figs 2.71B,C; 2.72A)
2. If the pelvis is oblique, there could be:
   a. an anatomical (true) LLD (Fig. 2.72B), or
   b. a functional lengthening of the leg as the result of an 'upslip' or 'rotational malalignment' (Figs 2.73A-D).

In sitting and lying supine or prone

If the pelvis is now level, this suggests an anatomical (true) leg length difference as the cause of the obliquity seen in standing. The LLD itself will still be evident in prone and supine-lying but all the pelvic landmarks will now be symmetrical in these positions (Fig. 2.72B). If the pelvic obliquity persists when sitting, with the iliac crest now elevated either on the same side or opposite to what is seen in standing, pelvic malalignment is probably present (Figs 2.73A-D, 2.76B). A less likely cause is a side-to-side difference in the actual height of the innominates that may become evident after pelvic fracture(s) or with impaired development (e.g. a hemi-pelvis; Fig. 3.87).

BONY LANDMARKS OF THE PELVIS

In practice, assessment depending on comparison of the pelvic landmarks may not be entirely accurate because of imbalances in muscle tension or strength, congenital or acquired side-to-side differences of

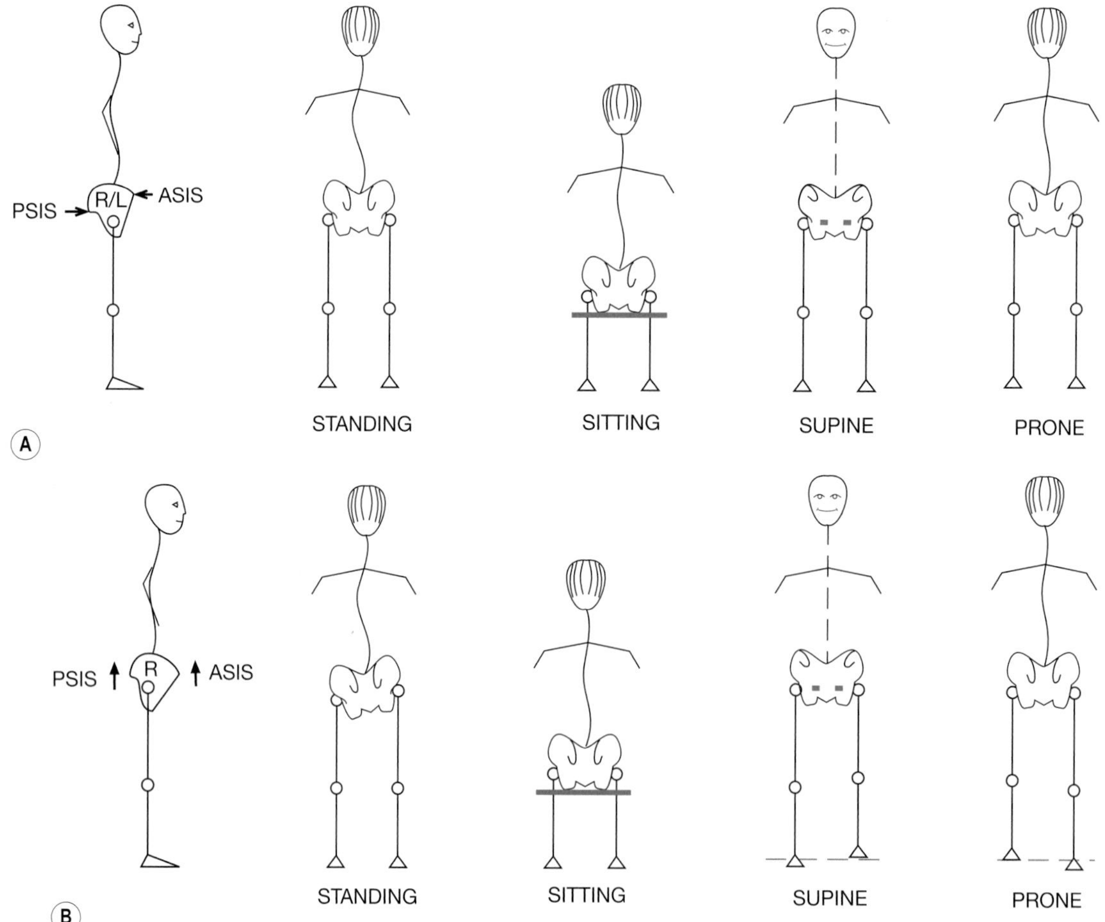

Fig. 2.72 Effect of leg length on the aligned pelvis. (A) Aligned: leg length equal. (B) Aligned: an anatomical (true) LLD (right leg long - pelvis up on right when standing, level sitting and lying). ASIS, anterior superior iliac spine; PSIS, posterior superior iliac spine.

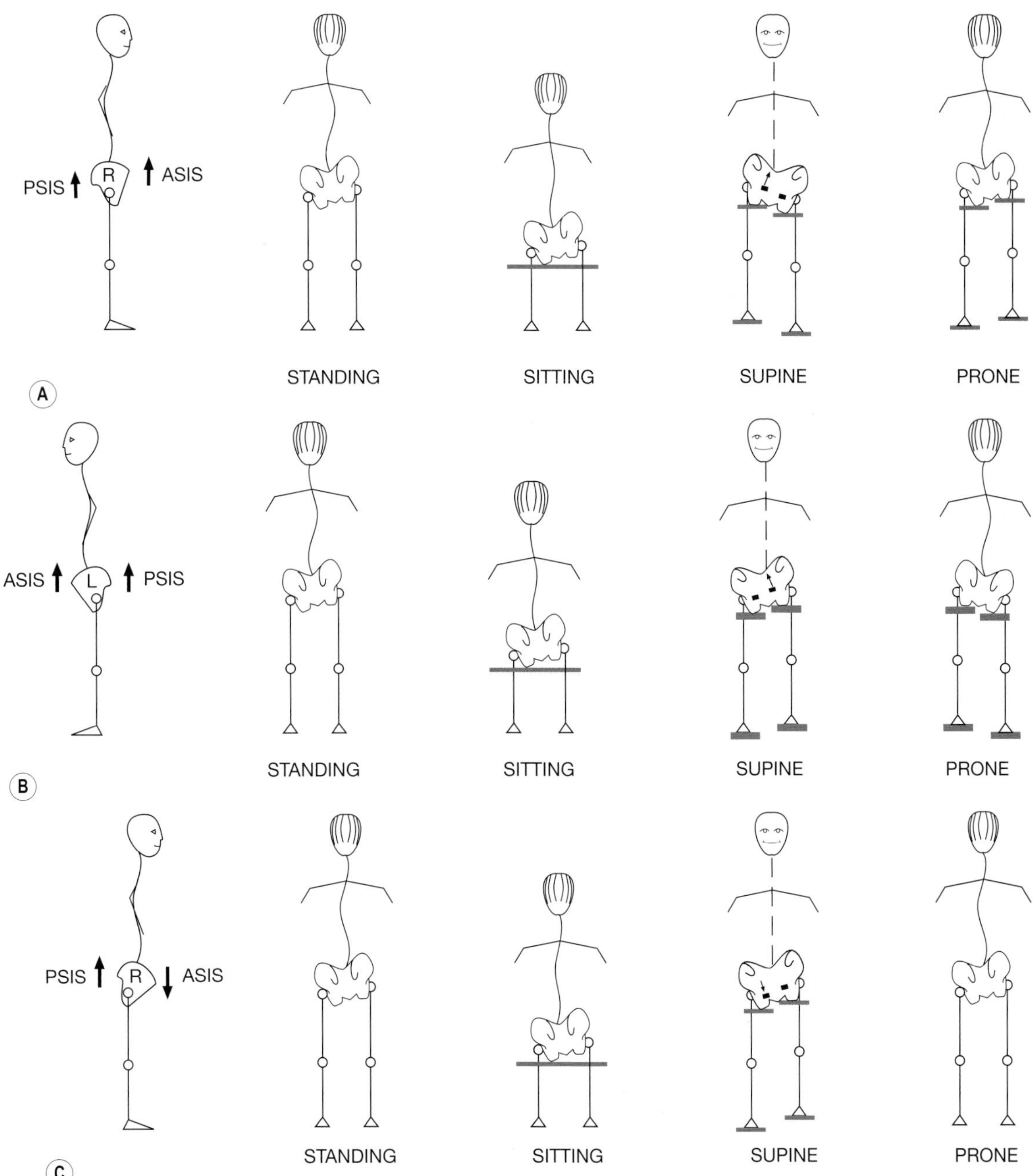

Fig. 2.73 Pelvic obliquity related to malalignment (some typical changes noted in standing, sitting, lying). (A) 'Right upslip' (all right pelvic landmarks are up in all 3 positions). (B) 'Left upslip' (right iliac crest often up in standing and sitting; left definitely up in lying). In both (C) 'right anterior rotational malalignment' (most common pattern) and

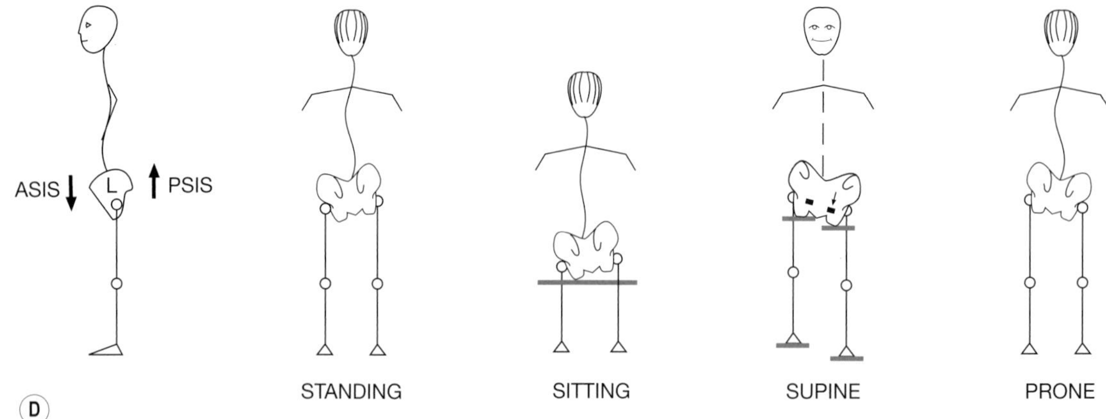

Fig. 2.73—cont'd (D) 'left anterior rotational malalignment' (less common pattern): all landmarks asymmetrical side-to-side, front-to-back. ASIS, anterior superior iliac spine; PSIS, posterior superior iliac spine.

bony contours, or a unilateral tendency to pronation or supination when weight-bearing.

> Attempts to establish the presence or absence of malalignment must never be limited to the assessment of landmarks alone but should be supplemented by the findings on examination for pelvic obliquity and leg length differences in various positions.

In alignment and with leg length equal

1. The iliac crests will be level when standing, sitting, and lying prone or supine (Figs 2.71, 2.72A).
2. The right and left ASIS and PSIS will be level when standing, sitting and lying. On a lateral view, the ASIS is positioned upward (craniad) relative to the PSIS by approximately the same amount on both sides.
3. The right and left superior and inferior pubic rami are level when lying supine or standing (Fig. 2.71C), the ischial tuberosities level in lying prone or standing (Fig. 2.71F).
4. The right and left ASIS and PSIS will be level in the coronal plane when assessed in supine- or prone-lying. Also, there is no rotation of the pelvis around the vertical axis (i.e. no rotation clockwise or counterclockwise; Fig. 2.9) or coronal axis (i.e. minimal or no tilting).

In alignment, with an anatomical (true) leg length difference

1. Only in standing are all landmarks elevated on the side of the long leg, with a uniform obliquity of the pelvic crests and superior pubic rami on clinical examination (Fig. 2.72B). A standing anteroposterior X-ray of the pelvis shows:
   a. a uniformly sloping obliquity of the sacral base, iliac crests and superior pubic bones, with no displacement of the innominates relative to the sacrum or of the pubic bones relative to each other
   b. a difference in the height of the femoral heads on standing views of the pelvis, which amounts to the true LLD (Fig. 2.74A).

Sacroiliac joint 'upslip'

On the side of the 'upslip', there is a simultaneous elevation of all the pelvic landmarks, anteriorly and posteriorly. Unlike in the case of the anatomical LLD, where the obliquity gradually slopes upward to the long-leg side in standing, one is dealing here with an obliquity that is actually disrupted on the side where the innominate has translated upward relative to the sacrum.

'Right upslip'

There is an upward displacement of the right ASIS, AIIS and pubic rami anteriorly, the PSIS and ischial tuberosity posteriorly (Figs 2.61A, 2.73A, 2.82). The

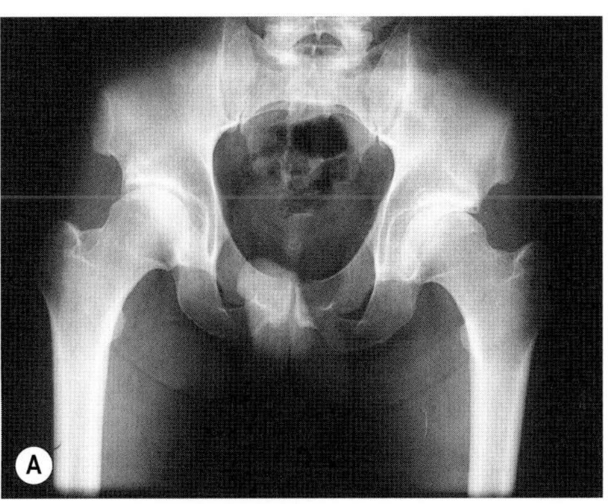

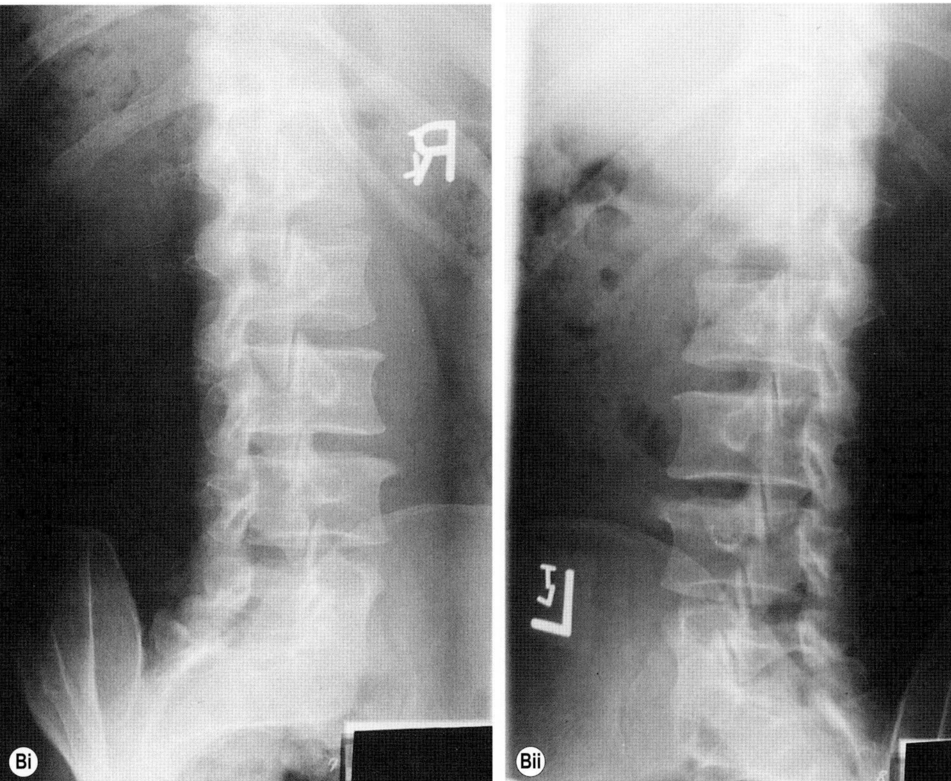

Fig. 2.74 X-ray: standing view of a person with anatomical (true) leg length difference - right leg long. (A) A-P view: right femoral head higher than left; note the uniform obliquity of the superior pubic rami (inclined to right; no displacement at symphysis pubis) and the similarity in appearance of R/L hip/sacroiliac joints and lesser trochanters. (B) (i) Right and (ii) left oblique views: the facet joints appear to be of uniform width except for right L4-L5, narrowed by what appear to be osteoarthritic changes.

right superior pubic ramus usually shifts upward by 3-5 mm, sometimes more, relative to the left one; this difference can be appreciated as a step deformity at the symphysis pubis on palpation and on X-ray. The right leg is pulled upward passively with the right innominate, so that it appears to be shorter than the left leg when the person is lying prone or supine (Fig. 2.73A); this shortening usually amounts to some 5-10 mm. In standing, however, the iliac crest is often elevated on the side of the 'upslip' so that the right leg appears to be the longer one in that position. In fact, this elevation of the right iliac crest frequently persists during sitting, when the pelvis would be expected to tilt down on the right to fill the space between the ischial tuberosity and seating surface created by the right innominate having moved upward relative to the sacrum. This finding may be due to factors such as:

1. some rotation of the pelvis in the coronal plane
2. asymmetric increase in muscle tension or actual spasm, which should also be suspected whenever there is persistence of an 'upslip' (e.g. involving ipsilateral quadratus lumborum, psoas major/minor; Fig. 2.62)

'Left upslip'

The iliac crest often appears up on the right side in standing (as if the pelvis is dropping down with the left leg being 'short') and in sitting (as if to fill in the gap between the ischial tuberosity and surface). The 'upslip' is most easily appreciated on examination in the supine and prone positions, in which case the left leg is noted to be shortened and the left ASIS, PSIS, pubic bone, iliac crest and ischial tuberosity have translated upward along the vertical plane relative to the sacrum and these same landmarks on the right side (Fig. 2.73B).

'Rotational malalignment'

Anterior and posterior superior iliac spines (ASIS, PSIS)

With 'anterior' rotation of an innominate bone around the coronal axis in the sagittal plane, the ipsilateral PSIS moves upward (cephalad) and the ASIS and pubic bone downward (caudad); whereas on 'posterior' rotation, it is the ASIS and pubic bone that moves upward and PSIS downward. The anterior or posterior rotation of the innominate on one side is usually compensated for by the contrary rotation of the innominate on the opposite side, which has the effect of amplifying both the side-to-side and front-to-back asymmetry of the landmarks. One can usually make the diagnosis of a 'rotational malalignment' on the basis of this complete asymmetry of the ASIS and PSIS (Figs 2.42; 2.73 C,D; 2.76).

Pubic bones

With a 'right anterior, left posterior' innominate rotation, there will be rotational displacement of the pubic bones evident at the symphysis pubis:

1. the right pubic bone rotates anteriorly, the left posteriorly around the coronal axis
2. there is also some craniodaudal translation in the vertical plane, relative to each other: downward (caudad) with 'anterior', upward with 'posterior' rotation; there results a displacement at the symphysis pubis that is usually easily apparent both on clinical examination (Fig. 2.76C) and on anteroposterior X-rays of the pelvis (Fig. 2.75)

In other words, as a result of either 'anterior' or 'posterior' rotation of one innominate, all the bony landmarks of the pelvis end up completely asymmetrical in all positions of examination, both on anterior-to-posterior and side-to-side comparison.

'Outflare and inflare'

The landmarks primarily used to detect an 'outflare' and 'inflare' are the ASIS, PSIS and midline markers such as the umbilicus and symphysis pubis anteriorly and gluteal crease posteriorly.

In someone who is in alignment

1. anterior assessment in supine-lying
   a. right and left ASIS are level in the coronal plane

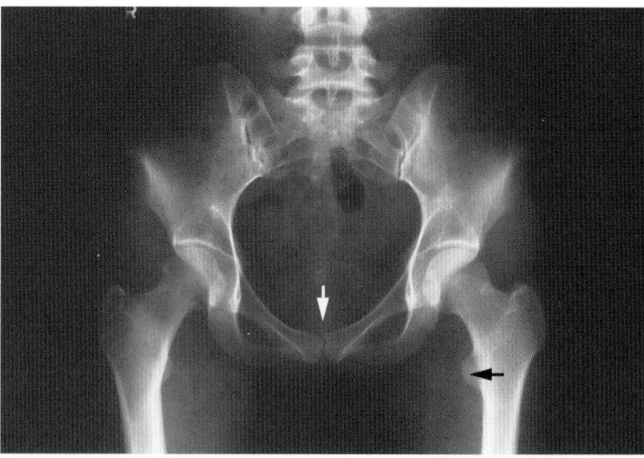

Fig. 2.75 X-ray: standing A-P view of the pelvis in a person with equal leg length and 'right anterior, left posterior' rotational malalignment. Note: (1) femoral heads level but pelvic crests oblique; (2) approximately 3 mm downward displacement of the right superior pubic ramus relative to the left at the symphysis pubis; (3) apparent asymmetry of the sacroiliac joints and lesser trochanters (the left appearing larger, the right smaller; compare with Figs 2.74A, 4.30A).

b. the thumbs placed on the tips of the ASIS are up an equal distance from the surface the person is lying on and a ruler or level ends up horizontal (Fig. 2.65)
c. right and left ASIS and PSIS are equidistant from centre (Figs 2.13Bii,Cii, 2.68, 2.69, 2.71Ei)
   i. anteriorly, one can use the umbilicus or an obvious central hairline (provided these have not been shifted off-centre by adhesions, scar tissue, organomegaly or masses), also the symphysis pubis, as a central marker (Figs 2.66-2.69)
   ii. the tips of the index or middle fingers meet in centre when the hands are rotated inward, with the thumbs anchored against the medial aspect of the ASIS to serve as a pivot point (Fig. 2.69)

2. posterior assessment in prone-lying
   - right and left PSIS are level in the coronal plane and equidistant from centre, with the gluteal crease usually serving best as a marker (Figs 2.13Cii; 2.71Ei)
3. the ASIS and PSIS and the pubic bones remain level in the coronal plane and there is no rotation around the vertical axis in the transverse plane on viewing the pelvis from front or back; therefore, there is no forward protrusion of the ASIS detectable on one side compared to the other when:
   a. lying prone or supine (Fig. 2.65)
   b. standing with the heels and back against the wall, or
   c. sitting with the buttocks and trunk pressed evenly into the back of the chair.

In someone with a 'right outflare, left inflare' (Figs 2.13, 2.64, 2.66):

1. the innominates have rotated clockwise around the vertical axis in the transverse plane
2. the right innominate flares outward, the left inward relative to the midline anteriorly
3. the right ASIS ends up away from centre in the supine position (Fig. 2.13Bi) and the right PSIS toward the centre when lying prone (Fig. 2.13 Ci); findings are reversed on the left side
4. a level shows the tip of the right ASIS to be comparatively lower (= 'outflare') than the left (= 'inflare') side in supine-lying (Figs 2.13Aiii; 2.64)
   - these same findings will also be evident in sitting and standing; in this example, a finger placed on the tips of the ASIS would show the left to be displaced forward, the right relatively backward in the transverse plane when the person or an examiner looks directly downward at the front of the pelvis

In someone with a 'right inflare, left outflare'

The opposite findings would be evident:

1. right ASIS is in toward, left away from the midline when lying supine; whereas right PSIS is out from and left in toward midline when lying prone
2. tip of right ASIS is higher, left lower on comparison, using a level or other technique

Diagnosis of 'outflare' and 'inflare' is simplified by the fact that, when lying supine and looking at the height of the tips of the ASIS:

RULE OF 4 'I's FOR DIAGNOSING AN 'INFLARE':

ASIS is 'HIGH' on the 'INFLARE' side and moved 'IN' toward the midline; treatment requires resisting attempts to push 'INWARD' with the knee on that side (**NOTE**: 4 words with an 'I' in them, demarcating that an 'INFLARE' is present on this side)

RULE OF 4 'O's FOR DIAGNOSING AN 'OUTFLARE':

ASIS is 'LOW' on the 'OUTFLARE' side and moved 'OUT' from the midline; treatment requires resisting attempts to push 'OUTWARD' with the knee on this side (**NOTE**: 4 words with an 'O' in them, demarcating that an 'OUTFLARE' is present on this side).

Treatment of 'outflare' and 'inflare' will be discussed in detail in Ch. 7.

'SITTING-LYING' TEST

This test affords an individual and those caring for patients a quick way of establishing whether malalignment is actually present and, if so, to find out whether there is a 'rotational malalignment', 'upslip', 'flare' or a combination of these, so that appropriate treatment can be initiated.

Leg length is compared by initially noting the level of the medial malleoli in the 'long-sitting' (sitting up with legs out in front, knees extended) and then 'supine-lying' positions (Figs 2.77A, 2.78A). Trying to compare the high points of the malleoli is sometimes diffcult, especially if the malleoli are

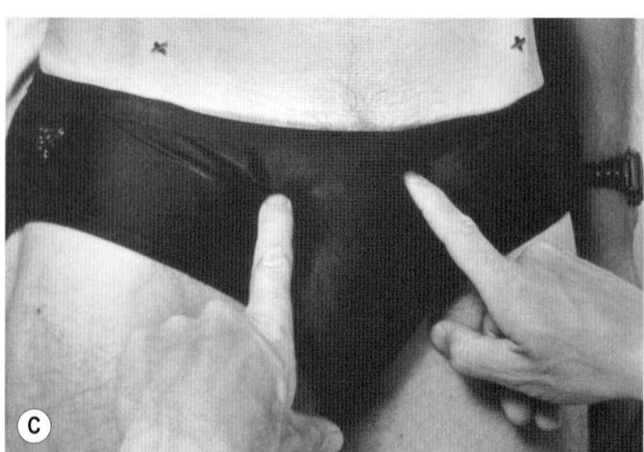

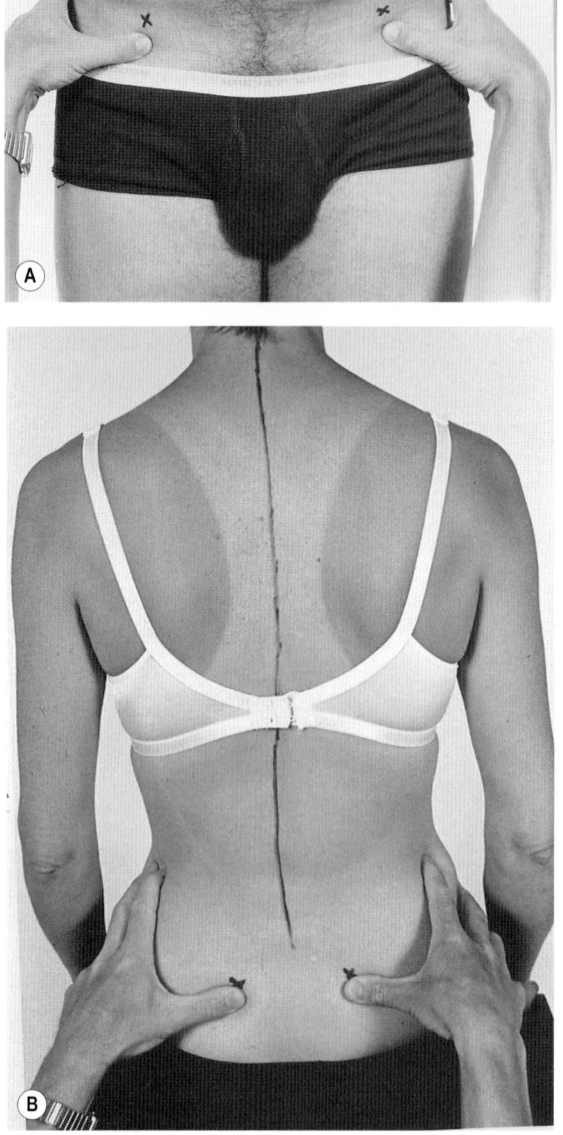

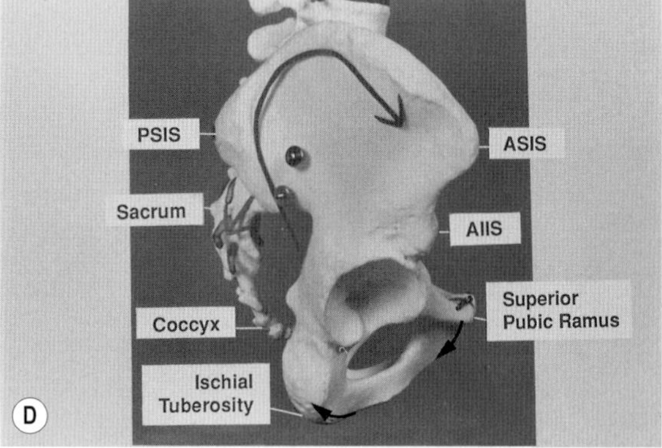

Fig. 2.76 'Rotational malalignment': 'right anterior, left posterior' innominate rotation in both subjects. (A) Asymmetry of anterior superior iliac spine (ASIS) (right down, left up). (B) Asymmetry of posterior superior iliac spine (PSIS) and iliac crests (right up, left down) in standing (also in sitting; see Fig. 3.86B); downward displacement of shoulder and brassiere on left. (C) Right superior pubic ramus displaced downward relative to the left. (D) Shift of the right pelvic landmarks relative to their left counterparts: right iliac crest, PSIS and ischial tuberosity moved upward; right ASIS, anterior inferior iliac spine and pubic ramus moved downward.

uneven in contour developmentally or as a result of injury, not very prominent or quite a distance apart (as seen, for example, in a person with 'knock-knees' or genu valgum). It is much easier, and more accurate, to compare the level of the thumbs placed in the hollow immediately below the medial malleolus on each side, directly overlying the medial ankle ligaments (Figs 2.77B, 2.78B). Point the tip of each thumb straight downward (distal phalanx vertical) so that you are now comparing the relative level of your interphalangeal joints (i.e. knuckles) which end up closer together and are more clearly demarcated than the malleoli, making side-to-side comparison more accurate. Remember to hold onto the ankles lightly - the thumbs are only serving you as a guide to compare side-to-side leg movement and length on sitting and lying. A common mistake is to hold on forcefully, at the risk of impairing free upward and downward movement of the legs, making the person tense up or causing actual discomfort.

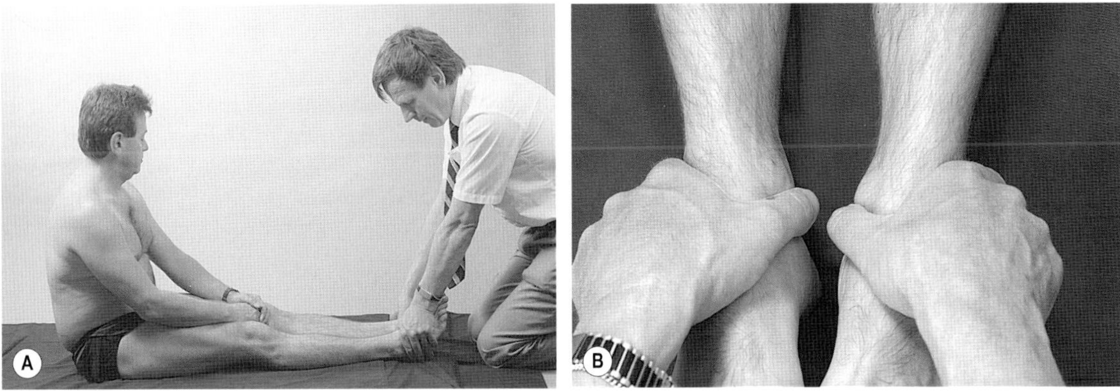

Fig. 2.77 Sitting part of the 'sitting-lying' test in male subject. (A) Long-sitting. (B) Left leg appears longer than the right.

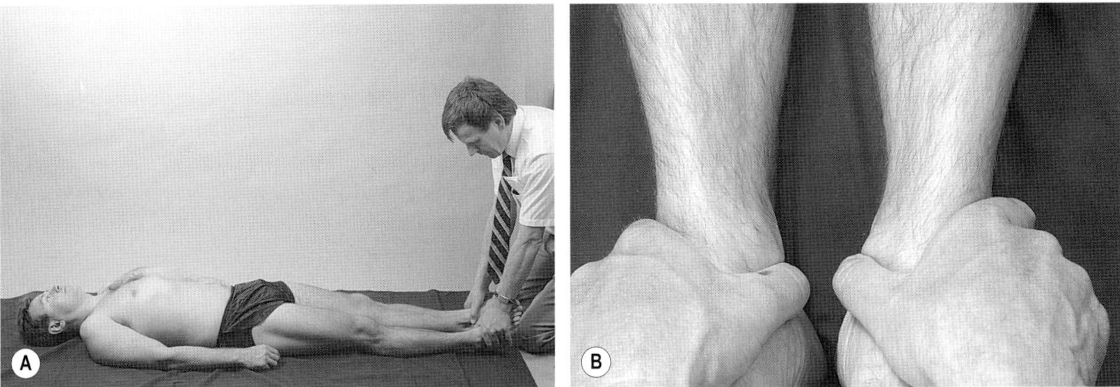

Fig. 2.78 Lying part of the 'sitting-lying' test in same subject. (A) Supine-lying. (B) There has been a shift in the leg length: the right leg has lengthened relative to the left leg (findings the reverse of those noted in Fig. 2.77B).

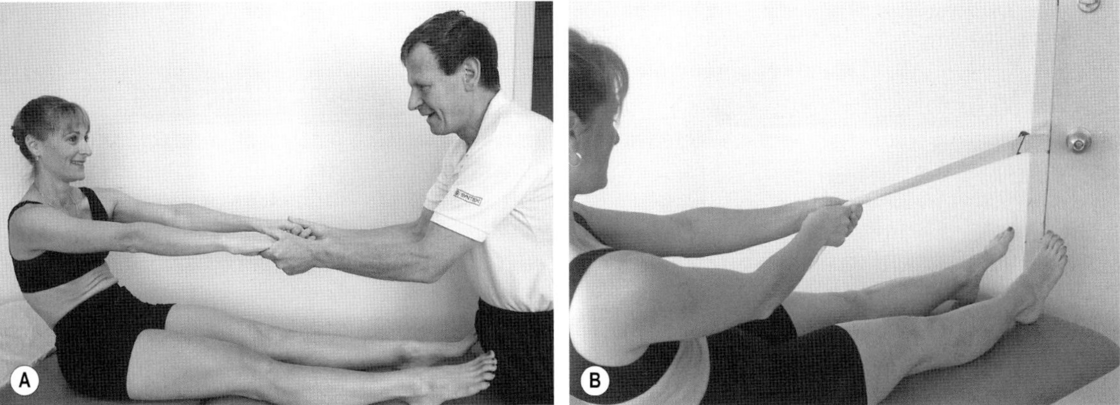

Fig. 2.79 'Sitting-lying' test: assisting sitting up to minimize contraction of any other muscles attached to the pelvic ring and decrease any error. (A) Assisted by a second person. (B) Subject using a strap or rope to pull up on (and let herself down with) while concentrating on detecting a leg length difference and any shift of the feet relative to each other on changing position.

At home, the test is best performed with the person lying on a firm bed, carpeted floor or even a table; a soft surface could interfere with the comparative movement of the legs on changing position from sitting to lying and may allow the pelvis and trunk to sink down unevenly. The heels must be able to slide without hindrance. If one or other heel gets caught up on the surface it will, in turn, shift the pelvis on that side and make the test invalid. A sheet covering the plinth or a towel placed under the heels will prevent them getting caught up on a vinyl or leather surface, especially if they are sweaty; alternately, the person can just keep their socks on for this test. If a smooth surface is not available at home, try lying on the floor; when out on the field, place a jacket under the heels, the smooth lining facing upward, which should allow the feet to move upward and downward more easily.

The person initially lies supine and is then asked to sit up. A shift of the pelvis or other error is less likely if the person avoids, as much as possible, activating leg, pelvic or trunk muscles that can influence movement of the pelvis; this can best be achieved:

1. on a 2-person test: having someone assist by holding on to the person's outstetched hands and gently pulling him/her up (Fig. 2.79A)
2. on a 1-person test: by pulling oneself up hanging on to a belt, strap or other anchored support (Fig. 2.79B).

During the motion of sitting up, concentrate on the movement of the feet - are the legs moving downward together (i.e. both lengthening)? Once you are sitting up, establish the relative leg length - are they the same length or is one leg longer than the other? The next step is to lie down, with the examiner's assistance or the aid of the support, while concentrating on whether:

1. the legs move upward together (i.e. shorten at the same rate)
2. if there is a short leg in sitting and the legs move up together on lying, is that leg short the same amount in both the sitting and lying positions?
3. one leg lengthens, the other shortens; that is, is there a shift in the relative leg length which reverses again on sitting up?

The manoeuvre is best repeated one or two times for confirmation of the findings observed initially. Sometimes initial findings may not match up with other changes detected on examination (e.g. shift of landmarks in a pattern typical of an 'upslip', 'outflare/inflare' or 'rotational malalignment') but, on repeat testing, are seen to change in a way that is consistent with the presentation of malalignment suspected as the person starts to relax and the pelvis and legs can move more freely. If a shift in length are suspected to be occurring on going from one position to another but proves hard to detect, consider doing the following:

1. with the person in long-sitting
   - using a ball-point or felt pen, make marks on the skin or socks directly adjacent to each other on the inside of the feet at the part where they come closest together; e.g. at the malleoli or the medial aspect of the 1st MTP joint (base of the first toe)
2. on lying-down
   a. does a difference in leg length become apparent, with the right and left marks separating?
3. if the marks did separate on lying down and the person then sits up:
   a. does this difference persist but remain exactly the same?
      - this would be in keeping with either an 'upslip' or a 'true' LLD)
   b. does the shift in the marks reverse, so that they come to match up again the way they were when initially drawn in sitting?
      - this would be in keeping with the shift that occurs with 'rotational malalignment'
4. are these findings consistent on repeating the 'sitting-lying' test once or twice?

Clinical correlation: 'sitting-lying' test

Barring excessive tension or contracture in the pelvic and hip girdle structures (e.g. unilateral contracture of quadratus lumborum or psoas major/minor pulling up on the ipsilateral innominate, with seeming 'shortening' of that leg; Fig. 2.62), the more common presentations on the 'sitting-lying' test are those described below.

Aligned, leg length equal

In supine-lying, the acetabula lie anterior and up (craniad) relative to the ischial tuberosities (Fig. 2.80A). On moving into the long-sitting position, flexion

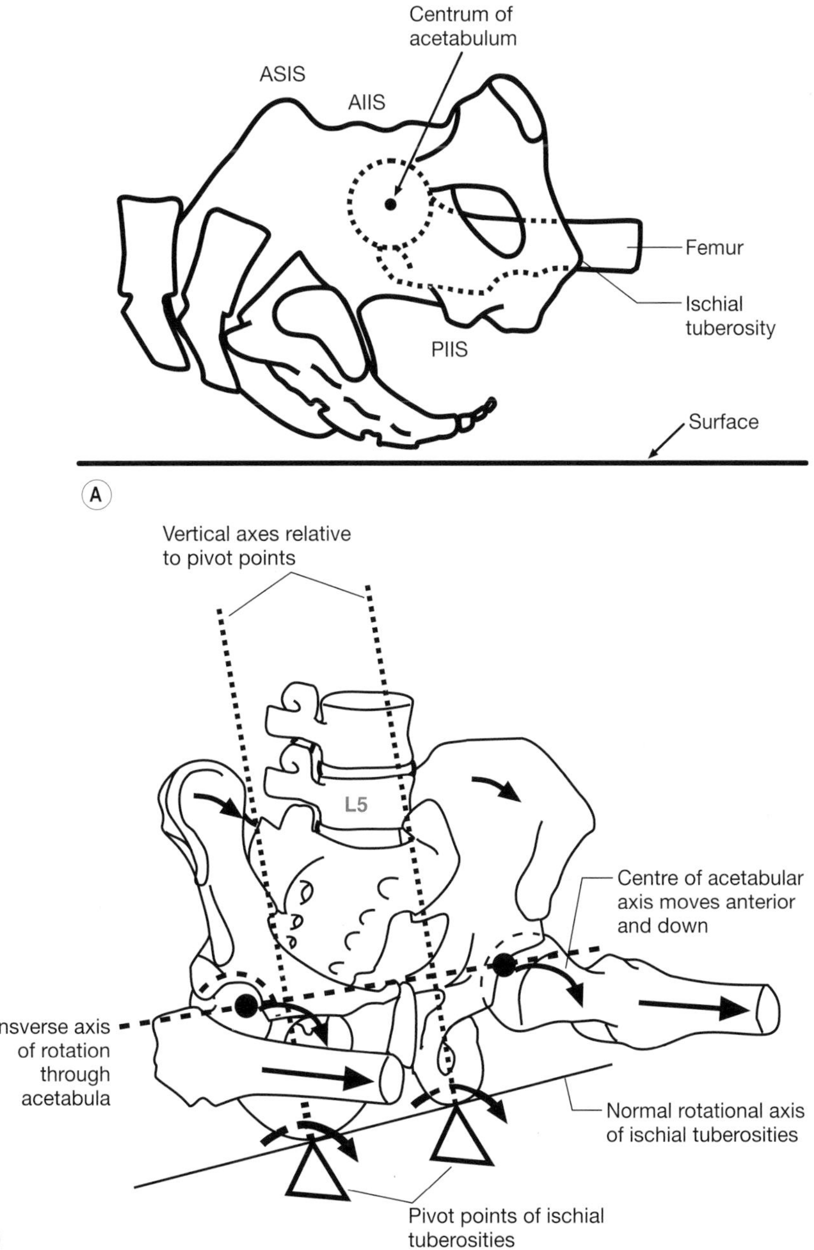

Fig. 2.80 'Sitting-lying' test: aligned, leg length equal and all landmarks symmetrical. (A) Supine-lying: the acetabula lie anterior and craniad relative to the ischial tuberosities. (B) Moving into long-sitting: the innominates pivot over the ischial tuberosities and the acetabula move forward and caudad, causing the legs to lengthen equally. ASIS, anterior superior iliac spine; AIIS, anterior inferior iliac spine; PIIS, posterior inferior iliac spine. *(Redrawn courtesy of DonTigny 1997.)*

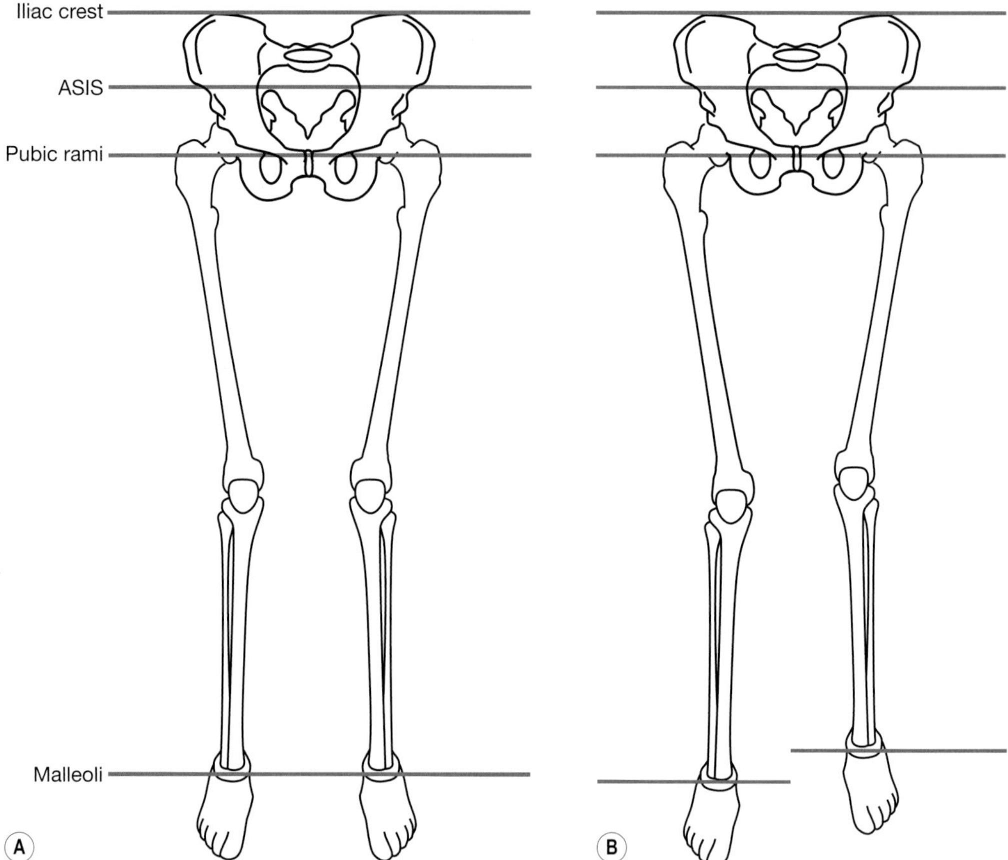

Fig. 2.81 'Sitting-lying' test: in alignment, the pelvic landmarks on the right match all those on the left. (A) Leg length equal: the malleoli match in sitting and lying. (B) Anatomical (true) leg length difference: right leg longer to the same extent in both sitting and lying. ASIS, anterior superior iliac spine.

occurs initially in the thoracic and then the lumbar spine, at which point the pelvic unit starts to tilt forward and eventually pivots over the now weight-bearing tuberosities as one unit. The acetabula are, therefore, moved even further anteriorly and also downward (caudad) so that the legs appear to lengthen to an equal extent (Fig. 2.80B). On returning to supine-lying, the pelvis tilts backward as one unit, the acetabula are moved in a posterior direction and upward (craniad) and the legs appear to shorten, again to an equal extent. The feet, therefore, move together: downward as the person assumes the long-sitting position, upward on supine-lying. The examiner's thumbs in the hollows just below the malleoli will match exactly in both positions (Fig. 2.81A). The pelvic landmarks are also all symmetrical in both prone and supine-lying (Figs 2.71, 2.72A).

'Outflare' and 'inflare'

Leg movement and lengthening/shortening are as for 'aligned, leg length equal', provided there is no coexistent true LLD and/or associated 'upslip' or 'rotational malalignment'. In other words, the legs are of equal length and move together, downward on long-sitting and upward on supine-lying.

Aligned, anatomical (true) leg length difference present

One leg is longer than the other (Fig. 2.72B). The pelvis, however, still rotates forward and backward around the coronal axis in the sagittal plane as one unit on long-sitting and supine-lying, respectively. Therefore, the legs and feet move downward and upward together and no change occurs in the length of either leg - the difference between the malleoli corresponds to the 'true' LLD and remains the same in both positions (Fig. 2.81B). All the pelvic

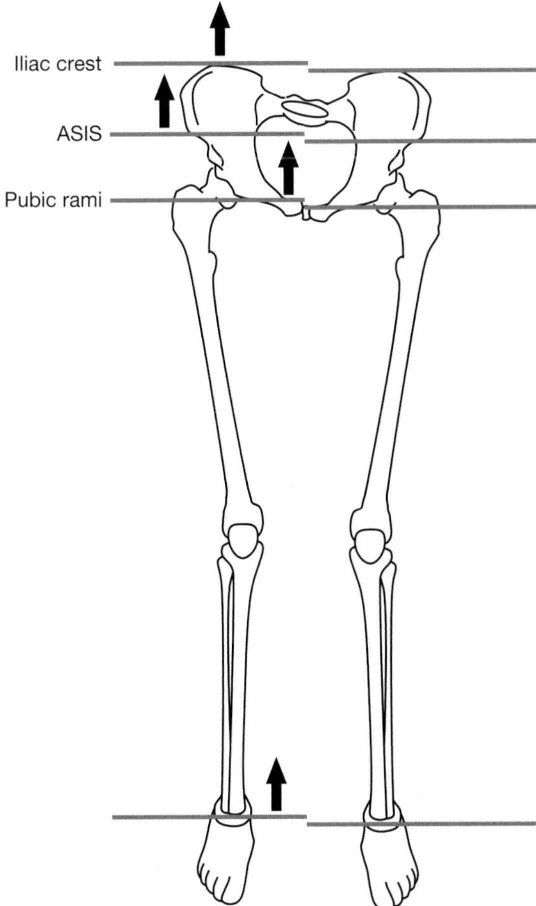

Fig. 2.82 'Sitting-lying' test: right sacroiliac joint 'upslip'. The right leg remains short to an equal extent in sitting and lying; the right anterior and posterior pelvic landmarks are all displaced upward on the right side relative to the sacrum and left innominate. ASIS, anterior superior iliac spine.

landmarks are higher on the side of the long leg in standing but level when sitting and lying.

Sacroiliac joint 'upslip'

With a 'right upslip', the right innominate is shifted straight upward (craniad) relative to the sacrum (Figs 2.73A, 2,82). The pelvis continues to move as one unit so that the legs still lengthen and shorten to an equal extent on long-sitting and supine-lying, respectively. The right leg will, therefore, appear to be shorter in both positions by at least the amount of relative upward shift that has occurred. However, that difference may be accentuated considerably by any reactive increase in tension of muscles in the ipsilateral flank and hip girdle region (Fig. 2.62). Similar to the situation with an anatomical LLD, the malleoli do not match, the difference remains the same in sitting and lying, and the feet move downward and upward together. The right anterior and posterior innominate landmarks, however, have all moved upward (craniad) (Figs 2.61A, 2.73A). The findings are the opposite for a 'left upslip' (Fig. 2.73B).

Sacroiliac joint 'downslip'

In the case of a 'right downslip', the right innominate will have moved downward relative to the sacrum, the right leg will be consistently longer in both long-sitting and supine-lying, and all the innominate landmarks on the right side will be displaced downward (caudad) relative to those on the left in both the supine and the prone position. The findings are the reverse for a 'left downslip'.

'Rotational malalignment'

When the person is in alignment, also with a 'true' LLD, 'upslip' or 'outflare/inflare' present, the pelvic ring moves as one unit on changing from sitting to lying or the reverse - any rotation around the SI joints is symmetrical. On sitting up, the pelvis pivots over the ischial tuberosities and rotates uniformly around an axis running through the acetabulae, causing them to move anterior and caudad so that the two legs lengthen to an equal extent (Fig. 2.80B).

With 'rotational malalignment', the pelvis no longer moves as one unit - there is now contrary rotation of the innominates around the coronal axis in the sagittal plane on sitting and lying. Assuming that the sacrum itself is still aligned (i.e. no sacral torsion, excessive nutation or counternutation), the following are the findings seen with:

'right anterior, left posterior' innominate rotation

1. in supine-lying
   Weight bearing is primarily on the dorsum of the sacral and coccygeal part of the pelvis (Fig. 2.80A). With the contrary rotation of the innominates, the right acetabulum will have been displaced downward (caudad) and posterior, the left upward (craniad) and anterior. There results a relative lengthening of the right and shortening of the left leg.
2. on moving up into the long-sitting position (Fig. 2.83), pressure is eventually exerted on:
   a. the anterior aspect of the ischial tuberosity of the right innominate, resulting in further

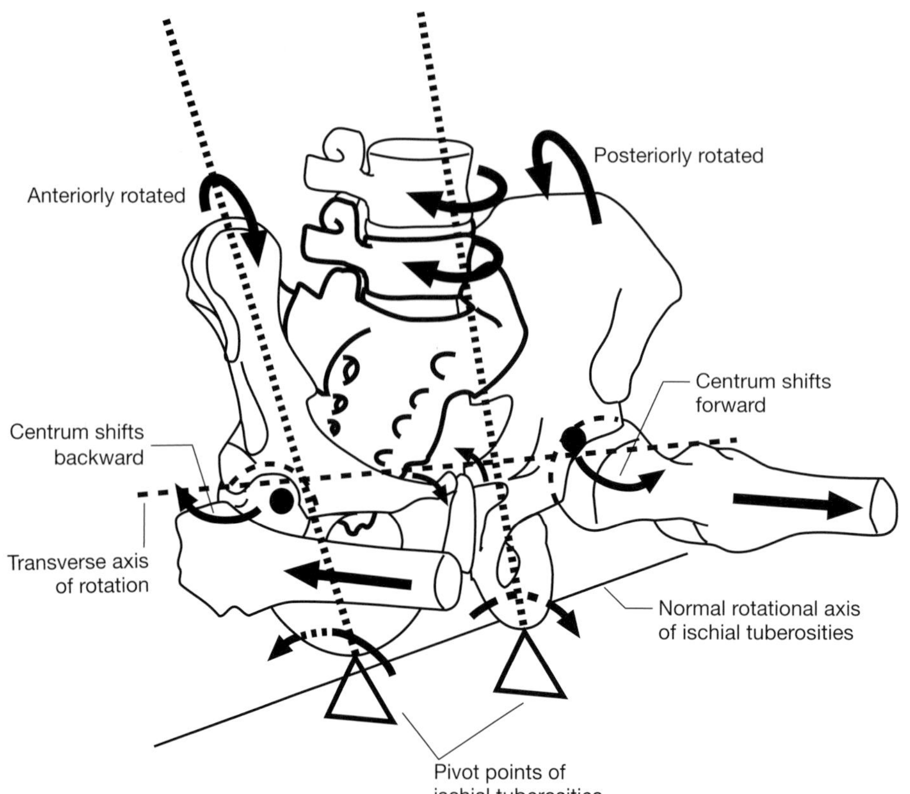

Fig. 2.83 'Sitting-lying' test: 'rotational malalignment'. Innominates have pivoted in contrary directions (right anterior, left posterior) and right ischial tuberosity is raised off the plinth, subjecting the left to increased weight-bearing. Centrum of each acetabulum moves in an opposite direction relative to the vertical and coronal axes, causing the right leg to shorten and the left to lengthen on long-sitting; the reverse occurs on supine-lying. *(Redrawn courtesy of DonTigny 1997; see also Fig. 2.80.)*

'anterior' rotation around the coronal axis to the point that the acetabulum is moved craniad, pulling the right leg up with it so that it appears to shorten

b. the posterior aspect of the ischial tuberosity of the left innominate, resulting in further 'posterior' rotation to the point that the acetabulum moves caudad, pushing the left leg downward so that it appears to lengthen

Pressure on these sites also causes some clockwise rotation of the pelvic unit around the vertical axis in the transverse plane, augmenting the apparent shortening of the right, lengthening of the left leg on sitting up.

In other words, there results a difference in leg length that changes on going from lying to sitting and the reverse. With a 'right anterior, left posterior' rotation:

1. on sitting up, there will be a relative lengthening of the left and shortening of the right leg; whereas
2. on lying supine, the reverse occurs so that the right leg now lengthens and the left shortens (Fig. 2.84).

'left anterior, right posterior' rotation

Findings opposite to those described above will be observed in someone with this pattern of 'rotational malalignment'.

If the innominates are indeed 'fixed' in a 'right anterior, left posterior' rotation:

1. the right superior iliac crest will now be higher than the left, with an obvious gap under the right ischial tuberosity and the seating-surface; whereas the left crest is lower so that the left ischial tuberosity ends up bearing more weight (Figs 2.73C, 6.4A,C)
2. not only does the right '**leg lengthen lying**' but there will also be a concomitant downward (caudad) displacement of the right anterior landmarks; i.e. the right anterior **landmarks are lower** (while those on the left will have moved upward) - the side-to-side difference is most easily discerned on comparison of right versus left ASIS and superior pubic bones (Fig. 2.76A,B). These changes, which together are indicative of the side of an 'anterior' rotation, are easily remembered by **'THE RULE OF THE 5 'L's**.

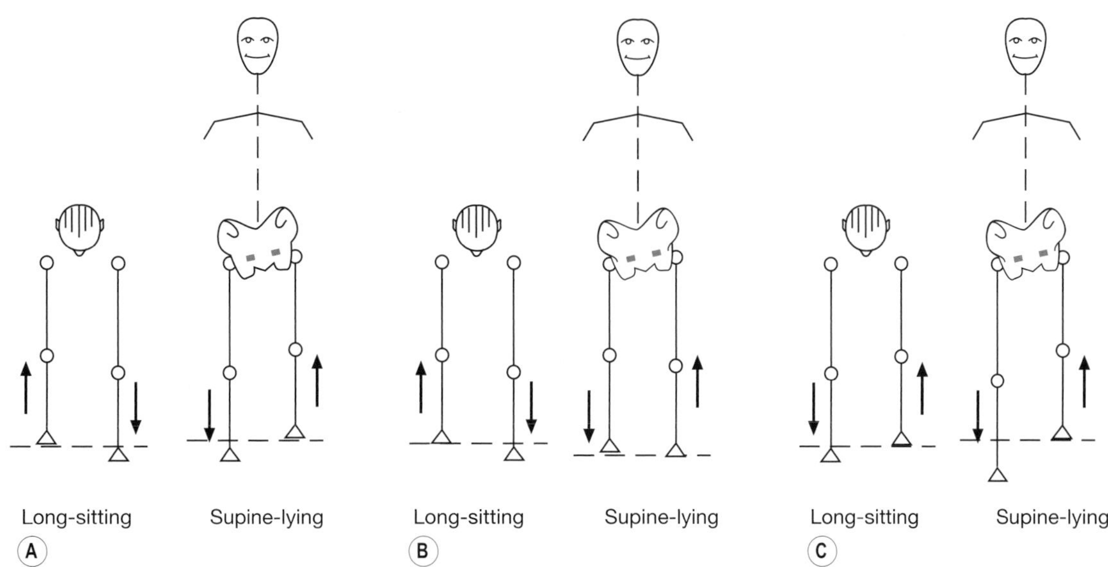

Fig. 2.84 'Sitting-lying' test: 'rotational malalignment' presentation. Suspect 'right anterior, left posterior' innominate rotation in all three cases, given the lengthening of the right leg relative to the left on moving from long-sitting to supine-lying. Note the asymmetry of the pelvic landmarks. (A) The right leg is shorter sitting, longer lying; this is the most common pattern. (B) The right leg is shorter sitting and still shorter, but less so, lying. (C) The right leg is longer sitting and, even more so, lying.

'THE RULE OF THE 5 'L's:

'**L**EG **L**ENGTHENS **L**YING, **L**ANDMARKS **L**OWER' = the side of the 'anteriorly' rotated innominate

Always keep in mind that there is just an apparent change in leg length on this test when 'rotational malalignment' is present. The emphasis is on detecting whether a shift occurs: any 'relative' shortening and lengthening of the legs on side-to-side comparison. For example, the right leg may be:

1. shorter than the left in sitting but longer in lying (Fig. 2.84A)
2. shorter than the left in sitting, still shorter but to a lesser extent in lying (Fig. 2.84B)
3. longer in sitting and even more so in lying (Fig. 2.84C).

In all three cases, there has been a relative lengthening of the right leg, consistent with a 'right anterior' rotation which could then be verified by noting that in each of these cases there is also asymmetry of all the landmarks on both anterior-to-posterior and side-to-side comparison, the anterior landmarks being lower on the right compared to left side (Fig. 2.76).

In someone with a 'left anterior, right posterior' rotation, the opposite leg length changes and pelvic asymmetries would be evident (Figs 2.73D, 2.85).

An underlying 'true' leg length difference will influence which leg actually ends up appearing longer or shorter in the long-sitting or supine-lying position when malalignment is present. However, at this point, the asymmetry of all the landmarks makes it impossible to discern the true leg length other than by a comparison of the femoral heads on a standing anteroposterior X-ray view of the pelvis (Figs 2.74A, 2.75). This problem is discussed in more detail under 'Functional leg length difference' in Ch. 3.

The difference in leg length detected on moving from one position to the other may be less than 5 mm or as much as 25-40 mm; most will show a change of about 5-10 mm. It must again be emphasized that when carrying out the 'sitting-lying' test, the actual length of either leg, or which leg is longer or shorter, is not what matters in the presence of a 'rotational malalignment'. What does matter is that:

1. there is a 'shift' - a relative change in leg length, suggesting 'rotational malalignment' is probably present
2. the right foot moves in a direction contrary to the left on this test

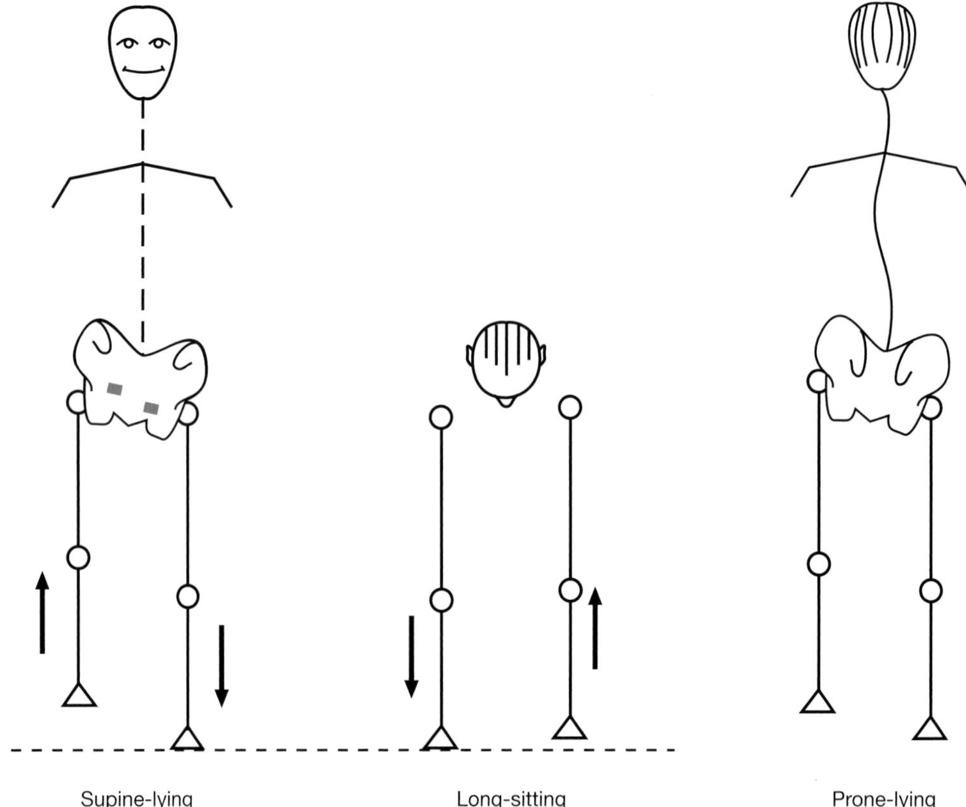

Fig. 2.85 'Sitting-lying' test: 'rotational malalignment'. Probable 'left anterior, right posterior' innominate rotation; confirm this by checking for asymmetry of pelvic landmarks; on side of 'anterior' rotation: Leg Legthens Lying, Landmarks Lower.

3. the side on which there is a relative lengthening of the leg on lying supine is likely to be the side of an 'anterior' rotation but this should always be confirmed by verifying that the anterior innominate landmarks on this side are, indeed, lower
4. all the pelvic landmarks are asymmetrical on anterior-to-posterior and side-to-side comparison in all positions of examination: standing, sitting and lying.

These four findings are pathognomonic of 'rotational malalignment'. However, false positives can occur with the 'sitting-lying' test for a number of reasons in a person who is actually in alignment and whose legs should lengthen and shorten to an equal extent on sitting and lying, respectively. For example:

1. Tightness of right gluteus maximus or hamstrings could impair anterior rotation on this side on sitting; if the left still rotates anteriorly normally, the left leg might appear to lengthen relatively more in sitting, then shorten on lying, so that it mistakenly appears that the right 'leg lengthened lying'
2. Tightness of right iliopsoas/rectus femoris could impair the normal posterior rotation of the right innominate on supine-lying. Pelvic tilt anteriorly is not impaired, so that the legs can lengthen the same amount on sitting-up. However, because right innominate posterior rotation is impaired by the tight muscles, there is relatively more left posterior rotation. The left leg will appear to shorten more than the right, again giving the mistaken impression that the right 'leg lengthened lying'.

In both cases, the 'sitting-lying' test suggests that, relatively, the right 'leg lengthened lying', giving the false impression that one is dealing with a 'right anterior, left posterior rotational malalignment'. However, the pelvic landmarks would be symmetrical and there would be no evidence of any findings typical of the 'malalignment syndrome' (Ch. 3).

It is for this reason that one must always check the position of the major landmarks (ASIS and pubic rami anteriorly; iliac crest, PSIS and ischial tuberosity posteriorly) to confirm the impression gained on the 'sitting-lying' test. To summarize, in regard to malalignment, the differential diagnosis to consider:

1. **when one leg is shorter by an equal amount in both sitting-up and lying-down**
   a. a 'true' LLD - all the landmarks are aligned; Fig. 2.81B)
   b. an 'upslip' - all these landmarks, both anterior and posterior, have moved upward on the side of the 'upslip' (Fig. 2.82)
2. **when leg length is equal**
   a. a pelvis in alignment - the landmarks are all symmetrical; Fig. 2.71)
   b. an 'outflare/inflare' presentation - there is counter- or clockwise rotation of these landmarks in the transverse plane and displacement relative to the centre (Figs 2.13, 2.64-2.68)
3. **when leg length shifts**
   a. suspect a 'rotational malalignment' (landmarks all asymmetrical) but
   b. rule out the person is not sitting or lying slightly asymmetrically with a wallet or other object in a back pocket or on account of a break in the plinth (Figs 2.107A, 2.108A, 2.114, 2.128, 2.129, 3.20A).

In order to reduce error, try to carry out the assessment of the landmarks in the same way each time, following the procedure outlined in Box 2.4. Which eye is dominant (Point 2, below) can usually be established quite easily:

1. hold up an index finger just in front of your nose so that it overlies a narrow mark, sign or other object some 5–10 meters away (e.g. fire alarm, clock, power pole).
2. close your left eye, leaving the right one open:
   a. if your index finger continues to overlie the object, you are probably right-eye dominant
   b. if your index finger moves to one side of the object, see what happens when you now close your right eye and leave the left one open
      - if the finger continues to overlie the object, you are probably left-eye dominant
3. if your finger shifts away from the object on closing either eye, consider your 'more dominant' eye to be the one that causes the lesser amount of shift when it alone is open

Therefore, if you are right-eye dominant:

1. approach the person with your right side adjacent to his or her side, whether they are lying supine or prone (Figs 2.66-2.69)

BOX 2.4 Assessing the anatomical landmarks

1. Whenever possible, face the person's front or back directly (Figs 2.76, 2.93, 2.95).
2. If this is not possible, try to approach the person so that you can place your dominant eye as close to his or her midline as possible (e.g. if you are left-eye dominant, sit with your left side next to the person lying supine or prone; Fig. 2.86).
3. Avoid looking at the landmarks at an angle, if at all possible, as this may hide/distort any differences.
4. Orientate right and left markers the same way in order to make side-to-side comparisons easier and more accurate. For example, the thumbs should both be:
   a. flexed 90 degrees at the interphalangeal joint when resting against the malleoli, tips pointing straight downward (Figs 2.77B, 2.78B)
   b. pointing straight upward (craniad), parallel to midline, when resting against the inside of the ASIS or PSIS to detect 'outflare' or 'inflare' (Figs 2.13B,C, 2.66, 2.68, 2.71Ei)
   c. aligned horizontally when resting against the lower part of ASIS, PSIS or along the superior pubic rami in order to detect a relative upward displacement or rotation (Figs 2.71, 2.76)

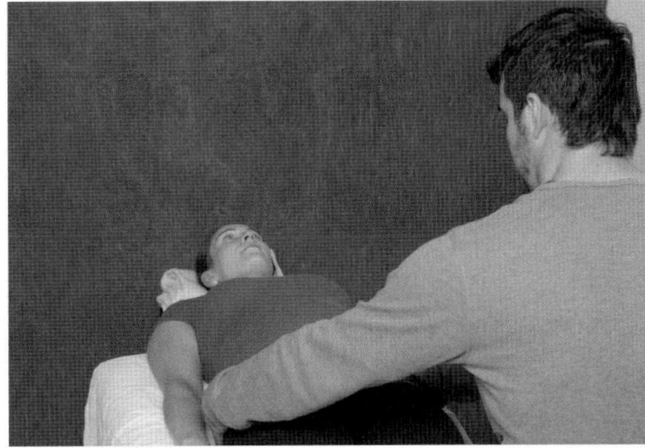

Fig. 2.86 'Left eye dominant' examiner sitting/standing to left of subject to bring his left eye closer to her midline.

2. sit on the side of the plinth (rather than standing and having to lean/twist forward), to decrease the angle between your eyes and the table; this helps to cut down any error on comparison of landmarks (especially those in close proximity, such as the pubic bones), or side-to-side differences in height and rotation
3. bring the right eye as close to the person's midline as possible, in order to increase the accuracy of side-to-side comparisons of landmarks

The opposite applies if you are left eye dominant (Fig. 2.86).

It is useful to get into the habit of standing or sitting by the person on the correct side, both to facilitate the assessment and to make it more accurate. This approach also proves valuable at the time of carrying out alignment corrections using muscle energy and other treatment techniques as it allows for quick feedback on whether or not realignment has been achieved (Figs 7.9Cii, 7.11, 7.13, 7.14).

TORSION OF THE SACRUM

Torsion of the sacrum refers to rotation of the sacrum relative to the innominates, around the three major axes (Fig. 2.9), the right or left oblique axis, or all of these (Box 2.1; Figs 2.10, 2.14, 2.21, 2.42, 2.88, 2.89). Sacral torsion is a natural part of daily activities such as reaching, throwing, walking and running. Torsion involves motion around these various axes and is governed by the movement of the trunk, pelvic bones and lower extremities. Normal sacral movement into nutation on initial trunk flexion, and nutation on extension, has been described above (Figs 2.11, 2.17, 2.18), as has movement around the oblique axes during the gait cycle (Figs 2.21, 2.41) and on unilateral facet joint impaction (Fig. 2.52).

The sacrum may actually become pathologically fixed so that there results a loss of motion into certain directions. The following are three of the more common reasons for the occurrence of such a loss of motion or 'fixation' of the sacrococcygeal complex:

1. a movement that inadvertently exceeds the physiological limit available in that direction
2. contracture of ligaments, capsules, fascia or other connective tissue that can affect the position of the complex; e.g. sacrospinous, long dorsal sacroiliac, sacrotuberous ligaments (Figs 2.4A, 2.5A, 2.19, 2.21)
3. asymmetrical impaction, as in a fall onto the right or left side of the complex
4. contractural shortening or excessive tension or spasm in one of the muscles that attaches to the sacrum or coccyx (e.g. piriformis; Fig. 2.46A)

The muscles primarily involved are the piriformis and iliacus. Piriformis originates from the anterior aspect of the sacral base; the diagonal direction of its pull rotates the sacral base posteriorly and down relative to the ilium. Iliacus rotates the ilium anteriorly, inward and down relative to the sacrum (Fig. 2.46). Either movement causes a wedging of the ilium against the anteriorly widening sacrum and would normally help to stabilize the SI joint; if excessive, however, it can result in a loss of mobility or even a complete 'jamming' of the already incongruous iliac and sacral surfaces (Figs 2.2, 2.3, 2.7B).

Sacral landmarks

The diagnosis of torsion around the vertical or one of the oblique axes can usually be made simply by observing 'the lie of the sacrum': comparing the position of distinguishing landmarks when the person lies prone.

1. position of the sacral base as judged by the sacral sulci

   The sulci are formed by the junction of the ala ('wings') of the sacral base with the ilium on either side. Locate the depression on each side at the junction of L5 and S1 with the tip of an index finger and then run the fingers outward at this level until they abut the medial edge of the posterior iliac crest (approximately 1.5-2.5 cm lateral to the midline, often clearly demarcated by an overlying dimple; Figs 2.6, 2.71A). Now gently push the tip of each index finger into the depression, or 'sulcus', formed at this junction of the sacrum with the pelvis (Fig. 2.87B -indicated by right index). The true depth of the sulcus is approximately 1.0-1.5 cm, usually reduced to about 0.5-1.0 cm by the overlying skin and subcutaneous tissues. The depth of the right sulcus should equal that on the left and lie level in the coronal (frontal) plane.
2. the inferior lateral angle (ILA)

   This is the corner formed at the point where the inferior part of the sacrum rapidly starts to taper toward its junction with the coccyx (Fig. 2.3A, 2.71Gi). It is usually easily palpable through the overlying soft tissues, 1.0-1.5 cm up and out from the sacrococcygeal junction (Fig. 2.71Gii).

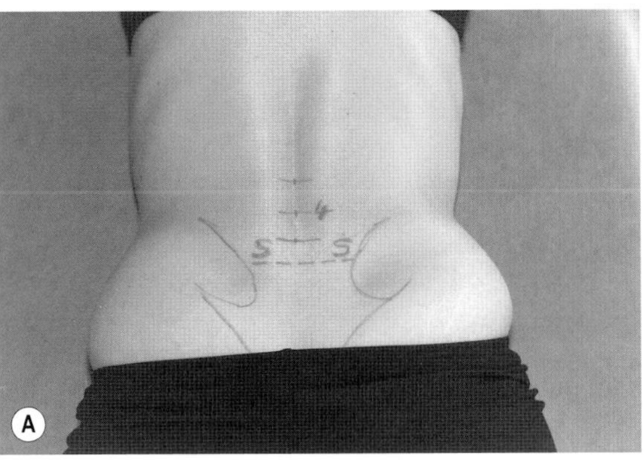

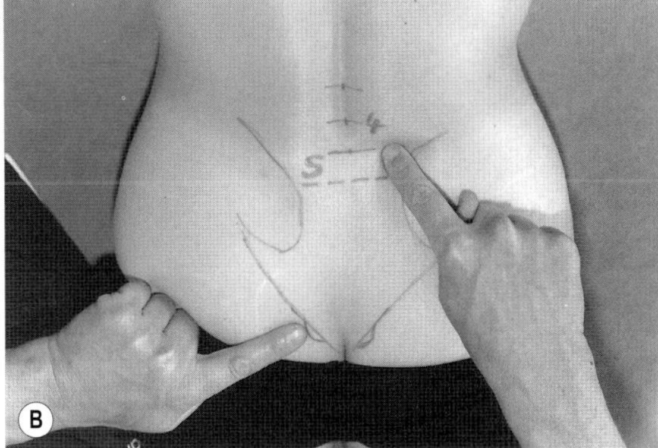

Fig. 2.87 Assessment of sacral landmarks in a prone-lying person. Note: the clinician with 'right eye dominance' should carry out the examination from the person's left in order to bring that eye closer to midline. (A) In alignment; the right and left sacral sulci (S) are of equal depth and level (as is the sacral base, demarcated by the dotted line); the solid line at '4' demarcates the L4 spinous process. (B) 'Left-on-left' rotation: the right index finger lies in the depressed right sacral sulcus, the left index finger on the ILA (the latter denoting the elevated left sacral margin; see also Figs 2.6, 2.71Gi)

3. the position of the sacral apex

   The sacral apex is the terminal part of the sacrum to which the coccyx attaches (Fig. 2.3A). Press the pulp of the index fingers or thumbs firmly down, through the soft tissues, onto the right and left lateral edges of this caudal part of the sacrum (just below the ILA). The fingers will normally lie at the same depth and equidistant from midline.

In the absence of rotation of the sacrum around the vertical axis or torsion around one of the oblique axes, comparison of right to left sacral base (sulci), sacral apex and ILA will show that these respective sites:

1. lie at an equal depth
2. are level in the coronal plane; that is, there is no relative displacement, upward (craniad) on one side and downward (caudad) on the other, except in the case of:
   a. a 'true' LLD, and then only when examined standing
   b. a functional LLD, as seen with an 'upslip' and 'rotational malalignment', where the pelvic unit as a whole tilts to right or left

However, it should be noted that whenever the sacral base is uneven on account of a 'true' LLD or malalignment, compensatory rotation around the sagittal axis can occur to the point that the person may present with the sacral base level in the coronal plane even though the LLD or malalignment persists (as discussed in Ch. 3; Fig. 3.90A,B).

Sacral torsion patterns

The following are some of the commonly occurring patterns of excessive or 'fixed' sacral torsion. The reader is referred to Richard (1986), Fowler (1986) and Greenman (1997) for further descriptions of these various forms and their effects on the lumbar spine.

'Left/left' or 'left-on-left' sacral torsion

The sacrum is fixed in forward rotation around the left oblique axis (Figs 2.21, 2.42, 2.50). Therefore, the right sacral sulcus (indicated by the right index finger in Fig. 2.87B) is depressed, the base having rotated anteriorly and downward (caudad); whereas the left sacral apex (left finger) and ILA is elevated, having rotated posteriorly and upward (craniad). The right ILA, like the right sulcus, also comes to lie anteriorly and caudad; the left ILA, posteriorly and craniad.

'Right/right' or 'right-on-right' sacral torsion

The sacrum is 'fixed' in forward rotation around the right oblique axis (Figs 2.14, 2.50, 2.52B). Findings are opposite to those seen with a 'left-on-left' torsion.

Rotation posteriorly around the left or right oblique axis

Rotation occurs in the direction opposite to that described for 'left-on-left' and 'right-on-right' forward rotations described above. The base rotates backward instead of forward around the left or right oblique axis, resulting in a 'left-on-right' and 'right-on-left' pattern, respectively (Fig. 2.88).

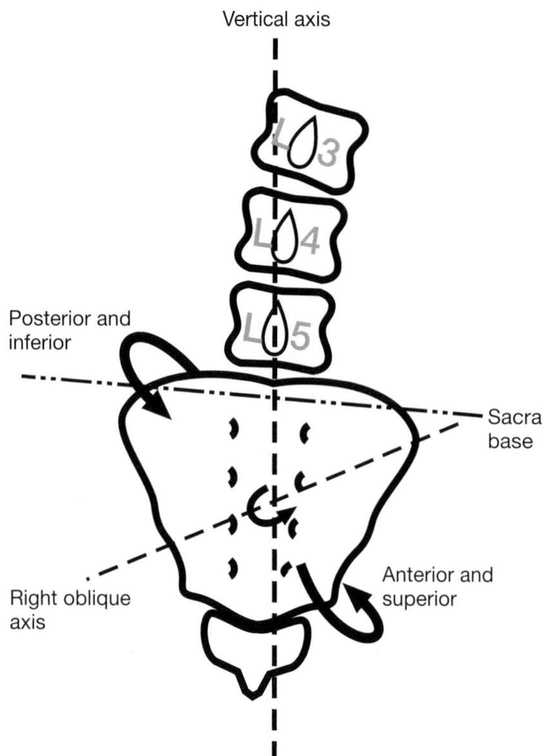

Fig. 2.88 Example of a 'backward' rotation: 'right-on-left' rotation around the right oblique axis.

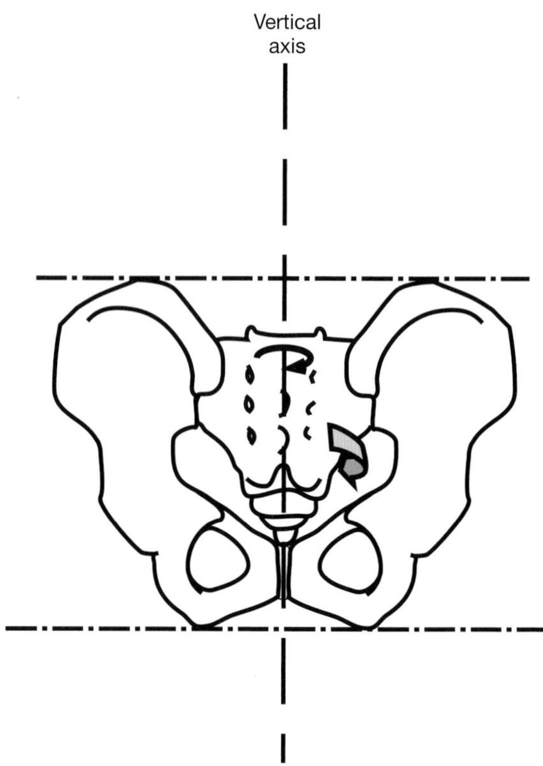

Fig. 2.89 Right unilateral anterior sacrum: rotation counterclockwise around the vertical axis.

Particularly significant is the fact that:

1. The forward rotations - 'left-on-left' and 'right-on-right' - accentuate the lumbosacral angle, increasing the lumbar lordosis and making the lumbar segment suppler.
2. The backward rotations - 'left-on-right' and 'right-on-left' - reduce the angle, and hence the lordosis, with a stiffening of the lumbar segment. Even worse, there may actually be formation of a lumbar kyphosis. These 'backward' presentations have been linked to distressing and seemingly unrelated problems (Richard 1986), including headaches and dysfunction of any or all of the following:
   a. gastrointestinal system (e.g. diarrhea alternating with constipation)
   b. genitourinary system (e.g. frequency, nocturia)
   c. menstrual cycle, and
   d. pelvic floor dysfunction

Right or left 'unilateral anterior sacrum'

The entire sacrum has rotated excessively to the right or left around the vertical axis in the transverse plane.

For example, a right unilateral anterior sacrum (i.e. sacral rotation counterclockwise; Fig. 2.89):

1. brings all the sacral landmarks anteriorly on the right and posteriorly on the left side
2. puts the following structures under increased tension:
   a. on the right side (sacrum in relative nutation)
      - anterior SI joint ligaments and capsule, also the sacrotuberous, sacrospinous, and interosseous ligament (Fig. 2.19A)
   b. on the left side (sacrum in relative counternutation)
      - posterior SI joint and long dorsal sacroiliac ligament (Fig. 2.19B)
3. jams the anteriorly-widening sacrum against the innominate on the left side.

Excessive rotation in the sagittal plane

As discussed further below ('Simultaneous bilateral SI joint malalignment'; see also Figs 2.11, 2.15-2.19), the sacrum presents in either:

1. excessive nutation, with the base fixed in an anterior position, and accentuation of the lumbar lordosis
2. excessive counternutation, with the base fixed in a posterior position, and flattening of the lumbar lordosis or even formation of a lumbar kyphosis.

Clinical correlation: sacral torsion

Unilateral anterior sacrum or sacral torsion around one of the oblique axes may occur in isolation or in addition to an anatomical (true) LLD or any of the three common presentations of malalignment. The sacral displacement may disappear completely on correction of the pelvic malalignment. However, as indicated above, if the sacral displacement persists it can continue to cause symptoms of its own and will require specific treatment measures (see Chs 7, 8).

CURVES OF THE SPINE AND VERTEBRAL ROTATIONAL DISPLACEMENT

It is rare to find a spine that is 'straight'. Most of us have some minor 'scoliotic' curves even when in alignment. 'Rotational malalignment' and an 'upslip' are usually associated with a more obvious scoliosis, which may simply be indicative of an attempt to compensate for the pelvic obliquity and to ensure the head ends up aligned as best as possible in all three planes so as not to compromise balance and vision. In addition, there may be one or more isolated vertebrae that are excessively rotated, or 'displaced', to the point they interrupt the particular segmental curve that they are a part of – cervical, thoracic or lumbar - and they stand out relative to the vertebra above and below. Such an apparent impingement of a vertebra between the adjacent vertebrae because of excessive rotation in a clockwise or counterclockwise direction (and the simultaneous side-flexion and extension or forward flexion) will henceforth be referred to as a '*vertebral rotational displacement*'.

To ascertain whether excessive curvature of the spine and/or rotational displacement of individual vertebra(e) is present, first examine the person from the back in standing, looking to see if the iliac crests, shoulders and inferior angles of the scapulae appear level or not (Figs 2.70, 2.90, 2.95A). Note any curvature(s) formed by the spinous processes. Is the spine straight, as it might be in someone who is in alignment? Does there appear to be one uniform curve or the more common double (or scoliotic) curve, with:

1. a lumbar component convex to one side, usually reversing around the thoracolumbar junction to give rise to a thoracic curve convex in the opposite direction (Figs 2.70, 2.72A, 2.73, 2.76B, 2.90)
2. the thoracic segment usually reversing proximally at about the cervicothoracic junction but sometimes as far down as the T4 or T5 level, to give rise to the cervical curve (Fig. 2.91).

Having the person bend forward brings the spinous processes into better relief and may make these curves more obvious. Alternately, asking the person to bring the scapulae together by contracting the rhomboid muscles may accentuate a curvature, particularly of the thoracic part of the spine, and help determine the proximal and distal points of reversal which form the cervicothoracic and thoracolumbar curves of the spine, respectively. Back extension tends to accentuate more the lumbar spine

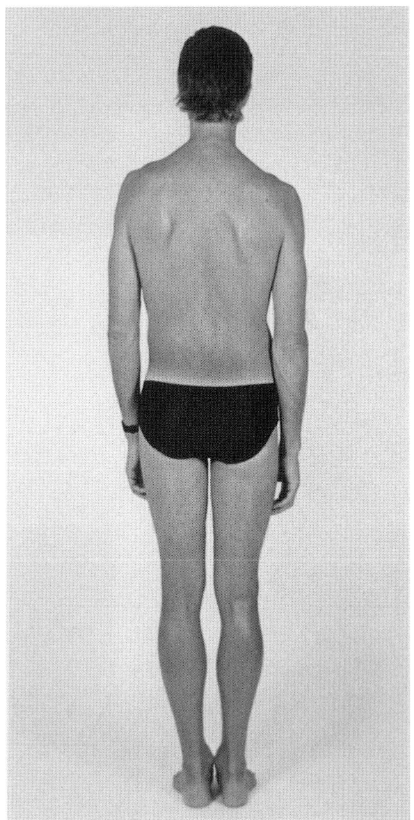

Fig. 2.90 Standing photo showing pelvic obliquity (iliac crest up on right), scoliotic curves (thoracic convex left, lumbar right) and depression of right scapula and shoulder. The right knee is partially flexed, as if the person were attempting to lower the pelvis on the high side.

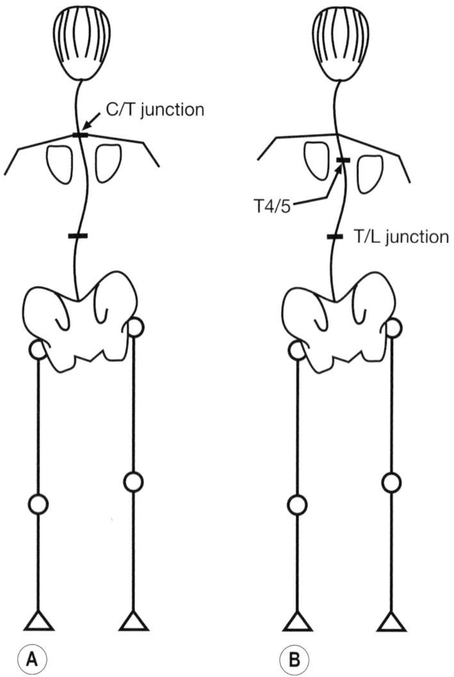

Fig. 2.91 Site of curve reversal at the proximal end of the thoracic spine. (A) More common: at the cervicothoracic (C/T) junction. (B) Less common: at the T4 or T5 vertebral level. T/L, thoracolumbar.

region (Fig. 2.120C). On side flexion, a completely flexible scoliotic curve will usually become one uniform curve; however, an interruption of this curve may still be evident on this manoeuvre, sometimes only on going to the right or left side, on account of:

1. the presence of pelvic malalignment and/or rotational displacement of one or more vertebrae
2. reactive muscle tightening or spasm to counter instability (e.g. joint laxity with ligament lengthening or osteoarthritis) and/or
3. pain from a structure being further strained or compressed by the manoeuvre (e.g. facet joints; Fig. 2.52B)

There may be failure of an area, or even an entire segment, to bend along with the rest of the spine. The lumbar segment, for example, may appear stiff as a rod on bending to one or both sides in someone whose thoracic segment still flexes easily to right and left (Fig. 2.92).

Next, examine the spine with the person sitting and do a side-to-side comparison of the level of the pelvic crests, shoulders and scapulae.

1. If the pelvis is now level, and any curves of the spine evident on standing have decreased or disappeared completely, these curves were

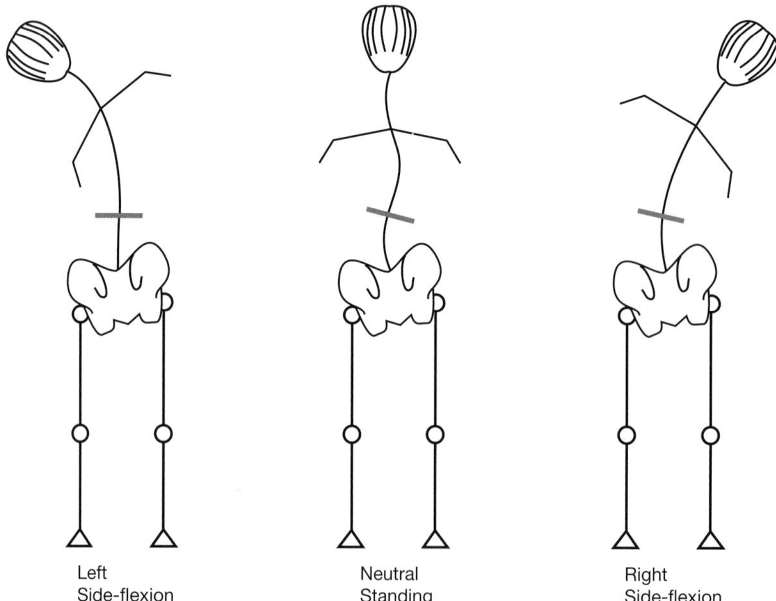

Fig. 2.92 Flexibility of the scoliotic curve noted when standing upright: flexibility of the lumbar segment is normal on right side-flexion but restricted on bending into the left.

probably 'functional', helping to compensate for the pelvic obliquity caused by an anatomical ('true') LLD (Fig. 2.72B).

2. At this initial stage of the examination, there may still be a residual, chronic increase in muscle tension that had been triggered by the LLD but may settle down with treatment, a heel raise (if indicated) and time to allow for further straightening of the spine.
3. Any residual curves may just represent the 'intrinsic' curves which most of us are blessed with, evident even when we are in alignment (Fig. 2.72A).

With the person lying supine, determine the slope of any persistent pelvic obliquity (Fig. 2.73A-D) and rule out the presence of an 'outflare/inflare' (Figs 2.13, 2.64-2.69). Then go on to a comparison of the right and left clavicle and ribs - these structures may provide some indication of the effect of a thoracic convexity or excessive rotational displacement of individual vertebrae on the anterior chest region. Tenderness and/or an actual anterior protrusion or recession of a clavicular joint may be indicative of a torsional effect on the clavicles caused by the malalignment that could, with time, result in further ligament laxity and, eventually, an actual subluxation or even dislocation of that joint (Figs 2.93A, 2.94B). Then apply light pressure to the 2nd to 11th right and left costochondral junctions individually - tenderness at one or more levels may be indicative of stress put on these joints by rotation of individual

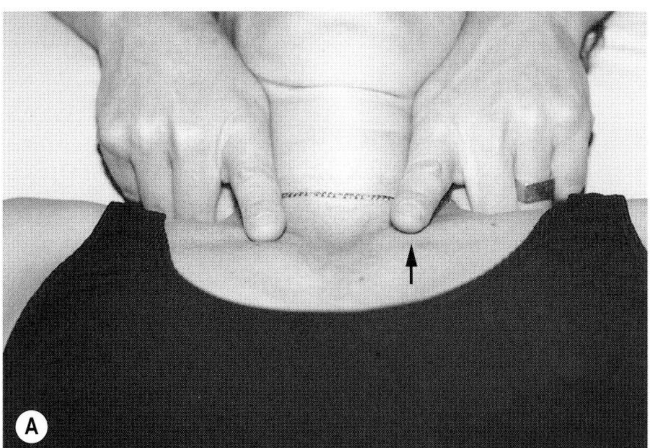

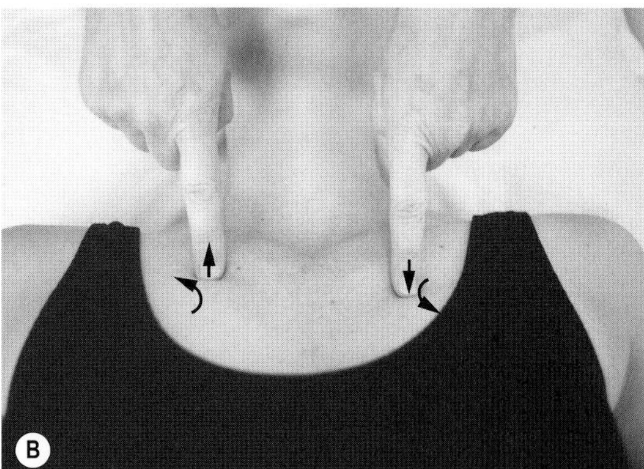

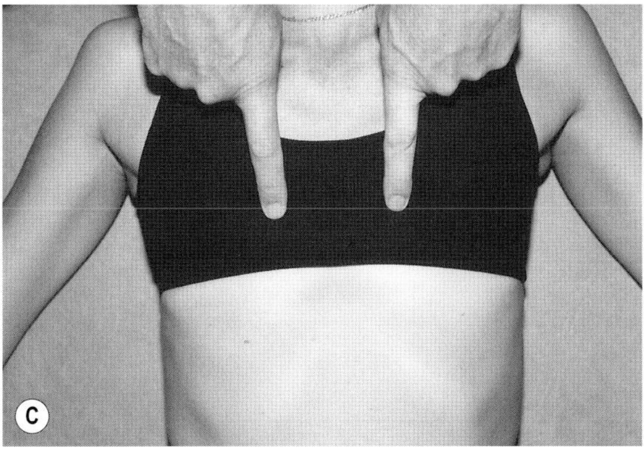

Fig. 2.93 Involvement of the ribs and clavicles with malalignment. (A) Posterior rotation of the left clavicle, resulting in anterior protrusion (and possibly eventual subluxation) at the left sternoclavicular junction, with the reverse findings on the right. (B) 1st to 4th, 5th or 6th rib level inclusive: showing the more commonly seen displacement of these upper left ribs downward and forward (anteriorly) relative to the right ones, which are displaced upward and backward (posteriorly) at these upper levels (thoracic convexity is to the left; see Figs 2.95, 3.15B). (C) 5th or 6th rib level (i.e. at or near the level of the apex of the thoracic convexity): the right and left ribs now match in both planes; the ribs below this level will show the right ones displaced downward and forward relative to the left ones, reflecting the change in direction of the thoracic curve below the apex.

thoracic vertebra(e) and the attaching ribs. The site of tenderness anteriorly can sometimes help localize a problem to a particular rib (e.g. subluxation) or vertebral level (which may turn out to be tender and/or displaced on examination of the spine itself). For example, tenderness of the 4th or 5th costochondral junction uni- or bilaterally is suggestive of a problem at around the T3-T6 vertebral levels of the spine (Figs 2.93C, 2.94A). However, there is not always a history of anterior chest discomfort or finding of costochondral tenderness in conjunction with an excessive vertebral rotational displacement.

The displacement of a clavicle or of one or more specific ribs on one side only (Fig. 2.93B), with or without tenderness over one or both sternoclavicular joints or any costochondral junction(s), can occur for a number of reasons. However, it may be seen simply as the result of these sites being put under increased biomechanical stresses by a functional thoracic convexity or a more localized problem, such as rotation of a clavicle or a specific vertebra (Fig. 2.94). In a person who has a left thoracic convexity, for example, when examined in supine-lying:

1. typically, the anterior chest cage shows the left 1st to 4th, 5th or 6th rib inclusive to lie 'anterior and down' a gradually decreasing amount on comparison to the right side; this is in keeping with the progressively decreasing 'right side-flexion, right rotation, and forward-flexion' of the upper thoracic vertebrae which, on the left side, pushes the ribs at these levels anteriorly and rotates them around the coronal axis while the opposite occurs on the right side - these changes account for the difference in their position at the costochondral junction on side-to-side comparison
2. either the 4th, 5th or 6th rib ends up level with their right counterpart
3. from this point down, the pattern reverses: the ribs on the right side now come to lie increasingly 'anterior and down' compared to the left ones; the point where this reversal occurs reflects the apex of the thoracic spine convexity.

Illustrated in Fig. 2.94 is the effect that an isolated excessive left rotational displacement of T5 has on the right and left ribs. The T5 vertebral body has rotated counterclockwise, left side-flexed as well as flexed forward. The 6th rib attaches to the inferior part of T5 vertebra at the costovertebral (C-V) joint and is actually affected more than the 5th rib. Overall effects of the T5 displacement include:

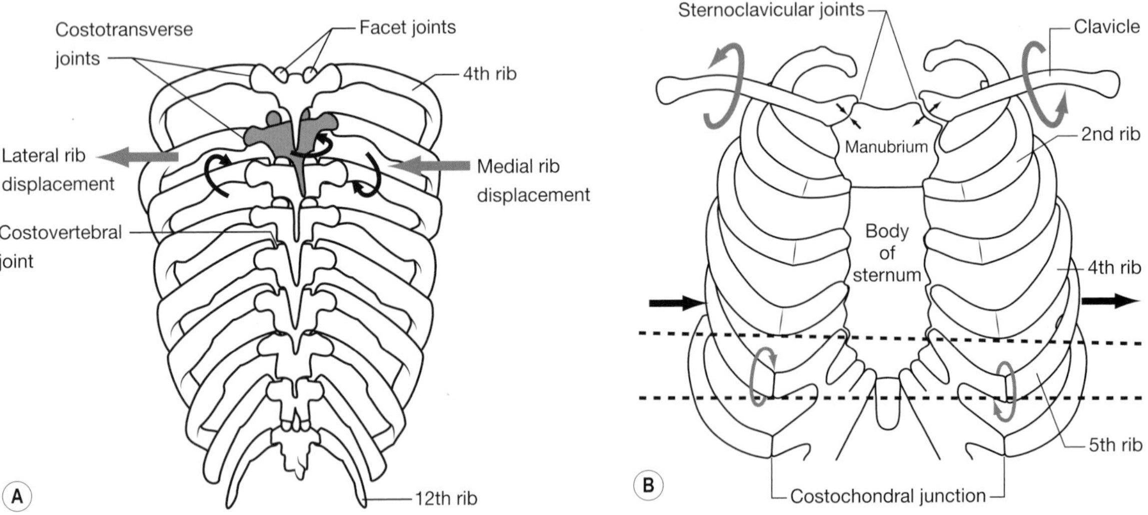

Fig. 2.94 T5 vertebral rotational displacement to the left, with simultaneous left side-flexion and either forward flexion or extension; i.e. a left 'FRS' or 'ERS' pattern, respectively (see also Figs 3.6, 3.13). (A) Posterior view: deviation of the T5 spinous process to the right, with contrary rib displacement and rotation; note the right facet joint compression, left 'distraction' or opening, and increase in stress on the costotransverse and costovertebral joints at this level. (B) Anterior view: stress on the bilateral 5th costochondral junctions through the ribs. Also illustrated are the typical opening and closing of the sternoclavicular joints caused by contrary rotation of the clavicles seen in conjunction with the compensatory scoliosis associated with pelvic malalignment.

1. on the right 6th rib
   a. pulling the rib upward (craniad) and medially at the C-V joint
   b. causing the rib to pivot around the transverse process (TP), at the costotransverse (C-T) joint
   c. posterior rotation of the rib around the coronal axis in the sagittal plane (as indicated by the arrow)
   d. pulling the right rib medially by its posterior attachments, with resultant distraction forces on the right C-V/C-T joints and, anteriorly, the C-C junction
2. on the left 6th rib
   a. displacement of the 6th rib downward and laterally at the C-V joint
   b. pivoting at the C-T joint, so that the rib rotates anteriorly around the coronal axis
   c. shifting of the rib backward and laterally, and
   d. compression forces on the left C-V/C-T joints and C-C junction.

Overall, stress is increased on the joints, capsules, and ligaments at all these anterior and posterior sites as well as the annulus, ligaments and disc itself because of T5 having rotated relative to the adjacent vertebrae.

Protrusion or recession of the anterior end of an isolated rib or ribs should raise suspicion of rib subluxation and/or possibly rotational displacement of a specific thoracic vertebra (Fig. 2.94), although these findings can also occur as a result of the ribs adjusting to an acute change in the thoracic convexity below the cervicothoracic level (Fig. 2.91).

Finally, look at the back with the person lying prone, his or her head resting in a face-hole or with the chin over the edge to prevent the upper spine from being twisted by a rotation of the head and neck (Fig. 2.95). Check the level of the pelvis and scapulae. If any curves are present, are they convex in the same direction as in standing and sitting? Again, does the upper thoracic curve start to reverse at the cervicothoracic junction, or at some point below (Fig. 2.91)?

To help to define these curves better, stand at the person's head and lay the pulp of your index fingers lightly against the right and left side of the protuberant spinous process of C7. Then run these fingers down alongside the thoracic and lumbar spinous processes and onto the sacrum. Note the direction in which the tips of your fingers point as they sweep downward and the sites at which their direction changes - usually at the apex of the thoracic and lumbar convexities (Fig. 2.95B-E).

Also note whether the smooth, contrasting curves formed by the spinous processes of the thoracic and lumbar segments are at any point acutely interrupted by a seemingly excessive rotational displacement of one or more of the vertebrae relative to the others. A rotation will henceforth be specified by the direction of rotation of the vertebral body. Examples of such a displacement include:

1. 'Left L4'

   Whereas Fig. 2.96A shows L4 aligned with L1-L5 to form a uniform lumbar convexity, this smooth curve is interrupted in Fig. 2.96B, with the body of L4 now 'left rotated'. Simultaneously running the index and middle finger along the right and left side of the spinous processes shows that of L4 deviating to the right; alternately, just one index or middle finger run alongside at about a 10-15 degree angle will
   a. bump into the bony protrusion of the L4 spinous process on the right and
   b. sink into a hollow created at this level by the L4 left rotation.
2. 'Left T5', 'Left T3'

   Findings for a 'left T5' rotation have been discussed above (Fig. 2.94A). In the case of a 'left T3', running a finger along the right and left side of the spinous processes from T6 upward shows a sudden right deviation of the T3 spinous process indicating that the T3 vertebral body has rotated to the left (counterclockwise) relative to the vertebrae above and below (Fig. 2.97A,B,C,E). A finger running alongside the spinous processes on the right side will abut the spinous process of T3 and be forced to move outward to get around it (Fig. 2.97D); whereas a finger on the left side would dip into the hollow created between T2 and T4 by rotation of that spinous process to the right.

The finger gliding past the level of the displaced vertebra may elicit a reflex contraction of the paravertebral muscles: the superficial and deep multifidi and adjacent erector spinae muscles. It may also cause outright pain and/or a spontaneous withdrawal reaction.

One can usually palpate, or even see, an increase in tension in the paravertebral muscles, and provoke pain from these muscles, also from the supraspinous, interspinous and facet joint ligaments, in particular.

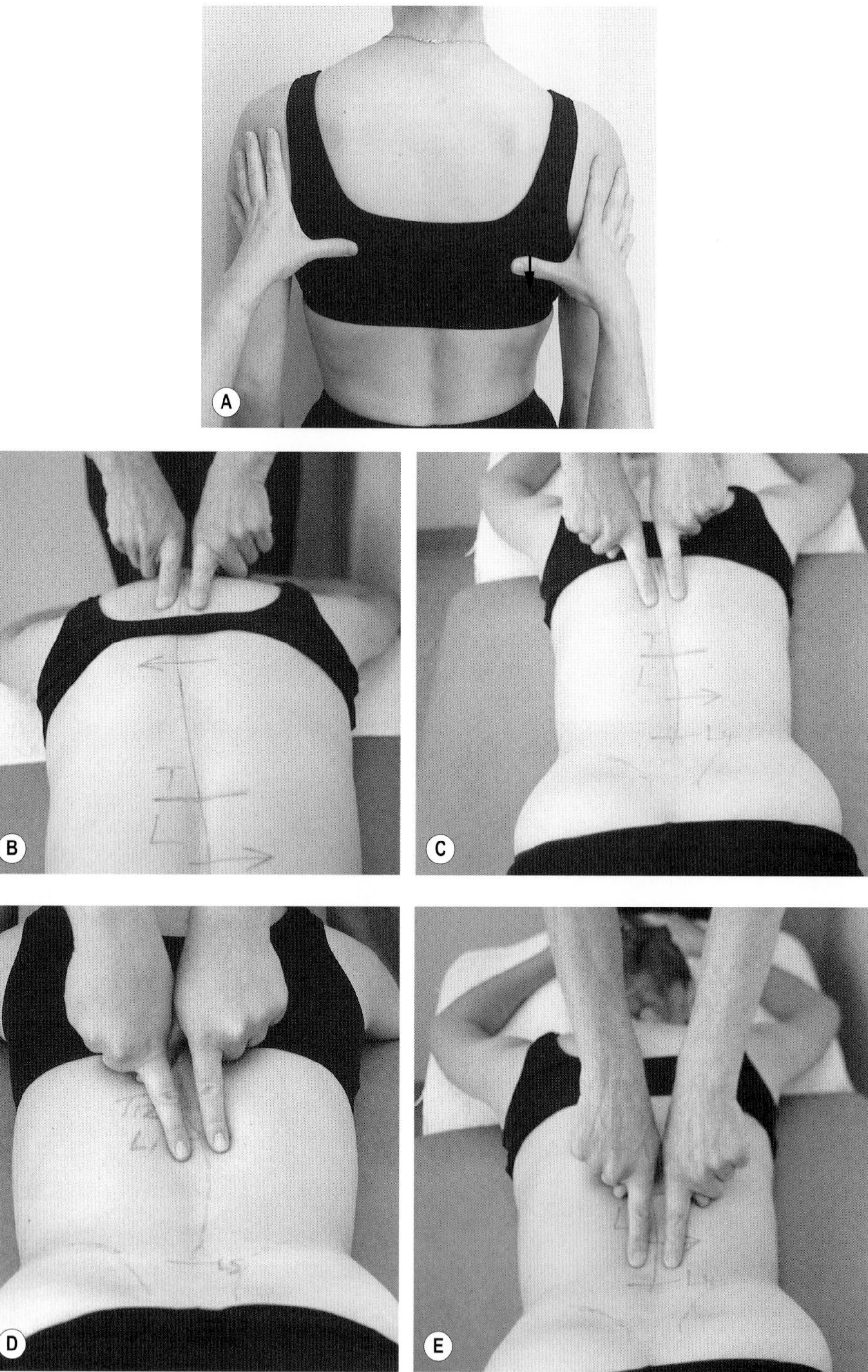

Fig. 2.95 Determining the direction of a thoracic and lumbar convexity. (A) In standing, downward displacement of the right scapular apex and the depressed right shoulder suggest (but do not confirm) a thoracic curve primarily convex to left (see also Fig. 2.91). (B) Left thoracic, right lumbar convexity (the apex of each curve is marked by a horizontal arrow); fingers alongside the spinous processes above thoracic apex - pointing to left. (C) Fingers below the thoracic apex - now pointing to right. (D) Fingers above lumbar apex - still pointing to right. (E) Fingers below lumbar apex - again pointing to left.

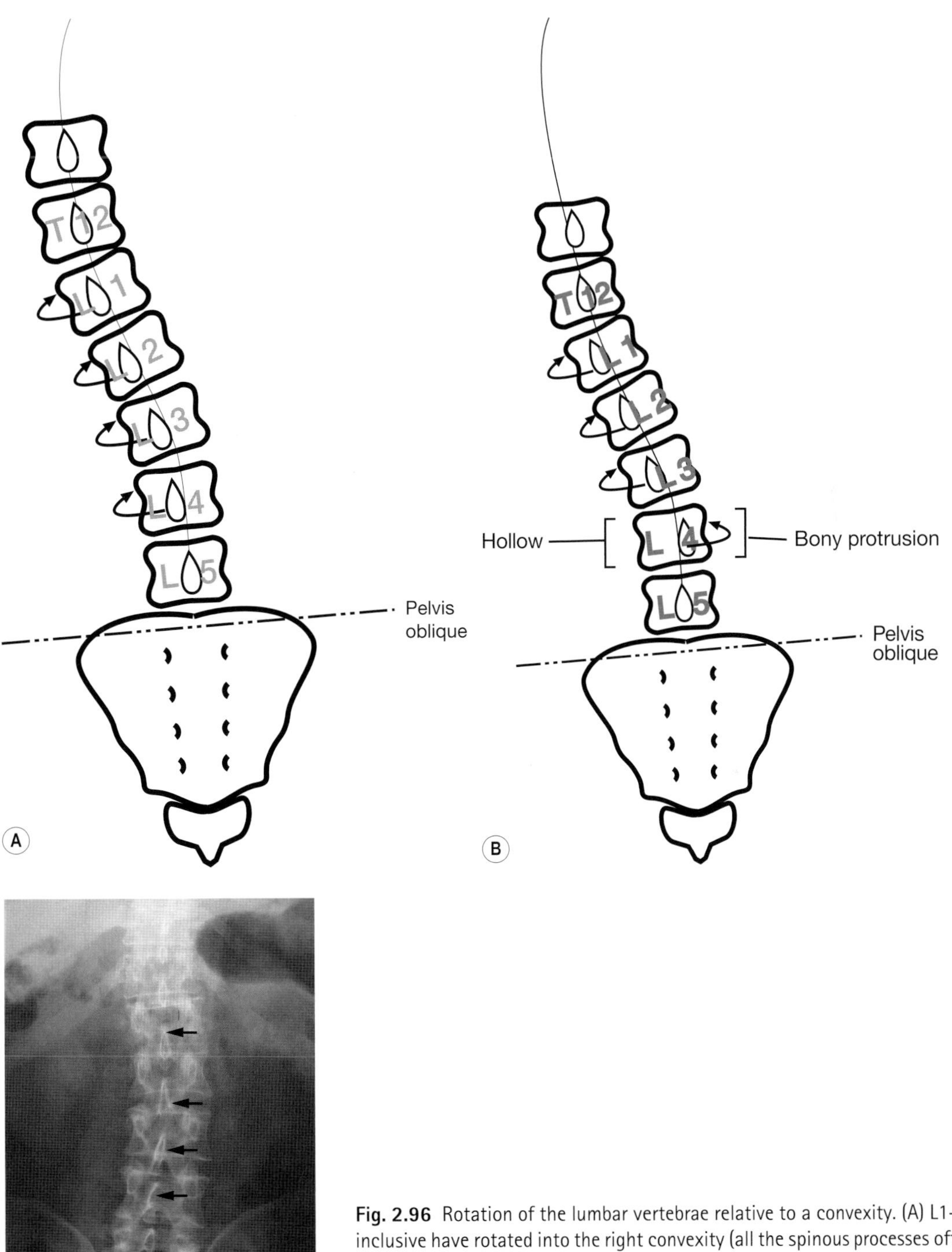

Fig. 2.96 Rotation of the lumbar vertebrae relative to a convexity. (A) L1–L4 inclusive have rotated into the right convexity (all the spinous processes off to the left of midline). (B) L4 vertebral rotational displacement to the left interrupts the continuity of vertebral rotation into the right convexity (L4 spinous process is now off to the right of midline). (C) X-ray: anteroposterior view of the lumbar spine showing typical L1-L4 inclusive counterclockwise rotation into a left lumbar convexity, with L5 spinous process almost back in the midline; there are changes indicative of an old L1 compression fracture.

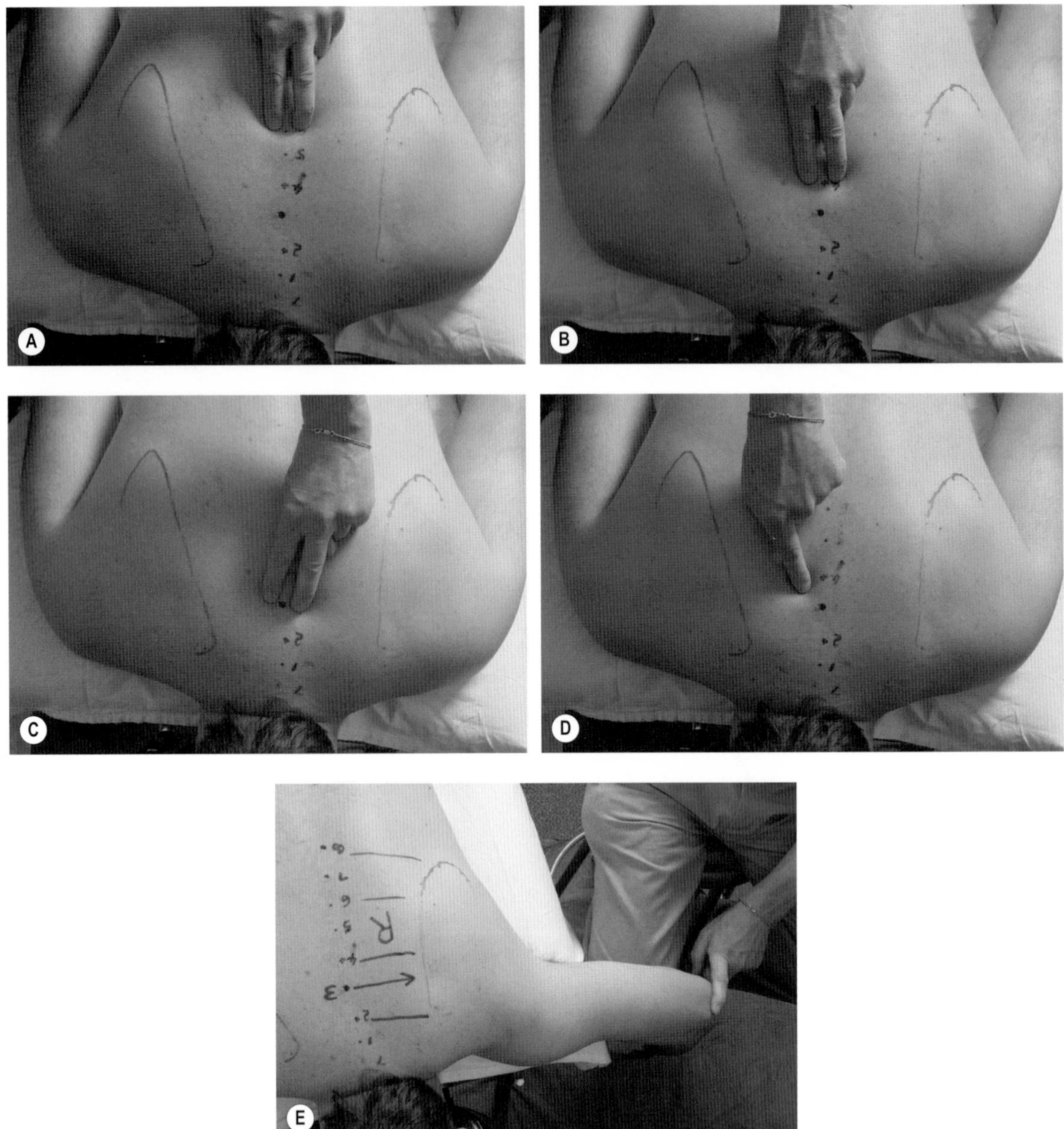

Fig. 2.97 Detecting a vertebral rotational displacement (see Figs 2.95, 2.96). There is a gentle curve of the upper thoracic spine segment, convex to left. (A,B) Index and middle fingers running upward (craniad) alongside thoracic spinous processes show T6,T5, T4 and T2,T1,C7 lying in line with this curve. (C) Fingers have to wind around T3 spinous process, which deviates to the right (= vertebral body rotated counterclockwise). (D) Index finger running along right side abuts on the deviating T3 spinous process; on the opposite side, there would be a 'hollow' detectable at this level. (E) Muscle Energy Technique (MET) to realign T3; arrow marks direction of pull generated on spinous process with left rhomboid contraction on resisted left elbow elevation.

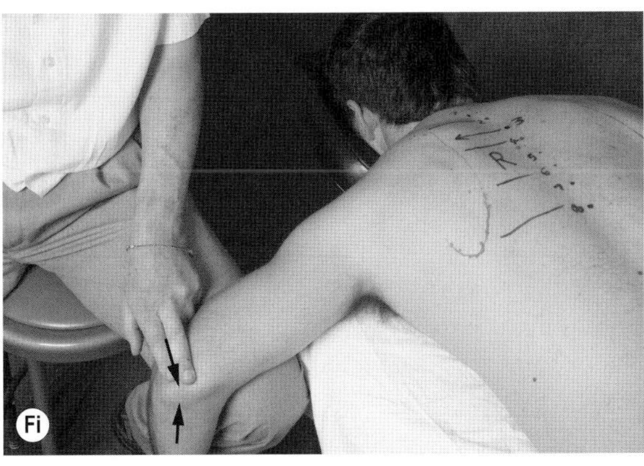

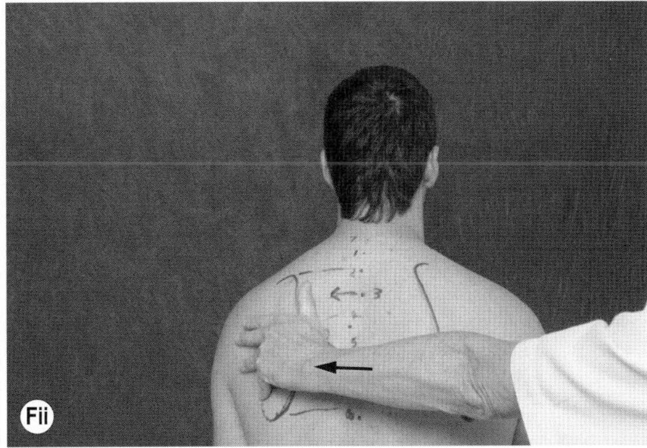

Fig. 2.97—contd (F) MET carried out by activating rhomboid (i) lying prone: blocking attempt to raise the elbow straight up toward the ceiling (ii) sitting: blocking attempt to move the scapula medially (see Chs 7, 8).

A force applied to the spinous processes in a posterior-to-anterior and right-left translatory direction may elicit pain from the displaced - and sometimes also immediately adjacent - vertebra(e) by stressing the soft tissues, intervertebral ligaments, capsules and facet joints in the vicinity (Fig. 4.20). It should, however, be noted that not all vertebrae that appear excessively rotated, or displaced, are symptomatic, prove painful on examination or even show an associated reactive increase in tension in the adjacent muscles.

Clinical correlation: curves of the spine

Anatomical (true) leg length difference

Compensatory scoliosis - usually a 'triple' curve, with a lumbar, thoracic and cervical component - is evident on standing. As the pelvis becomes level in sitting and lying (Fig. 2.72B), the curves are decreased, or sometimes even abolished, except at sites of any persistent rotational displacement of isolated vertebrae (Figs 2.94, 2.96, 2.97).

Sacroiliac joint 'upslip'

A right or left 'upslip' also results in obliquity of the pelvis, with formation of a compensatory scoliosis.

1. With a 'right upslip' (Fig. 2.73A), the pelvis is raised on the right side. The lumbar segment may be convex into either the high or the low side of the pelvis.
2. With a 'left upslip' (Fig. 2.73B), the obliquity may actually again be high on the right side in both standing and sitting but inclined up to the left in both prone and supine-lying, as expected. The direction of the curves remains constant in all positions, the lumbar curve usually convex to left and thoracic to right.

'Outflare/inflare'

Innominate rotation occurs around the vertical axis in the transverse plane so that, provided the leg length is equal, there is no pelvic obliquity. As in the case of someone with equal leg length, a scoliosis may still be present and is likely to be more obvious when standing.

'Rotational malalignment'

There is typically the triple curve with reversal at the thoracolumbar and cervicothoracic junctions. The curves usually persist in standing, sitting and lying prone but may change direction on moving from one position to another (Fig. 2.73C,D)

The pelvic obliquity is caused, in part, by:

1. contrary rotation of the innominate(s), with elevation of the iliac crest on the side of the 'anterior' rotation
2. an associated rotation ('tilting') of the pelvic unit around the sagittal axis in the coronal plane
3. the functional LLD

Which pelvic crest is higher or lower is, however, also influenced by other factors, including whether there is an underlying anatomical (true) LLD, a coexistent sacral torsion or an SI joint 'upslip'. It may, therefore, vary depending on the position of examination. Most prevalent is a consistent elevation of the right superior iliac crest. Perhaps it is this variability in the factors responsible for the pelvic obliquity that might explain why one also sees such variability in the curvatures evident on examination but it does not help to predict:

1. the presentation of scoliotic curves one might expect on examining someone with malalignment
2. whether the curves defined when standing will persist in sitting and lying, or
3. whether the curves will persist in sitting and reverse on lying prone

More important than noting a change of the particular curves in the various positions of examination is to accept that:

1. scoliotic curves are likely to be more obvious in someone presenting with a pelvic obliquity for whatever reason than if the pelvis were level, but in both cases are not necessarily of significance or the cause of any symptoms
2. emphasis should be on recognition and treatment of an underlying malalignment problem and any secondary symptoms
3. the curves are usually less pronounced in sitting and lying, particularly once realignment has been achieved

EXAMINATION OF THE SYMPHYSIS PUBIS

The examiner should note whether any of the following occur.

Pain on palpating or stressing the joint

The symphysis may be painful on direct palpation. Pain caused by joint distraction may indicate primarily a ligamentous or capsular problem as these are put under increased tension (Figs 2.98, 3.66). Pain caused by joint compression is more likely to indicate joint pathology (Figs 2.99, 2.100). Degenerative changes on X-ray and a positive bone scan could be in keeping with such pathology; certainly findings suggestive of 'osteitis pubis' can result with increased stress on the joint caused by sacroiliac and/or hip joint dysfunction and malalignment. However, degenerative changes are by no means pathognomonic for symptoms arising from the joint itself. Superoinferior translation gives information on joint stability; pain provoked in this way probably is less specific because the manoeuvre stresses both the symphysis pubis and SI joint, also attaching soft tissue structures (Fig. 2.101). Similarly, anteroposterior translation stresses both joints. These tests are more likely to suggest isolated symphysis pubis involvement if pain is experienced just in the midline anteriorly (Fig. 2.112B).

Disturbance of joint symmetry

The joint may actually be asymmetric but asymptomatic. Pain felt in this area may also arise from other nearby structures (e.g. adductor origin, pelvic floor muscles, ligaments) or have been referred to a pubic symphysis that is actually in alignment (e.g. from an SI joint or iliolumbar ligament; Fig. 3.46).

'Anterior' or 'posterior' rotation of an innominate bone does not occur without simultaneous rotation of one pubic bone relative to the other. Similarly, an 'upslip' or 'downslip' causes a simultaneous upward or downward translation, respectively, both at the SI joint and the symphysis pubis. The vertical displacement at the symphysis is usually some 3–5 mm and readily discernible:

1. on comparison of the level of the mid- or index fingers or lateral edge of the thumbs placed on the upper edge of the superior pubic ramus, 1.5-2.0 cm to either side of the midline (Figs 2.71C, 3.86D)
2. by appreciating a sudden drop or rise in the contour as one sweeps a finger along the upper edge from one side to the other
3. on the anteroposterior X-ray view of the pelvis (Fig. 2.75).

As indicated previously, this displacement is associated with an obliquity of the pubic bones that remains evident on standing, sitting and lying, in keeping with the obliquity of the whole pelvic unit.

Instability of the joint

Instability may become apparent as:

1. excessive gapping (greater than 5 mm) noticeable on joint palpation
2. excessive movement of the joint on subjecting it to translatory forces: superoinferior (Fig. 2.101) and anteroposterior (Fig. 2.112B)
3. suspicion of separation of the pubic bones on routine X-rays (see Fig. 2.75).

It should, however, be pointed out that even marked instability may not become readily apparent on clinical examination, or even routine anteroposterior views of the pelvis, especially when these are taken with the person lying supine. If instability is

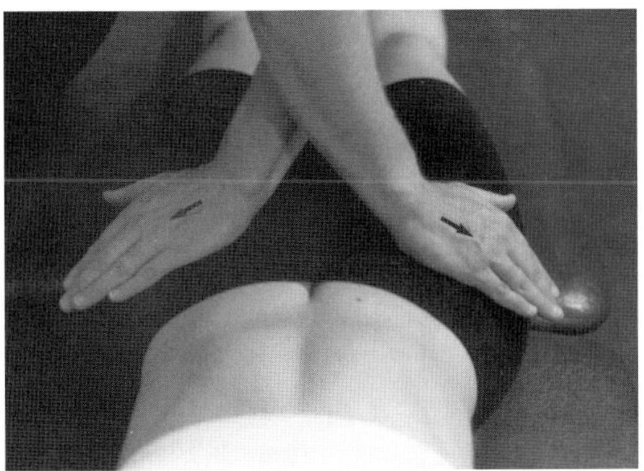

Fig. 2.98 Pain provocation test: transverse anterior distraction (symphysis pubis and anterior sacroiliac joint capsule and ligaments) with simultaneous posterior sacroiliac joint compression. *(Courtesy of Lee & Walsh 1996.)*

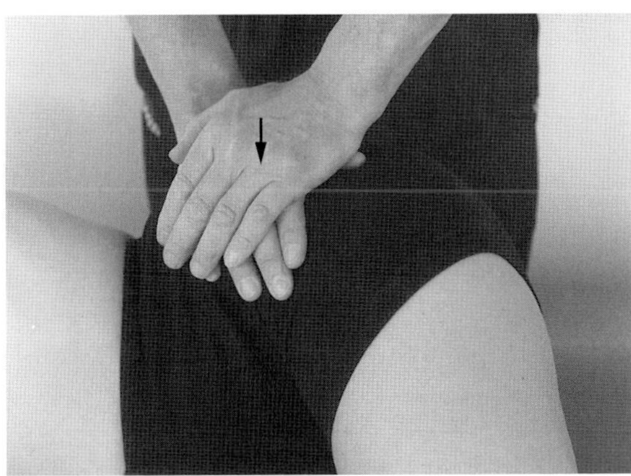

Fig. 2.100 Pain provocation test: anterior compression and posterior gapping achieved with a downward force on the upper innominate in side-lying. *(Courtesy of Lee & Walsh 1996.)*

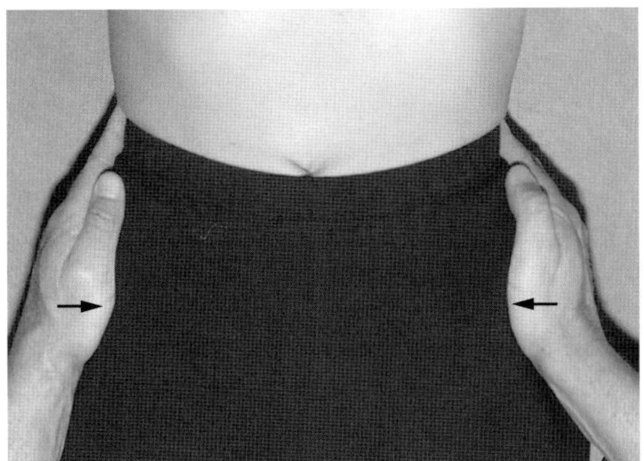

Fig. 2.99 Pain provocation test: medial compression of the innominates results in anterior compression and posterior distraction. *(Courtesy of Lee & Walsh 1996.)*

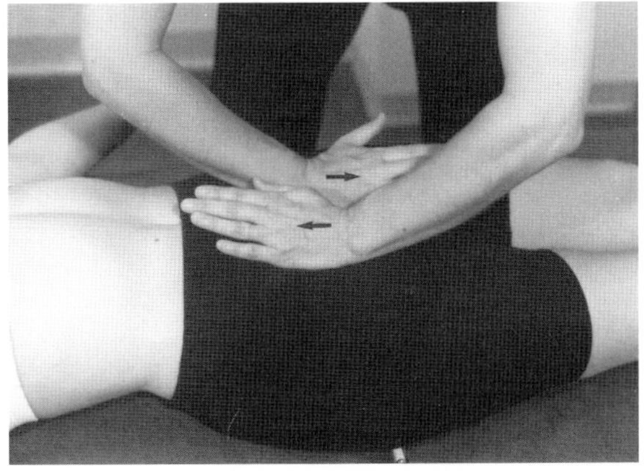

Fig. 2.101 Superoinferior translation test for the pubic symphysis. *(Courtesy Lee & Walsh 1996.)*

suspected, X-rays should be taken while stressing the joint, which can be achieved by:

1. carrying out an active straight leg raising test (see under 'Functional tests' below); this test has an advantage in that it can be carried out with the person lying supine (Figs 2.102A, 2.126A, 2.128)
2. maintaining a 'flamingo' or 'figure-4' position, standing alternately on the right and left legs, with the hip and knee of the opposite leg flexed and the foot resting against the weight-bearing leg at knee level (Fig. 2.102B)
3. standing on a stool and alternately letting one leg hang down while bearing full weight on the other one (Fig. 2.102C).

Clinical correlation: alignment at the symphysis pubis

Aligned, anatomical (true) leg length difference

With an anatomical long right leg, the right pubic bone lies higher than the left in standing (Fig. 2.72B). There is no actual displacement of the pubic bones relative to each other, just a uniform obliquity that inclines from left to right, which is evident on palpation and on a standing anteroposterior X-ray but abolished on sitting or on lying supine (Figs 2.74A, 2.81).

Sacroiliac joint 'upslip'

On the side of the 'upslip', there will usually be a 3–5 mm step-wise upward displacement of the

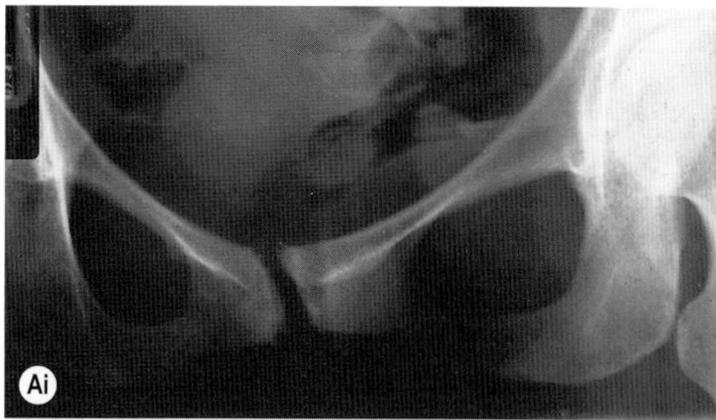

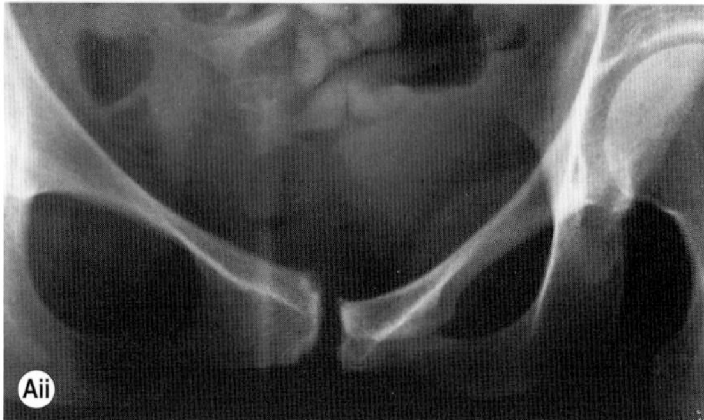

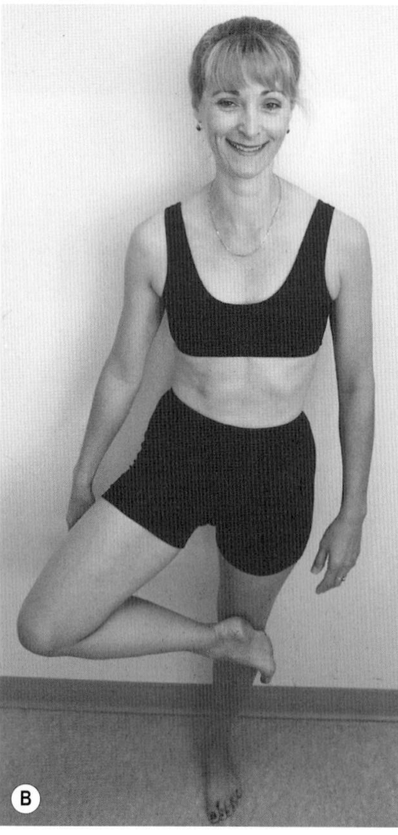

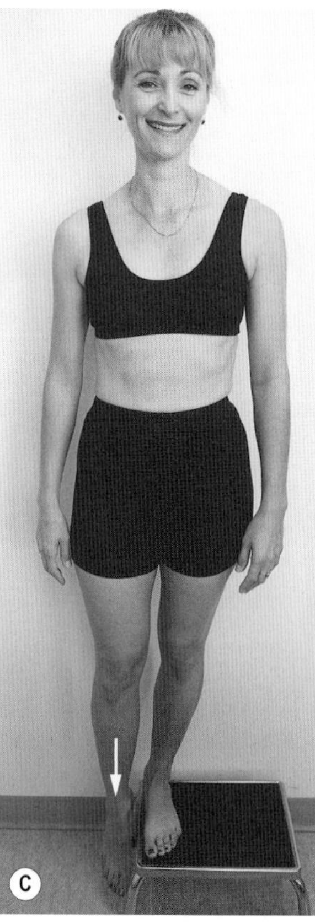

Fig. 2.102 X-ray diagnosis of symphysis pubis instability. (A) X-rays during 'active SLR' (ASLR) of a patient with a large displacement: (i) During ASLR of the right leg (reference side); (ii) During ASLR of the left (symptomatic) side. No malalignment of the pubic bones is seen during ASLR on the reference side. A step of about 5 mm is seen at the upper margins on the symptomatic side. The projection of the left pubic bone is smaller than that of the right, indicating an anterior rotation of the left pubic bone about an axis in the vicinity of the sacroiliac joint. *(Courtesy of Mens et al. 1997.)* (B) 'Flamingo' or 'figure-4' position likely to detect displacement of the left pubic bone relative to the right one when left SI joint is inadequately stabilized on left weight-bearing. (C) Left pubic bone is stressed by letting the right leg hang down freely suspended while bearing all weight on the left one.

pubic bone relative to that on the opposite side, with an obliquity inclined to the side of the 'upslip' in lying (Figs 2.73A,B, 2.82).

'Rotational malalignment'

With 'right anterior, left posterior' innominate rotation, the right pubic bone is shifted posteriorly and down, the left anteriorly and up. In addition to the contrary rotation of the pubic bones around the coronal axis, there is an actual downward displacement of the right pubic bone relative to the left evident at the symphysis (Figs 2.42, 2.73C,D, 2.75, 2.76C, 3.86D). 'Left anterior, right posterior' innominate rotation results in the opposite findings (Fig. 2.73D).

'Outflare/inflare'

The pubic bones are level but are subjected to compression/distraction stresses and may be tender/symptomatic.

HIP JOINT RANGES OF MOTION

As discussed in detail in Chapter 3, the hip ranges of motion are:

1. symmetrical in the person presenting in alignment or with an anatomical (true) LLD
2. asymmetrical in the presence of 'rotational malalignment', 'outflare/inflare' and an 'upslip' or 'downslip'.

Asymmetry of hip range of motion in the absence of pelvic malalignment, or in a pattern inconsistent with that typically associated with malalignment, should trigger a search for pathology involving the hip joint itself and/or specific soft tissues structures (see Appendix 3). Tightness of the acetabular anterior or Y ligaments, for example, will limit ipsilateral hip extension; a 'capsular pattern', with restriction of all joint ranges of motion, can result with generalized contracture of soft tissues and may be indicative of underlying hip joint osteoarthritis or of previous severe trauma with scarring.

ASSESSMENT OF LIGAMENTS AND MUSCLES

The examination for asymmetry and malalignment must include an assessment of tension and tenderness in the ligaments and muscles of the pelvic region and along the spine (Figs 2.4-2.6, 3.68). The sacrotuberous and sacrospinous ligaments, for example, are subjected to increased tension by sacral nutation and often prove tender to palpation (Figs 2.19A, 2.21). A spring test to briefly augment the nutation, and hence the tension, may provoke pain from these ligaments (Fig. 2.103A). Similarly, augmenting counternutation with anterior pressure on the apex of the sacrum may provoke pain from an already tense and often tender long dorsal sacroiliac ligament (Figs 2.5, 2.19B, 2.103B). There are patterns of muscles typically affected in terms of being tense

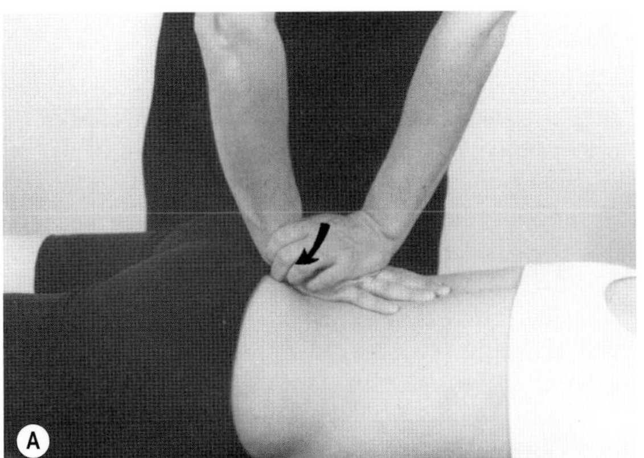

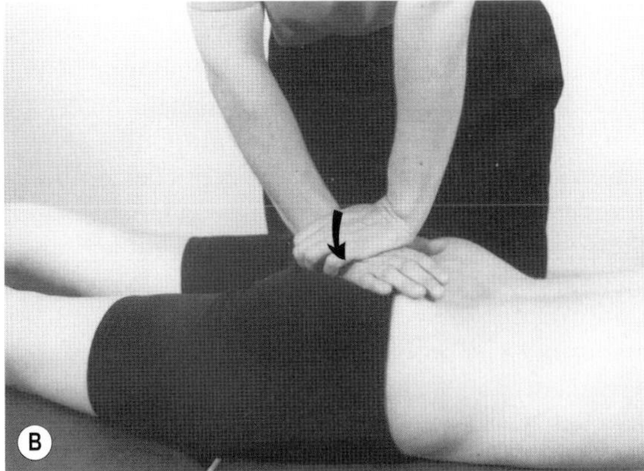

Fig. 2.103 Pain provocation tests for posterior pelvic ligaments, the hands applying an anterior force for 20 seconds. (A) Hands overlying the sacral base to enforce nutation and, thereby, increase tension in the sacrotuberous, sacrospinous and interosseous ligaments. (B) Hands overlying the sacral apex to enforce counternutation and, thereby, increase tension in the long dorsal sacroiliac ligament. *(Courtesy of Lee & Walsh 1996; see also Figs 2.5A, 2.19B.)*

and tender depending on the presentation at hand and, in the case of an 'upslip' or 'rotational malalignment', also a characteristic asymmetrical functional weakness distinct from a nerve root or peripheral nerve problem. The importance of these findings, both as a source of localized and referred pain and as a cause of recurrence of malalignment, is discussed in Chapter 3.

TESTS USED FOR THE EXAMINATION OF THE PELVIC GIRDLE

The assessment for malalignment requires an in-depth examination of the individual components – spine, pelvis and hip joints – and of the pelvic girdle as a unit. This section will concentrate on:

1. tests for mobility and stability
2. tests for ability of the unit to transfer load, remain stable and maintain balance when subjected to functional or dynamic stresses.

As Lee already pointed out so succinctly in 1992:

> *primary pathology of the lumbar spine can lead to secondary symptoms from the pelvic girdle. Alternately, primary pathology of the sacroiliac joint can lead to secondary symptoms from the lumbar spine*

The importance of the hip joints as part of this 'triage' has now been accepted. Because some of the tests for the pelvis also exert forces on the lumbosacral spine and hips, tests as selective as possible for these three individual segments must always be part of the examination. For example, activating external rotators of the thigh forces the femoral head forward, selectively increasing stress on the anterior hip capsule and compressing the structures lying immediately anterior: iliopsoas, pectineus, femoral nerve/artery/vein and others (Figs 2.104A,B, 4.14).

Over the past decade, the 'active straight leg raising' (ASLR) test has gained acceptance as being one of the more reliable ones for establishing whether there is indeed a problem with a pelvic joint, muscle or ligament and to help localize the site of pain origin. However, discussion will focus initially on other tests that have been used over the years and may:

1. increase a person's ability to assess a particular problem
2. be helpful in situations where factors limit what tests can be carried out safely and without aggravation; e.g. the site of injury, location and/or severity of the pain, or any limitation of mobility.

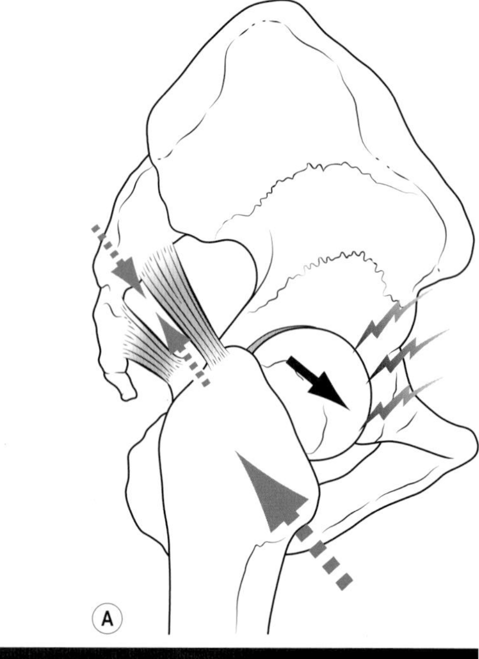

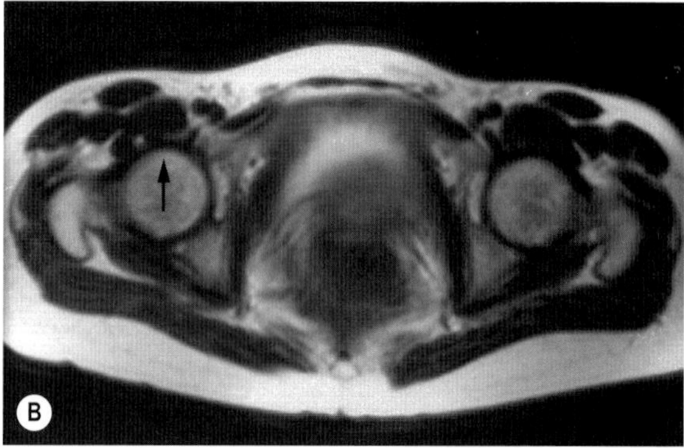

Fig. 2.104 Effects of femoral external rotation on hip joint and surrounding structures. (A) Overactivity of the deep external rotators of the hip pulls the greater trochanter posterior (large arrow) and forces the femoral head anterior. This position compresses the structures of the anterior hip and the subinguinal region. *(Courtesy of Lee 2007b; reproduced from Lee 2004a.)* (B) This is an MRI through both hips and the pelvic floor. Note the anterior position of the femoral head (arrow) and the resultant compression of the structures anterior to it. *(Courtesy of Lee 2007b.)*

The examination of gait, posture and the neurological, muscular and vascular systems is mentioned as appropriate throughout the text. For a more extensive coverage of these aspects, the reader is referred to Lee & Walsh (1996), Vleeming et al. 2007, Lee 2004a,b (e.g. 'Diagnosing the lumbosacral-hip dysfunction'),

Lee 2011 and authors concentrating specifically on neurovascular problems (e.g. Willard 2007).

TESTS FOR MOBILITY AND STABILITY

The following are tests commonly used to localize pain and to determine dysfunction of SI joint movement (e.g. hyper- or hypomobility, 'locking', or excessive rotation). Again, a caution is in order.

First, some of these tests are not specific for the SI joint itself because they also stress the hip joint, lumbosacral region or all three sites simultaneously. In order to better localize the pain, the examination should include tests that are more specific for stressing these sites individually.

Second, tests do not differentiate between pain arising from the joint itself, the supporting soft tissues or both. Compression tests are, generally, more likely to precipitate pain from the joint, distraction tests pain from the ligaments and capsule. The selective injection of local anaesthetic into the joint space or the ligaments may also be helpful in localizing the site of origin (see Ch. 7).

There may still be some value doing several stress tests in combination, especially if SI joint blocks under fluoroscopy are not available. Van der Wurff et al. (2006: 10) reported that, on comparison to fluoroscopically-controlled double SI joint blocks, a test regiment in which 3 or more of 5 non-invasive pain provocative tests proved positive was indicative that the pain was from the SI joint and could be 'used in early clinical decision making to reduce the number of unnecessary minimal invasive diagnostic SIJ procedures'.

Leverage tests

The following manoeuvres all depend on stressing the SI joint by using the femur like a lever to effect movement of the innominate bone. The femur can be used to rotate the innominate around the coronal axis, to move it in an anterior or posterior direction in the sagittal plane, or to adduct or abduct it relative to the sacrum. With the exception of Yeoman's test, all are carried out with the person lying supine. While leverage is here being discussed as a means of testing joints and soft tissue structures, it will be mentioned throughout the text from the viewpoint of how it can have detrimental or beneficial effects (see Ch. 7; Fig. 7.22)

First, with the hip flexed somewhere from 80 to 110-120 degrees to put the thigh at different angles relative to the innominate, push downward on the knee in order to move the femur, and hence the hip joint and innominate, in an anteroposterior direction (Fig. 2.105). There will be a simultaneous anterior rotational force of varying degree applied to the innominate, given that the acetabulum lies below the inferior transverse axis around which the wings of the ilia turn relative to the sacrum (Fig. 2.50)

Next, with the hip joint flexed to 90 degrees, the femur is passively adducted to stress the SI joint by forcing the anterior joint margins together and, at the same time, separating or 'gapping' the posterior joint margins to stress the posterior capsule and ligaments. The adduction force is applied with one hand on the outside of the knee while the other hand palpates the SI joint posteriorly to determine the amount of gapping (Fig. 2.106).

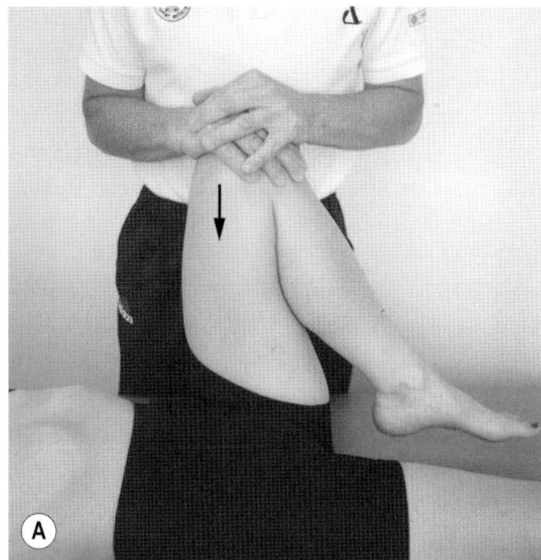

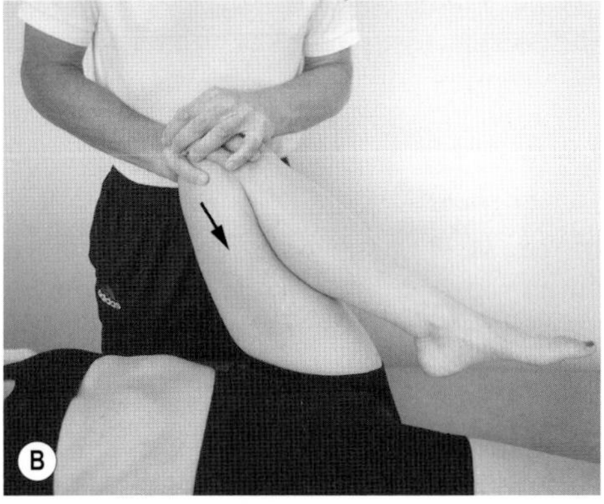

Fig. 2.105 Passive displacement of the innominate relative to the sacrum by a force applied through the femur. (A) Hip flexed to 90 degrees results in a more direct anteroposterior force. (B) Hip flexed to 110 degrees results in a relatively more anterior rotational force.

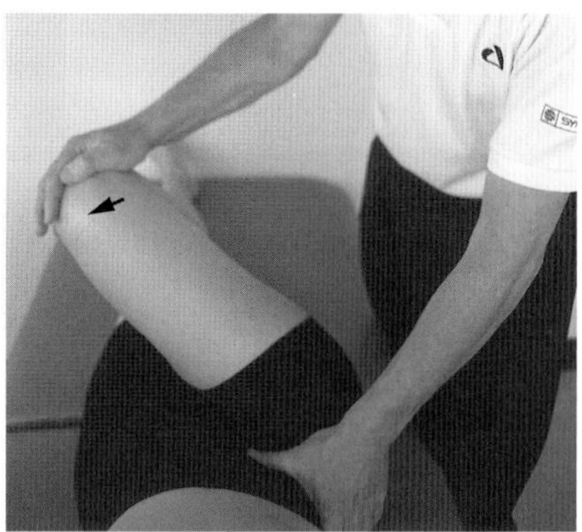

Fig. 2.106 Passive adduction of the right femur to 'gap' the posterior and compress the anterior aspect of the right sacroiliac joint.

Whereas gapping may be quite obviously increased or decreased from normal, always make a side-to-side comparison in order to determine any actual differences, in contrast to a generalized bilateral joint laxity or tightness that may be normal for that person. This test may not be tolerated when there is tenderness or spasm in muscles such as the iliopsoas and pectineus that are literally 'compressed' by the manoeuvre because it narrows the inguinal space. Alternately, posterior 'gapping' or distraction can be achieved by using a medial force applied to the ASIS of both innominates in supine lying (Fig. 2.99), or to the upper innominate in side-lying (Fig. 2.100).

Passive abduction of the flexed hip will gap the anterior part of the SI joint and stress the anterior capsule and ligaments; whereas the posterior aspect of the joint will be compressed.

Other stress tests, most of which also have a leverage component, can then be carried out.

Shear stress tests

1. ***anterior shear***

   This can be achieved with the FABER test (simultaneous hip Flexion, Abduction and External Rotation), also known as Patrick's or the 'figure-4' test. It has been commonly used to test for hip joint pathology and for restriction of range of motion, in particular external rotation (Figs 2.102B, 2.107A, 3.80). However, given that the hip joint lies caudad to the SI joint, this manoeuvre also turns the femur into a lever capable of:

   a. rotating the innominate posteriorly and externally (outward) relative to the sacrum,

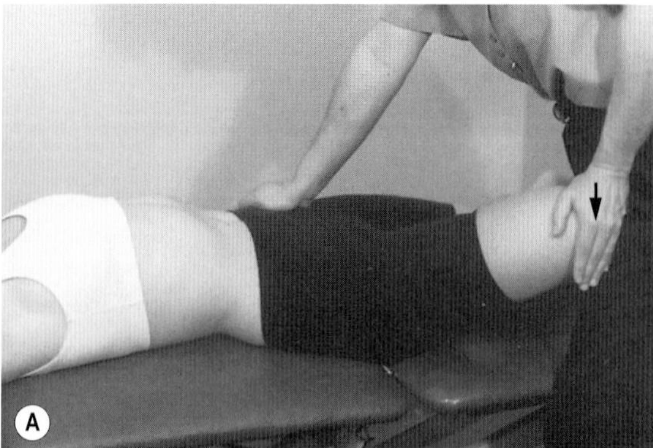

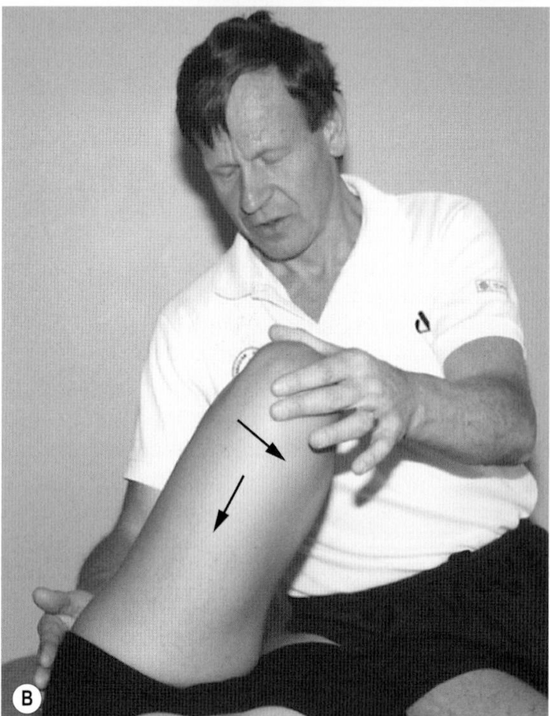

Fig. 2.107 Shear tests for the sacroiliac joint. (A) **FABER** manoeuvre (Flexion, **AB**duction and External Rotation). After finding the physiological limit of simultaneous movement in these directions, the femur is gently moved into further abduction and external rotation; at the same time, the contralateral innominate is fixed so that the flexed right femur becomes a lever capable of rotating the innominate externally and posteriorly through the hip joint. *(Courtesy of Lee & Walsh 1996; see also Fig. 3.80.)* (B) **FADE** (simultaneous Flexion, **AD**duction and External force) or **POSH** (**PO**sterior **SH**ear) test: the hip is flexed, the femur adducted and an axial force then exerted through the femur to push the ilium posteriorly relative to the sacrum.

and stretching the TFL/ITB complex and muscles in the anterior groin region (e.g. iliopsoas, pectineus, adductor origins)

b. effecting nutation and thereby stressing the sacrotuberous, sacrospinous and interosseous ligaments
c. compressing the SI joint posteriorly and opening it anteriorly, with stretching of the anterior SI joint capsule and ligaments
d. moving the ilium so it translates anteriorly relative to the sacrum while the pelvis is stabilized, with resultant shear stress on the anterior part of the SI joint.

2. *posterior shear*

   This can be effected with the FADE (simultaneous Flexion, Adduction, External force) or POSH (POsterior SHear) tests (Fig. 2.107B).

Hip extension tests

These are commonly used to stress the hip joint but progressive movement of the femur will eventually also stress the SI joint by rotating the innominate anteriorly in the sagittal plane.

1. *Yeoman's test*: passive unilateral hip extension, with the person prone (Figs 2.47B, 2.108A, 7.16)
2. *Gaenslen's test*: passive unilateral hip extension, with the person supine and the leg hanging over the side of the plinth (Fig. 2.108B).

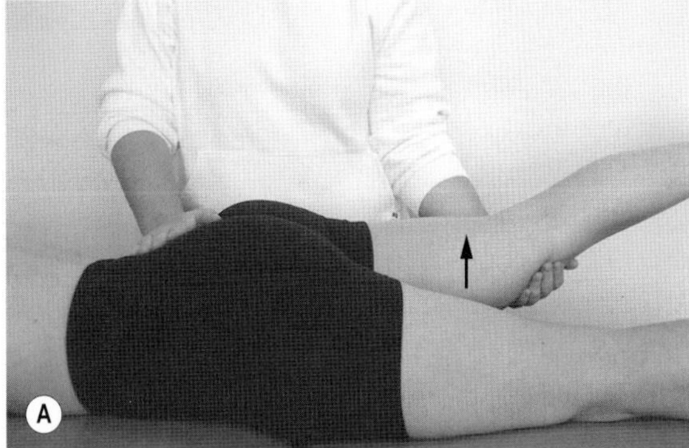

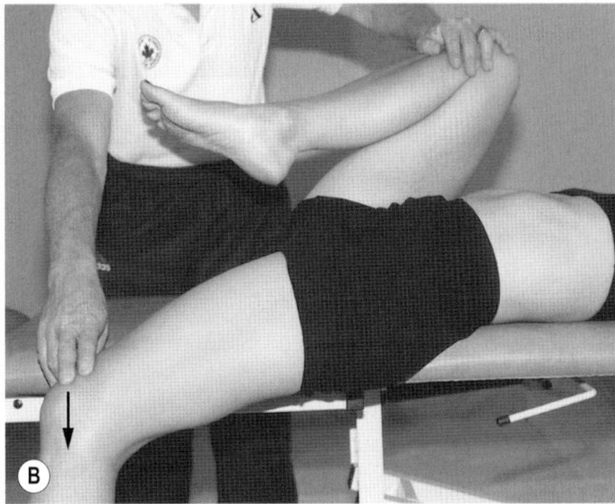

Fig. 2.108 Hip extension to effect anterior innominate rotation and stress the sacroiliac joint. (A) Right Yeoman's test (passive hip extension, prone-lying). (B) Left Gaenslen's test (passive hip extension, supine-lying).

Hip flexion tests

Passive straight leg raising, also hip flexion with the knee bent (Fig. 2.109), can both turn the femur into a lever arm. For example, on passive hip flexion of greater than 110-120 degrees, the femoral head engages the anterior acetabular rim and causes the innominate to rotate posteriorly in the sagittal plane (see Ch. 7). Any pain thus provoked, by stressing the SI joint itself and/or putting tender posterior pelvic ligaments under increased tension, may be confused with pain elicited by putting the sciatic nerve and nerve roots under stretch or by mechanically stressing the lumbar spine as it is forced into increasing flexion.

Wells back in 1986 suggested that some differentiation between a lumbar as opposed to an SI joint dysfunction should be possible. He felt that the SI joint is more likely to be the problem if the pain produced by a unilateral hip flexion test does not occur on carrying out the test on both sides simultaneously because the latter does

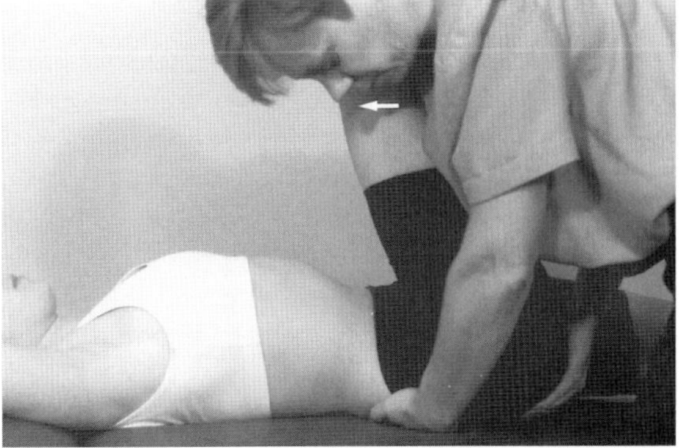

Fig. 2.109 Passive hip flexion, using the right femur to effect posterior rotation of the right innominate relative to the sacrum. *(Courtesy of Lee & Walsh 1996.)*

not produce the torsional stress on the SI joint that results with the unilateral test. Pain that persists on the bilateral test argues for a lumbar cause because the stresses on the nerves and lumbar spine are the same in both tests.

Spring tests

Pain originating from the hip joint proper may interfere with the interpretation of leverage-type tests and may even make it impossible to use them. One may be able to bypass this problem using passive mobility tests that attempt to shift either the innominate or the sacrum relative to the other, the aim being to assess the degree and quality of motion and to see whether the test provokes any symptoms.

Once the end of the passive range has been reached (= degree or quantity), the application of a gentle springing force provides further information regarding end-feel and symptom provocation (=quality). As Hesch et al. stressed (1992: 445), 'the spring test is . . . applied as a gentle force within the physiological range'. Findings run from excessive movement to varying degrees of impaired movement or absolutely no joint play or spring detectable. On all these tests, side-to-side comparison is imperative in order to detect a relative increase or decrease in mobility. The current teaching is that:

1. symmetry of findings is the norm
2. asymmetry is indicative of dysfunction

In other words, asymmetry - be it of joint stiffness, laxity or other 'abnormality' of motion - is more likely to present a clinical problem than if this stiffness, laxity or other change were found to be of the same degree (symmetrical) on side-to-side comparison (Buyruk et al. 1995b, 1999; Damen et al. 2002b; Buyruk 1997). The reader is referred to Lee & Walsh (1996) and Lee (1999; 2004a,b; 2011) for a more extensive description of the following spring tests.

Spring tests carried out with the person prone

Springing of the innominate in a posteroanterior direction creates a shear stress on the SI joint and allows for the localization of pain and the assessment of the amount of movement possible in the anterior direction.

The heel of one hand is placed on the innominate, directly on or alongside the PSIS; the heel of the other hand rests along the opposite border of the sacrum in order to stabilize the sacrum relative to the innominate (Fig. 2.110). After locking the elbow, bend forward with the trunk and apply a gradually increasing downward pressure on the innominate until all the slack in the soft tissues surrounding the SI joint has been taken up and the initial movement of the innominate stops. At this point, apply a quick, low-amplitude force directly through the outstretched arm to the hand and the underlying innominate.

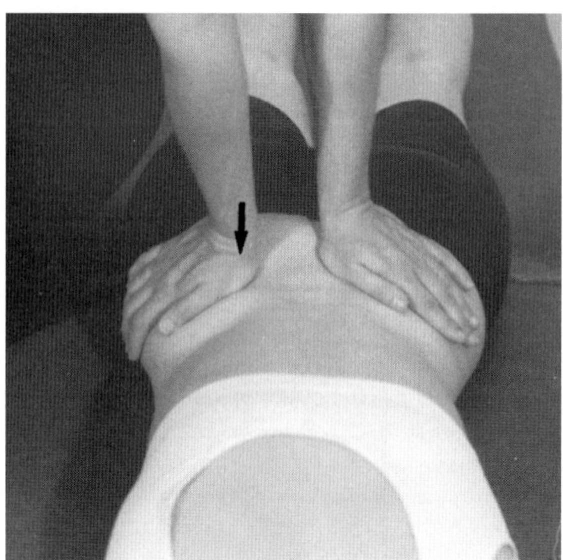

Fig. 2.110 Posterior-anterior shear stress on innominate relative to the sacrum: with the left hand on the far side of the sacrum for counterbalance, the right hand applies a quick downward force on the right innominate. *(Courtesy of Lee & Walsh 1996.)*

The above manoeuvre can be modified by placing the heel of the hand that rests on the innominate either just above or below the PSIS in order to produce an anterior or posterior rotational stress, respectively, on the innominate relative to the sacrum. The sacrum is stabilized by placing the heel of the other hand on the apex.

The SI joint and specific ligaments can be stressed selectively using a quick springing action to force the sacrum into increased nutation or counternutation, similar to the pain provocative tests using a prolonged force (see above and Fig. 2.103).

Pain may be provoked by stressing the SI joint in a longitudinal direction. The heel of one hand pushes on the apex of the sacrum in a cephalad (upward) direction as the heel of the other hand pushes caudad (downward) on the posterior iliac crest (Fig. 2.111A). Conversely, the heel of one hand exerts pressure in a caudad direction on the base of the sacrum as the heel of the other hand applies pressure against the ischial tuberosity to force the

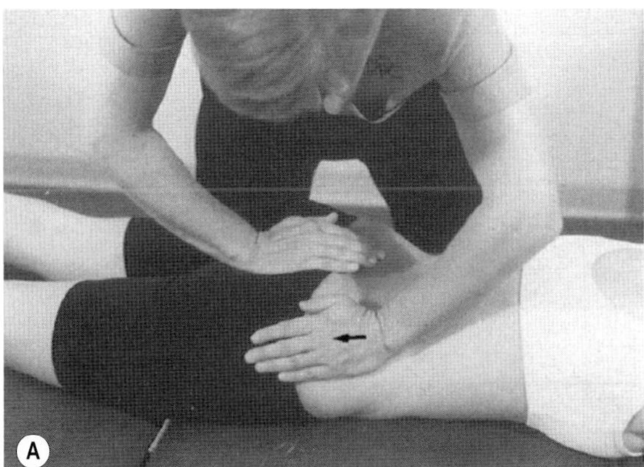

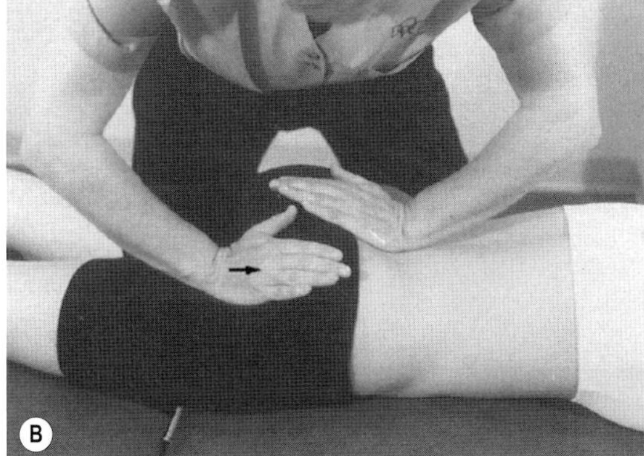

Fig. 2.111 Translation of the right innominate relative to the sacrum. (A) Inferosuperior: sacrum cephalad, innominate caudad. (B) Superoinferior: sacrum caudad, innominate cephalad. *(Courtesy of Lee & Walsh 1996.)*

innominate cephalad (Fig. 2.111B). If the sacrococcygeal joint or the coccyx itself is tender, it may be not be possible to perform these tests.

In another test, the fingers of one hand fix the ASIS and iliac crest while the heel of the other hand forces down on the ipsilateral side of the sacrum until end-feel is perceived (Fig. 2.112). A small amount of pain-free anteroposterior joint play in the sagittal plane can normally be detected. Alternatively, with the left hand steadying the sacrum, the right hand can apply a quick upward (posteroanterior) force on the innominate, with the person positioned either as in Fig. 2.112A or with the right hip in some flexion and the leg draped over the side (Fig. 2.112B).

Spring tests carried out with the person supine

Compression and distraction forces

These are modifications of the pain provocative tests discussed above, again with addition of a quick, low-amplitude stress on some of these tests once end-feel has been perceived on stretching the surrounding soft tissues (Figs. 2.98, 2.99, 2.101).

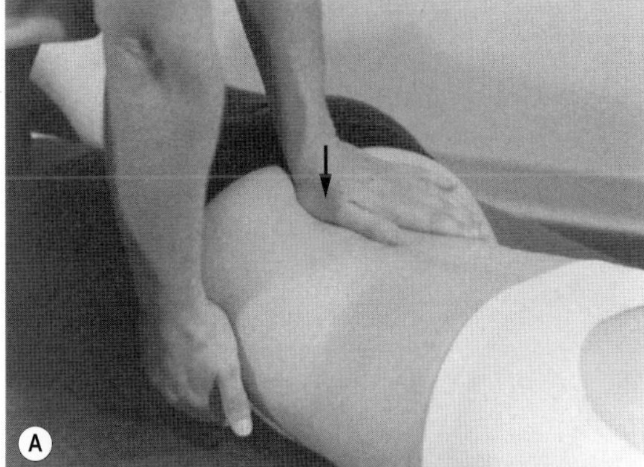

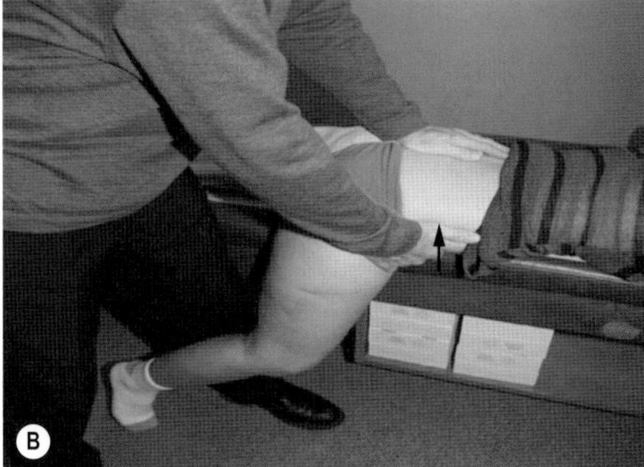

Fig. 2.112 (A) Posterior translation (innominate on the sacrum) - prone. Comparison of right to left side for detection of asymmetries is indicated. Here the right hand applied to the right anterior superior iliac spine and iliac crest fixes the innominate while a posteroanterior force is applied with the heel of the left hand to the ipsilateral side of the sacrum. Quantity and end feel of motion and the reproduction of symptoms are observed. *(Courtesy of Lee & Walsh 1996.)* (B) Lying prone with right leg hanging over the edge of plinth: anterior force [exerted by the left hand placed] on sacrum helps to stabilize the pelvis while sensing for movement at the SI joint when a posterior translatory force is applied [by the right hand] to the right innominate. *(Courtesy of Sweeting 2009.)*

Glide of the innominate relative to the sacrum

For the next three tests, the long and ring fingers are hooked around the medial edge of the posterior pelvic ring and come to lie in the sacral sulcus, where they can sense movement between the innominate and the sacrum. The index finger lies on the spinous process of L5 in order to sense the end of motion between the sacrum and the innominate.

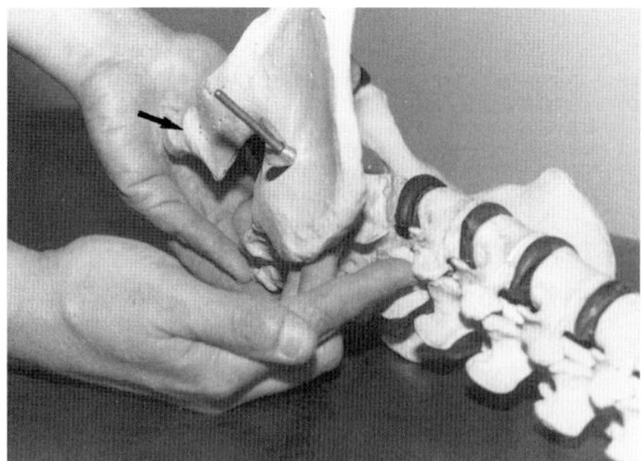

Fig. 2.113 Placement of the long and ring fingers in the sacral sulcus, and the index finger on L5 for sensing innominate movement relative to the sacrum. *(Courtesy of Lee & Walsh 1996.)*

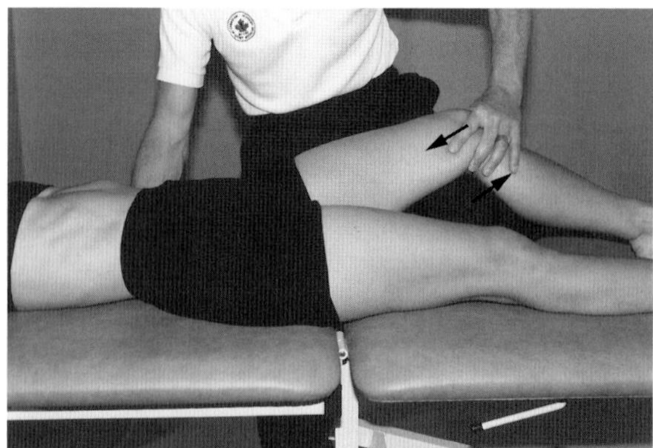

Fig. 2.114 Testing for left innominate movement relative to the sacrum in the craniocaudal or superoinferior plane, using pushing/pulling forces on the femur.

1. Anteroposterior plane

Increasing anteroposterior pressure is then applied to the anterior pelvic rim until end-feel is achieved, at which point the pelvic girdle as a unit starts to move laterally relative to L5 (Fig. 2.113). A note is made of:

a. the actual end-feel itself (well-defined, sloppy, etc.)
b. the amount of movement between the sacrum and innominate
c. whether there is any further displacement - and how much - of the innominate relative to the sacrum when a quick thrust is applied to the anterior iliac crest
d. whether these manoeuvres elicit any symptoms, and
e. how all the findings compare with doing the test on the opposite side.

2. Craniocaudal or superoinferior plane

For a test of the left SI joint (Fig. 2.114), the knee is about 20-30 degrees flexed, resting across a pillow or, if possible, across the examiner's knee (proped up on the plinth). With the right hand positioned to sense glide between the innominate and the sacrum, the examiner's left hand holds onto the distal end of the femur or patellofemoral region in order to apply a force, alternately:

a. pushing upward (cephalad)
b. pulling downward (caudad), an action that can be augmented by pressing his or her left knee against the posterior aspect of the proximal tibia.

3. Anterioposterior and rotational planes combined

The heel of the free hand applies pressure on the ipsilateral ASIS to create a translatory force in an anteroposterior direction until an end-feel is perceived, followed by a quick thrust to detect and evaluate any further displacement (Fig. 2.115A). The manoeuvre is then altered to assess the glide between the SI joint surfaces with rotation of the innominate in the sagittal plane:

a. by applying the force just above the ASIS (Fig. 2.115B) to effect anterior innominate rotation and relative sacral counternutation, which would decrease SI joint stability (Fig. 2.15)
b. by applying a force just below the ASIS (Fig. 2.115C) to effect posterior innominate rotation and relative sacral nutation, which should increase SI joint stability (Fig. 2.16)

If a leverage or spring test fails to provoke pain, that does not mean that the joint is functioning normally. The joint may, for example, be hypomobile or even immobile and yet be asymptomatic. It is now well recognized that it is often the joint that is still mobile that proves to be painful and may also be hypermobile, all this possibly because of the increased stress it is now subjected to as a result of the loss of mobility in the opposite joint. Always keep in mind that:

> *Mobility restrictions of the lumbar spine, pelvic girdle and/or hip joint will influence the function and motion of the adjacent regions. Often, all three areas require treatment and it is not rare for the most hypomobile area to be the least symptomatic.*
>
> (Lee 1992b; 475)

FUNCTIONAL OR DYNAMIC TESTS

The leverage and spring tests are passive tests for SI joint mobility and stability. The following tests try to assess, in particular, the ability to transfer load

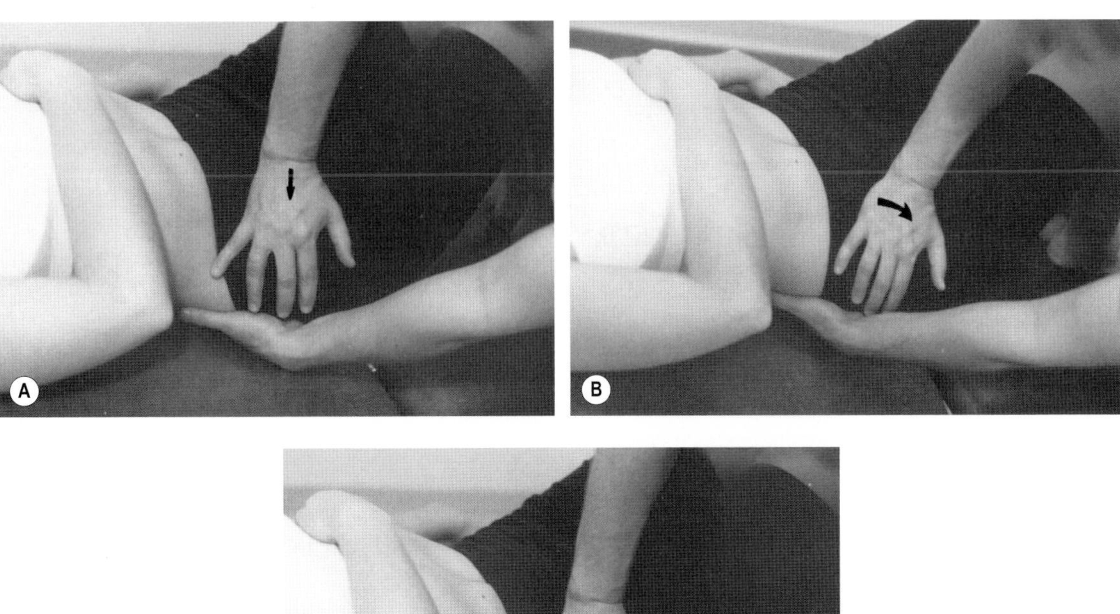

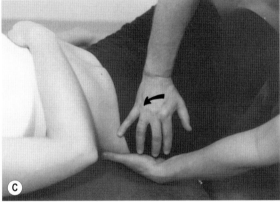

Fig. 2.115 Innominate movement relative to the sacrum. (A) Anteroposterior translation or glide: a posterior translation force is applied to the innominate and the motion is noted posteriorly. (B) Anterior rotation of the innominate requires an inferoposterior glide of the sacroiliac (SI) joint (a caudad force applied above the anterior superior iliac spine). (C) Posterior rotation of the innominate requires a superoanterior glide at the SI joint (a cephalad force applied below the anterior superior iliac spine). *(Courtesy of Lee 2004a.)*

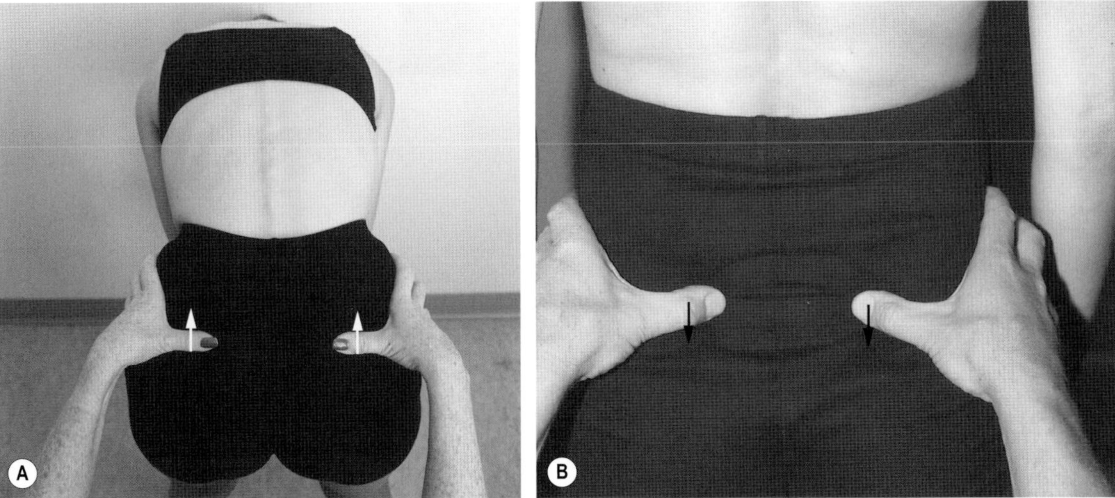

Fig. 2.116 Normal pelvic flexion/extension test. In standing (neutral position), the thumbs are on matching points - resting against the inferior aspect of the posterior superior iliac spines (PSIS; see also Fig. 2.71B). (A) On trunk flexion: the thumbs (= PSIS) move up an equal extent. (B) On trunk extension: the thumbs (= PSIS) move down an equal extent.

BOX 2.5	Functional or dynamic testing of the pelvic girdle

1. Gait analysis (see 'SI joint function during the gait cycle', above)
2. Lumbosacral tests in standing – bending forward and backward
3. Tests carried out weight-bearing on one leg, e.g. the Gillet (kinetic rotational); stork test
4. Active straight leg raising (ASLR) tests augmented by 'form' and 'force' closure

through the SI joints, such as occurs with day-to-day activities. These tests need to evaluate specifically:

1. the passive or 'form' closure system - articular and ligamentous
2. the active or 'force' closure system - myofascial
3. the control system - neural coordination.

Examples of the functional or dynamic tests commonly used are shown in Box 2.5.

Flexion and extension tests

These tests for movement of the lumbo-pelvic-hip complex and transfer of weight-bearing through the complex can be carried out with the person standing or sitting. If the person is seated, have him or her plant the feet on the ground or use a stool for support to improve stability and allow for maximum forward flexion of the trunk. When both SI joints function normally, and barring other influencing factors (e.g. a functional LLD or asymmetry of muscle tension), the movement of the L5 vertebral complex and movement of the sacrum and the ilia (= PSIS) on trunk flexion and extension is as one symmetrical unit rotating on the femoral heads (Figs 2.116, 2.117). A unilateral test will see a thumb placed on the sacrum rotate upward relative to that placed on the PSIS as the sacrum nutates on initial trunk flexion (Figs 2.17, 2.18, 2.118). The tests are carried out as described in Box 2.6.

One can encounter an abnormal sacral flexion/extension test for reasons other than dysfunction of movement of one or other SI joint. As Lee & Walsh already emphasized in 1996, these tests examine lower quadrant function in forward flexion and extension rather than being specific for SI joint mobility. For example, a positive forward-flexion test can result from unilateral restriction of flexion of the hip joint, piriformis muscle spasm or hypertonicity of the hamstrings (Lee 1992b, 2004a). The presence or absence of

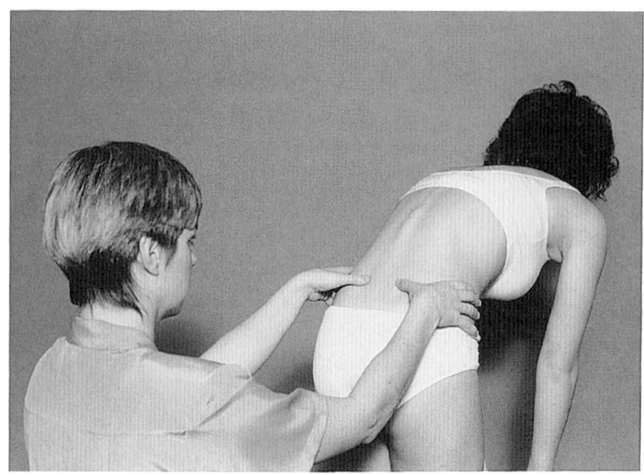

Fig. 2.117 Normal lumbosacral flexion/extension test. Thumbs on the transverse processes of the L5 vertebra travel an equal distance, upward on flexion and downward on extension. *(Courtesy of Lee 1999.)*

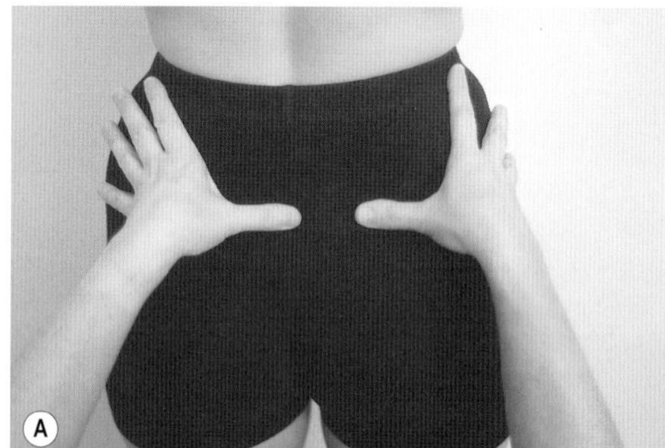

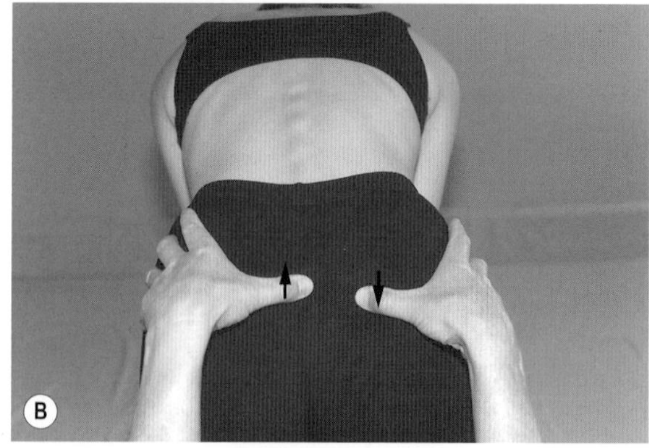

Fig. 2.118 Normal sacroiliac flexion/extension test. (A) Right thumb on the posterior superior iliac spine, left on the adjoining sacral base. (B) On the initial 45 degrees of flexion, the thumb on the sacrum has moved upward slightly relative to that on the ilium with movement of the sacral base into nutation and relative right innominate posterior rotation (see also Figs 2.17, 2.18).

BOX 2.6 Flexion and extension tests

1. A thumb is placed on the identical points on the ilium on each side (e.g. just inferior to the PSIS). The thumbs will move in unison to an equal extent once the sacrum and the innominates start to move together: upward on trunk flexion (Fig. 2.116A), downward on trunk extension (Fig. 2.116B).
2. L5 should also move symmetrically on these tests (Fig. 2.117): fingers placed on the transverse processes move forward and back together to equal extent in the sagittal plane and there is no evidence of any:
   a. rotation around the vertical axis (moving forward on one side and backward on the other in the transverse plane)
   b. side-flexion (moving up on one side and down on the other in the coronal plane).
3. One thumb is then placed on the ilium, against the inferior aspect of the PSIS and the other on the adjoining part of the sacral base (Fig. 2.118A).
   a. On forward flexion, the sacral base will normally move forward into nutation for approximately the first 45 degrees, with some approximation of the thumbs as the innominates flare out (Fig. 2.17A). Sacral nutation may eventually stop but the innominates continue to rotate anteriorly, with relative sacral counternutation (Fig. 2.18A). The stability of the sacroiliac joints is directly related to the range through which nutation can occur (Lee 1999, 2004a).
   b. On back extension, the sacrum normally stays in nutation relative to the innominates (Fig. 2.18C), with some separation of the thumbs.

such conditions will dictate the appropriate treatment. Carrying the test out in a sitting position will decrease, or even eliminate, some of the factors that affect lower quadrant function in standing.

Clinical correlation: flexion/extension tests

Sacroiliac joint 'upslip' and anatomical leg length difference
Neither an 'upslip' in isolation nor an anatomical (true) LLD is associated with evidence of movement dysfunction on the flexion/extension tests. With a 'right upslip', for example, the right PSIS remains higher than the left to an equal extent throughout the full range of flexion and extension carried out in either standing or sitting (Fig. 2.119B). Findings are similar when testing someone with an anatomical (true) long right leg but only in standing; whereas the PSIS and other pelvic landmarks will be level in sitting.

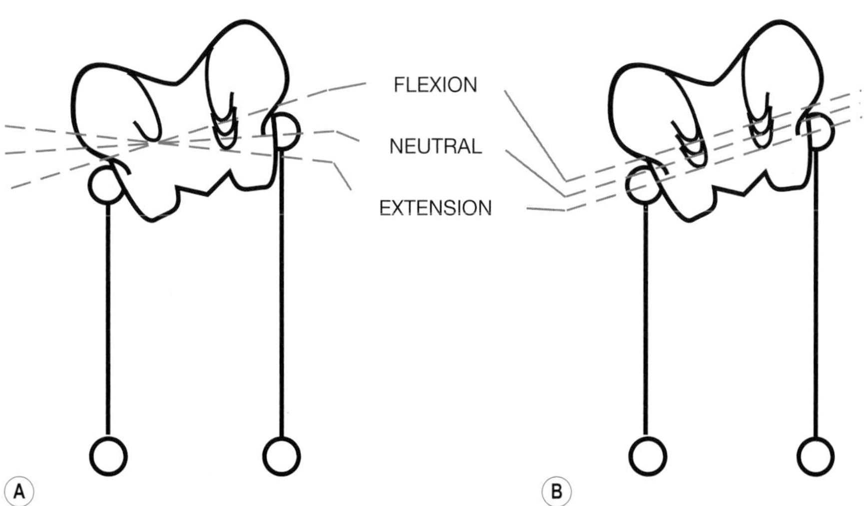

Fig. 2.119 Normal and abnormal changes in the position of the right relative to the left posterior superior iliac spine (PSIS) with trunk flexion and extension in standing. (A) With 'locking' of the right sacroiliac joint: excessive movement of the right PSIS upward with flexion, downward with extension relative to the left. (B) With an anatomical (true) leg length difference (right leg long) or a 'right upslip': the right and left PSIS will move upward and downward in unison and to an equal extent.

'Rotational malalignment'

Assuming an otherwise normal lower quadrant function, these tests will be abnormal when the excessive 'anterior' or 'posterior' rotation of an innominate bone has resulted in:

1. asymmetric movement of the pelvic ring on the femoral heads
2. a decrease of the amount of movement possible at one SI joint relative to the other, or even
3. a complete loss of movement, or 'locking', of one SI joint.

With 'locking' of the right SI joint, for example, the sacrum and the right innominate now move as one unit on trunk flexion and extension. Therefore, the right thumb will move relatively further than the left, upward on flexion and downward on extension (Figs 2.119A, 2.120). Remember that, with 'rotational malalignment', the right and left PSIS are usually no longer level in the neutral position, standing or sitting. To start with, the right may be noticeably higher or lower than the left. Therefore, with 'right anterior' rotation, and especially with a coexistent 'locking' of the right SI joint,

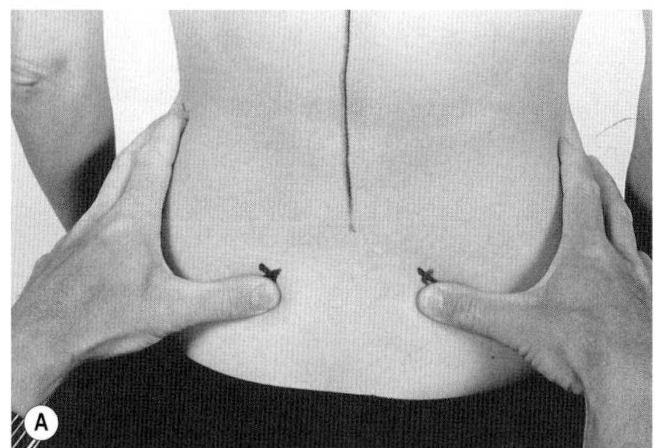

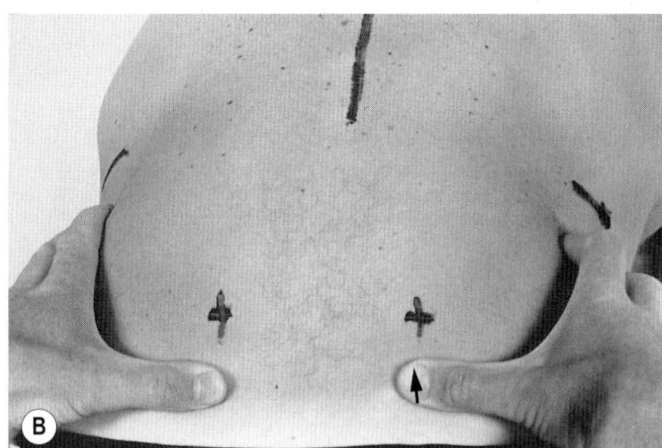

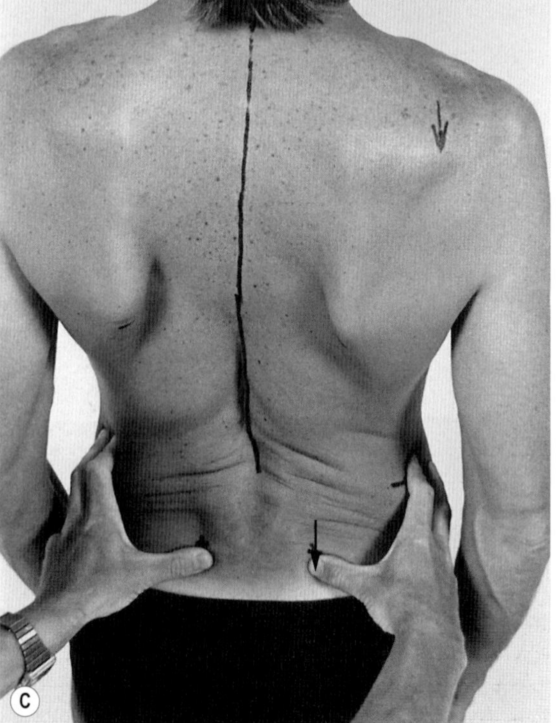

Fig. 2.120 Abnormal sacroiliac flexion/extension tests with 'rotational malalignment': right anterior and 'locked', left posterior. (A) In standing upright, the level of right posterior superior iliac spine (PSIS) is just above that of the left. (B) On trunk flexion: the right PSIS has moved even further upward. (C) On trunk extension: the right PSIS has moved below the left. Note: extension has accentuated the scoliotic curves, making the lumbar segment especially easier to discern.

comparison of the right and left thumb placed on the respective PSIS would show:

1. on forward flexion:
   a. a right PSIS that was lower than the left one to start with in the neutral standing position could end up level with or higher than the left
   b. if the right PSIS was already higher than the left one to start (Fig. 2.120A), the difference between them would increase (Fig. 2.120B)
2. on trunk extension:
   a. a right PSIS that was higher in the neutral position might become level with or end up lower than the left one (Figs 2.119A, 2.120C)
   b. if it was lower than the left to start with, the difference between them would increase.

Similar changes would occur on the flexion-extension test on comparing movement of a thumb placed on the PSIS to that of the other one placed at the same level on the sacrum (approximately at S2). In the person presenting with the 'left anterior and locked' pattern, the changes in relative PSIS movement would be the opposite to those discussed above for 'right anterior and locked'.

As with the 'sitting-lying' test, it is the relative change in position on these flexion-extension tests that is of prime importance to help diagnose the presence of a 'locking' of a joint and 'rotational malalignment' versus an 'upslip' (where the landmarks, though asymmetric, still move in unison and to an equal extent, as with a true LLD; Fig. 2.119B).

Ipsilateral kinetic rotational test (Gillet test, stork test)

The Gillet test is a test for:

1. the ability to balance while weight-bearing on one leg
2. the ability for parts of the pelvic girdle on the non-weight-bearing side to continue to undergo some rotation while those on the weight-bearing side become 'fixed' or stabilized as load is transferred through the pelvic girdle onto that leg.

The 'kinetic' tests can assess dynamic function of the pelvis with the person in the:

1. standing flexion phase
   a. ability to flex the hip on the non-weight-bearing side, to test ease of movement and mobility in the lumbo-pelvic-hip complex and, in particular, the SI joint
2. standing support phase
   a. ability to transfer a load through the low back, pelvis and hip onto the weight-bearing side
   b. ability of the pelvis 'to allow some intrapelvic rotation' (Hungerford 2002) while remaining stable in its starting position in both the coronal and sagittal plane (Hungerford et al. 2004)

Single-support 'kinetic' test

The full test entails assessing comparitive movement of the sacrum/innominates in the non-weight-bearing and support phase on active flexion and extension of the hip joint. For a test of the right side, the examiner initially places the right thumb against the inferior aspect of the right PSIS and the left thumb on the midline of the sacrum at the S2 level (Fig. 2.121A). The test is carried out as follows:

Right single non-weight-bearing phase

1. *'posterior rotational' or 'flexion' tests* (Fig. 2.121B)
   a. Right hip flexion to 90 degrees will normally cause the right innominate to rotate posteriorly relative to the sacrum. Therefore, the thumb on the right innominate will move downward relative to the left thumb resting on the sacrum (Fig. 2.121C). Flexion of the right hip higher than horizontal should result in further posterior rotation of the right innominate and downward displacement of the right thumb (i.e., right PSIS).
   b. With the right innominate posterior rotation, there will also be some simultaneous:
      i. left rotation of the sacrum around the vertical axis and torquing around the left oblique axis, as well as
      ii. left axial rotation of L5 coupled with side-flexion of the vertebral complex (Figs 2.21, 2.41).

The same test is then carried out on the left side for comparison to the movement seen on right hip flexion (Fig. 2.122). Comparative decrease of ease of

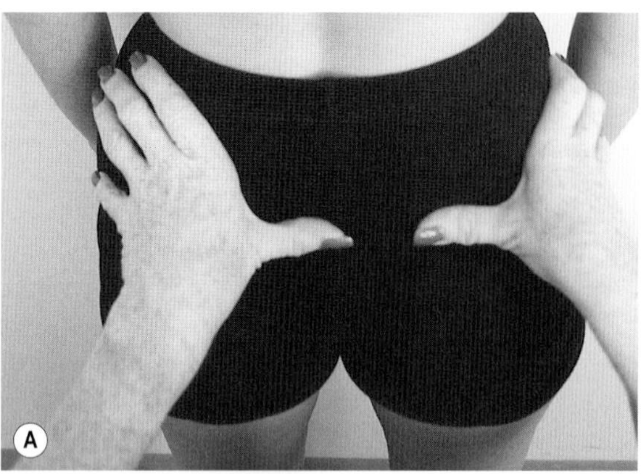

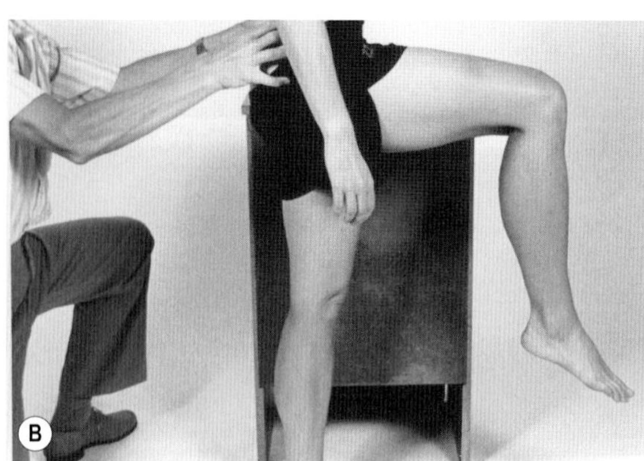

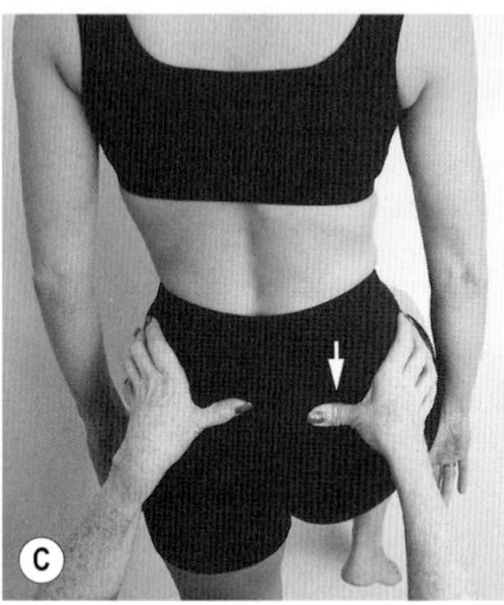

Fig. 2.121 Normal posterior kinetic rotational (Gillet) tests: hip flexion. (A) Starting position for the test on the right (the reverse of that seen in Fig. 2.122A). (B) Set-up for testing, with a side table to provide support should balance become a problem. (C) Right hip flexion: posterior rotation of the right innominate displaces the right thumb downward relative to that on the sacrum by an amount equal to that observed on carrying out the test on the left side (see Fig. 2.122B).

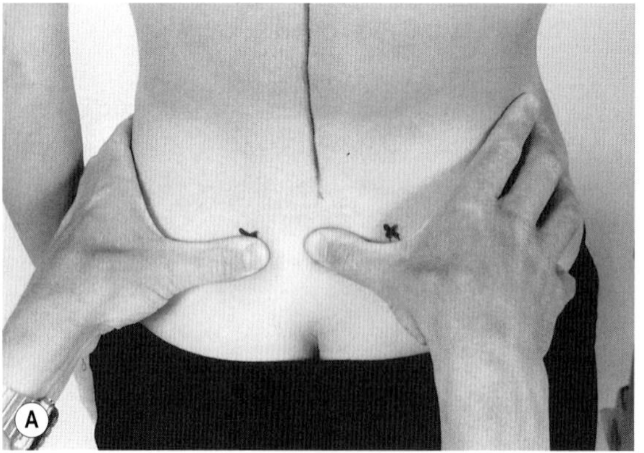

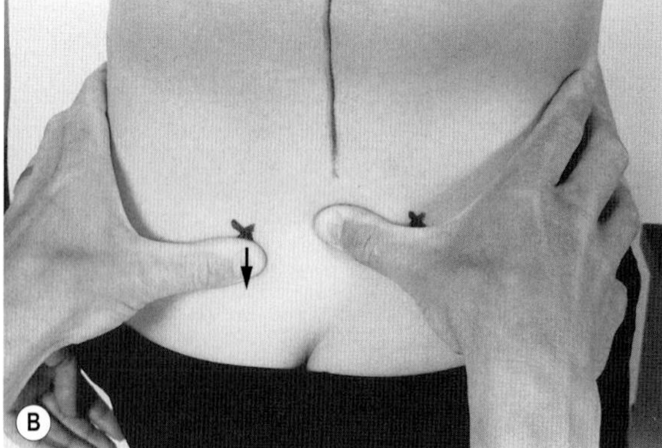

Fig. 2.122 Normal left Gillet test. (A) Starting position for the test: the left thumb placed against the inferior aspect of the left posterior superior iliac spine (PSIS), the right on the sacral base just lateral to the median sacral crest and level with the left thumb. (B) Left hip flexion: posterior rotation of left innominate displaces the left thumb (= PSIS) downward relative to that on the sacrum.

movement and/or abnormal movement may suggest impaired function involving the lumbo-pelvic-hip complex on one side.

2. ***'anterior rotational' or 'extension' tests***

   To test the right side, the person weight-bears on the left and increasingly extends the right hip joint (Fig. 2.123). Normally, this results in findings opposite to those seen on right hip flexion, namely: anterior rotation of the right innominate relative to the sacrum, with right axial rotation of the sacrum and right axial rotation and side-flexion of L5. The right thumb will move upward relative to the left one placed on the sacrum. Again, the left side is also tested to allow for comparison of range and ease of movement and mobility.

Right single-support phase

The stability required to turn the sacrum and an adjoining innominate into one unit capable of transfering weight through the ipsilateral SI joint depends in large part on:

1. alignment of the sacrum and ilium
2. intact, strong supportive ligaments
3. contraction of the muscles that stabilize that SI joint (e.g. iliopsoas, piriformis and gluteus maximus),

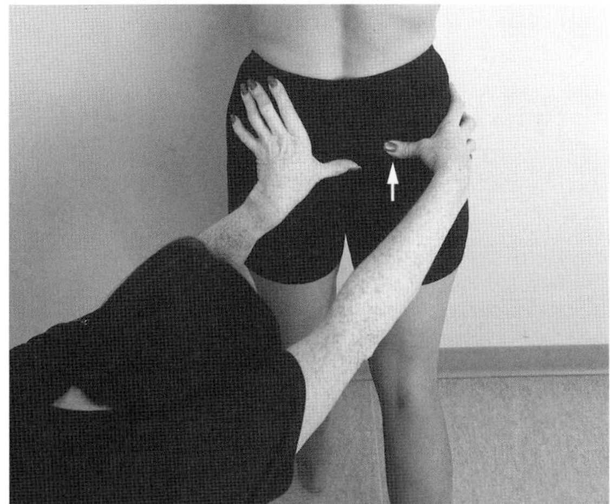

Fig. 2.123 Normal anterior kinetic rotational (Gillet) test: hip extension. Starting position for the test on the right side as in Fig. 2.121A (for the left: as in Fig. 2.122A). On right hip extension: anterior rotation of the right innominate displaces the right thumb (=PSIS) upward relative to the left one (resting on the sacrum).

4. the pelvis itself being properly aligned with the spine and femur

To test the single-support phase on the right side, place the right thumb below the PSIS and the left on the sacral midline at S2 level to start (Figs 2.121A, 2.124A). The pelvis functions best when in a vertical position relative to the femur, for weight transfer both through the pelvis and the hip joint. As the person raises the left leg and transfers weight entirely onto the right, 'the innominate should either move toward the vertical position (extend) or remain vertical relative to the femur' to maintain the stability of the unit (Fig. 2.124B). Therefore, when observing for any movement between the thumbs:

1. ***on a normal single-support test***

   There may be no movement at all or some downward movement of the right thumb, indicative of posterior rotation of the innominate relative to the sacrum (i.e., extension relative to the femur; Fig. 2.124B).

2. ***on an abnormal test***

   Changes indicative of 'failed load transfer through the pelvic girdle' (Hungerford et al. 2001, 2004; Hungerford 2002) include:

   a. the right thumb may move upward or outward, indicative of innominate rotation anteriorly or internally relative to the sacrum, respectively
   b. conversely, flexion of the innominate relative to the femur would signify failed load transfer through the hip joint and is recognized as 'a less stable position for load transfer through both the pelvis and the hip joint.' (Lee 2004a).

Comparitive kinetic tests: right versus left side

A normal posterior or anterior rotational test will show the amount of movement of the thumb on the right innominate to be equal to that detected on the left side. A positive (abnormal) kinetic rotational test can occur with movement dysfunction of the SI joint and may be partial or complete. There are, therefore, two possible findings when the dysfunction involves the right SI joint.

1. ***a completely abnormal test***

   'Locking' of the right SI joint is present and does not allow for any posterior rotation of the right innominate relative to the sacrum. For example, in the right 'posterior rotational' or 'flexion' test

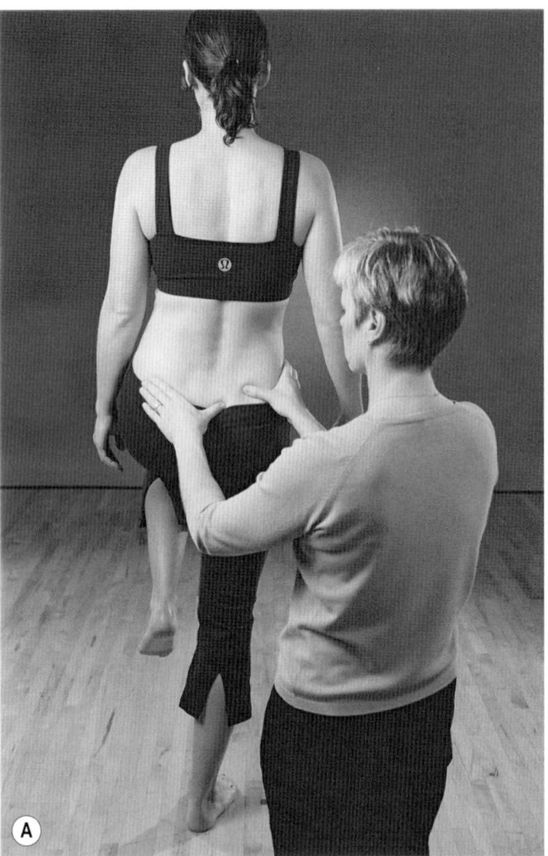

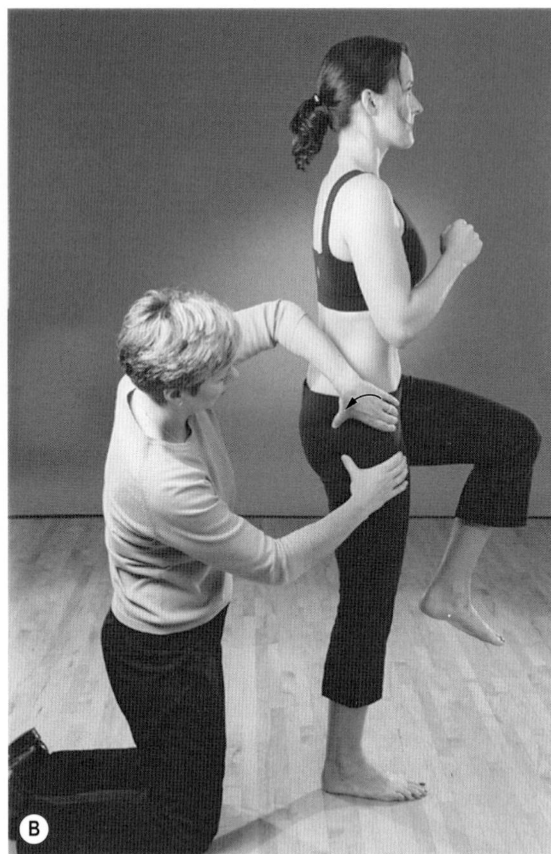

Fig. 2.124 Testing for ability to transfer weight through the hip and SI joint. In the one-leg standing test (single-support phase), the innominate should: (A) remain posteriorly rotated relative to the sacrum; (B) extend relative to the femur (arrow) or remain vertical. This is a stable position for load transfer through the hip joint. *(Courtesy of © Diane G. Lee Physiotherapist Corp.)*

shown in Fig. 2.125, the right thumb (PSIS) fails to move relative to the left (sacrum) on initial right hip flexion (Fig. 2.125A). On attempting to flex the right hip more than 90 degrees, the right thumb will actually begin to move upward (Fig. 2.125B). This finding is in keeping with the fact that further right hip flexion is accomplished by having the 'locked' sacrum and right innominate rotate as one unit, counterclockwise around the sacral axis in the coronal plane. The test will be normal on the left side.

2. ***a partially abnormal test***

   Limited movement between the right sacrum and innominate is possible, allowing some separation of the two thumbs, but perceptibly less on the right side compared to the freely-moving 'unlocked' left side.

A positive kinetic rotational test may also occur with intrinsic hip joint abnormality, lumbar spine scoliosis or leg length inequality (Bernard & Cassidy 1991) as well as with various lesions of the ipsilateral 'iliosacral' joint or the lumbar spine (Fowler 1986). Therefore, one should never rely on just one of the above test in isolation when attempting to establish the diagnosis of malalignment and SI joint dysfunction.

Clinical correlation: kinetic tests

1. Anatomical LLD, SI joint 'upslip' and 'outflare/inflare' The test is negative.
2. 'Rotational malalignment'

The test may be positive, with evidence of a partial or complete loss of SI joint mobility or 'locking' on one side. This 'locking' may resolve completely or

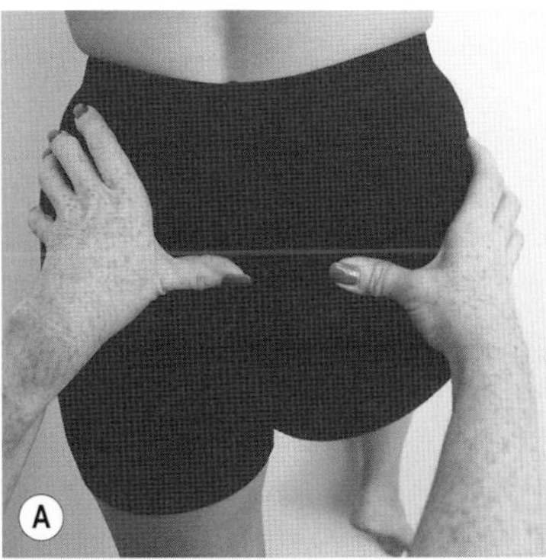

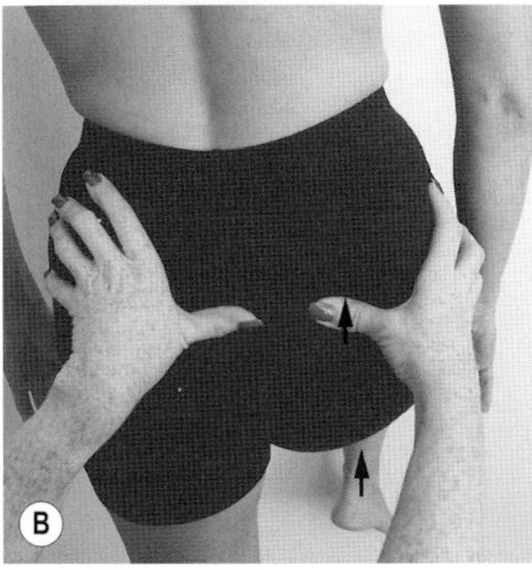

Fig. 2.125 Abnormal right kinetic rotational test (right sacroiliac joint 'locked'). (A) Right hip flexion: the right posterior superior iliac spine (PSIS) fails to drop down relative to the sacral base (relatively unchanged from Fig. 2.121A, view of person standing on both feet). (B) On increasing right hip flexion: the right PSIS actually moves upward - the sacrum and right innominate are moving together as one 'locked' unit, counterclockwise in the coronal (frontal) plane.

come back only rarely in the early course of treatment, even though malalignment of the pelvis is still recurring and any realignment achieved at any time during this stage is more likely to be maintained for only short periods of time.

EVALUATION OF LOAD TRANSFER ABILITY: ACTIVE STRAIGHT LEG RAISING

Active straight leg raising (ASLR), with or without reinforcement to engage the 'form' and 'force' closure mechanisms, can be used to:

1. evaluate the person's ability to transfer load from the trunk through the lumbosacral junction, pelvic girdle and hip joint to the lower extremity, either in prone or supine-lying
2. help localize pain originating from these regions

Right ASLR in supine-lying normally results in changes similar to those that occur during the gait cycle as the right leg swings forward, in preparation for heel-strike and weight transfer, namely:

1. posterior rotation of the right innominate and relative anterior rotation of the sacral base on the right, with sacral nutation, tightening of the sacrotuberous, sacrospinous and posterior SI joint ligaments (Figs 2.19A, 2.21), and stabilization of the right SI joint (DonTigny 1985)
2. a tendency of the whole pelvis to rotate around the vertical axis toward the raised right leg (Jull et al. 1993, 2000)
3. a simultaneous rotation at the lumbosacral junction in the opposite direction, with tightening of the right iliolumbar ligaments and a further decrease in movement of the right SI joint

Provided the local and global systems are functioning normally, the overall effect on carrying out a right ASLR is a stabilization of both the lumbosacral junction and the right SI joint, which in turn allows for a more effective load transfer from the spine to the leg on that side (Snijders et al. 1993a). In a stable pelvis, any adjustments are minimal; movement is limited to the hip joint (Fig. 2.126A). Increasingly strained movement of the lower extremity, pelvis or thorax suggests that there is a problem (Fig. 2.126B). Mens et al. in 1997 described how a decreased ability to actively straight leg raise while lying supine seemed to correlate with an abnormally increased mobility of the pelvic girdle, as evaluated by movement at the symphysis pubis on X-ray (Fig. 2.102A). In the attempt to improve pelvic stability, typical compensatory measures include:

1. activation of muscles in the local and global systems to stabilize the trunk, lumbosacral and pelvic regions (Fig. 2.126B)
2. initial internal rotation of the left leg, then rotation of the pelvis and finally thorax toward the side on which the ASLR is being carried out
3. Valsalva (breath holding) manoeuvre with abdominal distension (Fig. 2.127A), and sometimes obvious diastasis of the linea alba (Fig. 2.127B)
4. overactivity of external and internal obliques, with indrawing of chest cage and outflare of lower ribs, respectively, and overall limitation of lateral costal expansion on inspiration
5. overactivity of erector spinae, with thoracic spine extension

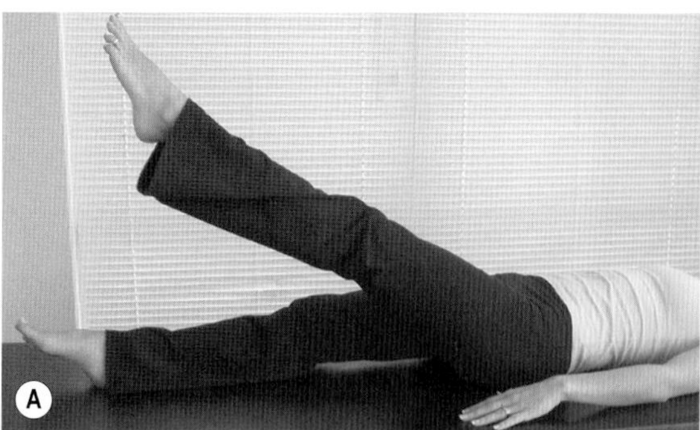

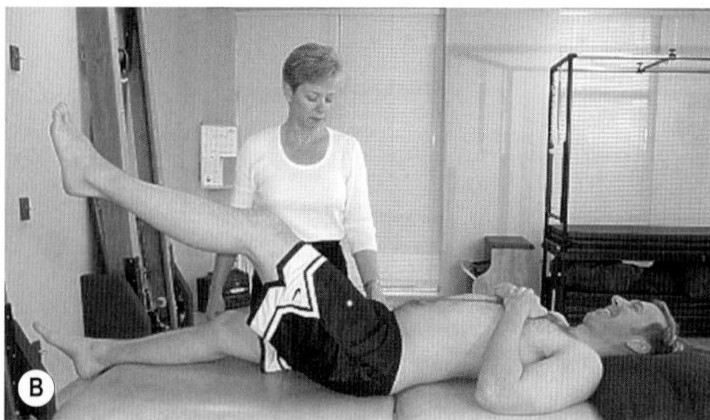

Fig. 2.126 Active straight leg raising (ASLR) used as a 'clinical test for measuring effective load transfer between the trunk and lower limbs' (p106). (A) An optimal ASLR. The only joint moving is the hip joint. The thorax, lumbar spine and pelvic girdle remain stable due to the co-activation of the local and global systems. (B) ASLR with loss of lumbopelvic stability - note the abdominal bulging, anterior pelvic tilt, and thoracic extension as well as the extreme effort required to lift the left leg. *(Courtesy of © Diane G. Lee Physiotherapist Corp.)*

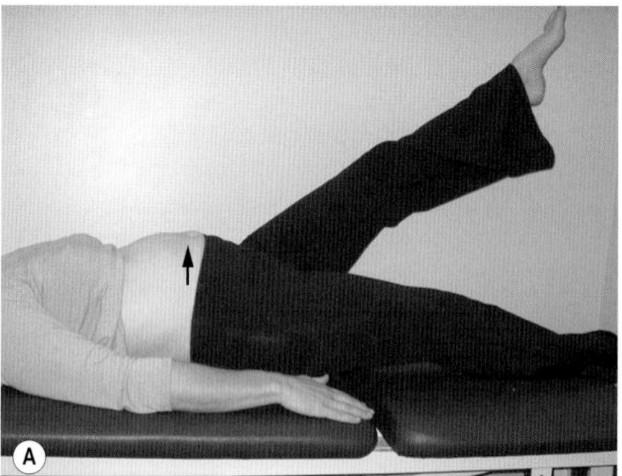

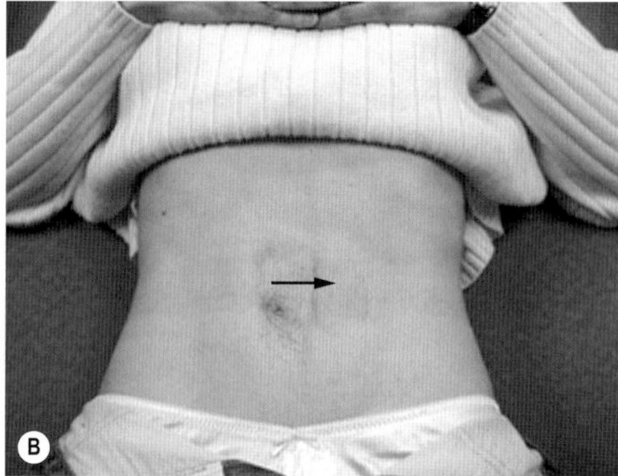

Fig. 2.127 Weakness of abdominal wall fascia and muscles. (A) ASLR with excessive abdominal bulging (arrow) on active straight leg raising and breath-holding: a Valsalva manoeuvre. (B) A large three-finger width diastasis of the linea alba. *(Courtesy of Lee 2004a.)*

Note is made of the following:

1. the degree of active straight leg raising (ASLR) possible on each side
2. the ease with which the ASLR is carried out (both as observed and as reported by the person)
3. any compensatory movements of the pelvis or trunk; these usually involve rotation of the pelvis and opposite leg toward the side of the leg being raised

The ASLR test is carried out both in supine and prone-lying. The person is initially observed performing a functional test, namely comparative unassisted straight leg raising, one leg at a time (Figs 2.128A, 2.129A). In the past, emphasis was on first observing the maximum hip flexion that could be achieved actively on each side and any obvious compensatory measures used in an attempt to improve that range of motion. ASLR was then repeated with addition of measures known to selectively reinforce 'form' and 'force' closure, noting particularly any uni- or bilateral increase in the maximum ROM achieved. Basing the test on evaluation of maximum hip flexion range, unfortunately, could be limited by problems other than SI joint instability, such as:

1. hip joint degeneration, contracture of surrounding structures (ligaments, capsule, muscles such as the hip extensors)

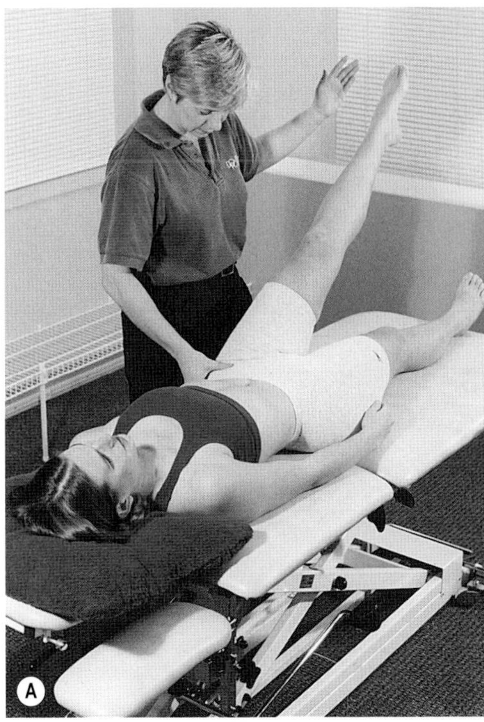

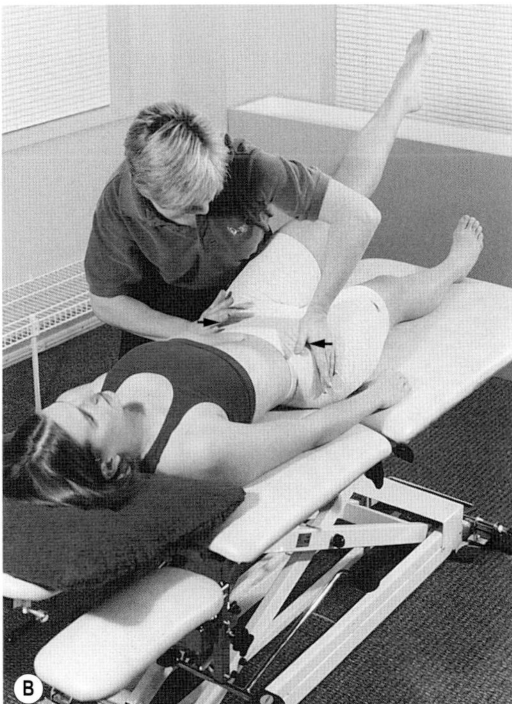

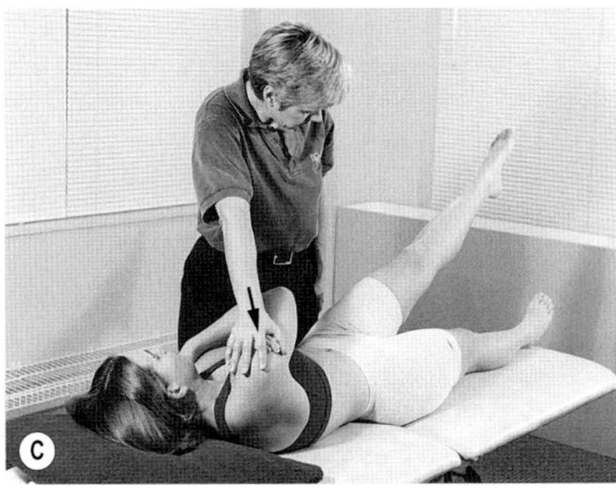

Fig. 2.128 Functional test for sacroiliac joint load transfer ability in supine-lying. (A) Functional test of supine active straight leg raise. (B) With form closure augmented. (C) With force closure augmented. *(Courtesy of Lee 1999.)*

2. pain elicited with pressure on a tender point as weight-bearing shifted across the sacrum/posterior innominate on doing the test
3. increasing tension in the posterior structures with posterior innominate rotation

More recently, stress has been on comparing the ease with which the ASLR test is carried out over a limited range (20-30 cm appears to be the norm) with and without re-enforcement measures (Mens 1999, 2001, 2002; Lee 2004a, 2007b; Richardson et al. 1999; Figs 2.128, 2.129). If dysfunction of load transfer through the pelvis is suspected, supplemental tests are indicated to define whether there is a problem attributable to the passive and/or active system ('form' and 'force' closure, respectively). Any improvement with addition of these measures would be suggested by:

1. an increase in the ease with which this manoeuvre is now carried out over the same range
2. a decrease in pain
3. a decreased need to rely on compensatory measures

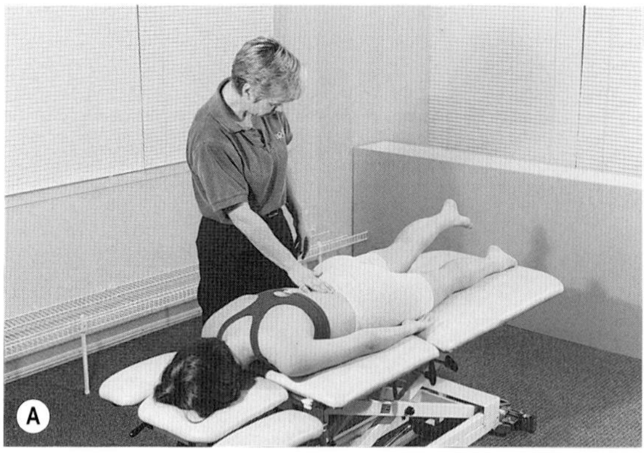

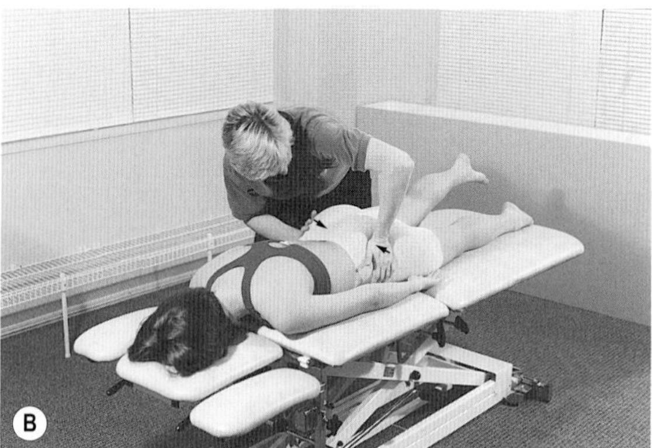

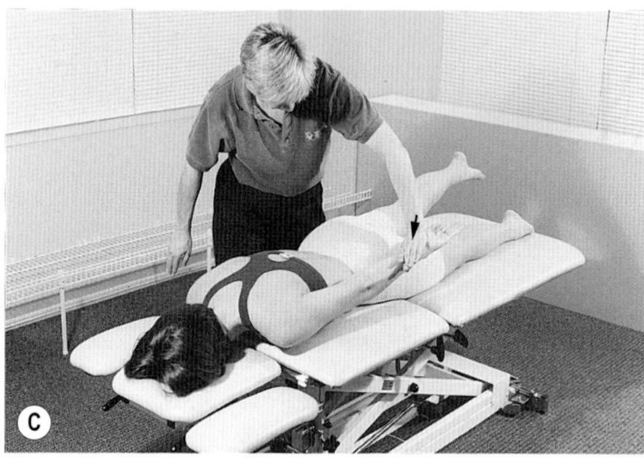

Fig. 2.129 Functional test for sacroiliac joint load transfer ability in prone-lying. (A) Functional test of prone active straight leg raise. (B) With form closure augmented. (C) With force closure augmented. *(Courtesy of Lee 1999.)*

Form closure (passive system) to supplement ASLR

An augmentation of 'form' closure which affects either the symphysis pubis or SI joint or both may be achieved with a medially directed compression force applied at different levels to the lateral aspect of the innominates. The repeat ASLR is carried out simultaneous with or immediately after application of the force (Figs 2.128B, 2.129B). Any improvement achieved suggests that the reinforcement has been able to partially or completely:

1. compensate for loss of the passive supporting system (e.g. joint laxity attributable to osteoarthritic degeneration and/or ligament lengthening or tear)
2. simulate the force produced by 'inner' and/or 'outer' core muscles; as documented by Lee (2004a, 2007b), some of the correlates of which sites were compressed and the muscles affected include:
   a. compression of anterior pelvis at level of ASIS bilaterally, simulating action of transversus abdominis (Fig. 2.128B)
   b. compression of posterior pelvis at level of PSIS bilaterally, simulating action of the sacral multifidi (Fig. 2.129B)

Effects evoked by compression at the pubic level (Fig. 130A), across the pelvis (Fig. 2.130B) and also by a decompression manoeuvre (Fig. 2.130C), are as illustrated.

The aim is to find 'the location where more (or less) compression reduces the effort necessary to lift the leg - the place where the patient noted: 'that feels marvelous!' (Lee 2004a: 107). This information can be useful in designing a sacral belt, compression shorts or combination (see Ch. 7) that:

1. actually applies pressure to a specific point or points in muscle, ligament or overlying bone that gives the most relief on the test, rather than applying uniform pressure at one level in the transverse plane (usually lying just below the ASIS), as has been the custom in the past (Figs. 7.34, 7.35).
2. applies selective medial pressure to the pelvic ring for effect; for example:

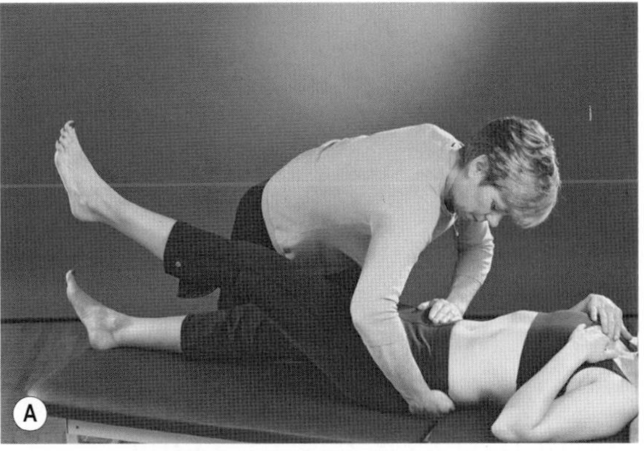

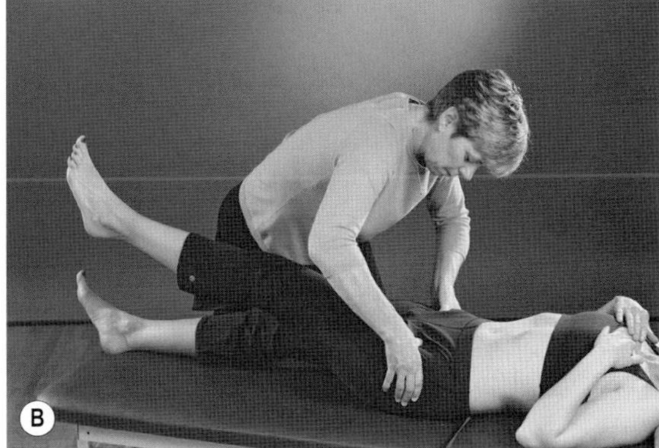

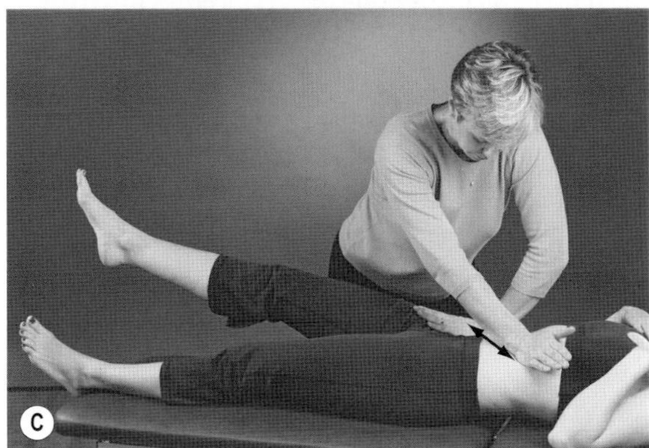

Fig. 2.130 (A) Compression of the right anterior pelvis and left posterior pelvis stimulates the action of the right transversus abdominis and the sacral multifidus.
(B) Compression of the anterior pelvis at the level of the pubic symphysis stimulates the action of the pelvic floor muscles.
(C) Decompression (lengthening) applied obliquely between the thorax and pelvis stimulates releasing the oblique sling system. The arrow indicates the direction of force applied by the therapist's hands. (See also Ch. 7 and Figs 7.34-7.36).
(Courtesy of © Diane G. Lee Physiotherapy Corp.)

a. to the innominates at a level above, at, or below the level of the ASIS to compress the anterior, decompress the posterior SI joint at that level bilaterally
b. to the lower innominate to put pressure on the pubic joint
c. to the innominates at points known to improve action in certain core muscles, if that has been helpful on the ASLR test; e.g. right ASIS and left PSIS, to stimulate the action of right transversus abdominis and left sacral multifidus (Fig. 2.130A)

'Force' closure (active, motor control system) to supplement ASLR

Improvement achieved by an augmentation of force closure suggests that the problem is primarily the result of a loss of strength in the supporting muscles, failure to coordinate muscle activation, or a combination of these.

Activating the 'inner core' system

ASLR is attempted while contracting transversus abdomini, multifidi, thoracic diaphragm and/or the pelvic floor muscles (Figs 2.28, 2.29, 2.53).

Activating the 'outer core' or global system

ALSR is repeated bilaterally to evaluate whether improvement has been achieved by activating parts of the global system on either side. For example, when testing the anterior oblique system, if the right side appears normal and only the left side shows improvement on reinforcement, it would suggest that there is a problem involving the left system that will hopefully respond to selective treatment.

1. *Anterior oblique system*
   After first carrying out left active straight leg raising in supine lying, the person is asked to repeat the manoeuvre immediately after having activated the anterior oblique system, or sling (Fig. 2.39). Activation is accomplished by fully flexing the right elbow, then reaching with that elbow over toward the left knee,

effectively flexing and rotating the trunk toward the left (Fig. 2.128C). Activation can be further augmented by resisting trunk rotation with pressure against the right anterior shoulder.

2. ***Posterior oblique system***
   After first carrying out the right ASLR in prone-lying, the person would then be asked to repeat hip extension immediately after having first extended and medially rotated the left arm against a steady resistance offered by the examiner (Fig. 2.129C). During this test, note is also made of the sequence of muscle activation: increasing resistance should first activate left latissimus dorsi, then augment tension in the thoracodorsal fascia to prime the rest of the posterior oblique system prior to actively extending the right leg starting with gluteus maximus and followed by the hamstrings, in particular biceps femoris (Fig. 2.35, 2.37).

SIMULTANEOUS BILATERAL SI JOINT MALALIGNEMNT

Discussion has been restricted primarily to the two major presentations, namely 'rotational malalignment' and SI joint 'upslip', both of which result in an asymmetric distortion of the pelvic ring and are associated with the 'malalignment syndrome' (Ch. 3). 'Outflare/inflare' lacks the features of the 'malalignment syndrome' but also causes a specific distortion, perhaps less dramatic, with some asymmetry and other biomechanical changes. For the sake of completion, brief mention must be made of some problems that relate to alignment but present with a symmetrical pelvic ring and also lack the features typical of the 'malalignment syndrome'. The diagnosis is often delayed or missed altogether because of a paucity of physical findings or difficulty in interpreting the signs and symptoms.

SYMMETRICAL MOVEMENT OF THE INNOMINATES RELATIVE TO THE SACRUM

Excessive simultaneous bilateral rotation of the innominates, either 'anteriorly' or 'posteriorly', and bilateral 'upslips' or 'downslips' can occur (DonTigny 1985, Richard 1986). These present primarily with signs of movement restriction in one direction, along with a displacement of the landmarks that, however, remains symmetrical and may, therefore, make any abnormality difficult to diagnose. Presentations to consider include:

Excessive 'bilateral anterior' innominate rotation

This presentation can occur if someone:

1. sustains an upward force through both lower extremities simultaneously when they are

Case History 2.1

A woman suffered a shear injury of her right sacroiliac joint when her right leg shot out in front of her on a wet floor and she landed primarily on her right buttock. The right sacroiliac joint was unstable in both the anteroposterior and craniocaudal planes, making it impossible to maintain any correction of the malalignment even for short periods of time. The results of active straight leg raising (ASLR) tests were as follows:

1. Right ASLR raising was to 40 degrees flexion in supine, 10 degrees extension in prone-lying, with pain felt in both positions; the values for the left were 70 and 30 degrees respectively, both pain free. Lateral compression (augmented 'form' closure) improved the values for the right side to 70 degrees supine and 30 prone, with report of a decrease in the associated pain; the values on the left side remained unchanged.
2. Activation of 'inner core' and the anterior and posterior oblique systems (augmented 'force' closure) failed to improve the values on either side.

The diagnostic impression was that of a shear injury of the right sacroiliac joint and a loss of 'form' closure, the instability probably being attributable to loss of the ligamentous support. 'Force' closure, derived from core muscle strength and coordination, appeared to be intact. The initial treatment consisted of using a sacroiliac belt and undergoing a course of prolotherapy injections to strengthen and tighten up the ligaments surrounding the right sacroiliac joint. Once ligamentous support had been regained, attempts at realignment and strengthening of the back, pelvic and hip girdle muscles were successfully resumed (see Ch. 7).

positioned with the hip flexed at, or nearly, the same angle (Fig. 2.51A)
2. falls onto the buttocks while the hips and knees are drawn up, so as to land on the anterior aspect of both ischial tuberosities simultaneously

There can result a bilateral restriction of hip flexion and straight leg raising, attributable to:

1. the mechanical limitation caused by impingement of the femoral head against the anteriorly rotated superior acetabular rims (Figs 2.47A, 2.109)
2. the increased tension in gluteus maximus, hamstrings and the posterior SI joint ligaments attributable to the increase in the distance between their origins and insertions
3. bilateral increase in hip extension, with the posterior rotation of the acetabular rim and relaxation of hip flexors (e.g. iliopsoas, TFL, rectus femoris)
4. a symmetrical upward movement of the PSIS bilaterally, making these landmarks more prominent
5. symmetrical downward movement and bilateral depression of the ASIS and pubic bones
6. sacral rotation into relative counternutation, a position of SI joint instability (Fig. 2.11B)

Excessive 'bilateral posterior' innominate rotation

This presentation can occur with a force that acts simultaneously:

1. upward on both lower extremities, when they are positioned with the hip in some extension to about the same degree bilaterally, or
2. onto the posterior aspect of the ischial tuberosities

There would result changes that are the opposite to those documented for 'bilateral anterior rotation' above; namely, relative sacral nutation (= stability) and simultaneous bilateral:

1. restriction of hip extension by the posterior rotation of the inferior acetabular rim and the increased tension in the hip flexor muscles
2. upward displacement of ASIS and pubic bones while the PSIS moves downward bilaterally

SACRAL ROTATION AROUND THE CORONAL AXIS

Some of the abnormal presentations involve excessive rotation of the sacrum around the coronal axis in the sagittal plane. For example, falling and landing on the sacral apex or the coccyx can rotate the base backward, into excessive counternutation; whereas a blow to the base can rotate it forward, into excessive nutation. Although landmarks are altered, their symmetry is preserved and that may be misleading. Richard (1986, p. 26) described the following:

'Bilateral sacrum anterior'

This lesion can result with hyperextension of the pelvis and spine. The sacrum becomes fixed in counternutation, with the base actually backward and the apex forward in 'flexion angulation'. The sacrospinous ligaments, which come to play the role of a pivot, are put under increased tension and are at risk of injury, as are the long dorsal sacroiliac ligaments bilaterally (Fig. 2.19B); whereas the pelvic floor muscles become hypotonic (Fig. 4.44C). The sacral sulci diminish or disappear, and the apex becomes less prominent. The lumbar lordosis is decreased or abolished, and the lumbar segment feels 'stiff' when one applies pressure to the spinous processes. The person may complain of back pain and difficulty in stooping forward.

The lumbosacral plexus bilaterally is put under increased tension (Fig. 4.15). A separation of iliacus and rectus femoris origins and insertions increases tension in these muscles bilaterally which, in turn, limits hip extension and decreases the space available for the exiting femoral and obturator nerves (Figs 4.14 and 4.15, respectively). There may be symptoms of bilateral groin discomfort and paraesthesias, suggestive of femoral and/or obturator nerve irritation, and the femoral stretch test may be positive.

'Bilateral sacrum posterior'

Excessive backward rotation of the apex and forward rotation of the sacral base (nutation) is sometimes seen following excessive forward flexion of the trunk and pelvis. It results in a uniform deepening of the sacral sulci and a uniform increase in the prominence of the inferolateral sacral angles and the sacral apex. The lumbar lordosis is increased; the lumbar segment feels supple and elastic when pressure is applied to the spinous processes. Resting pressure on the facet joints is increased and nerve roots may be compromised by a narrowing of the intervertebral foramina.

Tension in the sacrotuberous ligaments and hamstrings is increased by a separation of their origin and insertion (Fig. 2.19A); hip flexion is reduced, and all these structures, which may be tender to palpation, are now at an increased risk of injury. Pelvic floor dysfunction can be another complication as tension in the pelvic floor is increased with the apex rotating backward, especially if there is a coexistent excessive 'extension angulation' of the coccyx (see Fig. 4.44B). The person may complain of recurrent cramps in the hamstrings, and of pain from the lower sacral region and ischial attachments of the sacrotuberous ligaments.

These conditions are mentioned mainly to point out that there are other presentations involving rotation of pelvic structures that can be a major cause of debility. Unlike with an 'upslip' or 'rotational malalignment', however:

1. the symmetry of the landmarks is preserved
2. there is no associated 'malalignment syndrome'

THE STANDARD BACK EXAMINATION CAN BE MISLEADING

It cannot be emphasized strongly enough that the standard medical back examination is often completely normal in the person presenting with malalignment. Indeed, it may be expected to be normal depending on the scope of the examination, which usually will be limited to looking at the back and asking the patient to go through trunk flexion, extension, side-flexion and simultaneous extension with rotation to right and left, primarily to see if any of these provoke pain. There is less emphasis, if any, on whether there is a comparitive loss of range of motion, asymmetry of landmarks and/or limitation of a particular pattern of movement that would be in keeping with an underlying problem, such as malalignment (Ch. 3). The examination may include tests to stress specific joints (e.g. hips, facet joints, discs). However, if symptoms are due to an alignment problem, these manoeuvres may fail to provoke pain as these joints are not necessarily stressed:

1. by the underlying presentation of malalignment to actually becoming symptomatic, or
2. by the examiner to the point of provoking the pain

As will become increasingly evident in the following chapters, the different presentations of malalignment stress specific joints and soft tissues of the pelvis, spine and lower extremities, typically in an asymmetrical pattern. On doing the standard musculoskeletal examination, findings may be limited to noting tenderness in some ligament, tendon or muscle. Detection of such tenderness is too often misinterpreted as defining a localized problem (e.g. a 'bursitis' or a 'stretched' tendon or muscle). The examination does not necessarily stress the structures typically stressed by malalignment, or in such a way or hard enough as to actually provoke pain. Usually, in the standard examination, there is:

1. no comparison of the degree of tenderness, leave alone tension, detectable in the same structure on the opposite side
2. no search for the more global, but still specific, predictable patterns seen with involvement of the lumbo-pelvic-hip complex that define the various presentations of malalignment.

Evaluation of any abnormal patterns, if persued, is usually limited to observations that the pelvis is up on one side, one shoulder is lower than the other, the right or left leg is 'longer' (with no indication of whether this difference was seen in standing, sitting or lying) and failure to observe if a change in position altered the findings - all observations that would help establish whether malalignment is present and what particular presentation, to allow one to proceed with appropiate treatment.

Unfortunately, the fact that the limited standard examination has failed to elicit pain or establish that there are patterns of asymmetry signifying malalignment is present is often interpreted to mean that the person does not have a problem, when the real problem is that the clinician's examination skills are limited and, in fact, inadequate for establishing the diagnosis of malalignment. At the same time, it must be remembered that even if the examiner is familiar with the tests for malalignment, the diagnosis of this condition should be based on the findings on several forms of assessment, not just on the results of one or two tests alone. The examination should include an evaluation of:

1. leg length in more than one position
2. the typical patterns of asymmetry of landmarks, muscle strength and tension, weight bearing, joint ranges of motion as well as other aspects of the 'malalignment syndrome' (Ch. 3)

> Once the presence of malalignment has been established, one must avoid falling into the trap of automatically assuming that all of the person's complaints are attributable to the malalignment.

For those familiar with malalignment and the problems it presents, there is never any excuse for not carrying out at least a basic orthopaedic, neurological and vascular examination in order to rule out other pathology. Only this will allow one to determine, with some degree of certainty whether:

1. some or all of the person's symptoms are attributable to the malalignment
2. there is possibly an underlying/associated medical problem that is being covered-up by the the malalignment and
3. there is a need to proceed with other investigations and/or treatment efforts in addition to realignment

The intent of this chapter has been to provide a sound basis for the examination techniques that will be of help in recognizing whether a biomechanical problem such as malalignment of the pelvis and spine is present and could account for a person's complaints. Chapter 3 will present the 'malalignment syndrome': the secondary effects on the soft tissues and joints caused be two of the three common presentations: namely, 'upslip' and 'rotational malalignment'. Recognizing the features of this syndrome should further aid in making the distinction between problems caused by the malalignment, an underlying medical problem, or both.

Chapter 3

The Malalignment Syndrome

CHAPTER CONTENTS

DOI: 10.1016/B978-0-443-06929-1.00003-X

An 'upslip' or 'rotational malalignment' of the sacroiliac joint never exist in isolation: there are always associated changes involving both the axial and appendicular skeleton, the attaching soft tissues - capsules, ligaments, fascia, muscles, tendons - and the nerves. In addition to asymmetries of the skeletal and soft tissue structures, there is also a reorientation of the body segments from head to foot. The combined effect is henceforth referred to as the 'malalignment syndrome'.

CLINICAL FINDINGS COMMONLY NOTED WITH MALALIGNMENT

Malalignment syndrome will be discussed here in terms of findings on the physical examination that are commonly associated with the syndrome (Box 3.1).

The prevalence of malalignment, and of the three most common presentations, has been detailed in Chapter 2. Basically:

1. some 80-90% of adults present out of alignment
2. 'rotational malalignment' is by far the most frequently seen, in approximately 80%, either on its own or in combination with one/both of the other presentations
3. an 'upslip' presents on its own in about 10% and in combination with 'rotational malalignment' and/or an 'outflare/inflare' in another 5-10% of cases
4. 'outflare' and/or 'inflare' is present in approximately 45-50%, either in isolation or combined with one or both of the other types

The 'malalignment syndrome' itself is seen only in association with:

1. 'rotational malalignment'
2. an SI joint 'upslip'.

The discussion will focus first on the 'malalignment syndrome' specifically as seen in association with 'rotational malalignment', with reference to SI joint 'upslip' where appropriate. A separate section

BOX 3.1 Physical findings associated with the 'malalignment syndrome'

1. Asymmetry of pelvic orientation with any movement around the coronal, vertical and sagittal axes and in the three planes
2. Asymmetry of sacroiliac joint mobility
3. Pelvic obliquity and compensatory curvature, or 'scoliosis', of the lumbar, thoracic and cervical spine
4. Asymmetry of the thoracic and shoulder girdle ranges of motion
5. Asymmetry of lower extremity orientation
6. Asymmetry of foot alignment, weight-bearing and shoe wear
7. Asymmetry of muscle tension, strength and bulk
8. Asymmetry of ligament tension
9. Asymmetry of upper and lower extremity ranges of motion
10. Apparent (functional) leg length difference
11. Problems with balance and recovery

emphasizes the major similarities and differences in the presentation of the syndrome seen in association with an SI joint 'upslip', as compared with 'rotational malalignment'. There follows a discussion of the features of an 'outflare/inflare' presentation and how it differs from an 'upslip' and 'rotational malalignment'. Significant clinical correlations are indicated at the end of most of the subheadings. Reference is also made to Chapters 5 and 6 and Appendices 1–13 for a more detailed analysis of the sports-specific implications of this syndrome.

'MALALIGNMENT SYNDROME' SEEN WITH 'ROTATIONAL MALALIGNMENT

'Rotational malalignment' refers to the excessive 'anterior' or 'posterior' rotation of an innominate relative to the sacrum, around the coronal axis in the sagittal plane. The contralateral innominate usually compensates by rotating in the opposite direction. Furthermore, there may be:

1. torsion of the sacrum around the right or left oblique axis, which adds to the distortion of the pelvic ring (Figs 2.42, 2.50)
2. evidence of dysfunction of movement of the symphysis pubis or of one or both SI joints, which can range from hypermobility to various degrees of decreased mobility or even complete 'locking' (see Ch. 2).

DESCRIPTION OF 'ROTATIONAL MALALIGNMENT'

In order to prevent needless repetition, the following abbreviations will be used:

1. 'right (or left) anterior (or posterior)' rotation
   - referring to 'anterior' or 'posterior' rotation of the right or left innominate relative to the sacrum in the sagittal plane (Figs 2.10, 2.21, 2.42, 2.76)
2. 'right (or left) locked' on the kinetic rotational (Gillet) test
   - referring to 'locking' of the right (or left) SI joint (Figs 2.119, 2.120, 2.125)

'Right anterior, left locked', for example, would refer to a person presenting with 'anterior rotation' of the right innominate and 'locking' of the left SI joint; there will very likely also be a compensatory 'posterior' rotation of the left innominate. For illustrative purposes, reference is frequently made to 'right anterior and locked', which refers to the combination of 'right anterior rotation and locking of the right SI joint' because this is the most frequently seen of all these patterns of 'rotational malalignment' (see Appendix 1).

Clinical correlation

Localized pain may arise from one or both SI joints. Those with hypomobility or 'locking' of one SI joint not infrequently complain of pain from the region of the other, supposedly 'normal', SI joint. One explanation is that the pain is attributable to the increased stress placed on this 'normal' joint, its capsule and ligaments as it tries to compensate for the lack of mobility in the impaired SI joint (Figs 2.4, 2.5, 2.19).

The pain may also result from:

1. a passive increase in muscle or ligament tension; for example, the constant increase in tension in the right sacrotuberous and sacrospinous ligaments as long as a 'right posterior, left anterior' innominate rotation and torsion of the sacrum around the left oblique axis are present (Fig. 2.21)
2. a chronic increase in tension or even spasm in muscles that reflects:
   a. contraction to effect rotation of an innominate (e.g. iliacus; Fig. 2.46B,C) or sacral torsion (e.g. piriformis; Fig. 2.46A) as these muscles attempt to stabilize the SI joint(s) by bringing

the surfaces closer together, decreasing joint mobility or causing actual 'locking'

b. 'facilitation' of specific muscles occurring as part of the 'malalignment syndrome' itself (see 'Asymmetry of muscle tension' below).

Pain may also result from an increased or abnormal pressure on the malaligned, and hence incongruent, SI joint surfaces. Given the propeller-shape of this L-shaped joint, with the convex surface of one part of the ilium or sacrum fitting its concave counterpart, it is not hard to imagine how little displacement of one surface relative to the other is actually needed to result in stress on the joint (Fig. 2.3). Development of the convex iliac ridge and matching sacral concavity by the 3RD decade (Fig. 2.7B), also subsequently of other seemingly matching depressions and elevations or just degenerate changes will only further increase the stress that results with even minimal displacement of these joint surfaces whenever pelvic malalignment recurs. Bone scans may actually show increased and/or asymmetrical activity in the SI joints (Fig. 4.39). In the absence of any indications of an inflammatory condition, such as a seronegative spondyloarthropathy or ankylosing spondylitis, these abnormalities on the bone scan may simply reflect an increase in bone turnover triggered by an increase in pressure on the joint surfaces. Unless there is an actual inflammatory element, the abnormalities on the bone scans usually disappear with time as the pressure on the surfaces is finally relieved by keeping the joint in alignment.

Following successful realignment of a previously 'locked' joint, examination may now reveal hypermobility of that joint which can predispose to a recurrence of the malalignment and the 'locking'. The hypermobility may be indicative of ligament laxity, osteoarthritic joint degeneration, poor muscle support or control, or a combination of these. Ligament laxity may be the result of:

1. a previous severe sprain or strain of the ligaments, such as can occur with a shear injury to the SI joint sustained by falling and landing on one buttock or leg (Fig. 2.51B)
2. ligament lengthening that has occurred with time as the ligaments are:
   a. put under constant tension and gradually stretched by the distortion of the pelvic ring caused by the malalignment (Figs 2.19, 2.21, 3.65)
   b. repeatedly being submitted to quick stretches by some of the techniques used to correct the malalignment – especially high-velocity low-amplitude manipulations that make it difficult to judge the end-point and may result in repeated overstretching of the ligament - as compared to using a gentle low-velocity, high-amplitude manual therapy method, such as the muscle energy technique (see Chs 7,8).
3. generalized joint hypermobility, related to:
   a. a genetically-determined defect in the amount or quality of elastic tissue produced; this problem can vary in degree of severity and, at its worst, presents in the form of conditions such as the Ehler–Danlos syndrome
   b. an increase in relaxin hormone, sometimes as a result of a tumour but more commonly seen as a pregnancy progresses, usually from the 4th month on, subsiding gradually during the weeks post-partum but tending to remain elevated until breast-feeding is discontinued (Marnach et al. 2003)

The presence of generalized hypermobility other than during pregnancy is important to establish because these patients generally do not respond as well to realignment attempts, tend to lose correction more easily and are more likely to benefit from additional measures to maintain correction (e.g. foot orthotics, SI belts and ligament strengthening injections). Generalized hypermobility is more common in the group that repeatedly 'switches sides' and changes patterns of malalignment; for example, presenting with 'anterior' or 'posterior' rotation, 'upslip' or 'outflare/inflare' on different sides and in different combinations from one examination to the next, sometimes within hours.

A quick test to assess the degree of mobility is to have the person flex the wrist and then passively bring the thumb toward the volar aspect of the forearm (Fig. 3.1). In most tests, the thumb will end up parallel to the forearm. If the thumb is further away from the forearm (e.g. the person on the left in Fig. 3.1A), or if it ends up close to or even touching the forearm, the person may well have generalized joint hypo- or hypermobility, respectively. This should be confirmed by doing a more complete assessment of the amount of joint play possible on passive movement of other joints; for example, the 9-point Beighton scale may be appropriate (Beighton et al. 1999; Fig. 3.1B). A side-to-side comparison is also important to make sure one is not just dealing with laxity attributable to previous injury of specific ligaments on that side.

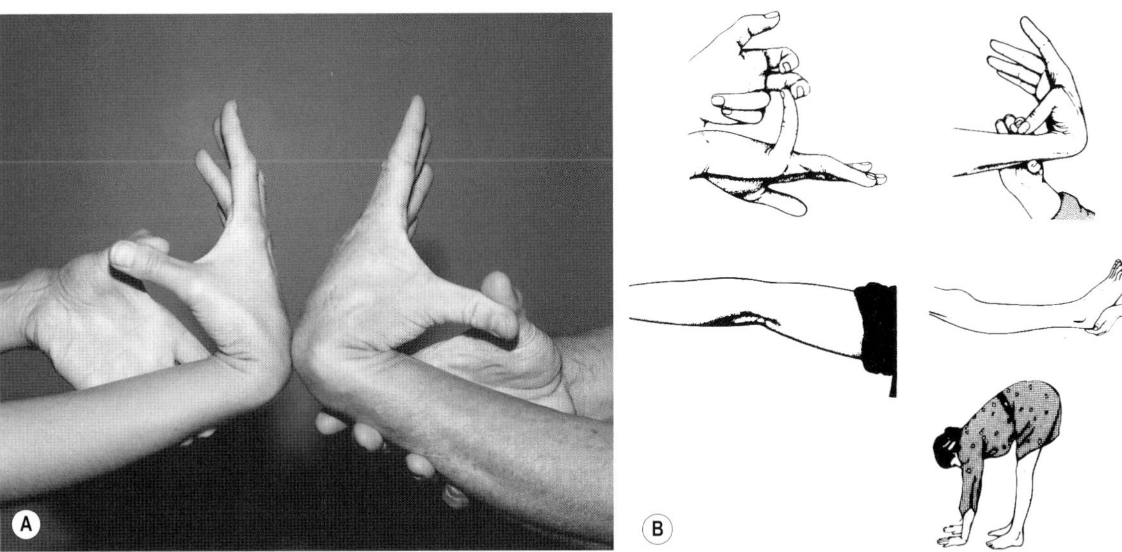

Fig. 3.1 Test for degree of overall joint mobility. (A) Mobility is relatively decreased in the person on the left, whose thumb actually points away, compared with the person on the right, whose thumb ends up parallel to the forearm (the usual finding with normal mobility). (B) 9-point Beighton scale for hypermobility: passive finger dorsiflexion past 90 degress (R/L); passive thumb apposition to the flexor surface of the forearm (R/L); hyperextension of the R/L elbow, the R/L knee beyond 10 degrees; trunk flexion to rest the palms on the floor (with the knees extended). *(Courtesy of Beighton 1999.)*

VARIANTS OF THE SYNDROME SEEN WITH 'ROTATIONAL MALALIGNMENT'

Malalignment of the pelvis, spine and extremities can result from a number of interacting causes. Postural distortion, for example, may result in a muscle imbalance but the distortion may itself be the result of such an imbalance. As Maffetone indicated in 1999, potentially more than one postural distortion can result from the same muscle imbalance. He gave the example of psoas major, indicating that inhibition of tension tone in this muscle on one side, for whatever reason, typically causes the pelvis to tilt. The pelvis usually rises on the opposite side, where psoas major is now in relative 'overfacilitation', the tension tone in the muscle being increased compared with that on the inhibited side (Fig. 3.2A). The effect would be to rotate the innominate anteriorly on the 'facilitated' side, raising the iliac crest. Maffetone, however, went on to say that:

> *... in many cases, the reverse is true and the psoas inhibition is found on the side of the elevated pelvis. This may depend on which problem was primary and which secondary, how the foot reacts, what other muscles are compensating, and other factors.*
>
> (Maffetone 1999: 88)

The reader is referred to works such as by Maffetone (1999) for a detailed discussion of the postural imbalances that can result with the 'inhibition' and 'facilitation' of various muscles.

This book will concentrate on two variants of the 'malalignment syndrome' seen in conjunction with particular patterns of 'rotational malalignment':

1. **the *'left anterior and locked"* pattern** (Fig. 3.3A)
   Individuals affected present with the left leg rotated externally (outward, away from midline) and the right internally (inward, toward midline), with a pattern of weight-bearing tending to left pronation and right supination. This relatively rare pattern (accounting for approximately 5% or less in an orthopaedic medicine practice) is seen in association with a combination of factors that most consistently involves 'anterior' rotation and 'outflare' of the left innominate and 'locking' of the left SI joint. It will, therefore, be referred to as the 'left anterior and locked' pattern.
2. **the *'more common'* rotational patterns** (Fig. 3.3B)
   Individuals affected present with the right leg rotated externally and the left internally, while

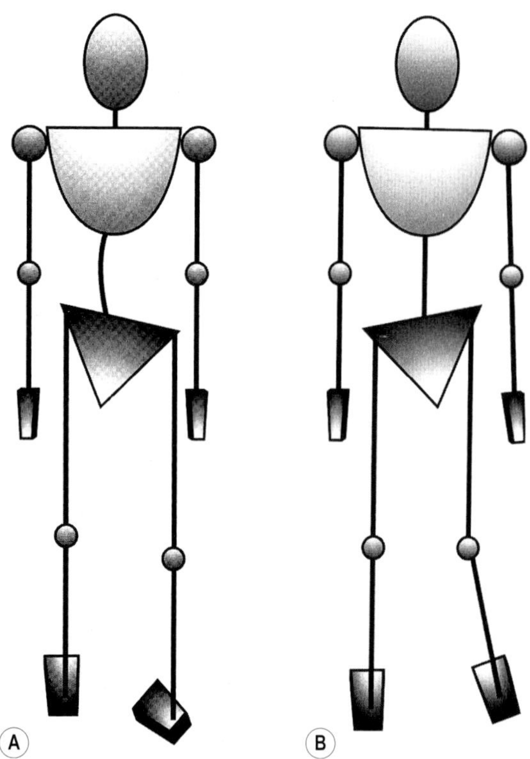

Fig. 3.2 Assessing static posture. (A) Psoas inhibition on the right may allow medial rotation of the ipsilateral foot with excess pronation. The lumbar spine is convex on the contralateral side (tight psoas). The pelvis may be lower (sometimes higher) on the ipsilateral side. (B) Right sartorius or gracilis inhibition may cause a posterior rotation of the pelvis, seen as an elevation of the ipsilateral side and genu valgum. *(Courtesy of Maffetone 1999.)*

weight-bearing tends to right pronation and left supination. The patterns can be made up of any combination of 'anterior' or 'posterior' rotation of either the right or left innominate, and 'locking' of either the right or left SI joint (excluding the rare 'left anterior and locked' pattern, mentioned above). These variations will henceforth be referred to as the 'more common' patterns as they account for about 90-95% of those presenting with 'rotational malalignment'.

The two variants of the 'malalignment syndrome' seen with the 'left anterior and locked' versus the other, 'more common', patterns of 'rotational malalignment' differ primarily from each other in terms of the associated pattern of:

1. asymmetry of joint ranges of motion
2. asymmetry of weight-bearing
3. asymmetry of muscle tension and strength

These differences will be highlighted in the discussion of the specific asymmetries.

ASYMMETRY OF PELVIC ORIENTATION IN THE CORONAL (FRONTAL) PLANE

> Pelvic obliquity is one of the most consistent findings seen with both 'rotational malalignment' and an 'upslip'

As indicated in Chapter 2, 'rotational malalignment' results in a complete asymmetry of the major pelvic landmarks (Figs 2.42, 2.73A,B, 2.76), both side-to-side and front-to-back, because of an asymmetry of the sacrum and the innominates with:

1. rotation around all 3 axes (Fig. 2.9)
   a. coronal = pelvic tilt (pelvic unit forward or backward) in the sagittal plane
   b. sagittal = pelvic obliquity (inclining up to the right or left side) in the coronal (frontal) plane
   c. vertical = pelvic rotation counter- or clockwise (right or left ASIS forward, respectively, in the transverse plane)
2. a possible simultaneous element of translation of the innominate(s) relative to the sacrum (at the SI joints) and/or to each other (at the symphysis pubis) in the three planes:
   a. coronal = medial-lateral and lateral-medial
   b. sagittal = posterior-anterior
   c. vertical = distraction-compression

Given the predominance of 'right anterior' innominate rotation, one is more likely to find elevation of the right than the left lateral iliac crest - approximately 80% versus 20%. One can, however, see the left crest elevated in conjunction with a 'right anterior' rotation. Which iliac crest is higher is determined not only by the direction of innominate rotation but also by factors such as:

1. the position in which the person is examined: with a 'right anterior' rotation, for example, the right iliac crest may be higher or lower in standing but will usually be higher in sitting and definitely in prone-lying; the most common pattern is shown in Figures 2.73C and 2.76B

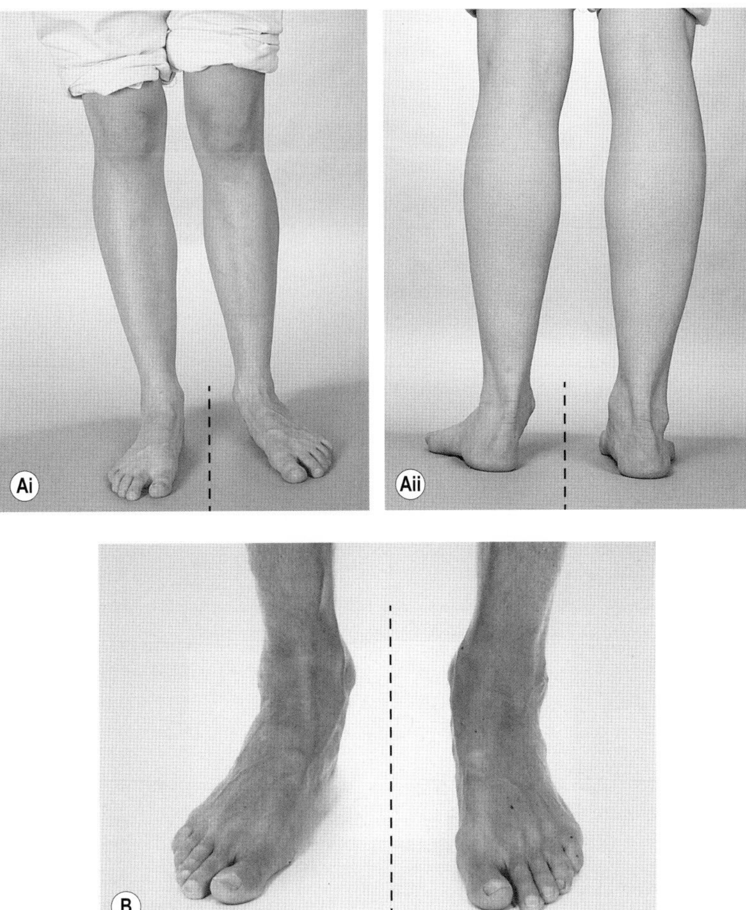

Fig. 3.3 Two variants of the 'rotational malalignment' presentation (see also Figs 3.22, 3.23). (A) With the rare 'left anterior and locked' pattern - the left foot turned outward from the midline and pronating, the right in toward midline and supinating: (i) standing and (ii) walking view. (B) With one of the 'more common' patterns: the right foot is turned outward and pronating; the left inward (may even cross the midline) and supinating (see Fig. 3.19Bii).

2. a coexisting anatomical (true) leg length difference (Figs 2.72B, 2.74A), 'upslip' or 'downslip' (Fig. 2.73A,B)
3. the direction of a sacral torsion, if present (Figs 2.10, 2.14, 2.42, 2.88)
4. the side of SI joint 'locking', if present (Figs 2.119-2.121)

As an example of these variations, a person with 'right anterior' rotation may have elevation on the left iliac crest in standing because of a true LLD, left leg long. In sitting and in lying prone, however, the crest may now be elevated on the right side because the effect of the LLD has been removed. Alternatively, someone with no LLD but a 'left anterior, right posterior' rotational pattern often has elevation of the right iliac crest in standing and sitting but elevation of the crest on the left side when lying prone and the typical findings on the 'sitting-lying' test in keeping with the 'left anterior' rotation; i.e. 'left leg lengthens lying, left landmarks (ASIS, pubic bone) lower'.

Clinical correlation: coronal (frontal) plane asymmetry

The difference in the elevation of the iliac crests is sometimes strikingly obvious and may be accentuated by the cut of a costume. The visual effect of this may distract from the aesthetic appearance. In disciplines such as dancing and figure-skating, this could conceivably affect the perception and judgement of style. In anyone, there may be mundane

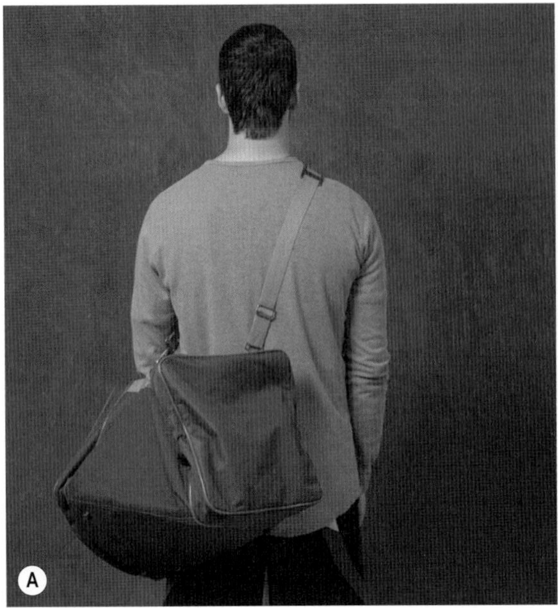

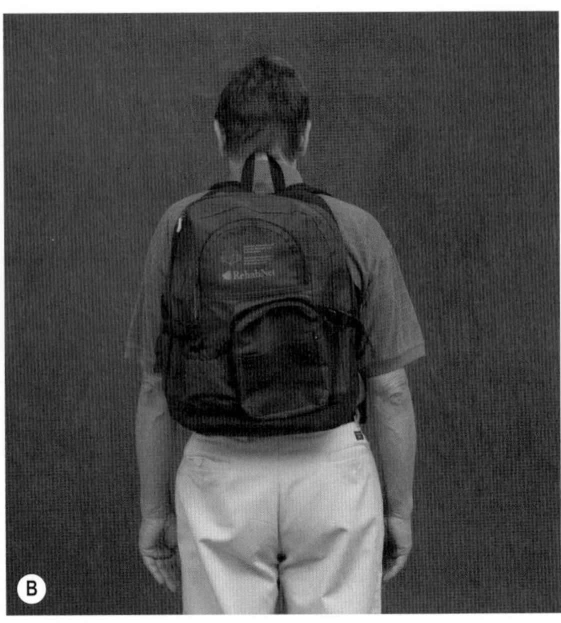

Fig. 3.4 An 'upslip' and 'rotational malalignment' typically result in one shoulder being lower (e.g. as a result of a compensatory scoliosis). (A) Bag carried on left repeatedly slips off lowered left shoulder; running the strap over the right side solves that problem but calls on a number of musculoskeletal adjustments (note person leaning into the right side). (B) Straps across both shoulders, as with a backpack, distribute the weight more evenly, decrease the need for adjustments and help counter recurrences of malalignment.

problems related to clothing, straps or belts repeatedly slipping down or even completely off on one side, just as objects carried over the 'lower' shoulder will tend to slip off (Figs 2.70, 2.76B, 2.90, 2.95A, 3.4).

Sitting is likely to present problems. The ischial tuberosities are at different levels: raised on the side of the 'anterior', lowered on the side of the 'posterior' rotation (Figs 2.76D, 6.4). With a 'right anterior' rotation, the right ischial tuberosity can easily end up 1 cm off the seating surface, the weight now borne primarily by the left tuberosity. The person often talks of 'sitting more on one buttock than the other' or 'off to one side' and may get relief simply by putting a hand, small pillow or a magazine under the raised tuberosity to fill the gap when riding (see Ch. 6), driving, flying, or travelling by other means, or in any other situation where they are sitting for a longer period of time.

Sitting increases the pressure on the lower tuberosity and creates a shearing force on the ipsilateral SI joint by pushing the innominate upward relative to the sacrum. In addition, the ischial tuberosities serve as the insertion of the sacrotuberous ligament and the origin of the hamstrings (Figs 2.5, 2.6, 2.21). These structures are more vulnerable to direct pressure at this site on the side of the 'posterior' rotation, especially when sitting in a slouched position or on a hard surface. Slouching or sitting in a bucket seat allows the pelvic ring - the innominates and sacrum - to tilt posteriorly as a unit, further increasing pressure, especially on the ischial tuberosity and the PSIS on the side of the posteriorly rotated innominate. Aside from using a hand, cushion or magazine between the raised ischial tuberosity and the seat to actually fill in the gap created by the 'anterior' rotation, the person may have found that he or she gets comfort by:

1. increasing the general amount of cushioning under both buttocks, allowing the lower one to sink in further than the higher one - memory foam is ideal for this (Fig. 7.42)
2. placing a cushion under the thighs, ahead of the ischial tuberosities; better still, a pillow that is tapered down from buttocks to thighs (which also shifts weight-bearing forward, more under the thighs)
3. continuously shifting weight-bearing from side-to-side to off-load the tender ischial tuberosity

None of these methods may work very well, especially when the person has to remain seated for a longer period of time in a confined space or when the seating area is small and hard, such as a church pew, a rowing shell or a bicycle seat. In riding, a lowered left ischial tuberosity may increase pressure on the horse's left paravertebral musculature, by digging into the muscles directly (bareback) or through the saddle (Fig. 6.4A). The increased pressure can cause a reflex increase in tension in these muscles so that the horse starts to appear 'stiff' on that side, hesitating or eventually even refusing to veer to the right on command (see Ch. 6).

Given all these situations in which the iliac crest is higher or lower, often changing from one position to another, it is important not to lose sight of the overall picture and realize that these variations in height call for tests which are more definitive and consideration of a differential diagnosis that, at this point, includes 'rotational malalignment' or an 'upslip', an anatomical (true) or a 'functional' LLD.

ASYMMETRY OF PELVIC ORIENTATION AND MOVEMENT AROUND THE VERTICAL AXIS IN THE TRANSVERSE PLANE

With 'rotational malalignment', the pelvic unit often appears rotated counterclockwise, around the vertical axis in the transverse plane some 5–10 degrees, rarely more. This probably relates to the fact that 'right anterior, left posterior' rotation, which tends to twist the pelvic ring in a counterclockwise direction and brings the right ASIS forward and the left backward, is by far the most frequently noted pattern. Therefore, the pelvis is more likely to jut out a bit at the front on the right side and recede on the left when the person is standing (Fig. 3.5A). Rotation in this plane will, however, also be influenced by the position of examination. Consider the example of the person who has such seemingly obvious right forward rotation in standing. When he or she goes to lie prone on a hard plinth, the protruding right ASIS will be the first to contact the plinth and will be forced posteriorly. In this position, therefore, the pelvis could now look level, or the right PSIS may even end up protruding backward compared to the left, as if the pelvis had rotated clockwise in the transverse plane.

> In the presence of 'rotational malalignment', active and passive rotation of the pelvis in the transverse plane is usually restricted into the side of the posteriorly rotated innominate.

Restriction into the side of the 'posterior' rotation can occur for the following reasons:

First, counterclockwise rotation of the pelvis in the transverse plane seen normally during the walking cycle - right ASIS forward with right 'swing' leg - occurs with the simultaneous contrary rotation of the innominates: right posterior and left anterior (Figs 2.12, 2.21, 2.22, 2.41). The pattern is reversed with clockwise rotation on swinging the left leg forward.

Second, when there is 'rotational malalignment' with the right innominate seemingly held in 'anterior', and the left in 'posterior' rotation, clockwise rotation is increased in part due to the fact that the malaligned innominates can rotate further from their resting position in the directions needed to allow this particular movement (Fig. 3.5B). The left one, which starts off rotated posteriorly, can rotate anteriorly through more degrees until it reaches the end of available range in the sagittal plane than if it had started from its normal position. Similarly, the anteriorly rotated right innominate can rotate posteriorly through more degrees until it reaches the end point in that direction. Also, on account of the wedging of the sacrum, the left innominate already flares slightly inward, the right outward. Overall, this translates into more degrees of clockwise rotation.

Conversely, counterclockwise rotation is limited by the fact that the innominates are already rotated part way into the directions required for them to move into for this manoeuvre (Fig. 3.5C). Namely, the right is already rotated anteriorly and the left posteriorly, restricting further movement into these directions required for counterclockwise rotation.

To assess rotation around the vertical axis in the transverse plane, ask the person to stand with the inside of the legs or feet just touching. Sit behind, your feet resting against the outside of his or her feet and, with your knees and calves gently press the lower part of the person's legs together in order to minimize any rotation that might otherwise occur through the lower extremities. With the arms crossed on the chest, he or she should let the trunk, head, neck and upper extremities move with the pelvis as one unit to end point, first to right and then to left. Note and compare the amount of rotation possible from neutral. There is often the feeling of a sudden, hard stop to rotation of the pelvis into the side of the restriction, which the person may well sense.

A rotation of 40 degrees to the right and only 30 degrees to the left would, for example, not be unusual in someone with 'rotational malalignment' with 'right anterior/left posterior' innominate rotation (Fig. 3.5B,C). Discrepancies of greater magnitude can occur, the degree of limitation appearing to be proportionate to the degree of difference in 'anterior' versus 'posterior' innominate rotation. However, correction of the malalignment

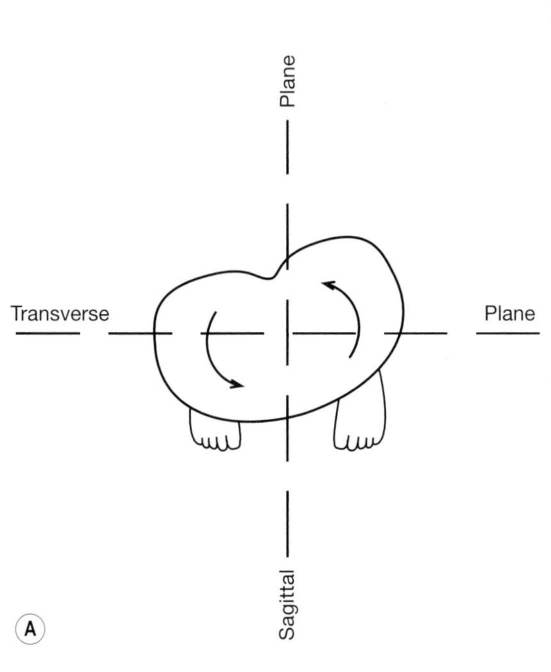

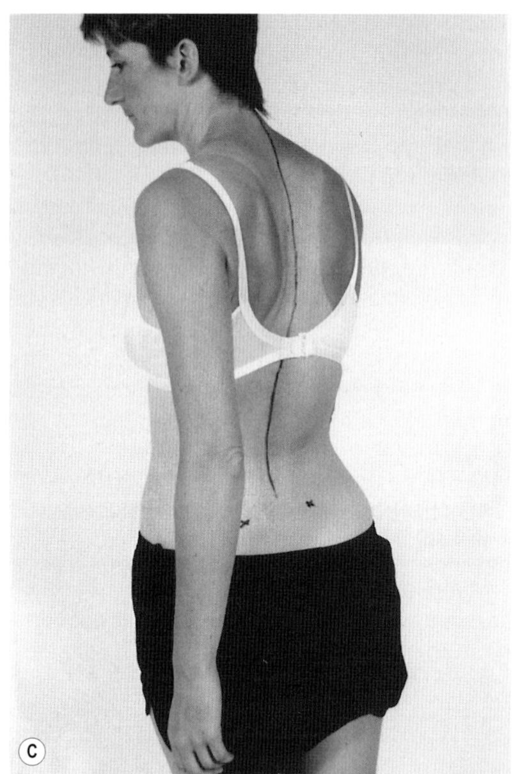

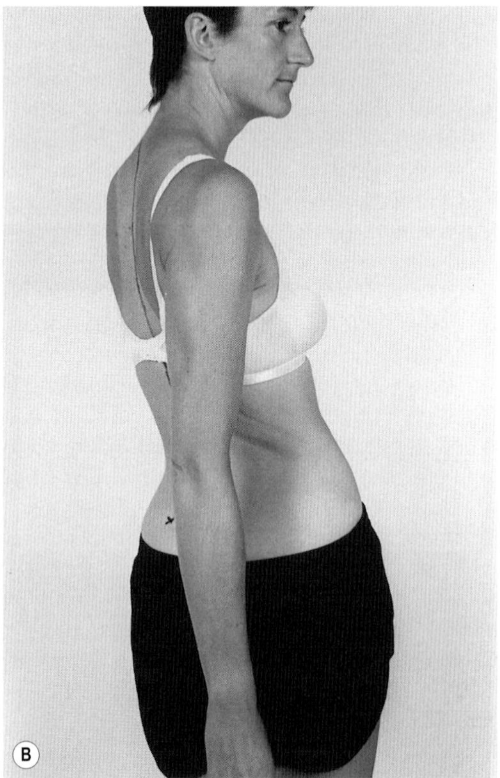

Fig. 3.5 Asymmetry of pelvic rotation around the vertical axis in the transverse plane typically seen with 'rotational malalignment'. (A) Passive: standing - asymmetry, usually with some counterclockwise rotation of the pelvis (left side positioned relatively backward, right forward on a superior view); the trunk may rotate in the opposite or the same direction, with compensatory rotation of the head and neck to keep them in midline (not shown). (B) Active clockwise rotation to 40 degrees. (C) Active counterclockwise rotation decreased to 30 degrees (note the decreased facial, shoulder girdle and chest profile compared with Fig. 3.5B).

immediately removes this restriction and may now allow for an equal amount of rotation: 40 degrees to right and left, in the example given. The fact that rotation might actually now be 45–50 degrees or even more bilaterally suggests that other restrictive factors were operative prior to realignment, such as restriction caused by sacral torsion and/or rotation, asymmetry of muscle tension, and asymmetry of the hip ranges of motion (see below).

Clinical correlation: transverse plane asymmetry

This asymmetry interferes with the ability to execute turning manoeuvres that require pelvic rotation in the transverse plane when both feet are on the ground. The prime example is downhill skiing, in which turns are initiated in large part by movement of the pelvis in this plane, combined with shifting weight onto the appropriate edges. The skier is more likely to experience limitation on attempting a turn into the side of a posterior innominate rotation (see Ch. 5).

> Forced active or passive rotation on the pelvis into the side of the limitation is more likely to lead to soft tissue or even bony injury because the physiological and anatomical barriers will now be exceeded earlier.

The anatomical barrier defines the terminal range of joint motion; movement past that point results in disruption of tissue. The person (e.g. workman, skier or wrestler) presenting with malalignment is, therefore, at increased risk of injury whenever an opponent, a change in direction, or a collision forces the pelvis into that restriction.

Rotation of the spine occurs primarily through the thoracic segment. Whenever rotation of the thoracic segment is impaired, rotational stresses on the lumbar spine and the pelvic region are increased, making them even more vulnerable to injury if forced actively or passively into the direction of a restriction already caused by the malalignment. This can occur, for example, whenever:

1. the thorax is pinned to the floor, such as in wrestling (Fig. 5.36)
2. a gymnast restricts thoracic rotation by holding on to the apparatus with both hands while spinning or twisting the pelvis and legs (Fig. 5.11B,D).

Conversely, a restriction of rotation of the pelvic unit in one direction at the pelvic level may require a compensatory increase in the amount of rotation of the thoracic spine. Such an increased demand on the thoracic segment is more likely with activities that normally require a simultaneous rotation of both the pelvis and trunk while standing upright: with certain field events (discus, hammer, shot and javelin), on playing golf, baseball, and court sports, or simply reaching to the right or left (Fig. 2.44). The increased stress placed especially on the thoracolumbar (T/L) junction may account for the onset or aggravation of mid back pain, especially if these actions are a part of the person's work or sports activities. This issue is discussed further under 'Curvatures of the lumbar, thoracic and cervical segments' (see below).

ASYMMETRY OF SACROILIAC JOINT MOBILITY

Those presenting with 'right' or 'left anterior' rotation show SI joint mobility dysfunction, which may take any of the forms shown in Box 3.2.

BOX 3.2 Sacroiliac joint movement dysfunction

1. 'Locking': jamming of the innominate and sacrum against each other on one side, (e.g. excessive 'anterior' rotation of an innominate) can result in a loss of movement between the two, so that they now move together instead; on the affected side, this results in:
   a. excessive upward and downward movement of the PSIS on trunk flexion and extension, respectively (Figs 2.119, 2.120)
   b. a failure of the landmarks to separate on the 'kinetic rotational' or Gillet test (Fig. 2.125)
   c. no movement being discernible on SI joint 'spring' stress tests (Figs 2.110–2.112)
2. Partial 'locking', which results in:
   a. some upward and downward movement of the PSIS relative to the sacrum on trunk flexion and extension, respectively, and the kinetic rotational and stress tests, but less than what occurs on comparison to the normal side
3. 'hypermobility' or 'laxity':
   a. defined as excessive movement around one or more axis and/or in the anteroposterior, craniocaudal or medial-lateral transverse plane(s) (Figs. 2.114, 2.115)
   b. detectable uni- or bilaterally on the stress tests

Hypomobility or outright 'locking' may be caused by excessive rotation of an innominate relative to the sacrum, a reflex increase in muscle tone or a combination of these.

The person who had 'rotational malalignment' with 'locking' or decreased mobility of one SI joint on initial examination may present for reassessment with the malalignment still evident even after having undergone a course of manual therapy treatments. At this time, possible findings include the following:

1. the previously noted hypomobility or actual 'locking' may still be detectable on the same side; also, sometimes these problems may actually have 'switched' sides
2. more likely than not, movement on lumbosacral flexion, extension and kinetic rotational tests will now be found to be normal (i.e., 'locking' resolved)
3. the side previously felt to be hypomobile may now turn out to be hypermobile, suggesting a possible underlying problem of ligament laxity, joint osteoarthritis, muscle weakness, impaired control or a combination of these that was previously hidden by the 'locking'.

Achieving correction of the 'rotational malalignment' usually re-establishes normal movement on flexion/extension and kinetic rotational tests, and may serve to expose an underlying problem of hypermobility.

CURVATURE OF THE LUMBAR, THORACIC AND CERVICAL SEGMENTS

What follows is an abbreviated discussion of how the resting curves of the spine are influenced by:

1. side-flexion of the spine and/or rotation of the pelvis and spine
2. malalignment of the pelvis and excessive rotation of individual vertebra(e) or a vertebral segment.

The interested reader is referred to extensive discussions of this aspect by Lovett 1903; Fryette 1954; Gracovetsky and Farfan 1986; Richard 1986; D Lee 1992b, 2004a, 2011).

In 1903, Lovett pointed out that:

1. the spine is a flexible rod that is already bent in one plane (sagittal) to create the lumbar lordosis and thoracic kyphosis
2. the rod, therefore, cannot be bent in another plane (e.g. coronal or 'frontal') without twisting at the same time.

> Therefore, in the absence of congenital or traumatic abnormalities of the vertebrae (e.g. hemivertebrae or stress fractures), the lateral curves of the spine are formed by rotation of the vertebrae of a respective segment: the lumbar, thoracic and cervical.

This feature was explored further by Gracovetsky and Farfan (1986). They reported that when one tries to superimpose a lateral curve on the pre-existing lumbar lordosis and thoracic kyphosis, the following occur:

First, the components of the lumbar spine are twisted. For example, on side-bending the trunk to the left, the bodies of vertebrae L1–L4 inclusive rotate to the right, into the convexity formed. Their spinous processes, therefore, rotate to the left, toward the concavity formed (Figs 2.42, 2.96, 3.6, 4.6, 4.24). This rotation is accompanied by simultaneous side-flexion of the vertebrae into the concave side, as well as either extension or forward flexion; that is, as discussed in Ch. 2, there is movement in all three planes (Figs 2.42, 2.52B, 2.94, 2.96).

The combination of **F**orward flexion, **S**ide-flexion and **R**otation constitutes the so-called '**FSR** movement'; should extension occur, the result would be an '**ESR** movement'. These patterns are delineated by the so-called 'laws' of Fryette (1954). A vertebra may become excessively rotated to the right or left and/or into extension or flexion, and become 'stuck' in that position. Movement in one facet joint will then be pathologically restricted, causing the vertebra to rotate around that facet on flexion or extension (Figs 2.52B, 2.94A).

In other words, the overall effect is normally 'a locking one and so plays a safety role. Where the physiological limit has been exceeded, to reverse this mechanism will be the key to the treatment of one part of the lower back syndrome' (Richard 1986).

Second, it is harder to predict the direction of vertebral rotation in the thoracic segment, which is affected by the attaching ribs, the overlying scapulae and soft tissue attachments. The clear-cut correlation that exists in the lumbar segment is missing. The central thoracic vertebrae are more likely to rotate into the convexity (Fig. 3.6); the upper ones are less likely to do so (Lee 1992b).

Third, during normal gait, there is a continuous change in the convex/concave curve patterns

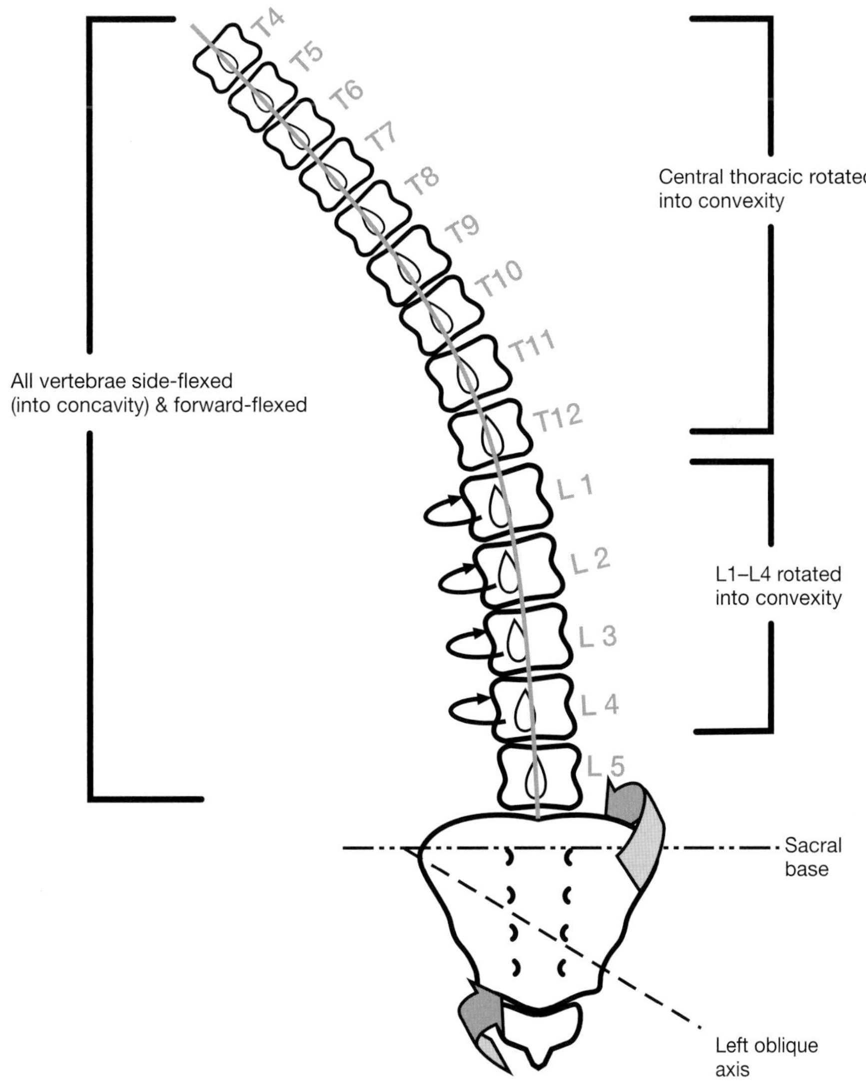

Fig. 3.6 Changes that occur normally in the vertebrae and sacrum on left side-bending: right rotation, forward flexion and left side-flexion.

seen in the thoracic and lumbar spine, changing in direction on right and left swing-through to weight-bearing back into swing-through phase of the cycle while the pelvis and thorax rotate in opposite directions in the transverse plane, balanced by contrary movement of the arms (Fig. 2.41). During normal gait, therefore, there is a matched rotation of the pelvis and spine which helps to balance body weight while the head remains centred throughout.

Effect of malalignment on the spine

Someone who is in alignment and has equal leg length may have a straight spine but, more likely, some minor 'intrinsic curves' when standing. 'Rotational malalignment' results in a pelvic obliquity attributable both to the rotation around the sagittal axis and to the shift of the iliac crests: up on the side of the 'anterior' and down on the side of the 'posterior' innominate rotation. Assuming a pelvic obliquity, right side up and left down: if the spine remained straight and perpendicular to the pelvis, the head would end up off-centre, leaning to the left, something that would disturb the visual and balancing mechanisms. A person usually will automatically form compensatory lateral curves of the spine so that the head ends up in centre, vertical and with the right and left eyes and ears level. Unfortunately, the compensatory curves can exacerbate any 'intrinsic curves'. Also, as indicated above:

1. The spine cannot accommodate without simultaneous rotation of the vertebrae in the thoracic and lumbar segments.
2. The curve formed in the thoracic segment is usually opposite in direction to that formed by the lumbar vertebrae, resulting in the typical double curve, or 'scoliosis' (Figs 3.7A, 3.8, 2.70, 2.90, 2.91, 2.95, 2.120C).
3. The lumbar and central thoracic vertebral bodies appear to rotate into the respective convexity of these curves (Fig. 3.6).
4. X-Rays will show this typical double, 'scoliotic' curve, with a reversal at the thoracolumbar junction (Figs 4.6, 4.31) and possibly also noticeable aggravation of any 'intrinsic' curves on comparison to X-rays taken when the person is in alignment.

If the cervical spine simply continued in the trajectory of the thoracic curve, the person would be walking about with the head and neck still half-cocked, leaning toward the side of the thoracic concavity! Among other things, this would continue to upset the balancing mechanism, which is dependent on visual and vestibular input and also, in large part, on proprioceptive signals arising from the muscles and joints in the neck region and the rest

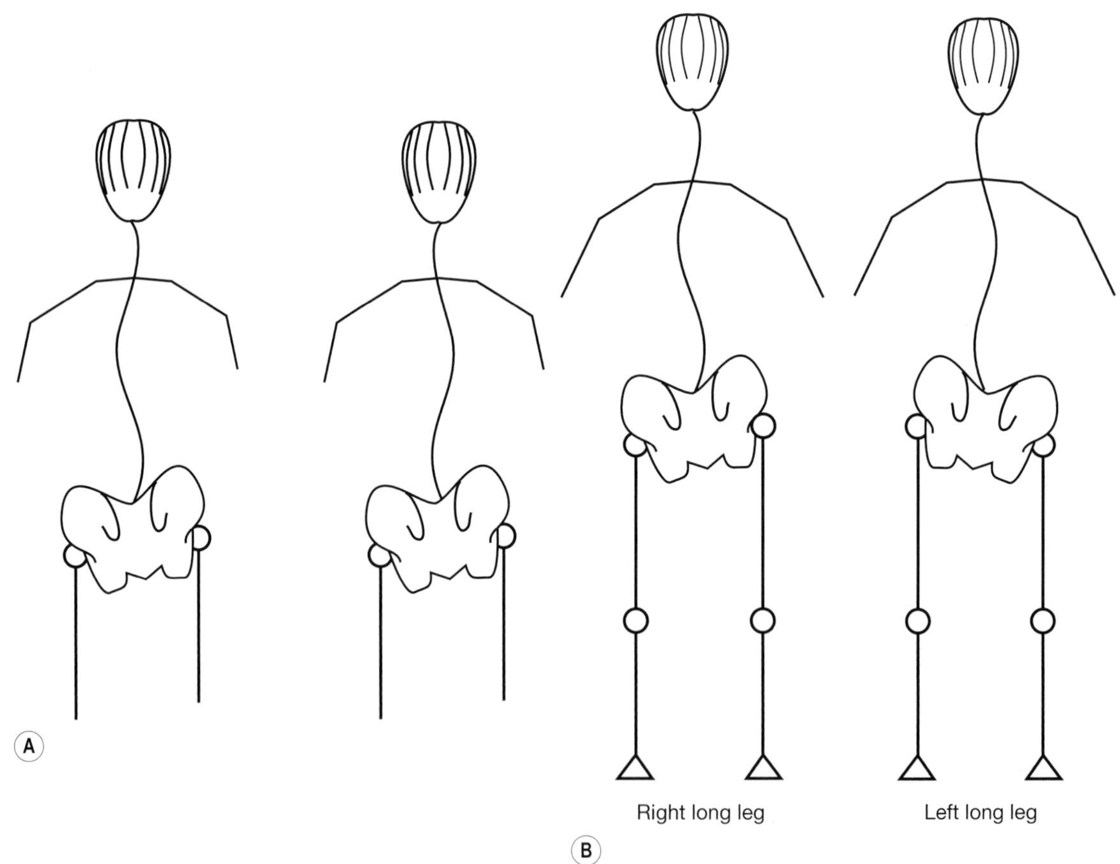

Fig. 3.7 Typical patterns of scoliosis (standing). (A) Patterns seen with 'rotational malalignment' and associated pelvic obliquity (inclined to the right side in the majority). (B) Scoliotic curves commonly seen with right and left anatomical (true) leg length difference.

of the body. The brain could have difficulty dealing with the additional sensory input generated when the head and neck are set at an angle.

There is, therefore, a further reversal in the curvature of the spine in order that the head will, hopefully, end up straight and in midline. This reversal usually occurs at the level of the cervicothoracic junction (Fig. 2.91A). It may, however, start as far down as T4 or T5, which accounts for a large number of those people with a very obvious curvature of the lower and mid-thoracic segment convex, for example, to the right yet with the shoulder and scapula dipped down on the right side instead of the left, as might be expected (Fig. 2.91B). Reversal occurring in the upper thoracic region creates another stress point and may account for reports of interscapular and upper back discomfort. Also, there is likely to be a constant increase in tension or outright contraction in muscles attempting to straighten the cervical spine and avoid any rotation of the head and neck.

The direction of the curves associated with 'rotational malalignment' (or an 'upslip') may differ depending on whether the person is examined standing, sitting or lying prone. The curves are probably best regarded as an adaptation of the spine to the interaction of several factors, including the direction of sacral torsion, the pelvic obliquity, the lateralization of 'anterior' and/or 'posterior' innominate rotation and SI joint 'locking', and the presence of any lengthening having occurred with prolonged stretching, or increased tension or actual contracture of soft tissue attaching to the pelvis, ribs and spine. More important than defining the direction of these curves is to determine if there are any factors that may have resulted in formation of the curves, including malalignment of the pelvis or rotation of individual vertebrae, that can be treated using manual therapy (see Ch. 7).

When the person is lying prone or supine, there is also the passive torquing of the pelvis and/or thorax that results from the plinth pushing upward on any bony point that has been rotated forward or backward (e.g. shoulder, ASIS or PSIS). If we assume that a person presents with 5–10 degrees of forward rotation of the pelvis on the right side, and a contrary rotation of the trunk so that the left shoulder ends up forward: on lying prone, the contact of these protruding points with the surface results in a force that torques the pelvis clockwise and the thorax counterclockwise. This may account for a reversal of the curves sometimes evident in prone-lying compared with those seen in standing and sitting.

When one looks at the combination of pelvic obliquity and the pattern of the thoracic and lumbar curves, the pattern is least likely to change from standing to sitting to lying prone if the anterior innominate rotation and 'locking' are both on the right side (Fig. 3.8A). With the 'left anterior and locked' pattern, the obliquity will change from the right side usually being higher in standing and sitting, to the left being higher when lying prone; whereas the curves may remain the same or change on going from one position to another (Fig. 3.8B). When the 'anterior' rotation is on one side and the 'locking' on the other, the curves are likely to change on lying prone; whereas the pelvic obliquity may stay the same, but this is not predictable (Fig. 3.8C).

Interestingly, the curves associated with an anatomical LLD in standing appear to be no less predictable than those associated with 'rotational malalignment'. That is, one may find a lumbar convexity into either the side of the long or short leg. This is in keeping with the literature, which suggests that the curve formed by the lumbar spine is usually convex to the long-leg side, but also warns of frequent exceptions.

However, as stated before, more important than determining the actual thoracic and lumbar curves in the various positions is to determine what is the reason for the curves - idiopathic scoliosis, LLD, malalignment, or some other underlying cause? - to help decide if and what treatment is indicated.

Biomechanical effects of the curves

The normal movement patterns possible at the lumbar, thoracic and cervical segments of the spine are unique to each segment. They are determined, in large part, by the orientation of the facet joints. Contributory factors include the inherent lordosis and kyphosis of the segment, the characteristics of the attaching soft tissues, the thickness and diameter of the discs, and any limiting factors suggestive of encroachment on a neural arch or nerve root. In the thoracic spine, there are also the limitations imposed by the chest cage (see Chs 2, 4).

> Malalignment, be it 'rotational malalignment' or an 'upslip' or 'downslip', has the effect of superimposing lateral spinal curves; that is, curves in the coronal (frontal) plane

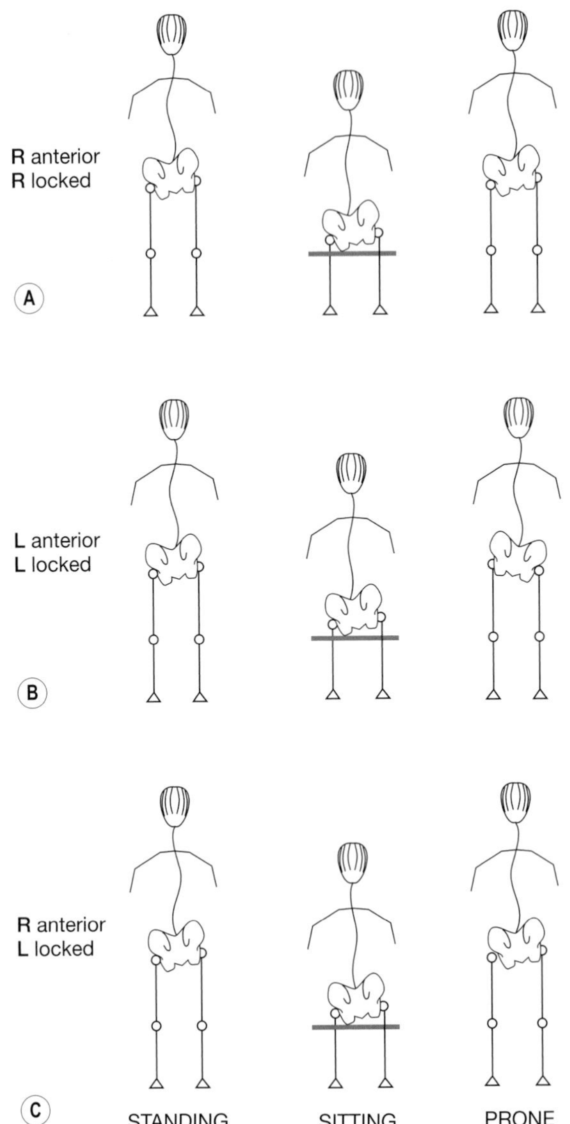

Fig. 3.8 Common patterns relating pelvic obliquity and scoliotic curves to the presentation of 'rotational malalignment'. (A) 'Right anterior, right locked'. (B) 'Left anterior, left locked'. (C) 'Right anterior, left locked'. NB: in (B), right pelvic crest is raised in standing and sitting, the left up in prone-lying; (C) shows a reversal of the scoliotic curves sometimes seen on moving from standing or sitting to prone-lying.

Needless to say, the overall effect is complex. What follows is a strictly biomechanical analysis that ignores the influence of muscles, ligaments and myofascial attachments. The reader is referred to Worth (1986), Grieve (1986a) and Gilmore (1986) for a more detailed analysis of movements of the cervical, thoracic and lumbar spine respectively, and to Lee (1993a, 1994a, 1994b) for an analysis of '*in vivo*' thoracic spine movement.

Study results and clinical correlations primarily for the lumbar, thoracic and cervical spine will be discussed together, in keeping with the fact that the spine should be considered as one unit and that pathology in one segment also affects the other segments.

The lumbar segment of the spine

The lumbar facet joints are oriented almost in the sagittal plane. This allows primarily for flexion and extension of this segment, while limiting side-bending and rotation.

As indicated above, the 'laws' of Fryette (1954) dictate that the formation of a right lumbar convexity on left trunk side-flexion is normally associated with:

1. the rotation of L1–L4 inclusive into the convexity; in this case, to the right (Figs 2.96A, 3.6, 4.26); there is also a simultaneous opening of the facet joint on the right and narrowing on the left (Fig. 2.52)
2. forward flexion of the lumbar segment
3. side flexion to the left

Clinical correlation: lumbar segment

The overall biomechanical effects of a lumbar convexity with malalignment superimposed, and possible clinical correlations, include the following:

1. *decreased movement, or even 'locking', of the lumbar segment*
   With time, this may exceed the safety role of the locking that occurs physiologically with normal side-flexion of the trunk.
2. *narrowing/degeneration of a facet joint space*
   This might explain the not uncommon scenario of a history of low to mid back pain:
   a. felt ipsilaterally on side-flexion into the side of the affected facet joint (e.g. lateral pelvic 'tilt'), or simultaneous extension and side-flexion (e.g. reaching down and to that side to pick up an object; baseball, rugby and other sports involving throwing and catching)
   b. felt contralateral to the direction of rotation especially when carried out with simultaneous extension of the trunk, as on a facet stress test or with similar manoeuvres during activities (e.g. reaching across to shelves - Fig. 2.44; playing golf and court sports - see Ch. 5); the extent of aggravation caused by the malalignment will become more obvious if the pain on the facet stress test decreases - or sometimes even disappears - following realignment
   Facet joint narrowing with or without degeneration might also be one reason why a person with malalignment repeatedly reports an increase in pain on attempting a posterior 'pelvic tilt' while lying supine: they are trying to flatten out a rotated lumbar segment when the overall flexibility is decreased and the facet joint surfaces are already approximated on one side because of the malalignment and may, therefore, not tolerate the further compression caused by this 'tilt' (see Fig. 7.2). Attempting to increase the lumbar lordosis (forward rotation of the pelvic unit in the sagittal plane, or 'anterior pelvic tilt') or side-bending into the side of the facet narrowing ('lateral pelvic tilt', in the coronal plane) would have a similar effect.
3. *narrowing of the disc and compression of the lateral vertebral margins on the side of the concavity*
   This constitutes a stress on both the disc and the vertebrae, with displacement of the nucleus pulposus and bulging of the annulus fibrosus toward the side of the convexity.
4. *widening of the joint margin on the side of the convexity*
   This widening, combined with the bulging of the annulus, puts the attachments of the annulus and ligaments to the adjoining vertebral margins under increased stress on the convex side.
5. *torsion of the annulus in a clockwise direction*
   Torsion would increase stretch on the oblique annular fibres and their nerve supply.
6. *narrowing of the disc anteriorly or posteriorly*
   a. Forward flexion compresses the adjacent vertebrae anteriorly. By forcing disc contents posteriorly, it can increase tension in the posterior longitudinal ligament and may contribute to any posterior or lateral bulging of the disc, possibly to the point of:
      i. touching the theca (dura) and causing typical 'cord symptoms'
      ii. accelerating disc and vertebral degeneration
   b. Spine extension compresses vertebrae posteriorly, forces disc contents anteriorly and increases tension in the anterior longitudinal ligament (Fig. 3.68).

The question is whether these stresses alone, or in combination, can initiate and/or accelerate the degeneration of the lumbar spine segment, including the deterioration of the annulus, with eventual disc protrusion. Certainly, the combination of axial rotation and simultaneous side-flexion was already identified by White & Panjabi (1978) as one of the worst forms of distortion to which the disc can be subjected, in terms of precipitating the degenerative changes that eventually lead to disc protrusion.

The thoracic segment of the spine

The superior facet joint surfaces are oriented increasingly backward, allowing primarily for medial and lateral rotation (around the vertical axis in the transverse plane) and side-flexion while limiting flexion/extension (Fig. 3.9). Movement in all three planes is restricted to some extent by the ribs and sternum.

There is disagreement over what exactly happens when one introduces a curve either by pure axial rotation or pure side-flexion of the thoracic segment. Lee (1993a: 20) in her clinical work noted that:

1. rotation of the trunk results in simultaneous side-flexion to the ipsilateral side
2. side-flexion produces contralateral rotation of the mid-thoracic spine; i.e., into the convexity
3. the biomechanics of the lower thoracic region are more complex as a result of 'some significant differences in the anatomy of this region', referring to the significaant transitional changes occurring between T11-L1 (Fig. 3.9).

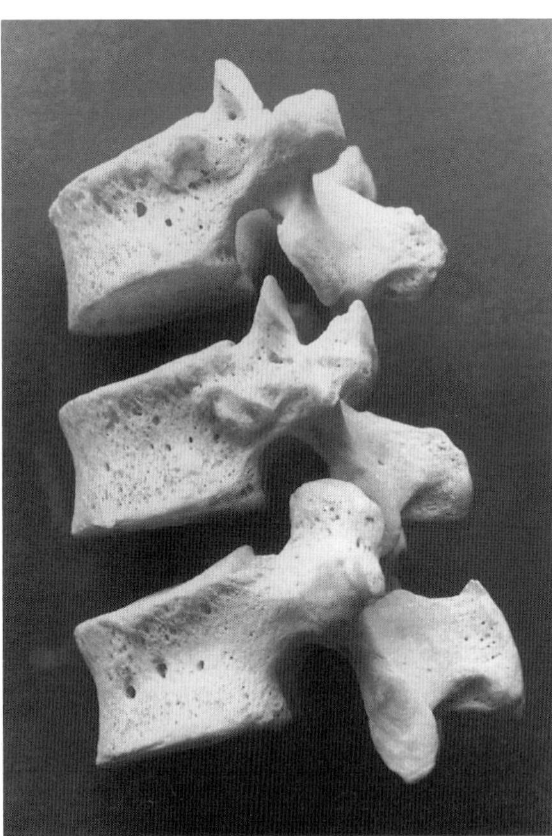

Fig. 3.9 Transitional facet joints at the thoracolumbar junction. The inferior facets of T12 (central vertebra) have a coronal and sagittal component; articulation with L1 (on the left) allows mainly flexion/extension, restricting axial rotation. The change in the orientation of the proximal T12 facets allows for axial rotation but starts to restrict flexion/extension.
(Courtesy of Lee 1994.)

Clinical correlation: thoracic segment

Presuming that there is a thoracic convexity to the right, the vertebrae are already side-flexed to the left and may be rotated to the right, into the convexity, in the central segment of the thoracic spine (Lee 1992b; Fig. 3.6). In that case, there will now be a limitation of further left side-flexion and of clockwise rotation around the vertical axis. Findings would be reversed with a thoracic convexity to the left.

Any limitation increases the risk of injury in daily activities, work and sports in which the trunk can be submitted to a rotational force, especially at a moment when pelvic rotation is either restricted (e.g. by standing with both feet firmly planted on the ground) or made more-or-less impossible (e.g. by sitting). These include:

1. ***an MVA, particularly in the case of a rear-end collision***
   - in countries driving on the right-hand side, the typical 3-point seat-belt does not restrain the right shoulder and the impact can result in excessive counterclockwise torquing of the driver's trunk
2. ***any torquing impact on the trunk imposed while the pelvis is stabilized***
   - for example, when sitting (especially with the feet secured on pedals or in stirrups, such as may be the case when cycling or riding a motorcycle or horse)
3. ***court sports***
   - in particular, tennis and other racquet sports (Figs 5.3, 5.4)
4. ***throwing sports***
   - with a rotational component of the trunk leading up to eventual release, while still more or less weight-bearing on both feet (e.g. hammer throw, discus and shot put; Figs 3.51, 5.30, 5.31)
5. ***rowing and other paddling sports***
   - from the symmetrical rotation of the thoracic spine required in open and flatwater kayaking to the more asymmetrical rotational strains imposed by canoeing, white-water kayaking and sweep rowing (Fig. 5.1).

In addition, the risk is increased in sports in which a person rotates the trunk either voluntarily or has it forced into the direction of limitation:

1. *passive forced rotation*
   - e.g. by an opponent in a sport (wrestling, judo, karate; Figs 5.35, 5.36), as the result of an impact (falls or a collision in a vehicle) or from a collision with an opponent or a fixture (court sports, hockey, soccer)
2. *in basketball*
   - excessive passive or active rotation of the trunk into the side of the limitation, such as may occur in the course of a lay-up, especially when the feet are still planted on the ground
3. *in golf*
   - for example, with a thoracic convexity to right and some of the vertebrae already rotated clockwise (into the convexity), there will be less leeway for a backswing to the right, and more for the down-stroke and follow-through to the left at these levels
4. *in gymnastics*
   - increased rotational forces through the thoracolumbar junction with rotational manoeuvres carried out while the trunk is relatively fixed (e.g. rotations of the pelvis and legs while the trunk is supported by the arms holding on to the bars; Fig. 5.11).

The thoracic spine is especially vulnerable in:

1. sports involving moving vehicles (e.g. bobsleds, the luge) and
2. MVAs, especially when safety restraints are limited to a lap belt (pelvic restraint) alone or the three-point system, with a strap across only one of the shoulders; these systems allow the unrestrained shoulder or shoulders to move forward or backward and torquing of the trunk on the fixed pelvis, possibly into one of the directions of limitation imposed by a coexisting malalignment.

The cervical segment of the spine

A number of patients present with neck pain in association with 'rotational malalignment' or an 'upslip'. In practically all cases, there is an increase in tension and tenderness localizing to the right neck muscles: upper trapezius, scalenes (Fig. 3.13), right paravertebrals and cervical erector spinae. This finding is not related to handedness nor to the direction of the curves of the spine. The curvature of the cervical segment is usually opposite in direction to that of the thoracic segment (Fig. 3.14). As indicated above, the point of reversal is sometimes as far down as T4 or T5 (Fig. 2.91B). At the level of reversal, wherever that may be, the adjoining vertebrae will rotate and side-flex but in opposite directions. Together, these factors create another stress point, and though the person may be asymptomatic, there is often tenderness to palpation at this site and in the adjacent tensed neck muscles (tending to involve particularly those on the right side: upper trapezii, scalenes, paravertebrals and erector spinae).

Neck range of motion (ROM) most consistently shows a limititation of right rotation and left side-flexion (Fig. 3.10). There are several factors that contribute to this asymmetry.

First, the malalignment of the pelvis and spine results in asymmetry of tension in all the skeletal muscles (see 'Asymmetry of muscle tension' below). As indicated, in the neck there is predominantly evidence of increased tension involving right upper trapezius, the scalenes, paravertebrals and cervical erector spinae muscles. Involvement of right upper trapezius, with its origin from the occiput, ligamentum nuchae and cervicothoracic spinous processes, would by itself limit right rotation by restricting any attempt to increase the distance between its origin and the insertions onto the 1st and 2nd rib while at the same time allowing for increased left rotation. Left side-flexion can be limited by tightness in any of these four muscle groups on the right side.

Second, the direction of the cervical curve is likely to be an important determinant. A lateral curve superimposed on the cervical lordosis will make it easier to move in some directions than others.

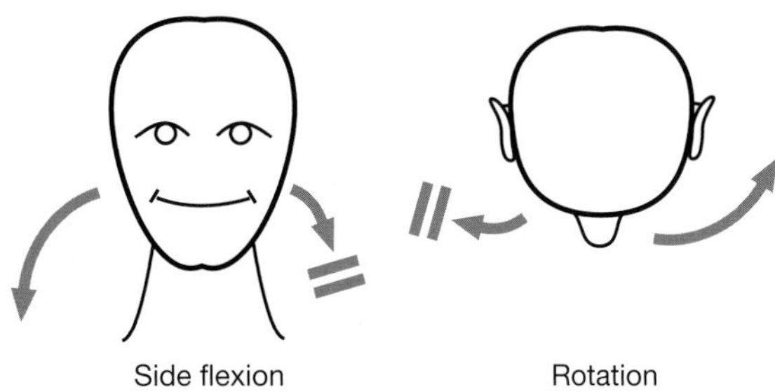

Fig. 3.10 Typical asymmetry of head and neck ranges of motion seen with 'rotational malalignment' or an 'upslip'.

Third, neck ranges of motion are also affected by rotational displacement of individual cervical vertebrae and the direction of the thoracic and lumbar curves. Such a displacement may be detected by:

1. having the person lie prone, head and neck looking over the edge of the plinth or through an opening to keep the head and neck straight and prevent further rotation of the cervical spine
2. presuming the right-handed examiner is standing at the head of the table, looking down toward the pelvis/feet (Fig. 2.95B,E), he or she would:
   a. Place the right index or middle finger on the right, the left one on the left transverse process (TP) to see if:
      i. they are at the same height off the table; i.e. level in the transverse plane (no rotation around the vertical axis evident)
      ii. the left TP is up, the right down relative to each other, indicating the vertebra has left-rotated; i.e., counterclockwise
      iii. the right TP is up, the left one down relative to each other, indicating the vertebra has right-rotated; i.e., clockwise
3. proceed downward from C2 to the thoracic vertebrae
   - note if the person indicates pain at any level; usually there is uni- or bilateral TP tenderness where one or more vertebrae have rotated, often also at the level(s) just above or below the rotated vertebra(e)
4. if any vertebrae have rotated, make sure these are attended to as part of the overall treatment, so that they end up back in alignment

In Figure 3.11, C1-T1 inclusive show some minimal rotation, into the left convexity. T2 and, even worse, T3 vertebrae have right rotated, going by the transverse process displacement on side-to-side comparison.

The neck ranges of motion usually become symmetrical again with correction of any vertebral/pelvic malalignment. For example, neck right rotation may be limited to 50 degrees, compared with a left rotation of 70 degrees, for a total of 120 degrees (Fig. 3.10). Following realignment, and barring any other pathology, the values will usually become equal at 70 degrees. The overall increase in the total range to 140 degrees probably reflects, in part, the relaxation of the neck and shoulder girdle muscles that occurs with the realignment of the vertebrae.

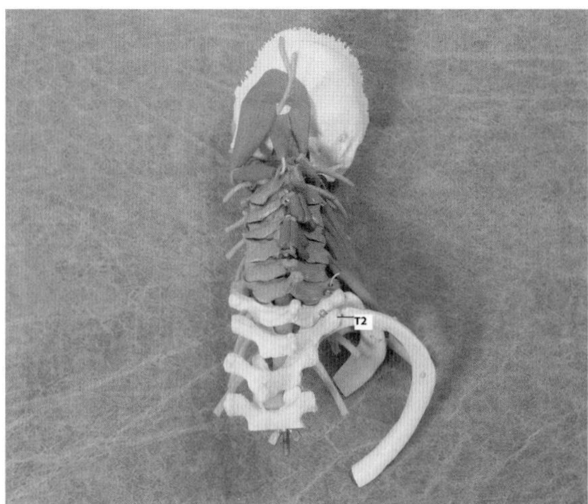

Fig. 3.11 Model of upper segment of spine demonstrates a minor cervical curve (convex to left - vertebrae left rotated) which is interupted by some T2 and exaggerated T3 vertebral displacement (vertebrae right rotated). Right T2 and T3 transverse process are displaced backward and will be more easily palpable than the left one, both in the prone position (as shown) and when lying supine.

Clinical correlation: cervical segment

Patients presenting with neck pain related to malalignment of the pelvis and spine sometimes have associated symptoms in the upper extremities. These include dysaesthesias and paraesthesias, which disappear with realignment only to recur as the malalignment itself recurs. Possible causes for these arm symptoms include the following:

Referral from structures in the neck that are being irritated because of the malalignment

1. increased tension or laxity involving ligaments or myofascial tissue, causing local or referred pain (see below).
2. stresses on articulations (compression or separation of surfaces; instability)

Increased curvature of the cervical spine, contrary rotation of C7/T1, rotation of individual vertebra(e) can cause symptoms from nervous tissue (spinal cord, dura, nerve roots) by putting these under increased tension or compressing them enough to cause irritation (e.g. by decreasing foraminal exit space on one side, especially if there is already an element of foraminal stenosis as seen with facet joint and/or disc degeneration and osteophyte formation).

Dysaesthesias or paraesthesias may be localized or referred from ligaments and myofascial structures in the neck that are lax or being put under increased stress on account of the malalignment. Evidence for actual root or peripheral nerve damage compression is usually lacking on neurological, electrodiagnostic or other investigations. Referral may be to the dermatome, myotome and/or sclerotome of the nerve innervating the structure affected by the malalignment. Figure 3.12 delineates typical patterns originating from the neck region; these include:

1. Curve reversal at the cervicothoracic junction cannot occur without rotation of vertebrae in opposite directions; here it affects C7 and T1 maximally. This puts increased stress on the intervertebral, supraspinous and interspinous ligaments joining the two vertebrae, and those attaching to the C7 and T1 transverse processes. The nerves innervating these ligaments and joints effected (e.g. facet joints) can cause pain at the base of the neck and/or paraesthesias on the medial aspect of the forearm and the fourth and fifth fingers, in effect mimicking a C8 root problem and/or even angina (Fig. 3.12A,Biv). The C7/T1 level can also refer to the C8 sclerotome at the medial epicondyle and mimic 'medial epicondylitis'.
2. A problem in the mid-cervical region can cause irritation of the C5 and/or C6 nerve roots, or referral to the C5 and C6 dermatome, resulting in symptoms that may suggest a C5 or C6 radiculopathy (Fig. 3.12A,Bii,Biii). There can also be referred pain to the sclerotome region on the lateral aspect of the elbow, symptoms that may lead to futile treatments for a problem erroneously diagnosed as a 'lateral epicondylitis'.
3. The upper cervical and occipital region can refer to various areas of the skull (Fig. 3.12A,Bi). For example, occiput-C1 refers to the frontal, also retro- and supraorbital region. C1-2, C2- 3 involvement can cause symptoms in the temporal region and behind the ear.
4. Trigger points that develop in the neck muscles can refer to the shoulder girdle, the anterior and posterior chest regions and the upper extremities (Travell & Simons 1983). Interestingly, these trigger point referral patterns can overlap with sclerotomal referral patterns originating from the ligaments attaching to the C7 transverse processes (Fig. 3.12A,Bv).
5. Other dermatomal/sclerotomal referral patterns are as shown in Fig. 3.12.

Irritation of cervical nerve tracts and vascular structures

1. The cervical roots and brachial plexus exit the neck region running through the cervical paravertebral muscles and then in between the anterior and middle scalene muscles, together with the subclavian artery; whereas the subclavian vein runs anterior to the anterior scalene (Fig. 3.13). The vessels and nerves then proceed through the thoracic outlet, formed by the clavicle and first rib. A chronic increase in tension in the scalenes and other surrounding muscles can narrow the space available to the exiting neurovascular bundle, both between the scalenes and in the thoracic outlet region, sometimes to the point of exerting direct pressure on these structures.
2. A rotation of the clavicle and the first rib caused by the malalignment can result in a further narrowing of the thoracic outlet (Fig. 3.13). Irritation of the nerve fibres as a result of increased tension or direct pressure on the nerve tracts and/or a compromise of their blood supply can cause symptoms and clinical findings suggestive of a nerve root, brachial plexus or peripheral nerve lesion. Tests for a 'thoracic outlet syndrome' may provoke paraesthesias, occasionally with an associated diminution or obliteration of the radial pulse. In the absence of a neurological deficit on examination, electrodiagnostic studies are usually normal. However, depending on history and other clinical findings, further investigations to rule out a 'thoracic outlet syndrome' may be appropriate.
3. The symptoms may be abolished by correction of the malalignment, with special attention paid to any coexisting rotational displacement of the cervical and upper thoracic vertebrae, the clavicle and the upper ribs (Fig. 2.94). Realignment may help simply by increasing the space available for the neurovascular bundle by:
   a. relaxing the surrounding muscles and re-establishing the normal spatial relationship between the vertebrae, clavicle and first rib
   b. decreasing tension, and hence irritability, in nerves within the ligaments and also in the autonomic fibres in this area.

Limitation of certain cervical spine ranges of motion

Any malalignment-related restriction of movement into a certain direction may affect performance, provoke pain and increase risk of injury. For

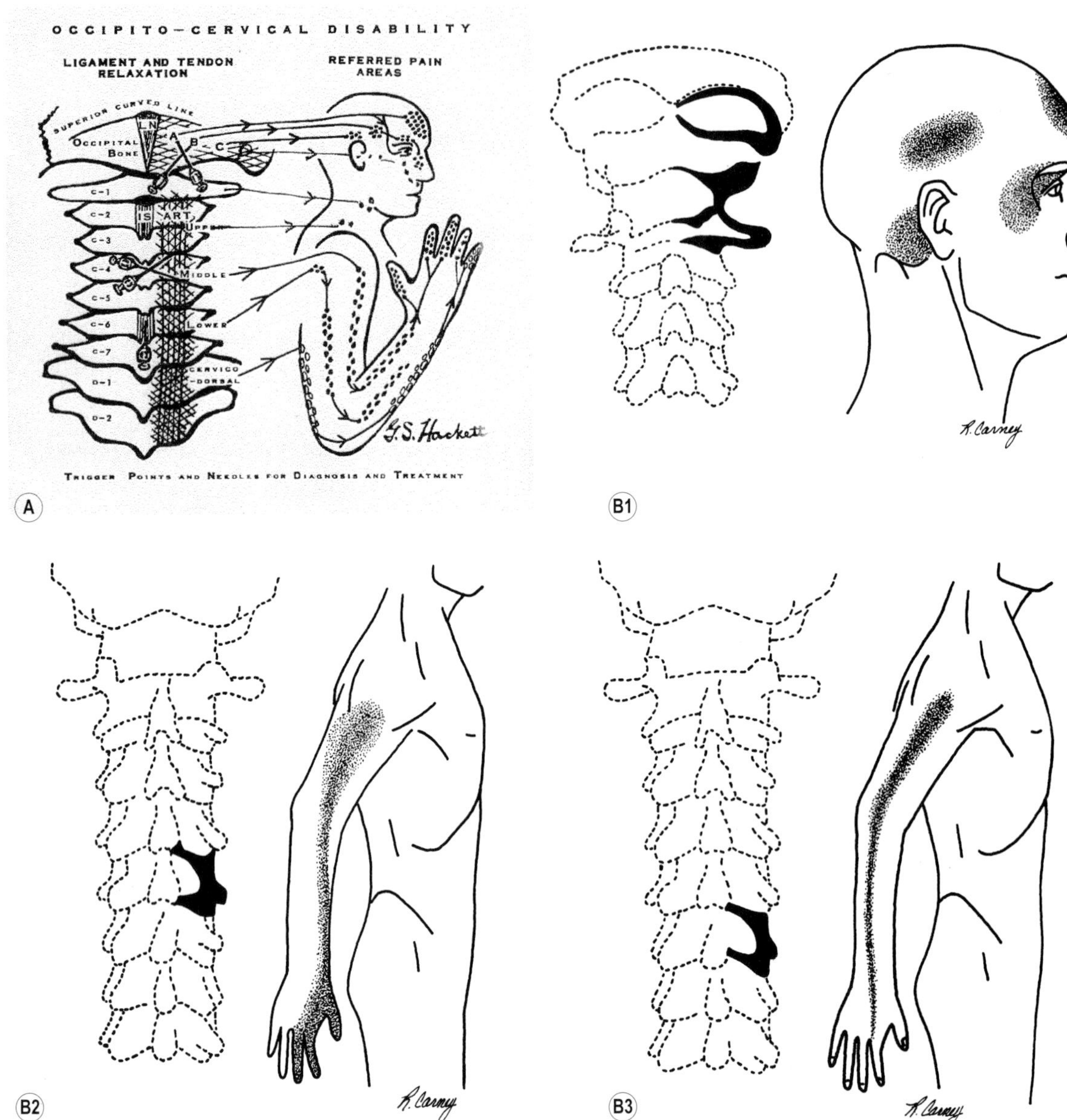

Fig. 3.12 (A) Typical referral sites from ligament and tendon relaxation in the occipital region and cervical spine. Note the referral from the cervicothoracic junction area to the medial aspect of forearm and the fourth and fifth fingers, which can mimic a C8 root pattern and angina; there is also C5 and C6 sclerotomal referral to the area around the lateral epiphysis. ART, articular ligaments; IS, interspinous ligaments; LN = ligamentum nuchae. *(Courtesy of Hackett 1958.)* (B) Myofascial attachments to bone have characteristic patterns of referred pain when injured. (1) Upper neck sites (occipitoatlantoaxial). (2) The C5 sclerotome, the thumb, is usually involved. (3) At the C6 sclerotome, the pain does not usually spread into the hand. (4) The C7 sclerotome, the fifth and often the fourth fingers are involved. (5) The up, front and back of the transverse process of C7 have important patterns. *(Courtesy of Dorman & Ravin 1991.)*

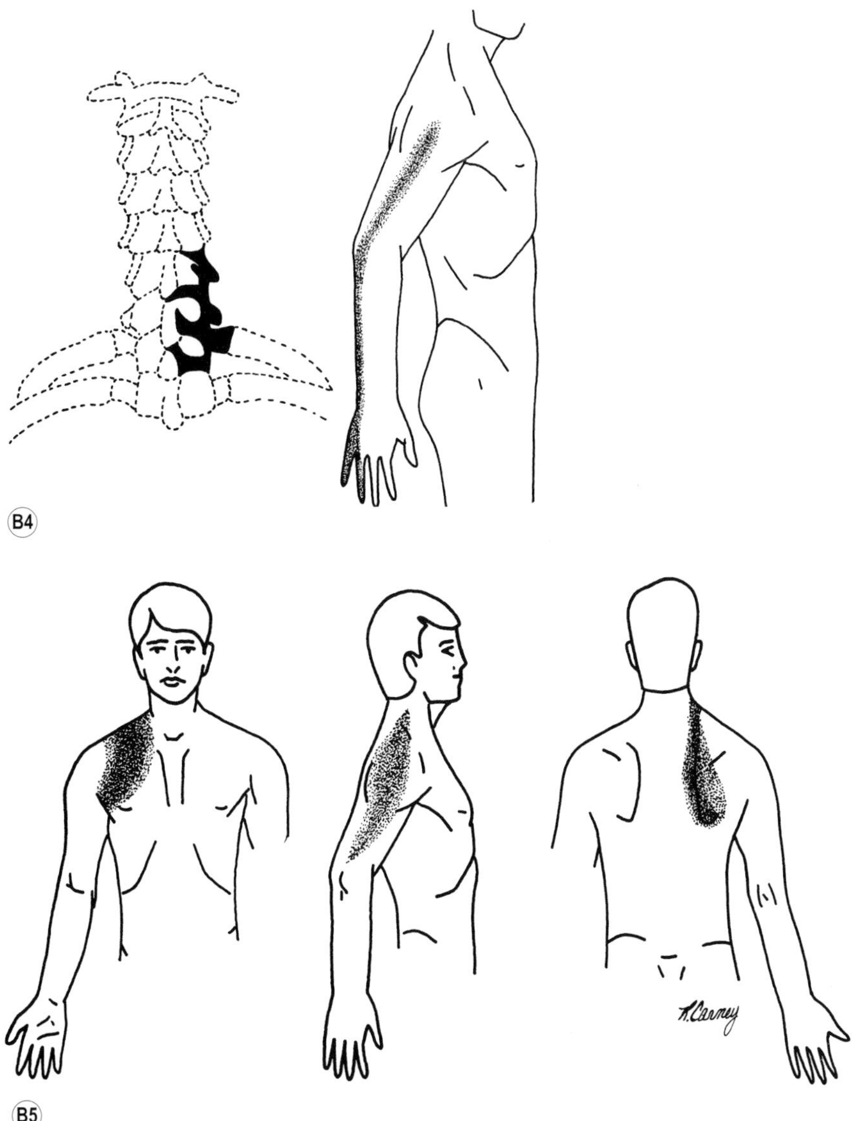

Fig. 3.12—cont'd

example, in some sports such as wrestling the athlete is at risk if an opponent moves the head and neck passively into such a restriction. Conversely, the increased range now available into the opposite direction may be advantageous and could also be a deciding factor of why we perform some activities one way and not the other. For example, in shooting, sighting is a combined movement of rotation and forward and side flexion. In someone who is right eye dominant and rests the gun/rifle against the right shoulder, having to rotate the head to the left and side-flex to the right would be even easier when malalignment is causing a restriction of right rotation and left side-flexion (Fig. 3.10). The same restriction would make it easier for someone doing the crawl, or freestyle swimming stroke, to turn the head to the left (see Ch. 5). Compared to breathing on the right, he or she would have to turn the trunk less or not at all on going to the left on alternate breathing, given the increased range of rotation available to that side at the head and neck. If lung capacity permits, they may prefer to breathe only

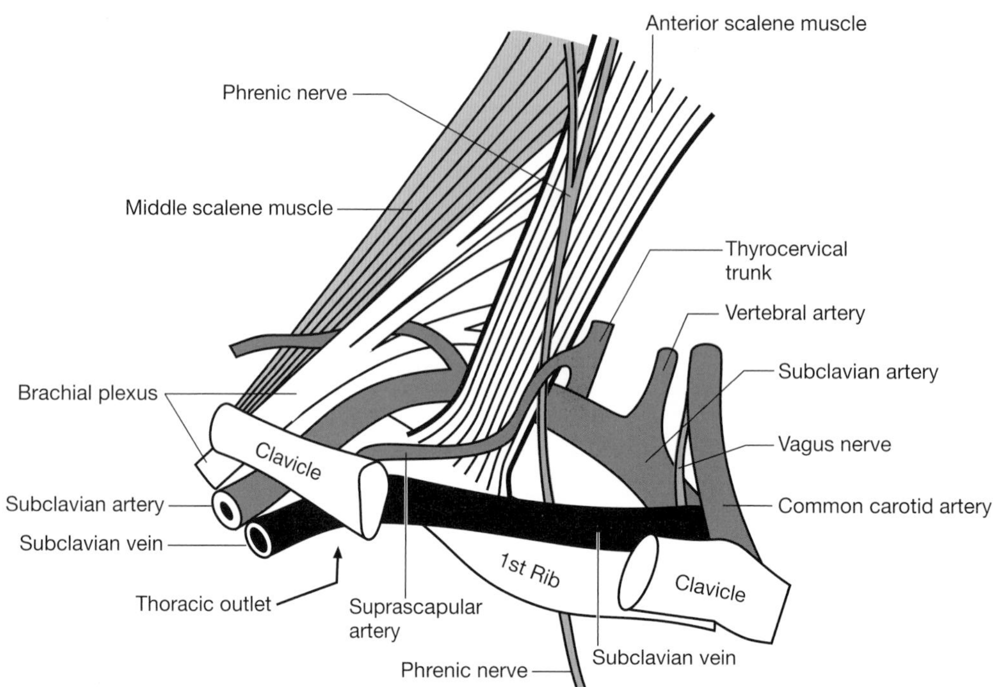

Fig. 3.13 Compromise of the brachial plexus of nerves and the subclavian artery can occur between a tense anterior and middle scalene muscle, or as they exit through the narrow thoracic outlet between the clavicle and underlying 1st rib. *(Redrawn courtesy of Pansky & House 1975.)*

on the side of increased neck rotation. Overall, breathing on just that side would mean less trunk rotation, or 'wobble', may be more energy efficient and result in increased speed.

Sites of curve reversal

The sites of reversal of the curves in the coronal (frontal) plane usually match those in the sagittal plane (Fig. 3.14). A lateral view of the spine from a cranial to caudal direction usually shows a change from a cervical lordosis to a thoracic kyphosis at the cervicothoracic junction, to a lumbar lordosis at the thoracolumbar junction, and a further reversal to a sacral kyphosis at the lumbosacral junction. The stress at these normal sites of reversal in the sagittal plane is, therefore, compounded by the fact that reversal of any lateral curves present usually occurs at exactly the same sites.

Stress is further increased at these points of curve reversal because the adjoining vertebrae are actually rotated in opposite directions. For example, in someone who presents with the pelvis in alignment and a lumbar curve convex to right and thoracic to left, L1 will most likely be rotated to the right, T12 to the left (Fig. 3.14C).

This twisting of vertebrae, combined with the changes in curvature, help to explain why tenderness and pain so often localize to the thoracolumbar and cervicothoracic junctions. However, the lumbosacral level is by far the most likely stress point to be tender on palpation and actually to be symptomatic, in large part as a result of the stress placed on:

1. L5-S1, which bears all the upper body weight
2. the L4–L5 level, which has to deal with the weight coming through L1-L4 and transfer it onto L5 and then S1; with the rotation of L1 to L4 inclusive into the convexity of a lumbar curve (Figs 2.96A, 3.6), these vertebrae come to act as a unit and are, therefore, less flexible, less capable of absorbing shock and hence impaired when it comes to dealing with any weight imposed from either direction
3. the L4-5 and L5–S1 level, especially if there is rotational displacement of either L4 and/or L5 relative to S1 (Figs 2.96B and 2.52, respectively)

Stress at sites of curve reversal may be further aggravated by the frequent occurrence of a vertebral

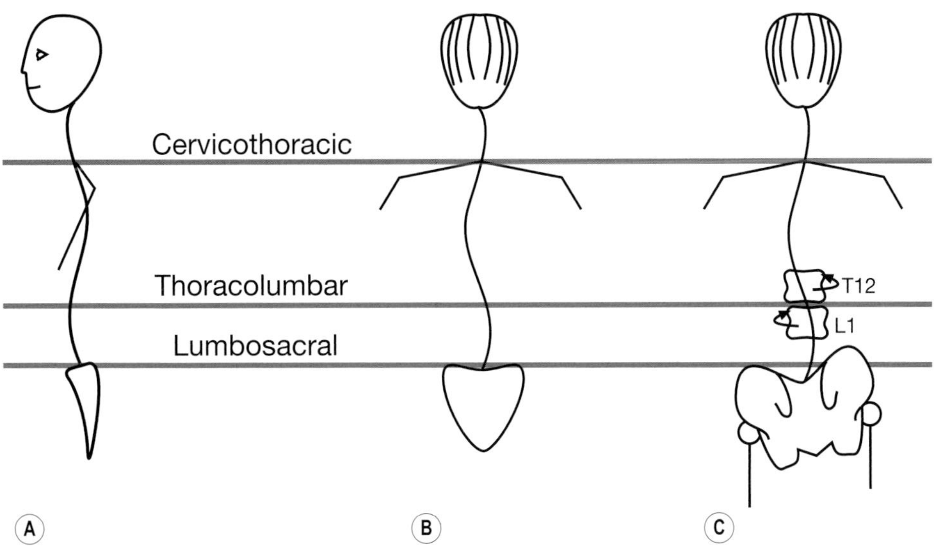

Fig. 3.14 Sites of spinal curve reversal and stress. Lateral and posterior views show matching sites of curve reversal in the sagittal and frontal planes respectively. Reversal at the thoracolumbar junction typically results in the rotation of T12 and L1 in opposite directions. (A) Lateral view; (B) posterior view; (C) thoracolumbar (T/L) junction. *(Redrawn courtesy of Pansky & House 1975.)*

rotational displacement at or adjacent to these sites of reversal: C7, T1, T12, L1, L4 and L5. An involvement of vertebrae at these levels often makes the immediate part of the curve reversal feel stiff and unyielding. Palpation is likely to reveal increased tone and tenderness in the paravertebral muscles running alongside. This may be a reflex increase in tension, in reaction to pain originating from the spine, or could reflect an attempt to stabilize this segment of the spine. Other mechanisms may, however, also be operative (see 'Asymmetry of muscle tension' below).

Pressure applied to the spinous processes repeatedly elicits a report of pain localized around T11,T12 and/or L1, L4, L5 or S1 areas, even though the person may not otherwise be aware of pain from these sites. However, if he or she actually do report discomfort from the spine, this is most likely to localize to:

1. a site of curve reversal, and hence of high stress
2. a site where one or more vertebrae have rotated excessively

Because of the altered biomechanics, these sites are not only more likely to be symptomatic but also more vulnerable to injury from either an acute sprain or strain of the area, or the stress of repetitive twisting and bending imposed by daily activities, work or participation in sports.

Clinical correlations: sites of curve reversal

Activities that demand increased motion of the spine in all three planes are more likely to trigger or aggravate pain from:

1. sites of vertebral rotational displacement
2. those sites already put under increased stress as a result of the compensatory curves formed with malalignment, especially where these curves change direction: the cervicothoracic, thoracolumbar and lumbosacral junctions.

Increased tension in the paravertebral muscles restricts those trunk ranges of motion which put these muscles under further stretch. Forward flexion is affected particularly by involvement of uni- or bilateral paravertebral, erector spinae and latissimus dorsi muscles; e.g. reaching forward; cycling, sculling (Fig. 5.6). Side-flexion in isolation, or combined with rotation (e.g. as in canoeing, rowing and kayaking; Fig. 5.1), will be limited by any increase in tension involving the contralateral paravertebral and/or shoulder girdle muscles. With 'rotational malalignment', it is seen to most often involve rhomboids, scalenes, upper trapezius, infraspinatus and teres minor on the right side (see 'Asymmetry of muscle tension' below).

Thoracolumbar curve reversal may also result in the 'thoracolumbar syndrome': irritation of the cutaneous sensory fibres from T12 and L1 giving rise to low back pain, with possible radiation to the buttock, abdomen and lateral thigh regions (see Ch. 4; Fig. 4.23).

ASYMMETRY OF THE THORAX, SHOULDER GIRDLES AND ARMS

Side-flexion of the trunk will normally have the effects listed in Box 3.3.

There is also an element of rotation of the vertebrae in the transverse plane. Whether rotation is directed into the convexity or the concavity seemingly depends on whether the initiating motion was either a pure side-flexion or a trunk rotation (Lee 1993a, 1994a, 1994b). Vertebral rotation rotates each set of attaching ribs in the same plane, pulling one posteriorly and pushing the opposite one anteriorly.

Rotational displacement of a specific vertebra or vertebrae has similar effects on the attaching ribs but in an exaggerated way, as discussed in Ch. 2 ('curves of the spine and vertebral rotation'). For example, left rotation and side-flexion of T5 can result in a rotational stress particularly on the sixth rib:

1. at the back
   a. posterior rotation of the right, and anterior rotation of the left rib, caused by the re-orientation of the costotransverse joints (right rib gliding inferior, left superior relative to the vertebral aspect of the joint)
   b. counterclockwise rotation in the transverse plane, so that there is some displacement of the lateral aspect, inward (medial) of the right rib and outward (lateral) of the left relative to the ribs above and below (Fig. 2.94A)
2. at the front
   a. these stresses are all transmitted anteriorly to the costochondral junctions, which may turn out to be just tender to palpation or actually outright painful (Fig. 2.94B).

BOX 3.3 Effects of trunk side-flexion on the ribs

1. Approximates the ribs on the concave side (Fig. 3.15A)
2. Causes some rotation of each pair of ribs in opposite directions (anteriorly on the concave, posteriorly on the convex side), a movement that appears to be determined by the fact that:
   a. after the motion of the ribs on the concave side has stopped, the thoracic vertebrae continue to side-flex slightly into the concave side
   b. this continued motion of the vertebrae causes the ribs on the concave side to glide upward, and the ribs on the convex side to glide downward, at the costotransverse joint
   c. the direction of this movement of the ribs is guided by the orientation of the costotransverse joint surfaces, translating into rotation: anterior on the concave and posterior on the convex side (Fig. 3.15B)

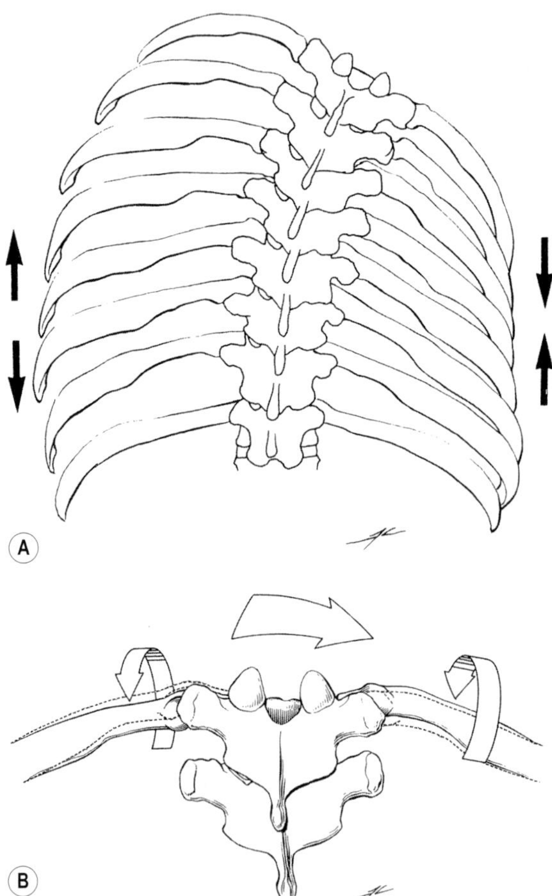

Fig. 3.15 Changes in the ribs associated with right trunk side flexion. (A) As the thorax side-flexes to the right, the ribs on the right approximate and those on the left separate at their lateral margins. The costal motion stops first, the thoracic vertebrae then continuing to side-flex slightly to the right. (B) In the vertebrosternal region, the superior glide of the right rib at the costotransverse joint induces anterior rotation of the same rib as a result of the curvature of the joint surfaces. The inferior glide of the left rib at the costotransverse joint induces posterior rotation of the same rib. *(Courtesy of Lee 1994.)*

Typical changes associated with 'rotational malalignment'

When the vertebrae are side-flexed into the concavity of a thoracic curve because of malalignment, there results a narrowing of the space between the ribs on that side. The lowest ribs may actually touch each other or the 11th will touch the lateral iliac crest on active side-flexion or sometimes just on deep breathing or even at rest. A lateral curving of the thoracic spine usually causes depression of the shoulder and scapula on the concave and elevation on the convex side (Figs 2.90, 2.91A). As described, when the thoracic curve begins to reverse as low as the T4 or T5 level, the shoulder may actually be lower on the side of the concavity formed by the proximal part of the thoracic spine (Fig. 2.91B). Also, in a person standing at ease, one may easily note some rotation of the entire thorax opposite in direction to that evident in the pelvis, so that the shoulder on one and ASIS on the opposite side appear forward rotated.

The overall effect is a combination of forward flexion, side-flexion and axial rotation of the thoracic vertebrae, maximal at the apex of the curve. The attaching pairs of ribs are displaced in opposite directions at each level in all three planes. This puts the rib attachments, both anteriorly and posteriorly, under some torsional stress and may result in tenderness and/or overt pain at these sites: the sternocostal and costochondral junctions anteriorly, and the costotransverse, costovertebral and facet joints posteriorly (Figs 2.94, 3.16).

Any coexisting rotational displacement of one or more vertebrae, especially in the upper thoracic spine, will compound the torsional stress on these sites at specific levels (Figs 2.94, 2.96B). Malalignment also creates a torsional force on the clavicles, increasing the stress on the acromioclavicular and sternoclavicular joints (Fig. 2.94B). Typical complaints and findings include:

1. ***anterior chest pain***: the pain can sometimes mimic angina; tenderness localizes to the sternoclavicular joint and/or the sternocostal or costochondral junction of the rib(s) involved
2. ***posterior chest, intercostal and/or 'mid back' pain***: recreated by stressing specific costovertebral and costotransverse joints
3. ***shoulder pain***: localizing to the acromioclavicular joint
4. ***tenderness over the lowest ribs***: especially when these impinge on each other and/or the lateral iliac crest

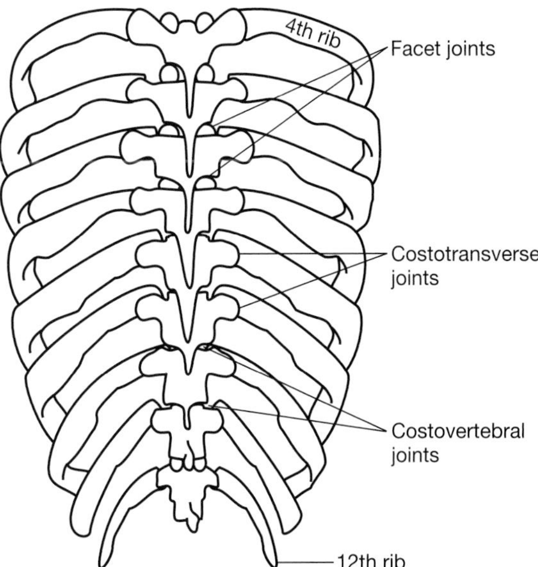

Fig. 3.16 Posterior rib cage structures put under stress by malalignment and vertebral/rib rotation (see also Fig. 2.94).

In the absence of a history of heart disease, trauma or evidence of an inflammatory process, these symptoms and signs may well be caused by the increased torsional stresses. Resolution on the correction of pelvic malalignment and rotational displacement of any thoracic vertebra(e) would substantiate the diagnosis.

One common presentation in standing is with some counter-rotation of the pelvis around the vertical axis, so that the right ASIS ends up slightly forward. The pelvic obliquity is most often with the right side up and the thoracic convexity runs opposite in direction to that seen in the lumbar segment - a thoracic curve convex right would usually be seen with a left lumbar convexity (e.g. Fig. 2.70). Frequently associated findings on examination of someone with 'rotational malalignment', some of which can be seen on Figures 2.70, 2.90, involve the following:

1. ***rotation of the thorax around the vertical axis***
   a. movement in the transverse plane is usually opposite in direction to that of the pelvis
   b. however, simultaneous rotation of the thorax into the same direction as the pelvis can also occur and results in both the pelvis and the shoulder appearing forward on the same side
2. assuming a thoracic right convexity and counterclockwise trunk rotation (Fig. 2.70):

a. *asymmetry of shoulder girdle reorientation*
   The left ends up retracted and depressed, the right protracted and elevated
b. *asymmetry of scapular reorientation*
   The left is rotated counterclockwise, sometimes to the point that the medial border appears to 'wing' and studies are initiated for a suspected weakness of mid-trapezius, the rhomboids or serratus anterior or a possible long thoracic nerve injury

3. *asymmetry of the glenoid fossae*
   Depression of the left shoulder and counterclockwise rotation of the left scapula reorients the left fossa downward and posteriorly; whereas on the elevated right side, the fossa ends up pointing more upward and anteriorly.
4. *asymmetry of glenohumeral ranges of motion (ROM)*
   Reorientation of the thorax and shoulder girdles and asymmetries of muscle tension (see below) alter the ranges possible at the shoulder joints. The typical pattern includes:
   a. a decrease in right internal, left external rotation (as illustrated by the values recorded on assessment in Fig. 3.17A)
   b. a decrease in left extension (Fig. 3.17B).
5. *asymmetry of other upper extremity ranges of motion*
   Malalignment can also result in an obvious asymmetry of some of the distal joint ROMs. For example, a typical finding is a 5–15 degree

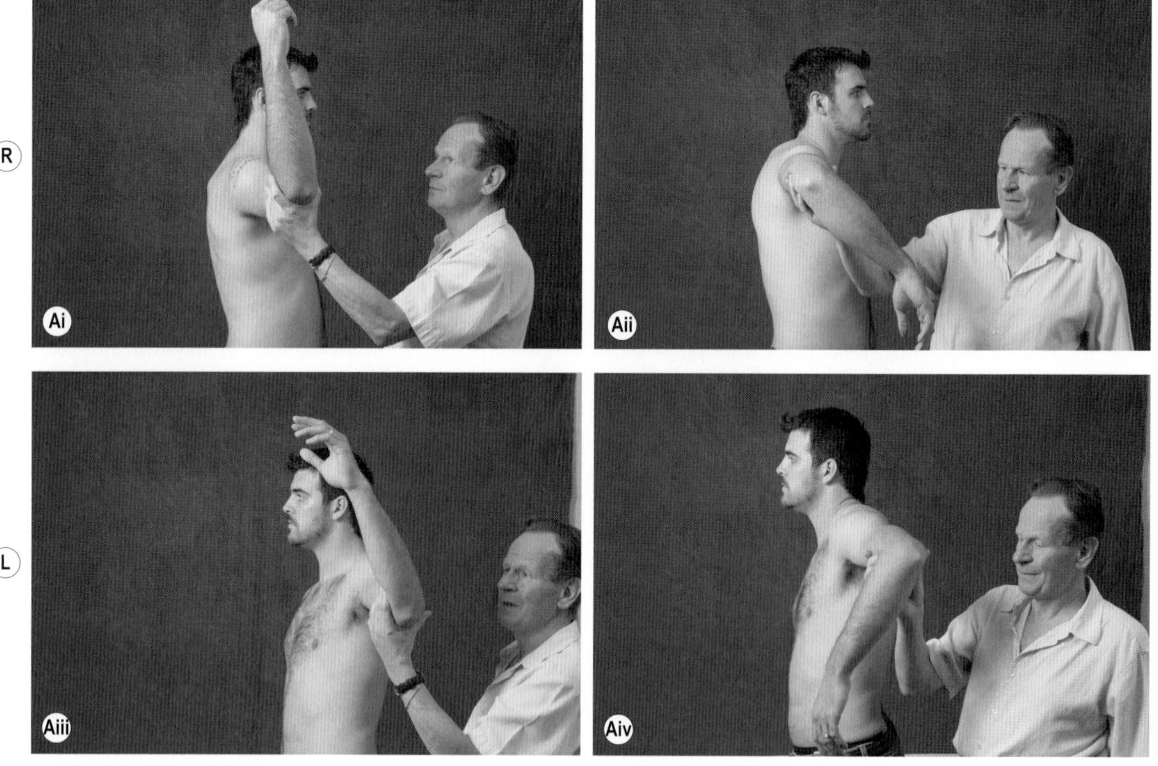

External rotation	Internal rotation	Combined ROM
Right = 95 degrees Left = 75 degrees	Right = 50 degrees Left = 70 degrees	Right = 145 degrees Left = 145 degrees

Fig. 3.17 Typical asymmetries in upper extremity ranges of motion seen with the 'most common' patterns of 'rotational malalignment' and an 'upslip'. When testing external and internal rotation - the relaxed arm is being supported by the examiner at the elbow to allow it to rotate freely (see Ai–iv); forearm pronation and supination - the elbows are steadied against the side (see C, D). (A) Decrease of right internal and left external rotation; the combined range, however, remains the same bilaterally.

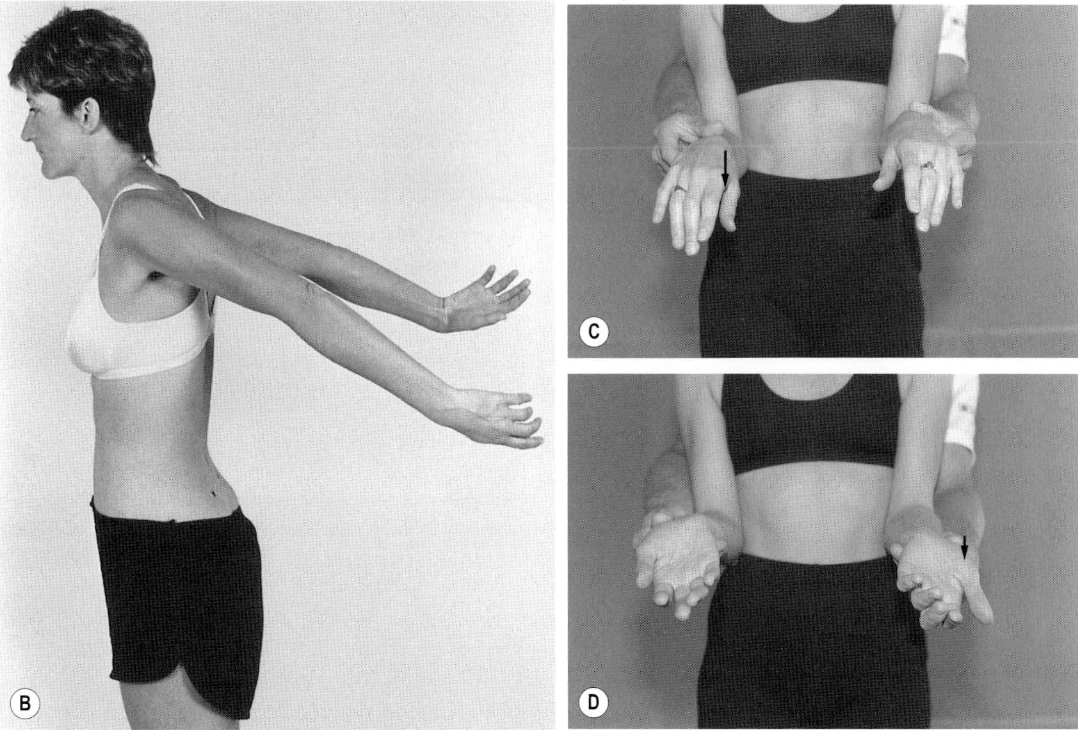

Fig. 3.17—cont'd (B) Limitation of left extension. (C) Limitation of left forearm pronation. (D) Limitation of right forearm supination.

limitation of left forearm pronation (Fig. 3.17C) and right supination (Fig. 3.17D).

6. ***asymmetry of strength***

   Malalignment usually results in an asymmetry of strength in the shoulder girdle and upper extremity muscles. Detection of the weakness is dependent on the position of examination (Maffetone 1999) and may not be as easily or as consistently apparent as the asymmetrical weakness detectable in the lower extremities (see 'Asymmetry of lower extremity muscle strength' below). Side-to-side differences are usually more obvious in the proximal muscles, especially anterior deltoid, supra- and infraspinatus and can disappear dramatically on realignment.

Clinical correlation: thorax and shoulder girdle

The asymmetry of thoracic and shoulder girdle alignment and ranges of motion, also of the strength and tension of the muscles in this area, increases the stress on the shoulder joint and rotator cuff complex bilaterally. The stress on the acromioclavicular and glenohumeral joint tendons, ligaments and capsules increases the likelihood of developing shoulder pain and may predispose to impingement, acute or chronic sprain, and joint wear and tear with early degeneration.

For example, the increased downward slant of the glenoid fossa on the side of the depressed shoulder decreases the passive support that the shelf formed by the lower rim usually provides for the humeral head. The capsule and cuff are now constantly subjected to increased gravitational traction forces which may be offset by the chronic reflex contraction of the shoulder girdle muscles attempting to stabilize the humeral head in the socket. Supraspinatus is particularly well suited for this task, which may explain the frequent report of pain from the right supraspinatus on neck rotation and the localization of supposed 'neck spasms' and tenderness to this muscle. These mechanisms may also play a role in the development of a complicating supraspinatus tendonitis, impingement, calcific tendonitis and subacromial bursitis.

Asymmetrical shoulder ROMs may affect performance, notably in work activities that depend on a full range of motion and result in stress on the joint by repeatedly having to hold on to and lift objects (e.g. carpentry, painting), those stressing the whole shoulder girdle in combination with movement of the trunk (e.g. throwing sports; Fig. 3.18) or those requiring a normal range of motion in combination with full and symmetrical muscle strength (e.g. weight-lifting, gymnastics, diving, synchronized swimming, the symmetrical strokes in swimming and rowing events). However, a specific asymmetry could prove useful in certain situations; for example:

1. when the increase in extension is on the dominant side (Fig. 3.17B)

   This may help in certain of the throwing sports in which the ability to generate velocity is dependent on an initial extension of the throwing arm at the shoulder (e.g. baseball, football and athletic events). The overhand throw, for example, begins with the throwing arm abducted, externally rotated and fully extended (Figs 3.18, 3.51, 5.31). An underarm throw begins with a backswing of the throwing arm, as far as extension at the shoulder will allow. In the side-arm throw used for the discus, the throwing arm is again initially fully extended
2. when finding oneself repeatedly requiring maximum range on use of the arm in one or more directions to reach further or while working within confined spaces

The asymmetry may prove costly in sports that require symmetrical arm extension for propulsion. As indicated in Ch. 5, if the left arm cannot extend as far as the right, the swimmer using the butterfly or elementary back stroke can compensate by:

1. limiting right arm extension to maintain symmetry of stroke force
2. rotating the trunk counterclockwise to increase the amount of extension possible on the left side, to the point where symmetry of stroke-force can be achieved; active trunk rotation, however, increases energy requirements and may cause a wobble and increase resistance to the water - both adaptive techniques could result in slowing.

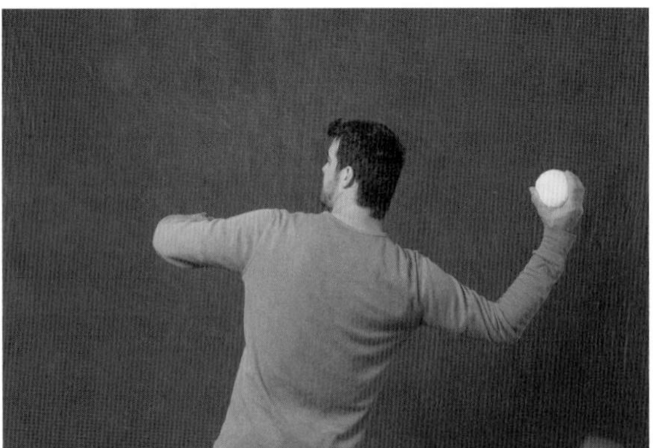

Fig. 3.18 Increased external rotation as a result of the asymmetry of shoulder ranges of motion seen with malalignment (Fig. 3.17A) may be of help if it occurs on the side of the throwing arm.

ASYMMETRY OF LOWER EXTREMITY ORIENTATION

Most people who are in alignment have their lower extremities in some external rotation, both feet pointing outward some 10–15 degrees relative to the midline (Fig. 3.19A). A small number have their legs in 'neutral', the feet pointing straight forward, and some are 'pigeon-toed', both feet pointing inward. Barring the effect of previous injuries, foot orientation relative to the midline is usually symmetrical in all three cases.

> 'Rotational malalignment', on the other hand, results in an asymmetrical orientation of the lower extremities: one leg undergoes some external and the other internal rotation.

There are many factors that can result in such a rotation. For example:

1. 'Facilitation' of the right gluteus maximus and/or piriformis, with simultaneous 'inhibition' of right tensor fascia lata, frequently seen in those with one of the 'more common' patterns of 'rotational malalignment', results in forces favouring outward rotation of the right leg; whereas the 'facilitation' of the left TFL/ITB complex and 'inhibition' of left external rotators favours internal rotation of that leg (see 'Asymmetry of muscle strength' below).
2. Pain on the lateral side of the foot, as may occur with a 'cuboid subluxation' (see below; Fig. 3.85A), may make a person change their gait pattern by increasing pronation and

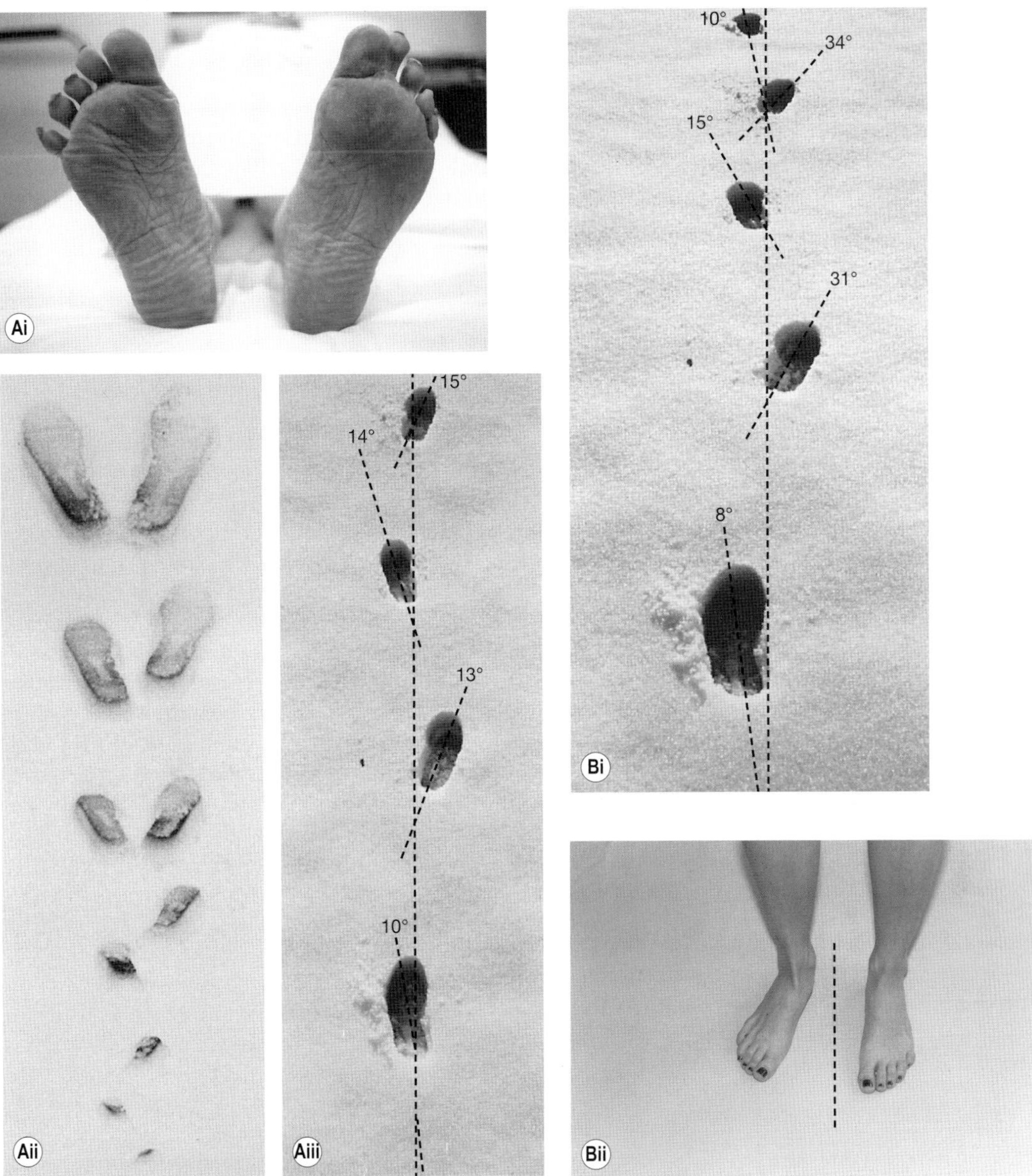

Fig. 3.19 Lower extremity rotation associated with malalignment. (A) Aligned: legs externally rotated to nearly equal extent relative to the midline: (i) lying supine; (ii) walking on snow; (iii) running on snow. (B) Malalignment present (one of the 'more common' rotational patterns or an 'upslip'): the right leg has undergone external, the left internal rotation: (i) running on snow (the same person as in Fig. 3.19Aii and Aiii, but before realignment): the right foot turned out considerably more than the left; B(ii) left internal rotation to the point at which the left foot actually crosses the midline and points to the right.

external rotation on that side, to shift weight-bearing medially and away from the painful lateral site.

Whatever the underlying cause may be, we appear eventually to be left with some consistent patterns of malalignment relating to lower extremity orientation and weight-bearing and associated asymmetries, as discussed in this chapter. For ease of recognition, the two main findings in regard to lower extremity orientation as related to the presentation of 'rotational malalignment' at hand are:

1. with the 'most common' patterns of 'rotational malalignment'

   The right lower extremity has rotated externally and the left internally (Figs 3.3B, 3.19B); typically, there is an associated passive:

   a. outward rotation of the right foot relative to midline to a varying degree; it is not unusual to see the right foot pointing out as much as 30–45 degrees from the midline
   b. inward rotation of the left leg toward the midline, sometimes so far that the foot has actually crossed the midline and ends up pointing to the right side (Fig. 3.19Bii).

2. with the 'left anterior and locked' pattern

   There is 'left anterior, right posterior' innominate rotation and 'locking' of the left SI joint: the right lower extremity has rotated internally and the left externally (Fig. 3.3A); typically, there is an associated passive:

   a. outward rotation of the left foot relative to the midline to varying degree
   b. inward rotation of the right foot toward, or possibly even across, the midline.

These patterns of leg rotation are readily apparent in most when walking behind them or observing their gait while carrying out specific tests in the clinic. The final pattern will be influenced by other factors that affect movement of the limbs and weight-bearing, such as a natural tendency to pronation or supination (discussed below; Fig. 3.33). In some, the exaggerated leg rotation in opposite directions may be more readily apparent when they are:

1. relaxed and lying supine or prone (Fig. 3.20)
2. asked to walk on the heels or toes, hop on the toes of one foot at a time, or run at increasing speed on a treadmill (Fig. 3.24A,B)

At the extreme, if the leg that has rotated internally has done so to the point that the foot actually crosses the midline (Fig. 3.19Bii), the person may appear to be walking almost sideways; in this case, alternately leading with the inside of the externally-rotated pronating right foot and then the outside of the internally-rotated, supinating left foot.

Clinical correlation: lower extremity orientation

The asymmetrical orientation of the lower extremities seen with the 'malalignment syndrome' is one of the major factors contributing to the asymmetry of lower limb biomechanical function. Other factors, including asymmetry of weight-bearing, muscle strength and tension, also affect orientation and influence the biomechanics of standing and walking. These are discussed in more detail below.

In those with one of the 'more common' rotational patterns and the associated clockwise rotation of the lower extremities, the heel of the out-turned right foot can now more easily strike – unintentionally - against the inside of the left foot or calf, usually just above the medial malleolus (Fig. 3.21Aii). Similarly, the toes or the tip of the shoe of the in-turned left foot can catch more easily against the medial aspect of the right shoe or the posteromedial aspect of the right calf (Fig. 3.21B).

Proof of such contact becomes more readily apparent when playing or running on a wet surface, when dirt and water tend to mark these sites.

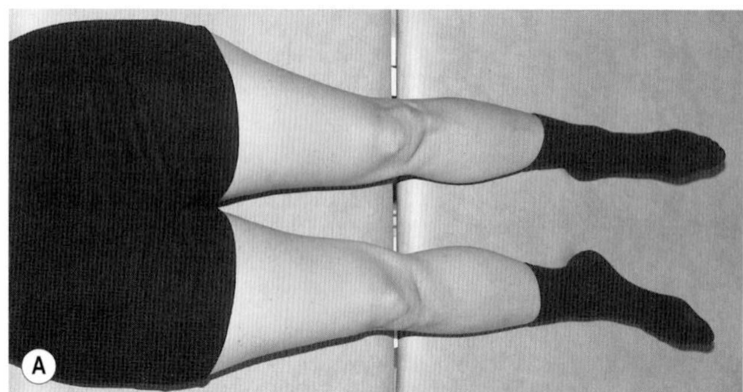

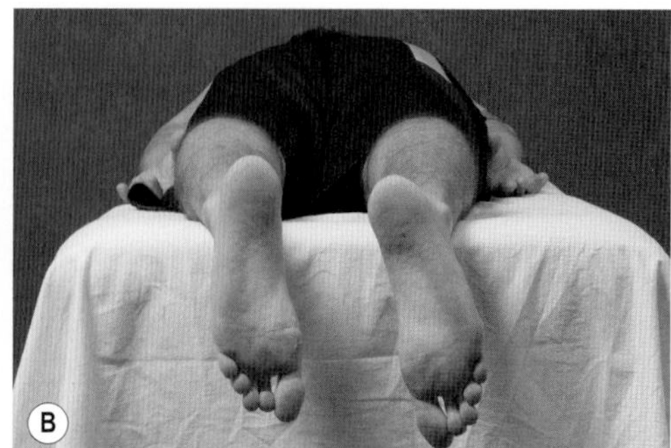

Fig. 3.20 Typical right external and left internal rotation of lower extremities evident in relaxed (A) supine- and (B) prone-lying.

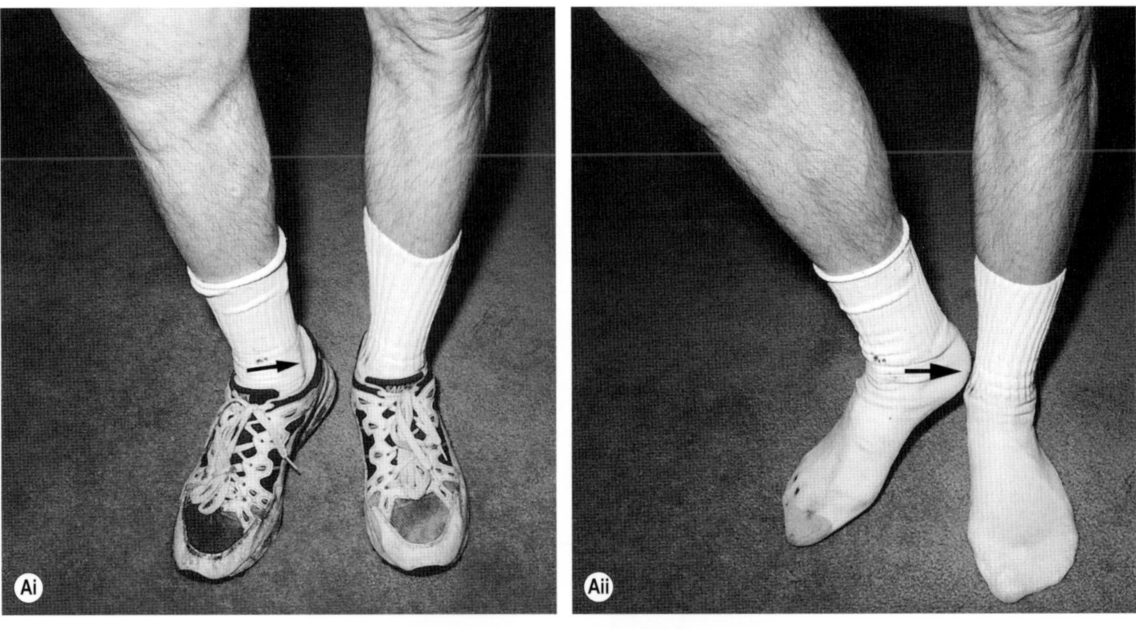

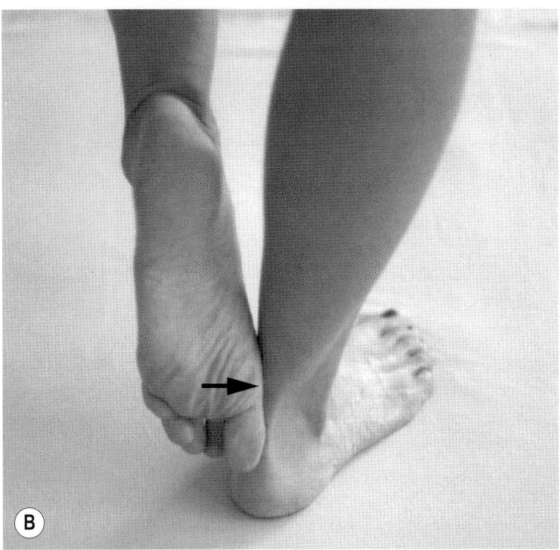

Fig. 3.21 Malalignment with increased right external, left internal rotation. (A) Right heel (i) strikes at or above the left medial malleolus, (ii) marking the inside of the left sock or calf. (B) The tip of the left foot catches the posteromedial right Achilles tendon and/or medial calf.

Contact may briefly upset the person, or even cause them to trip and fall at times. Tripping as a result of malalignment may pose more of a problem for children, given their generally decreased coordination and balance compared to adults.

The opposite findings and associated problems are seen with the 'left anterior and locked' pattern of rotational malalignment.

ASYMMETRY OF FOOT ALIGNMENT, WEIGHT-BEARING AND SHOE WEAR

It cannot be stressed enough that 'rotational malalignment' and an 'upslip' both cause a shift that often results in a striking asymmetry of the weight-bearing pattern. The direction of this shift is related, in part, to the pattern of lower extremity rotation (Figs 3.3, 3.22, 3.23B, 7.1):

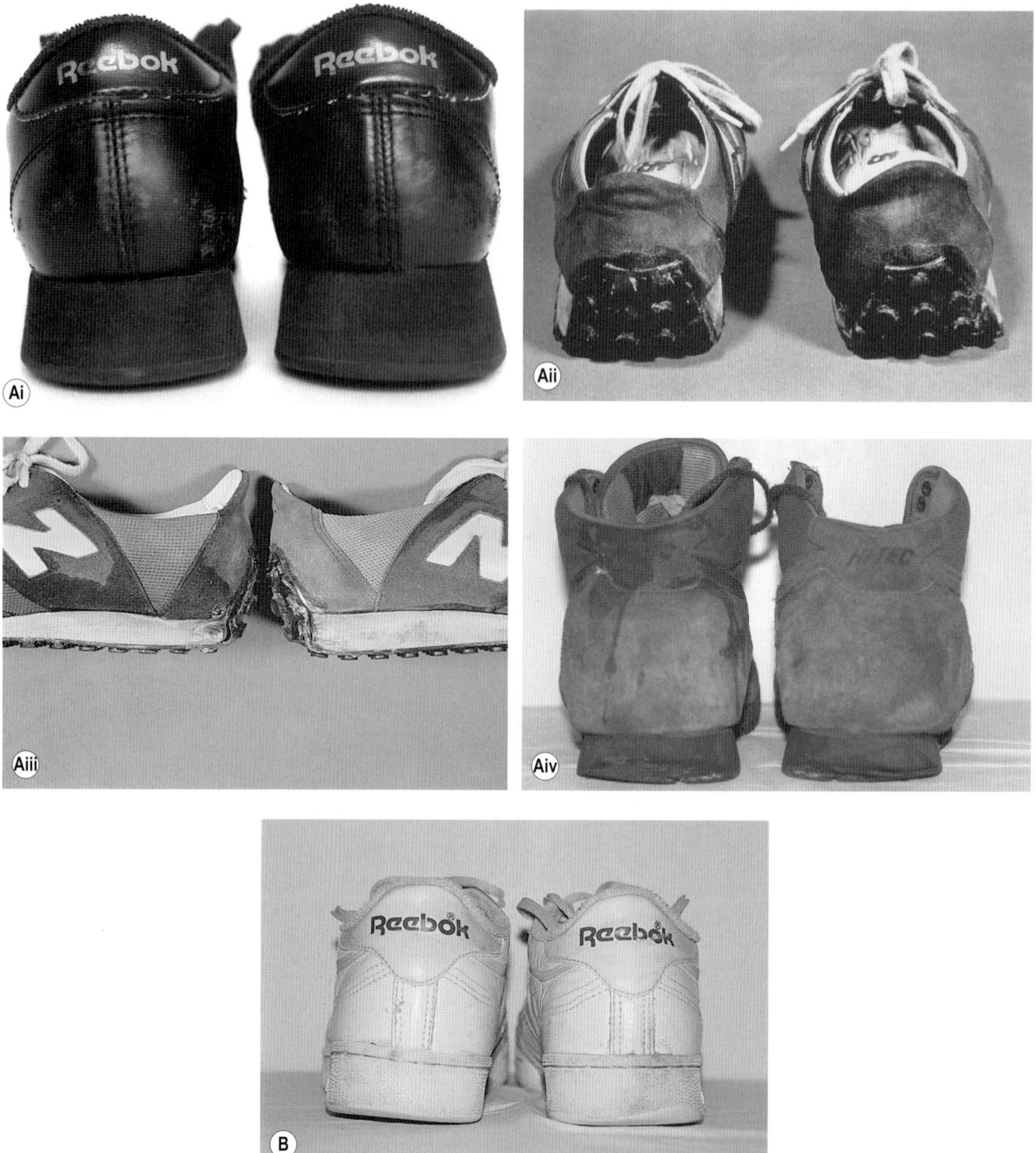

Fig. 3.22 Heel cup collapse reflecting a shift in weight-bearing with malalignment. (A) With the 'more common' patterns of 'rotational malalignment' and an 'upslip': heel cups collapse toward the left side with the tendency to right pronation, left supination: (i) walking shoes; (ii) running shoes after 6 weeks of 100 miles per week; (iii) lateral view of same running shoes - note the compression of the right medial heel material; (iv) boots. (B) 'Left anterior and locked': the left heel cup leans noticeably into the right, reflecting the underlying tendency to left pronation and right supination.

1. to the inside of the foot on the leg that has rotated externally; there may be an obvious collapse into pronation
2. to the outside of the foot on the leg that has rotated internally; there may be an obvious collapse into supination

Which leg rotates inward or outward is in turn related to the pattern of 'rotational malalignment': right outward and left inward with the 'more common' patterns, the opposite with 'left anterior and locked'.

Given the fact that most people show one of the 'more common' patterns, with rotation externally of the right and internally of the left lower extremity, the weight-bearing typically noted on observing gait and shoe-wear is that indicative of a tendency to right pronation and left supination (Fig. 3.22A). The opposite findings will be apparent in those with the relatively infrequently seen 'left anterior and locked' pattern (Fig. 3.22B).

Gradations between these extremes are possible. For example, in the person with one of the 'more common' rotational patterns who is seen to:

1. pronate on both sides
   - the tendency to pronate will be more marked on the side of the externally rotated leg (Fig. 3.23A)
2. supinate on both sides
   - the tendency to supinate will be more marked on the side of the internally rotated leg (Fig. 3.23B).

In other words, the actual weight-bearing pattern depends in large part on the presentation of the malalignment but continues to be influenced by the person's inherent tendency toward pronation or supination. The examiner must, therefore, look at the attitude of the feet both at rest and on weight-bearing when out of alignment and, subsequently, once realignment is being maintained, to verify that person's 'true' pattern (Fig. 3.33).

The detection of asymmetry can be improved by having him or her walk on the heels and toes, hop on one foot, and walk or run at increasing speed on a treadmill. When a person with one of the 'more common'

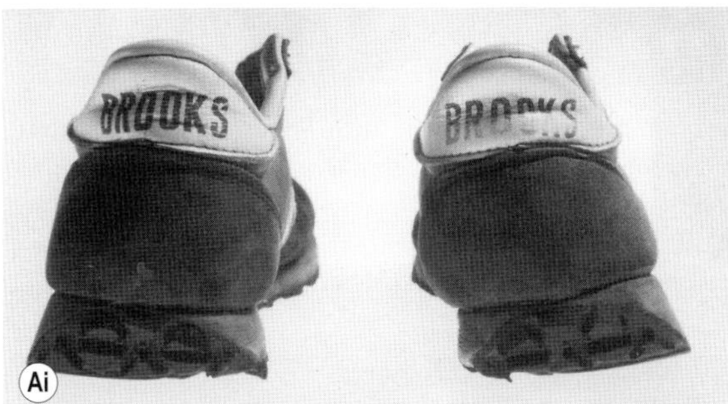

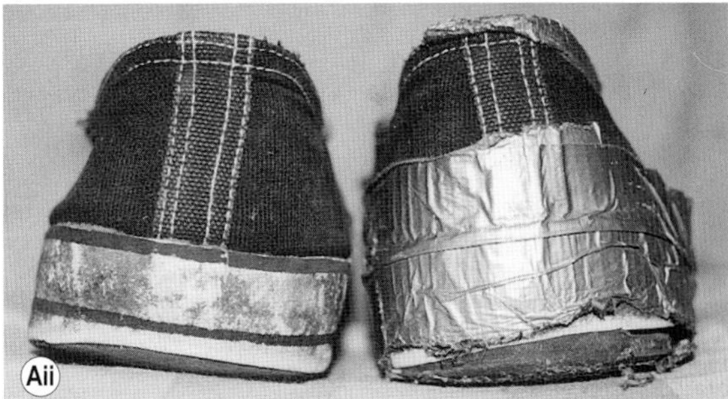

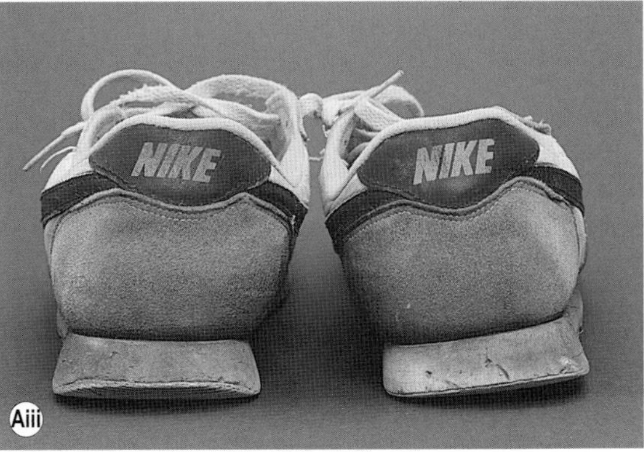

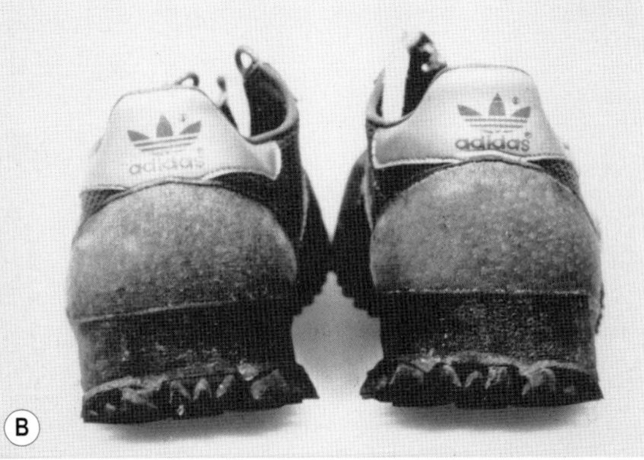

Fig. 3.23 Patterns of heel cup collapse reflecting the shift in weight-bearing seen with the 'more common' patterns of 'rotational malalignment' and an 'upslip'. (A) With bilateral pronation: (i) worse on the side of external rotation (right); (ii) marked right pronation leading to desperation measures using duct tape to reinforce the heel cup medially; (iii) typical running shoes (see also Fig. 3.32B). (B) With bilateral supination: worse on the side of internal rotation (left).

patterns of 'rotational malalignment' toe-walks, hops, or even just walks in high-heeled shoes, the right heel will typically be observed to 'whip' inward as the foot tends to collapse into pronation; whereas the left heel will stay vertical if that foot maintains a neutral position, or may actually whip outward as the foot collapses into frank supination (Fig. 3.24A,B).

On an analysis of a pair of day shoes or running shoes, the asymmetry can often be verified by the pattern of midsole compression, of wear on the heels and soles, and of collapse of the heel cup and uppers. A quantitative assessment of side-to-side differences is also possible. For example, the asymmetry of weight-bearing that occurs in a person with one of the 'more common' patterns and a tendency to right pronation and left supination, can be evident on:

1. a static topographical map of the soles made standing on the spot (Fig. 3.25A)

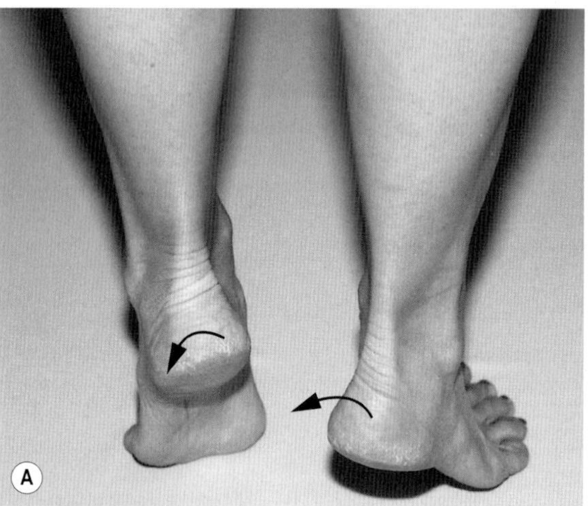

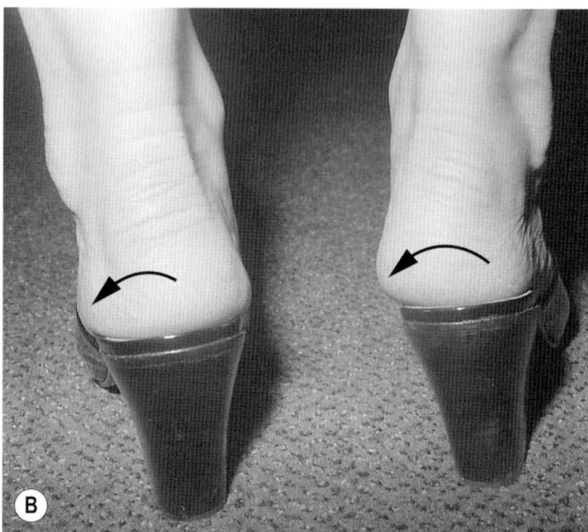

Fig. 3.24 Toe-walking accentuates the asymmetry of weight-bearing in the person with one of the 'more common' patterns of 'rotational malalignment' or an 'upslip'. (A) Inward whip and collapse of the heel (calcaneal eversion) on the right (pronating) side; positioning in neutral or even a whipping outward of the heel (calcaneal inversion) on the left (supinating) side. Note the markedly increased external rotation of the right leg compared with the left. (B) A similar pattern evident walking on high heels: the right heel pronates to the point of shifting inward (partially off the heel support), the left leaning slightly outward.

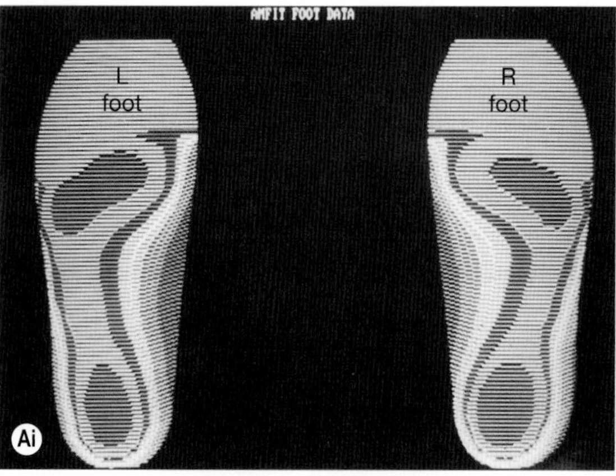

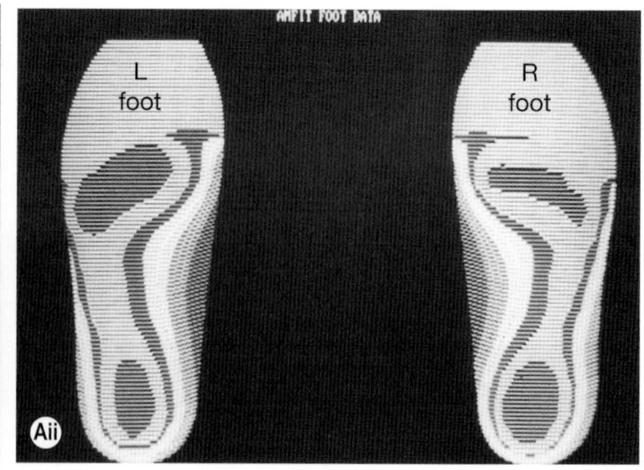

Fig. 3.25 Quantitative assessment of weight-bearing pattern. (A) Static topographical pattern of the sole of the foot on weight-bearing, recorded by air pressure sensors (Amfit Inc. CAD/CAM orthotic fabrication system). (i) Malalignment - an asymmetrical pattern results: note the increased width of the left medial grey bar (denoting the highest part of the medial longitudinal arch), in keeping with the tendency toward left supination. The width of the right bar, on comparison, has decreased with the collapse of the arch as a result of pronation. (ii) Realignment - increased symmetry of pattern: note the almost identical width of the right and left medial grey and white bars at the midsection of the arch.

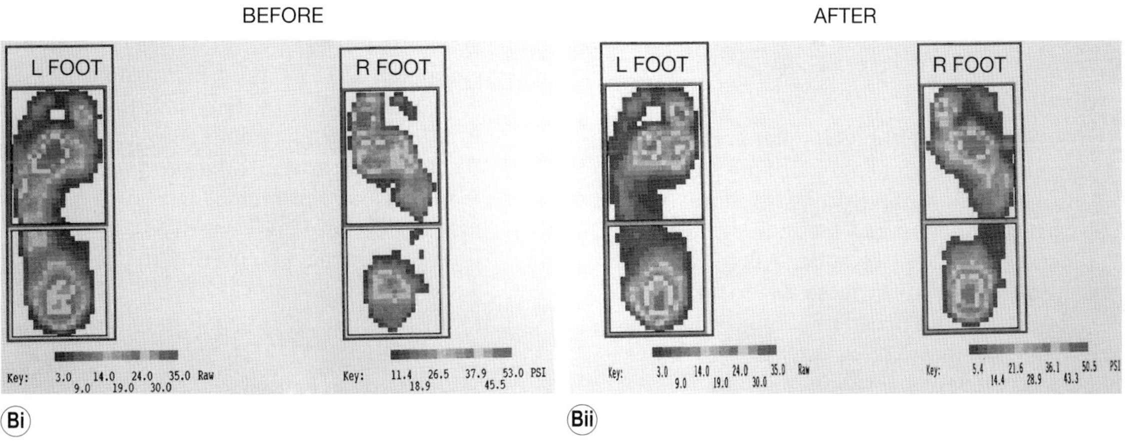

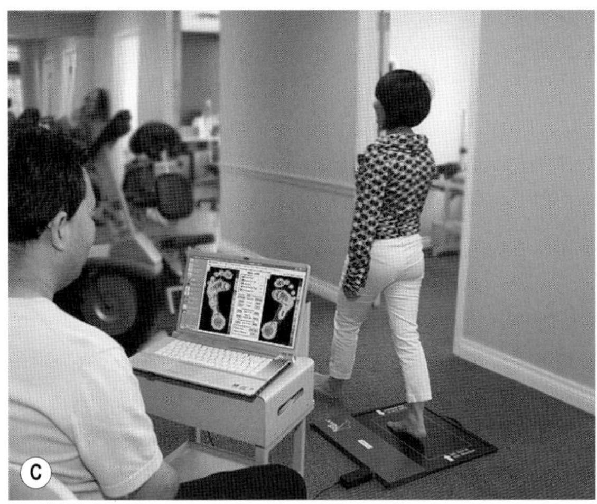

Fig. 3.25—cont'd (B) Dynamic pattern of weight distribution, recorded by 960 electronic measuring points within a 'sensor mat' in the shoe, which scans the foot in motion 30 times per second throughout stance (Footmaxx ™). The relative amount of weight borne is indicated by shading - maximal being black. (Bi) with malalalignment present - asymmetrical weight-bearing pattern reflecting the tendency toward right pronation and left supination: the right transfer of weight from the heel to the forefoot is 'disconnected' and overall less forceful; the left foot pattern shows more weight-bearing laterally and on the ball of the foot. (ii) on realignment - the pattern is much more symmetrical: the right foot now shows the weight-being transferred from heel to forefoot in a 'connected' pattern, with increased concentration on the heel, midfoot and ball of the foot regions; the left shows shift medially, considerable weight-bearing now being evident in the heel and medial midfoot areas. (C) Current dynamic method: a woman walking barefoot across a computerized mat (Footmaxx ™); more-or-less symmetrical display on screen is in keeping with the fact that realignment was achieved prior to her carrying out this test.

2. a dynamic pressure pattern made when walking or running (Fig. 3.25B) and
3. computerized weight-bearing patterns now commonly used to fit someone for orthotics (Fig. 3.25C)

These methods can show the right medial and left lateral shift: the left medial longitudinal arch will be deeper because of the tendency to supination; whereas the right arch will tend to flatten with pronation. These methods also offer one way of recording the return to the person's normal, and usually more symmetrical, weight-bearing pattern that occurs with realignment (Fig. 3.25A,B).

Attitude of the feet

Attitude of the feet: weight-bearing

1. **when in alignment**

   When non-weight-bearing, the feet of most people who are in alignment are suspended, more or less symmetrically, with the heels in varus angulation and the inner border of the foot up relative to the outside (Fig. 3.26Ai). This is true even for most of those who turn out to be supinators when weight-bearing; in only a small number of these - less than 5% - are the heels in neutral or actual valgus angulation at rest.

2. **when malalignment is present**

   With 'rotational malalignment', the attitude of the non-weight-bearing feet becomes asymmetrical. The most common finding, then, is an increase in the amount of heel, mid- and forefoot varus angulation on the side of the externally rotated lower extremity compared to the side of internal rotation (Fig. 3.26Aii). The relative findings are similar to those seen in a prone-lying person with right external rotation: the varus angulation of the right foot of about 20 degrees is relatively increased, compared to only 10 on the left (Fig. 3.26B). Factors contributing to this asymmetry at rest include:

   a. the asymmetric orientation of the foot and ankle joints
   b. the increased amount of inversion possible on passive movement of the subtalar joint on the side of external rotation (Fig. 3.27A,B)
   c. the asymmetrical tension in the muscles (see 'Asymmetry of muscle tension' below), those

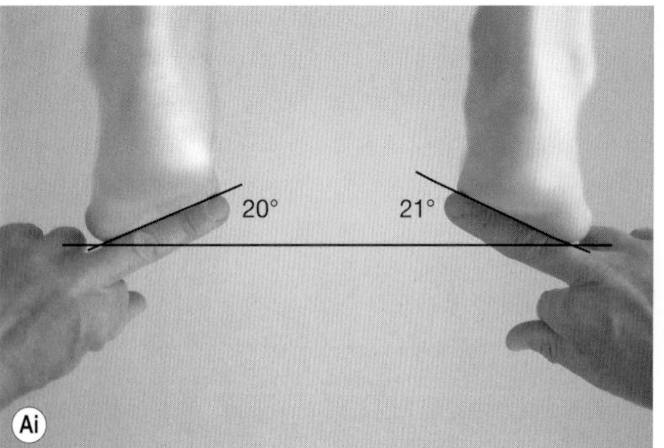

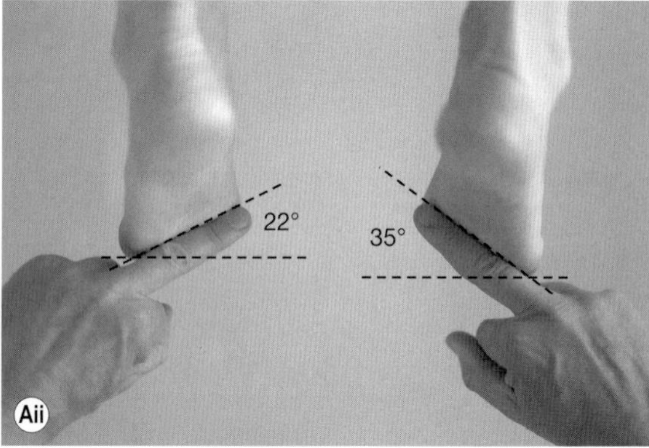

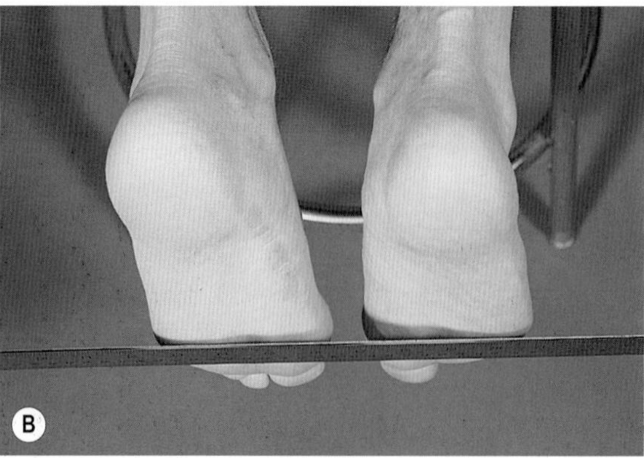

Fig. 3.26 Angulation of the feet at rest (non-weight-bearing). (A) Subject 1 (sitting): (i) in alignment: symmetrical varus angulation (20 degrees); (ii) with malalignment: the varus angulation is increased to 35 degrees on the right (the side of external rotation) compared with 22 degrees on the left (the side of internal rotation). (B) Subject 2 (prone-lying): with malalignment, varus angulation on the right is 20 degrees, versus 10 degrees on the left.

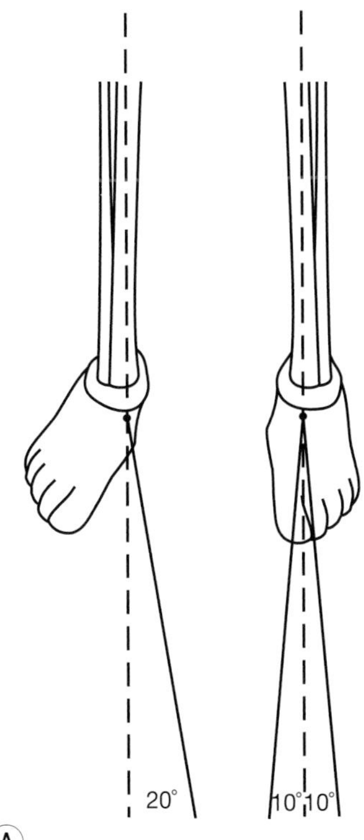

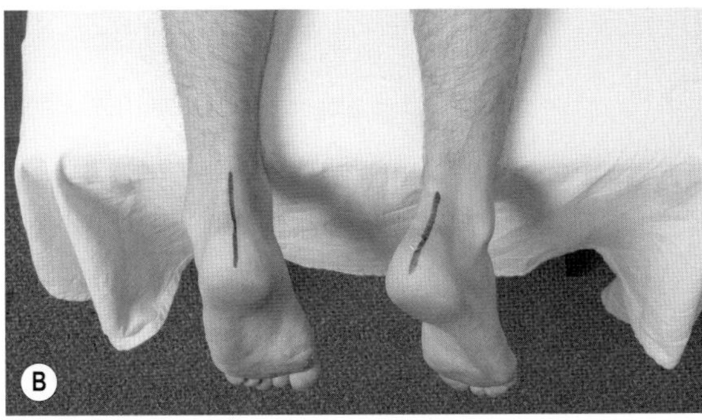

Fig. 3.27 Asymmetry of subtalar ranges of motion seen with the 'more common' patterns of 'rotational malalignment' or an 'upslip'. (A) With the person lying supine and the ankle 'locked' at 90 degrees, passive movement of the calcaneus typically shows: decreased right eversion (here 0 degrees versus left 10 degrees) and decreased left inversion (10 degrees versus right 20 degrees). Bilaterally, the combined range remains the same: 20 degrees. The right leg has rotated externally, the left internally. (B) Person with malalignment at rest, lying prone: right heel in obvious varus angulation while that on the left remains in near-neutral position.

with an 'upslip' or one or the 'more common' rotational patterns show increased tension in:

i. right tibialis anterior/posterior, tending to right foot varus
ii. left peroneus longus, tending to left foot valgus.

Attitude of the feet: weight-bearing

The varus angulation commonly seen when the feet are non-weight-bearing results in the following findings on weight-bearing:

1. **when in alignment**

   All of the non-weight-bearing foot is in varus and all of the lateral border, therefore, in a position to touch the ground first immediately on heel-strike. However, shoe wear initially occurs primarily on the posterior or posterolateral aspect of the heel and, as weight-bearing progresses anteriorly, more centrally and then underneath the ball of the foot, in a fairly symmetrical pattern (Fig. 3.28A,B; see 'Asymmetry of shoe wear' below). This wear pattern reflects the fact that, in preparation for weight-bearing, the feet are most often suspended in a varus attitude, and also with the ankles in neutral or slight dorsiflexion.

   Therefore, contact at heel-strike is more likely to occur first on the posterolateral edge of the heel, and that contact immediately initiates a force - supplemented by muscle action - that torques the foot and ankle into valgus; that is, toward medial weight-bearing and often frank pronation. This sequence of events, with the foot rolling inward, occurs so quickly that wear usually tends to be more obvious along the posterior rather than the posterolateral aspect of the heel (Fig. 3.28A,B). As weight-bearing shifts more medially and forward into the midfoot region, the subtalar joint and transverse metatarsal arch are literally 'unlocked' to help absorb shock. As the foot rises into plantar-flexion, weight-bearing is increasingly across or even lateral in the forefoot region and the calcaneo-cuboid-subtalar joints and midfoot progressively 'lock' in preparation for 'push-off' from the now relatively stable foot and ankle.

2. **when malalignment is present**

   Weight-bearing typically tends to be more posterolateral on the side of the externally rotated and more posterior on the side of the internally rotated lower extremity. In those

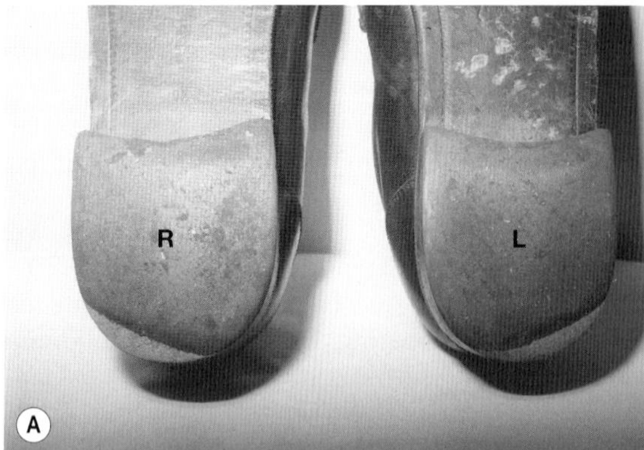

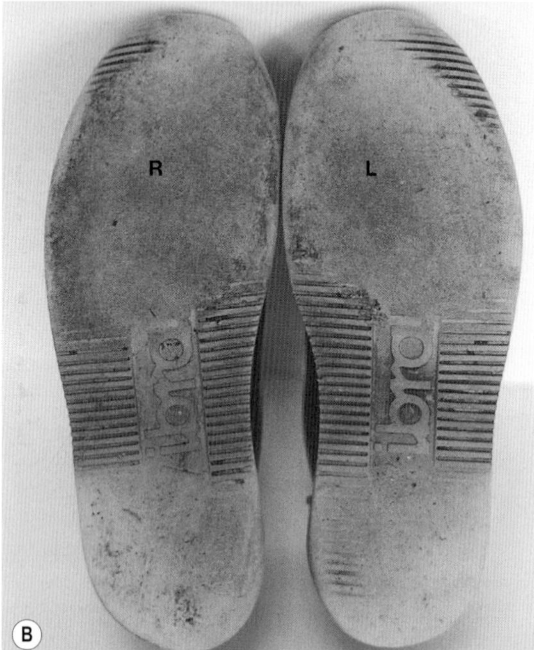

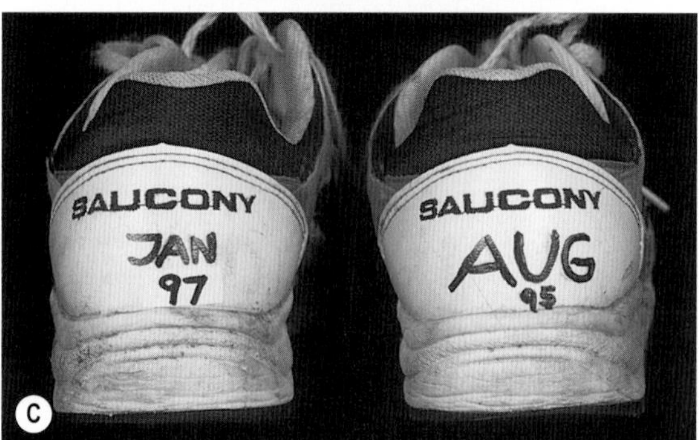

Fig. 3.28 Typical shoe wear pattern when in alignment. (A, B) View of heels and soles: heel wear is even and more posterior than lateral. (C) Posterior view: symmetrical width of heel and sole; heel cups lean inward 5 degrees, reflecting minimal pronation bilaterally, after 19 months wear!

with an 'upslip' or one of the 'more common' patterns of 'rotational malalignment':

weight-bearing on the right side

The increased varus angulation of the heel at heel strike results in:

1. initial contact and wear of the posterolateral to lateral aspect of the heel (Fig. 3.29A,B)
2. an accentuated medial torquing of the foot with increasingly more medial weight-bearing on progressing forward from the heel
3. tendency to pronation

The tendency to right pronation and medial weight-bearing appears to be in large part a passive phenomenon, the result of a number of factors initiated at heel-strike in most of us.

First, because of the varus angulation of the non-weight-bearing foot, the lateral edge of the heel is first to contact ground on weight-bearing; this has an outrigger effect, forcing the foot into neutral, or even valgus, following heel-strike.

Second, the more the right leg is in external rotation, the more the medial border of this foot comes to lie increasingly forward, especially when compared to what is occurring on the left side. On weight-bearing, there results a passive rolling from the lateral onto the medial aspect of the foot as it progresses from heel-strike to foot-flat.

Third, the pronation and associated eversion of the subtalar joint are also linked to an inward rotation of the tibia which, in turn, is linked to the external rotation of the femur. Inward rotation of the tibia, through a 'hinge-like' effect (Mann 1982), forces the calcaneus into further eversion: the varus angulation of the non-weight-bearing calcaneus changes to valgus on weight-bearing. This brings the axes running through the talonavicular and calcaneocuboid joints more into parallel and allows for more movement of the transverse tarsal joint (Fig. 3.30Ai,Bi). An unlocking of the metatarsals occurs, allowing the medial longitudinal arch to collapse as the foot simultaneously pronates, abducts and dorsiflexes and becomes increasingly able to absorb shock. As weight-bearing shifts forward, the sequence reverses to stabilize the foot in preparation for heel-strike (Fig. 3.30Aii,Bii).

Fourth, a further collapse of the right medial longitudinal arch may occur because of the malalignment-related functional weakness, or 'inhibition', of the right ankle invertors (tibialis anterior and posterior, which would normally help maintain the arch) and 'facilitation' of right peroneus longus (see 'Asymmetry of muscle strength' below).

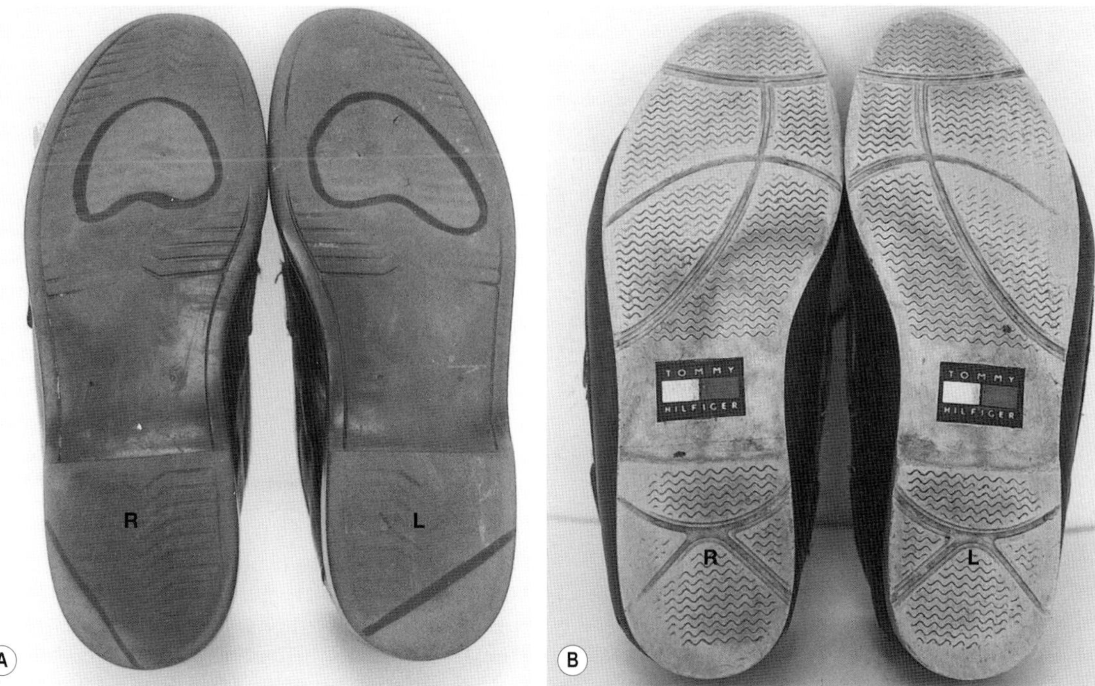

Fig. 3.29 Typical asymmetrical shoe wear pattern seen with malalignment, evident in the soles of pair (A) and (B). The right shoes both show increased wear: posterolaterally in the heel (reflecting the increased varus angulation at heel-strike), and medially in the forefoot (reflecting the tendency toward pronation). The left shoes both show generally increased wear involving a wider area posteriorly but also more medially than on the right (reflecting the comparatively decreased left varus angulation at impact; see also Fig. 3.26), and more laterally in the forefoot (reflecting the tendency toward supination).

Finally, any persistent limitation of the right subtalar eversion detected in supine lying may play a role (Fig. 3.27), provided this is still operative when the person is weight-bearing. As soon as all available eversion has been exhausted by the ways described above, further pronation and calcaneal eversion can be achieved by having the knee drop inward, allowing the foot and tibia to collapse inward more while predisposing to valgus angulation at the knee (Fig. 3.37: 'pronation').

weight-bearing on the left side

Initial contact is more uniform across the back of the heel, and the medial torquing force is diminished. Heel wear may be less marked but affect a greater area; there is usually less wear posterolaterally, tending to involve more the posterior aspect of the heel itself (Fig. 3.29). Weight-bearing forward to the forefoot remains relatively more lateral, reflecting the tendency toward supination.

The shift toward supination and lateral weight-bearing on the side of the internally rotated left leg is, for several reasons, probably also primarily a passive phenomenon, similar to the shift toward pronation on the side of the externally rotated right leg.

First, the tendency for the left foot to shift from varus to valgus is decreased or not even evident or actually reversed, in part due to the fact that the left non-weight-bearing foot is in less varus angulation at rest, rarely even in a neutral position.

Second, the internal rotation of the left lower extremity orients the foot more in the line of progression and may even cause the foot to actually cross the midline so that it now points inward (Fig. 3.19Bii):

1. the lateral border comes to lie increasingly forward, relatively speaking, ahead of the medial one
2. the foot will passively roll from the inner to the outer border on progressing from heel-strike to foot-flat or, depending on the amount of valgus angulation when non-weight-bearing, end up on the lateral aspect all along.

Third, because of the internal rotation of the femur, the tibia undergoes external rotation, and the

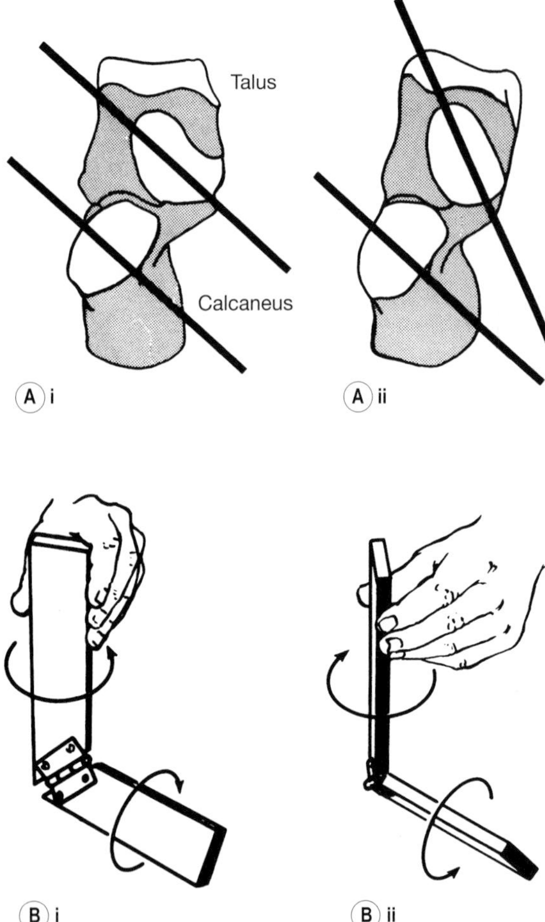

Fig. 3.30 Mobility of the foot and ankle. (A) Related to the axes of the transverse tarsal joint. (i) When the calcaneus is in eversion (e.g. pronation), the conjoint axes between the talonavicular and calcaneocuboid joints are parallel to one another so that increased motion occurs in the transverse tarsal joint. (ii) When the calcaneus is in inversion (e.g. supination), the axes are no longer parallel, and there is decreased motion and increased stability of the transverse tarsal joint. (B) Model of function of the subtalar joint as it translates motion from the tibia above to the calcaneus below: (i) inward rotation of the tibia causes outward rotation of the calcaneus (= eversion), (ii) outward rotation of the tibia causes inward rotation of the calcaneus (= inversion). *(Courtesy of Mann 1982.)*

hinge-effect causes the subtalar joint to reorient so that the calcaneus is passively forced into further inversion on weight-bearing. The axes of the transverse tarsal joint diverge; motion at this joint is decreased, locking the metatarsals and increasing the stability of the longitudinal arch (Fig. 3.30Aii,Bii). Weight is transferred forward either in a direct line from the heel to the toes, consistent with a neutral pattern of weight-bearing, or along the lateral border of the foot if the pattern is one of frank supination (Fig. 3.25A,B).

Fourth, once all the available range of calcaneal inversion attainable by the above ways has been achieved, any demands for further inversion can involve the knee dropping outward into neutral alignment or frank genu varum (Fig. 3.37-'supination').

Fifth, a further collapse of the lateral longitudinal arch may occur because of the malalignment-related weak and 'inhibited' left ankle evertors - peroneus longus, brevis and tertius - being unable to counter the increase in tension and strength in the 'facilitated' right tibialis anterior and posterior.

As a result of these factors, the shift in weight-bearing commonly seen in association with the 'more common' rotational patterns is one tending inward on the right and outward on the left. In 15–20%, the right foot will actually end up overtly pronating, and the left overtly supinating (Figs I.1 - in Introduction 2002; 3.22A). If there is obvious persistence of bilateral pronation, it will be more pronounced on the right side to varying degrees (Fig. 3.23A); if there is bilateral supination evident, it will be more obvious on the left to some degree (Fig. 3.23B). The reverse of these findings is seen with the 'left anterior and locked' pattern.

Sloping of the supporting surface will dramatically affect the shift in weight-bearing. The more common shift to right pronation, left supination (Fig. 3.31A) will be accentuated whenever the right foot is higher relative to the left on a surface sloping down to the left; for example, when running against traffic in Canada and the USA, or with the traffic in the UK, NZ, Australia (Fig. 3.31B). The runner may already have found that this tendency to shift into pronation on one side, supination on the other can be decreased, and the stability of the feet increased, by running or walking with the right foot on the 'down side' relative to the left (Fig. 3.31C).

Asymmetry of shoe wear

The shoes alone are just as important an indicator of the weight-bearing pattern as is watching the person walk up and down the hallway, preferably both when barefoot and when wearing shoes. Look at a pair of shoes worn for several months during the day and, if possible, one for some sports activity or just 'loafing around'. In the case of an athlete,

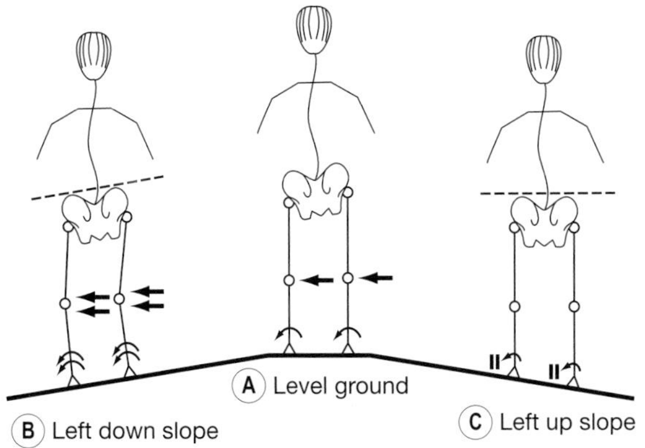

Fig. 3.31 The effect of a slope on the malalignment-related tendency toward right pronation, left supination on level ground. (A) Usual shift to left seen with an 'upslip' and the 'most common' patterns of 'rotational malalignment'. This shift is (B) accentuated on a slope declined to the left and (C) decreased on a slope inclined to the left.

running shoes worn in training and competition are more likely to help determine what happens at higher workloads and speeds when participating in his or her chosen sport. It will also help discover the occasional person who pronates when walking and changes to neutral or even progressively increasing supination on running, or shifts the opposite way - from supination to pronation.

High-heeled shoes may not be very helpful because the heel cup, sitting up on a pedestal, may too easily sway in either direction along with the heel itself. Usually the higher the base of the shoe, the less the support, sometimes seemingly amounting to no more than the straps. The point of heel contact is often too small to determine the true impact pattern on the sole. Observing someone walk when wearing high heels may, however, still reveal the asymmetry typical of malalignment, with the heel tending to fall inward or even over the medial edge of the base on the pronating side and outward or even over the lateral edge on the opposite, supinating side, similar to what may be seen on toe-walking (Fig. 3.24A,B). The stiff ankle section of a boot will sometimes yield enough to accurately reflect the asymmetry of weight-bearing forces, with inward or outward collapse of the heel-section (Fig. 3.22Aiv). However, the lower part of the boot usually tends to be very stiff - often reinforced with metal in the toe section and back toward the heel to varying degree - making the uppers more likely to collapse in either direction.

Heel cups and uppers

The pattern of heel cup collapse will often allow one to deduce:

1. that malalignment is very likely present
2. whether the malalignment is likely to be:
   a. the 'left anterior and locked' pattern
   b. one of the 'more common' patterns of 'rotational malalignment' or an 'upslip' (although it cannot distinguish between these)
   c. the person's probable inherent weight-bearing pattern: pronation or supination, although this presumption is tentative until re-examination of weight-bearing can be carried out once alignment is actually being maintained (see Fig. 3.22Ai,Aii compared to Fig. 3.33).

Patterns of wear typically associated with 'rotational malalignment' are described in Box 3.4.

With the 'more common' patterns of 'rotational malalignment', a force from the right appears to have displaced the heel cups - and sometimes quite obviously also the uppers - toward the left side (Fig. 3.22A). With the 'left anterior and locked' pattern, a force from the left appears to have displaced them toward the right side (Fig. 3.22B). The final pattern will depend on the effect of the malalignment-related forces on the person's inherent weight-bearing pattern. Again, this inherent pattern should be confirmed on follow-up gait assessment and examination of a new pair of shoes once alignment has been maintained for 2–3 months.

> In summary, the heel cup and uppers of the shoes have a windswept appearance, reflecting the shift in weight-bearing that occurs in a person with 'rotational malalignment' (also an 'upslip'): from 'right-to-left' with the 'more common' patterns, and 'left-to-right' with the 'left anterior and locked' combination.

Heel, sole and midsole wear patterns

Wear of the heel, sole and midsole often reflect the shift in weight-bearing. The following findings are typical of the 'more common' rotational patterns.

Heel

Right heel contact wear tends to involve primarily the posterolateral aspect (Fig. 3.29A,B). As discussed above, this reflects the combined effect of the external rotation of the right leg, comparatively increased varus angulation and the slight dorsiflexion of the

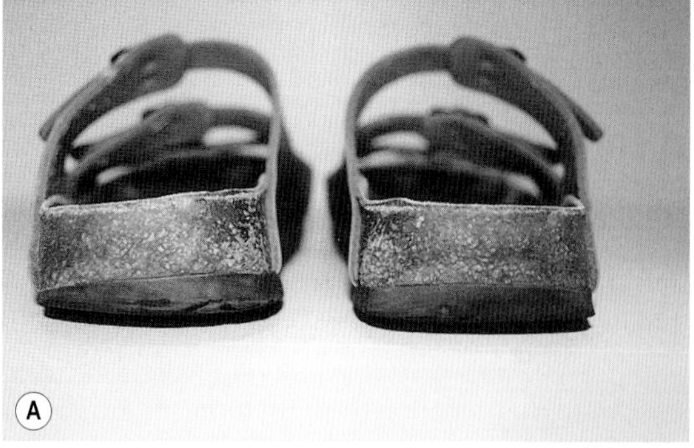

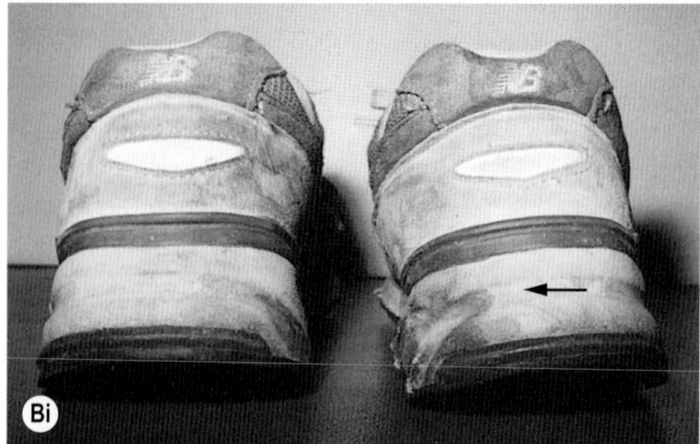

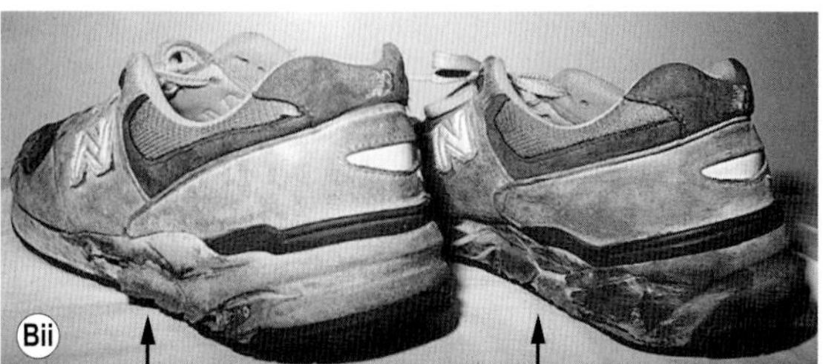

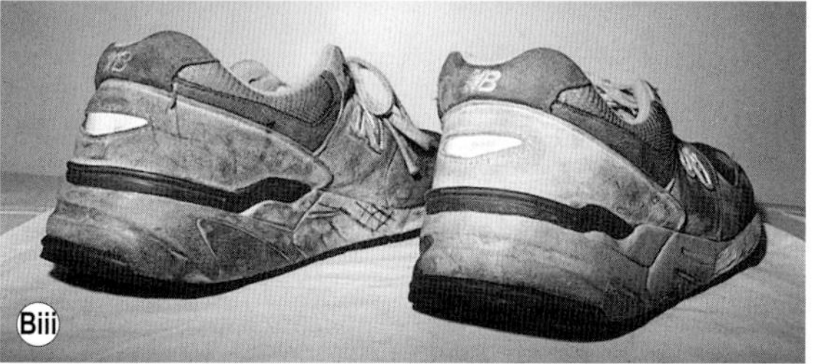

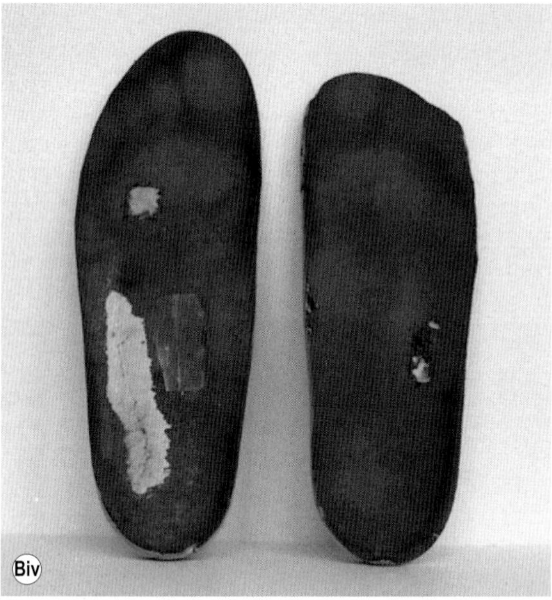

Fig. 3.32 Asymmetry of midsole compression and wear caused by malalignment is evident from heel to forefoot: the right medially from a tendency to pronation, the left laterally from a tendency to supination. (A) Birkenstock sandals: compression of the right medial and, more markedly, left lateral heel and sole. (B) Double-density, straight-last running shoes intended to counter pronation: (i) pronation more marked on the right, with deterioration (compression) of the right heel medially (arrow); (ii) view from the left: deterioration of the right inner and left outer midsole (arrows); (iii) view from the right: the left inner and right outer midsoles are both intact; (vi) top of insoles show markedly asymmetric wear (the person has deliberately cut front of right insole back to accommodate a 'cock-up' toe deformity; see Fig. 4.16A).

right foot just prior to heel-strike. In essence, these lower the posterolateral part of the shoe so that it is first to contact the ground (Fig. 3.26) and is likely to show more wear of the heel at this site (right shoe in Fig. 3.29). The greater the external rotation and varus angulation, the more lateral the initial heel wear; also, the more quickly the shoe will torque into a medial weight-bearing position. Left heel wear, in contrast, shows the impact to involve more the posterior aspect of the heel, given the relative decrease in varus angulation at heel-strike.

Midsole

Because the right foot can switch from the lateral impact to medial weight-bearing so quickly, a compression of midsole material on the medial aspect can occur as far back as the heel and go on from there to involve the mid- and forefoot section of the shoe (Figs 3.22Aiii, 3.32Bi,ii). In contrast, the left

BOX 3.4 Asymmetry of shoe wear (heel cups/uppers) typically associated with 'rotational malalignment'

'More common' patterns of 'rotational malalignment'

1. The typical wear of shoes seen reflects the tendency to right pronation and left supination, with frank inward collapse of the right and outward collapse of the left heel cup and upper, respectively (Fig. 3.22A).
2. Other findings commonly seen that are still in keeping with this shift on weight-bearing are:
   a. bilateral inward collapse but worse on the right (Fig. 3.23A)
   b. bilateral outward collapse but worse on the left (Fig. 3.23B).

These wear-patterns reflect the effect of the malalignment on what may turn out to be the person's inherent weight-bearing pattern when in alignment; namely, bilateral pronation or supination, respectively (Fig. 3.33).

'Left anterior and locked'

The classical finding seen is one of frank inward collapse of the left and outward collapse of the right heel cup and upper as a result of the forces tending to left pronation and right supination, respectively (Fig. 3.22B).

midsole material tends to compress and deteriorate more on the lateral aspect, usually most markedly in the heel (Fig. 3.32Bii).

Forefoot

Right sole wear is more central (under the ball of the foot) or even more medial, reflecting the rapid switch from varus at heel-strike to valgus by foot-flat (Fig. 3.29A,B). Depending on the degree of supination, the wear of the left sole in the forefoot section (ball of the foot) may be relatively less medial, more likely central (Fig. 3.29A) or even lateral (Fig. 3.29B).

Predicting weight-bearing following realignment

In those who are in alignment, the heel cups and uppers tend to collapse inward bilaterally to some extent in those who are pronators and outward in those who are supinators, while maintaining more of a vertical position in those with a neutral pattern of weight-bearing. In a few, the hindfoot pronates and the forefoot supinates, or vice versa, in which case the direction of collapse of the heel cups is opposite to that of the uppers.

When malalignment is present, the amount and direction of collapse of the heel cups and uppers can sometimes be a fairly reliable indicator of the inherent pattern of weight-bearing that will emerge on correction. When both shoes show an inward collapse, the person may well turn out to be a true pronator; when both show an outward collapse, a true supinator (Fig. 3.23). However, these assumptions do not always hold true. For example, those who pronate bilaterally - albeit asymmetrically - when out of alignment may actually turn out to have a neutral or even lateral weight-bearing pattern, with frank supination evident following realignment (Fig. 3.33). In other words, the person's true weight-bearing pattern may not become evident until the malalignment has been corrected.

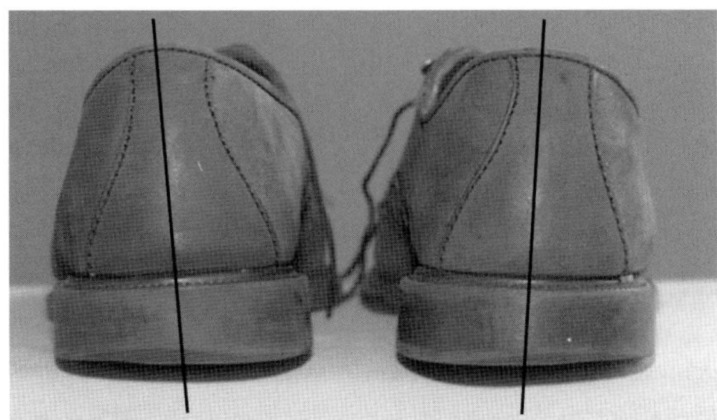

Fig. 3.33 This person has a pattern of right pronation, left supination evident when malalignment is present (see runners worn then; Fig. 3.22A). On realignment (shown here), he has reverted to his natural weight-bearing pattern of bilateral, symmetrical supination (both heel cups lean out 5 degrees).

Pitfalls to consider when assessing shoe wear

It must be remembered that the design of the shoe itself may influence the weight-bearing pattern or there may be excessive wear in a certain way for reasons other than malalignment. This may interfere with the assessment.

Increased heel and sole width

Increased heel and sole width may predispose to pronation. Assuming that the non-weight-bearing foot is in a varus attitude, the more the sole flares out and extends past the margins of the heel cup and the upper, the earlier it makes contact with the ground. In effect, it comes to act like an outrigger that can quickly flip the foot toward medial weight-bearing and pronation. The Nike LDV-1000 marketed in the 1970s serves as an unfortunate reminder of this (Fig. 3.34). The intent of the especially wide, outflaring heel and sole of this running shoe was to provide a larger base to land on; in theory, to thereby improve the stability of the foot and counter any tendency toward excessive pronation. Instead, the outwardly extending heel created an 'outrigger' effect that had exactly the opposite result in many: it increased the tendency to pronation because their feet were not positioned in neutral but actually in a varus attitude at heel-strike (Fig. 3.26A,B). The lateral border of the shoe, which served as an extension of the foot, merely came to touch the ground earlier and acted as a lever to flip the foot into pronation even sooner and more forcefully than would have occurred when barefoot.

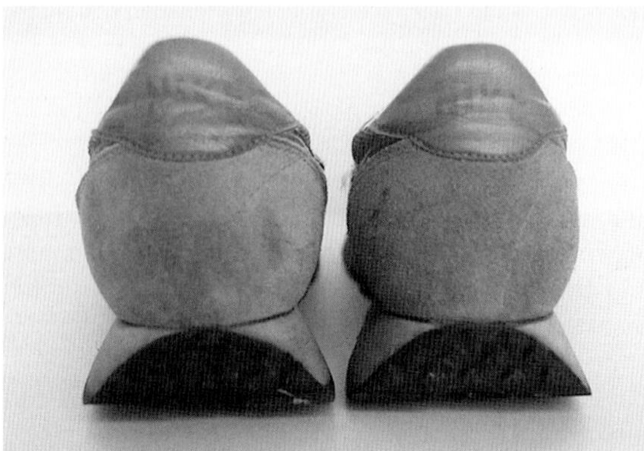

Fig. 3.34 Nike LDV-1000 running shoe with an 'outrigger-type' heel and sole intended the counteract pronation.

A wide heel and sole could conceivably also aggravate a problem of supination if the medial border made contact with the ground first. For this to happen, the non-weight-bearing foot would have to be in a valgus attitude, something that is seen much less frequently.

'Pronator' shoes: 'double-density midsole', 'straight' last

There continue to be a plethora of running shoes on the market intended specifically for pronators (Fig. 3.32, also shoe marked 'L' in Fig. 3.35A,B). Most of these have a medial reinforcement in the form of high-density midsole material - the so-called 'double-density midsole' – to reinforce the shoe medially and counteract any tendency toward excessive pronation; the grey and black material on the medial aspect of the left shoe is an example of this more supportive, and hence more rigid, material

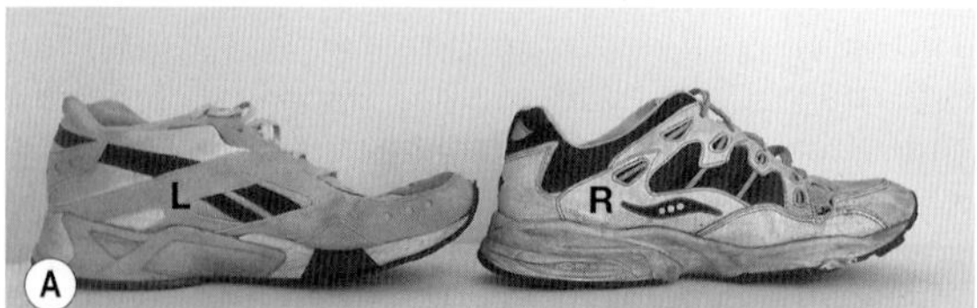

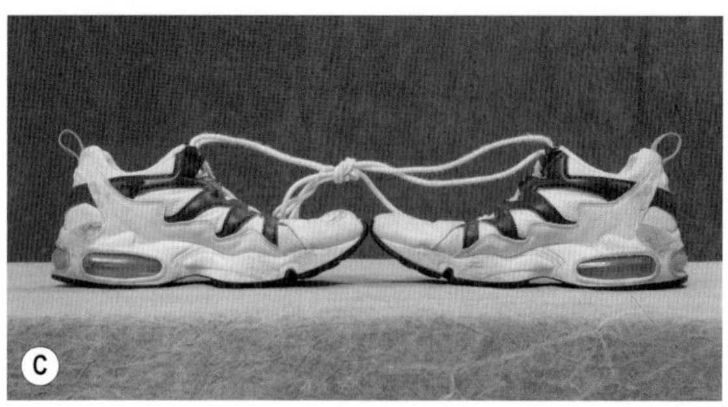

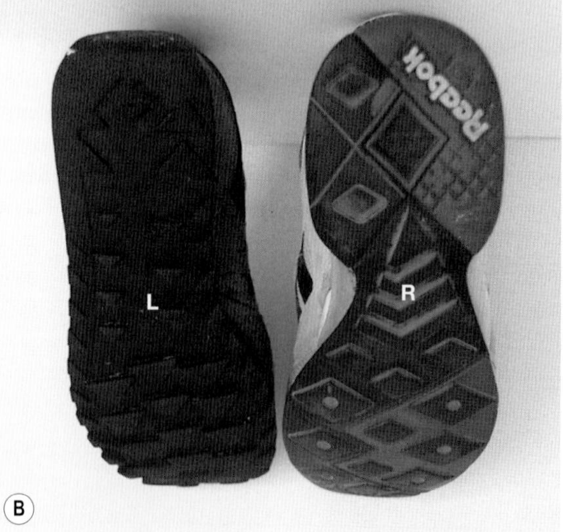

Fig. 3.35 Running shoes: modifications of the (A) midsole and (B) last. The shoe on the left is for a pronator: 'double-density' midsole (note medial reinforcement with the more dense gray material) and a 'straight last' (the medial arch filled in for extra support) to counteract medial arch collapse. The shoe on the right is for a supinator: uniformly thicker 'single-density' or 'neutral' midsole, for extra shock absorption, and a 'curved last' (with an indent or 'waist' at the medial arch level), which also allows for some collapse of the medial arch to increase the flexibility of the foot and, thereby, its ability to absorb shock. (C) View of medial aspect of a pair of runners: single-density midsole (uniform material throughout) for a supinator, with raised rearfoot and aircushion intended to improve shock absorption on heel-strike (see text).

(Fig. 3.35A). A 'straight last' sole, one with the sole filling in the space underlying the medial arch, provides further support to prevent medial longitudinal arch collapse (shoe marked 'L', showing uniform black sole on Fig. 3.35B).

These concepts of a medial reinforcement and straight last were first incorporated in the Brooks Chariot in the 1970s. In the presence of malalignment, running shoes conceived along these same lines may be helpful if the person still pronates, to some extent, bilaterally (Fig. 3.23A). If, however, he or she pronates on one side and maintains a neutral position or actually supinates on the other, this type of shoe could create problems on the side that supinates because:

1. the medial reinforcement will further increase the tendency toward supination by acting like a medial raise and countering any inward collapse of this foot
2. the ability to absorb shock and deal with ground reaction forces is further impaired by:
   a. the foot being forced toward and maintained in a more rigid, supinated position
   b. the increased density (= increased rigidity) of the medial midsole material
3. the inability of the medial longitudinal arch to collapse, often compounded by addition of a transverse arch reinforcement that is now a standard feature of most running shoes

The picture is often further complicated by provision of orthotics intended for a 'pronator', with addition of identical modifications bilaterally and with the casting having been done in a non-weight-bearing position (see 'orthotics' below).

Excessive shoe wear with time, positioning or injury

Excessive wearing down of the medial or lateral part of the heel and sole, and/or excessive inward or outward collapse of the heel cup and upper for whatever reason (e.g. breakdown attributable to prolonged use), will eventually predispose the person to an exaggerated degree of medial or lateral weight-bearing, respectively. Exaggerated shoe wear may eventually also hide the actual weight-bearing pattern, asymmetrical though this may be. If there is an underlying injury, shifting weight-bearing to off-load a painful area may result in atypical collapse and sole wear that could possibly provide a clue as to the site of the injury but is less likely to indicate whether malalignment is indeed present.

Factory-related changes

The actual shape of the shoes when they leave the factory may sometimes be misleading. A common variant is the new pair that already has the heel cups set in 5–10 degrees of varus; this could mistakenly suggest that the person is a supinator even though the shoes have hardly, if ever, been worn (Fig. 3.34). The angulation may even be greater on one side than the other, suggesting that malalignment is present when that is not the case.

Habits and ergonomics

Wear of the shoe may reflect a habit or way of using the shoe in a vocational or avocational setting rather than forces attributable to malalignment. The right shoe may, for example, have collapsed outward from operating the car gas or brake pedal with the foot in a varus attitude while pivoting with the heel on the car floor. Seeing such a lateral drift of the right shoe in a driver with one of the 'more common' patterns of 'rotational malalignment' or an 'upslip' would be completely out of keeping with the direction of the typical asymmetrical forces; namely, toward pronation on the right. In such cases, an examination of shoes not worn for driving is more likely to show the changes in keeping with those predicted for the presentation of malalignment at hand.

Walking or running on a slope or in a circular pattern

Repeatedly walking or running in the same direction on a road with a pronounced downslope from the centre, or along the side of a hill, will eventually collapse the uphill shoe inward and the downhill shoe outward in someone who is in alignment (Fig. 3.36). Running repeatedly around tight curves in the same direction (e.g. on a track) results in asymmetrical forces and eventually shoe wear patterns that may erroneously suggest that malalignment is present in someone who is actually in alignment.

Walking versus running

Remember that a person may pronate when walking but supinate when running or vice versa! Therefore, always ask to see both a pair of day shoes and those worn for athletic activities.

Rotational versus straight-line sports

The asymmetrical forces created by malalignment express themselves differently in those activities with a rotational component compared to those involving straight-line progression. The pattern of weight-bearing may, therefore, be different from one activity to another. The wear pattern of the

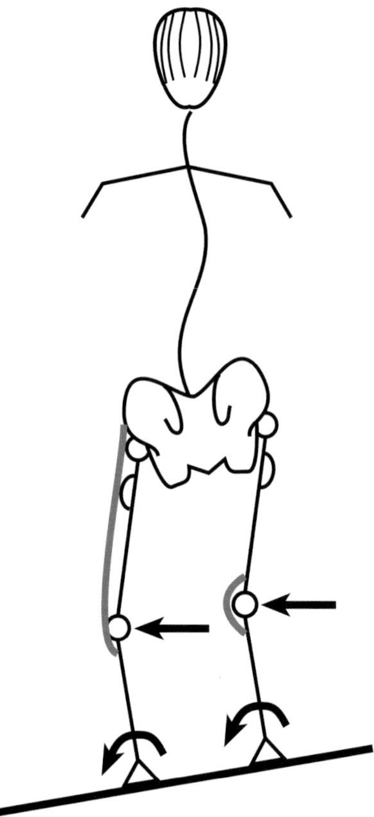

Fig. 3.36 In someone who is in alignment, repeated walks/runs on a slope banked upward to the right can eventually result in: (1) a pattern of heel cup collapse that mimics that seen with an 'upslip' and the 'more common' patterns of 'rotational malalignment' (see Figs 3.22A, 3.31B); (2) increased tension in the soft tissue structures - left lateral (e.g. tensor fascia lata/iliotibial band complex), right medial (e.g. medial collateral ligament); (c) left medial and right lateral joint line and compartment pressure - to the point at which these may become symptomatic (see Figs 3.37, 3.41).

shoes worn for these activities may reveal these different stresses.

Remember that if the examination findings and the impression gained from looking at the shoes do not seem to match up, ask to see some day shoes worn for different activities and a pair of running shoes.

A final observation on weight-bearing

Over the years, the author continues to be struck by the fact that, in those who are in alignment, a neutral to supination pattern of weight-bearing seems to be almost as prevalent in clinical practice as is pronation. One study (Schamberger 2002) looked at 120 patients as they presented consecutively at the office and subsequently for follow-up after treatment. The findings warrant repeating here as there continues to be a problem recognizing those who supinate compared to those who pronate. On the initial examination, 96 (80%) of these patients proved to be out of alignment. The findings of this study as they relate specifically to the examination of weight-bearing on walking, heel- and toe-walking, and hopping were as follows:

1. of those with malalignment evident on initial exam (n = 96):
   - 35% : pronation bilaterally
   - 8% : supination bilaterally
   - 35% : a 'neutral' pattern of weight-bearing bilaterally, with no obvious tendency to pronation or supination
   - 17% : a 'right pronation, left supination' pattern
   - 5% : a 'left pronation, right supination' pattern
2. on the first reassessment following realignment (n = 96):
   - 45% : pronation bilaterally
   - 11% : a 'right pronation, left supination' pattern
   - 11% : supination bilaterally
   - 33% : a neutral weight-bearing pattern

In other words, with realignment there was a 10% increase in the number of those with definite bilateral pronation, from 35% to 45%; whereas the combined total of those in a neutral position or actual supination remained relatively unchanged at 44%. Asymmetry of gait was still apparent in 11%, which could probably be expected to decrease as a more symmetrical gait pattern was gradually re-established and more and more muscles finally relaxed once alignment was being maintained.

Time and time again, patients who have been known to be in alignment for some time have presented with 'lateral' symptoms (e.g. tensor fascia lata/iliotibial band [TFL/ITB] tenderness, greater trochanteric pain and recurrent ankle inversion sprains). They had previously been diagnosed as being 'pronators' and had, therefore, been provided with 'double-density' running shoes and often also rigid or semi-rigid orthotics posted medially to equal extent; e.g. 2 degrees on the medial aspect of the forefoot, hindfoot or both, bilaterally. They were usually being referred because their 'lateral' symptoms had persisted or worsened despite these measures. On examination, they now turned out to have a neutral or even supination pattern of weight-bearing.

Persistence of 'lateral' symptoms was attributed to lateral traction forces, primarily attributable to:

1. their inherent lateral weight-bearing pattern
2. continued use of runners and orthotics intended to counter pronation

The following course of treatment proved adequate therapy for most:

1. an appropriate course of ankle strengthening exercises and lateral stretches, combined with
2. a simple change to a running shoe with features to increase shock absorption (Fig. 3.35C; shoe marked 'R' in Fig. 3.35A,B):
   a. a sole and midsole of uniform thickness and density (= 'single-density') and
   b. a 'curved last' to allow the foot to drop inward and 'unlock'
3. in some, addition of a soft-shell orthotic with a lateral raise, for further improvement of shock absorption and to accentuate the shift toward more medial weight-bearing, respectively.

'Pronation' became a powerful buzzword in the 1970s and 80s, to the point at which it definitely delayed general recognition of the supination pattern. Indeed, though 'supination' appears to have entered the vocabulary of most sports specialists and we have, hopefully, reached the stage where individuals no longer declare that 'there is no such thing as supination' at a medical meeting, even now there is a dearth of shoes made to specifically accommodate the needs of those that do supinate. A recent assessment of running shoes found the number made specifically for supinators compared to pronators still lagged drastically behind (10-20% at best versus 80-90%, respectively), despite the fact that the combined number of those that supinate or have a neutral pattern of weight-bearing is nearly the same as those that pronate.

In summary, since the mid-1970s, there has been an overemphasis on the recognition of pronation and the problems associated with it. As a result, pronation became more eagerly sought - and probably more readily recognized - than supination. Given this background, and the fact that excessive pronation on one side is not an uncommon feature with 'rotational malalignment' (and also an 'upslip'):

1. the pronation pattern is often very obvious on one side so that it stands out and, therefore, tends to catch the eye more easily - witness this author's experience of erroneously being treated for a 'problem of pronation' when actually supination was evident on the left side on examination of weight-bearing when walking and the wear pattern of the running shoes: right heel cup obviously collapsed inward, and the left one outward (Fig. 3.22aii)
2. the coexisting neutral or even frank supination pattern on the opposite side can easily be ignored as attention is diverted toward the pronating side
3. in those who pronate bilaterally, any asymmetry in the degree of pronation on comparing the right and left side is likely to go unrecognized unless the examiner is aware of the problem of malalignment and actually seeks out these asymmetries (Fig. 3.23A).

Clinical correlation: foot alignment, weight-bearing and shoe wear

The shift in weight-bearing that occurs with malalignment results in an asymmetry of forces in the lower extremities that predisposes to the injuries typically associated with pronation and supination.

On the side of external rotation and pronation

1. *increased tension in structures on the medial aspect of the leg* (Fig. 3.37)
   a. groin pain and/or medial thigh pain (irritation or strain of the origin, muscle mass or insertion of pectineus, gracilis, sartorius and the adductor group
   b. medial collateral ligament and medial plica of knee
   c. snapping of the medial plica and vastus medialis tendon across the medial femoral condyle
   d. increased tension on muscles running across the medial femoral condyles to tibial insertions (adductors, gracilis, sartorius)
   e. medial shin splints from periosteal irritation and inflammation along the tibialis posterior origin
   f. medial ankle ligaments (especially anterior tibiotalar)
2. *peripheral nerve involvement* (Fig. 3.38A)
   a. traction injury to the posterior tibial (running through the posterior tarsal tunnel), saphenous and distal (medial) deep peroneal nerves
   b. posterior tarsal tunnel syndrome, with irritation from the increased traction forces or actual compression of the nerve or its terminal branches (plantar nerves) by tightening of the overlying ligaments and flexor retinaculum

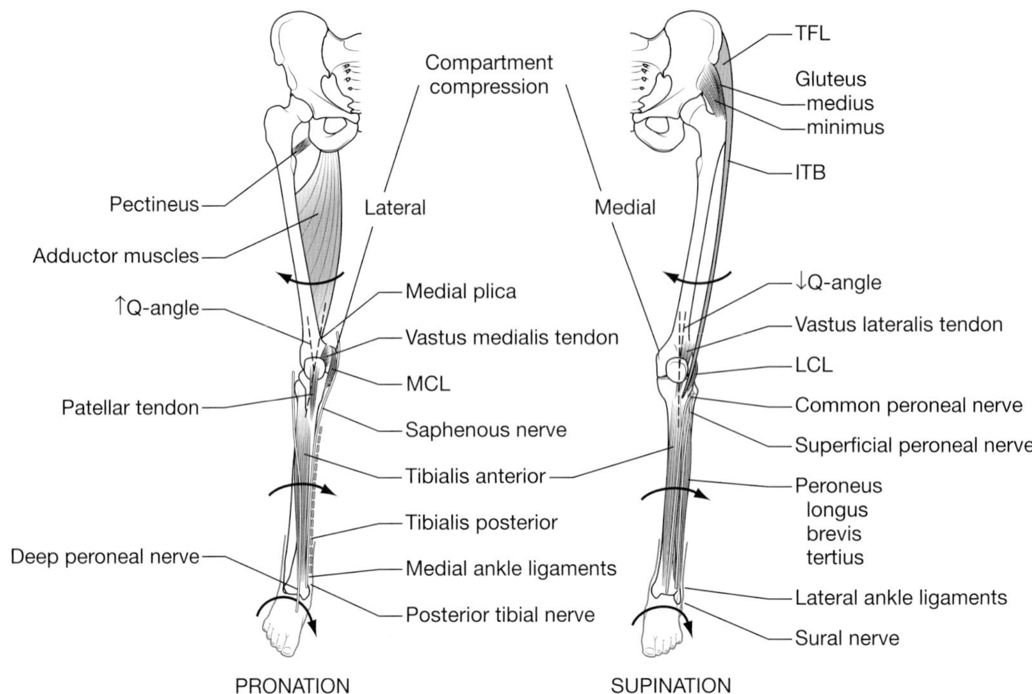

Fig. 3.37 Structures put under stress by a right pronation, left supination shift with malalignment. MCL/LCL, medial/lateral collateral ligament.

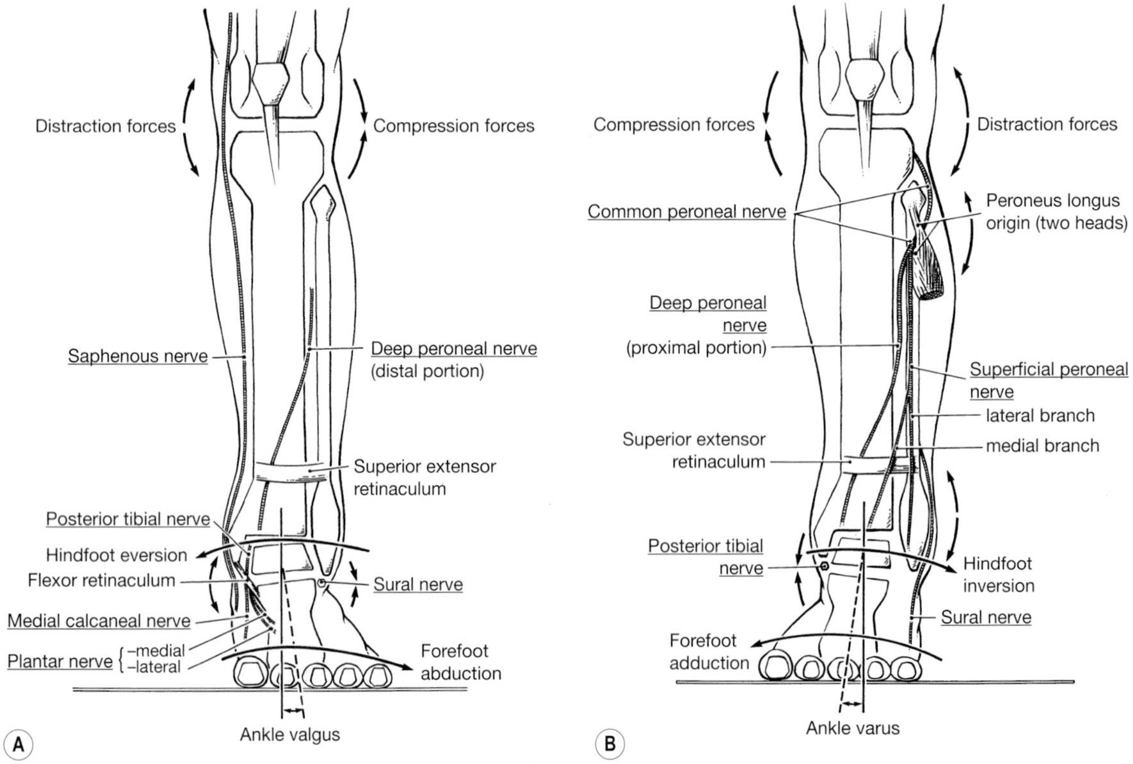

Fig. 3.38 Peripheral nerves in the left leg affected by a shift in weight-bearing. (A) Nerves affected by pronation forces. (B) Nerves affected by supination forces. *(Courtesy of Schamberger 1987.)*

c. compression injury of the sural nerve at the lateral ankle

3. *increased tendency to valgus angulation at the knee*
   a. increased pressure in the lateral knee joint compartment
   b. increased Q-angle and lateral tracking of the patella, pressure in the patellofemoral compartment and tension in the patellar tendon and its insertion into the tibial tubercle
   c. irritation of the saphenous nerve
   d. strain on muscles crossing the medial tibial condyle (gracilis, sartorius, semimembranosus and semitendinosus)
4. *increased pressure on the medial aspect of the foot with the medial shift in weight-bearing*
   a. precipitation or aggravation of problems relating to a hallux valgus, rigidus and limitus
   b. acceleration of first metatarsophalangeal joint degeneration, medial bunion formation
   c. sesamoiditis
   d. plantar fasciitis - usually worse on the medial aspect - on the basis of:
      i. excessive traction attributable to calcaneal eversion and collapse of the medial longitudinal arch with pronation
      ii. increased dorsiflexion possible on this side (Figs 3.75, 3.84)
   e. in the case of bilateral Morton's toes, a unilateral aggravation of stress on the second and third metatarsal heads with callus formation (Fig. 3.39Bi), tenderness and/or outright pain (metatarsalgia) or even stress fracture
5. *Achilles tendonitis on the basis of excessive traction, attributable to*:
   a. the separation of origin and insertion that occurs on weight-bearing because of:
      i. calcaneal inversion (collapsing into valgus; Fig. 3.40)
      ii. the increased ankle dorsiflexion usually possible on this side (Figs 3.75, 3.84).

On the side of internal rotation and supination

1. *increased tension in the lateral structures of the leg* (Figs 3.37, 3.38)

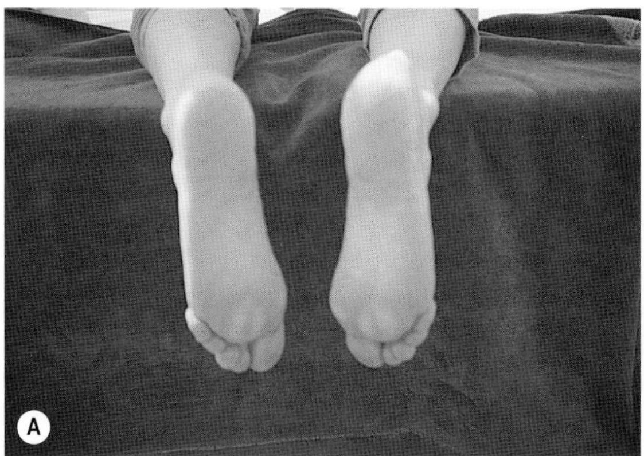

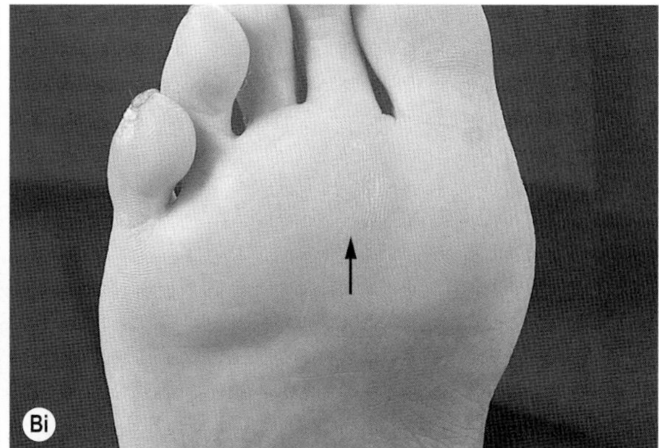

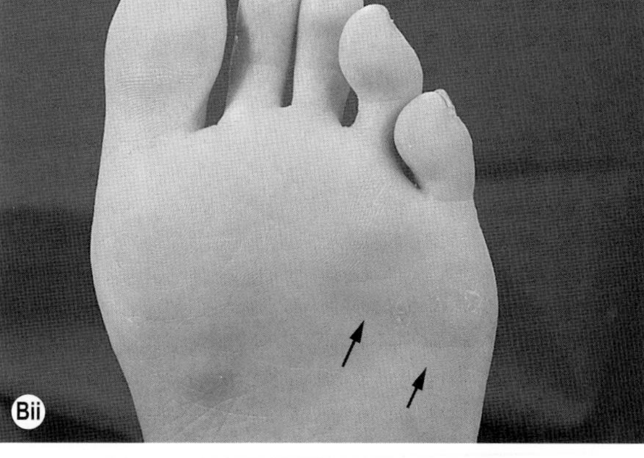

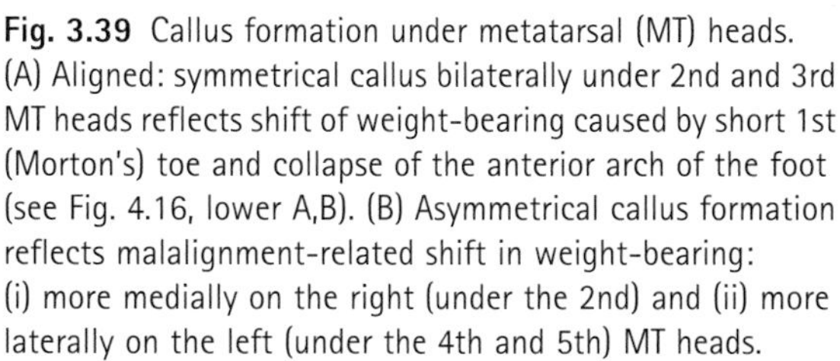

Fig. 3.39 Callus formation under metatarsal (MT) heads. (A) Aligned: symmetrical callus bilaterally under 2nd and 3rd MT heads reflects shift of weight-bearing caused by short 1st (Morton's) toe and collapse of the anterior arch of the foot (see Fig. 4.16, lower A,B). (B) Asymmetrical callus formation reflects malalignment-related shift in weight-bearing: (i) more medially on the right (under the 2nd) and (ii) more laterally on the left (under the 4th and 5th) MT heads.

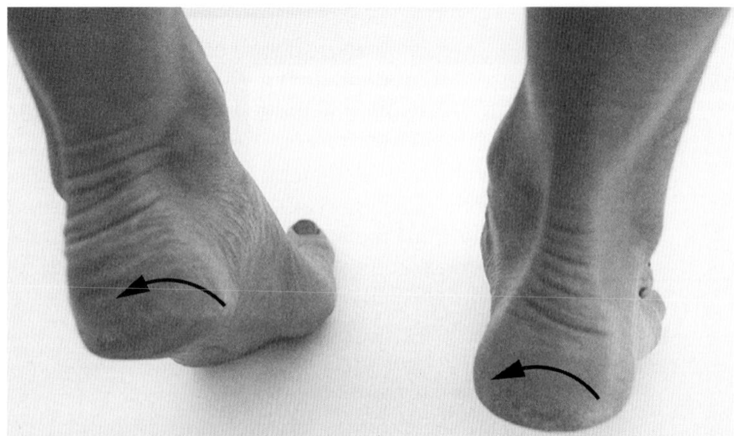

Fig. 3.40 Increased tension in the right Achilles tendon, reflecting external rotation of the right leg, heel collapse inward (pronation) and increased knee valgus angulation; the narrowing of the right tendon compared with that on the supinating left side is accentuated by toe-walking (see also Fig. 3.24A).

a. stress on the lateral sling (hip abductors - gluteus medius/minimus, TFL/ITB complex - and peroneus longus)
b. bursitis (TFL/ITB going across greater trochanter and lateral femoral condyle; Fig. 3.41)
c. lateral shin splints (tendonitis or sprain involving tibialis anterior and/or peroneal muscle group)
d. lateral ankle ligaments.

2. ***Peripheral nerve involvement*** (Fig. 3.38B)
   a. traction injury to the lateral femoral cutaneous nerve (meralgia parasthetica; Fig. 4.13), the common and superficial peroneal nerves and the sural nerve
   b. compression injury of posterior tibial nerve in the tarsal tunnel
3. ***tendency to varum at the knee***
   a. increased pressure in the medial knee joint compartment
   b. traction on the lateral (fibular) collateral ligament and lateral muscles (vastus lateralis, popliteus, biceps femoris insertions, lateral gastrocnemius origin)
   c. snapping of vastus lateralis across the lateral femoral condyle.
4. ***increased rigidity of the foot and ankle***
   a. an impaired ability to dissipate ground forces, predisposing to the development of plantar fasciitis, Achilles tendonitis and stress fractures.
5. ***increased weight-bearing on lateral aspect of the foot***
   a. painful callus formation, fourth and fifth metatarsalgia, and metatarsal stress fractures (Fig. 3.39Bii)

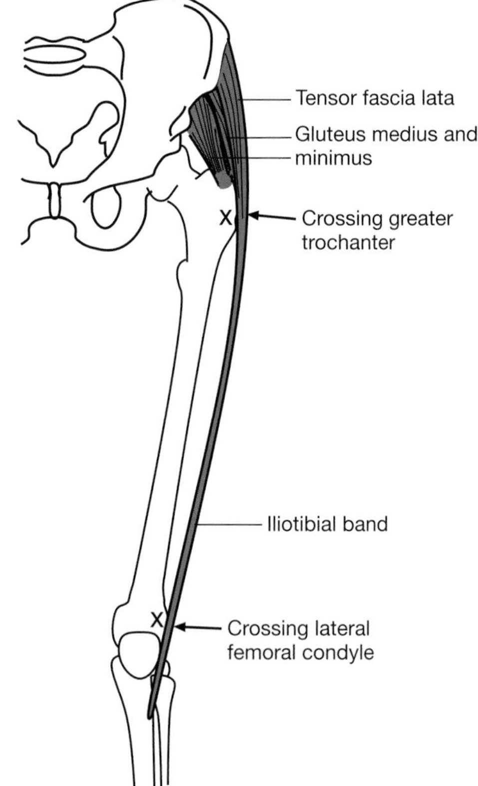

Fig. 3.41 Tensor fascia lata/iliotibial band complex spanning the greater trochanter and lateral femoral condyle - common sites of irritation and 'bursitis'.

   b. Morton's neuroma: typically, irritation of the natural thickening at the junction of the medial and lateral plantar nerve branches, usually lying in the space between the 3 rd-4th MTP heads, a space which is further narrowed on lateral weight-bearing (supinating; see Fig. 4.16B)

c. ankle inversion sprains

Problems relating to pronation and supination will be discussed in further detail, as appropriate, in other sections of this and the following chapters.

ASYMMETRY OF MUSCLE TENSION

Normally-functioning muscle has a resting 'tone' and is non-tender when relaxed. On gentle palpation, the tips of the fingers can sink into the muscle easily, and the pressure elicits no pain. Concentrate on the feel of the muscle being palpated and compare the resting tone, or tension, to that of the muscle(s) immediately adjacent and on the opposite side. In addition, look for reactive muscle tensing, a tell-tale sign that the muscle, its nerve supply or the vertebral segment to which it belongs may be in trouble.

Muscles are meant to contract and relax. Relaxation results in an increase in blood flow, allowing for optimal clearance of waste and delivery of oxygen and nutrients. Contraction decreases blood flow and impairs clearance of waste. A contraction of only 60% of maximum has been shown to stop blood flow into and out of the muscle completely (McArdle et al. 1986). Conditions that cause an increase in tension in a muscle over a longer period of time may eventually interfer with the normal function of that muscle and result in tenderness and pain.

Some of the muscles of the 'inner' and 'outer' core are constantly contracting and relaxing to ensure stability and balance at 'rest', also in preparation for dealing with a superimposed contraction of peripheral muscles so these can initiate and carry out a specific action precisely and safely (e.g. pitching a baseball; Figs 3.51, 5.31). This underlying muscle activity is at only about 5% demand and not likely to precipitate discomfort as it alternately works and rests different parts of a muscle complex. However, in someone presenting with 'rotational malalignment' or an 'upslip' there is a constant increase in tension - contraction at a higher demand level - seen in muscles in an asymmetrical pattern. This finding means that the muscles involved are always working to some extent, implying a constant increase in energy expenditure and production of waste occurring at a time of diminished blood flow. At the same time, a constant traction force is being exerted on the muscle origin and insertion. Given this persistent increase in tension, the muscle bulk proper and/or the fibro-osseous junctions will become tender to palpation and eventually outright painful. The term 'chronic tension myalgia' seems appropriate to describe this condition because the pain itself is myofascial in origin, involving the muscle itself, the neurovascular bundle, the enveloping fascia and the fibro-osseous junctions. We will first look at the problems of 'chronic tension myalgia' and 'trigger points' before going on to discuss findings relating to muscle tension that are particular to malalignment.

Chronic tension myalgia

The person with chronic tension myalgia may not even be aware that he or she is constantly tensing these muscles, seeing it is often an automatic response aimed at decreasing movement of a painful site or stabilizing what may turn out to be an unstable joint. A vicious cycle often ensues - the reflex increase in tension causes more pain which further increases the tension. At this stage, it is often still possible to interrupt the cycle simply by relaxing the muscle, temporarily stopping the pain or stabilizing the lax structure(s). Strengthening of 'inner' and 'outer' core muscles for stability and mobility, appropriate stretching, a progressive cardiovascular training program and stress reduction, in conjunction with massage, electrical modalities (e.g. transcutaneous electrical nerve stimulation), acupuncture or trigger point injection may be adequate treatment.

Whatmore & Kohli in 1974 postulated that the chronic contraction eventually fatigues the physiological mechanisms that sustain the contraction. When the energy reserves of the individual fibres drop below a critical level, 'fatigue spasm' ensues: the fibres remain involuntarily shortened. Persistent fatigue spasm can lead to a fixed shortening of muscle fibres that is maintained by 'physicochemical processes' within the fibres. Muscle fibres atrophy at the same time that the fibrous content of the muscle increases. These changes can sometimes be appreciated as tender, localized areas of crepitus on palpation and may be visualized by techniques such as MRI and Real-Time US or RTUS (Chs 4, 7). Once the condition has reached this stage it becomes much harder, sometimes impossible, to reverse.

Muscle trigger points

Myofascial pain associated with chronic tension myalgia is not to be confused with myofascial trigger points (Ch. 4). By definition, trigger points are very localized areas of hyperirritable tissue usually found within a taut band of skeletal muscle or the fascia surrounding or invaginating the muscle. A trigger point can, for example, localize to an excessively active muscle spindle. Trigger points are painful to compression and can give rise to characteristic referred pain patterns, tenderness and autonomic phenomena (Travell & Simons 1983, 1992; Fig. 3.45). Chronic tension myalgia and trigger points can coexist but trigger points in a muscle are not felt to result from a chronic increase in tension (Travell & Simons 1983).

Malalignment-related increase in muscle tension

In the presence of malalignment, a chronic increase in muscle tension can result for the four main reasons listed in Box 3.5 and will now be discussed in some detail.

Increased distance between origin and insertion

In association with malalignment, such an increase can result for two main reasons:

1. *A spatial reorientation of the bones has occurred*

   This point is best illustrated by 'anterior' and 'posterior' rotation of the innominates around the coronal axis in the sagittal plane and the effect of such rotation on the tension specifically in hamstrings, iliacus and rectus femoris (Figs 2.59, 3.42).

   'Anterior' rotation of the right innominate moves the right ischial tuberosity posteriorly and upward, effectively separating the hamstring origin from its insertions into the proximal tibia, and increasing tension in this muscle complex. Gluteus maximus is similarly affected, with separation of the iliac crest and greater trochanter. Alternately, the 'right anterior' rotation effectively moves the anterior iliac crest downward and approximates the iliacus origin to its insertion into the lesser trochanter, thereby decreasing tension in that muscle; pectineus, TFL, rectus femoris and the adductor complex are similarly effected.

   'Posterior' rotation of the left innominate has the opposite effect by lowering the ischial

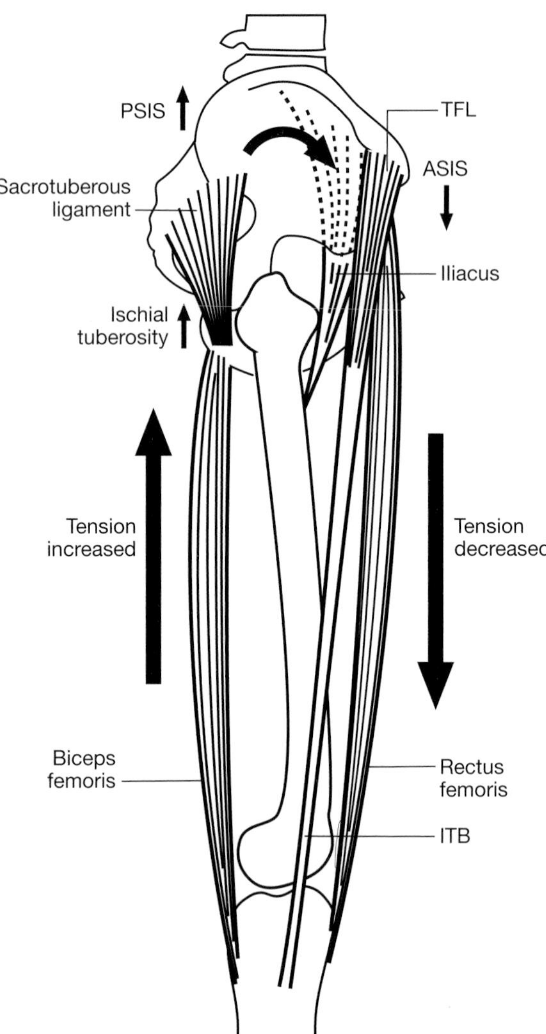

Fig. 3.42 Change in tension resulting from the shift of the origin toward or away from the insertion with right innominate anterior rotation (e.g. tension increased in biceps femoris and decreased in iliacus and rectus femoris). The reverse changes occur with right posterior rotation. PSIS, posterior superior iliac spine; ASIS, anterior superior iliac spine; TFL, tensor fascia lata; ITB, iliotibial band.

BOX 3.5 Malalignment as a cause of chronic increase in muscle tension

1. The malalignment has increased the distance between the muscle's origin and insertion.
2. The malalignment *per se* is associated with an autonomic increase in tone - or 'facilitation' - of specific muscles.
3. The increase in muscle tension is an attempt to splint
   a. an area that is painful
   b. a joint that is unstable

tuberosity and elevating the anterior iliac crest, thereby helping to relax the hamstrings while increasing tension in iliacus, pectineus, TFL, rectus femoris and the adductors on that side.

2. ***The distance between origin and insertion varies with the shift in the pattern of weight-bearing***
   Pronation, as discussed above, increases the distance along the inner part of the leg, from foot to groin, and increases the tension in the muscles on this medial aspect. Supination increases the distance along the outer part, from the foot to the iliac crest, and increases the tension in the muscles on the lateral aspect. This shift in weight-bearing typically associated with malalignment can actually result in symptoms and signs related to the stresses of pronation on one side and supination on the other (see 'Asymmetry of foot alignment, weight-bearing and shoe wear' above).

   The remarks regarding the increase in muscle tension caused by the separation of origin and insertion also apply to the ligaments on the side affected (see 'Asymmetry of ligament tension', below).

Autonomic increase in tone or 'facilitation' of specific muscles

Both 'rotational malalignment' and an 'upslip' are associated with an autonomic increase in tone in specific muscles, in a predictable asymmetric pattern that cannot be attributed simply to the separation of an origin and insertion (Fig. 3.43). On examining the person lying supine, muscles most consistently involved are:

1. on the right side - cervical paravertebrals (superficial erector spinae), scalenes, upper trapezius, infraspinatus, teres minor, piriformis and hamstrings
2. on the left side - hip abductors, TFL/ITB complex, iliopsoas, peroneus longus and gastrocnemius/soleus.

The increase in muscle tone usually reverts to normal, partially or completely, as soon as the malalignment has been corrected, suggesting that it may be related to an asymmetry of signals arising from structures that are affected by the malalignment on the right and left side. The TFL/ITB complex serves as a good example of this. When 'rotational malalignment' or an 'upslip' is present, the right complex remains relaxed and will usually allow

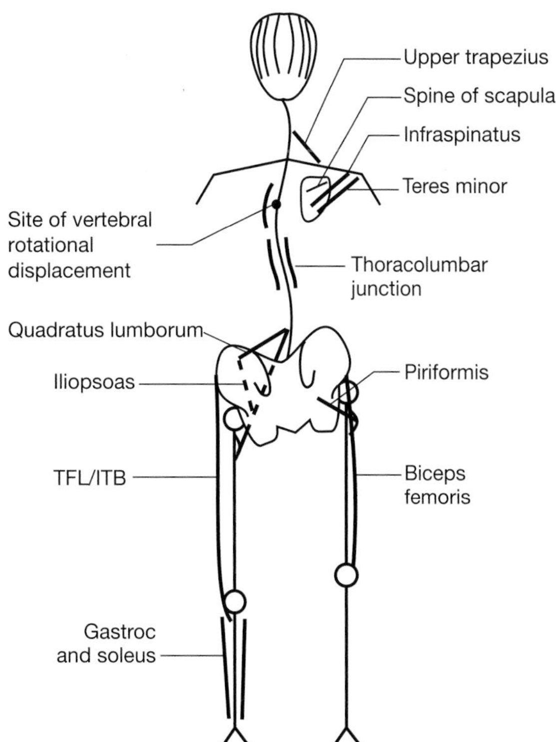

Fig. 3.43 Typical sites of increased muscle tension and tenderness resulting with a vertebral rotational displacement (e.g. mid-thoracic and T/L junction). The drawing also indicates the typical lateralization of increased tone ('facilitation') seen with pelvic malalignment; if the muscle involved shows increased tone bilaterally, the one indicated here is usually the one affected more severely. T/L, thoracolumbar; TFL/ITB, tensor fascia lata/iliotibial band; QL, quadratus lumborum.

the knee to come close to, if not completely onto, the plinth on Ober's test (Fig. 3.44Ai); whereas the complex on the left is tense and holds the knee at a variable distance up in the air (Fig. 3.44Aii). Following realignment, the tension in the left complex decreases immediately, usually allowing the left knee to come down as far as the right one (Fig. 3.44B). Occasionally, the right knee now ends up slightly higher than on initial assessment but matches the level to which the left has dropped. Factors to consider when trying to explain why the right knee might come up slightly would include:

1. the mechanical repositioning of the right acetabulum, so that it now matches that present on the left
2. a balancing of tone in the right compared to left hip girdle muscles

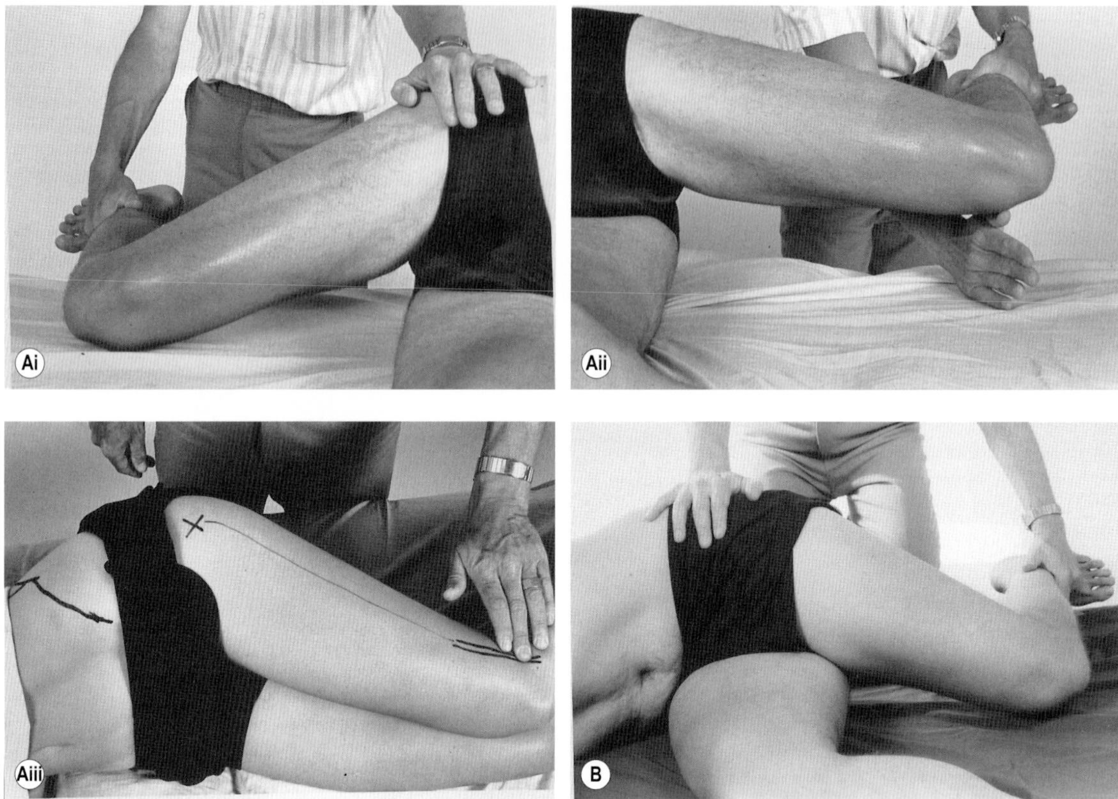

Fig. 3.44 Ober's test for limitation of hip adduction: primarily by tight short abductors (e.g. gluteal muscles) with knee flexed, long abductors (e.g. tensor fascia lata/iliotibial band or TFL/ITB) with knee extended. (A) In this person with an 'upslip' or a 'rotational malalignment': (i) the right adducts to touch the plinth; (ii) left adduction is limited compared to the right; (iii) the 'facilitated' left TFL/ITB complex proves consistently tense (and usually tender along part or all of its length). (B) Following realignment: left adduction now equals right.

The following are some possible mechanisms to consider in trying to explain these phenomena.

First, pelvic malalignment results in an asymmetry of proprioceptive signals arising from the joints. Possibly, the asymmetry of such signals could cause an increase or decrease in excitatory or inhibitory signals. However, as with muscle weakness (discussed below), the muscles showing the increase in tone tend to be consistently the same regardless of the presentation of malalignment. For example, this increase in tone consistently involves the left hip abductors and TFL/ITB complex (Figs 3.41, 3.43), regardless of whether:

1. the malalignment is in the form of 'rotational malalignment' or an 'upslip'
2. the 'anterior' innominate rotation or the 'upslip' is on the right or left side
3. there is a 'rotational malalignment' combined with an 'upslip'
4. there is an associated 'locking' of an SI joint

Therefore, asymmetry of proprioceptive signals (at least those from the pelvic/lumbosacral region) does not offer a plausible explanation.

Second, the above findings argue more for a cause at the spinal segmental or cortical level (Korr 1978). The increased tension may reflect segmental muscle 'facilitation' or 'inhibition'. The malalignment may itself have evolved as a result of such asymmetrical signals to the muscles arising from some other, more proximal site - the spinal cord, brain stem or the brain itself.

T12 or L1 vertebral rotation displacement, for example, is usually associated with an increase in tone ('facilitation') in the psoas major on one side, and relaxation ('inhibition') of this muscle on the opposite side, which would result in:

1. asymmetrical forces capable of causing not only malalignment of the pelvis but also more distal effects in its role as:
   a. an external rotator and hip flexor that influences the alignment of the lower extremities and also
   b. a stabilizer of the SI joint to effect load-transfer across the lumbo-pelvic-hip complex and to safeguard weight-bearing (Figs 2.46B,C, 2.62).

The segmental dysfunction may act on the muscle directly or affect muscle tone (and strength) indirectly by interfering with cortically-mediated motor control.

Third, some of the central effects of articular mechanoreceptor stimulation pointed out by Wyke (1985: 75) may be operative (see also Ch. 7: 'orthotics'). These include the nociceptor afferent activity arising from the type IV receptor system within the joint capsule and the fibres of the intrinsic joint and spinal ligaments. A pain-suppressive effect normally occurs with 'activation of the apical spinal interneurons', producing 'presynaptic inhibition of [this] nociceptor afferent activity'. Perhaps with the distortion of joint surfaces, tendons, ligaments and capsules associated with malalignment, there is an excessive stimulation of type IV receptors to the point at which activation of interneurons becomes inadequate, resulting in a failure of pain suppression at a segmental level. The increased tone in the paravertebral and more distal muscles may, therefore, reflect a problem at the spinal segmental level.

Finally, the malalignment, whatever its presentation, may induce rather non-specific signals related, possibly, to stretching and/or irritation of the dura and its continuation as the meninges. This stretching could result with any twisting of the spine, which would lengthen the distance between the forum magnum and the dural insertion as the conus medullaris and filum terminale at about S2 level (Ch. 8). Twisting is part of the compensatory scoliosis that occurs in reaction to the pelvic obliquity seen with 'rotational malalignment' and an 'upslip'. Rotational displacement of individual vertebrae (Figs 2.52, 2.94, 2.96B) may also end up irritating the dura. Signals originating from the dura and meninges as a result of these stresses, in turn, are suspected of having a general effect of stimulating or suppressing cortical motor signals to certain motor spindles, and inducing 'facilitation' or 'inhibition' of muscles, respectively.

Tension increased in an attempt to splint a painful area

The muscles in the vicinity of a painful area usually show an increase in tension. This may occur as a reaction to irritation of the nociceptive fibres. It may also be a reflex attempt to splint the painful area in order to prevent any movement that might worsen the pain. Malalignment automatically stresses a number of structures, especially the joints of the spine and pelvis. These sites can eventually become a source of irritation or pain that is aggravated by movement or any further stress that results with activity. It is not unusual to find increased tension (and tenderness) in the muscles capable of decreasing or preventing the movement of these painful areas. There is, for example, often splinting of the paravertebral muscles immediately adjacent to a rotationally displaced vertebra and at sites of curve reversal, especially the thoracolumbar junction.

Tension increased in an attempt to stabilize an area

Malalignment is frequently associated with joint instability for various reasons (see Ch. 2). Laxity of the ligaments, which allows for a recurrent rotational displacement of one or more vertebrae, results in a recurrent or chronic increase of tension in the paravertebrals and any other muscles that can effectively stabilize that segment. The instability of SI joints that can occur with sacral and innominate rotation or an 'upslip' typically result in a reactive increase in tension in the three prime muscles that can stabilize these joints: gluteus maximus, piriformis and iliopsoas (Figs 2.5, 2.46 2.62).

> In summary, in the presence of 'rotational malalignment' and/or an 'upslip', there is an increase in tension in certain muscles which may be:
> 1. active, such as a reflex response to pain or instability
> 2. passive, as seen with biomechanical changes that increase the distance between the muscle origin and insertion
> 3. secondary to a mechanism, segmental or cortical, that affects the muscle spindle setting and results in an asymmetric pattern of increased muscle tone or 'facilitation'

As long as the malalignment is present, a muscle showing an increase in tension is unlikely to respond to stretching attempts or will do so with difficulty and sometimes with precipitation or aggravation of discomfort. Any gains made in lengthening are only temporary if the shortening is itself secondary to the malalignment. With time, these muscles, their tendons and points of attachment can become tender to palpation or overtly painful. The myofascial pain that results may remain localized, have a referred component or both. A persistent increase in tension secondary to malalignment increases the risk of sprain or strain of the affected muscles when used to carry out more demanding work or athletic activities. Conversely, realignment may greatly benefit the recovery of those who have suffered a sprain or strain, simply by removing that component of the increase in tension and pain which is attributable to the malalignment (Cibulka et al. 1986) and, finally, allow for a progressive stretching programme.

Muscles most consistently showing an increase in tension with malalignment

Studies of those presenting with malalignment give an indication of the prevalence of the muscles typically noted to show an increase in tension and/or tenderness to palpation, as illustrated in Fig. 3.43 above. The figures also reflect the involvement of muscles on either the right or the left side in a predictable asymmetric pattern. The following are the muscles most consistently affected.

The right piriformis muscle

In the study mentioned above (Schamberger 2002), of those presenting with 'rotational malalignment' or an 'upslip':

1. 58% showed an increase in tone in the piriformis
2. a unilateral increase the tension was six times more likely to involve the right than the left side
3. the majority also showed sacral torsion around an oblique axis, almost as often around the right as the left axis
4. the side of involvement could not be correlated to:
   a. the side on which the leg was externally rotated
   b. separation or approximation of the origin and insertion
   c. whether the person presented with an 'upslip', the 'left anterior and locked' or one of the 'more common' patterns of 'rotational malalignment'
   d. the pattern of sacral torsion, if present

Given the lack of correlation to the pattern of malalignment present or the side of external rotation of the leg and the fact that it can be present on either the right or left or both sides (Schamberger 2002), the increase in tension so frequently detectable in piriformis in clinical practice and research suggests this involvement is:

1. possibly on account of 'facilitation' of piriformis, though this might be expected to affect the muscle on one side only
2. more likely to reflect an attempt by piriformis to decrease movement of a painful and/or unstable SI joint (Figs 2.46A, 4.17)

Clinical correlation: piriformis

Increased tone and recurrent spasm in one or both piriformis muscles is often blamed for a failure to correct the malalignment initially or for the recurrence of malalignment following correction. Its oblique attachment to the sacrum normally plays a vital role in stabilizing the SI joint on the side of single leg stance but has also been implicated as a cause of SI joint 'locking' and sacral torsion (see Ch. 2).

Lying and sitting, especially when slouching or sitting in bucket seats, can put direct pressure on the piriformis muscle bulk and insertion and create problems particularly for those in whom these sites are already tender.

The increased tension in piriformis can result in buttock and lower extremity pain on the basis of:

1. referred pain, felt primarily in the posterior thigh region (Fig. 3.45)
2. compromise and irritation of the sciatic nerve or its components; the problem of 'piriformis syndrome' and 'sciatica' are discussed in Chapter 4 (Fig. 4.17).

Piriformis involvement can contribute to the deep pain associated with pelvic floor dysfunction, with increased tension and acute tenderness evident on palpation of piriformis per rectum or vagina (Chs 4, 7; Fig. 2.53B).

The left hip abductors and TFL/ITB complex

Left gluteus medius, gluteus minimus and TFL, with its continuation as the iliotibial band, show an involvement in practically all persons with an 'upslip' or 'rotational malalignment' regardless of the pattern of presentation (Figs 3.44Aii,iii, 3.77). Peroneus longus may also be tense and tender. Pain in the region of the left hip, greater trochanter and lateral thigh and knee is certainly one of the more

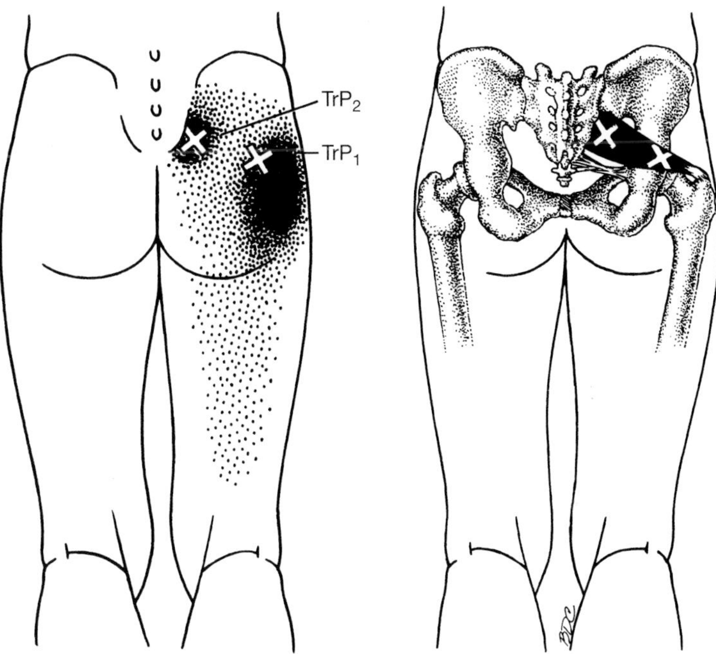

Fig. 3.45 Composite pattern of pain (solid and stippled pattern) referred from trigger points (TrPs; marked by X) in the right piriformis muscle. The lateral X (TrP1) indicates the most common TrP location. The stippling locates the spillover pattern that may be felt as less intense pain than that of the essential pattern (solid black). Spillover may be absent. *(Courtesy of Travell & Simons 1992.)*

common presenting complaints, less often pain felt more distally from the lateral 'calf' region. Increased tone in the TFL/ITB complex is readily detected. Tenderness to palpation is most likely to be found over the distal part on the left side, notably in the left ITB, less often along the full length of the ITB, the TFL and the hip abductor origin and muscle mass. Any increase in tension in the left hip abductors will, of course, contribute to the limitation of left hip adduction found in most (Fig. 3.44; see 'Asymmetry of lower extremity ranges of motion' below).

The TFL/ITB complex flexes, abducts and internally rotates the thigh. Therefore, one is most likely to reproduce the pain by first passively extending, adducting, and externally rotating the leg, to put the complex under increased tension, and then resisting the person's attempt to internally rotate that leg. Any increase in tension, passively or actively, strings the hip abductor/TFL complex more tightly across the greater trochanter, and the distal ITB across the lateral femoral condyle, increasing the chance of developing painful inflammation and/or bursitis at these sites (Fig. 3.41). The increase in tension and frequent lateralization of symptoms to the left side seen with malalignment is likely the result of a combination of factors, including:

1. 'facilitation' in left hip abductors (Figs 3.43, 3.44Aiii)
2. mechanical forces; e.g. being strung across the greater trochanter and lateral condyle (Fig. 3.41)
3. reaction to:
   a. shift to left lateral weight-bearing in those with an 'upslip' or one of the 'more common' rotational patterns, increasing the distance between origin and insertion of the lateral muscles and ligaments (Figs 3.37, 3.41)
   b. an underlying left-sided pain:
      i. local; e.g. from the left hip/SI joint
      ii. global; e.g. from muscles of the lateral 'sling' attempting to stabilize the left hip/SI joint (Fig. 2.40)
      iii. referred; e.g. from left iliolumbar ligament to the greater trochanteric sclerotome underlying this complex (Fig. 3.46)
4. in those with the 'left anterior and locked' pattern: the simultaneous external rotation of the left lower extremity, which increases tension by separating the TFL/ITB complex origin and insertion
5. the functional weakness of the left hip abductors consistently found in association with malalignment (see 'Asymmetrical functional weakness of lower extremity muscles' below); weak muscles also fatigue more easily.

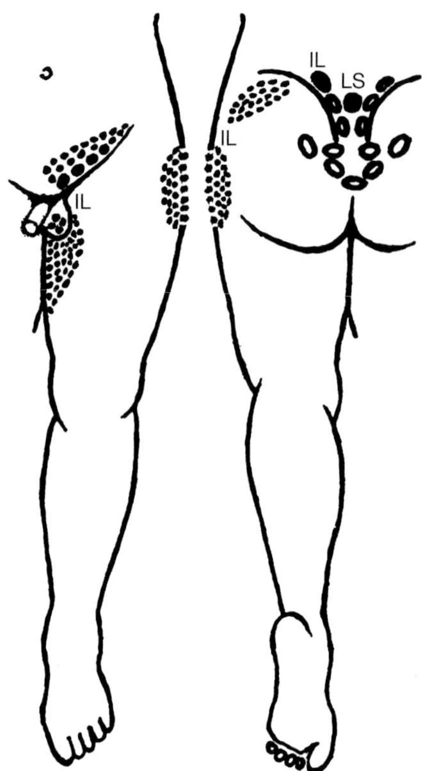

Fig. 3.46 Typical sites of referred pain from the left iliolumbar ligaments (IL), which are being irritated as a result of lumbosacral (LS) joint instability: the groin, the anterior medial upper two-thirds of the thigh, the lower abdomen above Poupart's ligament, the testicle in the male, the vagina in the female, the upper buttock beneath the crest of the ilium and the upper outer thigh. *(Courtesy of Hackett 1958.)*

Increased tension and tenderness in the left hip abductors, and tenderness over the greater trochanter and ITB, are all more prevalent with the 'more common' patterns and especially when 'right anterior' innominate rotation is present; whereas either bilateral involvement or no involvement at all is more likely to be associated with the 'left anterior and locked' pattern of rotational malalignment. The finding of a bilateral increase in hip abductor and/or ITB tone and tenderness should trigger a search for other factors capable of increasing tension in these lateral structures (Fig. 3.47).

First, passive contracture of the TFL/ITB complex can occur on the side on which the origin and insertion have been brought closer together (e.g. usually on the right side while an 'upslip' or one of the 'more common' rotational patterns is present). When such a contracture of the right complex has developed, outright pain may be triggered by any activities that suddenly increase tension in this complex, such as walking on a slope with the right leg on the downhill side (Figs 3.47A, 3.31C). Similarly, contracture of peroneus longus can occur and result in pain from anywhere along its length on being stressed this way.

Second, one should look for conditions that increase the distance along the lateral aspect of the lower extremity:

1. the person having a natural tendency toward a neutral to supination pattern of weight-bearing bilaterally, which may already stress this complex when aligned and even more on one side when out of alignment (Figs 3.23B, 3.47B)
2. genu varum, which may predispose to supination and strings TFL/ITB across the lateral condyle (Fig. 3.47C)
3. genu valgum, in which the acute inward angulation of the femur effectively strings the TFL/ITB across the greater trochanter (Fig. 3.47D)
4. orthotics with an unnecessary or excessive medial posting (raise) to the point of causing or aggravating the tendency to supination (Fig. 5.39)
5. a supinator wearing shoes intended for a pronator (Fig. 3.35).

Following realignment, onset of tightness and/or discomfort in the previously seemingly 'normal' (usually right) hip abductors and TFL/ITB complex is not unusual and may reflect:

1. this complex having undergone contracture by being put in a relaxed, shortened position while malalignment was present; on realignment, the right complex is now being put under increased tension and needs to stretch out to regain its normal length
2. the person's true weight-bearing pattern actually being one of supination (Fig. 3.33).

He or she should be advised that symptoms related to an increase in tension and tenderness precipitated by realignment are self-limiting; they usually last no more than 2 to 4 weeks, as the contracted soft tissues gradually adapt to the now symmetrical stresses that are inherent to being in alignment.

Clinical correlation: hip abductors and TFL/ITB complex

The TFL/ITB complex functions to abduct-flex-internally rotate the thigh. As discussed, contracture of the complex with shortening of the muscle fibres and fibrous tissue could occur with a chronic

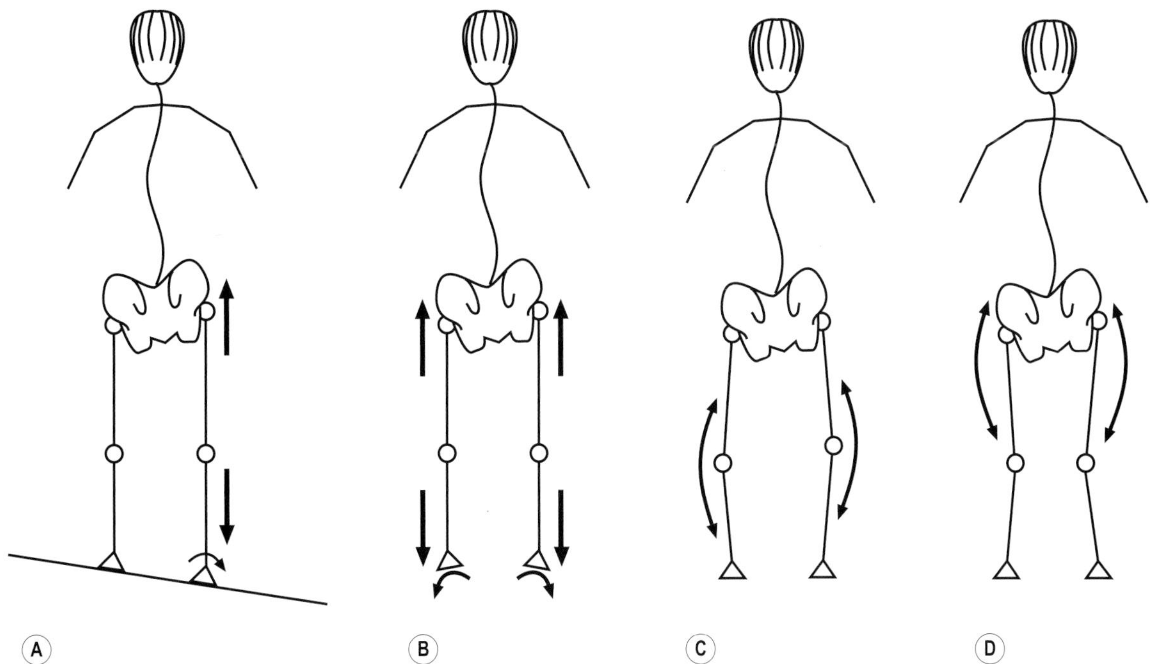

Fig. 3.47 Factors that can further aggravate a malalignment-related increase in tension and/or contracture in lateral structures (e.g. tensor fascia lata/iliotibial band or TFL/ITB). (A) Right leg 'downhill', when contracture of the right TFL/ITB has occurred with shortening. (B) Tendency to bilateral supination. (C) Genu varum. (D) Genu valgum.

increase in tension, constant contraction of the muscle or just being put into a shortened, relaxed position for a longer period of time. Tightening would result in limitation of hip adduction-extension-external rotation. There will usually be a comparative limitation on attempts to cross or 'scissor' the leg on the affected side, or to be able to sit cross-legged with the knees equidistant off the floor (Fig. 3.48).

> Given this uniform limitation of left hip adduction, it will usually be harder to cross the left leg over the right when sitting on a chair (Fig. 3.48B) or sitting cross-legged on the floor (Fig. 3.48C)

Problems with work and sports may arise because:

1. there is an actual physical limitation to adduction range
2. adduction past a certain point provokes pain by further increasing tension in the hip abductors/TFL/ITB complex and may result in an actual sprain or strain.

This limitation of ROM is, in part, also caused by the loss of left external rotation seen in those with one of the 'more common' rotational patterns or an 'upslip' (see 'Asymmetry of lower extremity ranges of motion' below; Fig. 3.77), in contrast to the relative increase in right flexion, abduction and external rotation (see FABER test; Figs 2.107A, 3.80).

Other activities that may be affected by a limitation of adduction can become quite obvious in sports and dance routines, including:

1. lateral movement of the body, as in running sideways or with cutting movements
2. certain steps in ballet and dance, and a number of routines in synchronized swimming, floor exercises, on the balance beam and other types of gymnastic apparatus (see Ch. 5)
3. figure skating, particularly whenever the trailing left leg has to be brought forward and acutely adducted to become the leading leg, to allow riding on the left outer edge when executing a clockwise circle; or in speed skating, whenever it becomes the trailing leg, adducts and goes into extension (see Ch. 5; Fig. 5.17)

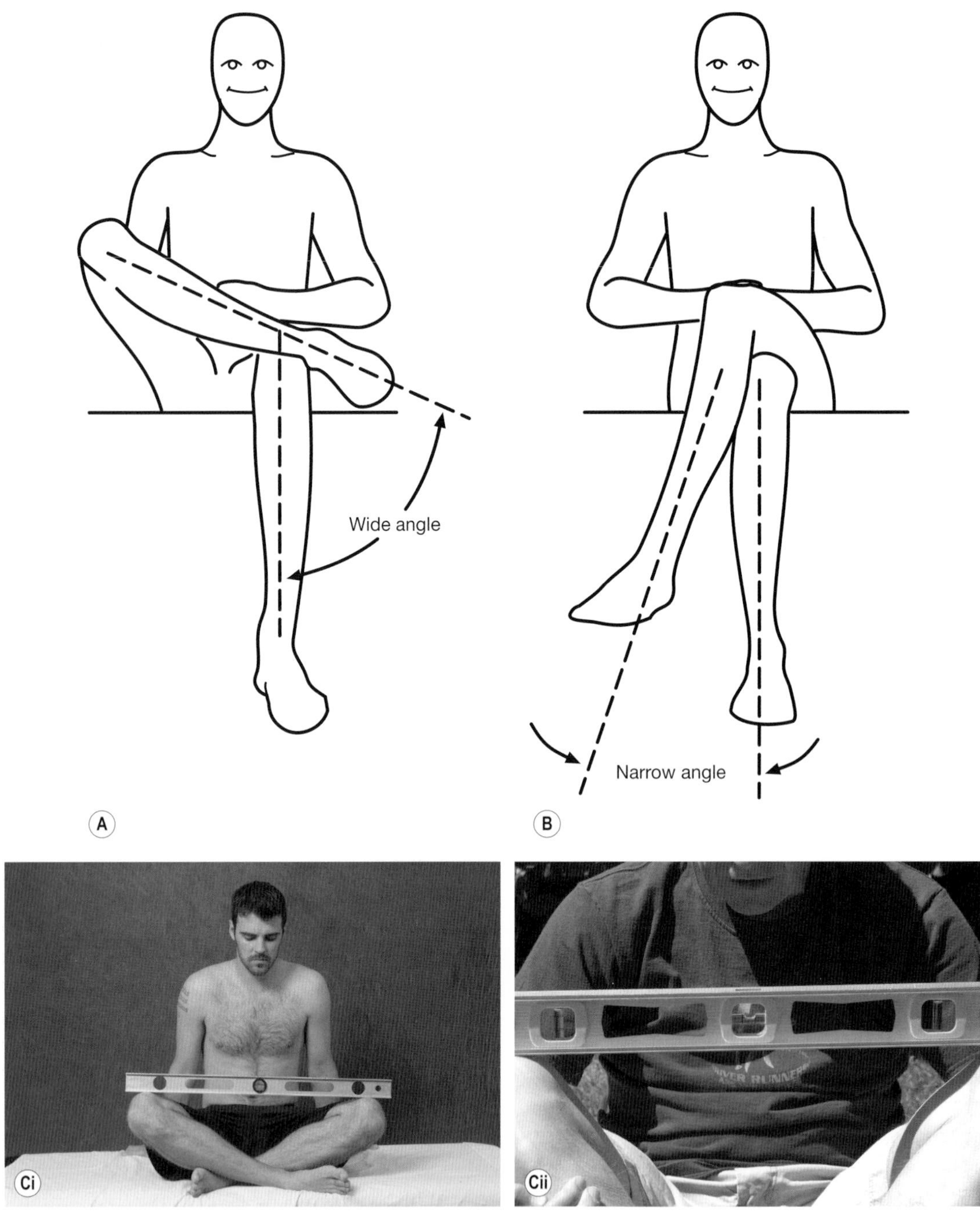

Fig. 3.48 A typical malalignment-related decrease of left hip external rotation and adduction can result in: (A) increased ease of crossing the right over the left leg; (B) a problem crossing left over right leg in sitting. *(Redrawn courtesy of Vleeming et al. 1997.)* (C) This problem can also become evident in cross-legged sitting: (i) 'left anterior' rotation present; impairs right external rotation (level up on right); (ii) 'right anterior, left posterior' rotational malalignment with decreased left external rotation possible (level up on left).

4. horseback riding, in which a limitation of adduction may interfere with the ability to apply pressure against the flank with the inside of the thigh or knee in order to control and guide the horse and where inability to symmetrically adduct the thighs to secure one's seating may compromise the ability to maintain stability and form (see Ch. 6).

The thoracic paravertebral muscles

Increased tone and tenderness to palpation most consistently involve the paravertebral muscles on either side of the lower half of the thoracic spine, the erector spinae and semispinalis thoracis, and less often iliocostalis and longissimus thoracis (Figs 2.37, 2.38). Most often affected is the segment running from about the level of T3, T4 or T5 down to T12/L1. Less frequently, involvement is localized to one or both sides of the mid-thoracic (T3–T7) region or the thoracolumbar junction, sometimes limited to an area immediately adjacent to the level of a vertebral rotational displacement.

The tense muscles are usually palpable like thick 'ropes' under the subcutaneous tissue, the amount of tenderness often maximal along the site of irritation or injury. There may also be obvious crepitus, suggesting chronic muscle tension has resulted in some muscle fibre atrophy and increase in fibrous tissue (see 'Asymmetric muscle tension', above and Ch. 8).

Clinical correlation: thoracic paravertebral muscles

On clinical examination, the person may complain of tightness and pain in the affected paravertebral muscles whenever the tension in these muscles is increased further as they are stretched with trunk forward flexion, rotation and/or side-flexion; also, whenever reflex contraction is triggered by a certain manoeuvre. Extension should relax these muscles but can sometimes trigger reactive splinting or spasm by increasing:

1. a lateral or anterior disc bulge or protrusion
2. the pressure on adjacent posterior vertebral edges or an already tender facet joint (Fig. 3.68)
3. foraminal narrowing, with secondary root irritation

The examination for range of motion should be carried out not only in standing but also in sitting, the latter to stabilize the pelvis and allow one to more selectively stress the thoracic and lumbosacral regions (Fig. 3.49). The most common finding, in sitting, is a restriction of trunk rotation by some 5–15 degrees on one side, usually into the direction of the thoracic convexity (Fig. 3.49B).

The restriction may reflect the fact that there is probably already a rotation of the central thoracic vertebrae into the convexity (see Ch. 2; Fig. 3.6). In the presence of an underlying thoracic convexity to the left, for example, the central vertebrae may already have rotated counterclockwise into the convexity, limiting their ability to rotate further to the left.

Other factors must, however, be operative, given that a restriction to the left can also be seen in association with a right thoracic convexity. For example, there may be an element of uni- or bilateral increase in tension involving segments of the thoracic paravertebral muscles (see above).

Excessive work routines or overtraining in a sport are more likely to bring on a sensation of pulling, discomfort, or outright pain from tense contralateral paravertebrals on side flexion, on trunk rotation while sitting or on first bending forward and then twisting the trunk to the right or left. This tightness and discomfort is more likely to become a problem with work or sports activities requiring repeated trunk flexion and/or rotation (e.g. facets of construction work, painting, kayaking, canoeing, gymnastics, martial arts, golfing and throwing sports). Typical of soft tissue, the symptoms will be maximal on starting the activity; e.g. on awakening and after having rested or maintained one position for a longer period of time. The symptoms may gradually subside as the muscles warm up with use and can again accommodate to being stretched but they may recur again as persistence with the activity results in muscle fatigue and a further increase in tension, obvious on palpation, and discomfort from the origin, muscle mass and/or insertion.

Range of motion will be limited in any direction of movement that further increases tension in these already tense and tender structures; attempts to move past that point can trigger muscle spasm or cause actual damage. This may happen inadvertently in the course of executing a manoeuvre that requires movement into one of the restricted ranges (e.g. torquing and side-flexing when lifting; a lay-up twist in basketball) or if the trunk is passively forced past a restriction (e.g. as in wrestling; Fig. 5.35).

The lumbar and sacral paravertebral muscles

Between L1/L2 and L4, the paravertebral muscles are often relaxed and non-tender, even in the presence of malalignment, pelvic obliquity and compensatory scoliosis. Pain is more likely to be elicited on

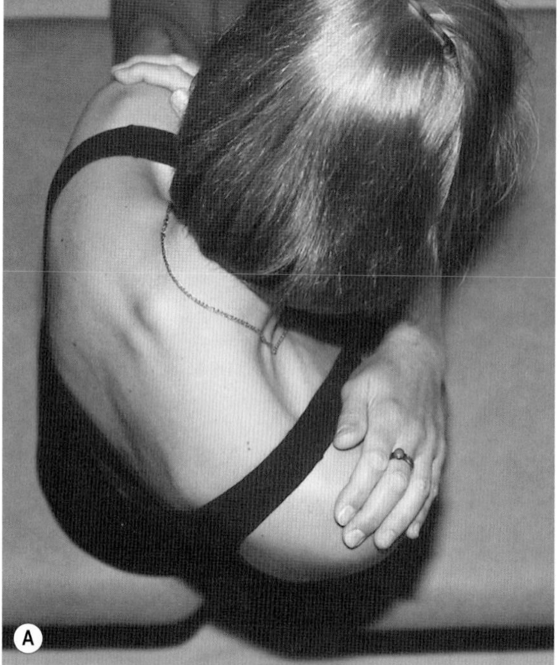
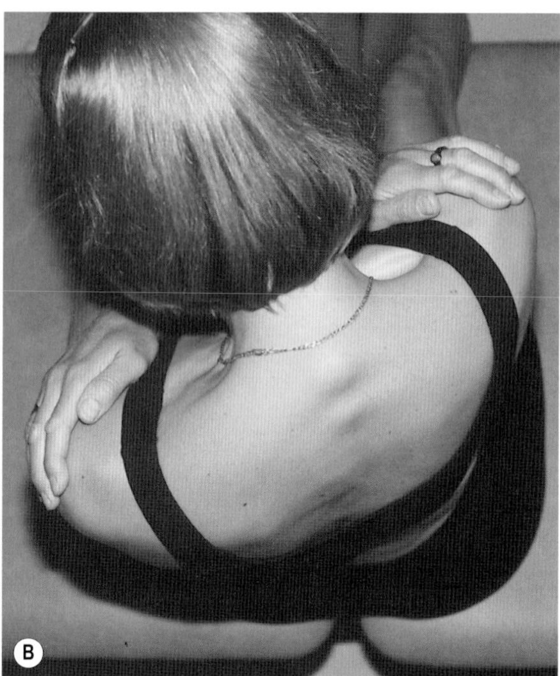
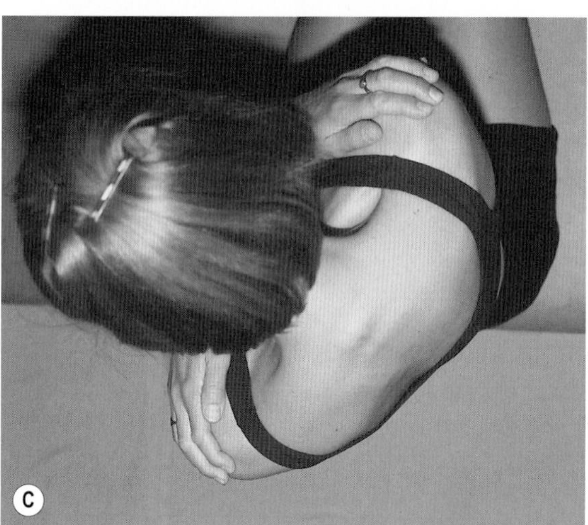

Fig. 3.49 Trunk rotation in sitting, to stress the thoracic structures. Restriction to the left may relate to the fact that the subject has a left thoracic convexity (as evident in Fig. 2.95B) with a counterclockwise rotation of the central thoracic vertebrae into the convexity, limiting further rotation into that direction (see also Figs 3.5, 3.6, 4.31B). (A) Right rotation to 45 degrees. (B) Left rotation limited to 35 degrees. (C) On realignment, left came to equal right rotation, with improvement to 55 degrees now evident bilaterally!

palpation of the lumbosacral junction area. Persistent increase in tension and/or tenderness between L1-L4 levels, if present, should raise suspicions that one might be dealing with splinting in reaction to some underlying pathological condition. The following need to be considered:

1. rotational displacement of any of the lumbar vertebrae
2. instability, often involving L4 and/or L5
3. pain attributable to facet joint or disc degeneration, spondylolisthesis, partial lumbarization or sacralization with pseudo-joint formation, disc protrusion or lateral recess stenosis (Ch. 4).
4. irritation of nerve fibres, from whatever cause; e.g. spondylotic narrowing of a foraminal opening, causing irritation of the exiting anterior or posterior root or the medial branch of the posterior primary ramus that innervates the facet joint
5. a pathological problem (e.g. abdominal mass, compression fracture, malignancy or metastases)

In a patient with known instability of L4 and/or L5 who presents with an episode of severe pain of acute onset in the lumbosacral region, often with recurrence of malalignment - one must always rule out rotational displacement of L4 and/or L5 which can itself cause:

1. unilateral impaction of a L5-S1 facet joint (Fig. 2.52B)
2. complicating sacral torsion and/or sacral rotation around the vertical axis (Fig. 2.52A,B).

Both problems described can, in turn, cause rotation of an unstable innominate or of the pelvic ring as a unit to the point of causing actual malalignment of the pelvic ring. However, the real problem is the rotational displacement of L4 and/or L5 and its secondary mechanical effects on the pelvic unit, all of which may then be perpetuated by:

1. reflex lumbosacral muscle spasm, triggered by pain and/or instability in this region
2. the pelvic malalignment itself

Quadratus lumborum

Increased tension in quadratus lumborum may be implicated in the recurrence of an 'upslip', 'rotational malalignment', vertebral rotational displacement or combinations of these.

First, attachments to the twelfth rib and the posterior iliac crest allow this muscle to pull the innominate upward (Fig. 2.62).

Second, origins from transverse processes of L1-4 and insertions posteriorly into the superior iliac crest and iliolumbar ligament exert:

1. an anterior rotational force on the innominate
2. a lateral and rotational force on these vertebrae, which may play a role in determining the direction that a compensatory curve of the lumbar spine will take.

Alternatively, rotational displacement of any of these vertebrae may increase tension in the muscle on one side and allow that on the opposite side to relax. For example, the frequently noted left rotation of the L1 vertebral complex (spinous process turned to the right) seen with an 'upslip' and 'rotational malalignment' may play a role in increasing tension in the attaching left quadratus lumborum. 'Facilitation' of this muscle on the left, 'inhibition' on the right side may be another factor (Figs 2.62, 3.43).

The iliopsoas muscle

The three components of this conjoint muscle are all strategically placed (Fig. 2.62). Psoas minor originates from the sides of the vertebral bodies of T12 to L5 and inserts into the superolateral aspect of the superior pubic ramus. Psoas major originates from the transverse processes of L1 to L5 and inserts into the lesser trochanter. Iliacus comes off the upper iliac fossa, iliac crest, anterior sacroiliac ligament and base of the sacrum; one part of it inserts into the tendon of psoas major, the other directly into the lesser trochanter (Figs 2.46A,B, 2.59, 2.75). Iliopsoas as such flexes the hip joint and externally rotates the femur; whereas, when the pelvis is stabilized (as in sitting), a side-to-side difference in tension of the individual components can result in the effects described in Box 3.6.

Increased tension in iliopsoas is felt to be one of the main reasons for the recurrence of malalignment after correction (Grieve 1983). Traction forces on the innominate could, for example, predispose to:

1. 'anterior' rotation (e.g. increased tension in iliacus)
2. 'posterior' rotation (e.g. increased tension in psoas minor)

BOX 3.6 Effects of increased tension in left iliopsoas muscle

When weight-bearing:

1. *Psoas major:* forward flexion, right rotation and left side-flexion of one or more vertebrae
2. *Psoas minor:* an upward shift of the ipsilateral left pubic bone, with or without posterior rotation of the left innominate
3. *Iliacus:* starting with left heel-strike and during left stance phase, progressive anterior rotation of the left innominate in the sagittal plane, combined with some sacral rotation around the left-on-left oblique axis; the overall effect during gait would be to gradually increase left counternutation and decrease SI joint stability on proceeding to left toe-off and into swing-through (Figs 2.21, 2.41)
4. *Conjoint iliopsoas:* external rotation, adduction of the femur, as well as upward traction force on the ipsilateral innominate
5. *Psoas major and minor:* an increase in the lumbar lordosis

When non-weight-bearing:

The combined effect is one of hip flexion (e.g. when clearing a leg through the swing phase), external rotation and adduction of the leg.

3. 'upslip' (e.g. increased tension in psoas minor in particular but also all 3 components as a unit exerting an upward force on the innominate - directly, with psoas minor pulling on the pubic tubercle and indirectly, with the femoral head being pulled upward into the hip socket
4. simultaneous 'rotational malalignment' and an 'upslip'

Intermittent spasm of the iliopsoas can account for the frequent report of a lancinating pain felt in the groin, often so severe that the person stops the activity in which he or she is engaged until the pain subsides (Wells 1986). When iliopsoas is involved alone or in conjunction with pectineus, frequent findings on clinical examination include the following.

First, active or passive adduction of the femur may be limited because it provokes pain by compromising the space available for an already tender iliopsoas exiting through the narrow femoral triangle, lying just anterior to the femur and acetabular rim.

Second, iliopsoas is more often tender just on the left side or worse on the left than right. This finding is frequently seen in the presence of the much more common 'left innominate posterior rotation' and 'left lower extremity in internal rotation'. Both of these biomechanical changes increase tension in the components of iliopsoas by separating their origin and insertion: posterior innominate rotation increasing tension in iliacus, internal leg rotation in iliopsoas (an external rotator). The fact that iliacus inserts, in part, into the tendon of psoas major will increase tension in that muscle as well. However, sometimes tenderness on exam is restricted to right iliopsoas, indicating that other factors may be operative; for example, there may be a reactive tensing of right iliopsoas to stabilize and/or decrease pain from the right SI joint.

Third, passive left hip abduction is also limited in nearly all of those with 'rotational malalignment'. An increase in tension in iliopsoas may be one factor contributing to this limitation but it does not explain why this limitation occurs on the left side regardless of what particular pattern of 'rotational malalignment' or 'upslip' (right/left) is at hand. However, it may relate, in part, to the fact that more than 80% of people seen with 'rotational malalignment' have one of the 'more common' rotational patterns. These patterns all have the associated 'right external, left internal' rotation of the lower extremity, which can decrease tension in the right iliopsoas and increase it in the left one simply by causing an approximation and separation of the muscle origin and insertion, respectively.

Problems involving the left adductors would also have to be considered, including:

1. 'facilitation' of the muscle group
2. 'posterior' innominate rotation (pulling upward on the origin from the pubic bone and ischial tuberosity)

However, there is no acetabular reorientation of the acatabulum with an 'upslip'. Also, there is no change in the biomechanical arrangement of the adductor muscle group other than it having been moved upward as one unit along with the innominate and the femur.

Possible explanations for the more frequent finding of increased tension/tenderness in left iliopsoas include:

1. Malalignment may 'facilitate' left iliopsoas.
2. The malalignment of the pelvis may itself be the result of increased tension in one or more components of iliopsoas, such as can be triggered by T12, L1 or L2 rotational displacement (Maffetone 1999; Fig. 3.2).
3. The left SI joint may actually become hypermobile as a result of the increased stress imposed if the right joint is 'locked' or hypomobile for other reasons; left iliopsoas would contract in an attempt to stabilize the now hypermobile left SI joint.
4. Reorientation of the acetabula - this is less likely to play a role, given that the limitation of passive left hip abduction in supine lying is seen to occur with either 'right' or 'left anterior rotational malalignment'.
5. With a left 'upslip', the femoral insertions of left psoas major and minor are actually moved upward passively, which would be expected to decrease tension in these muscles and should allow for a relative increase in left hip abduction compared to the right side. However, the reverse is usually found on examination.

With either 'rotational malalignment' or an 'upslip', increased tension and tenderness can be found in iliopsoas bilaterally, in which case it is usually significantly worse on the left than the right side. Bilateral involvement may be attributable to attempts to stabilize both SI joints and to cope with the increased workload that results from the change in weight-bearing stresses with any pelvic and femoral reorientation.

Again, the 'facilitation' of left iliopsoas on a spinal segmental or cortical basis seems a more probable explanation.

Clinical correlation: iliopsoas

The increased tension in iliopsoas on either side increases the chance of sustaining a sprain or strain of this muscle and/or avulsing the lesser trochanter. For example, an increase in tension in left iliacus resulting with left posterior innominate rotation makes injury of this muscle more likely with quick abduction manoeuvres, such as occur in hockey games when the goalie does the 'splits' or hyperabducts the leg on the side of the restriction (Figs 3.50, 5.21).

Iliopsoas is also more vulnerable in its role as an external rotator to any increase in tension that results with activities calling for passive internal rotation of that extremity when the foot is planted on the ground. For example, this may occur:

1. in a right-handed pitcher wearing cleats:
   a. on the right side, as he or she winds up by rotating the trunk/pelvis clockwise and weight-bearing on the more or less 'fixed' right leg
   b. on the left side, as he or she unwinds by rotating counterclockwise to release the ball while weight-bearing on the 'fixed' left leg (Figs 3.51, 5.30, 5.31)

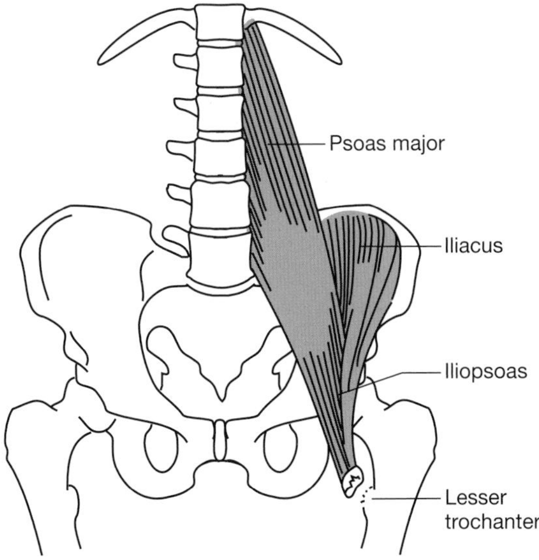

Fig. 3.50 Avulsion of the left lesser trochanter.

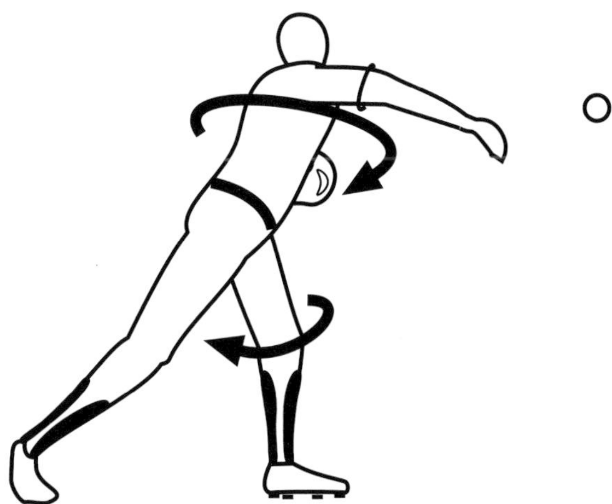

Fig. 3.51 Passive internal rotation of the weight-bearing left leg as the right-handed pitcher unwinds counterclockwise to release the ball (see also Figs 5.30, 5.31).

2. in a speed or figure-skater circling counter-clockwise:
   a. on the left leg, as he or she starts to adduct the right leg while balanced on the outer edge of the 'fixed' left skate (Fig. 5.17).

Anterior innominate rotation depresses the superior pubic ramus, increasing tension in the attaching psoas minor and exerting a traction force on its origins from T12 to L5. The result is a rotational stress on these vertebrae, augmenting the lumbar lordosis and limiting trunk extension.

Unilateral groin pain of sudden onset, with or without a history of injury (e.g. a fall landing hard on one or both feet, abduction of that leg), with increase in iliopsoas tension limited to or worse on that side, may require investigations to rule out problems such as an iliopectineal bursa, a strain or tear of iliopsoas or an acetabular labral tear (Fig. 4.2).

Rectus femoris

Rectus femoris originates from the anterior inferior iliac spine and the anterior rim of the acetabulum; it inserts into the base of the patella and indirectly into the tibial tubercle by way of the patellar tendon. This muscle, therefore, can act to flex the hip and/or extend the knee, making it ideal for the correction of 'rotational malalignment' using a muscle energy technique (see Ch. 7). Anterior innominate rotation will decrease tension in the muscle by bringing its origin closer to its insertion; whereas posterior rotation will increase tension by separating these sites (Fig. 3.42).

Clinical correlation: rectus femoris

Increased tension in rectus femoris results in an ipsilateral limitation of hip extension (Wells 1986b). Assuming tightness of the left rectus femoris, the restriction can be compensated for by:

1. increasing stride length and decreasing the stance phase on the left side
2. increasing the lumbar lordosis to encourage the tendency of the innominate to rotate anteriorly, the acetabulum backward to allow more left extension
3. increasing the amount of pelvic rotation counterclockwise around the vertical axis in the transverse plane; as the left leg moves through stance phase and progressively more into extension, it pulls on the tight rectus femoris and helps rotate the pelvis increasingly counterclockwise (Fig. 2.12)
4. increasing plantar flexion of the left ankle and foot to help increase the stride-length of that leg

Rectus femoris on the side of a posterior innominate rotation is at increased risk of sprain or strain with sudden or excessive hip extension, especially if there is a simultaneous eccentric or concentric contraction of the quadriceps. This can occur, for example, when coming out of the blocks on a sprint start. Extension of the hip is coupled with an initial eccentric contraction of the quadriceps to help extend and stabilize the knee of the driving leg throughout stance phase (Fig. 3.52A:1–5). A concentric contraction is superimposed at a time when the rectus femoris is already under maximal tension at the end of the stance phase and the extreme of hip extension, in order to help initiate hip flexion (Fig. 3.52B:5,6).

The upper trapezius muscle

As indicated above in the discussion on the neck region, there is usually an asymmetrical and apparently autonomic increase in tone involving the right upper trapezius alone or the right more than the left. Similar findings for right cervical paravertebrals and scalenes, probable biomechanical effects of the spinal curves and the clinical correlations have been cited above under 'The cervical segment of the spine'.

ASYMMETRICAL FUNCTIONAL WEAKNESS OF THE LOWER EXTREMITY MUSCLES

In those presenting with malalignment, manual assessment of muscle strength will usually reveal weakness in some upper and lower extremity muscles, which may be attributable to:

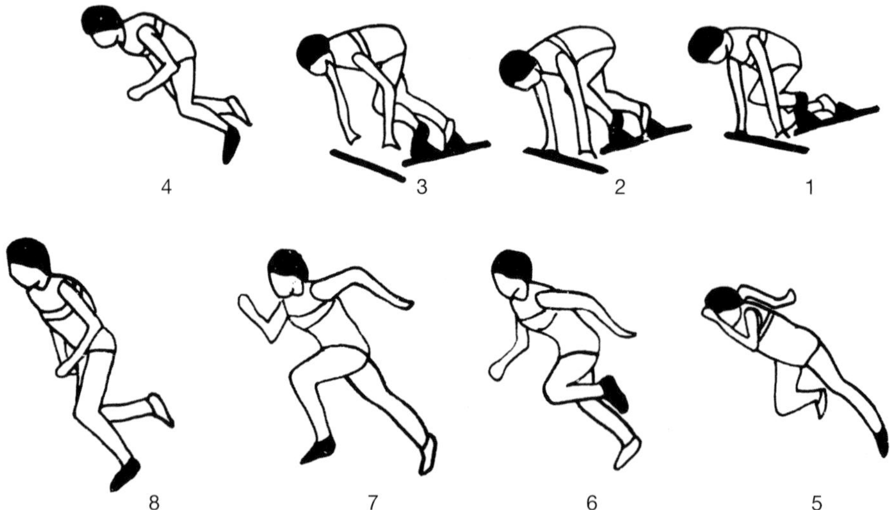

Fig. 3.52 Sprint start. The athlete who has increased resting tension in the left rectus femoris because of 'left posterior' innominate rotation (see Fig. 3.42) is at increased risk of injuring this muscle on a sprint start as tension is increased further with: (A) initial eccentric contraction to help to advance the pelvis and simultaneously steady the knee as it extends to provide the force for pushing off from the blocks (1–4); (B) superimposed passive stretching with acceleration as the pelvis (origin) continues to move forward and the hip extends, further separating origin and insertion (5); then concentric contraction (hip flexion, 6); (C) eccentric contraction to help to stabilize the knee as the foot comes to weight-bear again (7) and the hamstrings contract to straighten the knee for the next push-off (8). *(Courtesy of Paish 1976.)*

1. an asymmetrical 'functional' weakness
2. a reorientation of the muscle fibres
3. a loss of muscle bulk
4. pain (perceived or subconscious).

An example of upper extremity weakness seemingly related to pain is a giving-way of rhomboids and infraspinatus, a wrist flexor or extensors or even more distal muscles (e.g. FDL, APB), usually bilaterally, as a result of perceived or subconscious pain around the shoulder region. Pelvic malalignment results in increased stress on cervicothoracic or upper thoracic curve reversal sites (Figs 2.91, 2.94) and often a chronic increase in tension and tenderness involving cervicothoracic and shoulder girdle muscles: paravertebrals, scalenes, trapezii in particular. There may be a problem such as T4 or T5 rotational displacement or development of trigger points in this upper area. On testing distal upper extremity muscles, apparent weakness and giving-way could be, in part, attributable to the person tensing up these proximal muscles further to stabilize the neck and shoulder girdle. Unfortunately, increased activation of these muscles can irritate structures that are already being stressed, sites of vertebral displacement or trigger points. However, the seemingly 'weak' distal muscles may prove to have full strength - 5/5 – when re-tested with the forearm resting on a table or otherwise supported, the shoulder girdle muscles positioned so that they are completely relaxed throughout the test.

Weakness of the lower extremity muscles seen in association with malalignment presents in a surprisingly consistent, asymmetrical pattern (see Appendix 4). This weakness has been referred to as a 'pseudo-weakness' but is probably more appropriately called a 'functional' weakness', one that usually disappears immediately once realignment has been achieved. With few exceptions, a consistent pattern of this functional weakness is seen in association with the an SI joint 'upslip' and the 'more common' patterns of 'rotational malalignment'; a similar asymmetrical weakness has also been noted with the 'left anterior and locked' pattern. In other words:

1. the presence of the functional weakness correlates with the fact that malalignment of the pelvis is present
2. The malalignment may be either in the form of:
   a. a right or left 'upslip', or
   b. a 'left anterior and locked' or one of the 'more common' patterns of 'rotational malalignment'
3. Given that this functional weakness appears consistently in the same distribution, it appears to be determined primarily by factors other than the actual presentation of malalignment: inhibition at a spinal segmental, brain stem or cortical level need to be considered.

In order to allow for comparison of one side to the other or of one subject to another when testing a specific set of muscles:

1. the person should be standing, sitting or lying in the same way relative to the examiner
2. whenever possible, the examiner should be standing the same way in relation to the right and left component of the pair of muscles being tested and use the same hand or fingers to carry out each test.

In order to establish the presence and the extent of a 'functional' weakness, muscles must be tested in a consistent way to ensure validity of comparison by:

1. testing each pair of muscles with the person in the same position
2. applying resistance:
   a. to the same location in reference to the bony landmarks
   b. with the same hand or number of fingers
   c. at the same angle

For example, the ankle evertors (peroneus longus and brevis) are best tested with the person supine to stabilize the trunk, pelvis and legs and to minimize proximal muscles co-contraction and movement of any limbs as the person is asked to move the foot 'down and out' against resistance. The examiner preferably stands opposite to the side being tested (Fig. 3.53A,B). Initial resistance is applied with the hand and 2nd to 5th fingers hooked around the lateral border while the thumb encircles the dorsolateral aspect of that foot; if that can overcome the evertors on one or both sides, resistance can then be applied with 4, 3, or sometimes even just 2 fingers to determine the 'breaking point' and allow for an accurate side-to-side comparison. When malalignment is present, the difference between the two sides is usually quite easily detected on the first test.

Muscles like the extensor hallucis longus (EHL; Fig. 3.55A) make it possible to apply gradually increasing resistance of equal extent to both sides

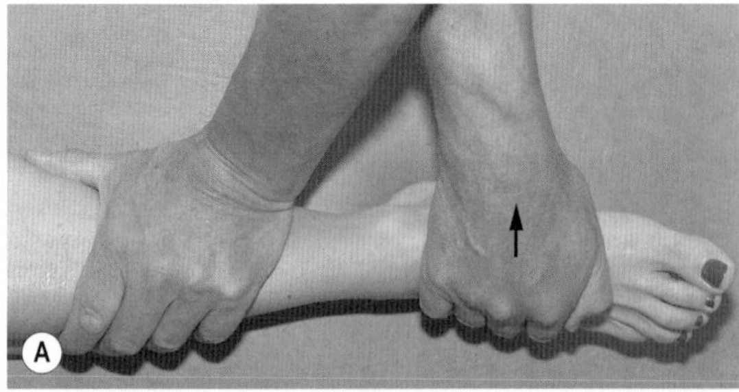

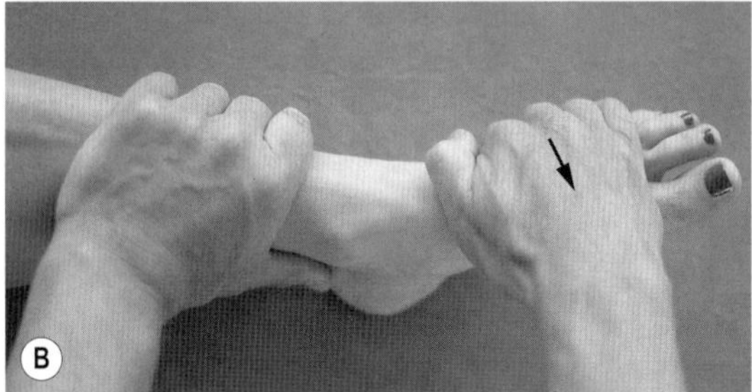

Fig. 3.53 Testing the strength of peroneus longus and brevis (ankle evertors: 'down and out'). (A) Right (consistently strong). (B) Left (consistently weak). NB: here the right hand is used to offer resistance; whenever possible, the same hand should be used at the same angle when testing each side to make right/left comparison more accurate.

simultaneously by hooking the opposite mid- and/ or index finger around the proximal phalanx of the extended first toes and then leaning increasingly backward, feet planted on the ground. At some point, the EHL on one side gives way and the first toe - typically the right when malalignment is present - collapses into flexion. Provided there are no painful degenerative changes, weakness on account of nerve injury, or other physical problems affecting the first toe, this test is one of the easiest to do and great for helping establish whether:

1. an 'upslip', 'rotational malalignment' or both are likely to be present (but it cannot distinguish which type or pattern is at hand)
2. treatment has been successful in achieving realignment, in which case strength will now equal that on the left side
3. treatment has been only partially successful, given that there is persistent comparative weakness of right EHL; examination may show correction of 'rotational malalignment' is incomplete, or reveal an underlying 'upslip' that now needs to be treated to achieve return to full strength

For some muscles (e.g. hip abductors, hamstrings and iliopsoas), the accuracy of comparison can be increased by applying resistance progressively more proximal or distal to a marker like the patella or popliteal fossa to help find this comparative 'breaking point' (Fig. 3.55B-E).

The side-to-side difference can sometimes be surprising: 1–1.5 grades less on the Oxford scale of 5 is not unusual. Right tibialis posterior (ankle inversion) might, for example, show a weakness with strength often being graded at only 3.5 or 4; whereas its left counterpart usually tests at full strength (Fig. 3.54A). Peroneus longus (ankle

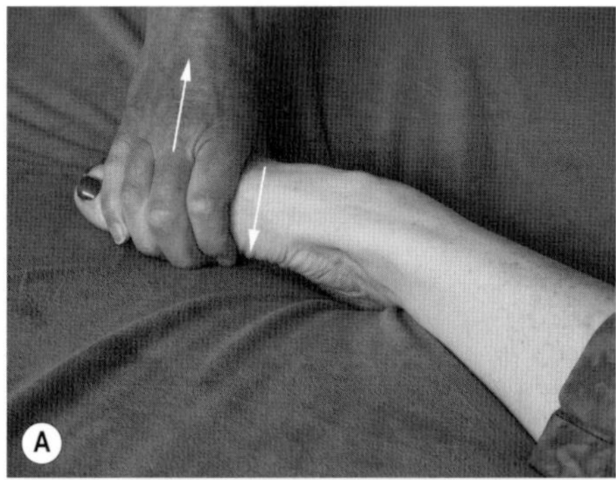

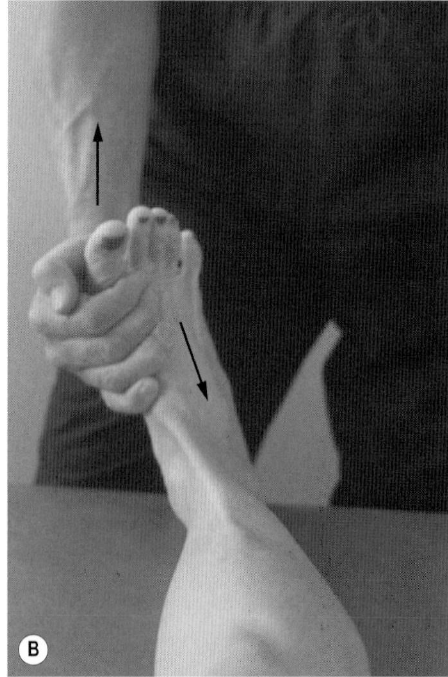

Fig. 3.54 Testing the strength of the ankle invertors. Both the right tibialis posterior ('down and in' - being tested in A) and right tibialis anterior ('up and in' - being tested in B) are consistently weak; whereas their left counterparts are strong.

eversion) will show a similar weakness but on the left side; whereas its right counterpart is considerably - and consistently - stronger, usually 5/5 (Fig. 3.53A,B).

Clinical and research findings: lower extremity muscles

The full pattern of this functional weakness seen in association with the 'more common' patterns of 'rotational malalignment' and an 'upslip' is described in Box 3.7.

Those who are out of alignment may display:

1. in 5-10%: the full pattern of asymmetric functional weakness in the lower extremity muscles, which includes right hip extensors and left hamstrings (see Box 7)
2. in 90-95%: an asymmetric pattern of weakness (sparing the right hip extensors and left hamstrings, which appear to have 5/5 strength bilaterally on manual testing)
3. seemingly no weakness in some other large muscle groups but, as indicated below, a comparative side-to-side weakness is likely to become apparent on mechanical testing (e.g. right quadriceps)

The muscles that prove weak most consistently are:

1. on the right side - the hip flexors, ankle invertors (tibialis anterior and posterior) and extensor hallucis longus (EHL)
2. on the left side - the hip abductors and ankle evertors

The weakness is consistently most pronounced in the right ankle invertors, left ankle evertors and right EHL (e.g. 3+ to 4/5). As indicated, right hip extensors and left hamstrings are more likely to show full strength but when weakness is evident on manual testing, it is frequently in this lower range of 3+ to 4; whereas their counterparts - left extensors and right hamstrings, respectively - are consistently 5/5 strength.

BOX 3.7 Patterns of functional weakness seen with the 'upslip' and 'rotational malalignment' presentations

1. ***Left ankle evertors (peroneus longus and brevis):*** tested lying supine, foot going 'down and out' (Fig. 3.53A,B)
2. ***Right ankle invertors (tibialis posterior and anterior):*** tested lying supine; foot 'down and in' and 'up and in', respectively (Fig. 3.54A,B)
3. ***Right extensor hallucis longus:*** EHL can be tested bilaterally simultaneously, with the person lying supine, 'big toes up'; the examiner can cross arms to permit hooking the middle and/or index fingers around the proximal phalanx of the opposite first toes and then lean backward to apply fairly symmetrical resistance until EHL gives way on one side (Fig. 3.55A)
4. ***Left hip abductors (gluteus medius/minimus and TFL):*** tested in side-lying, with the hip joint in neutral alignment so that the leg is in line with the body and the knee straight (for TFL) or in some flexion (for the gluteals); 'raise the leg up', against the resistance applied using a hand placed at, or just above or below, the knee joint (Fig. 3.55B)
5. ***Left hamstrings:*** tested in prone-lying with the knee flexed to 90 degrees; 'bend the knee' against a resistance to flexion applied to calf at mid-point or progressively more distally if necessary (Fig. 3.55C)
6. ***Right hip flexors (iliopsoas, rectus femoris, pectineus):*** tested in sitting, with legs over the edge of the plinth and the knees flexed to 90 degrees; resistance to 'raise the knee up' applied initially to the distal thigh, more proximally as needed for proper comparison to left (Figs 2.46B,C, 2.62, 3.55D, 4.2)
7. ***Right hip extensors (primarily gluteus maximus):*** tested in prone-lying, the knee 90 degrees flexed; 'raise the leg up' against a resistance applied initially to the distal thigh, more proximally as needed (Fig. 3.55E)
8. ***Left hip rotators:*** tested in either supine-lying, hip and knee flexed to 90 degrees, or prone-lying (see Figs 3.78, 3.79), knees flexed 90 degrees and, if possible, leg in midline to start; resistance is applied to distal tibia or ankle to counter an attempt to 'rotate the lower part of the leg':
   a. outward (testing internal rotation; Fig. 3.55F)
   b. inward (testing external rotation; Fig. 3.55G)
9. ***right hip adductors:***
   a. raising leg straight upward while in right side-lying, knee straight and the leg in line with the body, against a resistance applied at or around knee joint level, or
   b. pushing the knee in toward centre against a resistance applied to the inside of knee while sitting with the hip and knee flexed (contraction of left adductors is evident in Fig. 3.55H)

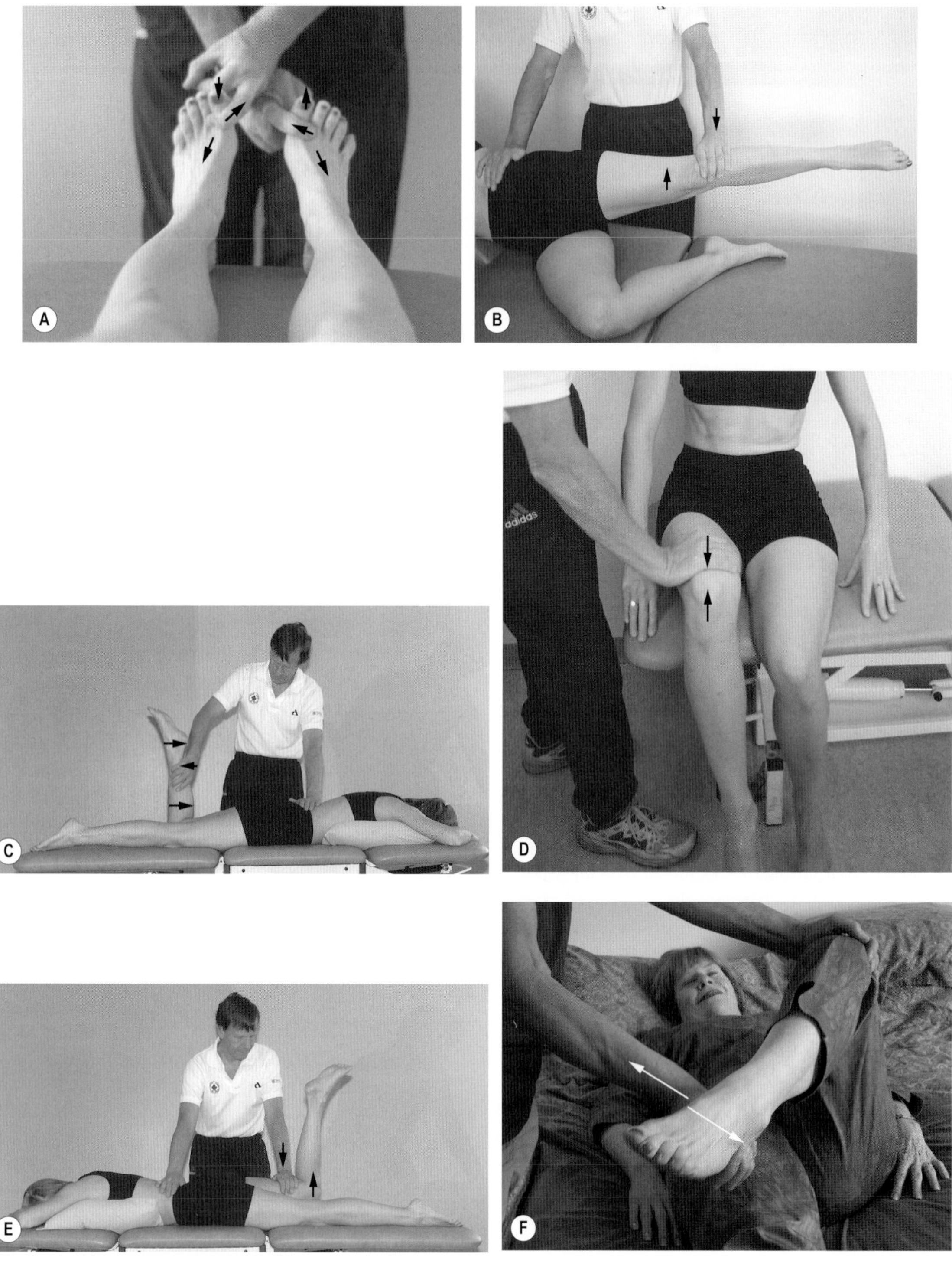

Fig. 3.55 Other muscles that typically give way because of the functional weakness seen with 'rotational malalignment' or an 'upslip': (A) right extensor hallucis longus (note: the examiner, applying progressively increasing symmetrical forces, has already overcome right EHL while the left remains strong); (B) left hip abductors and tensor fascia lata/iliotibial band complex; (C) left hamstrings; (D) right hip flexors; (E) right hip extensors; (F) right internal rotators (shown: testing the strong left ones)

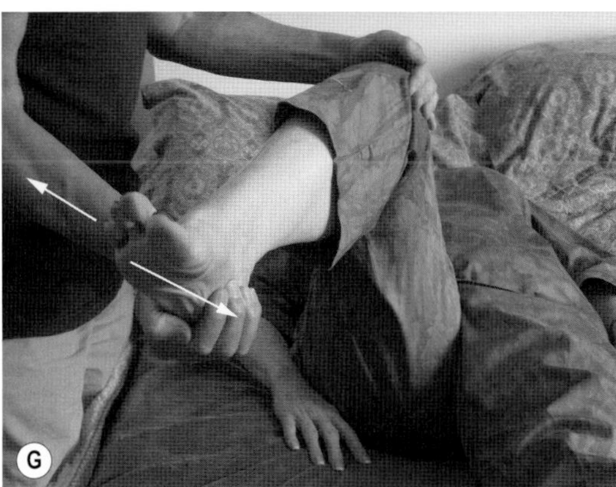

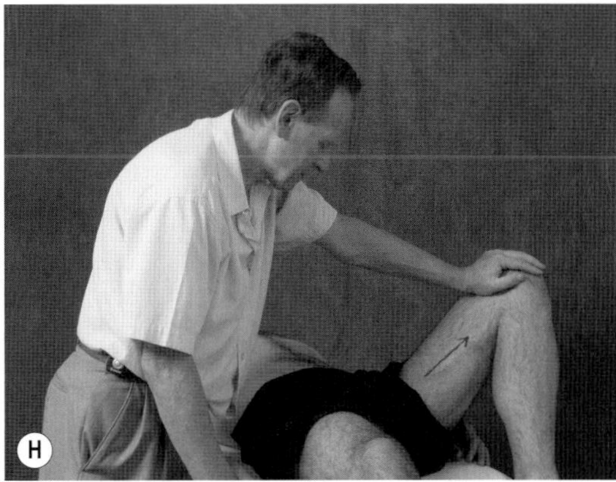

Fig. 3.55—cont'd (G) left external rotators (shown: testing the strong right ones); (H) left hip adductors (arrow overlying contracted muscle here indicates reversal of direction of pull - on origin from left pubic bone - to correct a left 'inflare' using MET).

Some muscles (e.g. quadriceps and triceps surae) are consistently strong on manual testing but this may be more a reflection of the inherent strength of these muscles which the examiner just cannot overcome in the person being tested. For example, when there was no right quadriceps weakness apparent on manual testing, the muscle turned out to be so strong that any side-to-side difference in strength could be detected only by doing dynamometer studies (Sweeting et al. 1989). These same studies showed that:

1. both the endurance and the power of the 'involved' leg muscles can be reduced in the presence of malalignment, and both can increase immediately following realignment
2. the increase in strength post-manipulation may be greater for an eccentric than a concentric quadriceps contraction; the latter will frequently not improve at all.

Other dynamometer studies have also shown a significant asymmetry in quadriceps strength on a side-to-side comparison before realignment, the right being weaker than the left (Hershler et al., unpublished data, 1989). The same effects described in the above studies, with recovery of muscle strength, were recorded immediately following correction of the malalignment. Clinically, muscles previously found to be weak will also show an appreciable increase in strength on manual retesting immediately following correction. Any side-to-side difference will either have disappeared completely or have decreased significantly. Ankle invertors and evertors, hamstrings and hip flexors and extensors usually retest at 5/5 bilaterally.

The left hip abductors are more likely to show some persistence of weakness but rarely of the same degree as before. Interestingly, they will usually show a gradual increase in strength on subsequent examinations until finally testing at 5/5 some days or even weeks after the initial correction, provided that alignment is being maintained in the interval. For example, improvement was recorded on dynamometer studies in an athlete who had shown an increase in left hip abductor force and endurance on an isometric fatigue test immediately after realignment, with a further increase in strength detectable on retesting after alignment had been maintained for 4 months; the left hip abductors were, however, still comparatively weaker than the right, even after that length of time (Hershler, personal communication, 1989). Herzog et al. (1988) reported a significant difference in force on comparing initial gait trials conducted to those carried out later on in a rehabilitation program aimed at the correction of sacroiliac dysfunction.

In other words, the changes relating to muscle strength and to weight-bearing forces on comparative gait trials are not necessarily apparent immediately post-realignment, or only better to some extent, compared to the improvements that become manifest on retesting as alignment is being maintained.

The time it takes for these changes to materialize may relate to the time it takes:

1. for the body to adapt fully to the realignment, with the elimination of any residual asymmetries in tension and the resolution of any contractures
2. to achieve full pelvic and spinal alignment, with the elimination of any change in tension attributable to 'facilitation' and 'inhibition' and/or persistent proprioceptive changes

Other observations in regards to return of strength in left 'hip abductor, TFL/ITB' complex include:

1. the inhibitory effect on the muscles on the left side may be more persistent the longer the malalignment has been present
2. conversely, weakness of the left complex seen in association with malalignment may be more likely to resolve quickly - and realignment more likely to be maintained - in the younger population where the problem is less likely to have been present for as long a period of time.

The author's clinical experience points to those in their 20s and early 30s and, with amazing consistency, also those on the maternity ward who:

1. have just gone through a major, unresolved trauma to the pelvic floor region (e.g. tissue tears, possibly a caesarian or other surgery)
2. have a history of recent onset or worsening of a pre-existing problem of back, groin or leg pain in the peri-natal period (Fig. 3.56)
3. nevertheless, will undergo successful reversal of the malalignment in over 90%, using gentle, modified muscle energy techniques (see Ch. 7), and
4. in 80-90%, maintain the pelvic realignment in the subsequent days despite the ongoing demands on the musculoskeletal system - healing of the pelvic floor, carrying and lifting the infant in awkward positions, muscle tension and emotional stress - that would usually cause an older person to go back out of alignment!

Recurrence of malalignment despite specific treatment attempts calls for a search of problems such as complications relating to the tissue injuries sustained during the delivery (e.g. failure to heal, infection, separation of the symphysis pubis; Fig. 2.102A) and a possible home assessment to help detect and modify any unwanted ways they are using to cope with the infant (e.g. excessive bending and torquing with lifting and transfer techniques; one-sided feeding and carrying).

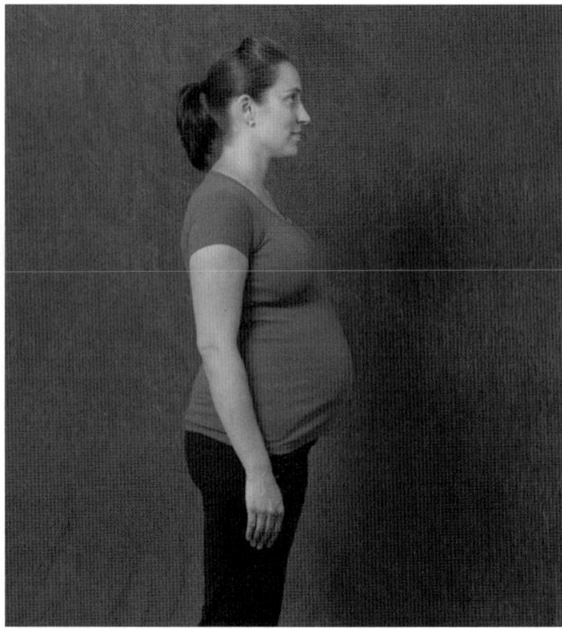

Fig. 3.56 Pre-partum low back pain is largely attributable to increased stress on the lumbosacral region as the lumbar lordosis increases in an attempt to compensate for the weight gain and anterior shift of the centre of gravity. This stress would be compounded by coexistent malalignment of the pelvis and/or spine.

Of note in this regard is the fact that the time when pelvic realignment and stability are finally being maintained is often marked by the onset of an increasing problem of recurrent vertebral rotational displacement, particularly likely to involve vertebrae in the thoracic and cervical spine segments. It may require ongoing treatment for some weeks or even months before stability of these spinal segments is finally achieved.

Any residual bilateral ankle muscle weakness will usually be symmetrical and in keeping with the true weight-bearing pattern that becomes evident once the person stays in alignment:

1. in those who turn out to be true pronators when aligned, there may be persistent weakness of bilateral ankle invertors - tibialis anterior and tibialis posterior
2. in those who turn out to be true supinators when aligned, there may be persistent weakness of bilateral ankle evertors; in particular, peroneus longus.

This residual weakness will usually respond to strengthening of the specific muscles involved.

Considerations: asymmetry of muscle strength

The following are some points to consider when trying to explain the pattern of asymmetrical functional weakness seen in association with an 'upslip' and 'rotational malalignment'.

The pattern cannot be attributed to laterality

With laterality, any increase in right or left upper and lower limb strength, muscle bulk and circumference are fairly consistently noted to be on the dominant side. There has not been any correlation of laterality of handed- or footedness, or of eye or ear dominance, to the actual presentation of malalignment; e.g. right or left 'upslip' or the various patterns of 'rotational malalignment' or 'outflare/inflare' (discussed below).

The pattern does not correspond to a nerve root or peripheral nerve lesion

There is usually a weakness involving muscles in both lower extremities, in an asymmetrical pattern that consistently involves muscles supplied by different nerve roots and/or peripheral nerves. In addition, electromyographic (EMG) and nerve conduction studies are normal (see 'Case history 3.1').

The pattern may relate to the relative leg length

Dorman et al. (1995) consistently found a weakness in the hip abductors on the side of the long leg, which corresponded to the side of the anterior innominate rotation. The side of the weakness could be changed simply by using a manual therapy manoeuvre to switch a posteriorly-rotated innominate to one in anterior rotation with a seemingly long leg. The fact that the strong abductors were found on the short leg (i.e. posteriorly rotated) side seemed to correspond to the increasing contraction detectable in these muscles to enhance 'force' closure when this was crucial to ensure stability of the SI joint in anticipation of heel-strike.

Given the amount of movement possible at the SI joints in various studies, the anterior rotation of one and posterior rotation of the other innominate were calculated to result in as much as 7.22 mm of difference in leg length in standing. The side-to-side difference in dynamic abductor strength observed in standing and walking could relate to abductor 'facilitation' or 'inhibition' and/or lever arm lengthening or shortening. During the gait cycle (Fig. 2.41), abductor facilitation on the side of the posteriorly rotated innominate - and hence short, swing leg side - would again be in keeping with an attempt to stabilize the SI joint in preparation for heel-strike.

However, on testing hip abductor strength in a static position (Fig. 3.55B), the author consistently notes the weakness to involve the left hip abductors, regardless of whether there is a left anterior or posterior innominate rotation present, or a functional left short or long leg in supine lying or standing. Admittedly, the person is tested only once or twice before and after the initial realignment, and the isometric resistance is applied to the leg at the 'breaking point' - usually found to coincide with the hand applied across or just proximal or distal to the patella. The lever arm of the leg would be increased if the leg is longer and/or whenever the resistance is applied at a more distant level. This could help explain the consistent finding of decreased abductor strength on the long-leg side by Dorman et al. (1995), who applied resistance down at the ankle level and would have had a greater magnification effect on the side of the longer lever arm as compared to that obtainable on the short-leg side. Also, there was no apparent assessment of strength in the short (gluteus medius/minimus) versus the long abductors (TFL/ITB complex).

The pattern may relate to impaired proprioception or kinaesthetic awareness

As proposed by Guymer in 1986, the pattern may be an expression of a 'proprioceptive adaptation' that has occurred as a result of the asymmetry of the joints. One manifestation of this 'adaptation' could be the frequently noted inability of the person to contract one of the weak muscles on command. This happens, for example, quite often when asking the person for an isolated contraction of the left peroneal muscles in order to evert and plantarflex the left ankle. He or she may eventually muster a fairly good contraction when given some tactile, visual and/or verbal feedback. The term 'functional weakness' has been used because the weakness is found to disappear immediately on correction of the malalignment (Janda 1986; Sweeting et al. 1989). Janda suggested some mechanisms to explain what has also been termed a 'pseudoparesis', including:

1. the impaired 'facilitation' of a muscle segment
2. an impaired sequencing of muscle contraction
3. an asynchrony of muscle contraction
4. an asymmetrical proprioceptive input from the muscles and joints.

'Pseudoparesis' probably entails a combination of these factors. 'Facilitation' and 'inhibition' are referred to throughout this text, and there is frequent mention of 'impaired sequencing' and 'asynchrony' of muscle contraction. It is, perhaps, this last suggestion regarding 'asymmetric proprioception' that is the most appealing as an explanation of why the strength, and perhaps also the tone, should be affected so readily by simple realignment procedures. The blatant weakness in the right extensor hallucis longus (EHL) may, for example, be reversed simply by squeezing the right tibia and fibula together at the level of the ankle; the weakness recurs as quickly as the pressure is released (D. Grant, pers. comm. 2000). Nerve endings associated with proprioception have been found in a wealth of structures: thoracodorsal fascia (Willard 1997, 2007; Panjabi 1992a,b), supra- and interspinous ligaments (Jiang et al. 1995), ligamentum flavum (Yamashita et al. 1990), muscles surrounding the facet joints (Cavanaugh 1997), the joint capsule (McLain 1994), and the joint surface itself (seemingly triggered by a variation in load - Avramov 1992). There is also an increasing documentation of impaired proprioceptive awareness (O'Sullivan et al. 2003) and lumbar segment postural control (Mok et al. 2004b) in patients with LBP that may be attributable to deficient innervation of the lumbar fascia (Bednar et al. 1995) and may contribute to difficulties encountered on attempting motor control retraining of local muscles in patients with LBP (Richardson 2004; Barker & Briggs 2007).

If, however, an asymmetry of joint proprioceptive signals was the cause, one would expect the pattern of this functional weakness to differ depending on the presentation of malalignment, given that joints are stressed differently in one presentation compared to another. For example:

1. the pattern of weakness is the same in those with a right or left 'upslip' and any of the 'more common' patterns of 'rotational malalignment', despite these considerable variations in alignment of the joints in the legs and pelvis
2. the 'more common' pattern of 'right anterior/left posterior' innominate rotation disorients pelvic and lower extremity joints in completely the opposite way compared to what is seen with the 'left anterior/right posterior' pattern. However, the pattern of asymmetrical weakness was not found to be consistently the opposite in one compared to the other (Schamberger 2002). The left hip abductors were the most obvious exception, being noticeably weaker than those on the right in as many of those with one of the 'more common' patterns of rotational malalignment or an 'upslip' as in those with the 'left anterior and locked' pattern (84% versus 82%, respectively).

Asymmetry of the joints, and hence asymmetry of the proprioceptive signals arising from the joints, does not seem to offer a full explanation for any differences (or lack thereof) in the pattern of asymmetrical functional weakness seen in association with the 'more common' patterns of 'rotational malalignment' and an 'upslip'.

Over the past decade, there has been an increasing realization that impaired muscle segmental 'facilitation', sequencing and/or asynchrony of contraction can result in problems such as failure of tension to resolve or muscles in the 'inner' and 'outer' core segments to activate properly, so that an individual may have difficulty achieving the stabilization of the pelvis and spine that would then allow him or her to carry out an intended action (e.g. simply maintaining balance when standing; or one more intricate, like throwing a ball; Figs 3.51, 5.31). Methods such as Real-Time Ultrasound visualization, surface- or intramuscular EMG have proven especially helpful for detecting problems of this kind, also for localizing muscles such as the mulifidi that are in spasm, show contractural changes, have atrophied, fail to activate in a proper sequential pattern, do not activate at all or possibly just on one side. Some of these techniques have also been helpful in providing feedback to teach patients how to overcome the problem at hand (see Ch. 4; Figs 4.46, 4.47).

The pattern may reflect dysfunction at the level of the spine, brain stem or cortex

More specifically, the dysfunction may involve a spinal segment and its associated dermatome, myotome and sclerotome, a theory advanced by Korr back in 1978. Segmental dysfunction could cause muscle weakness by interfering with centrally-mediated motor control, which depends on the appropriate inhibition or facilitation of the segment and, in turn, affects muscle tone. Decreased tone is associated with weakness, increased tone with increased strength.

The pattern may reflect impaired cerebrospinal fluid circulation

The answer may well lie in the hands of those therapists using the craniosacral release method for the treatment of alignment-related disorders (see Chs 7, 8). It is postulated that the malalignment reflects a disturbance of the normal pulsating flow of cerebrospinal fluid anywhere along its course. The disturbance, it is felt, comes in large part from an imbalance of tension affecting the dural sheath, or 'theca', which surrounds the cord and the individual nerve roots and is, in reality, an extension of the meninges running from the foramen magnum down to the filum terminale which inserts at about the S2 or S3 level and into the coccyx. The increased tension on the dura and meninges may actually be caused by a twisting of the spine and/or pelvis, which would increase the distance between the cranial origin and distal insertion. The twisting can result with rotational displacement of individual vertebra(e), segmental rotation seen with a pelvic obliquity and scoliosis, and sacral rotation (e.g. sacral torsion, excessive counternutation; Figs 2.11B, 2.21) and coccygeal anterior displacement or excessive flexion (Fig. 4.44).

However, these asymmetries of the spine, pelvis and lower extremities can be corrected with therapy restricted to working on the dural attachments at the foramen magnum and/or the sacrococcygeal insertions, without ever touching the musculoskeletal structures such as rotationally displaced vertebrae or the lumbo-pelvic-hip joint complex affected by the malalignment. Certainly, the results lend strength to the argument that the musculoskeletal asymmetries seen are themselves in large part the result of changes in tension involving the dura and meninges and the neural tissues that they enclose. Those skilled in craniosacral release are adept at sensing even minor fluctuations in muscle tone that occur in tandem with the pulsations of the rhythmic flow of cerebrospinal fluid; for example, the palpable waxing and waning of tone felt in the external and internal rotators of the extremities. Treatment is aimed at re-establishing the cranial rhythm and the normal, symmetrical cycle affecting tone in opposing muscle groups.

The normal rhythm is very obviously tied into a fluctuating increase and decrease in tone, alternately affecting the extensors and flexors throughout the body. An asymmetrical increase in tone in these opposing sets has been linked to a disturbance of the rhythmic, pulsating CSF flow. If the disturbance can result in a fluctuating asymmetrical tone involving either the external or internal rotators throughout the body, a similar mechanism might perhaps result in an asymmetry of muscle strength from head to toe. However, malalignment does not simply result in weakness in a whole set of muscles (e.g. either all the external or all the internal rotators). Rather, malalignment consistently:

1. presents as a pattern of opposites, regardless of the type of 'upslip' and/or 'rotational malalignment' actually at hand ('right' or 'left anterior' rotation etc)
2. affects rotators, extensors and flexors on the right and left side but in an asymmetrical pattern
3. presents with the same strength-weakness pattern; for example, in the lower extremities one notes the strong left internal, right external rotators and the weak left external, right internal rotators (see Box 3.7).

Nonetheless, craniosacral treatment aimed at re-establishing the cranial rhythm and the normal, symmetrical cycle that regulates tone in the muscles may be able to achieve alignment and symmetry of muscle strength, often where other treatment methods have failed. It remains to deduce the actual way in which the phenomena of the craniosacral rhythm (CSR) and malalignment are interlinked:

1. does disturbance of the CSR result in asymmetric muscle tension which, in turn, can cause the pelvis and spine to go out of alignment, with a secondary asymmetric change in strength?
2. does the craniosacral treatment simply reestablish normal dural-meningeal tension, allowing for return of the normal rhythm and, with it, a symmetry of muscle tone that allows the bones to slide back into alignment?
3. in others, is it the reverse sequence?
   a. do they first go out of alignment for whatever reason (e.g. a fall, inadvertent lift)?
   b. secondarily cause a disturbance of the CSR with resultant asymmetry of muscle tension and strength?
   c. respond to realignment using one of the simpler techniques like MET, and with that manage to re-establish the CSR?

The pattern may reflect a lateralization of motor dominance

Approximately 70% of us are left and 15% right motor dominant; the other 15% seemingly have equal involvement of both the right and left cortex. Could an asymmetry in motor control at the cortical level result in the asymmetry in muscle strength? If that were so, one might expect a different pattern of weakness in those who are right compared to left motor dominant but so far only one consistent pattern of weakness has been evident in the positions of testing. The prevalence of the rare exception, found in association with the 'left anterior and locked' malalignment pattern, amounts to around 5%, nowhere near the figure of 15% given above for the 'right dominant' group. However:

1. the total of 85% obtained by adding up those who have a one-sided (right or left) motor dominance is close to that of the 80-90% overall presenting with malalignment (Ch. 2)
2. there remain approximately 10-15% with apparently equal motor dominance; these figures are in the same range for those who present in alignment and have no history of treatment for a previous problem of malalignment
3. at the farthest level of influence, the myotome and eventually the motor unit itself (Fig. 8.2), the difference may reflect the 85-90% who show asymmetry and the 10-15% who are symmetrical in terms of tension and strength

The lateralization of motor dominance could certainly be one of the factors that determines why one person consistently goes out of alignment in one pattern (e.g. the rare 'left anterior and locked') and another in one of the 'more common' patterns of 'rotational malalignment', or an 'upslip'. Rather than being the 'cause' of a uniform pattern of weakness, an asymmetry in motor dominance may be more likely to influence the symmetry of muscle tone and secondarily contribute to the recurrence of a specific presentation of malalignment.

The pattern may be the result of a combination of some of the factors postulated above

Segmental or cortical factors may, for example, decrease the strength in left hamstrings by decreasing the spindle setting or inhibiting the firing of the spindle. Conversely, they may have the opposite effect on the right hamstrings, which consistently show increased tension to palpation and prove strong. The actual degree of weakness could be modified by:

1. a change in the length-tension ratio, which occurs with any change in the distance between the origin and insertion (Fig. 3.42)
2. asymmetrical proprioceptive input from the right and left side, resulting in a difference of motor control in paired muscles
3. subliminal or perceived pain that interferes with mustering a full contraction.

In summary, the craniosacral technique itself is another manual therapy method that can sometimes achieve lasting realignment of the pelvis and spine where other approaches have failed. Simply achieving realignment by any of these techniques may result in return of symmetrical muscle tone and strength. While none, unfortunately, provide an explanation of how the asymmetry came about in the first place, the segmental and cortical propositions and the craniosacral theory seem the most appealing (see Ch. 8).

Clinical correlation: functional weakness

Workers and athletes sometimes complain of one leg being weaker or feeling unstable on weight-bearing, fatiguing more easily or feeling sore after activity. For example, those who work in crawl spaces or with one leg in a full squat and the other extended (e.g. electricians, plumbers, and those in construction) may find it easier to support weight on the right or left leg and prefer to push themselves up to standing on that leg. Cyclists may note decreased strength on one side when pushing down on the pedal. Weightlifters doing a dead lift from a squatting position may feel awkward or report a weakness on one side compared to the other (Fig. 5.33). Runners can experience one leg fatiguing more readily and the muscles on that side feeling 'sore' as if from overuse (see 'Introduction 2002'). Swimmers may feel that one leg is not as effective as the other when kicking. Ice skaters and gymnasts may mistrust one leg because of a recurring sensation of giving way or unsteadiness on single-leg support activities and when landing on that leg (see Ch. 5). The preponderance of those with complaints relating to the right leg may just be a reflection of the increased prevalence of an 'upslip' and the 'more common' patterns of 'rotational malalignment' (notably, the 80% prevalence of the 'right anterior/left posterior' pattern) as opposed to the much less frequently seen 'left anterior and locked' combination (5%).

The pattern of asymmetrical functional weakness is not in keeping with involvement of any specific nerve root(s) or peripheral nerve(s) (see Ch. 4). Certainly, any weakness out of keeping with this asymmetrical, non-anatomical pattern should trigger a closer search for an underlying neurological lesion. Otherwise, if there are no suggestions of such a lesion by history or on clinical examination, and examination findings are limited to the asymmetrical weakness, the approach should be:

1. to correct the malalignment first, then
2. to re-examine strength to see if eliminating the malalignment-related functional weakness has unmasked a residual 'true' unilateral weakness restricted to a muscle or muscles supplied by a specific root or peripheral nerve
3. if so, to initiate appropriate further investigations and treatment.

The 'Case History 3.1' serves to illustrate this point.

ASYMMETRY OF MUSCLE STRENGTH – OTHER FACTORS TO CONSIDER

Asymmetry of strength related to muscle reorientation and bulk

In the presence of an 'upslip' or 'rotational malalignment', asymmetry of bulk has been most easily detectable in the quadriceps, and specifically in vastus medialis. It is usual for quadriceps to test at full strength manually, which is not surprising given that this muscle ranks as one of the strongest in most people. (see 'Asymmetrical functional weakness of lower extremity muscles', above).

Obvious wasting of the vastus medialis appears to correlate to the side of 'anterior' innominate rotation. In addition, those with one of the 'more common' patterns, and hence external rotation of the right lower extremity, are more likely to show relative wasting of the right and hypertrophy of the left vastus medialis (Fig. 3.57).

A difference in bulk of vastus medialis can be readily documented objectively using techniques such as the laser scanner for mapping the surface topography (Fig. 3.58A). The difference has usually decreased dramatically, or may no longer be apparent, on reassessment after alignment has been maintained for some 4–6 months and without having performed any specific routines aimed at strengthening the wasted vastus medialis (Fig. 3.58B).

Differences in the bulk of quadriceps components may reflect the fact that malalignment results in an asymmetry of both the tension and the

CASE HISTORY 3.1

A 42-year-old recreational runner presented with a history of gradually increasing, non-radiating low back pain aggravated by lifting, bending and running. On examination, malalignment with a 'right anterior and locked' presentation was evident with outward rotation of the right leg and pronation of the right foot and ankle. Weakness (4 to 4+ of 5) was asymmetrical, limited to extensor hallucis longus, hip extensors, tibialis anterior and posterior on the right and the hip abductors and peroneus longus on the left.

Left root stretch tests (Lasègue's straight leg raising, or 'bowstring', and Maitland's 'slump' test; Fig. 3.75) were questionably positive; otherwise neurological examination was normal. An examination of the back was unremarkable except for localized soft tissue tenderness and a report of pain with posteroanterior pressure to the spinous processes in prone-lying, the pain being confined to the L5 and S1 vertebral level. X-rays showed a moderate L5–S1 disc space narrowing.

Correction of the malalignment was easily achieved but failed to decrease the back pain even temporarily and could never be maintained for more than a few days. More significant was the finding that when the athlete was re-examined while temporarily in alignment, the weakness was limited to the left hip abductors and ankle evertors, the previously weak muscles on the right side now all 5/5 full strength. Further investigations were prompted by:

1. the persistent weakness when in alignment, restricted to the muscles on the left side with both L5 and S1 root innervation
2. the questionably positive left root stretch tests
3. the failure to respond symptomatically to a correction of the malalignment
4. the failure to maintain alignment.

A computed tomography scan showed a large L5–S1 posterolateral disc protrusion impinging on the left S1 root, and electromyography studies were in keeping with a left S1 radiculopathy. Denervation activity, which one can see with ongoing axon degeneration, was restricted to muscles in the left S1 anterior myotome and the left paravertebral muscles at the level of S1 and S2, consistent with compression and involving both the left anterior and posterior S1 root, respectively. Following a resection of the disc protrusion, the back pain resolved completely, realignment was now maintained, and full strength returned eventually to the left S1 innervated muscles.

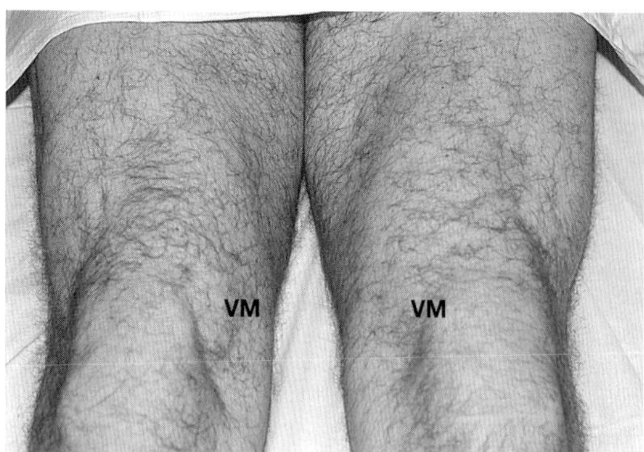

Fig. 3.57 Quadriceps asymmetry in a person with malalignment ('right anterior, left posterior' innominate rotation): wasting of the right and hypertrophy of the left vastus medialis (VM).

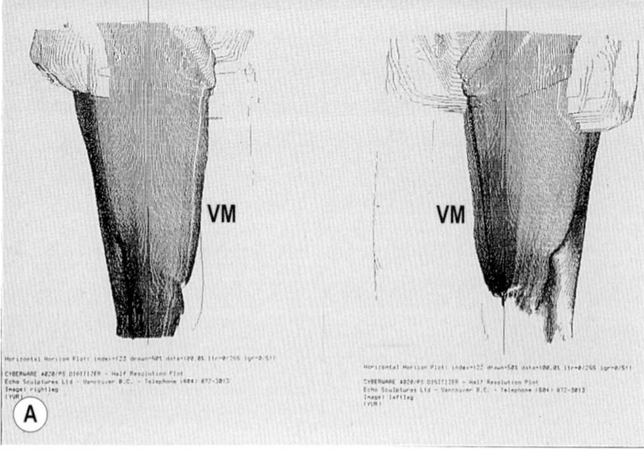

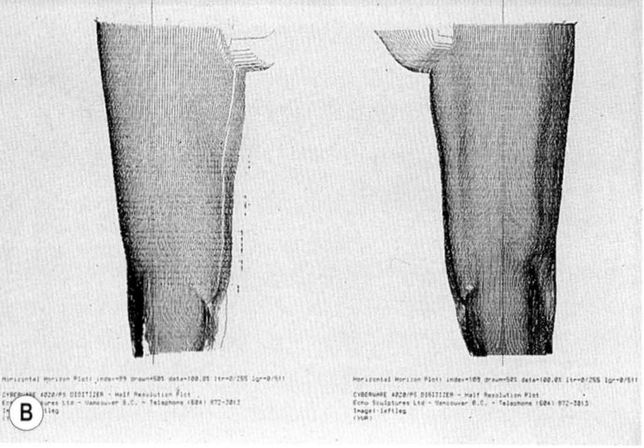

Fig. 3.58 Quadriceps bulk delineated with a laser scanner. (A) Asymmetry of vastus medialis (VM) with malalignment ('right anterior, left posterior' rotation): right wasted, left hypertrophied. (B) Almost symmetrical VM bulk within 4 months of maintaining alignment and return to regular activities (i.e. no selective muscle strengthening).

orientation of the fibres in these muscles and these, in turn, affect the strength of a contraction:

1. changes in tension

   'Anterior' rotation of the innominate, for example, approximates the rectus femoris origin and insertion, thereby decreasing tension, inhibiting muscle spindle firing and hence the strength of the contraction that the muscle can muster (Fig. 3.42). Vastus medialis could be affected secondarily because of its invaginations with rectus femoris. Posterior innominate rotation would have the opposite effect by increasing tension in rectus femoris. 'Facilitation' of the left and 'inhibition' of the right quadriceps would also affect tension.

2. orientation of muscle fibres

   The fibres in the various components of the quadriceps muscle are oriented at different angles to the midline (Fig. 3.59). Changing the angulation of these fibres will, in turn, affect the ability of each component to contribute to the strength of a contraction aimed at extending the knee and flexing the hip to advance the leg in the sagittal plane. Factors that can effect such a change include:

   a. external rotation (Fig. 3.60, right leg)

   The right quadriceps muscle as a whole ends up being oriented outward, away from midline, something that would decrease its ability to contribute to forward progression. In addition, the fibres of some of the quadriceps components end up being oriented at an increased angle to the line of progression. This effect will be maximal for muscles whose fibres are already angled more obliquely to the sagittal plane (e.g. vastus medialis and lateralis), as opposed to those more in line with the plane of progression (e.g. rectus femoris and vastus intermedius). Increasing external rotation, for example, causes the bulk of vastus medialis to face more and more forward and out; the fibres of the muscle come to pull at an increasing angle to the sagittal plane, decreasing their ability to contribute to this movement.

The increased tendency to pronation at the foot, an inward (valgus) collapse at the knee and outward drift of the patella further changes the orientation of the muscle fibres unfavourably. While the increased valgus angulation may increase tension in vastus medialis, it also puts

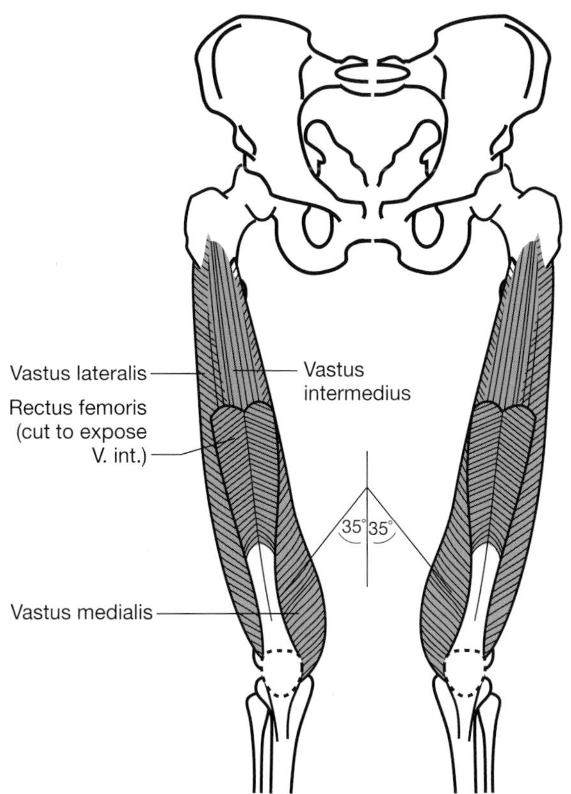

Fig. 3.59 The symmetrical angulation of vastus medialis fibres relative to the sagittal plane when the person is in alignment.

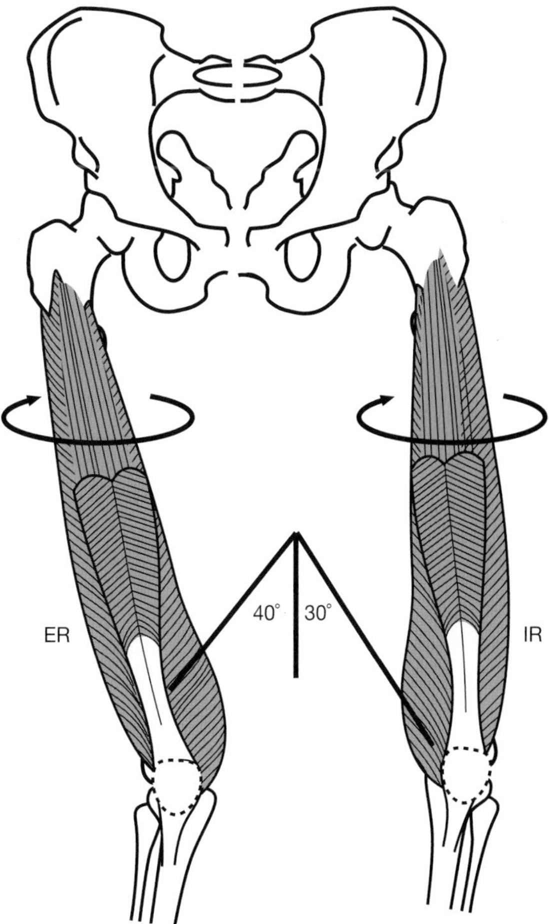

Fig. 3.60 The asymmetrical angulation of vastus medialis fibres seen with an 'upslip' and the 'more common' patterns of 'rotational malalignment': the right is increased with the external rotation and valgus angulation, the left decreased with the internal rotation and varus angulation.

this muscle at a further disadvantage as it now pulls on an increasingly lax rectus femoris that no longer sits directly over the foot (see Ch. 5). The combination of some of these changes would contribute to decreased stability of the right knee joint when landing on that extremity and during the stance phase.

b. internal rotation (Fig. 3.60, left leg).

The quadriceps complex, specifically the fibres of vastus medialis (probably also lateralis) are oriented more favourably relative to the line of progression because internal rotation brings the foot and leg more in line with the sagittal plane, as does any tendency to genu varum. Also, the foot and knee are stabilized somewhat during the weight-bearing phase, the knee sitting more directly over the foot and both pointing increasingly straight ahead (Figs 5.10, 5.13D).

c. tendency to genu valgum with pronation, genu varum with supination (Fig. 3.37)

When wasting of vastus medialis is present, one must always be sure to rule out other pathology, given that this muscle is notorious for being the most likely, and usually the first, to show wasting with painful afflictions of the knee and hip, in particular, and of the lower extremity in general.

Clinical correlation: asymmetrical muscle bulk

Reorientation of the medial and lateral components of the quadriceps muscle away from the sagittal plane on the side on which the lower extremity rotates externally with malalignment may:

1. decrease their ability to contribute to advancing the leg in the sagittal plane

2. result in a more rapid fatiguing of these muscles which, in turn, would contribute to:
   a. the muscles becoming sore as with overuse, even on running shorter distances than would previously have caused them to feel this way (e.g. feeling discomfort on the side of the external rotation after running only 20 km; whereas it might still take a marathon to provoke the same symptoms on the side of internal rotation; see 'Introduction 2002').
   b. that leg feeling weak and/or unstable
   c. an increasing tendency to valgus angulation at the knee, attributable in part to vastus medialis being weaker and fatiguing more rapidly
3. these changes, in combination with other factors cited, such as the tendency to pronation of the foot and lateral tracking of the patella, predisposing to the development of patellofemoral compartment syndrome and patellar tendonitis (which are typically much more common, or more severe, on the right side, in keeping with the number presenting with increased external rotation of the right leg; Fig. 3.37).

Unilateral quadriceps wasting will cause or aggravate an imbalance of strength involving the right versus the left quadriceps, and of the quadriceps versus the hamstrings on the same side. Imbalances involving these strong muscles are probably best detected using dynamometric studies (see above; personal communications: Sweeting 1989b, Hershler 1989). Clinically, the person afflicted with such a strength imbalance may report an occasional 'giving way' of the leg involved, more likely on going up or down stairs where quadriceps play an especially significant role. Some learn to anticipate the problem and are able to prevent a fall as the knee buckles while other are not as fortunate. If such imbalances are present, they also put the worker or athlete at increased risk of sustaining a muscle sprain or strain, especially if the activity requires repeated lifting, torquing or squatting. This problem involving the knee is quite distinct from feeling a sudden 'giving way' proximally, seemingly in the 'hip' region but that may actually be attributable to an SI joint instability: the so-called 'slipping clutch syndrome', discussed below (Dorman 1994, 1995; Dorman et al. 1998).

The question is whether malalignment affects the other muscles of the extremities, pelvis and trunk in a similar way, changing their orientation and, therefore, their ability to muster an optimal contraction and maintain their bulk. For example, a person may report feeling that the 'buttock' on one side feels 'smaller' compared to the other side. Examination sometimes show less muscle bulk: gluteus maximus and/or piriformis, in particular, may indeed feel smaller and also are often more tense and tender on the side indicated. There may be other, less obvious, differences in bulk involving the muscles around the buttock and hip girdle regions that are hard to appreciate on examination (more likely to be evident on CAT scan or MRI) but which are, nevertheless, present and could be contributing to the feeling that one hip girdle or leg is just not as strong as, feels more unstable, or fatigues more easily than the other. A difference in the bulk and strength of piriformis, iliopsoas or any of the gluteal components could certainly have these effects.

For example, 'right anterior' innominate rotation for reasons other than iliacus contracture, would decrease tension and change the orientation of that muscle which could, in turn, result in decreased ability of iliacus to contribute to hip flexion and external rotation, actual wasting and fatiguing more readily compared to the psoas component (Figs 2.46, 2.62).

Also, as indicated above, it is the right hip flexors and, in a small number, extensors that turn out to be weak compared to the left side of those presenting with an 'upslip' or one of the 'more common' rotational patterns. A functional weakness combined with any discomfort from the SI joint or soft tissues on that side certainly could result in holding back on full weight-bearing on the right side and eventual disuse wasting of the quadriceps and other muscles on this side (e.g. gluteus maximus).

The wasted muscle(s) may or may not respond normally to efforts at selective strengthening as long as they continue to be at a disadvantage on account of the co-existing functional weakness caused by the malalignment. Following realignment, muscle bulk may actually increase simply with more normal use of the lower extremities during everyday activities and eventually come to equal that on the opposite side without the person ever having done any selective strengthening exercises (Fig. 3.58B). The addition of symmetrical strengthening, however, may help to maintain bulk on the normal, or sometimes even hypertrophied, side while speeding up recovery on the wasted side. Sometimes, feedback by the therapist or using measures such as Real-Time US may be necessary initially to get the person to learn how to initiate contraction of a specific muscle and finally allow them to get on with a progressive strengthening programme (Ch. 7).

In summary, in the case of weakness and/or decreased muscle bulk in someone presenting with 'rotational malalignment' or an 'upslip'; the differential diagnoses to consider include:

1. malalignment-related functional weakness, in the typical asymmetric pattern, which may well disappear in part or completely on initial realignment
2. weakness in keeping with a specific root or peripheral nerve injury
3. weakness resulting from a combination of malalignment and a root/nerve injury
4. disuse weakness and wasting secondary to:
   a. just being less active physically
   b. inability to initiate a contraction fully, or not at all, because of fear of triggering pain
   c. failure to contract in the proper sequence
   d. actual muscle fibre atrophy, with eventual excessive fibrous tissue replacement
   e. unfavourable reorientation of muscle fibres

ASYMMETRY OF LIGAMENT TENSION

Ligaments should feel neither lax nor excessively taut, and they should not be tender. A side-to-side comparison is invaluable for determining any differences. Malalignment can increase tension by:

1. increasing the distance between the origin and insertion (Fig. 3.42)
2. increasing tension in a muscle that attaches to, or is in continuity with, the ligament

One example of the latter is the increased tension in left ITB seen with the 'facilitation' of left hip abductors and TFL (Fig. 3.41).

Another example involves the sacrotuberous (ST) ligament. Pansky & House (1975) found this ligament to be one of the origins of the long head of biceps femoris. Previous reference has been made to Vleeming et al. (1989a,b) who reported attachments running to the sacrotuberous ligament:

1. from the thoracolumbar (dorsal) fascia (Figs 2.37, 2.38)
2. in the form of muscle fibres from piriformis and gluteus maximus
3. as partial or complete continuity with the lateral head of biceps femoris in some 75% of cases (Figs 2.6, 2.21, 2.22).

In the majority, therefore, traction applied to gluteus maximus above or biceps femoris below could increase tension in the sacrotuberous ligament, and vice versa.

A persistent increase in tension in a ligament has four undesirable consequences.

1. The ligament eventually lengthens and fails to provide adequate support (e.g. left sacrospinous in Fig. 3.65B).
2. The ligament ultimately becomes painful.
   a. Pain most consistently localizes to the ligament origin and insertion which probably relates to the fact that histological studies show the highest concentration of neurological structures (e.g. pressure-sensitive corpuscles, proprioceptive sensors, nociceptive axons and other pain fibres) to lie in the region of the fibro-osseous junctions (Hackett & Henderson 1955).
   b. Chronic tension results in elongation, irritation and inflammation, particularly of the nerve structures within the ligament. The nerve fibres cannot elongate as quickly nor as much as the elastic components of the ligament and are, therefore, put under excessive stretch before elongation of the elastic elements has reached its limit (Hackett 1958; see Ch. 8).
   c. Prechtl & Powley (1990) showed how lumbosacral ligaments and other connective tissues are innervated by small-calibre, primary afferent fibres that can send nociceptive stimuli to the spinal cord. When irritated, these same fibres can also secrete pro-inflammatory neuropeptides capable of initiating peptide release and a chain of events leading to eventual tissue inflammation and oedema. Connective tissue structures in this region are also supplied by sympathetic efferent axons capable of releasing catecholamines.
   d. A balance between these two neural systems is thought to be important to the 'maintenance of the integrity of the lumbosacral ligamentous structures' (Willard 1995: 53). The balance can presumably be upset with chronic excessive tension in the ligaments, which may help to explain why ligament inflammation and pain often fail to settle down until normal tension has been re-established by correction of the

malalignment; the posterior pelvic ligaments are a prime example of this phenomenon (Fig. 2.5A).

e. The blood supply to the ligaments is already poor in comparison to the flow to other tissues and would be further compromised by any increase in tension and the associated catecholamine release with irritation of the sympathetic system.

3. An elongated, irritated and inflamed ligament can become a source of aberrant proprioceptive signals and referred pain symptoms (Hackett 1958). Trigger points can also develop in ligaments (Travell & Simons 1983, 1992).
4. Pain from a ligament results in a reflex increase in tension in adjacent muscles in an attempt to decrease movement in that area and thereby prevent further irritation of that ligament. A viscious cycle may evolve if the muscle splinting helps maintain the increased tension in the ligament so that it continues to be a source of painful irritation which, in turn, perpetuates the increase in muscle tension. If the splinting is asymmetrical, it will predispose to the recurrence of malalignment. Chronic splinting eventually leads to development of myofascial pain and chronic tension myalgia, a complication that may explain why in some patients the pain from the ligament(s) persists even after the strain on the ligament(s) has been removed on realignment and there is no evidence of ligamentous laxity. Persistence of actual inflammation of the ligament may be another reason (Ch. 7).

Ligaments typically affected by malalignment

'Rotational malalignment' (and also an 'upslip') most consistently affects the sacrospinous and the four major posterior pelvic ligaments on each side: the sacrotuberous, iliolumbar, long (dorsal) sacroiliac and posterior SI joint ligaments (Figs 2.4, 2.5A, 2.19). Also involved are the interosseous ligaments within the SI joints (Figs 2.4B, 2.13Aiii) and those supporting the symphysis pubis (Figs 2.4A, 3.66). The altered biomechanics can increase tension in specific lower extremity ligaments as well, sometimes to the point that they, too, become tender and even symptomatic. Typical of these are the lateral ligaments of the knee and ankle on the supinating side, and the medial ligaments on the pronating side (knee forced into varus and valgus angulation, respectively; Figs 3.37, 3.81). Following is a discussion relating to specific pelvic ligaments as they are affected by 'rotational malalignment' or an 'upslip'.

The iliolumbar ligaments

The iliolumbar ligaments originate from the transverse processes of L4 and L5 (Fig. 2.4A). The insertion includes:

1. a superficial component, onto the medial aspect of the posterior iliac crest at the level of L5 and S1
2. a deep component, with a fairly broad attachment along the anteromedial part of the ilium.

Overlying muscle, subcutaneous tissue and fat may preclude palpation of the origin and midpart in most but localized pressure can usually evoke pain from one or both transverse processes and the superficial insertion, all of which are usually directly palpable.

The ligaments can be put under increased tension by separating origin and insertion. For example, the right iliolumbar ligament would be put under stretch by:

1. contralateral (left) trunk side-flexion
2. active or passive 'right posterior' innominate rotation (Figs 2.47A, 2.115C), which moves the insertion further away
3. sacral nutation, which accentuates a lumbar lordosis and moves the L4/L5 origin forward relative to the iliac insertions Fig. 2.103A)
4. simultaneous trunk extension and right rotation; the latter may cause pain by compressing the left joint surfaces (positive left facet stress test) but if pain is evoked from the right side, it may indicate involvement of the right iliolumbar ligament which is being stressed as the L4/L5 transverse process origins are rotated posteriorly, away from the iliac insertions (Fig. 2.4A)

Involvement of the iliolumbar ligaments is suggested by:

1. tenderness on direct palpation of the tips of the L4 and L5 transverse processes, the ligaments themselves and/or the superficial insertions
2. pain on one or more of the selective stress tests outlined above

The iliolumbar ligaments needs to be considered in the differential diagnosis of pain in the region of the greater trochanter and lateral thigh:

1. referred pain

   A normal bone scan, and a failure of an injection of local anaesthetic into the soft-tissues surrounding the trochanter to bring even temporary relief, should suggest the possibility that one is dealing with pain to the lateral hip/thigh on a referred basis. The iliolumbar ligament sclerotome includes the greater trochanter. Malalignment, if present, may result in 'facilitation' and aggravate both local and referred unilateral ligament pain. If realignment alone fails to bring complete relief, the injection of local anaesthetic into the ligament itself should be tried (Fig. 3.46). The deep insertions may be difficult to reach other than with a 75–90 mm needle under fluoroscopic control. Surgery around the greater trochanter plays absolutely no role if the problem is one of pain referred to this region (see Ch. 7).

2. trochanteric bursitis

   Tenderness, oedema and increased warmth is maximal overlying the greater trochanter. Pain may localize there or radiate around and/or down the lateral thigh. Injection of local anaesthetic decreases or abolishes pain temporarily; anti-inflammatories (possibly including a trial of cortisone injections) or prolotherapy to stimulate collagen formation and strengthen the underlying tendon may be required for long-term relief (see Ch. 7). Resection of the bursa may be in order.

3. a combined problem of trochanteric bursitis and malalignment

   Injection around the area of the trochanter will probably bring only partial relief limited to the duration of the anaesthetic; in that case, cortisone injection around the bursa needs to be coordinated with realignment, and possibly also injection into the ligament itself, in order to achieve complete relief.

4. meralgia parasthetica

   Fibres from L2 and L3 form the lateral femoral cutaneous nerve (LFCN; Fig. 4.13), which can run into problems anywhere along its course along the back of the abdomen, then medial to the ASIS, under the inguinal ligament and finally, as the anterior and posterior terminal branches, to supply sensation to the proximal and distal postero- and anterolateral aspect of the thigh.

5. 'thoracolumbar syndrome'

   Irritation of the lateral branch formed by the posterior cutaneous fibres (originating primarily at the T11, T12 and L1 level) can result in hypersensitivity of the skin overlying the trochanter, which may be decreased with an injection of local anaesthetic into the skin but is completely abolished with a block of the lateral branch itself (see Ch. 4; Fig. 4.23A3,B3).

The sacrotuberous ligament

The sacrotuberous ligament has an extensive origin from the PSIS of the ilium, the 4th and 5th transverse tubercles of the sacrum and the lateral border of the sacrum and coccyx (Figs 2.5A, 2.6, 2.19A, 2.21, 3.61, 3.64). It inserts into the superior rim of the inner ischial tuberosity but may be in direct continuity with biceps femoris or, indirectly, by way of fascial connections to the hamstring origin (Pansky & House 1975; Vleeming et al. 1989a,b). The sacrotuberous origin is especially vulnerable in that:

1. 'posterior' rotation of the innominate, sacral torsion and nutation, and coccygeal rotation all increase the distance between its origin and insertion (Fig. 2.21)
2. both an 'upslip' and an 'anterior' innominate rotation increase tension in the ipsilateral long (dorsal) sacrotuberous ligament, which originates from the PSIS (Figs 2.5A, 2.19A)
3. tension in the ligament will be increased by active contraction of the hamstrings, gluteus maximus and/or piriformis, depending on the amount of continuity or fascial interconnection present between the ligament and these muscles; the ligament is also put at increased risk of injury by any passive increase in tension in these muscles, such as occurs with straight leg raising, stretching, squatting and jumping activities.

It is, therefore, not surprising that the sacrotuberous ligament is tender to palpation in the majority of those presenting with malalignment. In approximately 90%, the tenderness localizes to the origin alone; a small number (5-10%) have tenderness localizing along the length of the ligament and/or to its insertion or to all three sites but rarely just to the insertion (Schamberger 2002). A side-to-side difference in tension may be apparent on palpating the ligament with the person lying prone (Fig. 3.61A).

The sacrotuberous ligament referral pattern comprises primarily the posterior thigh and calf and the area around the heel - the calcaneal sclerotome - and to a large extent overlaps that of the sacrospinous ligament (Fig. 3.62).

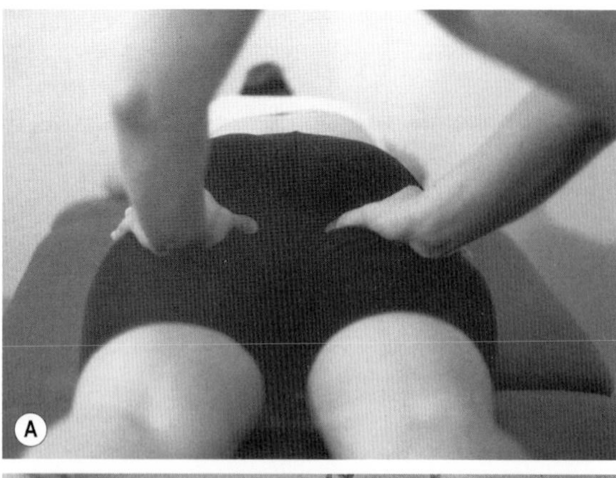

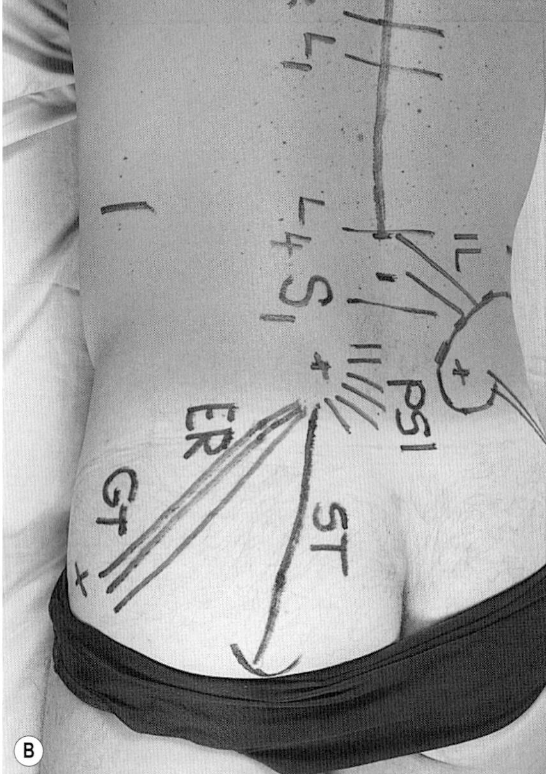

Fig. 3.61 Sacrotuberous ligament tension (see also Figs 2.5A, 2.6, 2.19, 2.22). (A) Comparative assessment of tension and tenderness in the right and left sacrotuberous ligaments. *(Courtesy of Lee & Walsh 1996.)* (B) Surface outlines showing the position of the left sacrotuberous (ST) ligament and other structures: L4-SI, vertebrae; IL, iliolumbar ligaments; PSI, posterior sacroiliac joint ligaments; ER, external rotator (piriformis); GT (x), greater trochanter (gluteus maximus insertion).

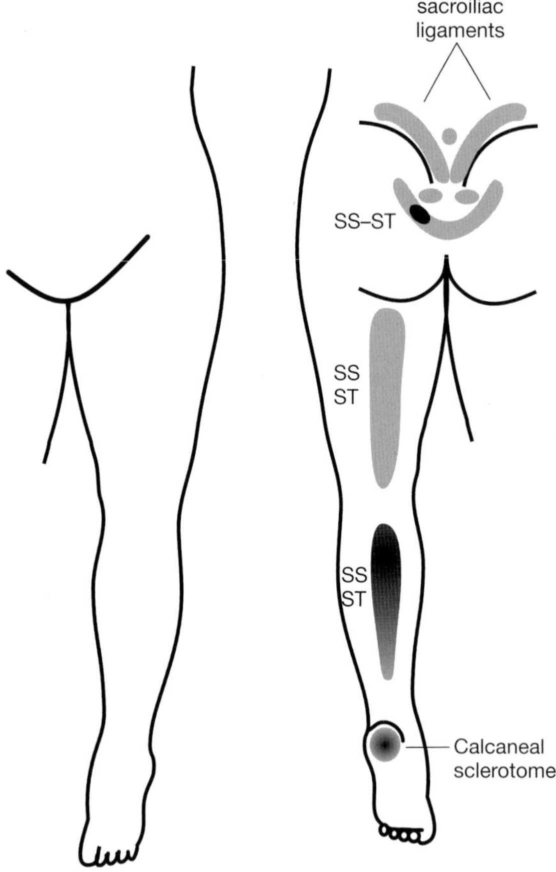

Fig. 3.62 Overlapping pain referral patterns of the sacrotuberous (ST) and sacrospinous (SS) ligaments. *(Redrawn courtesy of Hackett 1958.)*

The long (dorsal) sacrotuberous ligament

This lateral part of the sacrotuberous ligament originates primarily from the PSIS and joins the medial fibres originating from the sacrum to insert into the ischial tuberosity or continue in part or whole as biceps femoris. The connections to the sacrotuberous ligament and possibly biceps femoris make it more vulnerable to an increase in tension on sacral nutation and innominate anterior rotation, respectively (Figs 2.5A, 2.19; see below). Palpation may detect increased tension and tenderness of just this lateral aspect of the sacrotuberous ligament; whereas the referral pattern to the posterior thigh, calf and heel region overlaps that of the sacrospinous ligament (Fig. 3.62).

The sacroiliac ligaments

The downward and medial slant of a large part of the sacroiliac ligaments makes them particularly well suited for:

1. helping to transfer weight between the sacrum and the innominates
2. absorbing the shock associated with any downward movement of the sacrum relative to the innominates, such as occurs when landing on one or both feet.

Specific ligaments in this complex include the following:

The short posterior sacroiliac or 'dorsal' ligaments
These ligaments span the upper, middle and lower parts of the SI joint. Their origin runs from the PSIS to the posterior inferior iliac spine (PIIS) of the ilium; the insertion is onto the first three transverse tubercles of the sacrum (Figs 2.4B, 2.5A, 2.51). They are most easily palpated deep to the contours of the posterior pelvic rim ('PSI' on Fig. 3.61B). Tension in these ligaments is increased with any displacement of the ilium relative to the sacrum. Referred pain patterns from the superior and inferior segments are shown in Fig. 3.63.

The long posterior or 'dorsal' sacroiliac ligament
This distinct ligament has its origin primarily on the PSIS, running caudally and medially to insert into the posterolateral aspect of the sacrum at about the S3 level (Figs 2.5A, 2.19B). The S1, S2, and S3 posterior nerve root fibres, which help to innervate the posterior SI joint ligaments, are at risk of irritation or even compression with any increase in tension in the medial and lateral components of this ligament as these nerve fibres run laterally, traversing between these two components. The position of the ligament allows it to play a role in helping limit:

1. counternutation of the sacrum (Fig. 2.19B)
2. torsion of the sacrum around an oblique axes; torsion around the right oblique axis, for example, results in nutation of the left side with relaxation, and simultaneous counternutation of the right side with tightening of the right long dorsal ligament (Fig. 2.14)
3. 'anterior' rotation or an 'upslip' of the innominate (Fig. 2.19B).

Excessive movement in these directions probably accounts for the fact that the origin of this ligament is typically one of the most tender sites when malalignment is present. Pain attributable to excessive counternutation can sometimes be temporarily relieved by applying pressure to the base of the sacrum with the heel of the hand, forcing the sacrum into nutation and decreasing the tension in this ligament (Fig. 2.103A); pressure on the sacral apex to effect sacral counternutation typically aggravates the pain (Fig. 2.103B). The suspected role of the ligament in the causation of LBP and peri-partum pelvic floor pain as been extensively investigated (Vleeming et al. 1996; Vleeming et al. 2002).

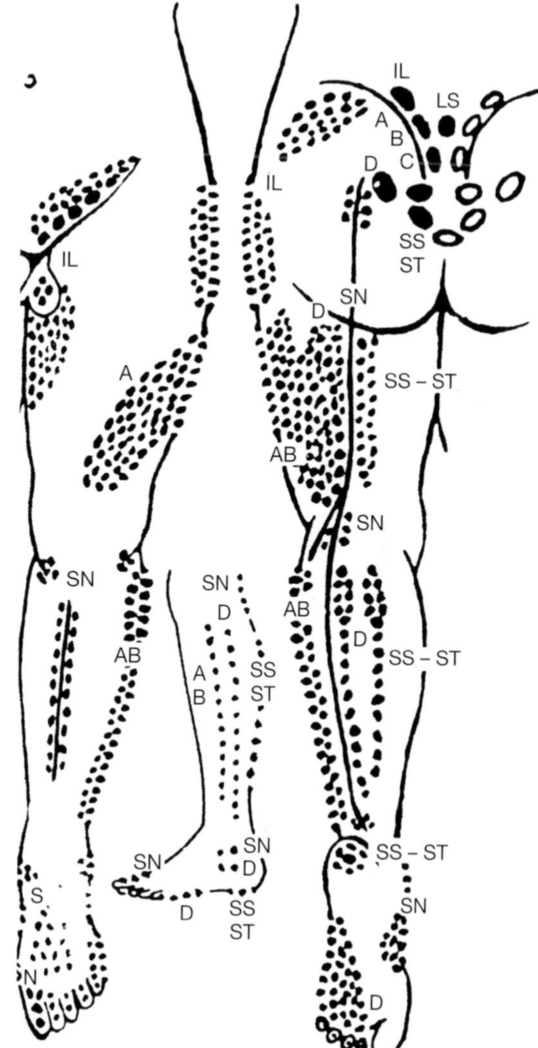

Fig. 3.63 Referral patterns from the posterior sacroiliac ligaments. From the superior segments: 'Relaxation of the ligaments of the lumbosacral (LS) and upper portion of the sacroiliac articulations (A and B) occur together so frequently that their referred pain area from the iliolumbar ligament and AB are combined in one dermatome.' From the inferior segments (C and D): 'Relaxation occurs together so frequently that their referred pain areas from . . .D and . . .SS–ST [sacrospinous–sacrotuberous] are combined in one dermatome.' SN, sciatic nerve. *(Courtesy of Hackett 1958.)*

The interosseous sacroiliac joint ligaments

These are short fibres running between the tuberosities of the sacrum and ilium. They lie deep to the posterior SI joint ligaments and cannot be palpated directly (Figs 2.4B, 2.13Aiii). They are put under increased tension and may become a source of pain with any displacement of the sacral and iliac joint surfaces relative to each other, as occurs with 'rotational malalignment', an 'upslip' or 'downslip', shear injury or excessive nutation or counternutation.

The anterior sacroiliac joint ligaments

These cross the anterior part of the joint, running from the anterolateral sacrum to the ilium (Figs 2.4A,B, 2.13Aiii). They are relatively sparse on comparison to the posterior pelvic ligaments (Ch. 2).

In summary, because of their attachment to the sacrum on one side and the ilium on the other, tension is increased in some or all of the above sacroiliac ligaments by:

1. upward or downward translation
2. 'anterior' or 'posterior' rotation of one bone relative to the other
3. 'outflare' and 'inflare' (discussed below)
4. sacroiliac joint gapping and other selective stress tests (see Ch. 2)

The sacrospinous ligament

The sacrospinous ligament originates from the posterolateral aspect of the sacrum and coccyx, inserts into the ischial spine, and thereby creates the greater sciatic foramen superiorly and the lesser one inferiorly (Figs 2.4A,B, 2.5A, 2.19A, 2.53B, 3.64). Its origin and insertion are approximately equidistant bilaterally in someone who is in alignment (Fig. 3.65A). Posterior rotation of the innominate separates the origin and insertion, increasing tension and often resulting in marked tenderness; anterior rotation brings the origin and insertion closer together, relaxing the ligament on this side by putting it into a shortened position (Fig. 3.65B). It is covered in large part by the sacrotuberous ligament and the buttock muscles and is, therefore, most easily palpated in its entirety by way of the rectum or vagina (Fig. 2.53B). Hesch et al. (1992) indicated that sacrospinous tenderness and hypotonus are often seen in association with ipsilateral symphysis pubis dysfunction. Involvement of these ligaments contributes to the 'deep' pain associated with pelvic floor dysfunction (see Ch. 4)

Ligaments spanning the pubic symphysis

The superior pubic ligaments connect the upper aspect of the pubic rami, the arcuate ligaments connect the rami inferiorly, and the interpubic

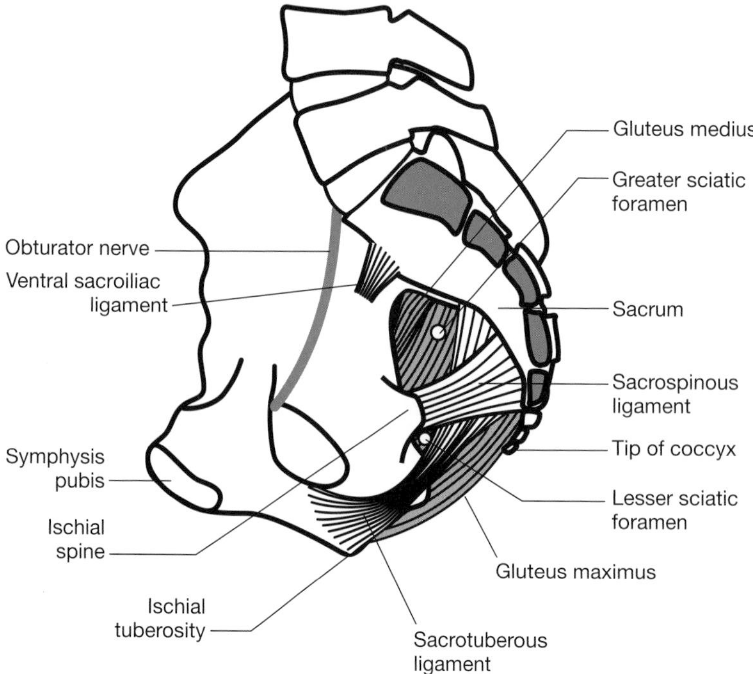

Fig. 3.64 Sacrospinous ligament on a lateral view from the inside of the pelvis. *(Redrawn courtesy of Grant 1980.)*

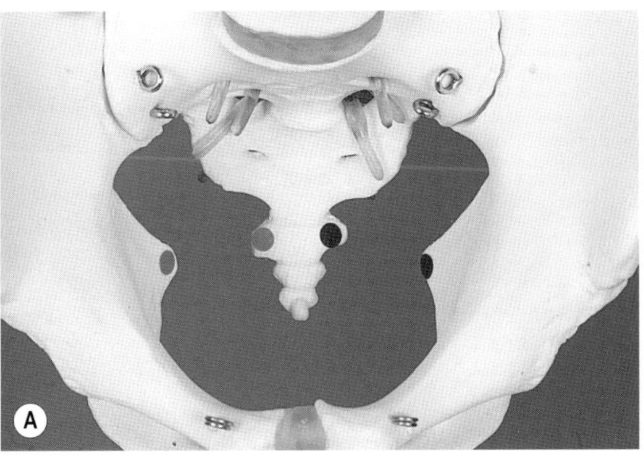

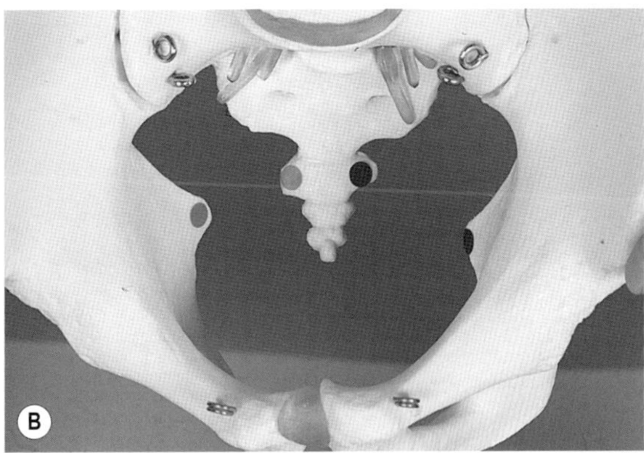

Fig. 3.65 Sacrospinous ligament origins and insertions on an anteroposterior view of pelvis. (A) Pelvis aligned: the distance between the right origin and insertion (light dots) is equal to that on the left (black dots). (B) 'Rotational malalignment' with 'right innominate anterior, left posterior' rotation: the origin and insertion are brought closer together on the right (light dots) and separated on the left (black dots). A similar change would occur with a 'right outflare, left inflare'.

ligaments run transversely across the fibrocartilaginous disc that is part of this amphiarthrodial joint (Figs 2.4A, 3.66). A displacement and/or torsion of one pubic bone relative to the other - as occurs with an 'upslip' and 'rotational malalignment' - creates stress on the ligaments and the disc (Figs 2.42, 2.75, 2.76C). Pain is felt in the region of the symphysis and/or may be referred to the testicles/vagina; it can also overlap with pain felt:

1. with inguinal ligament involvement
2. more laterally with involvement of the iliolumbar ligament (Hackett 1958; Fig. 3.63), or
3. when trigger points are evident in pectineus (Travell & Simons 1992; Figs 3.37, 4.2B).

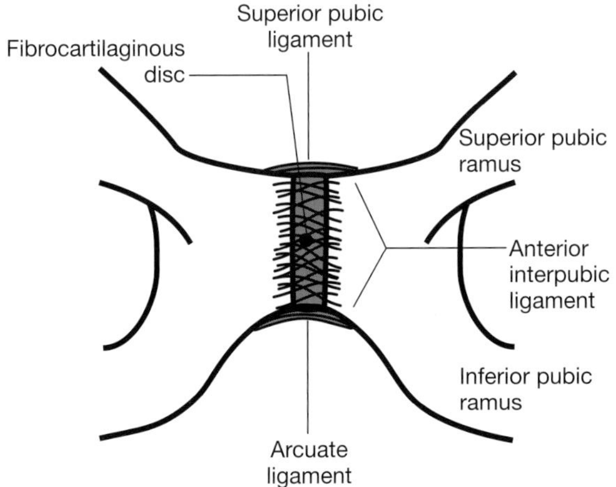

Fig. 3.66 Ligaments around the symphysis pubis.

The inguinal ligaments

One or both inguinal ligaments may be tense and tender in the presence of pelvic malalignment. Pain is usually felt in the groin region, tenderness being most acute at the insertion into the pubic tubercle (Fig. 2.4A).

The hip joint ligaments

The iliofemoral and pubofemoral ligaments (Figs 2.4A, 2.5A, 4.3) and the capsule especially are stressed by internal and external rotation of the lower extremities. Excessive tension can result in a 'deep' pain in the hip joint region and groin. Pain is referred primarily to the medial and posterior thigh, the lateral knee, the anterior shin and ankle, and the first toe (Fig. 3.67).

The intervertebral and sacral ligaments

The vertebral rotation that occurs with the formation of the compensatory curves of segments of the spine and excessive rotation of individual vertebrae predictably increases tension in specific ligaments and their nerve supply (Fig. 3.68). The ligaments that connect one vertebra to another include those running:

1. from one body to another: intervertebral, annular, anterior and posterior longitudinal, dural/thecal
2. between the posterior elements: the lamina and the transverse and spinous processes
3. across the facet joints

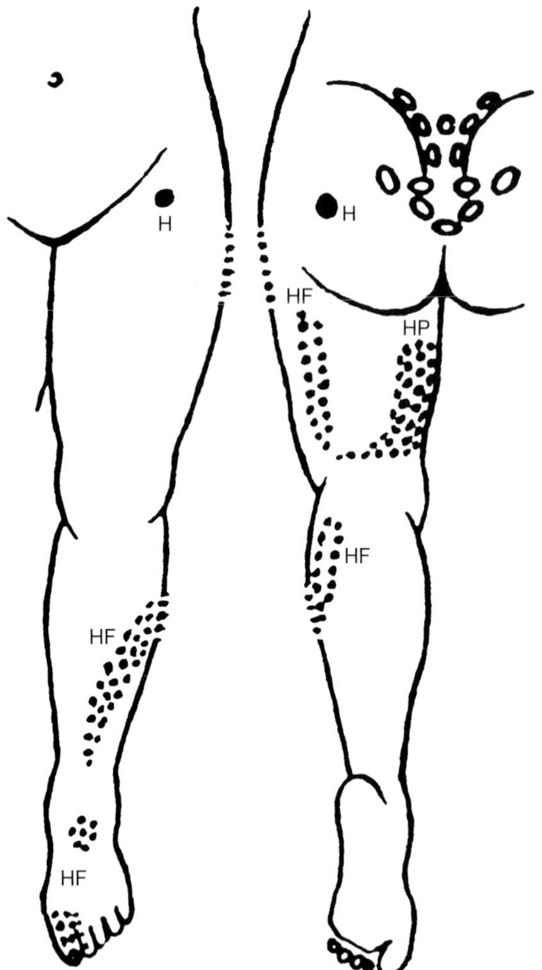

Fig. 3.67 Referred pain patterns from the iliofemoral and pubofemoral ligaments of the hip joint noted with hip joint instability [see also Figs 2.4A, 2.5A, 4.3]. H, location of the hip joint; HP, referral from the pelvic attachments; HF, referral from the femoral attachments. *(Courtesy of Hackett 1958.)*

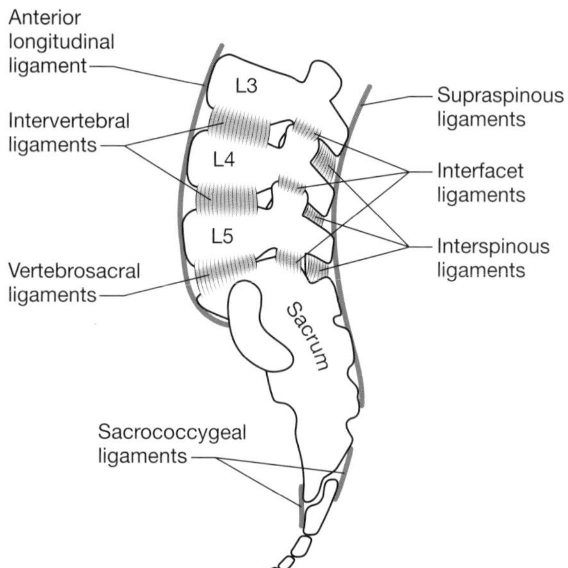

Fig. 3.68 Ligaments connecting the lumbar vertebrae to each other, the lumbosacral junction, and the 1st sacrococcygeal joint; (not shown: posterior longitudinal ligament).

Ligaments of the knee

The medial plica and medial collateral ligament

These are likely to be stressed on the side tending toward pronation and genu valgum, which increase tension in these ligaments (Figs 3.31, 3.36, 3.37). The problem will be on the right side in those with the 'more common' rotational patterns or an 'upslip', and on the left in those with the 'left anterior and locked' pattern.

The lateral collateral ligament

The lateral collateral ligament is likely to be involved on the side of lateral weight-bearing, supination or a tendency to genu varum, all of these tending to be a problem on the left side in those with an 'upslip' or one of the 'more common' rotational patterns (Figs 3.31, 3.36, 3.37)

The TFL/ITB complex

Tightness of this complex, typically seen on the left side, may restrict knee flexion because of its connections between the ITB insertion and the anterior capsule (Figs 3.37, 3.41, 3.44).

Ankle ligaments

Tenderness of these ligaments in the absence of injury may relate to a chronic or repetitive increase in tension attributable to malalignment. In keeping with an 'upslip' and the 'more common' rotational patterns (Figs 3.3B, 3.22A, 3.37), tenderness is more likely to involve the:

1. medial ligaments on the right side, given the tendency to medial weight-bearing and pronation; there may be simultaneous tibialis posterior tendonitis, irritation of the posterior tibial nerve or even an outright posterior tarsal tunnel syndrome detectable on nerve conduction and/or EMG studies (Fig. 3.38A).
2. lateral ligaments and extensor retinacula on the left side, given the tendency to left lateral weight-bearing and supination; there may be simultaneous

peroneus longus and brevis tendonitis, and occasionally peroneal and/or sural nerve irritation or even compression (Fig. 3.38B).

Clinical correlation: asymmetrical ligament tension

'Rotational malalignment' and an 'upslip' result in a predictable increase in tension in a number of ligaments which, with time, makes these ligaments more likely to become tender to palpation, to elongate and eventually to compromise joint stability and/or become a source of local as well as referred pain.

A ligament that has undergone contracture because of having been placed in a shortened position by the malalignment is now at increased risk of suffering a sprain or strain in the event of a sudden or unexpected superimposed stress which acutely increases tension in the ligament.

Any reflex muscle splinting intended to minimize pain originating from a ligament and to protect it against further abuse or injury, can unfortunately impair freedom of movement, result in complicating myofascial pain and also puts the muscle at increased risk of injury with sudden or excessive movement.

In addition, a ligament may fail in its role as a source of proprioceptive signals. The concept of ligament malfunction and recurrent injury is explored further under 'A problem with balance and recovery' below and in Ch. 5.

A common problem associated with malalignment is the limitation of standing and sitting tolerance - also described as the 'cocktail party syndrome' because the person has to move about continuously to evade discomfort - which is often attributable, in large part, to the painful posterior pelvic and pelvic floor ligaments in addition to related biomechanical problems previously discussed (see 'Asymmetry of pelvic orientation in the frontal plane').

Sitting in a slouched position tends to make matters worse by further increasing the tension in some of these ligaments. The straightening or even flexion of the lumbosacral segment, along with a tendency to posterior tilting of the pelvic unit exerts tension particularly on the iliolumbar and long dorsal sacroiliac ligaments. It may also result in pressure being exerted directly on a painful ligament - the sacrotuberous, sacrospinous and sacrococcygeal are especially vulnerable. Sitting upright, possibly with addition of a lumbosacral support to help maintain the lumbar lordosis, proves a simple preventative measure (Fig. 3.69). It will, however, put more pressure on the coccyx, in which case the addition of a coccygeal relief pillow may be appropriate (see Ch. 7; Fig. 7.43). Side-lying with the upper leg adducted and flexed at the hip puts the uppermost iliolumbar and posterior sacroiliac ligaments as well as the TFL/ITB complex under increased tension; simply limiting adduction by placing a pillow between the knees helps to counter these stresses (Fig. 3.70).

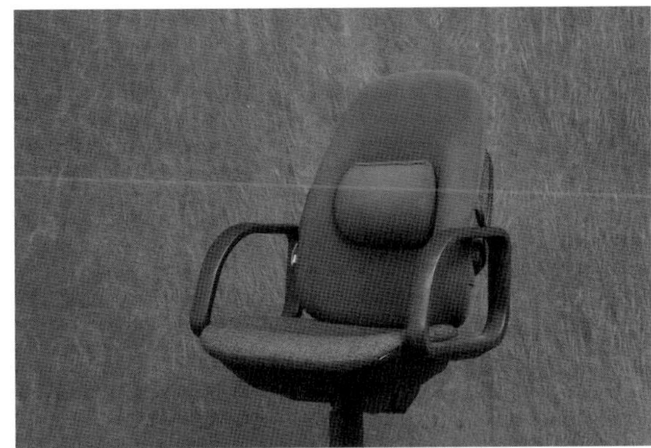

Fig. 3.69 Obus back support to prevent slouching; level of attached lumbosacral cushion is adjustable to help maintain the lumbar lordosis.

In some, the ligament pain resolves with time as alignment is maintained. In others, realignment alone fails to bring relief. This failure may be a reflection of the length of time required for these tissues to heal after what often amounts to months or even years of insult. There may also be an inflammatory component, given the good response to oral anti-inflammatory or injection with cortisone in

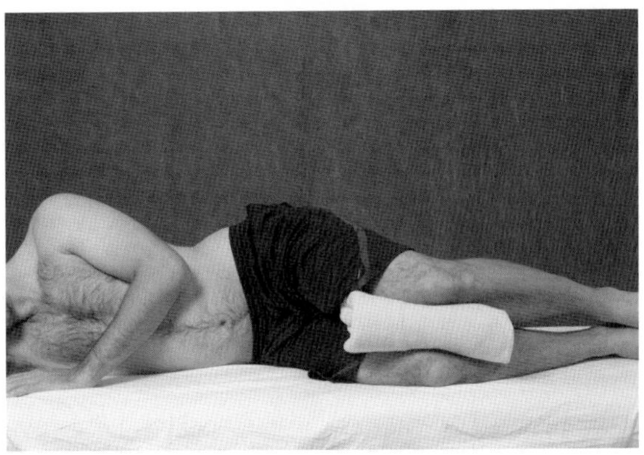

Fig. 3.70 Relief pillow between knees may help decrease pain from tight hip abductor/TFL/ITB complex by countering left leg adduction.

some (see Ch. 7). While the pain persists, it can severely limit a person's ability to participate in work or sports activities that:

1. require prolonged standing (e.g. construction, doorman, security, court sports) or sitting (e.g. reception, work on a computer, cycling, rowing)
2. repeatedly put the ligaments under increased stretch by squatting (e.g. certain tradesmen, weight-lifting), bending forward (e.g. cycling), twisting (e.g. working in small spaces, kayaking) or a combination of these (e.g. stocking shelves, rowing, canoeing).

ASYMMETRY OF THE LOWER EXTREMITY RANGES OF MOTION

One of the findings associated with 'rotational malalignment' is a consistent pattern of asymmetry of the lower extremity joint ranges of motion (Box 3.8; Appendix 3).

Some of these asymmetries can be explained on a purely mechanical basis. The example of hip extension and flexion (with the knee flexed) will help to illustrate this point (Box 3.8).

1. *Reorientation of the joint*

   'Anterior' rotation of the right innominate brings the anterior acetabular rim forward and down so that the mechanical blocking of hip joint flexion that occurs when the femoral head starts to contact the rim now occurs earlier and can limit right hip flexion (Figs 3.71Ai, 3.72B). The posterior acetabular rim on the right side will have moved backward and up, allowing increased extension before the mechanical blocking occurs (Figs 3.71Aiii, 3.72B). If there

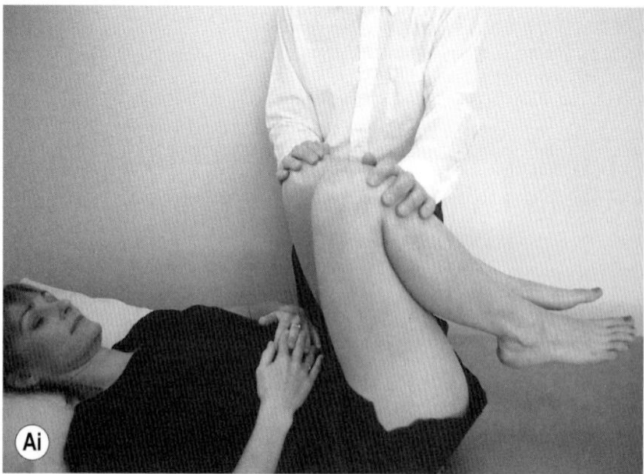

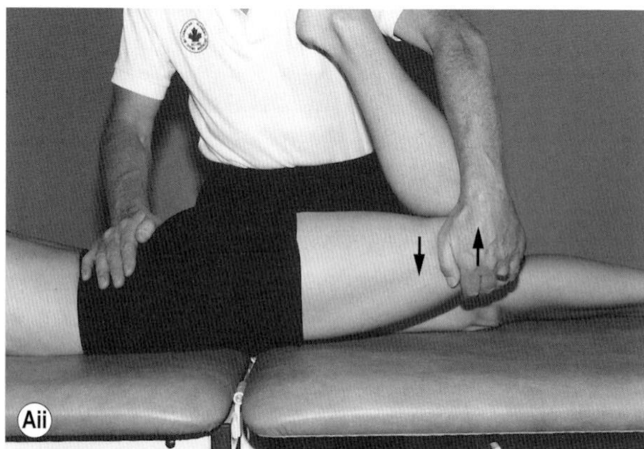

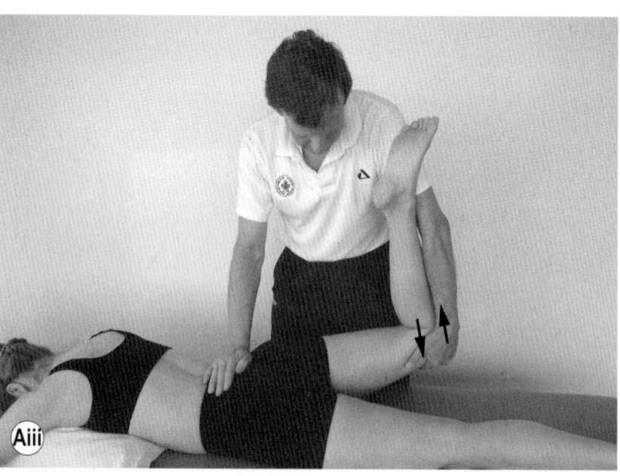

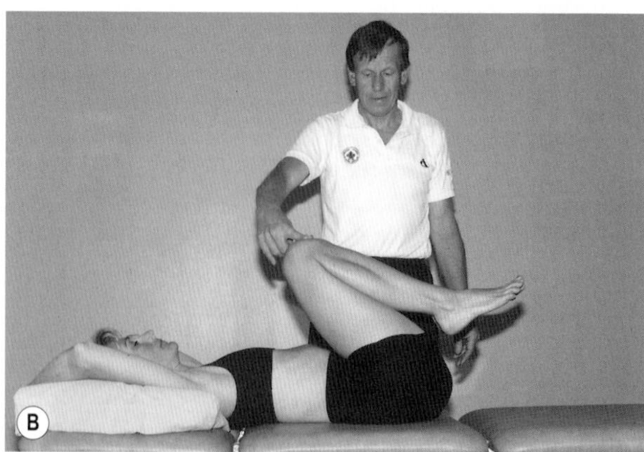

Fig. 3.71 Effect of alignment on passive hip flexion and extension, tested with knees in flexion. Note that, on realignment, there may be an overall increase in the flexion/extension range that cannot be attributed just to the realignment of the acetabula but probably relates, in part, to the re-establishment of normal muscle tension (see also Fig. 3.49). (A) With 'rotational malalignment' (right innominate anterior, left posterior): (i) limitation of right hip flexion (105 degrees) compared with left (115 degrees); (ii) limitation of left hip extension (10 degrees), compared with (iii) right of 25 degrees. (B) In alignment: hip flexion is now equal and actually increased to 130 degrees (and extension equal at 25 degrees).

BOX 3.8 Lower extremity ranges of motion with 'rotational malalignment'

1. Movement in any one plane of motion is restricted in one and increased in the opposite direction. For example, a typical finding with 'right anterior, left posterior' innominate rotation (Fig. 3.71) would be:

	Right	Left
Passive hip flexion (supine)	110 degrees	120 degrees
Passive hip extension (prone)	30 degrees	20 degrees
Total range:	140 degrees	140 degrees

   The findings would be the opposite for someone with 'right posterior, left anterior' rotation and similar (though reduced) with the knee extended (Fig. 3.72).
2. The total range of motion possible in a specific plane is, however, the same on both sides, provided there is no underlying pathology that could affect movement in that plane, such as ligament or joint deterioration, soft tissue contracture or impairment of neural control (Figs 2.23, 2.24). In the example above, the combined range possible in the right and left sagittal plane is the same: 140 degrees.

has been a compensatory 'posterior' rotation of the left innominate bone, repositioning of the left anterior and posterior rims allows for increased left flexion but decreases extension, by an amount equivalent to that seen on the right (Figs 3.71Ai and Aii, respectively, and 3.72 C). The findings will be the opposite with 'right posterior, left anterior' rotation. In both cases, the combined flexion/extension range of motion remains the same (90 degrees) on the right and left sides and would also be comparable to whenever the pelvis is aligned (Figs 3.71B, 3.72A).

2. *Displacement of origins and insertions*

   Right hip flexion, for example, is decreased by the increase in tension in the right gluteus maximus and hamstrings that results when 'right anterior' innominate rotation increases the distance between their origin and insertion. Simultaneous 'left posterior' innominate rotation will limit left hip extension by increasing tension in iliacus and rectus femoris through the same mechanism (Figs 2.59, 3.42).

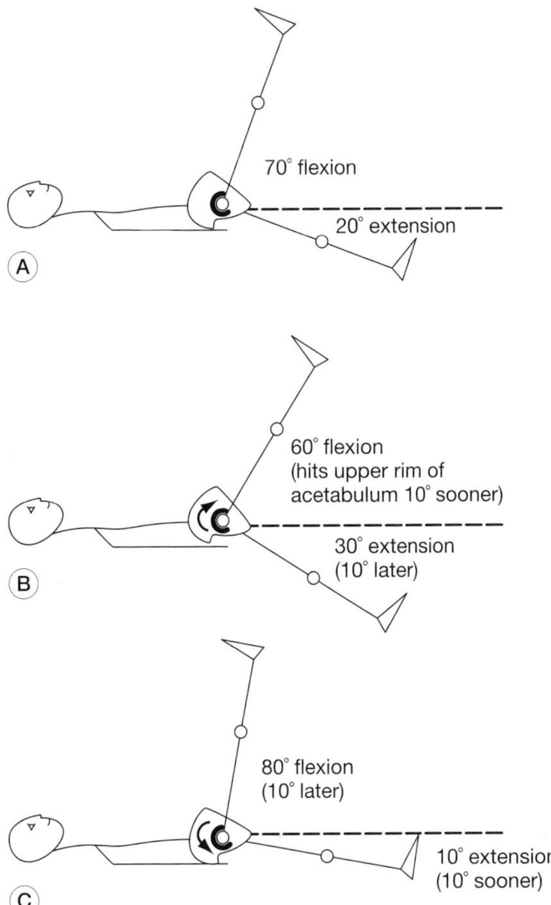

Fig. 3.72 Changes in right hip flexion/extension achieved, as a result of mechanical factors (reorientation of the acetabulum with innominate 'rotational malalignment': (A) normal orientation (pelvis aligned); (B) 'right anterior' rotation (C) 'right posterior' rotation. Barring other pathology, the combined range of motion remains 90 degrees in all three situations.

3. *Interaction between muscles, tendons and myofascial tissue*

   Right hip flexion can, for example, be decreased by any increase in tension in the sacrotuberous ligament which, in turn, results in an increase in tension in:

   a. biceps femoris, when it is in some continuity with the ligament (Figs 2.6, 2.59)
   b. a muscle such as piriformis (Figs 2.46A, 4.17) or gluteus maximus that is attached to the ligament directly or by way of fascial connections, also

c. proximally in the thoracolumbar fascia and contralateral latissimus dorsi (Figs 2.37, 2.38).

The asymmetry of some ranges of motion cannot be explained on a purely mechanical basis. Other factors, such as the autonomic increase in tension, or 'facilitation', that occurs in certain muscles, help to determine the differences noted (see 'Asymmetry of muscle tension' above and Fig. 3.43). There is, for example, the typical malalignment-related increase in tension in:

1. the left TFL, gluteus medius and minimus, which would help account for the almost universal restriction of passive left hip adduction (Figs 3.44Aii, 3.77)
2. the right hamstrings and piriformis, which would contribute to the limitation of right hip flexion (Fig. 3.71Ai)
3. left gastrocnemius, which is one factor that limits dorsiflexion of the left foot and ankle and probably also contributes to the limitation of passive left straight leg raising (Fig. 3.73A).

A distinctly different pattern of asymmetrical passive lower extremity joint ranges of motion can be documented in association with the different patterns of 'rotational malalignment':

1. the 'more common' patterns (Figs 3.71, 3.72)

   The one variation to be found within this group is a restriction of passive hip flexion on the right side in those with a 'right anterior' rotation (right hip extension increased), and restriction of flexion on the left side in those with 'left anterior' rotation (left extension increased).
2. 'left anterior and locked' patterns

   While the overall asymmetry of the range of motion is the opposite to that found in those with the 'more common' pattern having a 'right anterior' rotation, the one exception is that the limitation of hip adduction is on the left side in both.

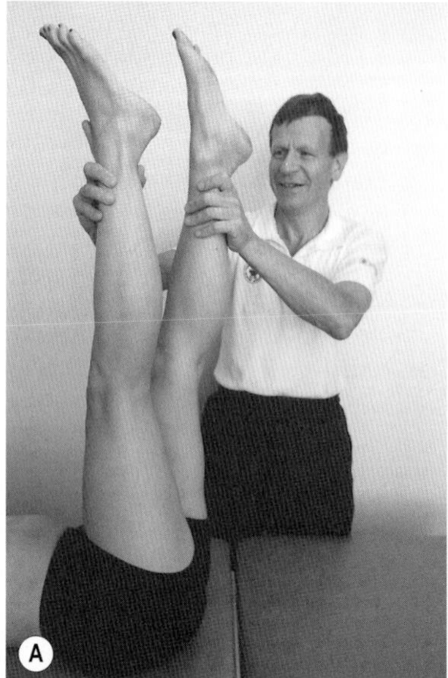

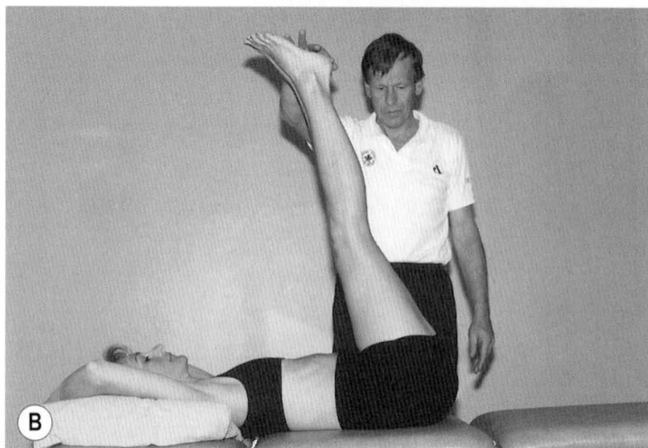

Fig. 3.73 Effect of multiple factors associated with malalignment resulting in asymmetrical passive straight leg raising. (A) With this person's 'rotational malalignment' present ('right anterior, left posterior'): right 95 degrees, left limited to 80 degrees. (B) In alignment: right and left now equal at 100 degrees.

Hip flexion and extension

As indicated above, 'right anterior, left posterior' innominate rotation results in a restriction of passive right hip flexion and left hip extension on carrying out these ranges of motion with the knees flexed (Fig. 3.71). The opposite pattern of restrictions is seen with 'left anterior, right posterior' rotation. Malalignment also affects active movement in these directions. The actual restrictions are, in part, determined by whether the pelvis is stabilized (as in sitting or lying) or free to move (as in walking).

In the person who is in alignment, all of the pelvic unit is free to tilt posteriorly around the coronal axis to increase the amount of hip flexion possible, as illustrated by the following examples:

1. The person is standing and kicks upward at a bag or opponent while keeping the knee straight. Simultaneous pelvic tilt posteriorly and some ipsilateral innominate posterior rotation increases hip flexion and allows the person to kick higher. Barring any other pathology, there should be no limitation of range on the right compared to the left side (Fig. 5.14A).
2. The woman sitting on the floor with her legs out in front and abducted (Fig. 3.74) can reach forward alternately to the right and left side to stretch the hamstrings and back extensor muscles. The pelvis is relatively 'fixed' by sitting on the floor. However, as the trunk flexes toward the right or left foot, the pelvis as a whole can still tilt anteriorly, increasing flexion at the hip joints by approximately the same extent on reaching forward to either foot (Fig. 3.74 B(i), C) or to both simultaneously (Fig. 3.74A).

The corresponding findings when someone presents with 'right anterior, left posterior' rotation are as follows.

1. He or she probably cannot kick as high with the right as the left leg when standing. Factors that contribute to this block to right active hip flexion include:
   a. rotation of the right anterior acetabular rim forward and downward creates a mechanical block (Fig. 3.72B)
   b. increased tension in the right hamstrings caused by the separation of origin and insertion, and the 'facilitation' usually seen on this side in association with the malalignment (Figs 2.59, 3.43)
   c. failure of the pelvis to tilt posteriorly as one unit
      i. the left innominate usually will compensate for a right 'anterior' rotation by rotating posteriorly, limiting the amount of further rotation possible into that direction
      ii. the right has rotated anteriorly and may be 'locked' as well, limiting efforts to achieve more posterior rotation on that side and capable of interfering with the simultaneous rotation of the sacrum required for the manoeuvre (Fig. 2.125)

   In the person with 'left anterior, right posterior' rotation, the restriction will be on attempting a left high kick.

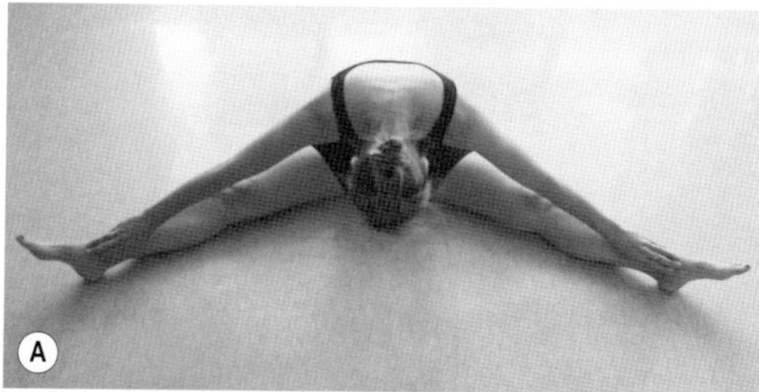

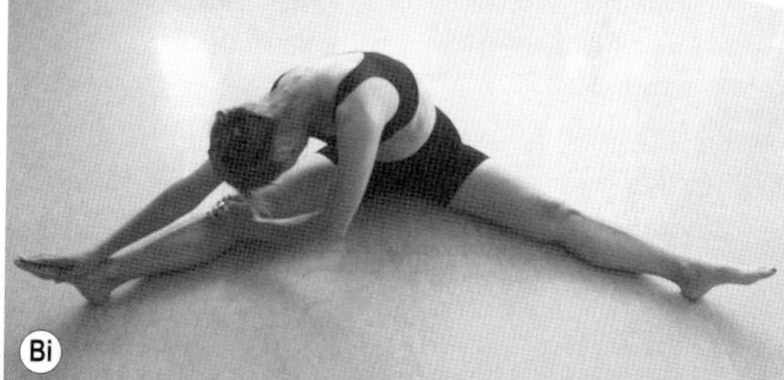

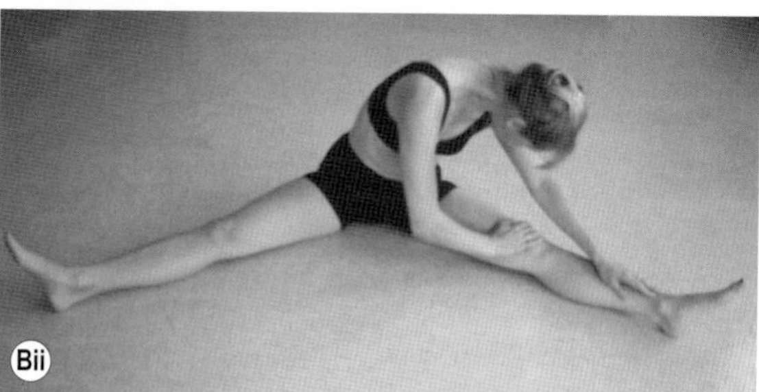

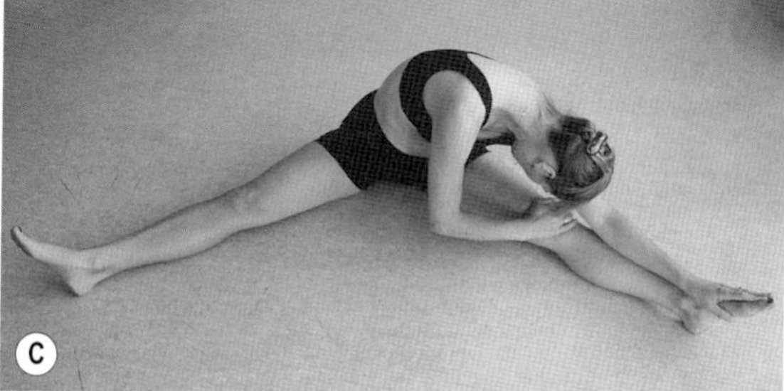

Fig. 3.74 Stretch of back extensors and hamstrings by reaching forward. (A) In alignment: symmetrical reach to both ankles/feet simultaneously, and to the right and left sides individually (not shown here). (B) With 'rotational malalignment' ('right anterior, left posterior'), reach to the left is impaired: (i) forehead 5 cm off right knee; (ii) forehead 25 cm off left knee. (C) On realignment: reach to the left now equals that to the right (Bi).

2. The woman sitting on the floor with her legs abducted cannot bring her forehead as close to the left knee as to the right, giving the impression that the left hip extensors and/or hamstrings are tighter than the right ones, limiting this movement (Fig. 3.74Bii).
   a. In effect, one might now expect more hip flexion to be possible on the left side (Fig. 3.72C), given that with the inomminate having rotated posteriorly:
      i. tension in these posterior muscles should decrease as the left origins and insertions have been brought closer together
      ii. the left anterior acetabular rim has rotated backward and upward, out of the way (Fig. 3.72C)
   b. The problem of limited left hip flexion, however, actually relates to the fact that:
      i. the pelvis has been 'fixed' with the left innominate posteriorly rotated; on attempted trunk and left hip flexion, the left innominate can no longer accommodate by rotating anteriorly around the coronal axis along with the rest of the pelvis, limiting hip (and thereby also trunk) flexion on the left side
      ii. there is an autonomic increase in tension in the left gastrocnemius (Fig. 3.43); 'facilitation' of this muscle accounts for some of the limitation of passive straight leg raising and ankle dorsiflexion on this side - the frequent report of tightness, sometimes even pain, tends to be maximal just above the popliteal region (near the gastrocnemius origins from the distal femur) but may also involve - or actually localize to - the musculotendinous junction of the Achilles tendon (Figs 3.73, 3.75Aii).

On the right side, the innominate is 'fixed' in an anteriorly rotated position. This simulates the anterior rotation of the pelvis that would normally occur with trunk flexion and allows the trunk to bend further forward on the pelvis. Relaxation of the right gastrocnemius by 'inhibition' could also play a role (see increase in right passive dorsiflexion in Fig. 3.84).

This side-to-side difference in trunk flexion can also be seen on Maitland's 'slump' test used for detecting nerve root and dural irritation (Fig. 3.75). The woman is sitting on the plinth, one

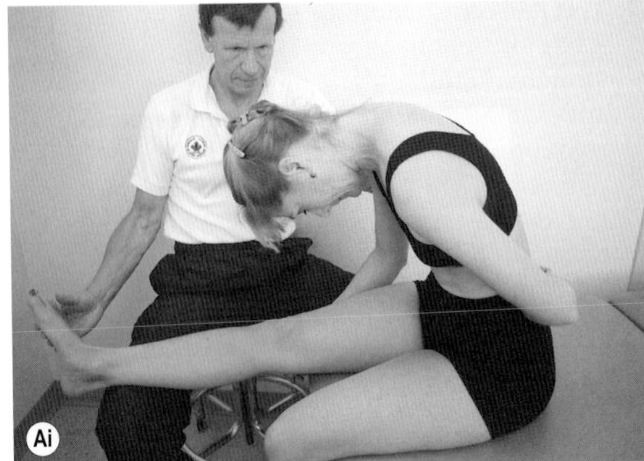

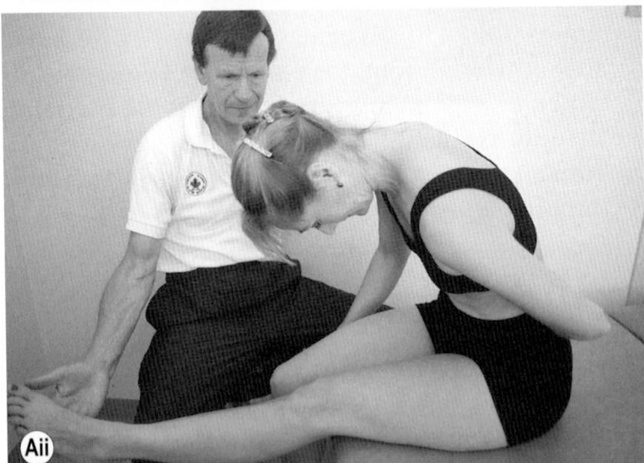

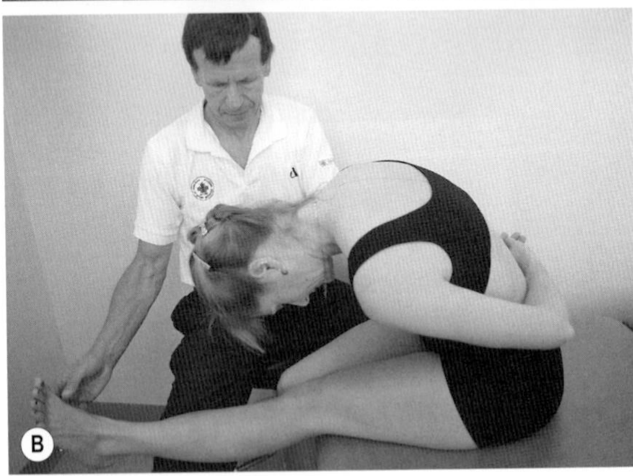

Fig. 3.75 Maitland's slump test for dural, root and peripheral nerve irritation. (A) With malalignment present ('right anterior, left posterior' rotation). (i) Right: relatively unrestricted trunk and head flexion (forehead 20 cm off knee); ankle dorsiflexion within 30 degrees short of neutral. (ii) Left: limitation of trunk and head flexion (forehead 28 cm off knee) and of dorsiflexion (45 degrees short of neutral). (B) In alignment: left trunk and head flexion improved and equal to the right; dorsiflexion increased bilaterally (15 degrees short of neutral).

leg out in front and supported at the ankle by the examiner in order to keep her hip approximately 90 degrees flexed and the knee in extension. She initially flexes the trunk and pelvis forward as far as possible to achieve the maximum degree of hip flexion - the point at which full passive knee extension can still be maintained. She is then asked to flex the head, following which the examiner gently moves the foot and ankle into passive dorsiflexion. Note is made if the test at any stage precipitated pain and/or parasthesias and, if so, whether the symptoms localized to a root or peripheral nerve pattern or were more in keeping with those typically felt with malalignment.

1. Whenever tightness, irritation or inflammation of the meninges, spinal cord, dura, nerve root or peripheral nerve structures is present, the head flexion superimposed on an already flexed trunk, and the subsequent ankle dorsiflexion, may provoke outright dysaesthesias (e.g. an electric shock sensation) from the low, middle or even upper back and neck region, and possibly down into the extended leg.
2. Mechanical compression of the anterior aspect of the vertebra(e) and/or of a degenerate disc occurring on trunk flexion may cause localized back pain, which is unlikely to be aggravated by the head flexion or dorsiflexion of the foot.
3. However, trunk flexion can increase the posterior bulging or actual protrusion of a disc and cause neurological symptoms that may then be aggravated by head flexion and foot dorsiflexion, both of which further increase tension in an already irritated spinal cord, dura or nerve root spanning the bulge or protrusion.
4. Carrying out a bilateral slump test, with both hips in flexion and knees in extension simultaneously, may fail to provoke mechanical symptoms but will continue to precipitate a neurological problem.

With an 'upslip' or one of the 'more common' rotational patterns, restriction of forward flexion of the trunk and ankle dorsiflexion is by far more common (80-90%) on the left side than the right on the slump test. Factors contributing to this include:

1. approximately 80% of those with 'rotational malalignment' have 'left innominate posterior' rotation (see Ch. 2)
2. there is typically 'facilitation' of some muscles (e.g. left gastrocnemius, quadratus lumborum) that can limit this movement; increased tone in the left gastrocnemius typically limits passive left ankle dorsiflexion and frequently provokes discomfort in the popliteal region and the calf (Figs 3.75Aii, 3.84).
3. any 'back pain' evoked often localizes to the ipsilateral hamstrings origin, buttock or lumbosacral region, reflecting the additional stress this test puts on the already tense and tender buttock muscles and ligaments (e.g. sacrotuberous ligaments put under tension by 'left posterior' rotation, sacral nutation), the distorted left SI joint and lumbosacral region.

Clinical correlation: hip flexion and extension

Those in situations that require running, jumping and high kicking may be aware of restrictions of hip flexion and extension which are, in fact, attributable to innominate rotation.

Restriction of hip flexion on the side of 'anterior' rotation

1. in standing

This restriction is, unfortunately, often mistakenly attributed to 'hamstring tightness' when the problem is actually the result of a combination of factors relating to changes in tension and the biomechanical forces that occur with the malalignment. Routine stretching is, therefore, unlikely to result in anything other than a temporary improvement until any increase in tension attributable to the malalignment is abolished with realignment.

The high kick is more likely to be restricted on the side of the 'anterior' rotation for the reasons cited above. The combined effect of these restrictions is to make a person more vulnerable to injuring the sacrotuberous ligament or the hamstrings, gluteus maximus or gastrocnemius when attempting a high kick, or when he or she tries to clear an obstacle in the course of duty (e.g. firefighting, police patrol) or a sport such as hurdling, with the 'wrong' leg leading.

2. in squatting

Malalignment results in an asymmetry of the lower extremities on squatting. The presentation depends on the underlying pattern of an 'upslip' or 'rotational malalignment'. For example, with a 'right anterior/left posterior' rotation, the restriction of right hip flexion may become evident on a full squat; so that the right thigh/knee may appear lower than the left (Fig. 3.76Bi). Pelvic rotation in the transverse plane and acetabular reorientation with innominate rotation (Figs 2.76D, 6.4B), also tightening of certain buttock muscles and ligaments (Figs 2.19, 3.42) are all contributing factors. The knee also appears to protrude further forward, as if the right thigh were longer than the left (Fig. 3.76Bi, Bii) and ends up relatively further out from midline compared to the left because of the tendency to right external rotation and abduction (Fig. 3.76Bi; see also FABER/FADE test: Figs 2.106, 2.107).

3. in lying supine

   The right thigh/knee tends to end up higher that the left (Fig. 3.76Bii).

Unfortunately, such asymmetry can prove costly, particularly in:

1. sports that reward the ability to squat fully and symmetrically; e.g. some gymnastic and weight-lifting events (Figs 3.76C, 5.21A)
2. situations where a combination of agility and ability to squat is essential, as it is for some hobbies such as gardening or when having to work close to the ground (e.g. laying carpet) or in confined spaces

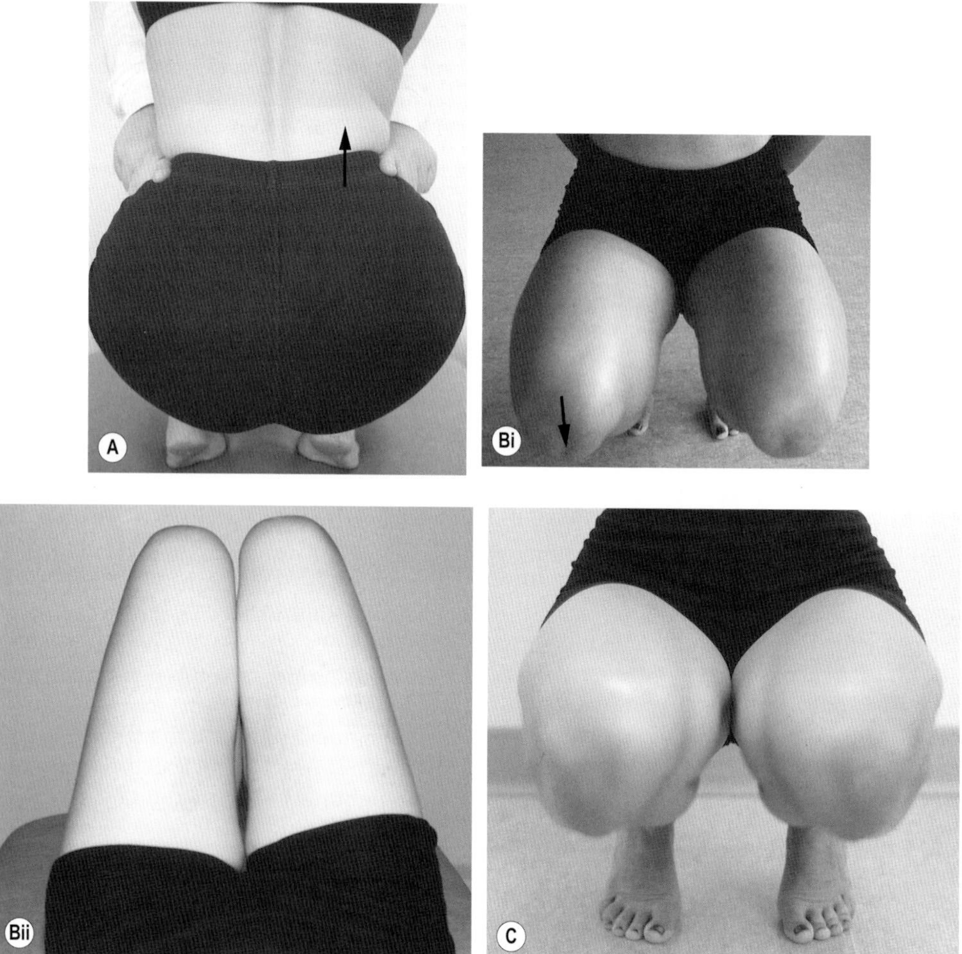

Fig. 3.76 Asymmetries with 'right anterior, left posterior' rotation noted on squatting. (A) Thumbs on iliac crests: right crest (and ischial tuberosity) up. (B) Thigh asymmetry: (i) right knee forward compared with the left one and lower partly due to decreased ability to flex the right hip (see also Fig. 3.71Ai) - it also tends to end up further out from midline; (ii) right knee higher than the left one (= forward on Bi). (C) Following correction, the pelvis is now level and the position of the knees again matches up.

Restriction of hip extension on the side of 'posterior' rotation

1. in standing

   Posterior innominate rotation creates a mechanical block to hip extension with the 'posterior and down' shift of the posteroinferior acetabular rim (Fig. 3.72C). The rotation also increases tension in rectus femoris, iliacus and its conjoint tendon with psoas major, by separating their origins and insertions (Fig. 3.42). The person may notice a decreased ability to extend the hip when the pelvis is supposedly free to move. Any increase in the lumbar lordosis to accommodate for the limitation of hip extension adds further stress to the lumbosacral region.

2. in prone-lying

   There may be associated discomfort, possibly felt just as a pulling sensation, localizing to the groin and/or anterior thigh region on that side with hip extension and on attempting to stretch these so-called 'tight' anterior muscles. Passive hip extension will be decreased (Fig. 3.71Aiii) and may provoke the person's symptoms of back and/or hip pain because of:

   a. pressure on the posterior acetabular rim
   b. leverage effecting anterior rotation of the left innominate, stressing the lumbosacral junction and the short and long dorsal sacroiliac ligaments (Figs 2.5, 2.19B)

A repeated or chronic increase in tension can result in myofascial pain and make these muscles more irritable, predisposing to spasms or 'cramping', which is sometimes felt as if someone had plunged a knife into the groin or the lateral aspect (or so-called 'gutter') of the abdomen. There is an increased risk of tearing the iliopsoas complex on excessive hip extension, abduction or combined manoeuvres. Rectus femoris is at increased risk of tearing in the following situations:

1. when the muscle is subjected to a further increase in tension by simultaneous hip and knee extension
2. on accelerating out of the blocks, rectus femoris on the side of the driving leg contracts eccentrically to counter any tendency to knee flexion and thereby help steady the knee as the hamstrings extend it, in preparation for push-off (Fig. 3.52A:1–4)
3. when there is a demand for a sudden increase in stride length, as occurs with acceleration and on jumping and negotiating obstacles
4. from mid-stance on, there is a progressive increase in tension passively as hip extension increases
5. when the muscle undergoes a lengthening (eccentric) contraction to control knee flexion and absorb shock, as occurs, for example, when jumping and landing on one leg
   - the lengthening contraction of rectus femoris allows for controlled knee flexion to help absorb ground forces; at the same time, the trunk may be thrown backward to help deceleration, increasing hip extension and passively increasing tension in rectus femoris at the same time by separating the muscle origin and insertion.

In walking or running, an 'upslip' or 'rotational malalignment' can result in an asymmetry of stride and a limitation of stride length for the same reasons that cause restrictions in stretching. A limitation of hip extension or flexion would, in effect, limit the leg going through a full stance or swing phase, respectively. Theoretically, this limitation could be compensated for by efforts such as increasing plantar flexion of the foot and ankle, or going into a supination pattern of movement on weight-bearing, to increase the length of the respective extremity. Both methods, however, raise the centre of gravity and, therefore, also increase the workload and decrease stability.

In an attempt to maintain a uniform stride length, either swing or stance phase may be changed to compensate for any limitation on the opposite side, at the cost of speed; alternately, one can increase stride frequency but this also is inefficient and results in having to cope with a larger workload. Compensation may be more likely to come about as a result of increased pelvic rotation around the vertical axis in the coronal (transverse) plane: either increasingly forward on the swing-leg side to counter a restriction of hip flexion, or backward on the stance-leg side to counter a restriction of hip extension (Fig. 2.12). Unfortunately, this adjustment:

1. comes at the cost of increased counter-rotation of the trunk, with simultaneous active external rotation of the swing-leg and passive internal rotation of the stance-leg, to keep them in the sagittal plane
2. may not be possible in the first place, or may be severely restrained by a concomitant 'outflare' and 'inflare', in which case the pelvis tends to rotate toward the side of the outflare (see Ch. 2; Figs 2.13, 2.64, 2.66)

Malalignment may be a factor determining the take-off leg in running or jumping events. Pole vaulting and the long, triple and high jumps, for example, involve a high kick and require an unrestricted range of hip flexion and extension, all of which can be affected by the malalignment. The high-jumper will likely lead with the side that can achieve maximum initial hip flexion combined with back extension (Fig. 5.12).

Hip adduction

Hip adduction is found to be restricted on the left side in practically all of those with the 'more common' patterns of 'rotational malalignment' or an 'upslip'. The restriction may occur primarily on the basis of the asymmetry in muscle tension that results with malalignment - specifically, the easily palpable increase in tension in the left hip abductors and the TFL/ITB complex, with the resulting limitation of left hip adduction evident on:

1. passive hip adduction, testing both the short and long hip abductors, carried out with the person supine and the hip flexed to 90 degrees (Figs 2.106, 2.107, 3.77)
2. Ober's test, testing mainly the short abductors in side-lying
   - in the vast majority, adduction is adequate to allow the right knee to come close to or actually touch the plinth (Fig. 3.44Ai); whereas left hip adduction is decreased relative to the right, so that the left knee comes to rest a variable distance up in the air but consistently further off the plinth than the right one (Fig. 3.44Aii)

Successful correction of the malalignment restores the symmetry of right and left hip adduction. When lying supine, the extent of left adduction now usually matches that recorded on the right side prior to realignment (45 degrees in Fig. 3.77A). On Ober's test, findings are similar, the left now matching the right. Occasionally, the right knee will turn out to be up a few degrees from the plinth compared to before, indicating a minimal decrease in adduction with realignment; however, more

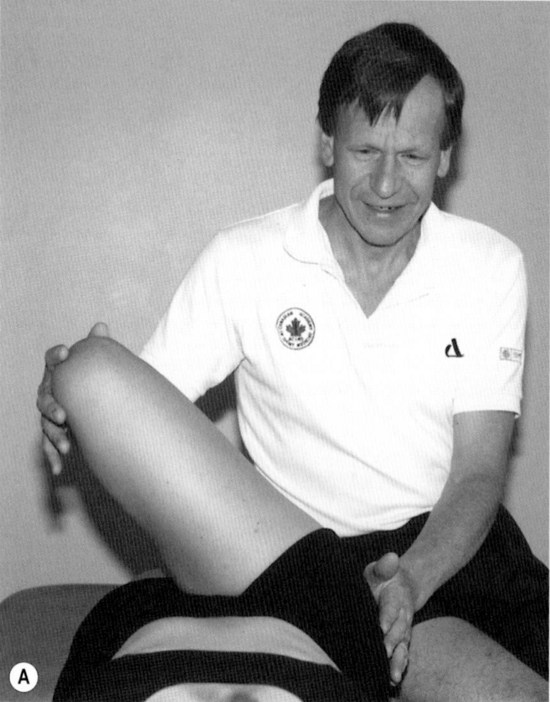

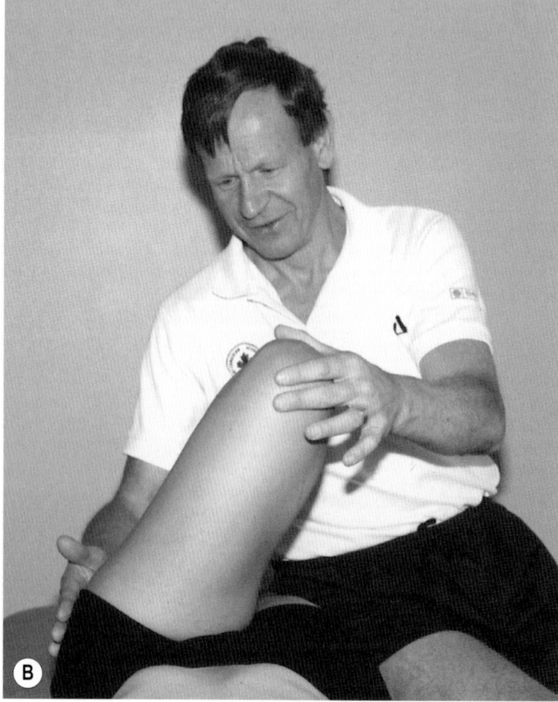

Fig. 3.77 Asymmetry of passive adduction of the flexed hip seen with an 'upslip' and the 'more common' patterns of 'rotational malalignment'. (A) Right here normal at 45 degrees. (B) Left decreased to 30 degrees.

important is the fact that the two sides now actually match up. Persistent asymmetry may indicate that:

1. the realignment was incomplete
2. there is a true element of tightness or contracture involving the hip abductors and/or TFL/ITB complex on that side
3. passive adduction is limited by:
   a. pain from the groin region caused, for example, by:
      i. excessive pressure sequentially on the acetabular rim, labrum and anterior SI joint region
      ii. compromise of a tender iliopsoas/pectineus muscle or iliopectineal bursa within the region of the femoral triangle (Figs 2.4A, 4.2)
   b. lumbosacral pain triggered by excessive stretching of painful posterior pelvic ligaments (e.g. in particular, the iliolumbar, sacrospinous and short/long dorsal sacroiliac ligaments)
   c. lateral hip pain caused by a tight TFL/ITB complex, sometimes snapping across the greater trochanter or exerting pressure on a co-existing trochanteric bursitis

Clinical correlation: hip adduction

If Point 3 is the case, the person may report pain from the groin, lumbosacral and/or sacroiliac region when passive adduction is carried out on examination. Other problems have been discussed in detail under 'left hip abductors' in the section on 'Asymmetry of muscle tension', above; in particular, relating to problems with control and seating when horseback riding, circling in skating, crossing the legs, cutting or turning corners, or simply sitting with the legs crossed (Figs 3.44, 5.17).

Hip abduction

Interestingly, abduction is also limited on the left side in the majority of people. The limitation may be caused by a number of factors, including:

1. the asymmetrical orientation of the hip sockets
2. the fact that, in the majority, this is the side of the 'posterior' rotation which, effectively, increases the tension in iliacus, gracilis and the adductor group by increasing the distance between their origin and insertion
3. 'facilitation' of left iliopsoas and the adductor group (see 'Asymmetry of muscle tension' above).

Clinical correlation: hip abduction

Goalies, especially in ice hockey, repeatedly use a rapid abduction of one or both lower extremities in the course of guarding the goal crease (Fig. 5.21B) . Limitation of abduction, typically on the left side, strains the joint and risks injury when abduction is forced (e.g. acetabular rim fracture, labral tear; Fig. 2.48). On the side of a 'posterior' rotation, there is an increased risk of spraining or straining the now tensed sartorius, adductor and iliopsoas or worse, avulsing the lesser trochanter (Fig. 3.50).

An asymmetrical abduction range may prove a limiting factor in speed-skating (Fig. 5.17) and ski-skating (Fig. 5.26A,B), in which full abduction is required to generate maximum symmetrical propulsion forces. In gymnastics and synchronized swimming, sports that repeatedly require a greater than normal amount of abduction, asymmetry may be costly in terms of performance and awards for style.

In horseback riding, the thigh on the side of reduced abduction is more tightly applied to the flank compared to that on the opposite side; attempts to compensate may come at the cost of disturbing proper seating and generating unwanted or inadequate control signals (see below and Ch. 6).

Hip external and internal rotation

When the person is in alignment, external and internal rotation of the right and left hip joints are symmetrical (Fig. 3.78A). An 'upslip' and the 'more common' rotational patterns show a restriction of right internal (Fig. 3.78B) and left external rotation (Fig. 3.79B). Barring underlying pathology, however, the total combined external and internal range available on the right and left sides will be the same. The 'left anterior and locked' pattern results in the opposite findings, with a restriction of left internal and right external rotation.

One might think that these restrictions are determined by the asymmetry in muscle tension. The findings associated with the 'more common' rotational patterns, for example, could easily result from the frequently detectable increase in tension in the right piriformis, an external rotator, and the left hip abductors and TFL/ITB complex, which are internal rotators. However:

1. it is these same muscles which most often show an increase in tension not just with the 'more common' rotational patterns but also with an 'upslip' and the 'left anterior and locked' pattern
2. reflex increase in tension in piriformis, gluteus maximus and iliopsoas - all external rotators - commonly occurs bilaterally as they attempt to stabilize the SI joint(s) and to decrease any pain originating from these regions.

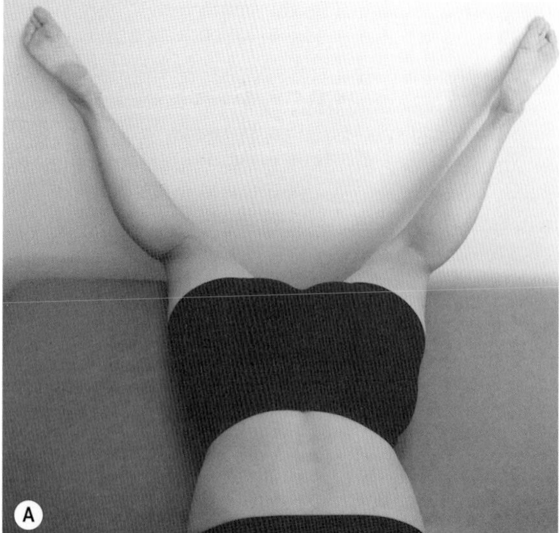

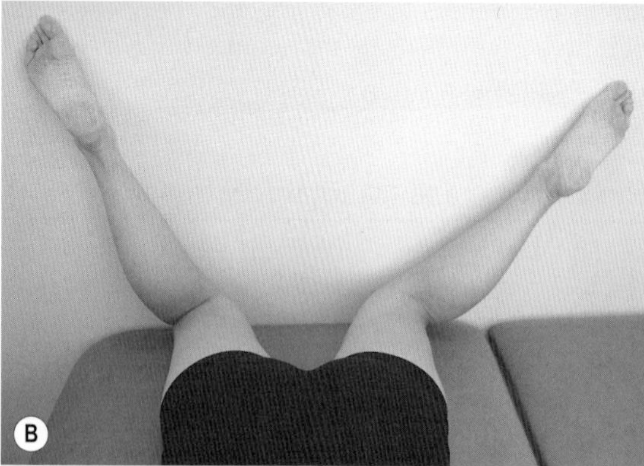

Fig. 3.78 Internal rotation (IR) of the hip. (A) In alignment: symmetrical (40 degrees). (B) With malalignment present: right decreased, left increased (30 degrees versus 50 degrees, respectively). In both situations: total equals 80 degrees.

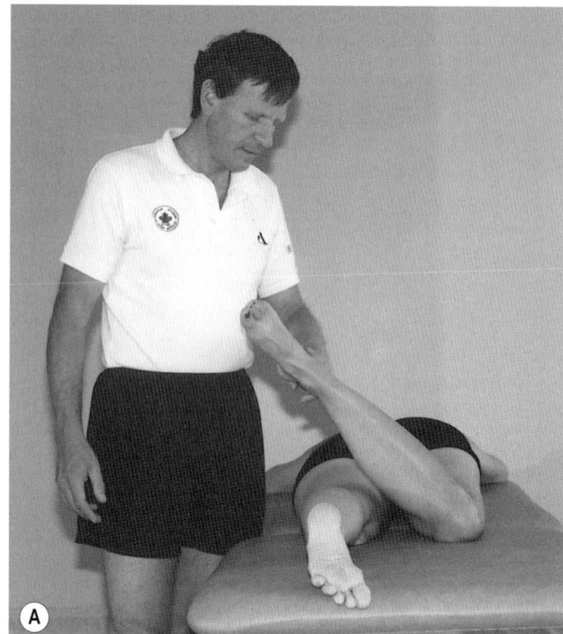

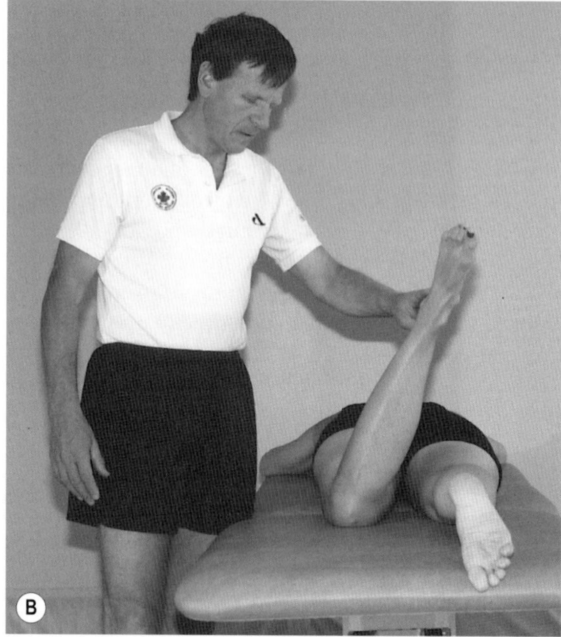

Figure 3.79 External rotation (ER) of the hip with malalignment. (A) Right of 45 degrees versus (B) left of 25 degrees. Prior to realignment, the total of right internal rotation (IR) of 30 degrees and ER (45 degrees) equalled the total of left IR (50 degrees) and ER (25 degrees); i.e. 75 degrees. The combined total improved to 85 degrees bilaterally when in alignment.

An asymmetrical orientation of the hip joints also fails to explain these findings, given that the pattern of limitation is the same regardless of whether the right or left innominate has rotated anteriorly. The exception is when 'left anterior' rotation is combined with 'locking' of the left SI joint. The combination of innominate orientation and SI joint mobility may, therefore, be one of the determining factors.

Clinical correlation: hip external and internal rotation

A modified Patrick's or FABER test for comparative hip ranges of motion allows the person a quick self-check on whether or not malalignment may be present (Fig. 2.107A). Lying supine, he or she lets the knees fall outward on either side while maintaining contact between the soles of the feet. The movement combines hip flexion, abduction and external rotation and also stresses the hip and SI joints (Fig. 3.80). Given that the malalignment results in asymmetry in all three ranges of motion, and barring any underlying pathology (e.g. hip joint degeneration; contracture of the capsule, muscles or other soft-tissues acting on the joint), one knee will typically fail to drop down as far as the other. The most common finding seen with an 'upslip' or one of the 'more common' rotational patterns is that the left knee ends up higher than the right, reflecting the restriction of left hip abduction and external rotation (Fig. 3.80A).

Unfortunately, the test does not help define the exact nature of the underlying malalignment, seeing that left external rotation is found to be decreased by both right and left 'anterior' rotation or an 'upslip'. The only obvious exception are those with the 'left anterior and locked' pattern, who show restriction of external rotation on the right side on FABER test. On realignment, the knees will again end up off the plinth to an equal extent (Fig. 3.80B).

External rotation is part of the lower extremity action in ski-skating, which is a part of traditional cross-country skiing and also a separate Nordic event (Fig. 5.26). It occurs in the trailing leg in speed-skating and is maximal as the blade reaches the terminal push-off point (Fig. 5.17). In those with one of the 'more common' rotational patterns or an 'upslip':

1. in these events, push-off may be impaired on the left side by the limitation of external rotation, compounded by the limitation of abduction and the impaired ability to dig in the inside of the left ski or blade, the latter because of the shift toward a left neutral to supinating pattern of weight-bearing (Figs 3.22A, 3.37)
2. the right, usually pronating, side may be able to dig in the inside edge but may run into problems holding this position because of a weakness and early fatiguing of the ankle invertors - tibialis anterior and posterior.

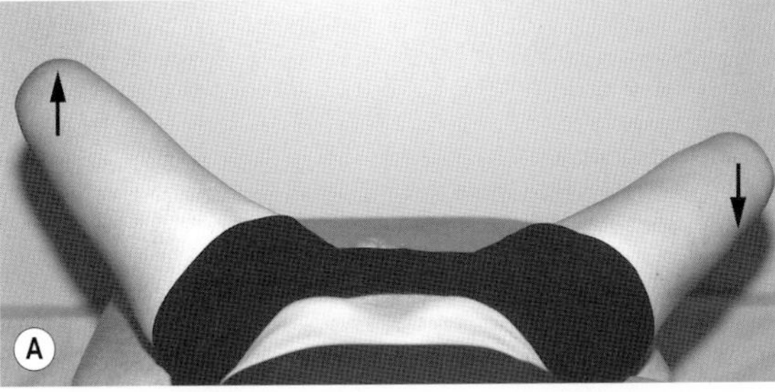

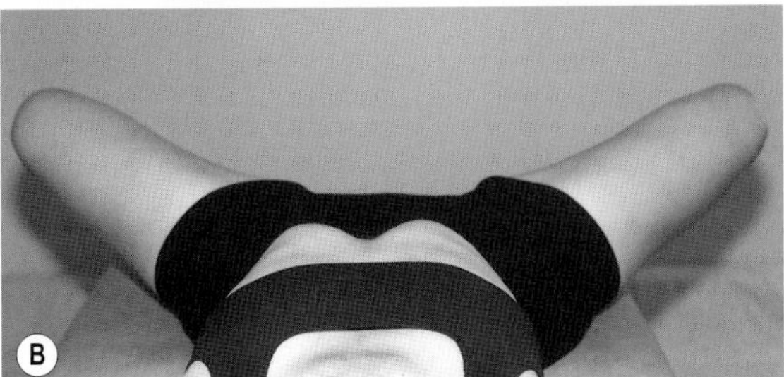

Fig. 3.80 Simultaneous bilateral flexion, abduction and external rotation (FABER test; Fig. 2.107A). (A) With malalignment: there is a restriction of these ranges on the left compared with the right side, so that the left knee ends up higher than the right. (B) In alignment: the left ranges now equal those on the right, and the knees end up level.

Crossing one leg over the other while sitting requires a simultaneous increase in adduction and external rotation in that leg. This becomes a particular problem with the 'more common' rotational patterns and an 'upslip', in which both left adduction and external rotation are restricted, making it harder to cross the left leg over the right (Fig. 3.48B). With the 'left anterior and locked' pattern, adduction is also restricted on the left; whereas external rotation is restricted on the right, so that crossing the legs may or may not prove more difficult on one side.

A restriction of internal or external rotation of a lower extremity may impair sweeping and kicking actions and is more likely to become a problem in soccer and similar sports. For example, with the hip and knee in flexion, a sweep or kick with the inside of the left foot may come to a sudden halt as the left external rotation range is reduced by the malalignment; the external rotator muscles are at risk of injury as they continue to contract though the motion has reached its end of range. When the action is one of sweeping or kicking outward with the right foot, a motion of internal rotation, it is the right internal rotators that are at risk as that range is exhausted earlier. If the player is unable to somehow compensate for such a limitation in range (e.g. trunk/pelvic side-flexion, or rotation in the transverse plane), the contracting muscles are at increased risk of injury.

Problems also arise when horseback riding. Limitations of left external and right internal rotation, in combination with a tendency toward left internal and right external rotation, interfere with the ability to achieve a secure seating position, or 'deep seat', and to use the thighs, knees and calves appropriately for signalling (see Chs 5, 6 and Fig. 5.37). Typically:

1. on the side of increased external rotation, and with the hip and knee in flexion, the thigh and

knee will tend to fall away from the horse's flank, the stirrup sweeps inward and it is the calf that ends up 'hugging' the horse's belly
2. on the side of increased internal rotation, the knee and thigh will come to be more closely applied to the flank; whereas the stirrup moves outward

These changes can result in misleading signals and interfere with control of the horse. The rider may appear crooked as he or she compensates by sitting asymmetrically in the saddle and this may interfere further with control, puts more strain on the rider and may be costly in terms of style.

The knee

> The knee appears to be an innocent bystander, subjected to stresses that arise from the various asymmetries associated with malalignment.

The most common finding in sitting and lying is that the patella rides high and squints outward on the side on which the leg has rotated externally (Figs 3.37, 3.81). When standing, those with an

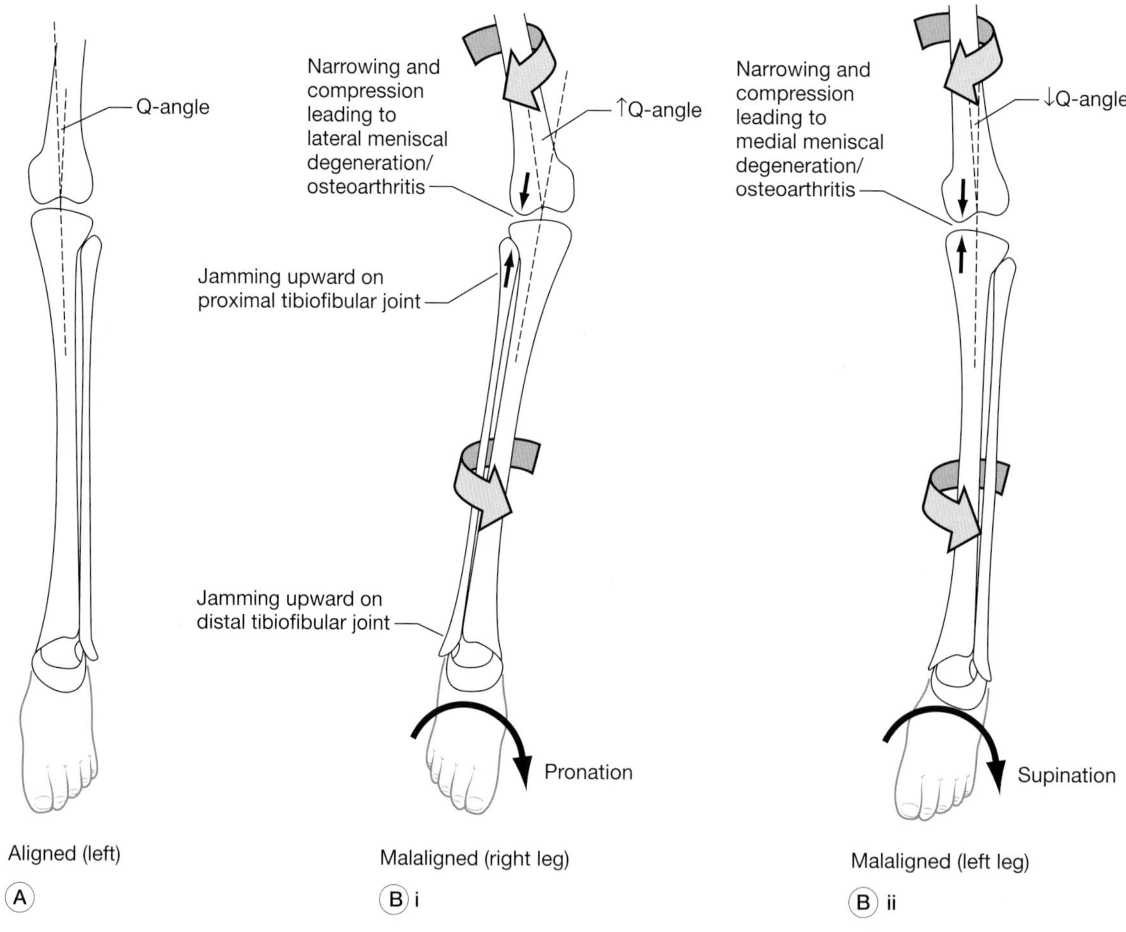

Fig. 3.81 Effect on Q-angle, pressure distribution in the knee joint compartments and tibiofibular joints with a malalignment-related shift to right pronation, left supination. (A) Aligned: there is a fairly uniform weight distribution through the medial and lateral knee compartments bilaterally (only the left is shown). (B) With malalignment (see also Figs 3.37, 3.38). (i) Right: increased pressure on the lateral compartment with the tendency toward pronation and knee valgus angulation (the Q-angle is increased). Excessive pronation can result in a forceful upward movement of the fibula and a jamming of the proximal tibiofibular joint (similar to what can result with an ankle eversion sprain). (ii) Left: increased pressure on the medial compartment with the tendency toward supination and knee varus angulation (the Q-angle is decreased).

'upslip' or one of the 'more common' rotational patterns may be seen to flex the knee on the high side of the pelvic obliquity, as if subconsciously trying to level the pelvis by this manoeuvre (Fig. 2.90). The knee flexion may also reflect the tendency to pronation on the side of external rotation, increasing both the knee valgus and flexion strain.

Unfortunately, flexing the knee when the foot is weight-bearing increases tension in the quadriceps mechanism, tending to pull the patella upward and increasing the pressure within the patellofemoral compartment. Other problems relating to weight-bearing include the following (Figs 3.37, 3.38):

Pronation

This accentuates any internal rotation of the tibia relative to the femur at the same time that the patella itself is being displaced upward by the increase in quadriceps tension and laterally by the relative external rotation of the femur and increase in the Q-angle. The combined effect is to increase the tension in the patellar tendon by separating the origin and insertion, and to offset the position of the patellar tendon relative to the groove, thereby further increasing the pressure especially within the lateral patellofemoral compartment. The increased tendency to pronation predisposes to valgus angulation of the knee, with:

1. increasing traction on the medial soft tissue structures (e.g. the medial collateral ligament, medial plica, vastus medialis tendon and saphenous nerve)
2. increased pressure within the lateral knee joint compartment (Figs 3.81Bi, 3.82-right leg).

Supination

This results in external rotation of the tibia relative to the femur and predisposes to varus angulation at the knee, increasing traction on the lateral soft tissue structures (e.g. the lateral collateral ligament, ITB and common peroneal nerve) and increasing the pressure within the medial knee joint compartment (Figs 3.81Bii, 3.82-left leg).

Rotation of the tibia relative to the femur

The contrary rotation of these bones associated with pronation and supination results in a torsional stress on the knee joint capsule itself, the menisci, and the anterior/posterior cruciate, collateral and interosseous ligaments, as well as on the proximal and distal tibiofibular joints.

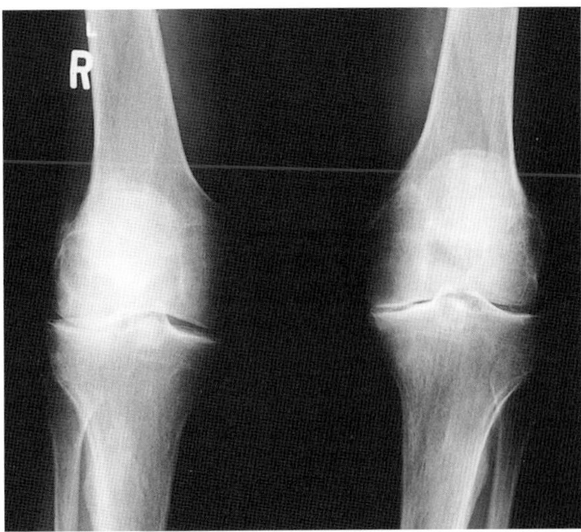

Fig. 3.82 Osteoarthritic changes of the knees as a result of a long-term pressure redistribution similar to what can occur with malalignment: accentuated wear of the right lateral and left medial knee joint compartments (see Fig. 3.81B).

Clinical correlation: the knee

In the person presenting with one of the 'more common' rotational patterns, with the pelvis high on the right side, a tendency to partly flex the right knee in standing, right pronation/left supination on weight-bearing (Figs 2.90, 3.37), typical complications include the following:

On the side of the 'externally rotated' right lower extremity

1. patellofemoral compartment syndrome
2. an increased risk of patellar subluxation or even dislocation
3. patellar tendonitis
4. right traction epiphysitis (Osgood–Schlatter's epiphysitis): if the tibial tubercle and tibia are not yet completely fused at the time they are being subjected to this increased stress, the irritation can stimulate increased bone turnover, which may result in an enlarged right tibial tubercle by the time growth has been completed; a chronic increase in tension in the tendon and/or direct pressure on the vulnerable epiphysis (e.g. with kneeling or on sustaining a contusion) can result in chronic epiphysitis and make this site an ongoing source of pain
5. increased traction on the right medial collateral ligament, which may cause tenderness, pain,

eventually elongation with joint instability and increased medial opening on valgus stress
6. inflammation of the medial collateral ligament, medial plica and vastus medialis; the increase in tension sometimes causes these to snap across the medial femoral condyle on flexion/extension movements of the knee
7. increased traction on right pes anserinus
8. paraesthesias or pain from irritation of the right saphenous nerve, vulnerable particularly where it crosses the medial tibial condyle and medial malleolus (Fig. 3.38A)
9. accelerated degeneration of the lateral knee joint compartment cartilage and meniscus (Figs 3.81Bi, 3.82-right leg).

On the side of the 'internally rotated' left lower extremity.

1. left lateral collateral ligament tenderness, pain, eventually elongation and joint laxity, with lateral joint line opening on varus stress
2. increased traction in the distal ITB, biceps femoris and the tendonous insertions of vastus lateralis lying in between; when under tension, one or all three structures may snap across the lateral femoral condyle repeatedly on knee flexion and extension, increasing the chance of developing ITB bursitis
3. upward traction exerted by the biceps femoris on its insertion into the proximal fibula, which can disturb the movement normally possible at the proximal, and also distal, tibiofibular joint
4. irritation of the common peroneal nerve or its branches (Fig. 3.38B)
5. accelerated degeneration of the medial knee joint compartment cartilage and meniscus (Figs 3.81Bii, 3.82-left leg).

In addition to the possibility of pain having been referred to the knee from the low back or hip regions (Figs 3.63, 3.67), always keep in mind the abnormal or exaggerated stresses that result with malalignment as an underlying cause of knee pain, instability or degeneration, especially when the person presents with:

1. unilateral knee problems in the absence of a history of trauma
   - right patellofemoral compartment syndrome is the most frequent complication, which relates to the majority presenting with one of the 'more common' patterns of 'rotational malalignment'
2. unilateral compartment involvement
   - osteoarthritis of the knee tends to affect more the medial, RA the lateral compartments bilaterally; whereas an 'upslip' or the 'more common' patterns of 'rotational malalignment' stress particularly the right lateral, left medial compartment

Tibiofibular joints

Normal movement at the proximal and distal tibiofibular joints is required to allow proper movement of the tibia, fibula, ankle and foot. There should be some glide possible in the sagittal plane (anterior-posterior) and vertical (cephalo-caudal) planes - with a sensation of giving way on passively moving or 'springing' these joints, usually more easily detectable proximally (Fig. 3.83).

A failure of one or both of these joints to move appropriately, or a difference in movement on side-to-side comparison, may indicate a problem. The anteroposterior glide of either joint can, for example, be impaired by a direct blow to the anterior or posterior aspect of the proximal or distal fibula. An acute ankle inversion sprain or the repetitive rolling outward on supination associated with malalignment would pull down on the fibula (Fig. 3.81Bii); whereas an acute ankle eversion sprain or the repetitive dorsiflexion, eversion and abduction of the pronating foot can force the fibula upward and may cause it to jam proximally (Fig. 3.81Bi).

Attempts at passive movement may elicit pain from the joint itself, the ligaments or both. Proximal

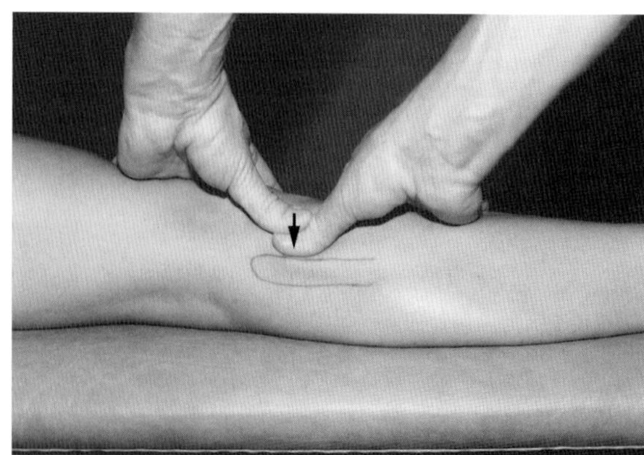

Fig. 3.83 Springing test for anteroposterior movement of the proximal tibiofibular joint.

joint pain calls for a check for undue tenderness or irritability of the common peroneal nerve, which innervates the joint and is at increased risk of entrapment, traction injury or both as it winds around the neck of the fibula (Fig. 4.11A).

The proximal tibiofibular joint

At this joint, the fibula normally glides anteriorly and upward on ankle dorsiflexion/pronation, and posteriorly and downward on plantarflexion/supination. It can get 'stuck' in an excessive upward or downward position with an ankle eversion or inversion sprain, respectively. The fibula is at risk of jamming against the lateral condyle of the proximal tibia as a result of:

1. upward traction forces; e.g. those exerted by biceps femoris and the lateral collateral ligament (both of which insert into the fibular head)
2. ankle dorsiflexion/eversion/abduction seen in association with pronation, which would push the fibula upward (craniad).

Aggravating factors such as these are frequently operative in the presence of malalignment. With the 'more common' patterns and an 'upslip' there is, for example, an increase in tension in right biceps femoris and tendency to right pronation, ankle dorsiflexion and eversion. The proximal end of the fibula may get jammed at the tibiofibular joint in an anterior and upward position while the distal end may be displaced posteriorly to the point of interfering with the function of the distal tibiofibular joint.

The distal tibiofibular joint

Movement at this joint is closely related to movement of the tibiotalar and, to lesser extent, subtalar joints. Valgus angulation of the tibiotalar joint, for example, can result in splaying of the space between the fibula and tibia, stressing the interosseous membrane. Dorsiflexion at the tibiotalar joint has a similar effect because of the wedge-shaped talus, wider inferiorly. Supination and increased ankle varus tense the fibulo-calcaneal ligaments and pull the fibula downward (caudad).

If the distal tibiofibular joint gets 'stuck', the ability of the calcaneus to evert or invert and of the foot to dorsi- or plantarflex are both impaired and the ankle becomes 'stiff'. The loss of ankle mobility, especially if associated with a downward displacement of the distal fibula, will also impair the internal and external rotation of the tibia that normally occurs with pronation and supination, respectively. In the presence of malalignment, a number of these factors are exaggerated and would predispose to development of ligament and joint discomfort and pathology.

The ankle (tibiotalar) joint

Dorsi- and plantarflexion of the foot reflect primarily movement at the tibiotalar joint in the sagittal plane, with contributions from the subtalar and distal tibiofibular joints. With an 'upslip' or any of the 'more common' rotational patterns, the right side shows increased dorsiflexion and decreased plantarflexion relative to the left (Fig. 3.84). These patterns are in keeping with the tendency toward right pronation (calcaneal eversion, forefoot abduction and dorsiflexion) and left supination (calcaneal inversion, forefoot adduction and plantarflexion).

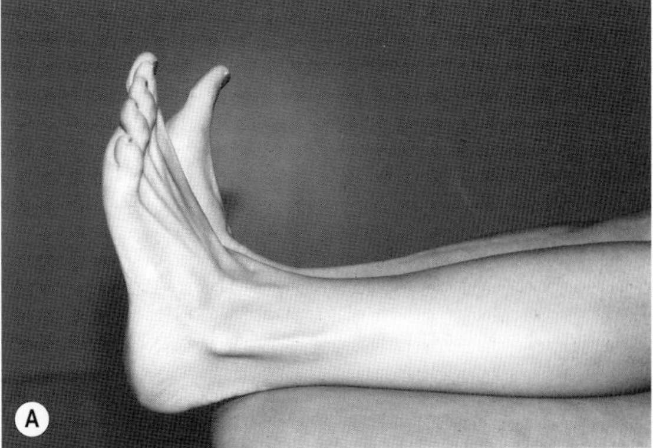

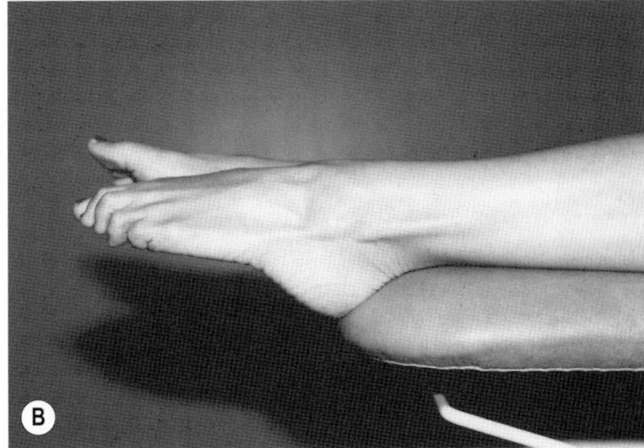

Fig. 3.84 Effect of an 'upslip' and the 'more common' patterns of 'rotational malalignment' on ankle movement. Relatively restricted of active/passive (A) left dorsiflexion; (B) right plantarflexion.

Findings are the opposite with the 'left anterior and locked' pattern: dorsiflexion increased on the left and plantarflexion on the right, reflecting the tendency toward left pronation and right supination, respectively.

When there is an exception to this pattern, consider:

1. a previous ankle injury that may have resulted in unilateral restriction of dorsi- and/or plantarflexion and often also limitation of subtalar eversion and/or inversion
2. actual degenerative changes or other pathology (e.g. spur formation, 'footballer's ankle; see below and Fig. 3.85B)
3. cuboid subluxation, which results in a stiff ankle with restricted motion in all four directions (see below; Fig. 3.85A)

Clinical correlation: tibiotalar joint

Propulsion with the flutter kick depends, in part, on the ability to plantarflex the foot. The asymmetry of plantarflexion seen with malalignment is probably one reason why some swimmers are unusually slow, fail to move forward or may actually move backward on doing the flutter kick while holding on to a board. Factors such as contrary rotation of the legs and the asymmetry of lower extremity muscle strength probably also play a role in creating this 'opposing propellers' effect (see Ch. 5).

Deep squats require a full range of ankle dorsiflexion, especially if the heels are to stay on the floor (e.g. working in a squat position; some gymnastic and weight-lifting routines). With an 'upslip' or 'rotational malalignment', dorsiflexion will be decreased on the side that tends toward supination. Once the limit of available dorsiflexion has been reached on that side, the following sequence occurs on attempting to squat further:

1. Tension in the tendo-Achilles complex on that side increases to the point at which attempts at further dorsiflexion begin to tighten up the plantar fascia and activate the 'windlass' mechanism sooner than normal.
2. Next, the heel begins to lift off the floor and weight-bearing is increasingly transferred to the forefoot as the foot and ankle are passively plantarflexed by this mechanism.

A person who is stationary and squatting to lift a weight may end up having to raise the heel right off the floor. Someone who is in motion (e.g. a floor gymnast) may end up:

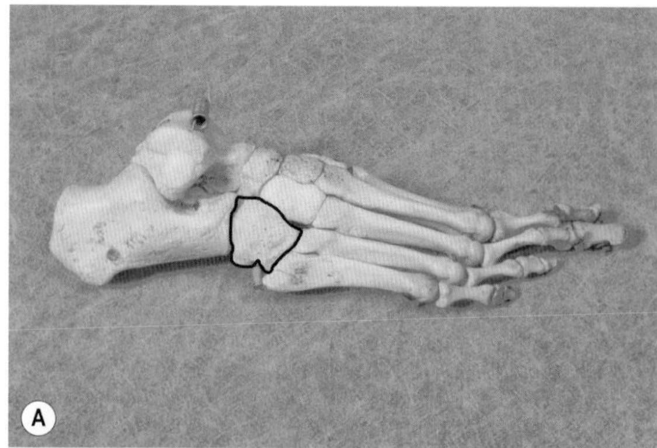

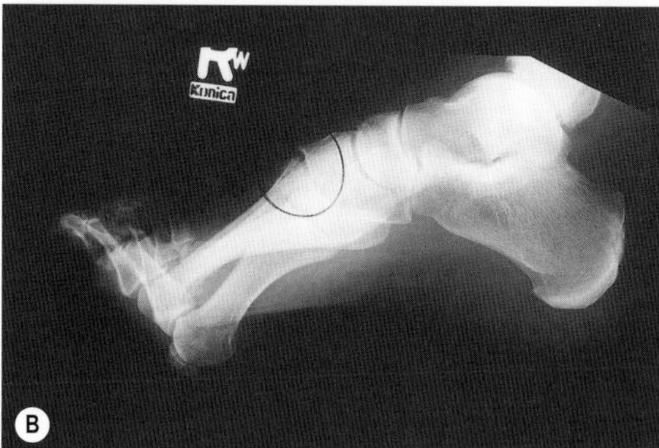

Fig. 3.85 (A) The cuboid bone (outlined in black) is prone to sublux from its position between the five adjoining bones of the mid and lateral foot, resulting in a 'stiff' ankle, with restriction of all ranges of motion and often also pain from the cuboid region. (B) Degenerative changes on the dorsum of the foot with an osteophytic spur projecting superiorly at the cuneiform-2nd metatarsal articulation, which can be precipitated or aggravated by malalignment: increased dorsiflexion can cause impingement, and increased plantarflexion excessive traction, at this site.

1. vaulting over the ball of the foot from mid-stance to toe-off or
2. collapsing into medial weight-bearing and pronation with that foot in an attempt to counter the tendency for the heel to come off the floor; that is, to counter the tendency to increasing plantarflexion and the associated rise of the centre of gravity

Both ways of compensating decrease stability and affect style. The increase in tension that results in the tendo-Achilles complex and in the plantar fascia with the premature activation of the 'windlass' mechanism increases the chance of developing painful inflammation (Achilles tendonitis or plantar fasciitis) or sustaining a sprain or strain of these structures.

The limitation of hip extension seen on the side of the posterior innominate rotation decreases the ability to lengthen that leg by extending the hip in late stance phase. The person can compensate by increasing plantarflexion of that foot in order to increase the leg length but this option will be limited on the side on which plantarflexion is already restricted:

1. on account of the malalignment, or
2. for other reasons (e.g. metatarsalgia, cuboid subluxation).

Activities calling on a maximum range of dorsiflexion or plantarflexion, such as competitive diving and dance routines, will be affected by any limitation (see Ch. 5).

A decrease in dorsiflexion range may become a limiting factor in cross-country skiing and especially telemarking, in which acute dorsiflexion accompanies knee flexion and hip extension of the back or inside leg when assuming the 'telemark' stance to execute a turn (Fig. 5.27).

In activities that require full dorsiflexion, the decrease of this motion seen on one side will cause an earlier transfer of weight to the metatarsal heads and an earlier impingement of structures on the dorsum of the foot (Fig. 3.84B). Stress would be maximal in work or sport routines requiring controlled ankle dorsiflexion when jumping and landing on one or both feet, such as may occur repeatedly during a work day in construction and in some field sports, also on jumping as part of a dance or floor routine or on a dismount. Anterior impingement of the ankle, a problem also known as 'footballer's ankle', particularly affects those playing Canadian or American football, soccer, or rugby on dry, hardened playing fields or artificial surfaces such as Astroturf (O'Brien 1992a). With time, the repeated stress can lead to problems: pain from irritation of the capsules, ligaments and bone, and from an acceleration of degenerative changes. The increased transfer of weight-bearing to the forefoot region may also contribute to the development of plantar fasciitis, metatarsalgia and metatarsal stress fractures.

The unilateral limitation of plantarflexion can result in contracture of the capsules, ligaments and tendons on the dorsum of that foot as these are no longer stretched fully as part of the daily activities. In ballet dancing, gymnastics and other activities that repeatedly require maximum available plantarflexion range, these contractures can result in the eventual formation of dorsal traction spurs (osteophytes) and other degenerative changes. Injuries such as marginal avulsion fractures are then more likely to occur on imparting a sudden or excessive stress to the dorsum of the plantarflexed foot (e.g. kicking a ball - or an opponent - with impact to the top of that foot, as in karate). The increase in plantarflexion on the opposite side - the left in those with an 'upslip' or one of the 'more common' rotational patterns - exerts unwanted traction forces on dorsal soft tissues and risks development of contractures of soft tissue structures on the sole of the foot (e.g. plantar fascia).

The subtalar (talocalcaneal) joint

The subtalar joint primarily permits calcaneal inversion and eversion relative to the talus. Some degree of abduction and adduction, as well as dorsi- and plantarflexion, is also normally possible. When examined lying supine and with the tibiotalar joint locked by holding the ankle in neutral (90 degrees), people presenting with an 'upslip' or one of the 'more common' rotational patterns show a restriction of passive right eversion and left inversion (Fig. 3.27A); whereas those with the 'left anterior and locked' pattern show a restriction of passive right inversion and left eversion.

Compared with the findings at rest, a gait examination of these people shows the tendency to pronate to be increased on the side that has the restriction of passive subtalar eversion, and the tendency to supinate to be increased on the side that shows the restriction of passive subtalar inversion. These changes suggest that restrictions of calcaneal inversion and eversion differ depending on whether the person is examined at rest (as described) or on weight-bearing, when other parameters, such as rotation of the femur and contrary rotation of the tibia and the amount of movement possible through the transverse tarsal joint and forefoot become the major determining factors (Figs 3.30, 3.37).

Clinical correlation: subtalar joint

Injury is more likely to result if either subtalar joint is forced into the direction of limited range, passively or actively, because the anatomical barrier will be reached earlier than usual.

Weight-bearing appears to reverse the restrictions at the subtalar joint so that the previously detected limitations of passive eversion and inversion at rest in neutral may not be of much consequence when the person is up and about (see 'Asymmetry of foot alignment, weight-bearing and shoe wear' above). On the gait examination of those with an 'upslip' or one of the 'more common' patterns of 'rotational malalignment', the majority show a noticeable calcaneal eversion on the right pronating side and a neutral or even frankly inverting calcaneus on the left supinating side (Figs 3.3B, 3.24 3.40). The opposite findings are evident with the 'left anterior and locked' pattern (Fig. 3.3A). With weight-bearing, however, there occur other changes that might make up for the restrictions of passive calcaneal eversion and inversion seen on non-weight-bearing with the ankle at 90 degrees to lock the tibiotalar joint.

First, there is the change in the axes running through the transverse tarsal (calcaneocuboid and talonavicular) joints (Mann 1982; Fig. 3.30), with:

1. divergence on the side of the internally rotated femur (=externally rotated tibia)
   a. this decreases the motion possible in these joints, locks the metatarsals and increases the stability of the longitudinal arch
   b. the end result is a tendency of this foot toward supination, adduction and plantarflexion; in other words, calcaneal inversion (Figs 3.3, 3.19Bii, 3.24, 3.30Aii, Bii)
2. parallel alignment on the side of the externally rotated femur (=internally rotated tibia)
   a. this increases the motion possible in these joints, unlocks the metatarsals and allows for a collapse of the medial longitudinal arch
   b. the end result is a tendency of this foot toward pronation, abduction and dorsiflexion, with calcaneal eversion (Figs 3.3, 3.19B, 3.24, 3.30Ai.Bi).

Second, a certain amount of inversion and eversion can occur at the tibiotalar joint and the joints of the forefoot.

Third, there is also the factor of how easily the knee can collapse into valgus on the pronating side and into varus on the supinating side. Any limitation of these motions - such as may occur with tightening of soft tissues, osteoarthritis or other pathology in the patello-tibial or tibiofibular joints - would increase stress distally and could exaggerate or decrease the normal motions at the ankle and foot or the already abnormal, asymmetrical ones noted when malalignment is evident.

Cuboid subluxation

In any assessment of problems that seem to affect movement of the tibiotalar and subtalar joint, a possible complicating cuboid subluxation needs to be kept in mind. This entity may occur on its own but is not uncommonly seen in conjunction with malalignment. Presenting features include:

1. report of pain over the lateral aspect of the foot, sometimes severe enough that the person shifts weight-bearing onto the forefoot to decrease the pain and counter any forces that might increase pressure on the cuboid and aggravate the subluxation
2. palpable downward (plantar) protrusion of the cuboid
3. acute tenderness over the margins of the cuboid and the adjoining calcaneus, navicular, cuneiform and 4TH and 5TH metatarsals which form the five adjoining joints that can end up getting inflammed and painful (Fig. 3.85A)

Treatment includes:

1. correcting pelvic malalignment and re-establishing normal gait, changes which on their own may allow the cuboid to slip back into alignment
2. forcing the cuboid back into proper alignment relative to the five surrounding bones, which can sometimes be achieved by:
   a. gently pushing upward from underneath the bone (toward the dorsum of the foot) with:
      i) both thumbs massaging the cuboid through the sole, or
      ii) tape across the sole, cinched up and anchored medially on the dorsum of the foot so as to create an upward force under the cuboid and perhaps also help shift weight-bearing medially
   b. manipulating the cuboid in an upward direction
      i) the patient stands on the good leg, holding on to a plinth or chair for balance
      ii) you hold on to the other foot, thumbs overlying the cuboid and fingers crossing over the dorsum; your hands also support the rest of that leg so that it can dangle down loosely, thigh vertical, knee flexed

iii) with a quick motion, bring the foot upward, ankle into neutral or slight dorsiflexion, and then 'snap' it downward into plantarflexion while your thumbs continue to apply an upward pressure on the cuboid; the procedure may have to be repeated
iv) there may be an audible 'pop' as the cuboid slots back into place; if successful, right and left ankle ranges of motion will become symmetrical again and the patient may feel immediate relief
v) unfortunately, there is a risk of you snapping one of your 1ST CMC or MCP joints with this manoeuvre, in which case there may again be an audible 'pop' and there will definitely be a sharp pain at the base of your thumb!

APPARENT LEG LENGTH DIFFERENCE

The basis of the 'sitting-lying' test has been discussed in Ch. 2 (Figs 2.77–2.85). Typical examination findings with an anatomical (true) LLD are listed in Appendix 6 and findings indicative of an LLD in combination with 'rotational malalignment' or an 'upslip' in Appendix 7 and 8. Unless otherwise indicated, the discussion that follows will be based on the premises that the person:

1. presents with an 'upslip' or one of the 'more common' patterns of 'rotational malalignment'
2. does not have an underlying anatomical (true) LLD.

The most common finding is that the right iliac crest is higher than the left when the person is standing (Figs 3.86A, 2.73, 2.76B,D, 3.8) which is not unlike the case of someone with an anatomically long right

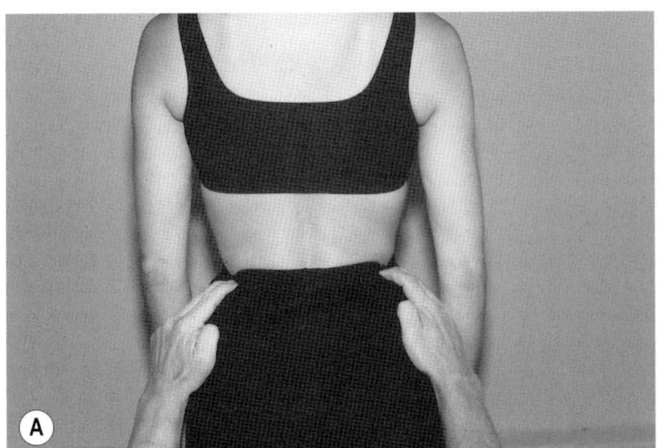

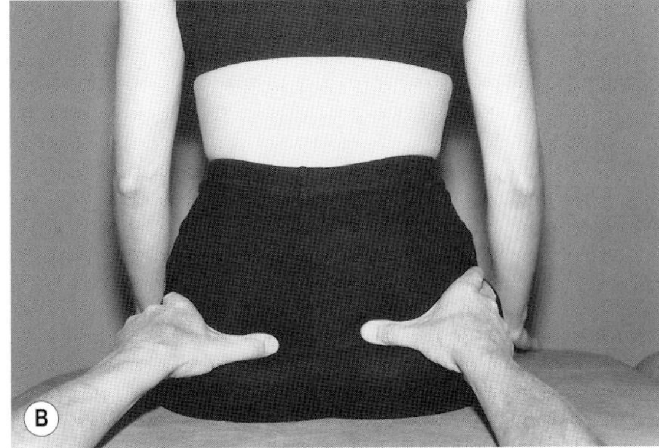

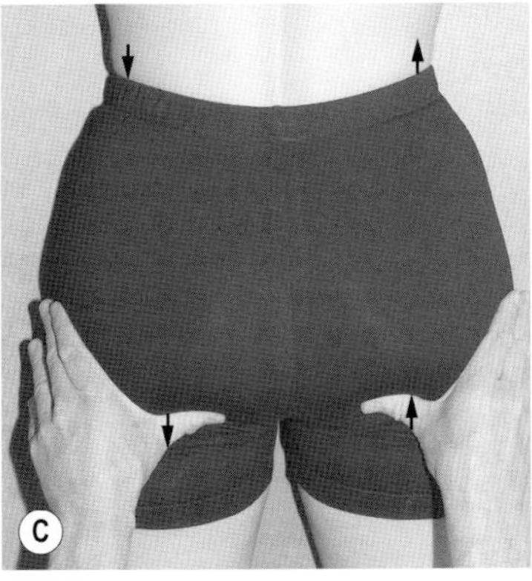

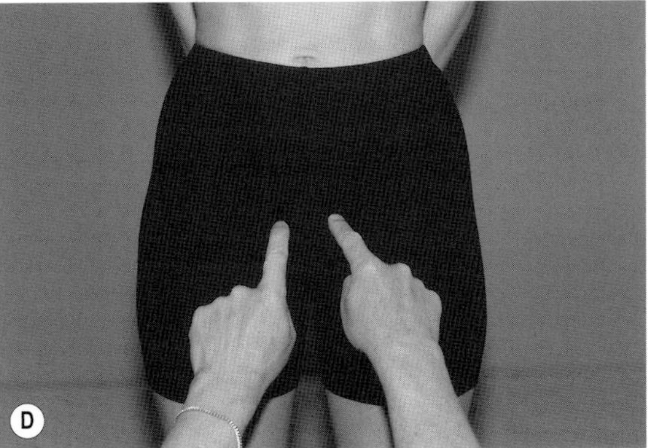

Fig. 3.86 A person known to have anatomically equal leg length when in alignment here presenting with pelvic malalignment ('right anterior, left posterior' rotation). Compared to the left side: (A) standing - right iliac crest up; (B) sitting - right posterior superior iliac spine (and iliac crest) up; (C) lying prone - right ischial tuberosity (and iliac crest) up; (D) standing - right pubic bone down.

leg (Fig. 2.72B). The pelvic obliquity will, however, persist in sitting (Fig. 3.86B), which is unlike the situation in those with an anatomical (true) LLD, whose pelvis would now be level (Fig. 2.72B). Though the obliquity in sitting may be opposite to that seen in standing (in this case, iliac crest now up on the left), it is more likely to be the same as in standing (i.e. up on the right; see Figs 2.73B,C; 2.76B). The fact that an obliquity persists in sitting indicates that:

1. the obliquity seen in standing is not simply caused by an anatomical LLD (although a concomitant underlying anatomical LLD could not be ruled out at this point)
2. malalignment ('rotational' and/or an 'upslip') is probably present.

A persistent obliquity may also result with a previous injury or asymmetrical growth of the right compared to the left innominate. When one examines those who are in or out of alignment, however, it is extremely rare to find developmental changes in the pelvic region that result in side-to-side differences of the magnitude of 1.0-2.0 cm that one commonly sees when malalignment is present (Fig. 3.87).

A knowledge of which iliac crest is higher when standing is not helpful for predicting which leg will be longer in long-sitting or supine-lying. Nor does it help to determine the side of an 'anterior' rotation or 'upslip'.

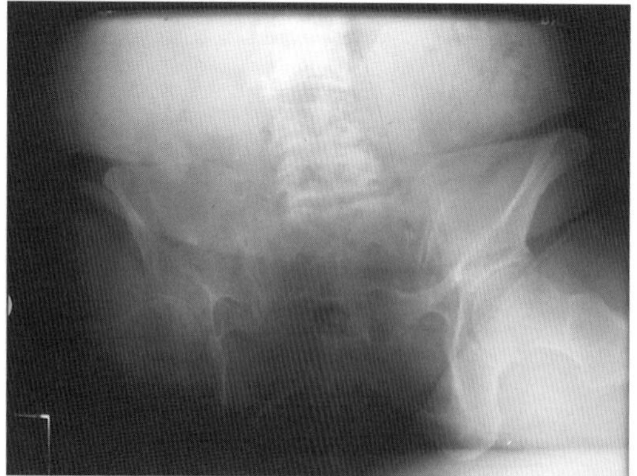

Fig. 3.87 This person is known to be in alignment but because of an underdeveloped left hemipelvis and hip joint (as the result of a left above knee amputation for tuberculosis at age 12), the left iliac crest appears 1 cm lower than the right when sitting.

Diagnosing leg length difference

From a diagnostic point of view, the apparent length of the legs, as noted in standing or in long-sitting and supine-lying, is of little importance in the presence of 'rotational malalignment' (Figs 2.77, 2.78, 2.84, 2.85). The right leg may, for example, be longer than the left in long-sitting and even longer in supine-lying (Fig. 3.88), but all this means is that there is probably an 'anterior' rotation of the right innominate that should then be verified by an assessment of the pelvic landmarks. It does not presuppose that the right leg is anatomically longer than the left! A typical example is that of the runner described in 'Case History 3.2'.

The 'long-sitting to supine-lying' test that shows a shift in leg lengths serves as a probable indicator of the presence of 'rotational malalignment' and helps to differentiate it from an anatomical (true) LLD and an 'upslip', although a co-existing anatomical LLD, 'upslip' or both cannot be ruled out. The test also affords the person or those doing the assessment an easy way of determining which side has rotated anteriorly or posteriorly. Knowledge of this is essential to allow one to then carry out the appropriate treatment techniques for the specific presentation and pattern of malalignment diagnosed (Chs 7, 8).

CASE HISTORY 3.2

A runner presented initially with low back pain. She was found to be in alignment but had an anatomical (true) LLD, the right leg 1 cm longer than the left (Fig. 3.89A). The back pain cleared with exercise and the provision of a right lift, initially 0.5 and eventually 1.0 cm in the heel, progressively tapered to the forefoot. Four months later, she returned complaining of pain in both the mid and low back region that had developed following a fall on ice. She was now found to have 'rotational malalignment', in a 'left anterior and locked' pattern. Despite the fact that she was known to have an anatomically longer right leg, the left leg was now 0.5 cm longer than the right in long-sitting; on lying supine, the left leg lengthened even more and ended up being 1.0 cm longer than the right (Fig. 3.89B). These findings were consistent with the 'left anterior' rotation, confirmed by finding complete asymmetry of the pelvic landmarks, and obviously said nothing about the anatomical (true) length of either leg.

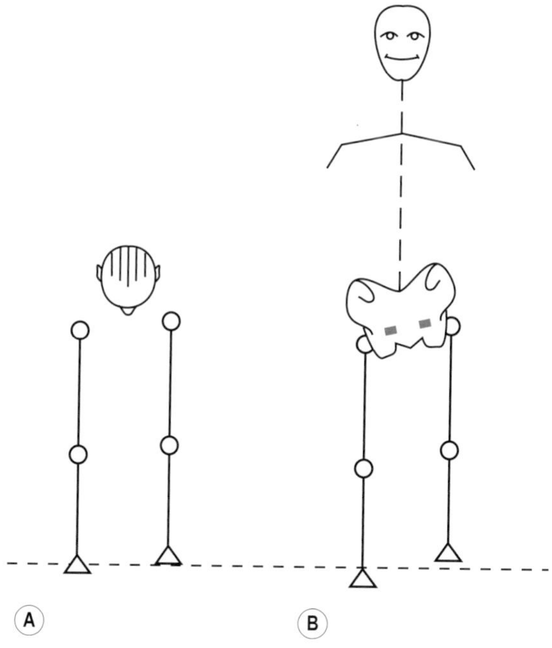

Fig. 3.88 Sitting-lying test: a change in functional leg length difference indicating probable 'right anterior' rotation. (A) Right leg longer in long-sitting. (B) Right leg even longer in supine-lying; i.e. right 'leg lengthened lying'.

Other factors to consider

It must again be emphasized that leg length *per se* is influenced by a number of factors, including whether there is a concomitant anatomical (true) LLD, sacral torsion, 'upslip'/'downslip', contracture or asymmetry of tension in the muscles and ligaments of the pelvic and hip girdle region.

> Differences in leg length of 2, 3 or even 4 cm can be attributable entirely to the presence of 'rotational malalignment', an 'upslip' or a combination of the two.

The fact is that differences as great as 2–4 cm may be observed to reverse completely on changing from the long-sitting to supine-lying position and yet, with realignment, most of these people will turn out to have legs of equal length! Remember that only 6-12% of us actually have evidence of an anatomical (true) LLD of 5 mm or more once in alignment (Armour & Scott 1981; Schamberger 2002).

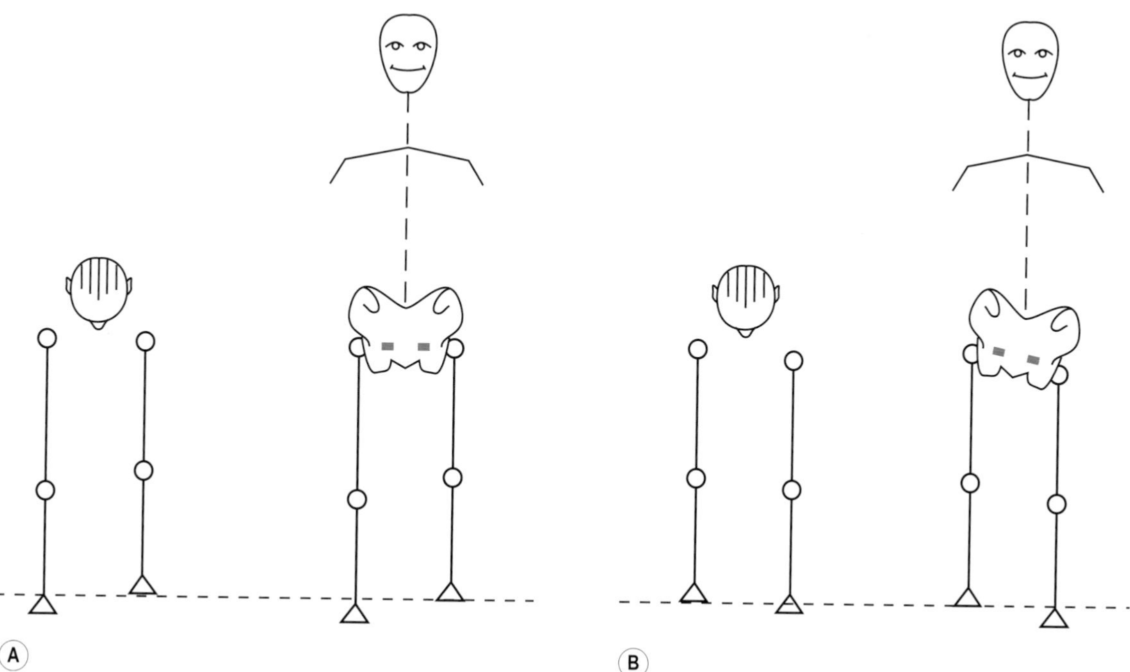

Fig. 3.89 Anatomical versus functional leg length difference (LLD) (see 'Case History 3.2'). (A) in alignment: anatomical (true) LLD with right leg longer than left by 1 cm, sitting and lying. (B) with superimposed 'left anterior' rotation: the left leg is now longer than the right by 0.5 cm in long-sitting and 1 cm when supine-lying.

The following basic approach is appropriate when dealing with a possible LLD:

1. As long as 'rotational malalignment' or an 'upslip' is present, a functional LLD will be present.
   a. There is, therefore, no point measuring leg length using the bony landmarks on the pelvis. In the case of someone with 'rotational malalignment', for example, measurement from the ASIS or PSIS to the medial malleoli, will be incorrect on both sides and on comparison of the right to left side. The ASIS and PSIS and, for that matter, any other pelvic landmark, will have changed position on one side compared to the other, not only in the sagittal but also in the coronal and vertical planes. At the same time, the asymmetrical reorientation of the right and left acetabulum has pushed the leg down on one side and pulled it up on the other. In other words, all the measurements will be inaccurate.
   b. Measuring from the greater trochanters to the floor in standing ignores any differences in the femoral head and neck and those due to displacement of the greater and lesser trochanters in opposite directions with the contrary internal/external rotation of the legs (Fig. 2.75).
2. If an anatomical (true) LLD is suspected:
   - one must first correct the 'rotational' (and any coexisting) malalignment and then carry out the measurements using the appropriate landmarks.
3. If the malalignment just cannot be corrected or there are ongoing complications (e.g. muscle spasm, joint laxity) that cause recurrence of malalignment in a symptomatic person, the following approach should be considered before trying to make up for the functional LLD with a lift:
   a. augment treatment aimed at settling down any complicating factors (e.g. pain, spasm); consideration of implementing one or more of the complementary techniques becomes even more important (Ch. 8)
   b. check the standing anteroposterior X-rays views to see if levelling of the sacral base has occurred in an attempt to counter the pelvic obliquity and compensate for the LLD (Fig. 3.90B).
   c. if compensatory sacral levelling has occurred, correction of the persistent pelvic obliquity with a lift under the apparently 'short' leg is contraindicated as it will actually unlevel the sacral base again, increasing the compensatory curves and the stress on the lumbosacral junction and spine (Fig. 3.90A).
4. If the sacrum is still unlevel, compensation either has not yet occurred or is incomplete. In that case:
   a. a lift to decrease or eliminate the residual pelvic obliquity may be helpful, aimed at levelling the sacral base, decreasing the stress on the lumbosacral junction and lessening any compensatory curves of the spine; in other words, aiming to achieve with the lift what would happen by sacral compensatory levelling (see Fig. 3.90B).
   b. an assessment of the LLD for the purpose of providing an appropriate lift should be made with the person standing, measuring from the lateral pelvic crest to the floor itself in order to minimize any error.

Clinical correlation: leg length difference

People are frequently told that one of their legs is 'long' or 'short'. The diagnosis is usually based on an examination in which the leg length was assessed in only one position; for example, looking at the iliac crest levels when standing or comparing leg length in long-sitting or when lying prone or supine. Lifts are sometimes prescribed on the basis of such a limited assessment. Problems may arise when the conclusions regarding leg length are based only on the following:

1. *comparison of the level of the pelvic crests done only in standing*

   The examiner might presuppose that the leg is short on the side on which the pelvic crest is low. A lift on the 'short' side might possibly be helpful because it will level out the pelvis and decrease the compensatory curves of the spine. However, if a compensatory levelling of the sacrum has already occurred, the addition of a lift on the side on which the pelvis appears low will only aggravate matters by causing recurrence of sacral base unlevelling, lumbosacral stress and the compensatory scoliosis (Fig. 3.90A).
2. *examination in either supine-lying or long-sitting only*

   Prescribing a lift on the basis of such a limited examination invites disaster.

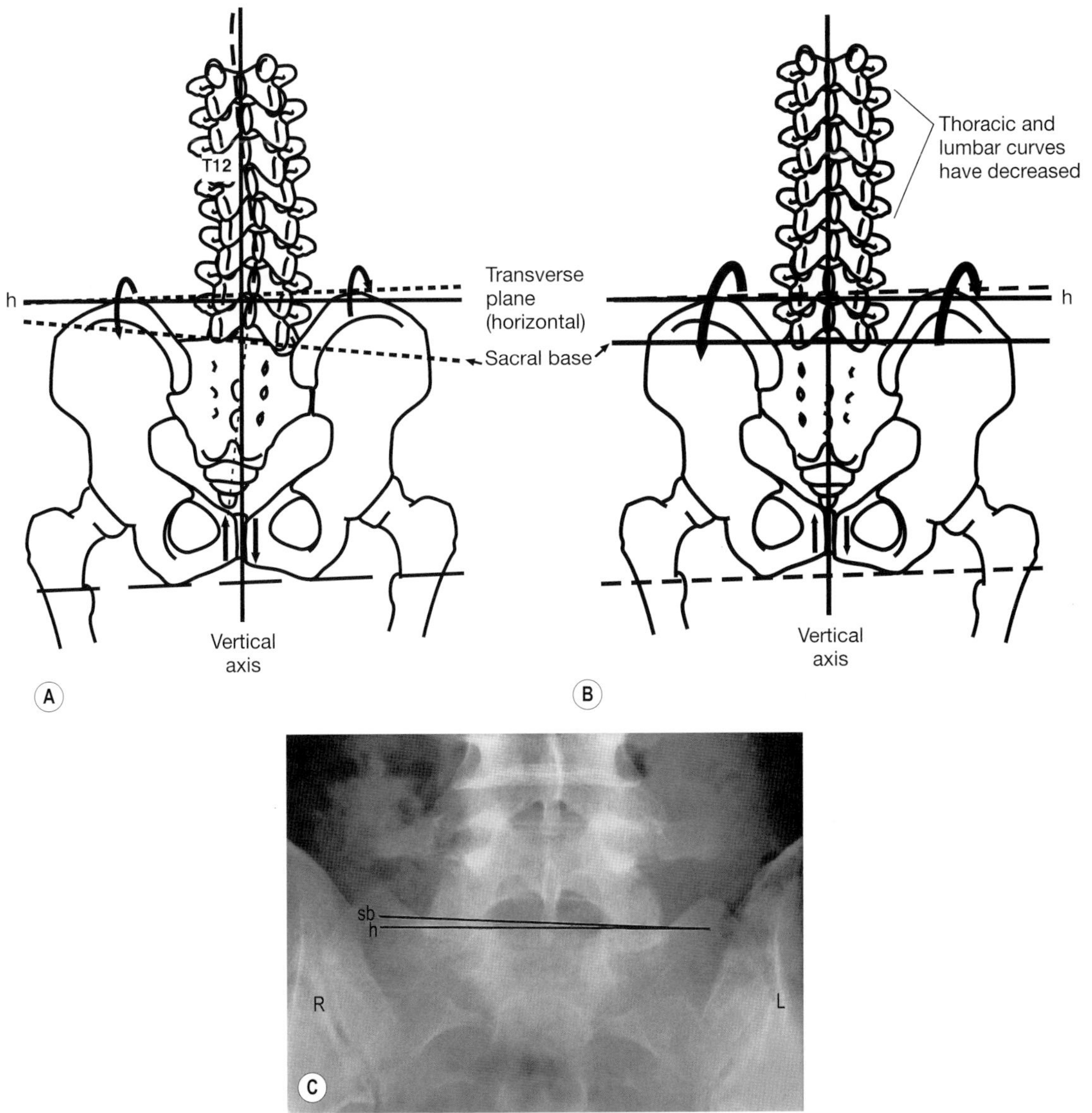

Fig. 3.90 Sacral adjustment to functional leg length difference caused by malalignment ('right anterior, left posterior' rotation). (A) Uncompensated: the iliac crests and the sacral base (upper and lower dashed line, repectively) are oblique (relative to 'horizontal' = line 'h'), and there is an accentuated compensatory scoliosis. (B) Compensated: although some obliquity of iliac crests persists (dashed line), the sacral base is now level and the degree of scoliosis decreased. (C) In this figure [A-P X-ray], the sacral base inclines to the [right] (black line sb, line h being the horizontal). Notice that the L5 vertebra appears to be side-bent to the right. This compensatory right side-bending of L5 effectively straightens the lumbar spine and there will be little remaining scoliosis. In this situation, the L5 vertebra will not function in a completely normal manner as some of its normal ranges of motion are used to correct the unlevelled sacral base. *(Courtesy of Ravin 2007.)*

It completely ignores the fact that when there is a concomitant malalignment of the pelvis, what seems to be the 'short' leg in one or both of these positions may actually become the 'long' leg in standing. It is, for example, not unusual to see the right leg shorter than the left in long-sitting and also shorter, but less so, when lying supine, yet to find the right iliac crest higher than the left when standing (Fig. 3.91).

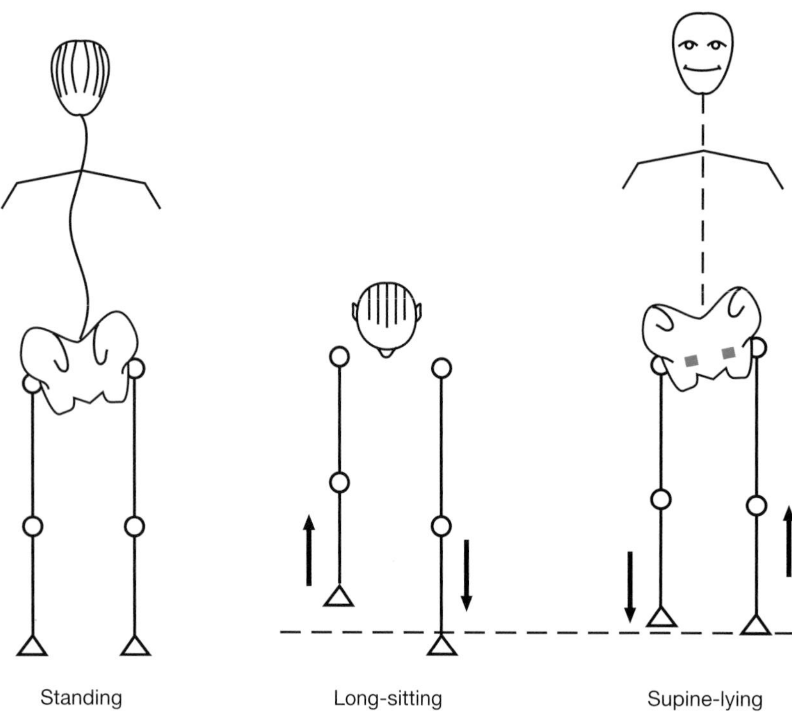

Fig. 3.91 The pelvis is high on the right side in standing. On moving from long-sitting to supine-lying, there is a relative lengthening of the short right leg, although it still ends up shorter than the left. This right 'leg lengthens lying' suggests a 'right anterior rotational malalignment' and can be confirmed by examination of the pelvic landmarks. An underlying anatomical (true) leg length difference (with the left longer than the right, or even the right longer than the left) cannot be ruled out at this stage but will become apparent on correction of the 'rotational malalignment' (and possible coexistent 'upslip').

This relative lengthening of the 'short' right leg on going from sitting to lying is in keeping with the diagnostic finding of right 'leg lengthens lying' which suggests that 'right anterior' rotation is present, to be confirmed by assessment of the landmarks (Ch. 2). The right leg will also be short in both long-sitting and supine-lying when a 'right upslip' is present, though the right side of the pelvis will turn out to be higher than the left in both the standing and sitting positions in most of these individuals. In both cases, prescribing a right heel lift on the basis of having looked at leg length only in the sitting or lying position will inadvertently result in a further increase of the pelvic tilt - right iliac crest up - and the compensatory curves, thereby increasing the stress that the pelvis and spine are already being subjected to because of the malalignment.

Following realignment, the prevalence of those with an anatomical LLD noted in the author's clinical studies - 12% in 1993, 10% in 1994 (Schamberger 2002) - is in line with study findings based on a comparison of the height of the femoral heads on anteroposterior pelvic X-rays taken while standing. Using this more accurate technique, for example, Armour & Scott (1981) found a prevalence of 10% in an adult population.

The tendency to pronate on one side is sometimes felt to be an attempt to compensate for a 'long' leg on that side. This may be true on the side of an anatomically long leg in someone who is in alignment. In those presenting with malalignment, however, the tendency to pronate does not always correspond to the side on which the pelvis is higher in standing but is more likely to be part and parcel of the presentation at hand:

1. on the right side in those with an 'upslip' or one of the 'more common' rotational patterns and associated external rotation of the right lower extremity, and
2. on the left side in those with the 'left anterior and locked' pattern and associated left external rotation.

Pronation that results in relative leg length shortening may also occur on the basis of:

1. isolated lower extremity muscle 'facilitation' or 'inhibition'; for example, 'facilitation' of peroneus longus/brevis and 'inhibition' of tibialis anterior/posterior
2. a medial shift in weight-bearing; for example, to decrease lateral foot pain (e.g. Morton's neuroma, stress fracture, cuboid subluxation)

Supination that appears to result in leg lengthening may occur on the basis of:

1. 'inhibition' of peroneus longus and 'facilitation' of tibialis posterior muscles
2. a lateral shift in weight-bearing to decrease medial foot pain (e.g. navicular fracture or subluxation; posterior tarsal tunnel syndrome)

The reader is referred to material specific to the topic of 'facilitation' and 'inhibition' relating to malalignment (e.g. Maffetone 1999). The emphasis here is on the fact that LLD seen in association with malalignment is usually part of a larger picture that can be readily divided into those with the conglomeration of findings typical of either (1) the 'left anterior and locked', or (2) an 'upslip' or one of the 'more common' patterns of 'rotational malalignment'. LLD is just one feature of the 'sitting-lying' test that allows for the ready detection and classification of these presentations.

In summary, it is of the utmost importance that the examiner assess leg length in several positions - standing, sitting and lying - to verify that a difference is indeed present and whether:

1. it is consistently the same on the 'sitting-lying' test, the legs moving down and up together, in which case the differential could be narrowed to an 'upslip' or anatomical (true) LLD
2. there is an actual shift in leg length on moving from one position to the other, in which case the diagnosis of 'rotational malalignment' must be considered and further clarified by correlation to the pelvic landmarks.

A PROBLEM WITH BALANCE AND RECOVERY

The asymmetries affecting the muscles, joints and lower extremities influence the ability to recover after having accidentally 'overshot' the mark or upset one's balance in some other way. Impaired balance and recovery may become strikingly obvious as a malalignment-related problem *per se* on taking the history and/or during the course of the examination.

Problems on static testing

On strength assessment of the ankle invertors and evertors, the person is instructed to move the foot 'up and in' (tibialis anterior), 'down and in' (tibialis posterior) and 'down and out' (peroneus longus and brevis). When malalignment is present, there is sometimes an obvious hesitation as the person tries to move the foot into one or more of these directions on command. The muscle or muscles that present a problem on attempting to initiate a specific movement are usually those which ultimately turn out to be weak in the asymmetric pattern of 'functional' weakness described above, affecting, in particular, the left ankle evertors and right ankle invertors (Box 7).

Not infrequently, the person cannot even muster a contraction of these muscles until given some tactile and/or visual cues, repeated verbal feedback and encouragement. One might, therefore, argue that impaired proprioception plays a role in the causation of this functional weakness. Other factors to consider are problems relating to 'facilitation' and 'inhibition', asymmetric strength, atrophy and impaired sequencing. For example, the person attempting right hip extension may contract hamstrings before gluteus maximus, instead of the proper sequence: gluteus maximus (to help stabilize the right SI joint and hip girdle) and then the hamstrings. Factors contributing to impair the sequencing probably include the fact that right gluteus maximus is inhibited (and actually proves weak in 5-10% on manual testing); whereas right hamstrings, notably biceps femoris, is usually 'facilitated' and strong (being 'set to fire', so to speak). In contrast, there is 'inhibition' and demonstrable weakness of the left hamstrings in these same 5-10% when tested in prone-lying (Fig. 3.55C). The question of 'causation', wasting and failure to contract has already been discussed at some length in relation to asymmetry of lower extremity muscle strength, tension and bulk (see above). In summary, as concerns right gluteus maximus, malfunction increases the burden on other muscles that can effect right hip extension and may be caused by:

1. true weakness
2. disuse weakness and even atrophy
3. failure to fire at all, or out of sequence
4. functional weakness

A problem with balance is more likely to become evident while carrying out the kinetic rotational (Gillett) test for SI joint mobility and load transfer, in which the person alternately ends up weight-bearing on one leg while flexing or extending the opposite hip joint (Figs 2.121-2.125)

On the Gillet test, when asked to bring the right knee up to horizontal and weight-bear just on the left, there should not be a moment's hesitation as the right thigh moves upward in the sagittal plane, the body weight being transferred and then balanced over a fairly straight left leg, with minimal Trendelenburg displacement evident (Fig. 2. 121B,C). The test is then carried out by flexing the left hip and having the right leg weight-bear. Alternatively, the person can carry out a one leg partial squat on their own, going down about 30 to 60 degrees (Peterson & Nittinger 2006; Fig. 3.92A) or may be called upon to bear all weight on one lower extremity during an activity (Fig. 3.92B). When right or left weight-bearing, is there any sensation of insecurity in that:

1. balance is a problem on one side?
2. coordination appears impaired?
3. one side seems to be weaker?
4. there is noticeable tightness or stiffness on comparing sides?
5. the manoeuvre provokes or worsens pain on the right or left side?

Comparatively, the manoeuvre causes a problem in a small number of people and is more likely to occur on left hip flexion: the now weight-bearing right leg is noted to adduct, the trunk and pelvis simultaneously swaying, the pelvis usually shifts outward (abducting) to the right while the trunk sways to the left (adducting) - a compensated Trendelenburg sign (Figs 2.58B, 3.93). Equilibrium is reached when the weight of the body is balanced over the right hip, with the leg somewhat adducted. These changes may indicate an attempt to compensate for impaired 'form' and/or 'force' closure which had resulted in right SI joint instability and/or difficulty transferring weight through the joint (Fig. 2.25). In this case,

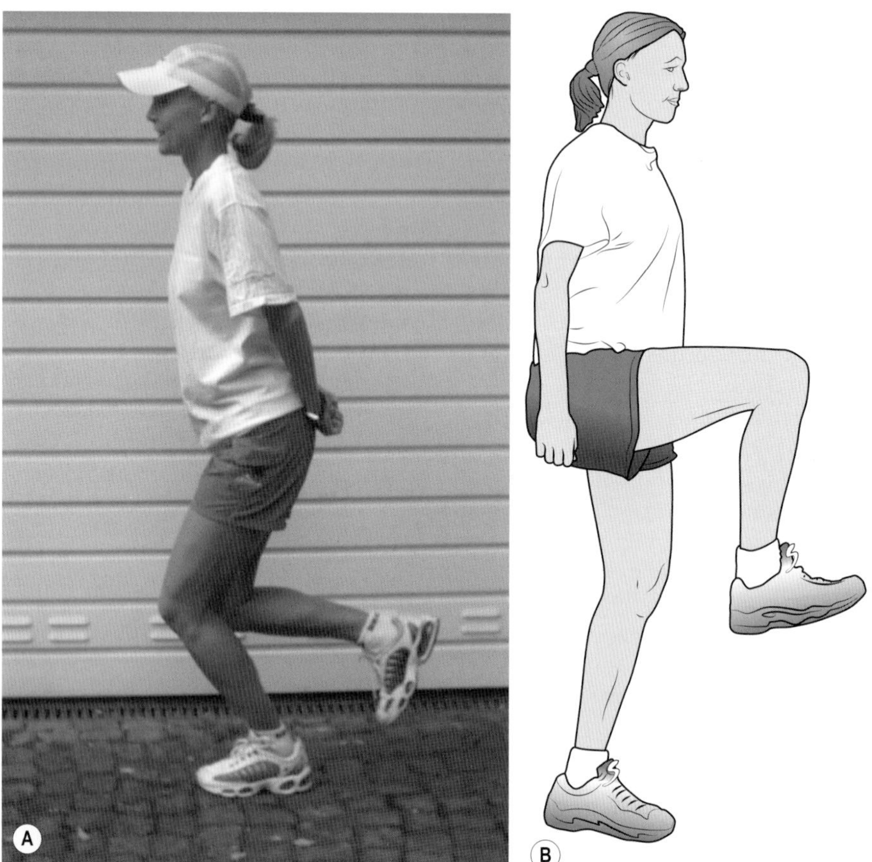

Fig. 3.92 (A) 'One leg squat' to determine side-to-side differences in balance, strength, pain, coordination and tightness/stiffness. (B) Test for lower extremity dynamic stability (balance). *(Courtesy Petersen & Nittinger, 2006).*

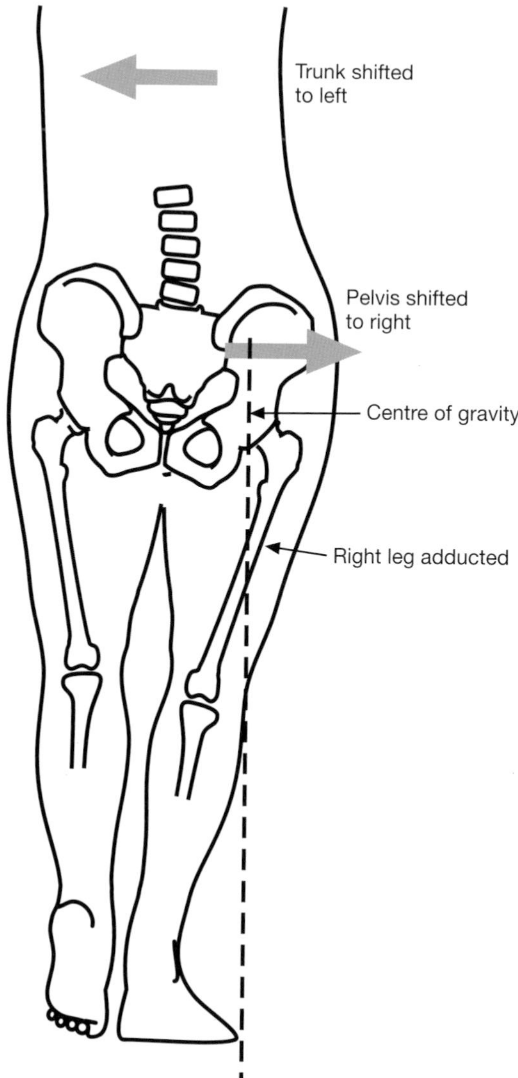

Fig. 3.93 Compensated right Trendelenburg gait. A problem with transfer of weight through the right sacroiliac joint as a result of impaired 'form' or 'force' closure is reduced or prevented by having the pelvis abduct and shift to the right, thereby increasing compression of the right sacroiliac joint and minimizing vertical shear stress through that joint (see also Figs 2.1C, 2.58).

vertical shear stresses and weight-bearing through the right SI joint are decreased by the pelvic abduction and by shifting the centre of gravity laterally, respectively. More weight is borne directly through the hip joint instead. Other possibilities to consider include:

1. the instability that results in the ankle and foot with right pronation and tendency to right knee valgus, and the functional weakness involving muscles that would normally be able to counter these movements
2. the increased stability of the left leg, with 'locking' of the foot and ankle as it moves into supination, and increasingly neutral or varus alignment of the knee joint

In some, the sway seen on raising the left knee may turn into an unmistakable wobble. They may even reach for support, suggesting that the right leg is weak or possibly that they are disorientated in terms of their position in space. A few are actually unable to carry out the manoeuvre at all. They may fail on repeated attempts and express the fear that they will lose their balance or that their right hip or knee will buckle and cause them to fall.

A person who appears to have instability on one side on the Gillet test may even report:

1. insecurity on walking, with evidence of an abnormal gait pattern (e.g. shortened stance phase on the insecure side)
2. problems more noticeable when coming down a slope or staircase, with the knee on the insecure side feeling 'wobbly' as that leg starts weight-bearing.

This problem of imbalance has so far been seen mainly on attempts to stand on the right leg alone in association with one of the 'more common' patterns of 'rotational malalignment', suggesting that the presence and side of the instability may be in some part determined by the malalignment. The limited number of times this phenomenon has been observed with the 'left anterior and locked' presentation may reflect the fact that this pattern is so much less prevalent than the 'more common' patterns (5-10% versus 80-90%, respectively) and that only a small number of those with 'rotational malalignment' actually admit to having a problem or show evidence of instability on examination. However, as indicated above, when it is evident it can present a very obvious handicap for some.

This instability cannot be explained entirely on the basis of the functional weakness, given that the pattern of asymmetrical weakness involves muscles in the hip girdles and legs on both sides. Other factors to consider include:

1. asymmetry of the lower extremity joint ranges of motion

2. an asymmetry of proprioceptive input from the pelvic and lower extremity joints and soft tissues
3. deficient kinaesthetic sensitivity of the ankle on the side of the instability (as discussed below); the knee and hip joint on this side could conceivably be affected in the same way
4. an asymmetry of weight-bearing, the instability being seen primarily on the side where the person tends toward pronation so that:
   a. the foot and ankle are 'unlocked' and more mobile
   b. the knee is placed under valgus stress and is no longer located directly over the foot
5. instability of the SI joint due to ligamentous or osteoarticular damage, muscle weakness, impaired neural control, possibly also presenting with a history suggestive of the 'slipping clutch' phenomenon (see below)
6. deficient segmental or central nervous system control.

Needless to say, a feeling of instability when weight-bearing on only one leg could invite disaster in certain jobs and athletic activities. The problem is more likely to become evident in a person working on uneven ground, up- or down-grade, or using stairs or ladders repeatedly, as in construction, roofing, and firefighting. Athletes probably learn to decrease the chance of this problem interfering with an activity by tailoring their style to decrease the detrimental impact of their specific problem. However, sometimes an activity dictates a movement pattern that is contrary to the one that would avoid this problem. Examples include unexpected weight-bearing, squatting and torsional demands on the body in a work-situation, such as a rescue operation, or specific routines demanded of an athlete that run counter to the way that he or she would find easier to perform (e.g. compulsory figures in ice skating; Fig. 5.19). Also, anyone presenting with this problem is liable to mishap should they accidentally be forced to lead with, take off from or land on the 'shaky' or 'weak' leg. Consider the predicament of the ice hockey player who inadvertently ends up having to bear all the weight on the 'wrong' (i.e. 'unstable' or 'weak') leg while making a turn, attempting to shoot the puck or avoiding a collision.

All of us have patterns of movement that we can carry out feeling strong and confident; other patterns we perform feeling weak and insecure. Some of that may be caused by laterality but the vast majority of those who have a problem balancing on the right-leg, for example, happen to be right-handed and right-footed and might be expected to have a stronger, more stable leg on that side. Following correction of the malalignment, the single-stance test is performed by most without hesitation or evidence of instability. This immediate improvement argues against the problem being one of laterality but makes it more likely to be attributable to one or more of the changes seen in association with malalignment.

Problems on dynamic testing: gait examination

Regular walking, including heel- or toe-walking, rarely presents a problem. However, attempting to hop on one foot while staying up on the toes may prove difficult, if not impossible, when the person is out of alignment. The problem is more likely to occur on the side that tends to pronate; the foot and ankle feel insecure and collapse inward - a definite medial whip of the heel is often evident (Figs 3.24, 3.40). In contrast, the foot on the side that tends to supinate provides a more stable base; toe-walking and single-leg hopping are carried out with greater ease and the heel usually remains in the midline (neutral) but may whip outward. This tendency for the pronating foot to whip inward and the supinating one outward, which may already have been evident on toe-walking, is more likely to become evident - or can usually be accentuated - when single-leg hopping on the spot. Better still, if the person is capable, have him or her hop away from you on one leg a short distance along a real or imaginary straight line, switching to the other leg at half-way to allow for side-to-side comparison.

Instability of isolated joints on walking or running

When asked about 'weakness', a person presenting with malalignment may recall a sensation of the hip or knee giving way but examination may fail to show any evidence of pathology; in particular, no instability of the hip or knee joint itself. The 'giving way' is sometimes preceded by a sharp pain, possibly originating from one of the soft tissues or nerves that is already in trouble as a result of the malalignment:

1. in the immediate vicinity of the knee joint (Fig. 3.38)
2. distant from the knee joint but able to refer to this area; for example, pain referred from the femoral attachments of the hip articular ligaments (Figs 3.67, 4.3).

This pain can cause a reflex relaxation of muscles responsible for supporting the joint and the feeling of the joint 'giving way'. Reflex relaxation of the quadriceps, for example, makes the knee buckle; an impulse capable of temporarily shutting down piriformis or gluteus maximus would have a similar effect on the hip joint, allowing it to collapse into flexion. The person may actually fall.

The 'slipping clutch' syndrome refers to the experience of an episodic 'giving way' of one leg, without any pain necessarily preceding this sensation (Dorman 1994, 1995; Dorman et al. 1998; Vleeming 1995a). The giving way occurs as the person first puts weight on the affected leg, often on getting up after sitting for a while but may also occur as that side enters the stance phase during what has been an uneventful walk prior to that point. The problem is felt to relate to a 'slight slippage due to failure of the force closure mechanism of the [SI] joint, which should occur normally at this moment' (Dorman 1997: 512; Fig. 3.94). Although 'force closure' is mentioned, the problem is probably caused by a combination of:

1. a failure of the muscles that would normally help to stabilize the joint ('force' closure), in that the contraction
   a. is inadequate, as in the case of actual muscle weakness
   b. occurs in an uncoordinated manner, as with impairment of neural control
2. a failure of the supporting ligaments, with a loss of the normal elasticity in the posterior sacroiliac ligaments ('form' closure) that may have been caused by:
   a. the constant tension they have been subjected to by the malalignment, or
   b. a definite injury, such as a ligament strain or tear, which sebsequently healed in a lengthened position because a co-existing malalignment problem was never corrected (Fig. 2.51B).

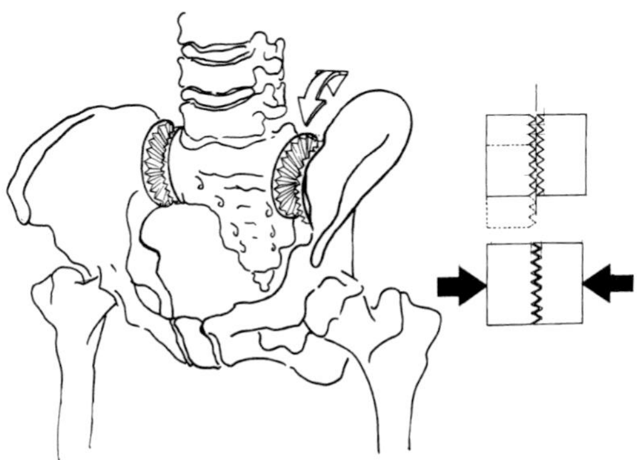

Fig. 3.94 Whimsical depiction of sacroiliac joints with friction device. Failure can result in what has been called a 'slipping clutch' phenomenon, with a sensation of something giving way in the hip girdle region. *(Courtesy of Vleeming et al. 1997.)*

Recovery is achieved through the combination of muscle strengthening and retraining for coordinated contraction, prolotherapy injections to tighten up the ligaments and simultaneous ongoing efforts at achieving and maintaining realignment (see Ch. 7).

Persons with a history of recurrent ankle sprains may not experience any pain preceding such a 'sprain', or the pain may occur only rarely. If tenderness is present, it may be limited to the lateral ankle ligaments, and rarely includes the peroneal muscles or tendons. There is sometimes an obvious precipitating event, such as stepping off a curb or onto a pebble, that causes the inversion or eversion to occur but the history often suggests that the ankle 'just gives way'. Ankle inversion sprains tend to be more common than eversion sprains, the left ankle being involved more often than the right.

He or she is usually diagnosed as having a 'chronically unstable ankle', with lengthening of the ligaments that is attributed to the previous sprains or strains. Ligament lengthening and ankle instability may certainly be evident on clinical examination. In the author's experience, however, that is very often not the case. In those presenting with one of the 'more common' patterns of 'rotational malalignment' or an 'upslip', passively moving the subtalar joint with the tibio-talar joint locked at 90 degrees - when a ligament laxity is most likely to become evident - consistently reveals an actual limitation of left inversion and an increase in eversion compared to the right side (Fig. 3.27). However, the shift in weight-bearing toward right pronation, left supination becomes apparent in standing or on walking. Also, in addition to the inability to muster a full-strength contraction of the right ankle invertors and left evertors, there may be an obvious difficulty with knowing how to move the right foot 'up and in' and 'down and in' and the left 'down and out' on command, a problem alluded to above and one that can usually be overcome by providing tactile and other types of feedback. These findings suggest that, in the absence of any obvious ligament laxity, it is the functional weakness, possibly in combination with impaired proprioception and kinaesthetic awareness, that is responsible for the feeling of instability and that results in a problem of insecure placement of the foot and ankle and a tendency to recurrent sprains.

This conjecture was supported by Lentell et al. (1992: 85), whose studies on subjects with chronically unstable ankles indicate that impaired balance is more of a proprioceptive problem than weakness of the ankle invertors and evertors. They reported that strength studies failed to show a significant difference between the involved and the uninvolved side. A modified Romberg test, however, revealed differences in gross balance between the two extremities in the majority of subjects. These authors concluded that:

> *muscular weakness is not a major contributing factor to the chronically unstable ankle [and that] the findings do support the presence of proprioceptive deficits associated with this condition*

Their advice was to make proprioceptive activities a primary consideration in the management of this problem.

Reports by others (Freeman et al. 1965; Garn & Newton 1988; Glencross & Thornton 1981) all remarked on the apparent proprioceptive deficits and the need to improve kinaesthetic awareness in these individuals. There was no indication that the subjects were classified in some way according to alignment status in any of these studies.

> Unfortunately, if a coexisting problem of malalignment is responsible for the 'functional' weakness and apparent proprioceptive impairment, carrying out activities intended to improve ankle strength and kinaesthetic awareness, without simultaneous correction of the malalignment, may fail to improve matters significantly or do so only temporarily, if at all.

Given that the ankle ligaments often do not show laxity in those presenting with malalignment, how can they 'malfunction' – in terms of impaired proprioception and kinaesthetic awareness – in order to actually lead to recurrent ankle inversion sprains? Suppose that the medial part of the runner's left foot has just landed on a rock or curb that inadvertently tilts the left foot into increased lateral weight-bearing. Such a forced inversion results in a sudden increase in tension in the lateral ankle ligaments and would normally trigger a barrage of proprioceptive signals to quickly activate the ankle evertors. The timely, strong contraction of these muscles would usually be adequate to counter any further inversion and avert possible injury. For some reason, however, the sequence fails in those with malalignment and an ankle inversion sprain or strain can result. The following are some explanations to consider:

There is a malalignment-related functional weakness of the left peroneal muscles

The strength of the actual contraction achieved may be inadequate because of the functional weakness.

A failure or delay of peroneal muscle contraction may be the cause

Perhaps the tendency to supination on the left, as part of the malalignment, puts the lateral ligaments constantly under stretch and 'fatigues' the stretch receptors so that when they are suddenly put under an even greater load, they fail to respond appropriately.

a. Some of the mechanoreceptors may no longer respond, or they may respond at varying rates, so that the duration of the signal is increased but its strength (amplitude) decreased. The signal generated may be too weak to trigger an 'all or none' contraction of the ankle evertors.
b. Alternatively, generation of the signal may be delayed to the point that by the time it finally triggers the muscle contraction, it is too late to be of use - the ankle inversion has already occurred.

There is a temporary ligament deafferentation

In those presenting with malalignment who do not have any evidence of ligament laxity, the feeling of instability and the weakness of the left ankle evertors usually disappears with realignment. The 'kinaesthetic deficit' in these persons may be occurring on the basis of a temporary deafferentation linked to the malalignment.

There is some joint instability secondary to the malalignment

With malalignment, there is frequently a detectable instability of one or both SI joints that is abolished or decreased with realignment (Figs 2.113-2.115). This phenomenon may affect other joints as well but may not be as easily detectable, or it may just not be looked for on the examination. The knee, for example, may be unstable on account of excessive varus or valgus angulation, the contrary rotation of the femur on the tibia, or the weakness of some of the stabilizing muscles. Similarly, these are factors to consider when trying to explain the apparent instability of some of ankle joints and recurrent inversion sprains.

The problem of recurrent right ankle inversion sprains as it relates to the mechanical factor of increased varus angulation at rest and, more important, just as the foot contacts the ground, has been discussed above (Fig. 3.26).

Clinical correlation: balance

Balance plays a major role in ensuring a stable landing on a jump or dismount. For example, when a gymnast sways momentarily on landing, or even has to take a small step to aid recovery, we talk in terms of the athlete having lost his or her 'footing'. Could it be that in some cases the problem is actually caused by an unstable leg, the one the athlete may also prove to have trouble standing on when carrying out the kinetic rotational (Gillet) or single-leg stance test? Maybe this leg sometimes simply 'gives way' when suddenly having to weight-bear on landing, or just feels insecure as a result of some of the factors cited above.

The 'slipping clutch' phenomenon offers another possible explanation. This 'loss of balance' may often be just another manifestation of how the changes associated with malalignment can interfere with athletic performance. It would be more of a problem in those sports in which the athlete has to land on one leg (e.g. figure-skating). In order to avoid the mishaps that might otherwise occur, this 'instability' could conceivably lead to a leg preference and/or a habit of approaching the task repeatedly from the same, more dependable side.

Sports such as fencing, karate and judo involve 'lunging' or rapidly moving one foot forward in a straight line (Figs 5.10, 5.13D). Maximum stability derives from placement of the knee directly over the advancing foot. A malalignment-related shift off centre to right or left decreases stability and may prove costly at a time when this foot is supporting most of the athlete's weight (see Ch. 5).

Some moves in sports such as karate and judo require a rapid rotation of the body while supported on just one leg. The 'roundhouse' kick, for example, requires balancing on one foot at a time when the body is rotating to develop the momentum required to deliver a good blow with the other leg (Fig. 5.14B,C). Again, the athlete may have a leg preference when it comes to making a turn supported on one leg. This preference is more likely to relate to a feeling of stability when supported on that leg, rather than leg dominance. Another factor may be the asymmetry of pelvic and lower extremity ranges of motion.

THE 'MALALIGNMENT SYNDROME' ASSOCIATED WITH A SACROILIAC JOINT 'UPSLIP'

Apart from 'rotational malalignment', the other common presentation of asymmetric malalignment associated with aspects of the 'malalignment syndrome' is the 'upslip': displacement of the SI joint surfaces by upward translation of an innominate, relative to the sacrum, in the vertical plane.

'Upslips' and 'downslips' have been discussed at length in Ch. 2. As indicated, a 'downslip' occurs less frequently than an 'upslip' and will not be discussed further, other than to summarize that typically:

1. the person has sustained a traction force injury to the extremity involved; for example, the body being thrown forward at a time when the foot on that side was still being held back in stirrups, stuck in mud, or otherwise restrained
2. the 'downslip' was missed on initial examination; it is usually discovered when the person fails to respond to treatment for what appears to be an 'upslip' of the opposite side, raising suspicions that eventually lead to a reassessment and, finally, treatment aimed at correcting the 'downslip'.

In one of the author's studies of 122 patients seen in succession at the office, none presented with a 'downslip' (Schamberger 2002). 12% presented with an 'upslip' alone; that is, all the innominate landmarks up and the leg short on that side. In 9%, an 'upslip' became evident following the correction of a 'rotational malalignment'. That is, while the innominate was shifted upward, the presence of the 'upslip' in these 9% was masked by a coexisting 'rotational malalignment', with the complete asymmetry of the landmarks and usually contrary rotation of the innominates (Fig. 2.61B). Therefore, the combined total of those presenting with an 'upslip' was 21%. An 'upslip' is also seen in 5-10% of those presenting with an 'outflare/inflare' and usually readily discernible on initial examination.

The 'malalignment syndrome' noted in association with an 'upslip' is, in large part, the same as that seen with the 'more common' patterns of 'rotational malalignment' and has been alluded to throughout the discussion above. Similarities and salient differences will be discussed briefly at this time under the same headings as for 'rotational malalignment'. Unless otherwise stated, it is assumed that leg length is equal; i.e. there is no associated anatomical (true) LLD.

Asymmetry of pelvic orientation with translation in the vertical plane

On the side of the 'upslip', the upward translation of the innominate relative to the sacrum results in an elevation of all the anterior and posterior bony landmarks - PSIS, ASIS, pubic rami and iliac crest - relative to those on the opposite side (Fig. 2.61A). This shift, which includes a 2–3 mm step deformity at the symphysis pubis, is best observed in supine- and prone-lying (Fig. 2.73A,B) and an anteroposterior standing X-Ray of the pelvis (though these findings should be apparent on clinical examination and only rarely require an X-Ray for diagnosis). The leg is short on the side of the 'upslip', best seen in supine or prone-lying and on the sitting-lying test (Fig. 2.73A,B). The high side of the pelvis in sitting or standing does not always correspond with the side of the 'upslip'. For example, with a 'right upslip', the iliac crest is high on the right side in standing, sitting and lying prone. Those with a 'left upslip' present with the left iliac crest high in lying; however, it is the right iliac crest that is usually high in standing, often also when sitting. These findings suggest that the 'upslip' may be associated with some rotation of the pelvic unit around the sagittal axis in the coronal (frontal) plane (Figs 2.9, 2.73B).

As indicated, approximately 10% of upslips exist in isolation; there is no rotation of the innominate involved around the coronal axis, nor is there any torsion of the sacrum. However, an 'upslip' can coexist with any one or all of the other presentations of malalignment: 'rotational', 'outflare/inflare', sacral torsion and vertebral rotational displacement. When the 'upslip' coexists with a 'rotational malalignment', the asymmetries caused by innominate rotation in the sagittal plane usually hide the presence of the 'upslip'. However, the upward translation on the side of the 'upslip' may either accentuate some of the asymmetries caused by the 'rotational malalignment', or make them less easily discernable. For example, in someone with a 'right anterior, left posterior' innominate rotation who develops a coexistent 'right upslip':

1. the step deformity of the pubic bones seen initially - down on the right relative to the left side (Figs 2.42, 2.76C) - may now appear decreased or no longer discernible because of the 'right upslip'
2. the rotational downward displacement of the right ASIS may now be less obvious, the upward displacement of the right PSIS accentuated on comparison to the left side (Fig. 2.61B)

Correction of the 'rotational malalignment' will reveal the underlying 'right upslip', with all right landmarks now up relative to those on the left (Fig. 2.73A).

Pelvic orientation and movement in the transverse plane

On standing, there may be some minimal rotation around the vertical axis evident, causing the ASIS to protrude slightly forward on the right or left side. However, the actual full range of motion in the transverse plane is symmetrical to right and left (unlike those with 'rotational malalignment', who show a restriction into the side of the 'posterior' rotation; Fig. 3.5C).

Sacroiliac joint mobility

The force that pushed the innominate upward (craniad) relative to the sacrum may actually have 'jammed' the SI joint in the vertical plane. However, there is usually no restriction of mobility evident on the sacral flexion and extension, kinetic rotational (Gillet) and SI joint stress tests.

Curvature of the lumbar, thoracic and cervical segments

There is an obliquity of the pelvis, usually high on the right side in standing and sitting, often even in those with a left 'upslip'. Studies on persons presenting with either a right or left upslip indicated approximately a 50/50 distribution in those with the lumbar curve convex to the right or left (Schamberger 2002). Regardless of the direction, the lumbar curve typically reverses at the thoracolumbar junction to give rise to a thoracic curve convex to the opposite side, with a further reversal that can happen somewhere in the upper thoracic spine but usually occurs at the cervicothoracic junction (Fig. 2.91).

As with 'rotational malalignment', asymmetry of head and neck movement typically includes a limitation of right rotation and left side-flexion (Fig. 3.10).

Asymmetry of the thorax, shoulder girdle and arms

The findings are similar to those seen with the 'more common' patterns of 'rotational malalignment'; for example, the right glenohumeral joint shows increased external and decreased internal rotation compared to the left (Fig. 3.17A).

Asymmetry of leg orientation and ROM

The pattern is similar to that described for the 'more common' patterns of 'rotational malalignment': external rotation of the right and internal rotation of the left lower extremity.

Asymmetry of foot alignment, weight-bearing and shoe wear

This is the same as seen with the 'more common' rotational patterns: a shift tending to right pronation and left supination.

Asymmetry of lower extremity muscle tension

The asymmetry that results with an 'upslip' appears to be in the same pattern as that associated with 'rotational malalignment'. There is, for example, increased tension in the left gluteus medius/minimus and TFL/ITB complex (limiting left hip adduction on Ober's test; Fig. 3.44) and in the right ankle dorsiflexors, left plantarflexors (Fig. 3.84). This would support the conjecture that the asymmetry of tension is not determined by the actual presentation of pelvic malalignment but more likely by spinal segmental or cortical factors.

The 'upslip' itself may be the result of an asymmetry in muscle tension. A 'left upslip', for example, can result from an increase in tension in the left quadratus lumborum or psoas major or minor (Fig. 2.62). This increase in tension may, in turn, be attributable to:

1. an underlying muscle injury

   For example, left quadratus lumborum can be stretched to the point of causing a sprain or strain by:

   a. reaching excessively forward and to the right, or
   b. picking up a weight from that awkward position, especially if the weight turns out to be heavier than expected (Figs 2.43, 2.44)
2. 'facilitation' of one or both of these muscles
3. irritation or actual injury of the nerve supply by vertebral rotational displacement (commonly involving L1 and less often L2 or L3 vertebrae)
4. a protective splinting reaction involving these muscles, such as may occur with pain from nearby ligaments (e.g. iliolumbar) or the SI joint that are being put under stress by the malalignment.

Asymmetry of lower extremity muscle strength

The asymmetry is similar to that found in association with the 'more common' rotational patterns (see Appendix 4).

Asymmetry of ligament tension

Tenderness of one or more of the posterior pelvic ligaments (iliolumbar, posterior SI joint and sacrotuberous) can be seen on one or both sides in association with a 'right' or 'left upslip'. Some ligaments will end up in a shortened position; for example, the iliolumbar ligaments on the side of the 'upslip' (Fig. 2.4A). With time, these 'shortened' ligaments may undergo contracture and feel especially 'tight' or even temporarily painful on correction of the 'upslip' until their proper length has finally been regained, usually within some 2–4 weeks of maintaining alignment.

The tension in several other ligaments will increase because the upward shift of an innominate relative to the sacrum separates their origin and insertion; they may undergo lengthening with time. Likely to be affected are:

1. the anterior sacroiliac ligament (upper part; Fig. 2.4A), and
2. the long (dorsal) sacroiliac ligament (Figs 2.5A, 2.19).

Asymmetry of lower extremity ranges of motion

Hip flexion and extension are usually both symmetrical but passive hip flexion and/or extension are occasionally decreased on the side of the 'upslip'.

The difference may be attributable to an increase in tension on that side, caused by reflex splinting and/ or just tightness in the ipsilateral hamstrings and rectus femoris, respectively. The other hip ranges of motion, and those at the ankles, are asymmetrical in the same directions as with the 'more common' patterns of 'rotational malalignment'.

Apparent leg length difference

On the side of the 'upslip', the leg is drawn upward passively, along with the innominate. Assuming an anatomically equal leg length, the person will now have a short leg evident on that side. The difference in length may amount to no more than 3-5 mm but is usually easily discernible in both long-sitting and supine-lying and does not change on going from one position to the other (Figs 2.73A,B, 2.82). Since an anatomical LLD in isolation will also present with one leg short by an equal amount in both positions, consider the steps outlined in Box 3.9 when trying to differentiate one from the other. In particular, the unilateral upward shift of all the pelvic landmarks and the asymmetry of lower extremity tension and strength seen with the 'upslip' will quickly help separate it from a 'true' LLD.

BOX 3.9 Effect of concommitant leg length difference on the diagnosis of an 'upslip'

1. The diagnosis of an 'upslip' should never be based simply on the finding of a leg length difference (LLD) that remains exactly the same on both parts of the 'sitting-lying' test; always check the position of the innominate landmarks as well, which will all be:
   a. displaced upward, both anteriorly and posteriorly, on the side of the 'upslip'
   b. in their normal position and symmetrical when one is dealing with an anatomical 'true' LLD alone.
2. A concommitant anatomical (true) LLD, long on the side of the 'upslip', could compensate for, or even exceed, the shortening of the leg that has occurred because of the 'upslip'; however, in sitting and lying all the pelvic landmarks remain displaced upward on the side of the 'upslip' compared to the sacrum and the opposite side while the pelvic obliquity persists.
3. The presence or absence of an anatomical LLD is best established after correction of the 'upslip' and rarely requires resorting to a comparison of the height of the femoral heads on a standing X-ray to do so.

COMMENTS REGARDING THE 'MALALIGNMENT SYNDROME' AND 'OUTFLARE/INFLARE' PRESENTATION

'Outflare' and 'inflare' have been described extensively in Ch. 2. It has also been repeatedly noted that the 'malaligment syndrome', as defined at the beginning of this chapter, is a conglomeration of signs and symptoms seen only in association with 'rotational malalignment' and an 'upslip'. To emphasize this point, here follows a discussion of key aspects that comprise the 'malalignment syndrome' and whether they feature in any way in those presenting with just an 'outflare/inflare' on its own. Again, it is assumed that there is no underlying anatomical (true) LLD unless specifically indicated.

Pelvic orientation and movement around the vertical axis in the transverse plane

Rotation of the right or left innominate around the vertical axis in the transverse plane - either individually or involving both - is a key feature of the 'flare' presentations. 'Outflare' and 'inflare' are called by the positioning of the anterior aspect of the innominates toward or away from midline. The ASIS is a especially well suited landmark for assessing such a change (Figs 2.13A,Bi). With clockwise rotation, the left innominate 'inflares' (i.e., the left ASIS moves toward midline) and the right 'outflares' (i.e., the right ASIS moves away from midline). This translates into the left ASIS:

1. ending up higher than the right ASIS when lying supine (Figs 2.13Aiii, 2.64A,B)
2. being positioned forward relative to the right ASIS in standing and sitting

Sometimes, the fact that there has been innominate rotation is easily - and more accurately - discernible on comparison of the height of the right and left PSIS and their distance from the midline crease when the person is lying prone; positioning of these landmarks will be the opposite to those on the front (Fig. 2.13Ci): the right PSIS is closer to midline (= 'right outflare') and the left further away (= 'left inflare').

The trunk may rotate along with the pelvic displacement, backward on the side of the 'outflare' and forward on the side of the 'inflare' but more often faces straight forward, like the feet, and thereby can make the presence of a 'flare' more easily evident to the person on self-assessment simply by looking straight downward at the anterior pelvic landmarks when standing or sitting.

A person with a 'right outflare, left inflare' may report that when walking quickly and even more likely when running, there is a sensation that:

1. the pelvis and trunk tend to rotate toward the side of the right 'outflare' (in keeping with the clockwise rotation of the innominate)
2. during the swing phase:
   a. there is an apparent 'block' to swinging the leg through on the right 'outflare' side, where backward movement of the innominate in the transverse plane now orients the hip joint more posteriorly and the femur can impinge earlier against the superoanterior acetabular rim
   b. it seems easier to swing the left leg forward (in keeping with the fact that on this, the left 'inflare' side, the hip joint is now oriented more anteriorly, with the superoanterior acetabular rim positioned further forward)

On full correction of the 'outflare/inflare', the person should no longer be aware of:

1. a 'block' on attempting to rotate the pelvic unit toward the 'inflare' side in standing
2. a problem achieving an unhindered swing-through of the leg on the 'outflare' side.

Pelvic orientation in the coronal (frontal) plane

The pelvis is level, given that leg length is assumed to be equal and there has only been rotation of the innominate(s) around the vertical axis in the transverse plane.

Sacroiliac joint mobility

No SI joint 'locking' and no instabilitiy relating simply to the 'outflare' and 'inflare' are observed (unlike 'rotational malalignment', in which the joint surface displacement alone can result in 'locking' or some joint instability in the absence of actual ligament laxity, joint degeneration or muscle weakness).

Curvature of the lumbar, thoracic and cervical segments

There will be a torsional effect on the lumbosacral junction and the spine resulting from any passive clockwise or counterclockwise rotation of the pelvic unit in the transverse plane with the 'flare'. Therefore, a lumbar convexity of varying degree, with reversal at points proximally (thoracolumbar, cervicothoracic) may be evident. However, given that the pelvis remains level with a 'flare' presentation and barring any underlying pathology (e.g. disc or facet degeneration, marked soft tissue contracture, muscle spasm), the curves are less marked than with an 'upslip' or 'rotational malalignment'.

Asymmetry of the thorax, shoulder girdle and arms

The thorax may compensate by rotating in the direction opposite to any pelvic rotation in the transverse plane so that the trunk ends up facing forward or just slightly the opposite way. Shoulder and arm ranges of motion are symmetrical, the shoulders are level and one usually does not see winging of the scapula just on account of the 'flare'.

Asymmetry of leg orientation and ROM

On the 'outflare' side, there is the 'backward and out' reorientation of the acetabulum: the now more forward-lying superoanterior acetabular rim is in a position to interfer with hip flexion and straight leg raising (SLR). On the 'inflare' side, the acetabulum comes to lie more 'forward and in', with the infero-posterior rim in a position to limit primarily hip extension.

The clockwise rotation of the pelvic unit typically seen with 'right outflare, left inflare' results in some passive leg rotation: the right externally, left internally. This may be evident when the person is at rest, lying prone or supine. The rotation is not likely to be noticeable when standing - the toes usually point forward - suggesting the change is minimal or that there has been some accommodation, as might occur with active contraction of right internal and left external rotators.

In summary:

1. The reorientation of the acetabula that occurs with 'right outflare' and 'left inflare' creates a block primarily to:
   a. right hip flexion and straight leg raising
   b. left hip extension
2. Clockwise rotation of the innominates results in some passive leg rotation in prone or supine-lying: the right externally and left internally, respectively. The reverse findings are seen on counterclockwise rotation with a 'left outflare, right inflare': passive right internal, left external rotation.

Asymmetry of foot alignment, weight-bearing and shoe wear

There is no aymmetry of these noted with an 'outflare/inflare' but they may be affected by inherent traits (e.g. whether the person is a pronator or supinator, has genu varum or valgum), or problems that can cause pain and alter weight-bearing (e.g. hallux varum or valgum, Morton's toe or neuralgia), independent of a 'flare' being present.

Asymmetry of lower extremity muscle tension

There is no indication of an asymmetrical pattern of tension, as seen with an 'upslip' or 'rotational malalignment'. However, when standing, weight-bearing on both feet, any rotation of the pelvic ring with a 'flare' will increase tension in some pelvic muscles by separating their origin and insertion while relaxing their partner on the opposite side. For example, rotation clockwise (that is, 'left inflare, right ouflare') passively increases tension:

1. on the left 'inflare' side - particularly in piriformis (Figs 2.5B, 2.46A, 4.17)
2. on the right 'outflare' side - in iliacus, adductors, sartorius, gluteus medius/minimus and the TFL/ITB complex

Asymmetry of lower extremity muscle strength

Muscle strength is symmetrical and full (5/5) in upper and lower extremities.

Asymmetry of ligament tension

Remember, one can have just a one-sided 'outflare' or 'inflare' present on its own. If so, the effect would be:

1. with a 'right outflare' only

   The pelvis on the right side 'opens up' like a book, so to speak: the innominate, 'hinged' at the SI joint, moves outward and opens the SI joint anteriorly while closing it posteriorly. The shift results in:

   a. increased tension in the ipsilateral deep iliolumbar ligament, also the anterior ligaments and capsule of the symphysis pubis and SI joint (Figs 2.4A,B, 2.5A, 3.64-3.66)
   b. decreased tension in the ipsilateral superior iliolumbar, sacrospinous, posterior SI joint, interosseous, long (dorsal) sacroiliac ligaments (Figs 2.5A, 2.13Aiii, 2.19B).
2. with a 'left inflare' only

   The front of the left innominate moves inward, closing the SI joint anteriorly while opening it posteriorly. The pattern of increased and decreased ligament tension is the opposite to that documented for a 'right outflare'.

The presentation of a combined 'right outflare, left inflare' would, therefore, result in an associated increase in tension as outlined and affect primarily the right anterior and left posterior ligaments, respectively.

Asymmetry of lower extremity ranges of motion

See 'Asymmetry of lower extremity orientation' above.

Apparent leg length difference

Leg length is equal, provided that there is no anatomical (true) LLD.

COMBINATIONS OF ASYMMETRIES: A SUMMARY

People not infrequently present with combinations of asymmetries and the findings on examination may at first be confusing. The choice of treatment and the prognosis very much depend on accurately diagnosing which of the 3 main presentations are at hand. Keep in mind the following:

'Rotational malalignment'

1. occurs in about 80% of those presenting with malalignment
2. of these, the right innominate is rotated anteriorly in 80-90% and the left in 10-20%

'Outflare' and 'Inflare'

1. occurs in 40-50%
2. there may be just a unilateral 'outflare' or 'inflare' in isolation but usually they present in combination (e.g. 'right outflare, left inflare')

'Upslip'

1. occurs in isolation in 10%

2. another 10% are found in combination with a 'rotational malalignment', 'outflare/inflare', or both
3. an 'upslip' is easily distinguished from a coexisting 'outflare/inflare' but may not become evident until a coexisting 'rotational malalignment' has been corrected

Changing presentation(s)

1. 5–10%, especially those who are hypermobile and patients during the early phase of their treatment, may readily switch from one presentation and/or side to another
2. for example, they can appear with:
   a. one, two or all three presentations of malalignment at one time,
   b. the same pattern, but with a reversal of sides, at another time, or
   c. combinations that, sometimes, are seen to change again within hours or days from those documented on the previous examination (e.g. 'right anterior rotation, left upslip' on one day, 'left anterior rotation, right upslip, right outflare/left inflare' on another)
   d. a coexisting sacral and/or vertebral rotational displacement, which may also occur in isolation and vary in type/direction/level involved on repeat examinations
3. this variability usually becomes less and less of a problem as:
   a. stability improves with core muscle strengthening (see Ch. 7)
   b. realignment is being maintained for increasingly longer periods of time, and
   c. the body tissues and brain start to adjust to being in alignment

Anatomical (true) LLD

1. found in approximately 10% of the population
2. it will affect the findings associated with a coexisting malalignment

Step-wise approach: reaching a diagnosis

The following approach should be helpful in trying to distinguish between the 3 main presentations and various combinations.

First, establish whether there is any pelvic obliquity in standing

1. if there is, and if it is abolished in sitting, the obliquity is most likely caused by an anatomical (true) LLD
2. a coexistent 'outflare/inflare' will still have to be ruled out (see below)

If the obliquity is not abolished in sitting, 'rotational malalignment' and/or 'upslip' is probably present

1. obliquity in sitting, unfortunately, is not helpful in differentiating between the two, or whether one or the other involves the right or left side; for example:
   a. someone with a 'left upslip' may actually show a high right posterior iliac crest in standing and sitting, and the left crest high only when lying prone (Fig. 2.73B)
   b. someone with 'right anterior' innominate rotation may show the left iliac crest high in standing and/or sitting but always the right crest up when lying prone
2. while the possibility that the persistent obliquity may be attributable to injury (e.g. fracture) or a developmental problem affecting the pelvis, hip and/or spine needs to be considered:
   a. these occur considerably less frequently than the 80-90% of the population presenting with malalignment
   b. they are very likely to become suspect as a problem from the history and clinical examination findings, in which case further investigations may be in order
   c. symptoms stemming from an injury or developmental anomaly are likely to be worsened by the stress imposed by a coexistent malalignment problem

Next, establish the differential diagnosis by carrying out tests for anatomical (true) LLD and the 3 main presentations

1. the 'long-sitting and supine-lying' test
2. side-to-side comparison of landmarks, and
3. assessment for any of the asymmetries that are part of the 'malalignment syndrome', seen only with an 'upslip' and 'rotational malalignment'; strength is particularly easy to check (eg. EHL)

A. an anatomically (true) short leg only

1. similarly to an 'upslip', the leg will be short to an equal extent both in sitting and lying as the legs

move together: downward on long-sitting, upward on supine-lying

2. however:

 (a) in standing, the pelvis will always be lower on the short-leg side, and

 (b) in sitting and lying, the right and left pelvic landmarks match up, being level both anteriorly and posteriorly.

3. the above findings will also be evident in someone presenting with a coexistent 'outflare/inflare' but would be hidden by an 'upslip' or 'rotational malalignment'

B. an 'upslip' only

1. on the 'sitting-lying' test, the legs will move downward and upward together but, on the side of the 'upslip', the leg will be short in both sitting and lying to an equal extent, and
2. all the anterior and posterior pelvic landmarks will have moved upward relative to the sacrum and opposite innominate
3. on having the person sit or lie down to remove the influence of the lower extremities on the pelvis, the pelvic obliquity that results with an 'upslip' will become evident in both positions; also noting that the anterior and posterior pelvic landmarks are up on the left side would support suspicions of a left 'upslip'.

C. a coexistent 'upslip' and anatomical (true) LLD

1. Aspects of the 'malalignment syndrome' are seen with the 'upslip'. A quick test of first toe extensor strength (extensor hallucis longus, or EHL), will show:
   a. comparative weakness on the right in someone with a coexistent 'upslip' (as occurs with a coexistent 'rotational malalignment'); whereas
   b. in someone whose pelvis is in alignment, the right EHL will prove full strength and equal to the left, regardless of whether there is a coexistent anatomical (true) LLD
2. cumulative or cancelling effect on leg length
   a. the shortening seen on the 'sitting-lying' test will be cumulative if the anatomical short leg is on the same side as the 'upslip'
   b. the difference in leg length on one side may cancel out that on the opposite side; for example, an anatomically short right leg may be offset by a 'left upslip', so that:
      i. there may no longer be a leg length difference evident in the long-sitting and supine-lying positions
      ii. the pelvis may now appear level in standing if the effect of the left 'upslip' cancels out that of the short right leg.

D. an 'outflare/inflare' only

1. the leg length is equal so that:
   a. the pelvis will be level in standing
   b. the legs move downward and upward together on the 'sitting-lying' test and their length matches in both positions
2. the innominate rotation around the vertical axis in the transverse plane:
   a. will bring the ASIS forward and in toward midline on the 'inflare' side (= ASIS high when supine), outward and away from midline on the 'outflare' side (= ASIS low when supine)
   b. remember the **Rule of the 4 'O's (= Outflare) and 4 'I's (= Inflare)**
   c. findings will be the opposite when using the PSIS as the landmark in prone-lying (Figs 2.13, 2.66-2.68)
3. there is no indication of the 'malalignment syndrome'; e.g. no asymmetry of muscle tension or strength, no shift in weight-bearing)

E. a coexistent 'outflare/inflare' and 'upslip'

Excepting the fact that the legs move together on the 'sitting-lying' test (downward with sitting, upward with lying) in both, there are some findings that can readily define the presence of each entity:

1. 'upslip': leg short to same extent on sitting-lying test, upward displacement of unilateral pelvic landmarks, pelvic obliquity in all positions, 'malalignment syndrome' present (e.g. comparative weakness of right EHL)
2. 'outflare/inflare': the key feature is that there is a definite rotation of the innominate around the vertical axis, with displacement of ASIS and PSIS evident, (described under Point D; Fig. 2.13); leg length equal

F. 'rotational malalignment' only

1. the difference in leg length changes on moving from the long-sitting to the supine-lying position; that is, there is a shift in leg length
2. the leg that lengthens on supine-lying indicates the side of a probable 'anterior' innominate rotation but this needs to be confirmed by finding:
   a. anterior landmarks (e.g. ASIS and pubic bone) are lower on that side as well; remember the **'Rule of the 5 'L's**:

Leg Lengthens Lying, Landmarks Lower = side of the 'anteriorly' rotated innominate

b. there is likely (but not necessarily) also a compensatory 'posterior' rotation of the opposite innominate
c. complete asymmetry of all the pelvic landmarks: right compared to left, anterior to posterior
d. findings of the 'malalignment syndrome' are evident

G. 'rotational malalignment' coexistent with an 'outflare/inflare'

1. 'rotational malalignment': pelvic obliquity, functional LLD, shift in leg length on sitting-lying test, evidence of the 'malalignment syndrome'
2. 'outflare/inflare': there is obvious displacement of the ASIS anteriorly and PSIS posteriorly
   a. relative to the midline, and
   b. in the transverse plane

H. 'rotational malalignment' coexistent with an 'upslip'

1. findings of the 'rotational malalignment' are readily apparent and may completely hide the presence of a concomitant 'upslip'
2. correction of the 'rotational malalignment':
   (a) may reveal the underlying 'upslip', which is then treated
   (b) rarely results in simultaneous resolution of the 'upslip'

I. combination of all 3 presentations: 'rotational malalignment', 'outflare/inflare', 'upslip'

The coexistent 'rotational malalignment' and 'outflare/inflare' can be readily defined (see Point H); whereas the 'upslip' may not become obvious until the 'rotational malalignment' has been corrected (see Points B, E).

IV. which leg actually ends up being the longer or shorter one on the 'long-sitting, supine-lying' test is irrelevant

1. the key is to determine:
   a. if there is a relatively short leg
   b. if it is short the same amount on sitting and lying - query 'upslip' or an anatomical (true) LLD
   c. if the leg length shifts - query 'rotational malalignment'
2. as indicated above, 'rotational malalignment' may coexist with an 'outflare/inflare' and may or may not be hiding an 'upslip', anatomical LLD or both
3. the findings of an anatomical LLD will be readily apparent with a coexistent 'outflare/inflare' (see Point I)

V. examination of the relative position of the pelvic landmarks in supine and prone-lying

1. with an anatomical LLD, right and left-sided landmarks will be symmetrical, anteriorly and posteriorly
2. an 'upslip' results in a relative upward shift of all the ipsilateral landmarks
3. 'rotational malalignment' results in a complete asymmetry of landmarks on anterior/posterior and right/left comparison
4. the landmarks for 'outflare/inflare' will appear displaced relative to midline and in the transverse plane (see Point D)

The next chapter will explore some of the pain phenomena and medical problems commonly seen in association with the 'malalignment syndrome'.

Chapter 4

The malalignment syndrome: Related pain phenomena and the implications for medicine

CHAPTER CONTENTS

DOI: 10.1016/B978-0-443-06929-1.00004-1

One facet of the 'malalignment syndrome' seen in association with an 'upslip' and 'rotational malalignment' is the asymmetrical stress on soft tissues and joints that can eventually result in predictable sites of tenderness to palpation. With time, or as the result of a superimposed acute insult, these tender structures may become the source of overt localized and/or referred pain symptoms. The altered biomechanics also results in some commonly recognized pain patterns, injuries and 'syndromes' being seen with increased frequency in association with malalignment; right patello-femoral compartment syndrome is just one example (Figs 3.37, 3.38, 3.60 and see below). Unfortunately, treatment is often limited to the specific site of tenderness or pain, or to the particular pain syndrome, because of a failure to realize that these are but part of a greater entity: the 'malalignment syndrome'. Correct the malalignment and the associated pain phenomena will often disappear spontaneously or with little additional treatment.

Some common clinical conditions (e.g. idiopathic scoliosis) are unfavourably affected by coexistent malalignment. In addition, symptoms resulting from malalignment can sometimes mimic clinical problems typically implicating one or more of the major organ systems of the body; in particular, the cardiovascular, rheumatological, orthopaedic and neurological. The confusion that can result when trying to establish a diagnosis may lead to needless and sometimes costly and even dangerous investigations that, in the end, still fail to come up with the right diagnosis and recommendations for appropriate treatment.

PAIN CAUSED BY AN INCREASE IN SOFT TISSUE TENSION

The malalignment-related increase in tension involving muscle, ligament, capsule or fascia can occur by different mechanisms. To summarize, those capable of increasing the vectored force in these tissues include:

1. an increase in the length-tension ratio with any increase in the distance between the origin and insertion
2. torsion of the vertebral, pelvic or appendicular bones relative to one another
3. 'facilitation' and 'inhibition', noted to affect specific muscles in an asymmetrical pattern
4. an attempt to splint a painful or unstable area
5. a 'functional' leg length difference (LLD).

The first four mechanisms have been discussed in detail in Chapter 3 under 'Asymmetry of muscle tension' (Figs 3.42–3.47). A functional LLD affects tension in both static and dynamic situations. Take the example of a person whose right side of the pelvis is higher than the left when standing. There may be an increase in tension in right hip abductor muscles and the tensor fascia lata/iliotibial band (TFL/ITB) complex because the downward drop of the pelvis on the left side increases the distance between the origin and insertion of these same structures on the right (Fig. 4.1A). When weight-bearing on the short left leg during a walk or run, the left hip abductors have to work harder to counter any drop of the pelvis on the right, perhaps even to raise the pelvis further on the right side in order to allow the long right leg to clear the ground without hindrance to swing-through (Fig. 4.1B).

Box 4.1 denotes the structures that most consistently show an increase in tension and/or tenderness as a result of these various mechanisms relating to an 'upslip' and 'rotational malalignment'.

With time, any soft tissue subjected to an increase in tension because of the malalignment is likely to become tender to palpation (e.g. sacrotuberous ligament; DonTigny 1985; Midttun & Bojsen-Moller 1986; Brendstrap & Midttun 1998). That structure may eventually develop an aching discomfort or become outright painful. Mechanisms that can precipitate what is often characterized as a deep, achy bone pain include:

1. a chronic increase in tension, particularly as it affects:
   a. the muscles, which are supposed to relax after a contraction, and
   b. the ligaments, whose nerve supply cannot elongate as easily nor as much as the elastic components (Hackett 1958; see Ch. 3: 'Asymmetry of ligament tension' and Ch. 8)
2. any additional increase in tension, as may occur with:
   a. an acute stress incurred with a sudden movement or load imposed
   b. a persistent or repetitive stress caused by a call for increased effort during work or an athletic activity (e.g. running up- and downhill or longer distances without having prepared with progressively demanding workouts)

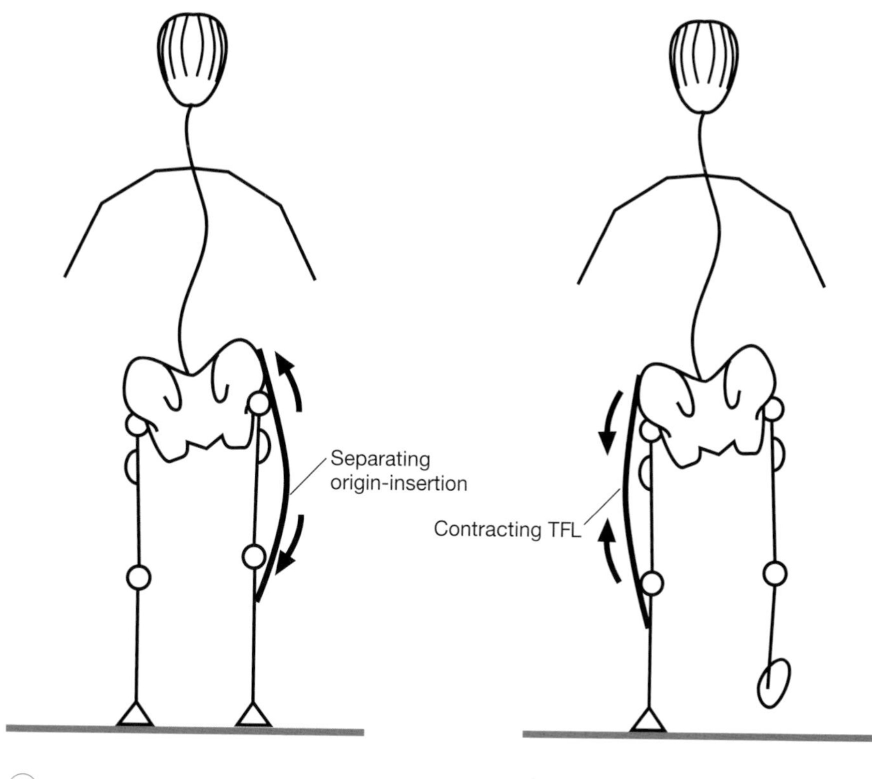

Fig. 4.1 Effect of functional leg length difference (right leg long in standing) on tension in the hip abductors and tensor fascia lata/iliotibial band complex. (A) Static: in standing, tension increases on the right side as the origin and insertion are separated and muscle contraction counteracts the drop of the pelvis to the left; the person can compensate by shifting the pelvis to the right (see Figs 2.58, 3.93). (B) Dynamic: when walking or running, tension increases on left weight-bearing as the left abductors contract to counter the drop of the right side of the pelvis and to help with clearance of the 'long' right leg.

BOX 4.1 Structures typically showing an increase in tension and/or tenderness with 'malalignment syndrome'

Muscles (Fig. 3.43)

1. right infraspinatus and/or teres minor
2. thoracic paravertebral muscles, especially those adjacent to sites of vertebral rotational displacement and curve reversal (e.g. the thoracolumbar junction)
3. piriformis, particularly the right one with 'right anterior' rotation present
4. iliopsoas, particularly the left one with 'left posterior' rotation present
5. the left hip abductors and TFL/ITB complex
6. the right hamstrings
7. the left gastrocnemius/soleus complex

Ligaments (Figs 2.4, 2.5, 2.6, 3.61–3.68)

1. the iliolumbar and sacrotuberous ligaments, and those crossing the posterior sacroiliac joint (often evident bilaterally)
2. the long dorsal sacroiliac ligaments (Fig 2.19B)
3. the lumbosacral intervertebral ligaments and facet joint ligaments

3. the tense structure being 'strung' over a bony or other elevation, possibly even 'snapping' across that prominence; e.g. the TFL over the greater trochanter and the ITB over the lateral femoral condyle (Fig. 3.41); iliacus, iliopsoas/pectineus and rectus femoris over the anterior femoral head and acetabular rim (Figs 2.46B,C, 2.59, 3.42, 4.2).

The long-term resolution of the pain from these structures will depend primarily on regaining normal muscle tone which, in turn, depends largely on achieving and maintaining alignment.

SPECIFICIC SITES OF PAIN RELATED TO MALALIGNMENT

The sometimes very specific and often predictable patterns of pain and tenderness to palpation seen in association with an SI joint 'upslip' and 'rotational malalignment' are primarily the result of the four factors outlined in Box 4.2.

Therefore, even though the person may be asymptomatic, examination will usually reveal tenderness localizing to the specific structures that are typically

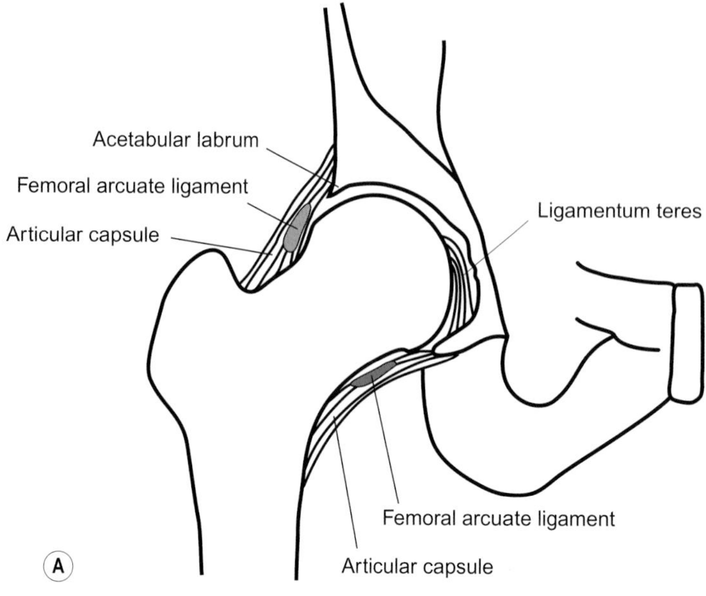

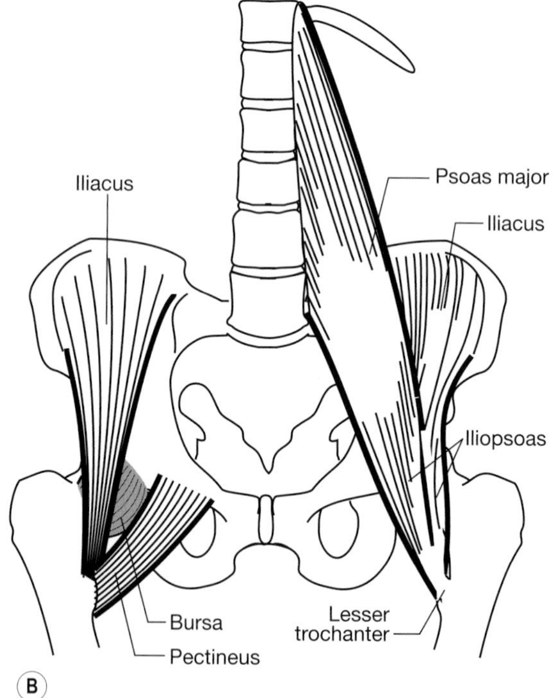

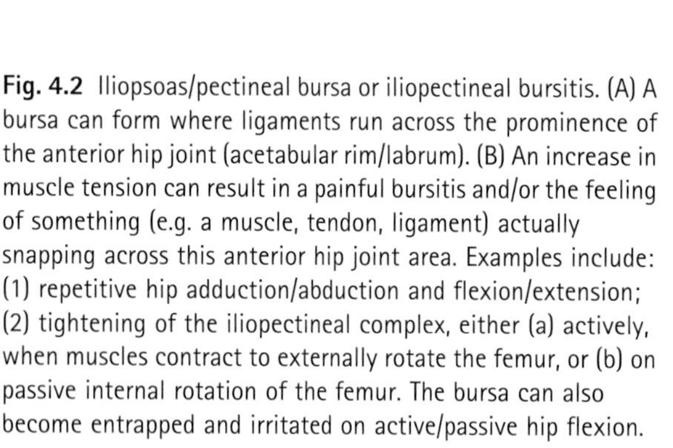

Fig. 4.2 Iliopsoas/pectineal bursa or iliopectineal bursitis. (A) A bursa can form where ligaments run across the prominence of the anterior hip joint (acetabular rim/labrum). (B) An increase in muscle tension can result in a painful bursitis and/or the feeling of something (e.g. a muscle, tendon, ligament) actually snapping across this anterior hip joint area. Examples include: (1) repetitive hip adduction/abduction and flexion/extension; (2) tightening of the iliopectineal complex, either (a) actively, when muscles contract to externally rotate the femur, or (b) on passive internal rotation of the femur. The bursa can also become entrapped and irritated on active/passive hip flexion.

BOX 4.2 Causes of pain on palpation seen with an 'upslip' and 'rotational malalignment'

1. a chronic increase in tension in a specific soft tissue structure (e.g. joint capsule, muscle, tendon or ligament)
2. unevenly distributed or excessive pressure within and around the joints, particularly those which are weight-bearing and/or subjected to a torsional stress by malalignment (e.g. the hip and knee joints; Figs 3.37, 3.60, 3.81, 3.82, 4.3)
3. an irritation or injury of nerve roots and peripheral nerves as a result of a chronic increase in traction, compression or a combination of these (Figs 3.12, 3.13, 3.37, 3.38 and 'Implications for neurology and neurosurgery' below).
4. a structure that is the source of referred pain to a distant site (Figs 3.12, 3.45, 3.46, 3.62, 3.63, 3.67, 4.8–4.10)

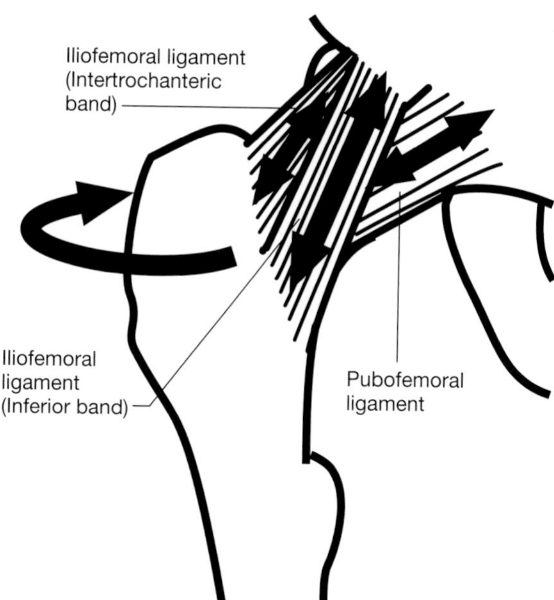

Fig. 4.3 Anterior hip joint capsule and iliofemoral and pubofemoral ligaments subjected to a torsional stress with malalignment-related external rotation of the right lower extremity (see also Figs 2.4A, 2.5A).

put under stress by the malalignment. He or she must be considered at increased risk of developing an overtly painful condition with any superimposed physical or mental stresses that inadvertently place additional demands on any of these sites.

EMOTIONAL STRESS

An acute emotional stress may trigger a 'fight or flight' reaction, with temporary release of epinephrine and an increase in muscle tone. A chronic emotional response, such as one provoked by a stressful life style and/or persistent pain, is associated with an increase in circulating stress-related neuropeptides and persistent increase in epinephrine and cortisol levels (Holstege et al. 1996; Sapolsky & Spencer 1997). One effect is to persistently keep the level of the resting muscle tone above normal.

Such an increase in tone in the pelvic muscles has been shown to increase compression of the SI joints (van Wingerden et al. 2001; Richardson et al. 2002) and would similarly affect hip joints if malalignment were present. Joint compression, in turn, may:

1. make the joints feel 'stiff'
2. precipitate or worsen joint pain
3. irritate joint nerve supply to the point of hypersensitivity; presumably, there is sensitization of both the peripheral and central nervous system fibres (Butler 2000; Butler & Moseley 2003, 2007; Moseley & Hodges 2005), also impaired output of sensory signals (e.g. proprioceptive) and misinterpretation of signals which, in turn, affects motor output

Emotional complications with regards to motor output may include:

1. muscle(s) triggered too easily and/or out of sequence because of the hypersensitivity to acetylcholine (see Ch. 3 and 'IMS', Ch. 8); hypersensitivity of nociceptive fibres results in a more readily evoked response with any further irritation of the joint, triggering reflex muscle contraction and worsening of the joint compression - in effect, initiating and perpetuating a vicious cycle
2. inadequate contraction as sensory signals may be scattered, not arrive in unison or be weak
3. increased tendency for 'flare-ups', with reflex spasm triggered more readily in reaction to a pain signal
4. problems on attempting a progressive rehabilitation programme; increasing the activity level now aggravates pain and triggers 'flare-ups' more easily
5. initially, intermittent avoidance of activity to avert these 'flare-ups' and pain; eventually, persistent

avoidance 'due to their fear of reinjury or an underlying belief that they are unable to perform because of their condition [fear avoidance]' (Vlaeyen & Linton 2000; Vlaeyen & Vancleef 2007).

PHYSICAL STRESS

Acute stress

Even a minor lifting or twisting action that exerts a further acute traction or compression force on an asymptomatic but tender structure may cause it to now become overtly painful. The person is often diagnosed as having sustained a 'sprain' or 'strain'.

Chronic or repetitive stress

The site may also become symptomatic when even a minor increase in stress is superimposed on a chronic or repetitive basis. A walker or runner with an 'upslip' or one of the 'more common' rotational patterns, for example, may be asymptomatic but on examination show increased tension and tenderness in the left hip abductors and TFL/ITB complex, attributable to the combined effect of the malalignment-related:

1. increase in tension in the left complex as a result of 'facilitation'
2. shift to left lateral weight-bearing, separating origin and insertion
3. functional weakness and tendency to fatigue more easily on this side

If that person now increases the number of miles walked or run on a surface with a slope banked downward to the left (e.g. running against the traffic in Canada or the USA, or with the traffic in the UK; walking clockwise on a hillside), there will be an accentuation of the left lateral shift, and the tendency toward supination and genu varum on this side (Figs 3.31, 3.36, 4.4A). The combination of increased mileage and left traction forces may, with time, make the already tender left hip abductors and TFL/ITB complex overtly symptomatic. Increasing the amount of up- and downhill running also puts more demand on this complex bilaterally; the more susceptible left complex is, however, again more likely to become symptomatic. Similarly, the left one is at increased risk with cutting actions (e.g. playing rugby, soccer or American football).

In essence, one is dealing with a type of 'overuse' injury. The person may get some relief on a slope banked upward to the left (Fig. 4.4B). Understandably, lateral traction forces are decreased with the left foot now on the upside and a straightening of the legs, possibly also some levelling of the pelvis which very likely is high on the right side because of the malalignment (Figs 2.72, 2.73, 2.76B). However, this practice should not be encouraged for safety reasons if it means running on a road going with the traffic.

Standard treatment measures that would be appropriate for a 'sprain' or 'strain' or a suspected 'overuse injury' are usually instituted. The injury in both cases may respond to such treatment, combined with rest, and the pain subside with healing.

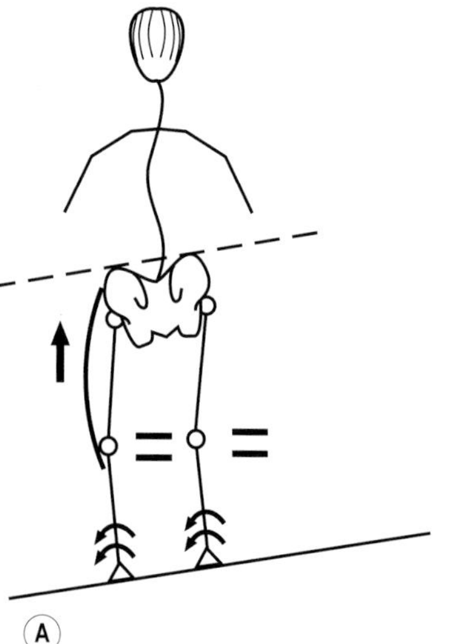

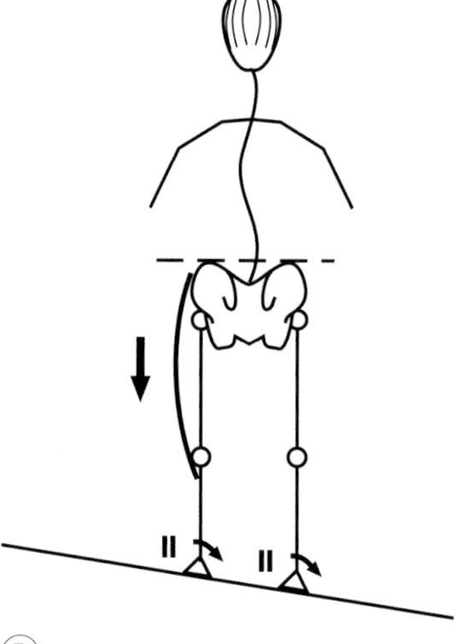

Fig. 4.4 Effect of a slope on the increased tension in the left hip abductors and tensor fascia lata/iliotibial band complex. Malalignment has already caused an increase in tension through 'facilitation' and the tendency to left supination. (A) Downslope to left increases the tension by accentuating supination. (B) Upslope to left decreases the tension by counteracting supination.

Unfortunately, if the malalignment is not corrected at the same time, the person remains at increased risk of having the same injury recur upon resuming the activity.

These injuries may actually fail to respond to standard treatment measures if malalignment persists or keeps on recurring.

> It appears that the persistence of chronic tension or compression forces attributable to malalignment can interfere with the ability of the tissue to heal following a superimposed acute or chronic injury.

In other words, recovery is slowed or may fail to occur until the stress caused by these forces is removed on realignment. Box 4.3 lists some ways in which the persistence of this stress could affect healing unfavourably.

BOX 4.3 Negative effect of malalignment stresses on healing

1. It interferes with the flow of blood needed for:
   a. the delivery of scavenger and repair cells, oxygen and nutrients
   b. the removal of damaged tissue and clearance of waste
2. Stretching a ligament results in excessive tension on nerve fibres long before the connective tissue components are affected because the nerve fibres have relatively less elasticity (Hackett 1956, 1958). The stretching can result in:
   a. irritation of the nociceptive axons, release of neuropeptides and initiation of a neurogenic inflammatory response (Willard 1995, 2007; see also Chs 7, 8)
   b. eventual frank hypersensitivity and even neuralgic pain, and
   c. aggravation of connective tissue degenerative processes.
3. The stresses relating to ongoing malalignment can then perpetuate these insults:
   a. to the nerves, with even relatively minor ongoing traction or compression forces risking development of a chronic painful condition
   b. to the bones and joints (e.g. disturbance of the nerve supply and constant compression of joint surfaces accelerates degeneration by interfering with cartilage nutrition and repair).

In summary, the recognition of the specific sites of tenderness and of the pain patterns typically associated with malalignment should:

1. raise suspicions that malalignment is indeed present
2. prompt a search for other features of the 'malalignment syndrome'
3. help to ensure appropriate treatment, the key component of this being realignment to remove any abnormal tension and/or compression forces and to promote healing.

COMMON PAIN SYNDROMES CAUSED OR AGGRAVATED BY MALALIGNMENT

A syndrome is a constellation of signs and symptoms attributable to a unifying cause. Although we may identify the syndrome and even recognize the cause, we must, however, always ask ourselves whether the syndrome or that cause may not be part of an even larger entity. A typical example is that of the person who presents with right knee pain of unknown origin. We may quickly arrive at a diagnosis of 'patellofemoral compartment syndrome' (PFCS) on the basis of the outward tracking of the patella on knee extension, a positive apprehension test and tenderness of the patellar tendon origin and the medial and lateral patellar facets. We have established patellofemoral compartment syndrome as the 'cause' of the pain but, in reality, it may amount to no more than having established the 'location' of the pain. We have not answered the questions of 'what caused the PFCS to develop in the first place?', 'why at this time?' and 'why on the right side and not the left, or bilaterally?'

If we look further, we might note that this individual pronates markedly with the right foot, causing the right knee to collapse into valgus on weight-bearing; whereas the left foot pronates less so, remains in neutral or actually supinates on toe-walking or hopping. The right lower extremity is in more obvious external rotation, the left less so or even in neutral or turned inward past midline (Fig. 3.19).

By looking beyond the right knee and at the kinetic chain, we have established the reason for the pain: excessive external rotation coupled with right pronation and increased valgus stress on the right knee, with an increase of the Q-angle and

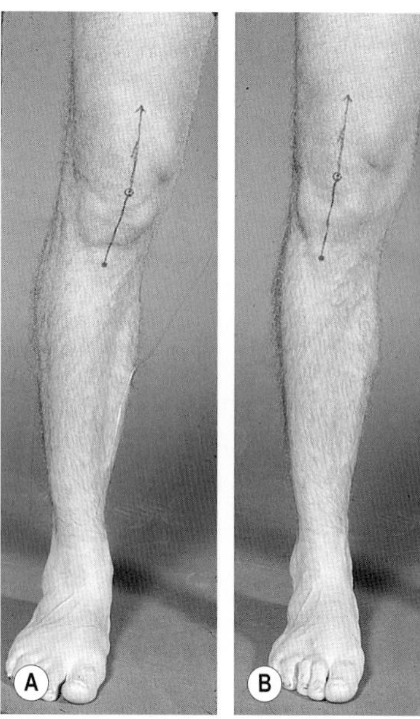

Fig. 4.5 Stresses predisposing to right patellofemoral compartment syndrome. (A) With malalignment: the tendency toward right pronation and knee valgus has here increased the Q-angle to 10 degrees. The right patella now tracks more laterally on knee extension, increasing the stress on the compartment. (B) On realignment: the Q-angle is reduced to almost 0 degrees; improved patellar tracking (relatively straight upward and downward) decreases the stress on the compartment.

lateral patellar tracking (Figs 3.37, 3.81, 4.5). The combined effect is an increase in tension in the right patellofemoral complex. Increasing the pressure with which the patella is forced onto the underlying femoral groove and condyles, and decreasing the accuracy with which the patellofemoral surfaces match up as the patella tends to track more laterally can eventually result in increased wear and tear, inflammation and pain.

Looking at the larger picture, namely the alignment of the pelvis and spine, we might find that he or she actually presents with an 'upslip', one of the 'more common' patterns of 'rotational malalignment', or both, and the resulting tendency to right external rotation, pronation and valgus stress. If the right side of the pelvis were higher than the left on standing - which it is in about 80% or more of those with a 'rotational' presentation and most of those with an 'upslip' - the increase in pressure within the right patellofemoral compartment could be compounded by:

1. keeping the right knee slightly flexed in an attempt to lower the pelvis on that side (Fig. 2.90)
2. secondary wasting of right vastus medialis (Figs 3.57, 3.58) that may relate to:
   a. unfavourable reorientation of the muscle fibres (Figs 3.59. 3.60)
   b. decrease in muscle tension with right quadiceps 'inhibition' and, if there is also right innominate 'anterior' rotation, approximation of the origin and insertion (Fig. 3.42)
   c. inability to muster as strong a contraction as usual, on account of these changes

MALALIGNMENT: IMPLICATIONS FOR MEDICINE

The patellofemoral syndrome discussed above did not represent just an isolated phenomenon but was an integral part of a larger entity, the 'malalignment syndrome', and so it can be with a number of other well-known medical conditions. In that regard, malalignment is of significance because it can:

1. aggravate an existing condition
2. mimic a medical condition
3. precipitate such a condition

The following are some examples from clinical practice that help illustrate these points.

1. Some clinical presentations may be unfavourably affected by coexistent malalignment. For example, someone with idiopathic scoliosis may become symptomatic only whenever the malalignment recurs (Fig. 4.6A). These symptoms presumably result from their attempts to cope with the malalignment-related changes. In particular, there is now the pelvic obliquity and compensatory scoliosis superimposed on their underlying condition. The altered biomechanics creates additional stresses on:
   a. the thoracolumbar and lumbosacral junctions, which probably accounts for their frequent complaint of mid- and low back pain whenever malalignment has recurred
   b. the facet joints and discs, as a result of any increase of L1–L4 rotation into the exacerbated lumbar convexity (Figs 2.96, 4.6A, 4.33)
2. Some of the structures that become tender and/or painful as a result of being put under increased

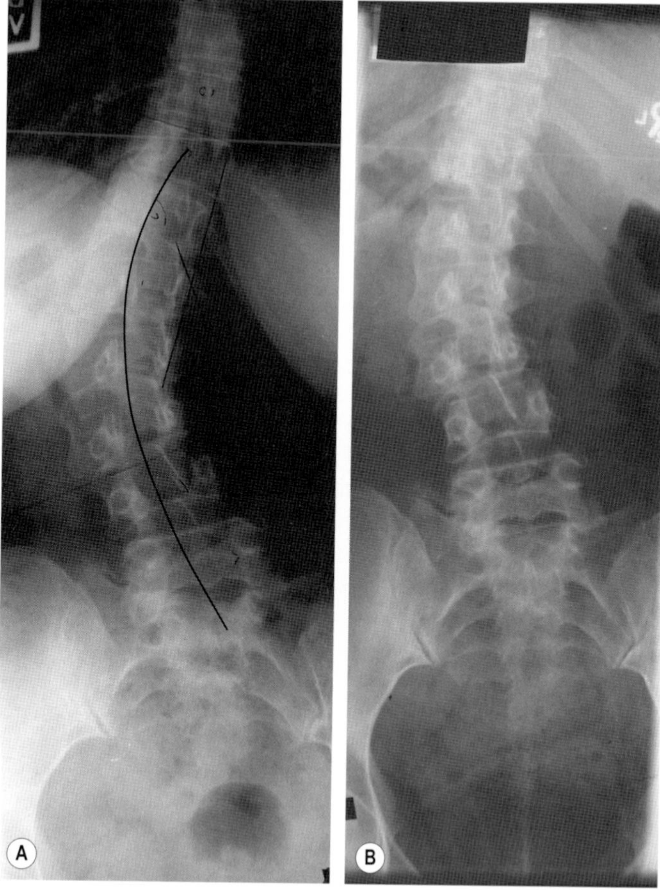

Fig. 4.6 A patient with advanced idiopathic scoliosis (a lumbar levoscoliosis of 37 degrees when in alignment). (A) With coexistent pelvic malalignment: the L1-L4 vertebrae have rotated into the marked left lumbar convexity to the point at which the spinous processes of T12, L1, and L2 successively overlie the right pars interarticularis of the vertebra below; that of L4 is starting to come back to the midline. The left lumbar facet joints have been opened, the right ones compressed. The pelvis is oblique, with the right iliac crest and sacral base lower than that on the left as a result of 'left anterior, right posterior' rotation. (B) With realignment: the L1-L4 rotation is less pronounced, and the T12-L2 spinous processes now lie distinctly separate from the right pars and comparatively closer to the midline. The opening of the left facet joints is not as marked, and the pelvis and sacral base is level.

stress, and certain of their common referral sites, are in close proximity to areas classically identified with problems in major organ systems. Both the deep iliolumbar and the anterior SI joint ligaments, for example, are capable of referring to McBurney's point and mimicking appendicitis (Fig. 3.46).

3. Malalignment-related symptoms may mimic some common pain phenomena. Irritation of myofascial tissue at the C4-C5 level, for example, can present like a 'carpal tunnel syndrome' yet nerve conduction tests will prove negative and symptoms disappear with vertebral realignment (Fig. 3.12Bii). In others, increased tension with narrowing of the thoracic outlet can affect the brachial plexus to precipitate an actual carpal tunnel syndrome (Fig. 3.13).

A failure to recognize these facets of the 'malalignment syndrome' runs the risk of causing confusion, which may result in investigations that are at best harmless, albeit perhaps not required, and at worst costly or dangerous and may lead to misdiagnosis and inadequate or even inappropriate treatment. The following discussion will concentrate on:

1. some of the more common pain phenomena and syndromes that may be attributable to malalignment or can be affected by the presence of malalignment, and
2. how these conditions may overlap with problems typically dealt with by some of the medical specialties.

IMPLICATIONS FOR CARDIOLOGY AND CARDIAC REHABILITATION

Chest pain of musculoskeletal origin is a complaint that can be related to malalignment, one that a cardiologist may have to differentiate from angina and other symptoms typical of coronary artery disease. In cardiac rehabilitation, musculoskeletal symptoms caused by malalignment are:

1. responsible for some of the more frequently encountered complaints that staff have to deal with in exercise classes on a day-to-day basis
2. one of the more common reasons for the temporary or permanent interruption of a patient's exercise programme.

CASE HISTORY 4.1 Mrs. O.J.

1. History: two myocardial infarcts in 1994; five-vessel coronary artery bypass graft in 1995; since then, occasional angina, brought on by effort and relieved by nitroglycerine spray
2. On referral: in alignment; no musculoskeletal problems noted
3. Course: 4 weeks after starting the programme, complained of interscapular pain when using the rower
4. Findings: T8 vertebral body right rotational displacement (spinous process to the left); acute pain on trunk extension, flexion and especially rotation while sitting, also with direct posteroanterior and medial pressure on the T8 spinous process
5. Treatment: realignment of T8 resolved the problem

CASE HISTORY 4.2 Mr. D.S.

1. History: myocardial infarct in 1997 at age 49; going on to uneventful five-vessel coronary artery bypass graft
2. On referral: no musculoskeletal complaints; malalignment of the pelvis and compensatory scoliosis but no indication of tenderness in muscles or ligaments typically put under stress
3. Course:
   a. managed to progressively increase the exercise level without a problem even though the malalignment had never been corrected
   b. shortly after graduating to a home program (including regular light weights and exercises with more of a torsional component), he presented with interscapular pain; in addition to the previously noted pelvic malalignment, examination now also revealed T4 and T5 rotational displacement and bilateral tender, tense adjacent paravertebral muscles
   c. pelvic and vertebral realignment resolved the problem and allowed him to resume an exercise program but avoiding any torsional stresses

The following case studies of patients enrolled in a cardiac rehabilitation program show that malalignment:

1. may not be a problem for the patient until he or she begins to exercise
2. may not be evident on initial examination but may develop with progressive increase in exercise, particularly if this now involves an asymmetric and/or torsional component

CASE HISTORY 4.3 Mrs. M.M.

1. History: myocardial infarct 1995, one-vessel coronary artery bypass graft in 1996; rehabilitation programme started in August 1996
2. Discharge clinic (1997): note was made that the programme had been interrupted from Dec. 18, 1996 to Jan. 29, 1997 because of 'low back pain', which had persisted and was now localized to the right 'buttock', pointing to the lumbosacral region or nearby underlying right sacroiliac joint
3. Findings: pelvic malalignment with 'right anterior' rotation, also T7 rotational displacement; tenderness localizing to the left 7th costochondral junction and the ligaments crossing the posterior aspect of the right sacroiliac joint; facet stress tests negative
4. Course: realignment of the pelvis and spine resolved the low back pain and allowed return to exercising

CASE HISTORY 4.4 Mrs. K.M.

1. History: pulmonary hypertension requiring the repair of an atrioseptal defect; for 3 months postoperatively, ongoing tightness of the sternotomy scar area and discomfort in the left anterior chest region, leading to $30,000 of repeat investigations (including cardiac catheterization), which were all negative
2. Findings: acutely tender bilateral 4th and 5th costochondral junctions (those on the left corresponding to her site of pain); left rotation of the T6 vertebra with displacement of the 4th, 5th and 6th ribs bilaterally (similar to the T5 vertebra rotational displacement in Fig. 2.94); malalignment of the pelvis and spine
3. Course: 'cardiac' symptoms resolved completely on realignment combined with massage of the anterior chest and thoracic paravertebral muscles

3. can result in needless investigation and ongoing patient discomfort as a result of failure to suspect malalignment in the first place.

Typical 'cardiac' presentations of malalignment

Those involved in the care of patients with coronary artery disease should bear in mind that malalignment can cause the following problems that may sometimes be confused with symptoms precipitated by coronary artery disease.

Back pain

Particularly important is back pain arising from the sites of stress caused by:

1. curve reversal (Fig. 3.14)
   a. mid back pain from reversal at the thoracolumbar junction
   b. upper back pain from the reversal that occurs most frequently at the cervicothoracic junction but may occur in the upper thoracic spine and is then more likely to become a problem that can lead to confusion with the symptoms of coronary artery disease (Fig. 2.91B)
2. rotational displacement of any of the thoracic vertebrae, T4 and T5 being the most likely to be involved and to cause pain by stressing particularly the costovertebral and costotransverse joints at these levels (Figs 2.94A, 3.15, 3.16).

Anterior chest pain that can mimic angina

There may be anterior chest pain from the irritation of one or more of the costochondral junctions:

1. irritation of a junction caused by rib rotation or subluxation that may occur in isolation (e.g. following trauma or with a severe cough) but is also seen in association with rotational displacement of one of the thoracic vertebrae and of the attached rib or ribs (Fig. 2.94)
2. in those who have undergone open heart surgery, the vertebral rotation may itself represent a complication of the rib displacement that occurred while carrying out the sternotomy; unfortunately, the rotational displacement has persisted and now perpetuates the rib displacement and rotational stress on the costochondral junction(s), long after the sternotomy has healed.

Anterior chest pain can also arise as the result of excessive rotation of a clavicle and increased stress on:

1. the sternoclavicular joint (Fig. 2.94B)
2. the acromioclavicular joint and the ligaments connecting the distal clavicle to the coracoid process, resulting in chest pain that is more anterolateral (Fig. 4.7).

Pain may radiate straight through to the anterior chest from the irritation of a disc, facet joint, costovertebral or costotransverse joint, or any other structure stressed by rotational displacement of one of the upper or mid-thoracic vertebrae; e.g. the ligaments coming off the C7 transverse process (Grieve 1986b; Fig. 3.12A,B5).

Recurrent right, left or central mid-chest discomfort may be attributable to increased irritability of the thoracic diaphragm and 'cramping' or spasm of that muscle triggered, for example, by:

1. irritation of the roots that form the phrenic nerve (C3, C4 and C5) by rotational displacement of one of the mid-cervical vertebrae, or irritation of that nerve anywhere along its course (Fig. 3.13)

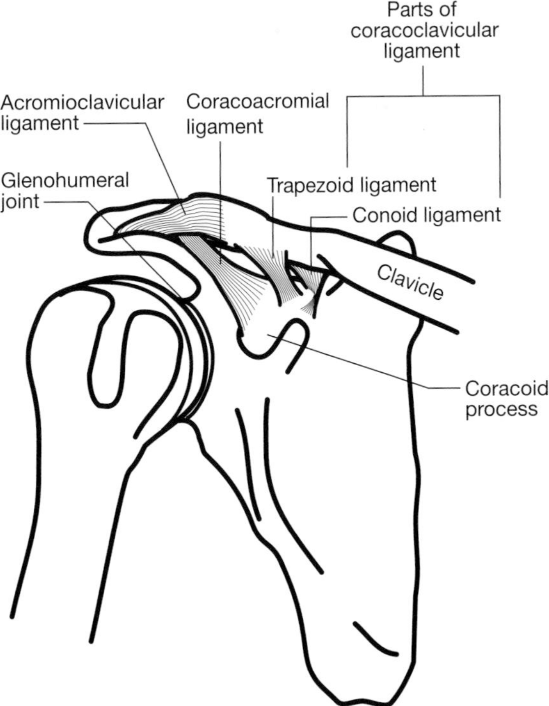

Fig. 4.7 The right acromioclavicular and lateral clavicular ligaments.

2. irritation of the autonomic nerve supply; e.g. triggering an excessive autonomic response because of irritation of the parasympathetic outflow tracts by cervical vertebral rotation or paravertebral muscle spasm
3. increased tension on the diaphragm muscle caused by:
   a. the shift of its origin(s) from the seventh to twelfth ribs that can occur with rotational displacement of any of these lower thoracic vertebrae
   b. attempts by the muscle to decrease pain and/or increase stability of a rib cage structure or the thoracic spine

Pain referred into one arm or to the jaw

Referral may occur from cervical spine ligaments and joints:

1. in the atlanto-occipital and atlantoaxial region:
   - to the jaw and skull (C2, C3; Fig. 3.12A,B1)
2. at the cervicothoracic junction:
   - mainly in a C8/T1 pattern, to the medial arm and forearm and the fourth and fifth fingers; this is more likely to occur when there is a rotational displacement of C7 and T1 in addition to the stress of curve reversal at this junction (Fig. 3.12A,B4) and it is capable of mimicking angina.

There may be myofascial pain and trigger points in the neck and shoulder girdle:

1. Localized pain from muscles, tendons, ligaments or fascia in this area may eventually develop with the chronic increase in tension that can result with malalignment (e.g. pectoral or intercostal muscles splinting a painful costochondral junction) and the development of trigger points within these tissues.
2. A number of the shoulder girdle soft tissues that are put under increased stress by malalignment can give rise to pain referred to the areas classically associated with angina; for example, a trigger point in latissimus dorsi can also refer along the inner arm and forearm, down to the fourth and fifth fingers (Fig. 4.8).

As part of the 'T3' or 'T4 syndrome' (see Ch. 5):

1. rotational displacement of any of the vertebrae in the T3 to T7 region but most often involving T3 or T4

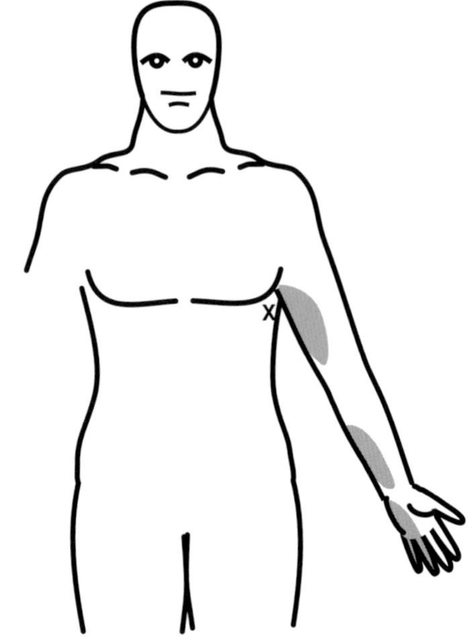

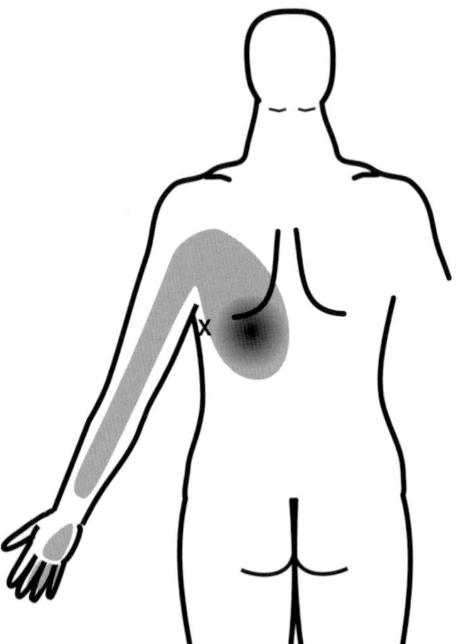

Fig. 4.8 Referral pattern from trigger points (X) in latissimus dorsi. 'Spill-over' into the arm (light grey) can mimic a C8/T1 root problem or angina. *(Redrawn courtesy of Travell & Simons 1983.)*

2. can result in referred pain that typically involves:
   a. the hand and fingers, and less often part or all of the arm, either uni- or bilaterally (in which case it is symmetrical) and/or
   b. parts of the head and neck (Fig. 4.9).

Angina coexistent with symptomatic malalignment

As indicated above, the person with malalignment may present with symptoms that can mimic angina. Like the general population, 80% of those with a cardiac condition can be expected to be out of alignment (see Ch. 2). Hence, there may be those who:

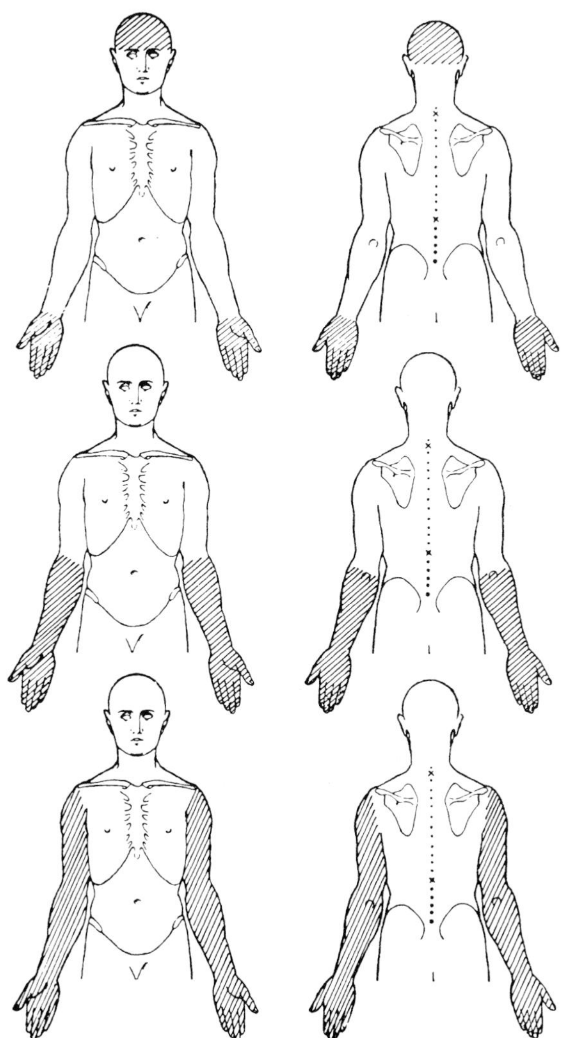

Fig. 4.9 'T3' or 'T4' syndrome: common areas of upper limb symptoms. The upper diagram shows classical areas of head pain. *(Courtesy of McGuckin 1986.)*

1. present with an apparent cardiac problem but whose symptoms are strictly on account of a malalignment problem
2. have symptoms caused strictly by their cardiac condition, while the malalignment remains asymptomatic in terms of not causing any 'cardiac-like' symptoms
3. have overlapping symptoms, caused both by the cardiovascular system and the malalignment

Typical of the latter presentation is the patient with known 'unstable angina' whose 'cardiac' symptoms may come on either at rest or with effort and may or may not respond to nitroglycerine spray, or do so incompletely or inconsistently. One must always rule out the possibility that this is not someone whose symptoms at any one time may vary because:

1. they actually do suffer from 'unstable angina', and the recurrence of the angina at any time triggers a further increase in muscle tension that can more easily precipitate symptoms from muscles that are already tense and tender because of the malalignment
2. the angina may itself be triggered by the increase in the cardiac workload and cardiovascular changes that occur as a result of pain caused by the malalignment (e.g. secondary increase in blood pressure and heart rate)
3. the symptoms are strictly on the basis of the malalignment, and hence can also come on at rest and will fail to respond to nitroglycerine.

Always remember to consider malalignment in the differential diagnosis when a patient presents with angina, particularly when there are features that do not exactly fit the 'cardiac picture' and there is possibly a musculoskeletal component.

When dealing with any patient referred for cardiac rehabilitation, examination of their musculoskeletal system should be part of the initial assessment, including a look at pelvic and spine alignment. Musculoskeletal complaints are common and a major cause for patients interrupting or discontinuing their exercise programme to get over some complication, particularly back, hip and knee pain. Malalignment makes it more likely for these complications to develop or become symptomatic. Those who are already out of alignment on entering an exercise programme are also at increased risk of becoming symptomatic or aggravating malalignment-related musculoskeletal symptoms. Becoming aware of malalignment, diagnosing it at the initial outpatient visit and treating it on a preventative basis (or at least keeping an eye on it as the patient starts in the programme) would go a long way toward making their participation in a cardiac rehabilitation programme less likely to be interrupted and more likely to be progressive and enjoyable.

DENTISTRY

As indicated in Ch. 3, malalignment affects the joints from the toes up to the head and neck. Temporomandibular joint involvement ranges from initial minimal displacement, which can progress to subluxation and frank dislocation as the capsule and supporting ligaments are gradually stretched beyond the point of being able to provide adequate support and the muscles can no longer compensate. There results a very obvious palpable, or even visible (and sometimes, audible) displacement of the mandible on opening and closing of the jaw. Constant protective splinting, primarily of the temporal and masseter muscles, eventually results in tenderness to outright pain from that joint region which may suggest involvement of the gums and teeth.

Rotational displacement of the upper cervical vertebra, with irritation or compression of C1, C2 and C3, can cause localized pain in the base and sides of the neck and referred pain and paraesthesias in the forehead, temporal and mandibular regions (Fig. 3.12A,Bi). This pain may be hard to differentiate from the gnawing, 'deep' pain sometimes associated with dental problems (Blum 2004a,b).

Unilateral excessive bite, or worse still, grinding of the teeth, has been identified as either:

1. the result of the asymmetry of the pelvis and spine seen with malalignment, or
2. an actual cause of that malalignment

Insertion of rubber or plastic 'spacers' on the side involved has been found successful in gradually shifting bite more to the opposite side as the thickness is progressively increased from an initial 3-5 mm until tests show bite to be equal on the right and left side. Selectively placing the spacers more anteriorly, posteriorly (e.g. over the molars) or in diagonal patterns may have the effect of creating rotational forces that can actually correct some presentations of malalignment.

Dental issues are discussed further in Ch. 6, in regard to how they can cause alignment problems in horses.

IMPLICATIONS FOR NEUROLOGY AND NEUROSURGERY

Malalignment can result in symptoms or signs that suggest an involvement of the neurological system, on the basis of:

1. patterns of referred pain and paraesthesias that may mimic a root or peripheral nerve distribution
2. nerve fibre traction or compression caused, for example, by shifts in weight-bearing, changes in the length-tension ratio, asymmetry in muscle tension and reflex spasm with narrowing of root and nerve outlets
3. weakness of the lower extremity muscles in a pattern that may be confused with a root or peripheral nerve lesion
4. seemingly positive root stretch tests which can mimic a root or plexus problem (Figs 3.45, 3.63, 3.67, 3.75, 4.10)
   a. by further stressing structures already tender as a result of the malalignment (e.g. the SI joints and posterior pelvic ligaments) and
   b. by provoking back or buttock pain, with radiation or referral to a leg

These patients are frequently referred for neurological or neurosurgical consultation and for electrodiagnostic studies. However, unless the consultant is aware of at least some of the common presentations of malalignment and their 'neurological' implications, none of these examinations and investigations are likely to be very helpful, other than to rule out a coexistent neurological lesion.

Once such a lesion seems to have been 'ruled out', the temptation is not infrequently to attribute the patient's persistent problems to a catch-all diagnosis such as 'mechanical back pain'. Worse yet is to inadvertently accuse the patient of malingering, or to attach some other unfavourable psychiatric 'label' (see 'Psychiatry' below), when in reality the patient's actual problem, namely symptoms and signs caused by the presence of the malalignment, has been overlooked because of a shortcoming in the clinician's diagnostic skills.

Referred patterns of pain and paraesthesias

Pain and paraesthesias can be referred to the dermatome, myotome and/or sclerotome, reflecting the innervation of the structure that is the actual source of these symptoms. Hackett (1958) deserves special mention for his exquisite work of mapping

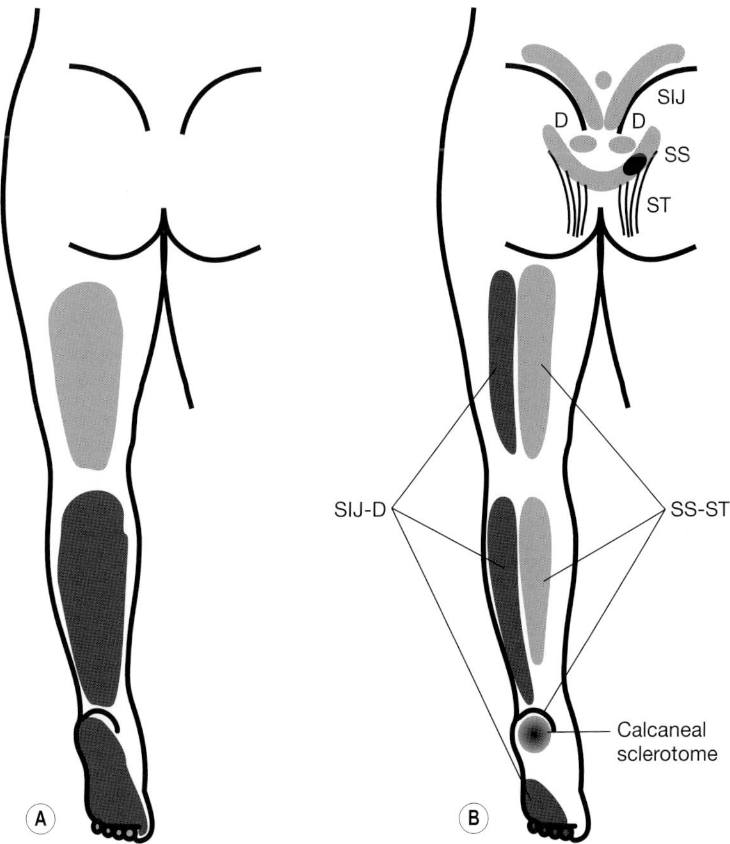

Fig. 4.10 Nerve root versus referred pattern of dysaesthesias. (A) S1 radiculopathy pattern. (B) Referred pattern from lower posterior sacroiliac (SIJ-D), sacrotuberous (ST) and sacrospinous (SS) ligaments associated with sacroiliac joint instability. *(Redrawn courtesy of Hackett 1958.)*

these patterns by injecting hypertonic saline into specific ligaments (Fig. 3.12A,B). Travell & Simons (1983, 1992) did much to clarify the referral patterns of trigger points. Patterns originating from deteriorating discs, facet joints and inflamed or impinged tendons have also been well documented (McCall et al. 1979; Mooney & Robertson 1976; Travell & Simons 1992).

The stress imposed on numerous structures by malalignment frequently results in referred symptoms. Particularly common are paraesthesias and/or dysaethesias in what may at first appear to be a 'non-anatomical' distribution in terms of not fitting a root or peripheral nerve pattern. For example, an area often involved is the anterolateral aspect of a thigh, which can reflect referral from the upper posterior SI joint ligaments (Fig. 3.63A). The person may report feeling pins and needles or numbness, a waft of air may prove 'irritating'. Sometimes, there is just a sensation that something is 'off', such as the touch of clothes simply feeling 'different' compared to the surrounding area or to the opposite side. The diagnosis of 'meralgia paraesthetica' may be contemplated but LFCN nerve conduction studies are normal (see below and Fig. 4.13).

More important, referral patterns can mimic a root or peripheral nerve problem. An S1 root injury, for example, can result in pain and/or paraesthesias in the posterior calf, the lateral aspect and sole of the foot and infrequently also the posterior thigh (Fig. 4.10A). The lower posterior sacroiliac, sacrospinous and sacrotuberous ligaments, which are mainly S1, S2 and S3 innervated, are capable of referring to all three sites, and this may raise suspicions of an S1 root lesion when the real problem is one of irritation or injury affecting one or more of these ligaments (Fig. 4.10B)

The pain and paraesthesias represent referred symptoms involving the S1 myotome (muscles in the calf, foot and posterior thigh, particularly the lateral hamstrings), dermatome (the skin overlying the posterior calf and the heel and sole) and sclerotome (which includes the weight-bearing part of the calcaneus; see 'Introduction 2002'). Symptoms are more likely to be on a referred basis, rather than from irritation or injury of the S1 root, when the neurological examination discloses the findings outlined in Box 4.4.

Significant points to appreciate when trying to differentiate between a nerve injury and referred symptoms include the following:

Location

Symptoms arising from injury to a specific root or peripheral nerve tend to be more or less constant in location, in keeping with the area supplied by the compromised nerve tissue. With referred symptoms, the location of the areas involved may also remain constant but the number of sites that are symptomatic at any one time may vary.

In the example involving the lower posterior sacroiliac, the sacrospinous and sacrotuberous ligaments (Fig. 4.10B), the patient may report that there is sometimes no pain at all, or there may be just heel pain; whereas at other times dysaesthesias are felt just in the posterior thigh or the posterior calf region. All three sites are, however, more likely to be involved together when the pain is 'really bad'.

In others with involvement of these ligaments, dysaesthesias may affect the posterior thigh first, and only if this gets worse will there eventually be pain also in the calf and finally in the heel and foot region - a domino-like effect which could also present in the reverse order: from the foot, up to the calf and then the thigh. There may be no pain felt in the ligaments that are the source of the referred pain but they are likely to prove tender to palpation.

BOX 4.4 Findings suggesting pain and paraesthesias on a referred basis rather than S1 nerve root irritation or compression

1. Full strength in the S1 myotome muscles or, if malalignment is present, the weakness that:
   a. involves S1 myotome muscles bilaterally, in the typical asymmetrical pattern; e.g. the right gluteus maximus (L5/S1) and tibialis posterior (L5/S1), the left hamstrings (L5/S2/S2) and peroneus longus (L5/S1)
   b. shows simultaneous asymmetrical weakness involving other myotomes, with overlapping of root innervation; e.g. right iliopsoas (L2,L3), quadratus (L2-4), and tibialis anterior (L4,L5); left gluteus maximus (L5,S1) and peroneus (L5,S1)
2. Normal pinprick and light touch sensation over the posterior calf and the sole, or responses to sensory testing that are somewhat variable or ill-defined ('non-anatomical')
3. Preservation of the ankle reflex
4. Negative root stretch tests or, with malalignment present, the symptoms evoked by these manoeuvres could be attributable to tender soft tissue or joint structures being put under further stress (e.g. the posterior pelvic ligaments, the posterior SI joint capsule or the joint itself limiting left Maitland's 'slump' test; Fig. 3.75)

Intensity

Referred pain is more likely to fluctuate in intensity from being very severe at one time to being just bothersome or not even present at another. Nerve pain is more likely to be constantly there, to get progressively worse with the increasing nerve irritation and inflammation associated with a traction or compression injury, and may get better gradually as these factors resolve.

Relation to activity and rest

Referred pain from the irritation of ligaments, fascia and other connective tissue structures is more likely to be a problem on getting up from lying or sitting, tends to get better on moving about but may worsen again when the activity is continued for a longer period of time. These soft tissues tend to contract when put in a relaxed, shortened position at rest and will, therefore, often be a source of pain on initially moving around until they have been stretched out again to full length. However, pain may recur as muscle fatigue sets in with continued activity: the muscles tire and tense up and, along with the ligaments and other connective tissues, are once more subjected to increased stress.

In contrast, pain arising from nerve tissue may settle somewhat with rest but may also worsen, often assuming a 'burning' quality at these times. This pain tends to get steadily worse with activity and may persist with rest and on lying down as, for example, with compression by a disc or metastases.

Pattern of weakness and wasting

Barring generalized disuse weakness and wasting in an extremity, a root or peripheral nerve injury usually results in weakness and wasting confined to the muscle(s) innervated by the affected root or nerve. A left S1 root lesion, for example, will result in weakness and wasting localizing to muscles in the ipsilateral S1 myotome.

In contrast, malalignment results in an asymmetrical pattern of weakness that involves muscles from several myotomes - L2 to S1 - on both sides in a pattern that is not consistent with either a root or a peripheral nerve injury (see Appendix 4). In the presence of malalignment, any weakness not in keeping with this asymmetrical pattern should raise suspicions of an underlying neurological lesion and call for immediate further investigations. If, however, there is no definite or only a questionable indication of an underlying neurological lesion, and there is no apparent contraindication to mobilization, the best thing is to proceed with realignment to:

1. remove any findings that are definitely attributable to the malalignment itself, and
2. help clarify whether or not there is an underlying neurological lesion localizing, for example, to a specific root or peripheral nerve.

In other words, the patient is re-examined after realignment to determine whether there is any sensory or reflex change or residual weakness and, if so, whether it conforms to a root or peripheral nerve pattern that may previously have been hidden by the functional 'non-anatomic' changes that are known to be part of the 'malalignment syndrome' (see 'Asymmetry of muscle strength', Ch. 3). Further investigations should be guided by these persistent findings.

Response to a block with local anaesthetic

A block will usually give temporary relief if a nerve root or peripheral nerve is the cause of the problem. Similarly, local anaesthetic should bring relief when injected into the structure that is the cause of any referred symptoms (e.g. the sacrospinous or sacrotuberous ligaments) but not when injected into the site of referral itself (e.g. the calcaneal region; see 'Introduction 2002').

Response to realignment

The correction of malalignment is unlikely to abolish the dysaesthesias associated with the actual irritation or injury of a nerve root or peripheral nerve but it may well decrease the pain by:

1. relieving the tension on the root or nerve itself; e.g. by bringing the root origin and terminations back into their normal position again
2. decreasing compression; for example, by decreasing tension in the muscles that the nerves have to pass between or through:
   a. brachial plexus through the thoracic outlet (Fig. 3.13) and lumbosacral through the femoral triangle (Fig. 4.14), respectively
   b. tibial and peroneal nerve components of the sciatic nerve coming through the greater sciatic notch to run between gluteus maximus and piriformis muscle, or actually through piriformis (Fig. 4.17)
3. decreasing tone by shutting off any 'facilitation'
4. increasing the space available (e.g. increasing foraminal openings or decreasing disc bulging or protrusion by decreasing vertebral rotational displacement, disc torsion and compression).

The abolition of pain and paraesthesias following realignment will help to confirm the referred nature of these symptoms. Complete relief of pain does not, however, always occur on realignment even when these symptoms are indeed strictly malalignment-related. If a ligament has, for example, been stretched for a long period of time because of malalignment, simply restoring the tension to normal with realignment may no longer be adequate to stop this ligament from continuing to be tender and an ongoing source of referred symptoms. Prolonged ligament stretching can cause ligament inflammation, excessive lengthening or even partial tearing. Nerve fibres are more likely to cause ongoing symptoms as they are at greater risk of injury, being unable to accommodate to the stretching as well as the elastic component, with complicating nociceptive inflammatory response and neuralgia (see above). Similarly, trigger points may fail to disappear with realignment alone. All can be an ongoing source of pain and referred symptoms until dealt with by additional means (Ch. 7).

Malalignment-related nerve injury

Malalignment particularly affects the peripheral nerves in the lower extremities by causing a shift in weight-bearing and accentuating the stresses caused by pronation and supination (Schamberger 1987). The shift in weight-bearing can result in excessive traction, compression or a combination of the two, which may be compounded by the functional LLD and a coexistent genu valgum or varum.

Peripheral nerves affected by medial shift (pronation)

A medial shift increases the tension primarily in the saphenous and posterior tibial nerves (Figs. 3.37, 3.38A). The common peroneal nerve may also be affected, in particular the deep peroneal branch (which wraps around the fibular head) and its sensory branch (which comes to lie progressively more medially distal to the anterior tarsal tunnel on its way to supply the first web space; Figs 3.37, 3.38A, 4.11A, 4.12A). Posterior tarsal tunnel syndrome can be caused by the medial traction forces on the posterior tibial nerve and its branches, compounded by compression within the tunnel as the medial restraining ligament (flexor retinaculum) is put under increasing tension (Figs 3.37, 3.38A, 4.11B). The sural nerve may be entrapped and compressed by excessive ankle eversion (Figs 3.38A, 4.12A).

Peripheral nerves affected by lateral shift (supination)

A lateral shift increases the traction forces distally on the sural nerve and the common peroneal nerve and its branches, especially the superficial peroneal nerve (Figs 3.37, 3.38B) and accessory peroneal nerve (if present), also proximally on lateral superficial sensory nerves such as the lateral sural cutaneous branch (Fig. 4.12A) and lateral femoral cutaneous nerve (LFCN; Fig. 4.13). The posterior tibial nerve can be entrapped and compressed as the space available within the posterior tarsal tunnel is compromised by excessive varus angulation (ankle inversion) that can occur with supination (Fig. 3.38B).

Other mechanisms of injury to nerves

Malalignment can result in irritation or actual compression or compromise of the blood supply to the nerves in the upper and lower extremities by several mechanisms.

1. **Narrowing of spinal/foraminal outlet for nerve root fibres**

   An 'upslip' or 'rotational malalignment' results in a pelvic obliquity and compensatory scoliosis. Assuming a right lumbar convexity, this would have been formed by left side-flexion and clockwise rotation primarily of L1-L4 vertebrae (Fig. 2.96A). Addition of simultaneous forward flexion would further increase the possibility of these changes:

   a. accentuating a disc bulge or protrusion into the right side of the spinal canal and/or foramen(a), and

   b. compromising the space for the exiting left nerve roots by decreasing the size of the left intervertebral foramena (while, at the same time, opening up those on the right).

   Symptoms of root compromise may occur whenever malalignment is present and may subside with realignment if the bulge or protrusion once again recedes and the foramina re-open, as is sometimes the case.

2. **Compromising the peripheral nerve and/or blood flow at sites of anatomical narrowing**

   A malalignment-related rotation of the bones, muscle hypertonicity and contracture can all compromise:

   a. *the posterior triangle of the neck*
   Dysaesthesias may be attributable to an increase in tension in the anterior and middle scalene muscles, which narrows the outlet for the mid-section of the brachial plexus and subclavian artery (Fig. 3.13)

   b. *the thoracic outlet lying between the clavicle and first rib*
   An increase in tension, particularly in the scalenes and subclavius muscle, also a rotation of the first rib and the clavicle relative to each other, can narrow the space available for the traversing lower section of the subclavian vessels and brachial plexus (especially the C8 and T1 fibres that constitute the medial cord of the plexus; Fig. 3.13)

   c. *the femoral triangle*
   A tense iliacus and psoas can push:
      i. the exiting ilioinguinal, iliohypogastric or LFCN against the medial edge of the anterior superior iliac spine (Fig. 4.13)
      ii. the LFCN against the inguinal ligament or the fascia lata (which it pierces), or
      iii. the femoral neurovascular complex anteriorly against the iliac fascia and inguinal ligament (Fig. 4.14)

   d. *the greater sciatic foramen*
   Piriformis contraction can narrow the exit route of the sciatic nerve or its tibial and/or peroneal nerve component (see 'Sciatica' and 'Piriformis syndrome' below; Figs 4.17, 4.18)

   e. *the pelvic floor*
   Tightness in the myofascial tissue compromises the space available for the lumbosacral plexus, the splanchnic, pudendal and genitofemoral nerves (see 'Gastroenterology' section, below; Fig. 4.15)

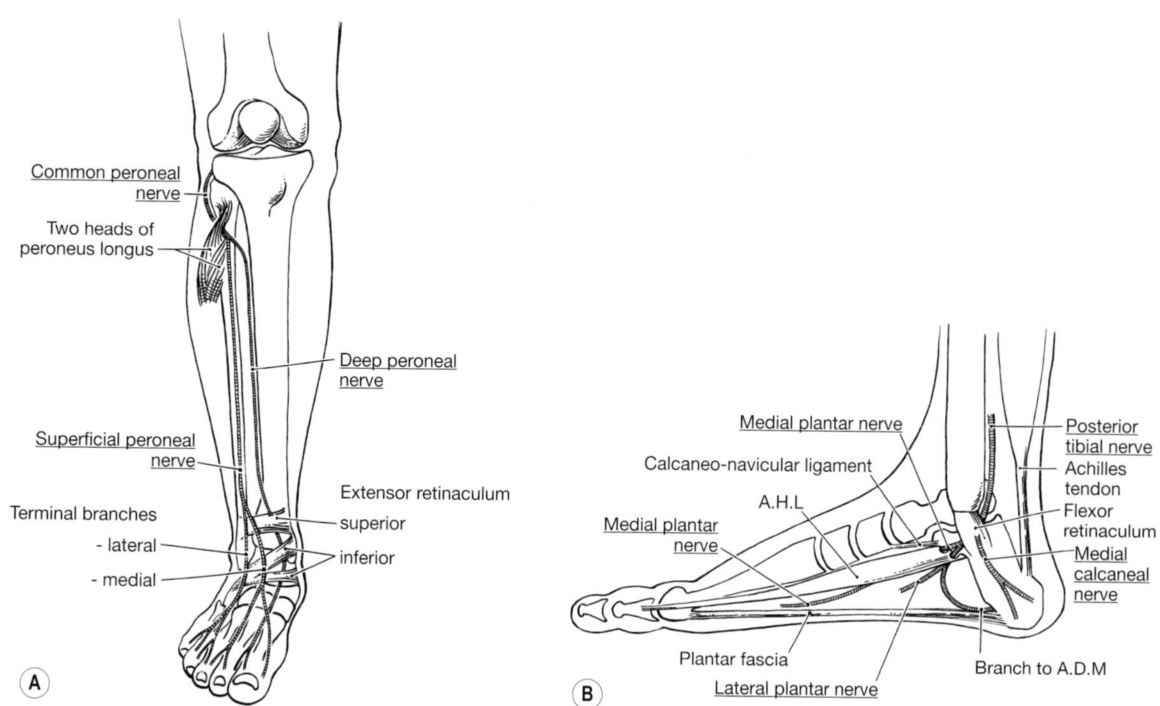

Fig. 4.11 Nerve structures put under tension by pronation. (A) Distal part of superficial and deep peroneal nerve branches; (B) Posterior tibial nerves, as seen on medial view of foot and ankle. AHL, abductor hallucis longus; ADM, abductor digiti minimi. *(Courtesy of Schamberger 1987.)*

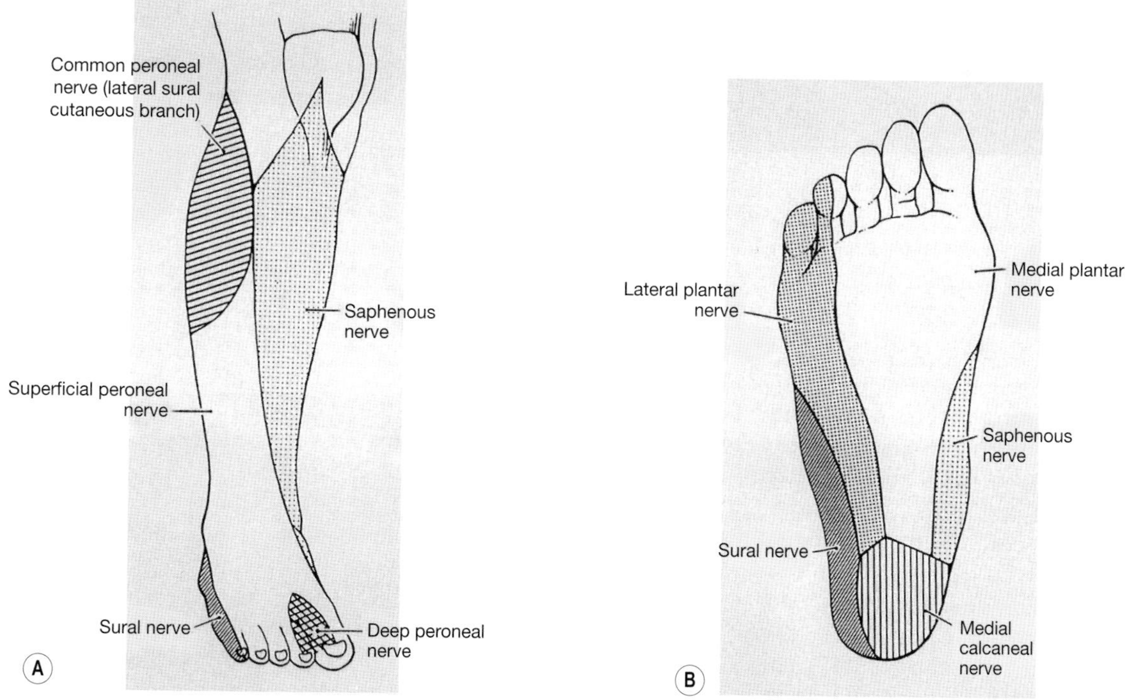

Fig. 4.12 Sensory distribution in the lower leg. (A) Anterior aspect. (B) Sole of the foot. *(Courtesy of Schamberger 1987.)*

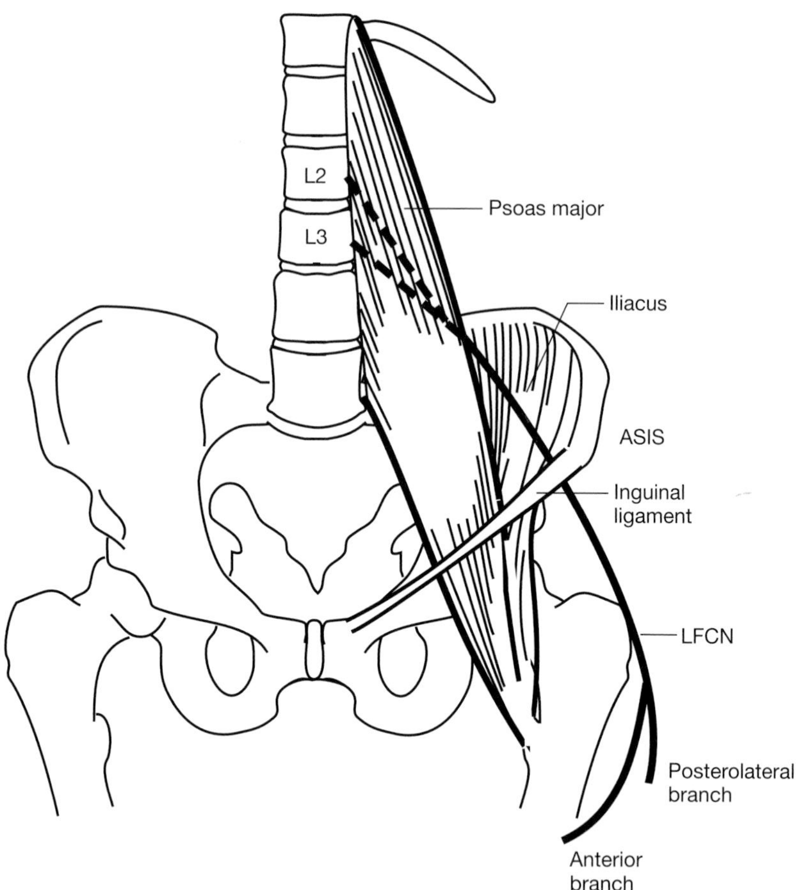

Fig. 4.13 Course of the left lateral femoral cutaneous nerve (LFCN), which supplies sensation to the skin of the anterolateral part of the thigh. Nerve irritation can occur: at its origin (the posterior roots of L2 and L3) and as it travels laterally lying between psoas major and iliacus, then running along the medial aspect of the anterior superior iliac spine (ASIS), under the inguinal ligament origin, and on to a point some 12 cm distally where it becomes superficial and divides into the anterior and posterolateral branches. Malalignment-related causes include: a) compression with increased tension in iliopsoas, left innominate 'posterior rotation' and/or an 'inflare'; b) traction forces caused by left innominate 'anterior rotation' and/or an 'outflare'; c) lateral traction forces (e.g. excessive hip adduction with genu valgum, supination, lower limb external rotation) at the (i) ASIS/inguinal ligament junction and (ii) the distal point where it is still relatively 'fixed' as it penetrates the subcutaneous layers.

f. *the long dorsal sacroiliac ligament*
The dorsal rami of S1, S2 and S3 can be compressed as they traverse laterally, lying between the medial and lateral components of a tight ligament (Fig. 2.19B).

3. **Compression of the interdigital nerves of the foot**

Pronation causes a collapse of the anterior transverse arch of the foot and angulation of the metatarsophalangeal (MTP) joints into extension. Metatarsalgia is common as a result of the increased weight-bearing on the central MT heads. In addition, the increased angulation of the central MTP joints and also the plantar digital nerves at this site can result in irritation or actual compression because of:

a. increased pressure on the nerve(s) against the edges of the deep transverse metatarsal ligaments
b. entrapment between the deep and superficial ligaments as the arch collapses and the forefoot splays, increasing tension in these ligaments and narrowing the space in between (Fig. 4.16)

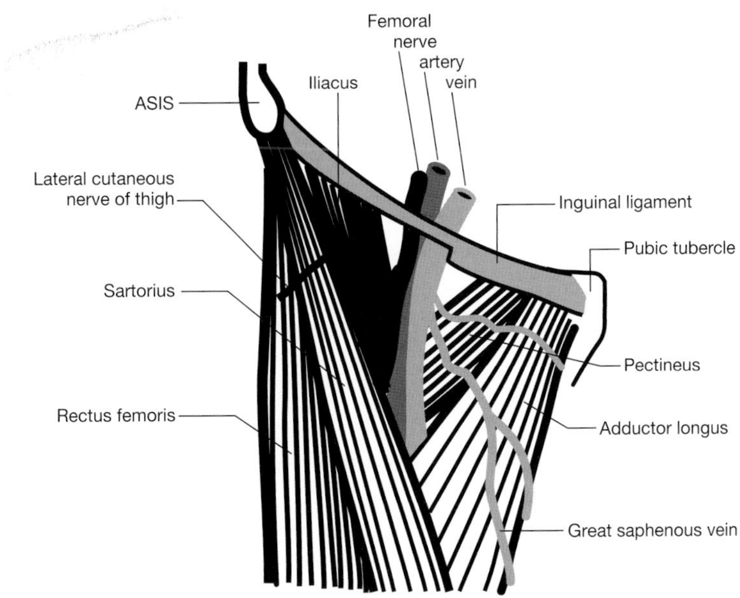

Fig. 4.14 Neurovascular structures at risk of compromise within the femoral triangle by any increase in tension, particularly in iliacus, psoas and pectineus. ASIS, anterior superior iliac spine. *(Redrawn courtesy of Grant 1980.)*

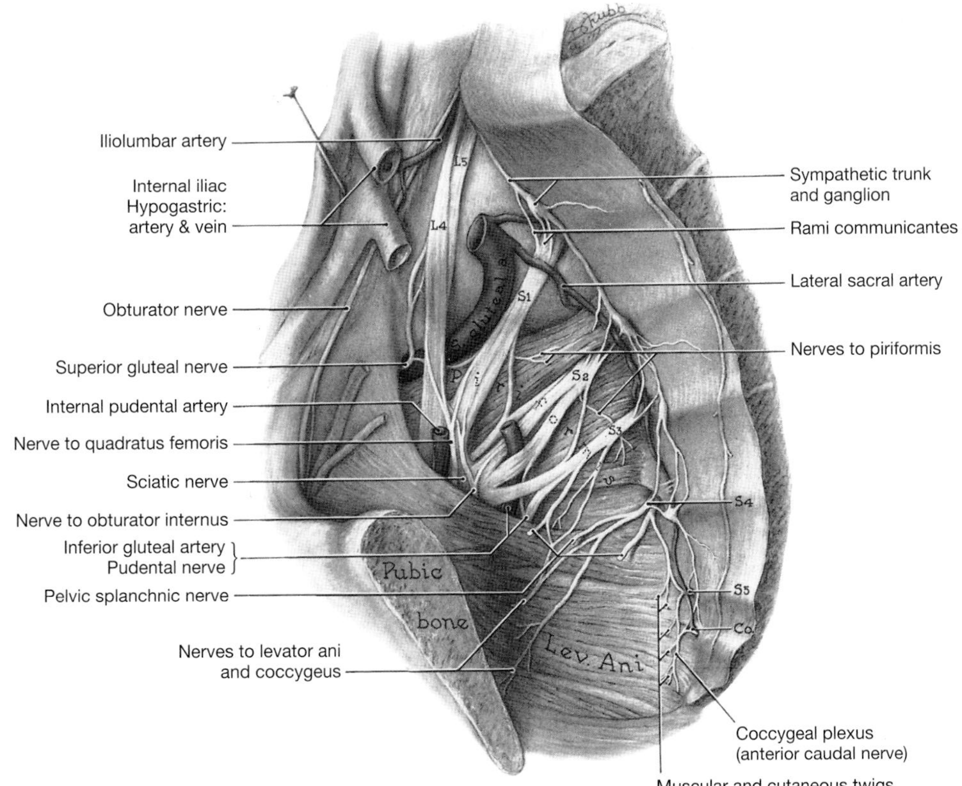

Fig. 4.15 Neurovascular structures of the lumbosacral plexus at risk of compromise by an increase in pelvic floor myofascial tissue tension. The autonomic nerve supply to the bowel and bladder from the S2, S3 and S4 roots exits as the pelvic splanchnic nerve, anterior to the sacrococcygeal joint region. *(Courtesy of Grant 1980.)*

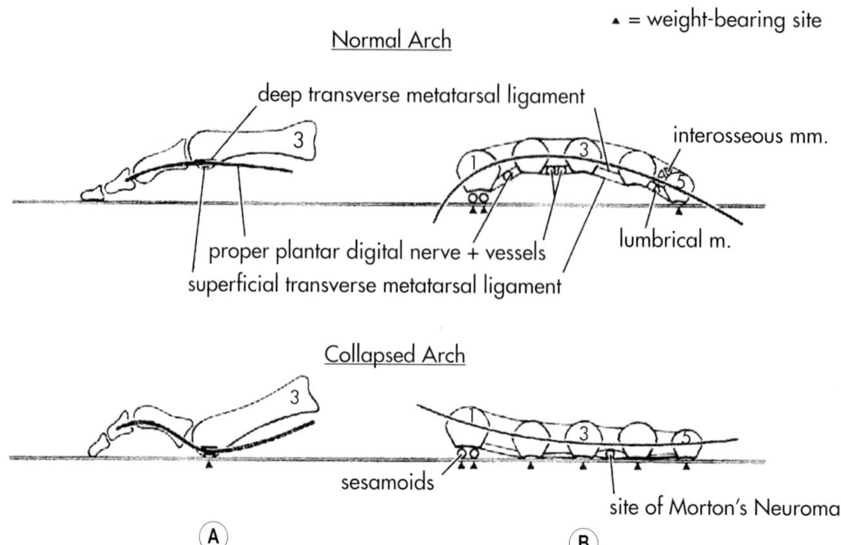

Fig. 4.16 Compromise of nerves in the foot with malalignment. Space for the plantar digital nerves between the central metatarsal (MT) heads is decreased on collapse of the anterior transverse arch (lower 'B') and as they are put under increased tension and 'squeezed' between the superficial and deep transverse MT ligaments by the associated 'cock-up' toe deformity (lower 'A'). The lower anterior view 'B' shows how a left lateral shift in weight-bearing (supination) could irritate the junction of the medial and lateral plantar nerve branches or an actual Morton's neuroma, usually located laterally, between the 3rd and 4th MT heads. *(Courtesy of Schamberger 1987.)*

The lateral shift in weight-bearing and tendency to supination can activate a latent Morton's neuroma by narrowing the space between the third and fourth metatarsal heads, squeezing the natural thickening typically formed at this site by the junction of a branch from the medial and lateral plantar nerve terminations of the posterior tibial nerve (Figs 3.38A, 4.11B). A neuroma on the left side is more likely to become symptomatic given that, in the vast majority with an 'upslip' or 'rotational malalignment', the shift is toward left lateral weight-bearing and supination (Figs 3.22A, 3.23, 3.24, 3.37). The problem would be compounded by collapse of the anterior transverse arch (Fig. 4.16B - lower part).

All of these nerves become more vulnerable to a traction or compression injury on the basis of:

a. activity-related repetitive minor increases in pronation or supination
b. an acute injury; for example, the excessive supination that results with an ankle inversion sprain acting on an already tense and irritable Morton's neuroma, LFCN, peroneal or sural nerve.

IMPLICATIONS FOR ORTHOPAEDIC SURGERY

The biomechanics of malalignment should be of particular interest to those practicing orthopaedic surgery. Discussion here will be limited to some specific orthopaedic entities that can result from or somehow be affected by malalignment.

Typical problems caused by the altered biomechanical stresses that result with malalignment are mentioned throughout this text and relate primarily to:

1. asymmetries of ranges of motion, especially those affecting the shoulder, hip girdle and joints of the lower extremities
2. asymmetries of weight-bearing, specifically those resulting in excessive unilateral pronation or supination, alterations of the gait pattern and secondary stresses on joints and soft tissue structures
3. asymmetries of muscle tension and strength

Iliopectineal bursitis

This bursa lies on the anterior aspect of the hip joint and usually communicates with the joint between the pubococcygeal and iliofemoral ligaments (Figs 4.2, 4.3). When inflamed, the bursa may become palpable just distal to the anterior inferior iliac spine and lateral to the symphysis pubis (Fig. 2.76D). Visualization by ultrasound or on magnetic resonance imaging may be necessary to confirm the diagnosis.

Inflammation has been associated with hip joint synovitis and osteoarthritis, as well as with an increase in tension in the overlying iliopsoas or pectineal muscles that may result in these muscles snapping repeatedly across the anterior aspect of the hip joint on hip flexion and extension (Figs 2.46B,C; 2.62, 3.42). Iliopectineal bursitis must be considered in the differential diagnosis of anterior hip tenderness and pain in the presence of malalignment, in which the frequent finding of an increase in tension in iliopsoas on one or both sides may be on the basis of:

1. an adaptive shortening or contracture having occurred on the side of an 'anterior' rotation, and which is now limiting hip extension
2. an increase in the length-tension ratio with separation of origin and insertion:
   a. on the side of a 'posterior' rotation, or
   b. with rotational displacement of one or more of its proximal origins (the transverse process and lateral aspect of vertebrae T12-L5)
3. reflex contraction or spasm in an attempt to stabilize a painful or unstable SI joint (Fig. 2.46B)
4. 'facilitation', typically noted with an 'upslip' and 'rotational malalignment'

Pain from the axial skeleton

The asymmetry of the spine seen as part of the 'malalignment syndrome' results in increased biomechanical stresses running the length of the axial skeleton (Box 4.5).

Upper extremity pain

Malalignment must be considered in the differential diagnosis of pain affecting the upper extremities, especially if the diagnosis proves elusive and the pain is resistant to standard therapy approaches. The following should be considered.

BOX 4.5 Malalignment-related biomechanical stresses on the axial skeleton

Distraction and compression

Capsules, discs and bony structures on the convex side of a curvature of the spine are distracted; whereas those on the concave side are compressed (Fig. 2.60).

Simultaneous vertebral rotation and side flexion

1. The four upper lumbar vertebrae usually rotate into the convexity and side-flex into the concavity (Figs 2.42, 2.96A, 3.6, 4.6, 4.24, 4.26).
2. The pressure distribution is altered, with an asymmetrical loading of the disc.
3. A torsional strain is imposed on the disc, annulus fibrosus and capsule, as well as the muscles and ligaments that attach to each vertebral complex (Figs 2.29, 3.68).
4. Relative to the direction of vertebral rotation, the facet joints are compressed contralaterally and distracted ipsilaterally (Figs 2.52B, 4.6, 4.31A, 4.32, 4.33)
5. All of these structures have sensory innervation and can, with time, become a source of localized and/or referred pain.

Curve reversal and interruption

Pain and tenderness localize in particular to the junctional (lumbosacral, thoracolumbar and cervicothoracic) areas and any sites of vertebral rotational displacement (Figs 2.91, 2.94, 3.14, 3.15)

Thoracolumbar junction involvement

This can mimic Maigne's 'thoracolumbar syndrome' (Fig. 4.23).

Lumbosacral nociceptor sensory fibre irritation

1. Those that supply the anterior longitudinal ligament, periosteum and anterior vertebral body have to ascend with the sympathetic fibres to finally gain access to the spinal nerve dorsal rami at the L1-L2 level (Fig. 4.15).
2. Irritation of these sensory fibres anywhere below this level can present as referred pain proximally, in the thoracolumbar region.

Asymmetries of ranges of motion

Stress is increased on upper extremity joints by the limitation of movement in specific directions. One most consistently sees, for example:

1. **at the glenohumeral joints**: a limitation of right internal and left external rotation (Fig. 3.17A), and of left extension compared to the right (Fig. 3.17B)
2. **at the elbow**: a limitation of left forearm pronation and right supination (Fig. 3.17C, D).

Referred symptoms of pain and paraesthesias

Cervical vertebral rotational displacement can cause referred symptoms in a dermatomal, myotomal or sclerotomal pattern involving the forehead, cheek, neck and shoulder region (C2-C5), and from the shoulder to the fingers (C5-T1).

Sclerotomal referral is often not recognized. C4-C5 and C5-C6 level rotational stress can, for example, result in a referral to the C5 and C6 sclerotomal sites along the lateral elbow region, capable of mimicking a lateral epicondylitis or 'tennis elbow' (Fig. 3.12A,B2,B3). An irritation of C8 and T1 (Fig. 3.12A,B4) can result in referral to sclerotomal sites along the medial elbow (capable of mimicking a medial epicondylitis or 'golfer's elbow'), the wrist and 4th and 5th fingers (presenting as 'angina'); also note that involvement of the C7 and C8 sclerotomal sites may refer just to the 4th and 5th fingers.

A failure of these sites to respond to standard physiotherapy treatment, injection of local anaesthetic or cortisone, or possibly other 'desperation' measures should raise concerns that the 'epicondylitis' pain, for example, is occurring on the basis of sclerotomal referral, and should prompt a search for a vertebral rotational displacement with localizing facet and/or soft tissue tenderness in the immediate region at the level(s) involved.

Thoracic compression/distraction/torsion

The clavicles are subjected to stresses of this type because they are part of the trunk and vulnerable to rotation and displacement with malalignment (Figs 2.93, 2.94B). Pain is likely to localize to the joints proper and to the securing ligaments: in particular, the sternoclavicular medially and the coracoclavicular laterally (Figs 2.93, 4.7). In comparison to the acromioclavicular joint, the sternoclavicular joint appears less capable of dealing with these stresses. The joint has some motion 'in almost any direction' (Pansky & House 1975) and is more likely to be tender on palpation and to develop a weakness of the anchoring ligaments that eventually allows a frank anterior subluxation of this end of the clavicle relative to the manubrial part of the sternum and the 1st and 2nd ribs. The ribs themselves are more likely to become a source of pain, especially as rib movement with vertebral rotational displacement subjects the posterior and anterior anchoring points to increased stress (costovertebral/transverse joints and costochondral junctions, respectively; see Chs 2, 3 and Figs 2.94, 3.15, 3.16). Increasing ligament laxity may eventually result in recurrent subluxation - with or without pain - of some ribs as well.

Pelvic and lower extremity joint pain and degeneration

LLD, whether anatomical (true) or 'functional', has been implicated in the acceleration of hip and knee joint degeneration. Campbell-Smith (1964) and Dixon & Campbell-Smith (1969) drew attention to 'long leg arthropathy', indicating that degeneration and pain are more likely to involve the hip joint on the long-leg side and the knee joint on the short-leg side. The effect of the functional LLD associated with malalignment is compounded by the asymmetry of lower extremity loading, attributable in large part to the shift in weight-bearing and one extremity tending to rotate externally, the other internally (Figs 3.81, 3.82). The effect of malalignment in terms of causing asymmetrical stresses on the hip, knee and ankle joints, and how these can become a site of localized and/or referred pain, has been discussed at length in Ch. 3.

Sciatica

In its strictest sense, 'sciatica' refers to a pressure neuritis, typically from a disc protrusion. There is irritation of the nerve root fibres or the nerve root sleeve, which gives rise to back pain and muscle spasm, as well as pain or sensory symptoms down the leg in the distribution of the affected root. As correctly indicated by Williams (1997: 350): 'The simplest definition for *sciatica* is back pain that *radiates* down one leg below the knee'. Nowadays, the term is more commonly used to refer to an entrapment of the sciatic nerve at the level of the sciatic notch, where it exits from the pelvis (Fig. 4.17). Compression at this site can result in intermittent paraesthesias, pain and/or weakness in the distribution of the tibial and/or peroneal nerve component These arise from the lumbosacral plexus as individual nerves and eventually lie together to form the sciatic nerve proper, the peroneal lateral to the tibial

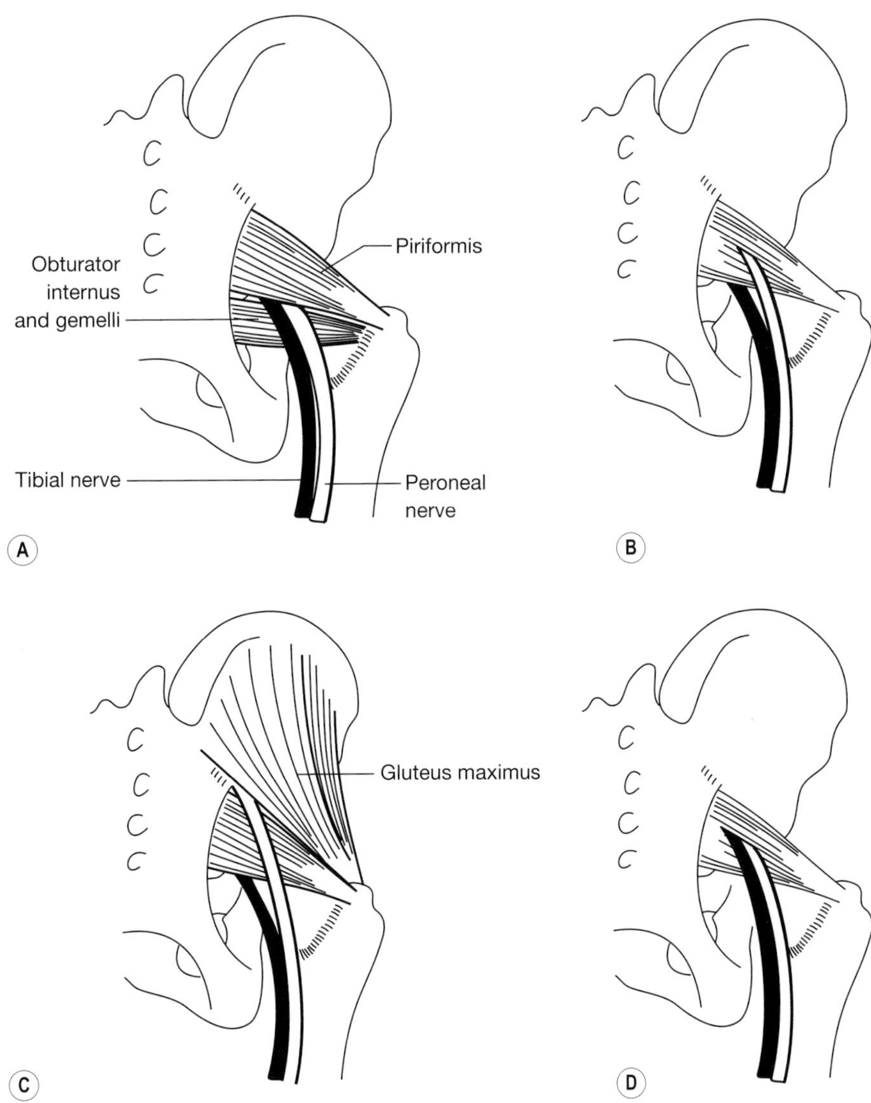

Fig. 4.17 Variations in the course of the sciatic nerve components on exiting from the greater sciatic foramen. Most often, they exit together just below the piriformis (A). An increase in tension in specific muscles can compromise the peroneal, tibial, or both components.

component. As Williams stated, symptoms will be felt '*below the knee*'.

The sciatic nerve leaves the pelvis by way of the greater sciatic notch. The piriformis muscle divides this foramen into a superior and inferior portion; the other borders of the inferior portion are comprised of the medial edge of the innominate laterally, the sacrotuberous ligament medially, and the upper edge of the sacrospinous ligament and ischial spine inferiorly (Figs 2.5A, 3.64, 4.17). Grant (1964) reported that, in 87.3% of 640 dissections, both the tibial and the peroneal division passed through this inferior portion, below the piriformis muscle (Fig. 4.17A). The peroneal component can actually pass directly through this muscle (Fig. 4.17B): 12.2% in Grant (1964), 20.77% of 130 dissections by Pećina (1979); or pass above it in a few (0.5% in Grant 1964), exiting between the superior border of piriformis and the inferior border of gluteus medius and minimus before joining the tibial component (Fig. 4.17C). Very rarely both components actually traversed the muscle mass together (Fig. 4.17D).

The lateral position of the peroneal nerve makes it more vulnerable to compression against the bony lateral border of the foramen. In the variants in which the peroneal nerve passes either through or above the piriformis muscle, this component is at increased risk of compression by contraction of the muscles that it traverses or adjoins. Piriformis functions as an abductor and external rotator of the lower extremity (Fig. 2.46A). Sciatic nerve entrapment can, therefore, occur:

1. acutely with a strong piriformis contraction
2. with a piriformis muscle sprain or strain caused by excessive and/or sudden passive internal rotation and adduction of the leg or if active external rotation/adduction are blocked (particularly if either occurs while tension in the muscle is already increased; e.g. piriformis in partial/full contraction at the time)
3. over a period of time, with repetitive activity that incorporates these same mechanisms

These actions increase the risk of injury to both the nerve and muscle in someone with the chronic increase in piriformis tension so often seen in association with malalignment because of:

1. separation of right piriformis origin and insertion, as would occur with an innominate 'inflare' (Fig. 2.46A), excessive sacral nutation and also internal rotation of a lower extremity
2. 'facilitation' resulting in an increase in the resting tone of the muscle
3. reflex contraction or just a reactive increase in resting tone, as it attempts to decrease pain and/or help stabilize the SI joint

The symptoms may be provoked on clinical examination using manoeuvres that combine passive traction (to increase tension in both piriformis and the sciatic nerve) with a simultaneous resisted active piriformis contraction, intended to compress the nerve (see 'piriformis syndrome' below). These separated effects can typically be achieved by:

1. passive hip flexion, adduction and internal rotation, to put nerve and muscle under maximum stretch (the FAIR manoeuvre; Fig. 4.18A,B) which can be augmented by simultaneously resisting active hip extension, abduction and external rotation
2. passive internal rotation of the supine-lying person's extended leg (Freiberg manoeuvre)
3. passive straight leg raising and internal rotation combined with a resisted contraction of the external rotators
4. resisted active hip abduction in side-lying or when the person is sitting

When piriformis is involved, these tests provoke pain that tends to localize to the buttock and spare the lumbar spine. When there is irritation of the peroneal or tibial component, pain and paraesthesias consistently involve the respective areas supplied by these nerves in the lower extremities (Fig. 4.12A,B).

In contrast, those presenting with malalignment frequently use the term 'sciatica' loosely to describe pain or paraesthesias felt primarily in the low back and/or buttock region and radiating a variable distance down the 'back of the leg'. On further questioning, the pain usually stops part-way down the thigh or at the knee, although sometimes it may go down into the calf and as far as the ankle. Symptoms in the foot are rare. When present, dysaesthesias often involve only part of the dorsum or sole in a non-anatomical pattern and a patient may be able to state quite definitely that any abnormal sensations in the foot do not appear to be continuous with those felt more proximally. In fact, typical of referred symptoms, the dysaesthesias:

1. may at times be felt only in the leg,
2. at other times only in the foot, and
3. sometimes in both sites simultaneously or not at all.

These phenomena are characteristic of referred paraesthesias and dysaesthesias, as discussed above (Figs 3.45, 3.63, 4.10). On closer examination, one is likely to find a malalignment-related increase in tension and tenderness of one or more of the structures capable of referring to the posterior thigh, calf, ankle and foot. The piriformis muscle itself and the sacrotuberous ligament are typical of structures that can be activated by the malalignment and, in turn, precipitate local and referred symptoms that come to mimic 'sciatica'.

Symptoms felt only a variable distance down the back of the thigh, occasionally into the calf or in a patchy pattern as far as the foot, are more likely to be occurring on the basis of referral from structures upset by the malalignment rather than being a true 'sciatica', especially if:

1. there is no evidence of a neurological deficit, and
2. root stretch tests and pressure applied over the sciatic notch do not suggest increased irritability of the sciatic nerve or its components and fail to recreate the patient's dysaesthesias; whereas pressure over the piriformis muscle itself, the sacrotuberous ligament and other structures known to refer in this pattern might do so.

Piriformis syndrome

Yeoman (1928) attributed 'sciatica' to inflammation of the anatomically adjacent SI joint and piriformis muscle where the sciatic nerve exits through the greater sciatic notch. As originally described by him, the 'piriformis syndrome' was precipitated by a traumatic injury to the sacroiliac and gluteal region. Specific signs and symptoms, with some modifications by Robinson (1947) and Papadapoulos & Khan (2004), include the following:

1. pain in the piriformis muscle and the region of the SI joint and greater sciatic notch, radiating 'down the leg' and causing difficulty in walking
2. markedly tender, palpable 'sausage-shaped' mass over the piriformis muscle (now often described as a 'pear-shaped' mass)
3. a positive straight leg raising test and positive Lasègue's sign
4. eventually gluteal muscle atrophy
5. typical aggravation of the symptoms by prolonged hip flexion, adduction and internal rotation, and by bending and lifting
6. an absence of findings in the low back and hip regions

Pace & Nagle (1976), reporting on a series of 45 patients diagnosed as having 'piriformis syndrome', noted that only half had a history of trauma, usually minor. Pain and weakness on resisting simultaneous abduction and external rotation of the thigh was one of the most consistent findings on clinical examination. They also commonly found a trigger point located within the piriformis that was responsible for a distinct tenderness on the lateral pelvic wall; pressure on this trigger point reproduced the original complaint(s). The point was located fairly high up and felt to correspond to the medial trigger point described by Travell & Simons (1992), the lateral one being located at the junction of the middle and distal third (Fig. 3.45). The symptoms were abolished with trigger point injections.

A tear of the piriformis muscle results in a circumscribed area that is acutely tender and probably localized most accurately by internal palpation (Fig. 2.53B). Nerve conduction and electromyographic studies may be abnormal because:

1. there is denervation activity indicative of injury to muscle fibres and ongoing healing
2. the tear and/or subsequent oedematous swelling has resulted in pressure injury to a nerve (e.g. the nearby tibial or peroneal nerve component; the nerve fibres from S1 and S2 that supply pirifomis directly; Fig. 4.15)

There may, therefore, be evidence of impaired nerve conduction, ongoing denervation and/or reinnervation changes suggestive of previous nerve injury (see below).

As indicated, piriformis originates from the sacrum (2nd to 4th segment), superior margin of the notch and the ST ligament; it inserts into the superior aspect of the greater trochanter (Figs 2.46A, 3.45). Piriformis comes to act primarily as an external rotator when the leg is straight and an abductor when the hip and knee are flexed. Ventral rami of the lumbosacral plexus (L4-S3) converge at the inferior border of piriformis to form the sciatic nerve, exit through the greater sciatic notch and divide into the peroneal and tibial components. In 12%, this division occurs more proximally or at the level of piriformis (Fig. 4.17), leading to the various patterns in which these components pass by or actually through the muscle. Whether or not these variations play any role in the 'pathology' of the 'piriformis syndrome' is uncertain.

There is ongoing disagreement whether the 'piriformis syndrome' indeed exists. Kirkaldy-Willis & Hill (1979) felt that 'pirifomis syndrome' was often under-diagnosed or mistaken for 'more common conditions such as facet arthropathy, sacroiliitis and radiculopathy'. Papadapoulos & Khan (2004) described the 'syndrome' as a constellation of symptoms, including low back and buttock pain with referral to the leg. However, questions continue to be asked whether:

1. 'piriformis syndrome' is a distinct clinical entity?
2. it involves:
   a. neuropathic pain from compression of the sciatic nerve entrapped by the piriformis muscle as it courses through the greater sciatic notch?
   b. myofascial pain from a tight, hypertrophied, tender piriformis, without nerve entrapment?

Fishman et al. (2002) felt the syndrome accounts for 6-8% of LBP and 'sciatica' in the USA. He has tried to improve the objectivity of criteria for the clinical diagnosis of 'piriformis syndrome' and selection of subjects to participate in research studies by using what have come to be known as 'Fishman's clinical criteria'.

Fishman's clinical criteria for 'piriformis syndrome'

1. tenderness at the sciatic notch
2. positive Lasègue's sign at 45 degrees
3. increased pain in the sciatic distribution with the thigh in the FAIR position (Flexion, Adduction, Internal Rotation)
4. electrodiagnostic studies negative for myopathy or neuropathy

However, as the authors of a recent review of the literature indicated, the diagnosis continues to be:

> *largely clinical and. . .one of exclusion. Herniated nucleus pulposus. . .facet arthropathy, spinal stenosis and lumbar muscle strain must be ruled out, although due to compensatory biomechanical factors it is possible for the piriformis syndrome to develop concurrently or as a sequelum of these other conditions.*
>
> (Kirschner et al. 2009: 11)

Reference to 'these other conditions' was limited to the four listed. Also, there was no description of any of the possible 'compensatory biomechanical factors' and, specifically, no mention whether pelvic and/or spine malalignment was looked for by the authors of any of the 11 papers on 'piriformis syndrome' reviewed. The subjects studied typically complained of buttock pain, possibly with 'ipsilateral radiation down the posterior thigh'; how far exactly, and in what pattern(s) was not specified. Of interest was the authors' mention that:

> *if weakness or sensory loss is elicited, the diagnosis of pirirformis syndrome becomes less likely, except in the more chronic presentations where secondary disuse atrophy may be present*
>
> (Kirschner et al. 2009:11)

There was no indication whether these findings were in keeping with a neurological problem, or whether the weakness documented was limited to the unilateral piriformis or muscles innervated by the peroneal and/or tibial nerve component.

As with 'sciatica', symptoms were aggravated by:

1. active external rotation, with contraction of the tender muscle (e.g. kicking a ball with the outside of the foot by externally rotating/abducting the lower extremity; skate skiing (Fig. 5.26)
2. passive internal rotation, which stretches the muscle

Diagnosis of 'piriformis syndrome'

Attempts to make the diagnosis more objective has led to recommendations regarding use of some 'confirmed' examination techniques and electrodiagnostic studies.

Physical testing

1. passive
   a. Freiberg's manoeuvre
      Passive internal rotation of the leg is intended to stretch the 'irritated' piriformis and provoke sciatic nerve compression (Beatty 1994); on Pećina's cadaver study, the manoeuvre was shown to compress the peroneal nerve passing through the muscle (1979)
   b. 'FAIR' manoeuvre (Fig. 4.18)
      Passive 'Flexion Adduction Internal Rotation' can trigger symptoms by putting the affected piriformis under stretch
2. active
   a. 'PACE'
      The patient is sitting and abducts the hip against resistance, to see if activating piriformis provokes pain.
   b. Beatty test
      The patient is lying in the lateral decubitus position, knee and hip flexed; abduction of the upper thigh to activate piriformis is likely to provoke:
      i. deep buttock pain in someone with piriformis syndrome
      ii. low back and leg pain in those with lumbar disc disease

Medical imaging

1. An MRI may help to rule out anatomic anomalies (e.g. accessory piriformis), bursa, or any surrounding structures that can play a role in nerve root, sciatic or distal nerve compression. For example, in a case reported by Stewart (2003), the MRI allowed for visualization of enlargement of piriformis and the sciatic nerve itself, with concomitant nerve compression.
2. CAT scan and ultrasound have been useful more for ruling out mass lesions capable of causing back or buttock pain and compressing the sciatic nerve: tumors, aneurysms, haematomas, endometriosis, infectious processes and complicating abscesses.

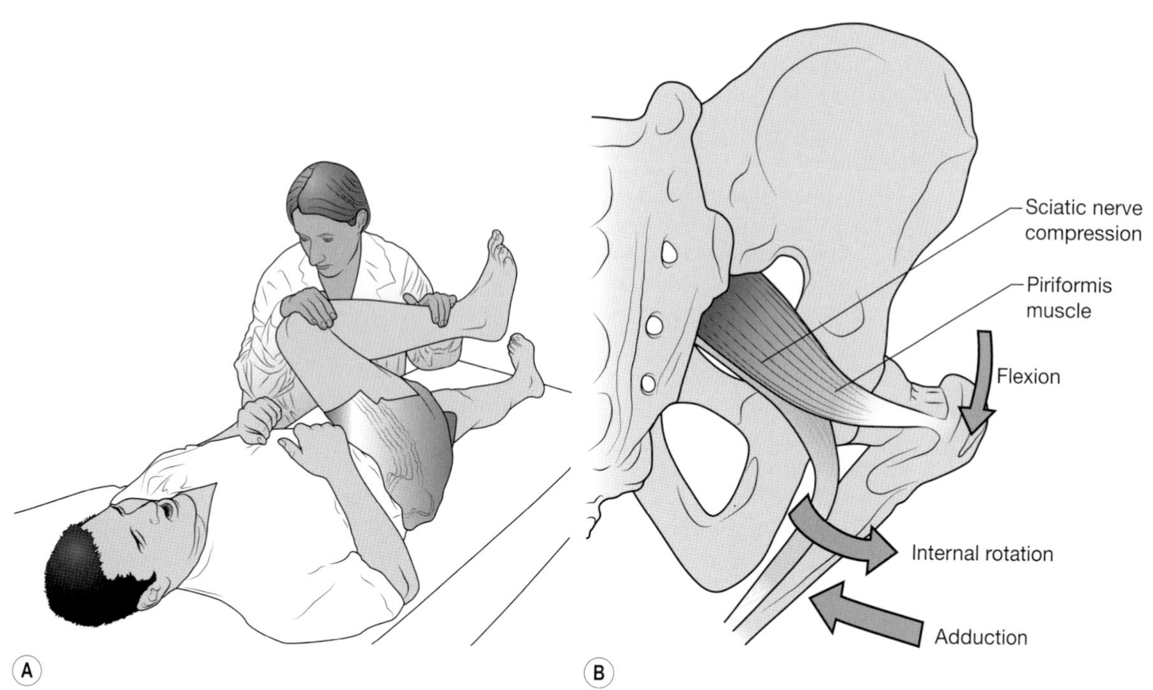

Fig. 4.18 Piriformis syndrome, diagnosis and treatment. (A) The FAIR manoeuvre: the examiner passively Flexes, Adducts and Internally Rotates the hip to see if this reproduces a complaint of buttock pain radiating down the leg. (B) The anatomy of the piriformis and surrounding structures in the FAIR position. The sciatic nerve is compressed with the hip passively flexed, adducted and internally rotated. *(Redrawn courtesy of Kirschner et al. 2009.)*

Electrodiagnostic studies

Nerve conduction studies (NCS) and EMG are usually normal. However, in the absence of an underlying myopathy, neuropathy or recent muscle injury (e.g. a tear or contusion) there can be findings consistent with nerve compromise or definite injury:

1. abnormal spontaneous activity on EMG may suggest:
   a. compression with ongoing death of peripheral nerve fibres; the muscles involved will help narrow involvement to the sciatic nerve itself or the peroneal and/or tibial components
   b. previous compression, with chronic denervation activity and/or motor potentials of large amplitude and increased duration, consistent with reinnervation
   c. a nerve root problem - this is less likely if the denervation activity is not limited to a specific myotome distribution and is absent on testing the paravertebral muscles supplied by the suspected root(s)
2. Nerve conduction studies
   a. SNAP or CMUAP: amplitude loss, indicative of the loss of nerve or muscle fibres, respectively.
   b. H-reflex latency: probably a spinal reflex, it can be triggered by electrical stimulation of afferent fibres in a mixed nerve and activation of motor neurons to the muscle mainly through a monosynaptic connection in the spinal cord. For example, the H-reflex elicited by stimulating the tibial nerve in the popliteal region is the electrical manifestation of the ankle jerk. It looks at the latency for sensory signals to ascend in the tibial nerve up to the spinal cord where they stimulate some S1 root motor fibres which, in turn, trigger a weak contraction of gastrocnemius; i.e. the S1 afferent and efferent components of the reflex arc, respectively. Slowing has been reported to occur on some of these H-reflex studies when carried out simultaneously with the 'FAIR' manoeuvre, in an attempt to compromise the nerve. This slowing of the latency has been used as a criterion for the diagnosis of 'piriformis syndrome', also for the selection of subjects to be included in research studies (Fishman & Zybert 1992).

c. Magnetic stimulation of L5 and S1 nerve root: one study showed significant slowing of the motor nerve conduction velocity in the gluteal segment of the sciatic nerve, but only for L5 (Chang et al. 2006).

Local anaesthetic injection

1. Lidocaine injection into the piriformis muscle has been effective both diagnostically, with relief of pain within minutes, and for treatment. Injection may be done blindly, using anatomical landmarks (e.g. the greater trochanter or acetabulum and the SI joint), but guidance using EMG, fluoroscopic myogram or these in combination has definite advantages (Fig. 4.19).
2. Lidocaine combined with a corticosteroid is often used for longer acting treatment effect.

Botulinum-A toxin injection

The toxin acts at the level of the muscle spindle and affects both motor and sensory pathways by inhibiting gamma motor neurons and blocking Type 1a afferent signals, respectively.

1. it presumably relieves pain by relaxing painfully spastic muscles
2. there are conflicting reports as to its effectiveness in treating myofascial pain seen with various medical conditions, including 'piriformis syndrome'

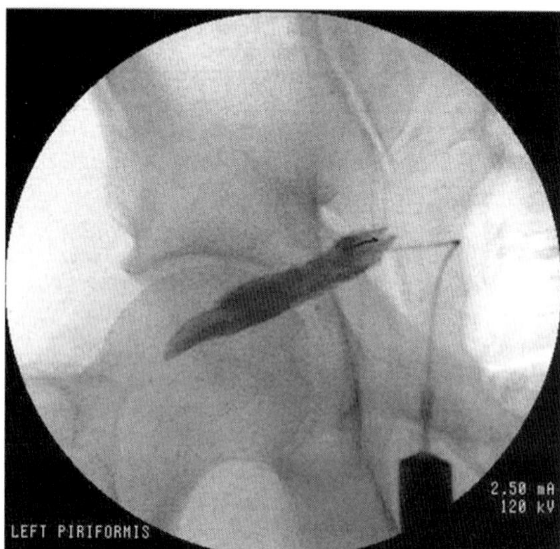

Fig. 4.19 Fluoroscopic myogram of the piriformis. Note contrast flow along the distribution of the piriformis muscle. *(Courtesy of Kirschner et al. 2009.)*

More recently, double-blind, randomized controlled trials by Fishman et al. (2002), Childers et al. (2006) and others have reported significant changes with the use of Botox compared to controls but variation in terms of injection (blinded or guided), pain assessment method (e.g. use of the VAS or 'SF Short Form'), use of supplementary physiotherapy treatment and other factors has made comparison of these studies difficult.

Standard treatment approach in the presence of malalignment

Kirschner et al. (2009) noted that the mainstay of treatment continues to be piriformis stretching 'aimed to correct the underlying pathology by relaxing the tight piriformis, and related muscle stretching to relieve nerve compression'. Suggestions from the literature included:

1. use of moist heat and ultrasound prior to stretching piriformis, which lies deep to gluteus maximus
2. subsequent stretching: hip and knee flexion, hip adduction and internal rotation of the thigh (i.e. as in the 'FAIR' manoeuvre), with the understanding that this could provoke pain during initial treatment sessions, given the stress the tender piriformis is subjected to by this manoeuvre
3. followed by 'lumbosacral stabilization' and 'myofascial release' (with no indication of the exact problem on hand that requires 'stabilization' or the actual treatment approach suggested)
4. if these methods and oral medications failed: consideration of one of the injection techniques

Many of those who have been labeled as having a 'piriformis syndrome' do not have a history of an acute or repetitive mechanism of injury that might have caused entrapment of the sciatic nerve, and their electrodiagnostic studies are normal. A large number, however, present with an 'upslip', 'rotational malalignment' 'flare' or combinations of these and show the typical increase in piriformis tension and tenderness; findings are more in keeping with:

1. a reflex increase in tension, or even spasm, in this muscle as it attempts to counter SI joint instability and/or discomfort (see Chs 2, 3)
2. an increase in the length-tension ration by separation of origin and insertion, as would occur on the side of an 'inflare' and with sacral nutation and 'posterior' innominate rotation
3. 'facilitation' triggered by the malalignment

Accompanying symptoms of pain and paraesthesias often lead to the diagnosis of a 'piriformis syndrome' with irritation of the sciatic nerve, even though the symptoms actually radiate only a varying distance down the back of the leg, usually not past the knee and very rarely involving the foot; that is, these symptoms are not in keeping with irritation or injury specifically to the peroneal or tibial nerve. They are more likely to arise on the basis of referral, originating from the piriformis itself, trigger points within that muscle, or from the nearby ligaments, hip or SI joint (Figs 3.45, 3.62, 3.67). The medial and lateral piriformis trigger points, for example, refer pain to the sacroiliac region primarily, the buttock in general, the hip joint posteriorly and occasionally to the proximal two-thirds of the posterior thigh, but neither to the posterior calf nor into the foot (Travell & Simons 1992).

In a person with 'rotational malalignment', a 'posterior' innominate rotation with relative sacral nutation separates piriformis origin and insertion. When combined with an 'inflare' of that innominate, it further increases tension in this muscle to the point of narrowing the space available for the sciatic nerve traversing the inferior part of the greater sciatic foramen. With time, a chronic increase in piriformis tension combined with such a narrowing of the outlet could admittedly result in some nerve fibre irritation, paraesthesias and pain down the leg and into the foot in the distribution specific for one or both components, in the form of a true 'sciatica'.

In most people presenting out of alignment, therefore, increased tension and tenderness of piriformis and the referred symptoms are very likely to be just another manifestation of the changes asociated with the malalignment, rather than a *bona fide*, isolated 'piriformis syndrome'.

In keeping with this assumption is the fact that the signs and symptoms usually disappear quite quickly on realignment. On the other hand, increased tension or spasm following an actual injury of piriformis has been implicated as one cause of the initial occurrence and subsequent recurrences of malalignment. The muscle originates primarily from the anterior sacrum/greater sciatic notch area, crosses both the SI and the hip joints, and inserts into the upper, posterior aspect of the greater trochanter (Figs 2.46A, 3.45). It is in a strategic position to exert rotational or traction forces on these structures. In addition, the increase in tension in the piriformis muscle typically noted with malalignment puts the person at increased risk of suffering an accidental sprain or strain of this muscle and presenting with a *bona fide* acute 'piriformis syndrome'. In this case, treatment of the piriformis injury in isolation, without simultaneous correction of the malalignment, is likely to prolong recovery and increases the risk of the injury recurring. Similarly, the 'standard' treatment methods for a 'piriformis syndrome' suggested above would be inappropriate:

1. anti-inflammatory medication, orally or by injection, likely will provide only temporary relief at best as they fail to correct the alignment
2. corticosteroids are used at the risk of increasing laxity of the musculotendinous junction and, in case of needle misplacement, the nearby hip and SI joint capsule and ligaments
3. when an increase in tension is caused by the malalignment being present, it is unlikely to respond to stretching, or will do so only temporarily unless the malalignment is corrected (see 'Asymmetry of muscle tension' and Ch. 7)
4. Botulinum-A toxin can decrease pain and muscle tension for approximately 3 months but during this time it will also cause piriformis weakening and atrophy (Childers et al. 2006); in someone with malalignment, that could interfere with the muscle's protective role in terms of trying to decrease SI joint pain, increase pelvic stability and help maintain alignment.

Summary: 'piriformis syndrome'

1. There very likely exists a 'piriformis syndrome' as a distinct entity, with the features described by Yeoman, Robinson and others. Diagnosis should depend on increasingly objective clinical and investigative studies.
2. All of the three common presentations of malalignment can affect pirifomis for various reasons, such as an increase in tension and trigger point formation. The symptoms and signs that result are part of the 'malalignment syndrome' and are similar to those felt to comprise the *bona fide* 'piriformis syndrome' (see Point 1) but they will usually decrease or resolve completely with realignment.

3. Presence of the 'piriformis syndrome' can precipitate malalignment and vice versa. The two can coexist and symptoms may overlap. Initial treatment should be aimed at realignment, including core muscle strengthening, stretching, and other measures, as indicated in Ch. 7. If there are residual findings attributable to an underlying 'piriformis syndrome', these may require addition of some of the specific treatments listed above (e.g. 'standard' physiotherapy approaches, medication and possibly injections) to completely resolve the problem.

'Thoracolumbar syndrome'

Back in 1972, Maigne already drew attention to the fact that 'low back pain erroneously attributed to lumbar or lumbosacral disease may well be caused by referred pain from the thoracolumbar junction' (1980: 393). In 1980, he reported on a series of 138 patients, all of whom complained of low back pain but whose pain originated from the transitional area of the spine, the thoracolumbar region (see Chs 2, 3; Fig. 3.9). Maigne was referring to the fact that T12 typically had:

1. superior facets that were oriented in the coronal plane, in keeping with the rest of the thoracic spine and allowing primarily for rotation
2. inferior facets that were oriented in the sagittal plane, in keeping with the lumbar part of the spine and allowing primarily for flexion and extension.

He felt that the syndrome was attributable to the resultant 'disharmony of movement', usually of T12 relative to L1, but also at times involving the vertebra above or below. This disharmony would eventually result in a painful facet joint on one side, and evidence of irritation of the cutaneous branches originating from the posterior roots of T11, T12 and L1 on the same side. The thoracolumbar level involved could be determined by:

1. applying pressure to and 'frictioning' directly over the facet joints lying about 1–1.5 cm from the midline (Fig. 4.20B)
2. applying lateral pressure to the spinous processes to further compromise the contralateral facet joints involved (Fig. 4.20A)

On dissection, the cutaneous branches were shown to descend in the subcutaneous tissue and end in the skin of the lower lumbar area. Typical findings on examination included a painful 'crestal point' (where these branches crossed the posterior iliac crest; Fig. 4.21) and acute tenderness on skin-rolling and pinching the subcutaneous tissue they supplied (Fig. 4.22). Subsequently, Maigne et al. (1986) and Maigne (1995) referred to these branches as the 'posterior branch' of spinal nerves T12 and L1, frequently with contributions from T11 and L2 (Fig. 4.23 A1,B1), at the same time drawing attention to two other 'cutaneous perforating' branches that could also be part of the 'thoracolumbar syndrome':

1. an *'anterior cutaneous perforating branch'*
   Formed by the anterior rami of spinal nerves T12 and L1 (Fig. 4.23 A2,B2), it innervates:
   a. the skin of the lower abdomen, the inner aspect of the upper thighs and the labia majora or scrotum (= *dermatome*)
   b. the lower part of rectus abdominis and transversus abdominis (= *myotome*; Fig. 2.31B)
   c. the pubis (pubic bone = *sclerotome*).
2. a *'lateral cutaneous perforating branch'*
   Formed by the anterior rami of T12 and L1 (Fig. 4.23 A3,B3), it innervates the lateral hip, thigh and occasionally also the groin region to a varying extent.

Maigne felt that irritation of these three cutaneous branches arising from the thoracolumbar junction area happened because:

1. the greatest degree of rotation and lateral flexion occurred at this level
2. a rotary twisting movement eventually resulted in a 'minimal vertebral displacement', usually of T12 relative to L1.

In 1980, Maigne reported how frequently in clinical practice pain elicited with pressure applied to the spinous processes and facets joints was limited to the T11-T12 or T12-L1 level. In 1995, his statistics indicated that this particular localization of tenderness to the mid back was found in approximately 30% of those presenting with 'back pain'. Failure to elicit pain radiating into the legs, the absence of scoliosis and of an antalgic spine, and a 'usually negative' straight leg raising test should raise suspicions that the problem was not in the lumbosacral but the thoracolumbar part of the spine. The clinical presentation could include any or all of the following:

Low back pain of thoracolumbar origin

The pain is described as being mostly chronic in type, although it can be acute in origin and felt as

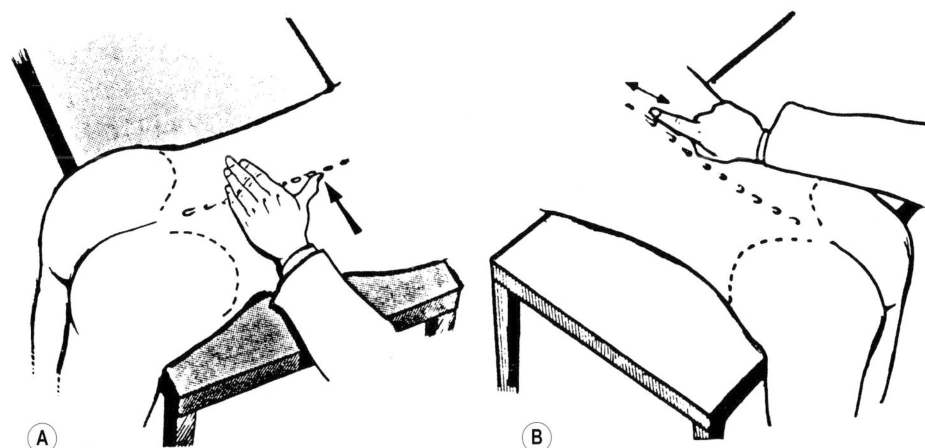

Fig. 4.20 Thoracolumbar syndrome: method of determining the thoracolumbar level involved. (A) Lateral pressure over the spinous process at the involved level is usually painful in only one direction - left or right. (B) Seeking the painful posterior articular point (facet joint) by pressure and friction 1 cm from the midline. *(Courtesy of Maigne 1995.)*

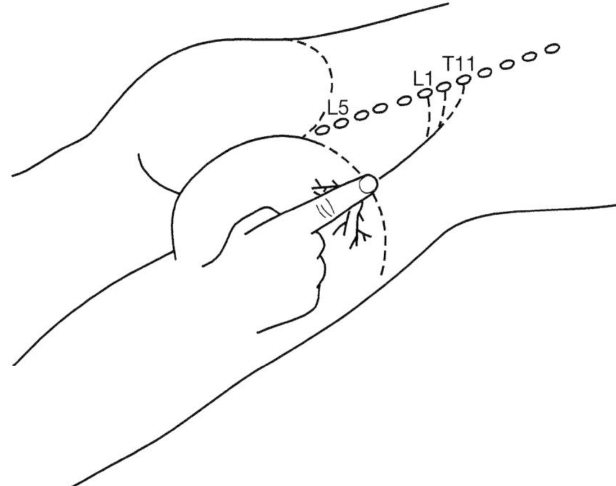

Fig. 4.21 Thoracolumbar syndrome, with irritation of cutaneous nerves formed by branches from T11, T12 and L1. The posterior branch, which ends in the skin of the posterior lumbosacral and buttock area, may be found by applying friction and pressure to the posterior iliac crest to seek the 'crestal point'. *(Redrawn courtesy of Maigne 1995.)*

such. It is usually unilateral and perceived in the sacroiliac, low back or buttock region, sometimes with referral to the lateral thigh (Fig. 4.23A1,B1). Patients never complain of symptoms in the thoracolumbar region. Clinical signs include:

1. at the posterior iliac crest point, a very tender site situated 7–10 cm lateral to the midline where the posterior branch crosses the crest
2. pain on skin-rolling (Fig. 4.22) as irritation of the skin innervated by the posterior branch can result in a limited area of cellulalgia in the upper buttock region; the skin becomes very painful and often feels thickened when rolled between the thumb and index finger
3. relief of the pain on manipulation or injection;
   - manipulation of the thoracolumbar region or the injection of local anaesthetic around selective facet joints in this area should relieve the presenting pain, allowing free movement and resulting in the disappearance of the crestal point and area of cellulalgia.

'Pseudo-visceral pain'

Involvement of the anterior branch can result in pain over the lower abdominal wall, groin or testicle (Fig. 4.23A2, B2):

> *It is experienced as a deep, tight pain, perfectly simulating visceral pain; . . . it is variable and episodic in nature and can occur at the same time as the back pain.*
>
> (Maigne 1995: 88)

If, however, it occurs at separate times, the patient may fail to associate the two pains and end up being seen by a gynaecologist for this part of the pain and an orthopaedic surgeon for the low back pain. Maigne went on to warn that persistence of these pains may lead to:

> *. . .multiple and sometimes extensive investigations. Minor abnormalities may be found which often lead to inappropriate surgical treatment.*
>
> (Maigne 1995:88)

This is, unfortunately, particularly true in the field of gynaecology.

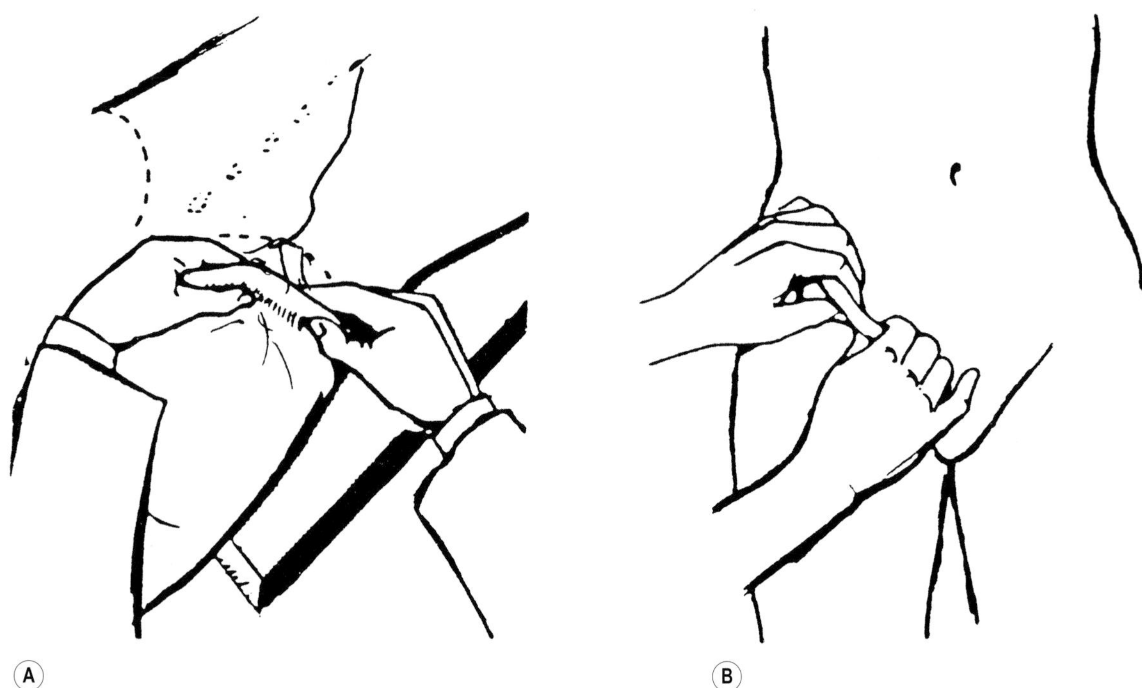

Fig. 4.22 Seeking painful subcutaneous tissue by pinching a skin fold supplied by a cutaneous branch and pulling and rolling it. (A) Cellulalgia from the posterior branch. (B) Cellulalgia from the anterior branch. *(Courtesy of Maigne 1995.)*

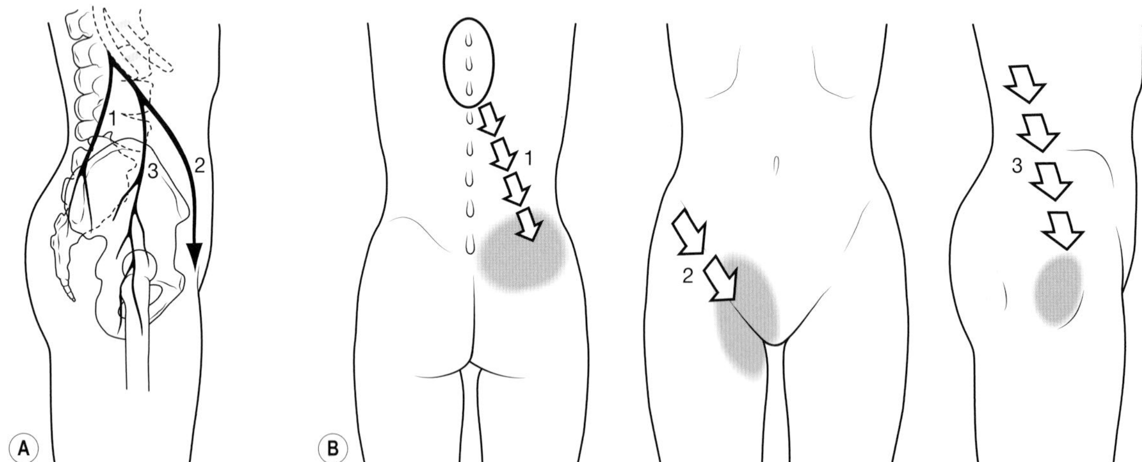

Fig. 4.23 Problems relating to the T12 and L1 cutaneous branches. A1,B1: Posterior branch: low back pain. A2, B2: Anterior branch: pseudo-visceral pain. A3,B3: Lateral perforating branch: pseudo-hip pain. *(Redrawn courtesy of Maigne 1995.)*

On clinical examination, the pseudo-visceral problem is characterized by an area of cellulalgia localizing to the lower abdomen and upper inner aspect of the thigh. The pain is unilateral and corresponds to the side of the back pain.

In one out of three cases, involvement of the anterior branch also results in a marked tenderness of the 'hemipubis' on one side, although the patient rarely complains spontaneously of pubic pain. The prevalence of this sign is increased in those engaged in sports that involve the abdominal and adductor muscles (e.g. hockey, soccer and tennis).

'Pseudo-hip pain'

Involvement of the lateral cutaneous perforating branches can cause pain in the greater trochanter region, sometimes in the groin, and may simulate hip pain (Fig. 4.23A3,B3). Pain evoked on compression of the overlying area of cellulalgia against the trochanter often leads to the mistaken diagnosis of 'trochanteric bursitis' but local injections (predictably) fail. Tenderness localizes to the point at which the cutaneous fibres cross the lateral iliac crest just above the trochanter, and to the area of cellulalgia that runs vertically between these two landmarks.

Mention is made here of the 'thoracolumbar syndrome' because of the large number of those who present with malalignment and who have tenderness localizing to the thoracolumbar junction. In a study of 96 individuals presenting with malalignment (Schamberger 2002), 76% had pain when pressure was applied to the spine; in 22% of these, the pain was limited to the thoracolumbar junction alone.

> An 'upslip' and 'rotational malalignment' will either cause or accentuate an already existing scoliosis, with lateral curvatures of the thoracic and lumbar segments that in most persons reverse at the thoracolumbar junction (Fig. 3.14B,C)

Any curvature of the adjoining part of the lumbar and thoracic segment is formed by the simultaneous side flexion and, in the lumbar and parts of the thoracic spine, rotation of the vertebrae into the convexity of that particular segment. The reversal of the curve, therefore, means the rotation of adjoining vertebrae in contrary directions at the point at which these segments meet. Even if the lumbar segment appears straight and stiff in the presence of malalignment, a change again usually occurs at the thoracolumbar junction, leading into a right or left thoracic convexity (Fig. 2.92). In that case, T12 would still end up rotated relative to L1 (Fig. 3.14C).

The usual reversal of the lumbar lordosis to a thoracic kyphosis that occurs at this junction in the sagittal plane can only add further to the stress at this level of the spine (Fig. 3.14A). In addition, T12 or L1 rank among the vertebrae that most often show rotational displacement in conjunction with an 'upslip' or 'rotational malalignment' (see Ch. 3).

Given that the thoracolumbar junction is one of the high-stress areas of our spine, particularly in the presence of malalignment, it is really no wonder that bony and soft tissue structures in this area prove to be tender on examination. The symptoms and signs of a 'thoracolumbar syndrome' could easily develop, even though the patient may be unable to recall a specific 'rotatory twisting movement' that might cause Maigne's traumatic 'minimal vertebral rotation'. Malalignment, for example, increases the stress on the T12-L1 facet joints because the rotation of these vertebrae in opposite directions results in:

1. compression of the facet joint surfaces on one side, possibly with a complicating:
   a. entrapment of the capsule and/or branches of the posterior root fibres innervating the joint
   b. foraminal narrowing or aggravation of a stenosis
2. distraction of the joint surfaces on the opposite side, which increases the tension on that joint capsule and nerve fibres (Fig. 2.52B)
3. irritation of the nerve fibres, including the cutaneous branches mentioned by Maigne.

The localized increase in tone and tenderness to palpation so frequently seen in the immediately adjacent paravertebral and erector spinalis muscles and limited to the thoracolumbar junction area may be no more than a reflex splinting of the muscles overlying a facet joint and/or disc structure that has become unstable or a cause of discomfort with the relative vertebral displacement. It could also be an indicator of a reactive increase in muscle fibre tone triggered by irritation of their nerve supply; in this case, the medial branch of the posterior root that innervates the multifidi, rotatores and interspinous muscles at each level (Fig. 2.29).

However, although the person with malalignment may show tenderness of these various sites and tissues in the thoracolumbar junction area, he or she may not be aware of discomfort in the mid back region, similar to the situation Maigne described for someone presenting with the 'thoracolumbar syndrome'. A number do show tenderness of one or more of the three cutaneous perforating sensory nerves where they cross the posterior and/or lateral pelvic crest, and hypersensitivity of the overlying skin, in keeping with a full-blown 'thoracolumbar syndrome'. Once alignment has been achieved and is being maintained, muscle tension and tenderness, along with other signs and symptoms localizing to the thoracolumbar, iliac crest, abdominal and hip regions, usually resolve fairly quickly (see Appendix 9).

Another form of 'thoracolumbar syndrome' has been blamed on irritation of either the L1 or L2 root, which contribute to the formation of the LFCN (L2, L3). It can present as:

1. deep abdominal pain with irritation near the root origin and where it runs posterior to psoas
2. anterior abdominal pain (lateralizing on palpation to where the LFCN runs medial to the anterior superior iliac spine), and
3. the distal symptoms of meralgia paraesthetica: anterolateral hip and thigh dysaesthesias in the distribution of the terminating anterior and/or posterolateral branches to the skin (Fig. 4.13).

Development of a 'thoracolumbar syndrome' has also been attributed by some to the hypermobility that can develop with increased stress on the thoracolumbar junction from loss of movement in the low or mid-lumbar segments noted with:

1. fusion of these segments (Paris 1990)
2. prolonged close-packing of the facets characteristic of an increased tendency to lumbar spine extension, seen with:
   a. the 'faulty lordotic posture' typical of those presenting with chronic pelvic pain (Baker 1998)
   b. excessive nutation of the sacrum and a secondary increase in the lordosis that occurs with a 'bilateral anterior sacrum' (see Ch. 2)
   c. an increasing lumbar lordosis to counter excessive lower abdominal girth or the weight of a growing fetus (Fig. 3.56)

Malalignment and coexistent conditions of the spine

Some common conditions involving the spine do not present any problems for most people; they are usually considered to be 'benign', albeit a possible cause of trouble in the future. The chance of these conditions becoming symptomatic is, however, increased by the stresses that malalignment imposes on the spine. The key, then, is to recognize the contributing role of the malalignment. Initial treatment should be aimed at achieving alignment rather than attempting to treat what may actually turn out to be a benign underlying condition once the superimposed stress has diminished or even disappeared on realignment.

'Scoliosis'

The word 'scoliosis' strikes fear in the hearts of parents and those children old enough to understand its implications: a gradually increasing C-curve or double curve, accelerated degeneration of the spine, deformity, limitation of activity and eventually complications relating to the spinal cord itself or to compromised function of the heart and lungs. The picture described is that of progressive 'idiopathic scoliosis'. The tentative diagnosis is often made at the time of a screening examination, usually confirmed later by someone with a special interest in this condition. And yet, how often do those familiar with malalignment see parents presenting with a child or teenager who has already been labeled as having 'scoliosis' but:

1. whose X-rays show no congenital malformations or bony anomalies, such as hemi-vertebrae or absent ribs, that would predispose to a progressive course
2. who by history and on review of the clinical records has no convincing evidence of such a progressive course, or at most only a few degrees change recorded over the years, and
3. who, on examination, proves to have no more than the compensatory, albeit perhaps accentuated, curvatures of the spine (Figs 2.42, 2.76B, 2.90, 2.120C, 3.5C), typically attributable to the pelvic obliquity caused by an underlying problem of malalignment?

The compensatory curves seen in association with malalignment, sometimes in conjunction with a complicating anatomical ('true') LLD, can easily measure up to 10, 15 or even 20 degrees, large enough perhaps for someone to think that the label 'idiopathic scoliosis' is appropriate (Figs 3.7, 3.8). In a large number of these children or teenagers, however, there is no indication of a progressive element on follow-up, and the curves can either be abolished or significantly reduced with realignment. Any residual curvatures then usually amount to no more than the average intrinsic curves of the lumbar and thoracic segments that may be typical for that child's age group.

It would save a lot of grief and worry if some of these children were not labeled 'scoliotic' until the malalignment was first corrected and the residual curvatures measured and followed for a year or two while maintaining alignment and strengthening the trunk and pelvic core muscles in particular, in order to see whether:

1. there is indeed a progressive element to these curves
2. the diagnosis of a progressive 'idiopathic scoliosis' is warranted, and treated accordingly.

> Even if the diagnosis of 'idiopathic scoliosis' is eventually felt to be appropriate, it is still in the child or adult's best interest to correct any pelvic malalignment or vertebral rotational displacement on an ongoing basis in order to remove that component of the curvature (and the associated stresses) which is strictly attributable to the malalignment (Fig. 4.6).

In the author's experience, a correction of malalignment of the pelvis has consistently been possible in those patients with a *bona fide* - and often advanced - idiopathic scoliosis, even when associated with curves up to 30–40 degrees. They typically present with a history of mid and/or low back pain of recent onset. Although realignment with levelling of the pelvis may not have resulted in an appreciable decrease in the measurement of the scoliotic curves, it has repeatedly brought about a decrease or even resolution of their pain, and an increased ability to pursue work and leisure activities. In these patients, correcting any recurrence of malalignment as quickly as possible is advisable, to avert recurrence of these complaints.

A scoliosis often first becomes apparent on examination when the person presents with symptoms. It is, however, this author's contention that:

1. the majority of those who are in their teens and older will present with malalignment and will probably have been out of alignment for some time, given that longitudinal studies already show a prevalence of 75% for malalignment in elementary school children (Klein 1973; Klein & Buckley 1968)
2. most would already have shown a scoliosis on routine examination when they were still asymptomatic
3. the scoliosis, in the majority, is of the non-progressive type and represents in part, if not entirely, an attempt to compensate for the pelvic obliquity attributable to:
   a. a functional LLD seen in all of the 80% plus who are subsequently noted to have an 'upslip' or 'rotational malalignment' (Figs 2.77, 2.78, 2.82, 2.84, 2.85)
   b. an anatomical (true) LLD seen in approximately 10%, in isolation or with a concomitant malalignment (Figs 2.72B, 2.81)
4. the malalignment has had a large part to play in the evolution of the pathological stresses on the thoracolumbar and lumbosacral junctions that eventually resulted in their specific symptoms
5. the compensatory component of the scoliosis will in most cases decrease or even disappear completely if correction of the malalignment is carried out early enough (Fig. 4.6). Persistent scoliosis, however, results in contracture of specific myofascial and ligamentous structures (Fig. 2.60). Therefore, the longer malalignment has been present, and the older the person, the more likely the compensatory component will be to persist or fail to correct completely on realignment.

Realignment combined with a stretching and strengthening program and possibly appropriate orthotics

CASE HISTORY 4.5

A 3-year old girl was seen regarding her 'scoliosis'. She was asymptomatic. On examination, malalignment was present with a 'right anterior, left posterior' rotation and functional LLD. There was a marked pelvic obliquity - the right iliac crest 1.5 cm higher than the left on standing, sitting and lying prone - and compensatory scoliosis evident. Realignment was easily achieved using muscle energy technique, following which the pelvis was level, the leg length equal and the previous scoliotic curves practically non-existent. If malalignment can be seen in children as young as this, and if there is no evidence of abnormality (e.g. hemi-vertebrae) on examination or X-rays, the question arises as to whether these children can eventually go on to develop a progressive 'idiopathic scoliosis' as a result of not having had treatment for a problem of malalignment - and the sometimes considerable associated compensatory scoliosis - earlier in life.

and trunk and seating supports should be the initial mainstay of treatment and may be all that is needed to relieve the symptoms. The person should be advised to keep asymmetric activities and those with a rotational component to a minimum, in order to avoid further stress on the already painful sites and to decrease the chance of recurrence of the malalignment, until pelvic and spine stability has improved and realignment is being achieved more easily and maintained for longer periods of time.

Spondylolisthesis

Spondylolisthesis, even an advanced spondylolisthesis of 25-50% (Grade 2), generally remains asymptomatic. The L5-S1 level is most often involved; a concomitant degeneration of the disc at this level is typical. An anterior displacement of L5 on S1 is most likely to render the L5 root symptomatic, by it being put under traction, becoming entrapped by a prominent disc bulge or protrusion, spinal stenosis or foraminal narrowing, or a combination of these factors.

Some persons may experience intermittent back pain with or without transient root symptoms. Exacerbations are more likely with activities that put an extension or torsional strain on the spine, such as working with arms above horizontal (e.g. stocking shelves), gardening, wrestling or playing court sports. Concomitant malalignment with compensatory scoliosis automatically increases the stress on a lumbosacral spondylolisthetic level, partly on account of the L1–L4 rotation into the lumbar convexity (Figs 2.42, 2.96, 4.6, 4.24, 4.31, 4.33). In addition, symptoms are likely to be aggravated by any coexistent instability of L4 and/or L5. Instability can develop eventually because of the increased stress on ligaments in this area that results from the combined effect of the spondylolisthesis, any disc degeneration and the stress superimposed by recurrent malalignment (Fig. 2.52).

Initial treatment should be aimed at stabilizing the lumbosacral area by combining realignment with a core muscle strengthening programme, the use of a lumbosacral support and possibly the addition of prolotherapy injections to strengthen the ligaments by stimulating collagen formation (see Ch. 7). The person should avoid activities with a rotational component to decrease the chance of recurrence of the malalignment. Surgery is not indicated until the effect of the above measures has had a fair trial or unless there is evidence of instability not amenable to conservative measures, an increasing scoliosis and/or spinal or foraminal stenosis with irritation or compression of the spinal cord or roots.

Unilateral lumbarization, sacralization and transverse process pseudoarthrosis

In all three conditions, the vertebra is anchored on one side (Figs 4.24-4.26). Even simple flexion and extension of the spine results in a rotational strain as the free side of the vertebra rotates forward and backward, respectively, to a varying extent, essentially pivoting around the congenital or developmental

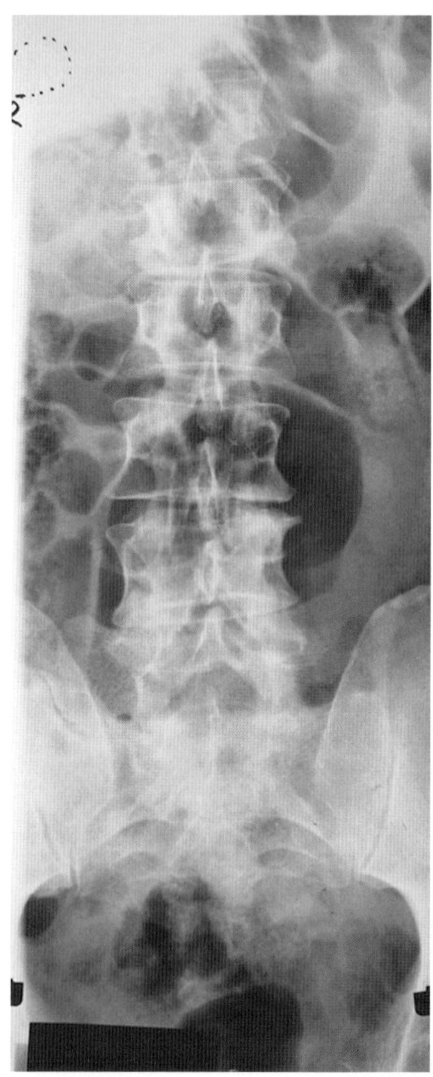

Fig. 4.24 Unilateral partial sacralization of L5, with the formation of a pseudoarthrosis between the right transverse process and both the ilium and sacrum. Malalignment is present, with pelvic obliquity, lumbar dextroscoliosis and L1-L4 rotation into the convexity. Asymmetry of the sacroiliac joint articular surfaces relative to the X-ray beam results in different parts of the joint showing on the right compared with the left side. Realignment resolved the right lumbosacral back pain.

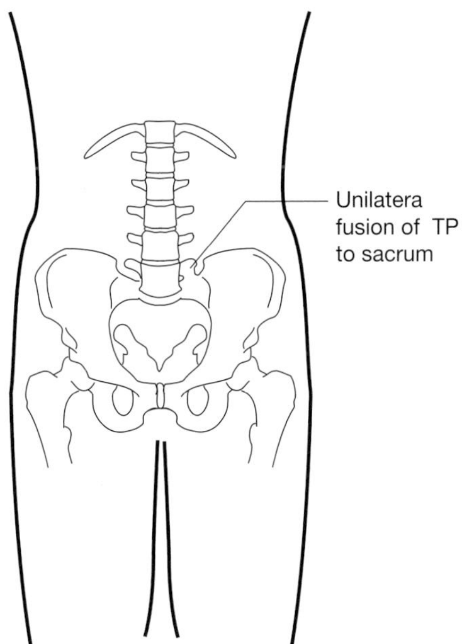

Fig. 4.25 Complete sacralization of left L5 transverse process (TP) in a person who is in alignment and standing.

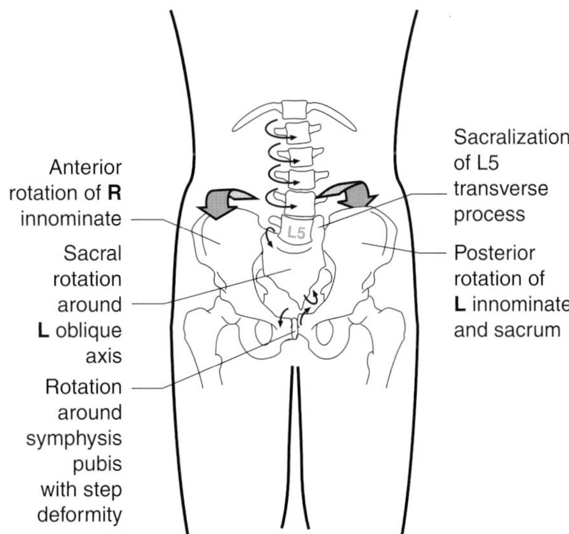

Fig. 4.26 Hinge-like effect of left L5 sacralization (see Fig. 4.25) on spine and pelvic motion when the trunk flexes forward.

unilateral pseudoarthrosis or fusion. The effects relating to malalignment are twofold:

1. spine forward-flexion, extension or side-flexion all cause torquing of this vertebral segment, with forces exerted on the vertebrae above and below (or L5 on the sacrum), and increasing the chance of malalignment occurring in the first place or recurring subsequently
2. even when just standing, sitting or lying, the pelvic obliquity and sacral torsion associated with a coexistent malalignment increase the torquing force constantly exerted on the lumbar vertebrae, especially at the L4-L5 and L5-S1 levels, and the chance of these segments becoming symptomatic.

In some, surgical fusion of the free side carried out while the person is aligned may be the logical procedure in order to stop any recurrence of the malalignment and allow symptoms to resolve. Unfortunately, fusion increases stress on the levels above and below, and can accelerate degeneration at these sites.

IMPLICATIONS FOR PSYCHIATRY AND PSYCHOLOGY

The patients seen by a psychiatrist or psychologist for 'problems of the mind' are not immune to malalignment and the associated neuromuscular problems. One is likely to have a detrimental effect on the other, so it would be in the patient's interest to find relief for problems that relate to a co-existent malalignment in order to improve their chance of resolving the emotional issues that they are trying to cope with. Mention has been made throughout the text of the interplay of mental and physical aspects as relates to the case of the 'malalignment syndrome'.

Stability: Active, passive, neural and emotional keystones

As alluded to in Ch. 2 (Figs 2.23, 2.24), Panjabi's 1992 conceptual model gradually found application to help explain the stabilizing system of the entire musculoskeltal system and not just that of the spine (Lee 1999). Over the past decade, there has also been increasing recognition of the role of emotional factors, how they interplay with the 3 keystones - active, passive and neural control - and are, therefore, capable of influencing and even causing musculoskeletal complaints (Fig. 2.27).

Stress

An increase in stress generated by fear, anxiety and other emotional issues results in a general increase in the 'resting' muscle tone. This stress also has a more definitive effect on muscles that have previously been injured or chronically 'tensed-up', as can occur in the form of:

1. reflex increase in muscle tone or spasm in reaction to problems caused by malalignment

2. muscles that sometime in the past showed increased tension in an asymmetric pattern on account of 'facilitation', change in length-tension ratio and other factors typically seen in conjunction with malalignment

The muscles that were involved then would be:

1. among the first to react to any increase in the emotional stress level
2. likely to cause a recurrence of the malalignment, associated musculoskeletal stresses and recurrence of previous complaints of discomfort, localized and/or referred pain

Hyperventilation and emotional states

Hyperventilation, whether precipitated by physical activity or emotional states such as apprehension, anxiety and fear, has been shown to interfere with the function of specific core muscles and to compromise spinal stability (see 'Implications for respirology' below). Alternately, hyperventilation appears capable of precipitating these emotional and somatic states in patients with known anxiety disorders and stress-related complaints (Hodges et al. 2001; Hodges et al. 2002).

'Abnormal' pain

A pain issue encountered in someone with emotional problems may appear 'abnormal' or be confused with other types of pain phenomena if the person working with the patient is not familiar with the pain patterns noted in conjunction with malalignment.

Referred pain

Those dealing with patients suspected of having psychological or psychiatric problems would be well served by a knowledge of common musculoskeletal referred pain patterns, and particularly those typically seen along with the other problems that are part of the 'malalignment syndrome' (Figs 3.12, 3.46, 3.63, 3.67, 4.8, 4.9, 4.10). A second opinion from someone familiar with malalignment may be worthwhile to allay or support suspicions that there is indeed an underlying neuromuscular problem. For example, there may be pain referred to a specific dermatome or sclerotome but, for lack of knowledge of these patterns, this is misdiagnosed as being in a 'non-anatomical' pattern, something that could affect the subsequent psychiatric assessment and treatment unfavourably.

Hysteria

The patient may complain of pain at a site that is commonly involved in someone presenting with malalignment. An example is the coccyx, one of the sites that:

1. can be injured directly and cause stresses on the pelvic ring that lead to recurrence of malalignment, or
2. may have become painful as a result of the stressful changes imposed secondary to the malalignment.

A sub-group of those presenting with 'idiopathic coccydynia' (see 'Coccydynia, pelvic floor dystonia and levator ani sydrome' below) may be suspected of having psychogenic pain or 'hysteria' if:

1. they have normal X-rays and findings on the static and dynamic studies of the coccygeal joints
2. the history and clinical examination is negative for pathology of the rectum and surrounding structures
3. their coccydynia presents as a constant pain, not relieved by sitting or lying down

Pain precipitated by emotional 'unwinding'

Samorodin (Schamberger 2002: 293) alluded to the analogy of a 'tangled telephone cord' to explain the basis of craniosacral therapy. Similar to the telephone cord, the body was noted to present a system that could:

> *...transmit, absorb or disperse the forces imposed on it...*
>
> *...the absorption or dispersion of forces has the most negative impact on the human body. The dispersion of a physical force through the body often arises from an acute injury such as a haematoma, strain, sprain or fracture. When the body absorbs the impact of a force or a 'stressor', the telephone cord analogy applies*

Malalignment belongs to the latter category of insults, or 'stressors', in that the body usually adapts to these initially. The sudden presentation of a 'dysfunction', with or without obvious precipitating cause, 'may be the result of the inability of the body to adapt to any further 'quantums' of absorbed energy common to the type of, and intensity of, ...activity [imposed]'. The 'dysfunction' may be triggered by inability to adapt to:

1. an acute increase in demand
   - e.g. going on a demanding hike without adequate preparation, or
2. repetitive insults
   - e.g. going travelling and having to deal with repeatedly lifting suitcases and using stairs

In the case of malalignment, examples of the adaptation and a possible subsequent 'dysfunction' include:

1. shortening (contracture) of muscle on the concave side of a scoliotic curve, with eventual inability to adapt to any further stresses imposed; for example, shortening to the point where the muscle can no longer lengthen completely, putting it at risk of suffering a 'dysfunction' in the form of a sprain or strain simply because it has reached the point where it is unable to deal with even a minor increase in tension such as might occur simply on leaning into the opposite (convex) side (see 'quadratus lumborum'; Figs 2.62, 2.43, 3.43)
2. an adaptive reflex increase in tension in an attempt to stabilize a joint and decrease pain, with eventual 'dysfunction' marked by development of a 'chronic tension myalgia', and a lowering of the overall pain level
3. adaptation involving a shift in weight-bearing and secondary change in joint alignment, presenting suddenly as a 'dysfunction' of the knee joint, with:
   a. onset of acute or chronic pain from the supporting capsule, ligaments or tendons and their nerve supply that have up to this point been able to cope with the increase in tension caused by the shift: MCL, LCL, ITB, to name a few (Figs 3.36 3.37, 3.38, 3.41, 3.81), or
   b. onset of pain from compression having caused advanced deterioration of specific structures (e.g. meniscus, cartilage; Fig. 3.81) or even osteoarthritic degeneration of a specific compartment (e.g. right lateral tibiofemoral involvement, resulting with right pronation and increased genu valgum; Figs 3.37, 3.82)

Standard physiotherapy treatment measures fail, similar to the way that, according to Samorodin (Schamberger 2002: 393):

> *stretching a tangled telephone cord does not reduce its tendency to tangle when the tension is removed but suspending the handset by its cord allows the system to unwind on its own*

The key is to find a treatment approach, such as craniosacral release, that may allow for such an 'unwinding' effect:

> *tissue unwinding re-establishes a more biomechanically efficient gait and movement pattern. Given that movement is inherently a function of the nervous system, efficient biomechanics lead to efficient nerve function* (393)

Those using these treatment techniques may seemingly 'unwind' patients who have failed to disperse stresses they have been subjected to in the form of an injury some time ago, or repetitive insults over a period of time. They now present with the impaired neuromuscular function, or 'tangle'. However, resolving the 'tangle' that is part of an obvious malalignment problem not infrequently precipitates an unexpected psychological response as realignment is achieved, indicative of the fact that there was indeed an emotional component to the initial injury or the repetitive insults that the person has 'bottled up', or 'absorbed', and never had a chance to deal with properly. Typical changes include:

1. a feeling of 'profound relaxation'
2. a sudden feeling of abandonment, with weeping and need for emotional support
3. a 'startle response', with screaming, swearing and sometimes flailing of arms and legs

It is as though the person is finally able to release and, hopefully, start to deal with unresolved psychological concerns. Those attending should be aware of what has likely happened, be able to provide the emotional support needed there and then, and possibly arrange for professional counseling if this appears indicated.

Post-surgical complications

Surgery is sometimes turned to as a last resort in those patients who have failed to respond to a conservative course of treatment. Measures seen in conjunction with malalignment include:

1. SI joint fusion
2. lumbosacral fusion
3. coccygectomy

As concerns the psychiatrist/psychologist, complications include:

1. With any surgery, there is the risk of entrapment of severed nerve fibres or formation of a neuroma within the scar. The nerve tissue may get irritated to the point that it becomes hypersensitive and an ongoing source of discomfort, paraesthesias or even neuralgic pain. A trial of an injection of local anaesthetic can quickly establish whether a full course of some 8 to 12 desensitization injections, done on a weekly or bi-weekly basis, may be worthwhile. Pain may resolve completely but can reappear some weeks or months later, in which case:
   a. a recurrence of the malalignment should be ruled out, as it may be increasing traction on

one of these vulnerable ligaments or scars, causing irritation of the nerve fibres trapped within to the point where hyperaesthesia again becomes a problem

b. a repeat course of injections could be considered to provide relief for a further, hopefully longer, interval.

2. 'phantom limb syndrome'

Maigne & Chatellier (2001) noted the possibility of this problem occuring in those that had undergone a coccygectomy which, as they pointed out, is indeed 'an amputation' (see 'Coccydynia' below).

The risk of 'labelling' and formation of ingrained mental concepts

Patients who are out of alignment often present with pain and musculoskeletal discomfort on examination. There may be trigger points that confuse the issue by causing referred pain (Fig. 3.45), a myriad of musculoskeletal problems, variation of the site or sites where the pain is felt to occur from one day to the next or even on the same day. In the case of an 'upslip' and 'rotational malalignment' there is, in addition, a functional LLD and a specific asymmetrical pattern of weight-bearing, weakness, tension and joint range of motion. Standard investigations are usually normal and there may be little to find on routine physical examination, which so often fails to include an assessment of alignment, never mind a look for some of the typical changes indicative of malalignment (see Chs 2, 3).

A psychiatrist/psychologist and, for that matter, anyone else treating a patient whose problems are caused, in part or completely, by an underlying 'malalignment syndrome' must be aware of three unfortunate but common complications.

Misdiagnosis

If the physician or therapist involved is not familiar with the presentations of 'malalignment', the risk is that the physical problems will escape detection or be misinterpreted and the patient misdiagnosed as having:

1. a non-descript 'entity', for want of a better 'diagnosis' for the physical findings at hand

   Typically, the patient is likely to have had one of these diagnoses firmly engrained in their mind: 'fibromyalgia', 'chronic tension pain', 'tension headaches', 'myofibralgia', 'rheumatoid condition', 'polymyalgia', to name a few of those commonly encountered in clinical practice.
2. depression, anxiety, or a problem with malingering

Mistreatment

A sincere effort at treatment on the patient's part may include a 'standard physiotherapy program' (see above), modified one-on-one or group exercises, instruction in a home program, counseling and, very likely, medications (analgesics, antidepressants, sedatives or other). Failure to improve may, unfortunately, be misinterpreted as 'malingering'. As long as the underlying problem - the malalignment - is present:

1. any attempt to stretch, strengthen and exercise, no matter how sincere, will probably result in only short-lived improvement (see 'treatment' above and Ch. 7) and could actually aggravate the musculoskeletal symptoms
2. the muscle relaxants, sedatives and analgesics may have only a temporary or no effect at all because they, just like the other attempts at treatment, do not resolve the underlying cause of the problems – the malalignment - and, unfortunately, may trigger or worsen any psychological factors.

The combined effect is to reinforce suspicions that the problem at hand is of an 'emotional' or 'psychological' nature, ignoring any physical component. A vicious cycle may ensue, impeding progress and delaying initiation of an appropriate treatment programme.

Complicating long-term misunderstanding, mislabelling, and hypochondriasis on behalf of the treated patient

If these patients eventually do present for assessment specifically of their musculoskeletal problems by someone trained in manual therapy, the diagnosis and complications of malalignment may become quite obvious. Instituting the appropriate course of treatment stands a good chance of finally achieving:

1. realignment
2. palpable relaxation of muscles, tendons and ligaments, with resolution of any reflex increase in muscle tension or triggering of spasms
3. stability of pelvis and spine, and
4. ability to finally progress with a strengthening and cardiac fitness program

However, despite finally progressing with a successful treatment programme and making obvious gains physically, a number of patients unfortunately are unable to overcome their long-standing concerns with pain and to rid themselves of an erroneously-applied label - be it 'fibromyalgia', 'chronic tension pain', or whatever - that they have carried for months or years and which by now has become firmly engrained in their mind to the point of interfering with their ability to get back to a normal way of life.

They see themselves as being 'stuck' with the detrimental aspects of the particular syndrome which, in their experience as a member of our society, usually proves difficult to treat and is likely to cause ongoing symptoms. Psychologically, the fear that they are at risk of re-triggering these symptoms may, unfortunately, cause them to hold back from engaging fully in activities in their daily life as well as the treatment programme advocated for the 'malalignment syndrome'. This long-term complication of having been 'mislabeled' will not necessarily disappear even though one makes them aware that the correct diagnosis has finally been arrived at and pointing out any beneficial changes that have actually been achieved with proper treatment in their case. It is at this stage that some further psychiatric or psychological counseling is in order, preferably by someone familiar with malalignment, to help them overcome this last, but often major, hurdle on their way to a full recovery.

IMPLICATIONS FOR RADIOLOGY AND MEDICAL IMAGING

An appreciation of the changes that occur with the natural development and aging of the SI joint, and the particular effects caused by malalignment being superimposed on the hip, pelvic, and lumbosacral regions, is essential for the proper interpretation of X-rays and scans of the axial and appendicular skeleton.

Radiographs (X-Rays)

Normal changes relating to development and to the asymmetries associated with malalignment can easily result in misinterpretation of what are essentially normal X-rays. To compound the problem, the patient with malalignment may have marked difficulty lying on a radiology table, trying to get a twisted pelvis, spine and extremities to accommodate to a hard, flat surface. This problem is similar to that of the patient who experiences increased pain on attempting to flatten the back doing the 'pelvic tilt' manoeuvre whenever he or she is out of alignment (Fig. 7.2).

Ideally, the radiologist is familiar with the changes attributable to malalignment and should be able to comment on the presence and, on occasion, the actual presentation of malalignment evident on the films.

Sacroiliac joints

The developmental changes that the SI joint undergoes have been described in detail in Ch. 2 and are summarized in Box 4.6. Even when a person is in alignment, certain aspects of the joint easily lend themselves to misinterpretation:

1. The roughening caused by formation of the physiologically normal intra-articular ridges and depressions; these findings:
   a. are felt to be a normal developmental phenomenon coincident with the time of adolescent weight gain and seemingly intended to increase joint stability and ability to transfer loads
   b. may be misread as 'osteophytes' or other changes that are then misinterpreted as being indicative of advancing SI joint degeneration (Cassidy 1992; Vleeming et al. 1990a; Figs 2.7, 4.34)

BOX 4.6 Development of the sacroiliac joint

1. The sacroiliac joint at birth is a planar joint, developing a thick layer of hyaline cartilage over the sacral, and a thin fibrocartilagenous cover over the iliac, surface in the ensuing years (Fig. 2.7A).
2. After puberty, the joint surfaces roughen with:
   a. the initial development of a crescent-shaped ridge running the length of the iliac surface and a matching depression on the sacral side
   b. the subsequent development of further irregularities and prominences, probably as an adaptation to adolescent weight gain and to improve load transfer (Fig. 2.7B).

2. the overlap attributable to the posterior-to-anterior widening of the sacrum in the sagittal plane (Figs 2.4B, 2.46D, 2.52A)
3. the change in angulation of the joint surfaces because of the:
   a. L-shape of the joint, with a short and a long arm
   b. anteroposterior and craniocaudal propeller-like features of these arms; e.g. sacral convex short, concave long arm, with the opposite shaping of the iliac surfaces so that they fit the sacral ones, and
   c. reversal on side-to-side comparison (Figs 2.2, 2.3A,B).

In a person who is actually in alignment, different parts of an SI joint become apparent depending on his or her position relative to the plane of the film (largely on account of Points 2 and 3) and the actual angle of projection of the beam (Figs 4.27, 4.28, 4.31-4.34).

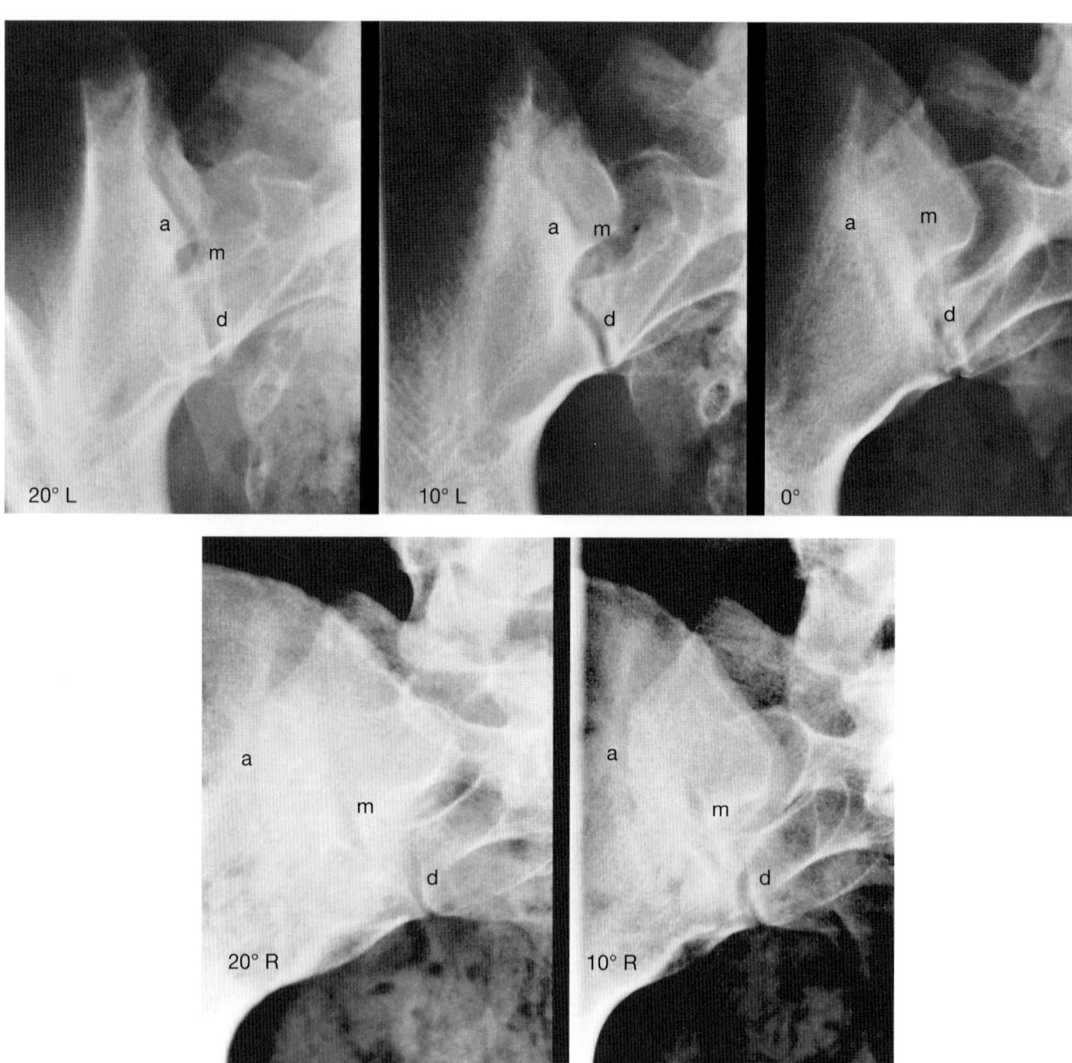

Fig. 4.27 The right sacroiliac joint seen from different angles in A-P projection: from 20 degrees left to 20 degrees right in 10 degree steps. The ventral (a), middle (m) and posterior (d) parts of the joint are seen. In the 20 degree left directed projection, all parts are superimposed. This projection is a simulation of a posteroanterior projection or an anteroposterior projection with the patient turned 25 degrees to the left, called the oblique position. *(Courtesy of Dyjkstra 2007.)*

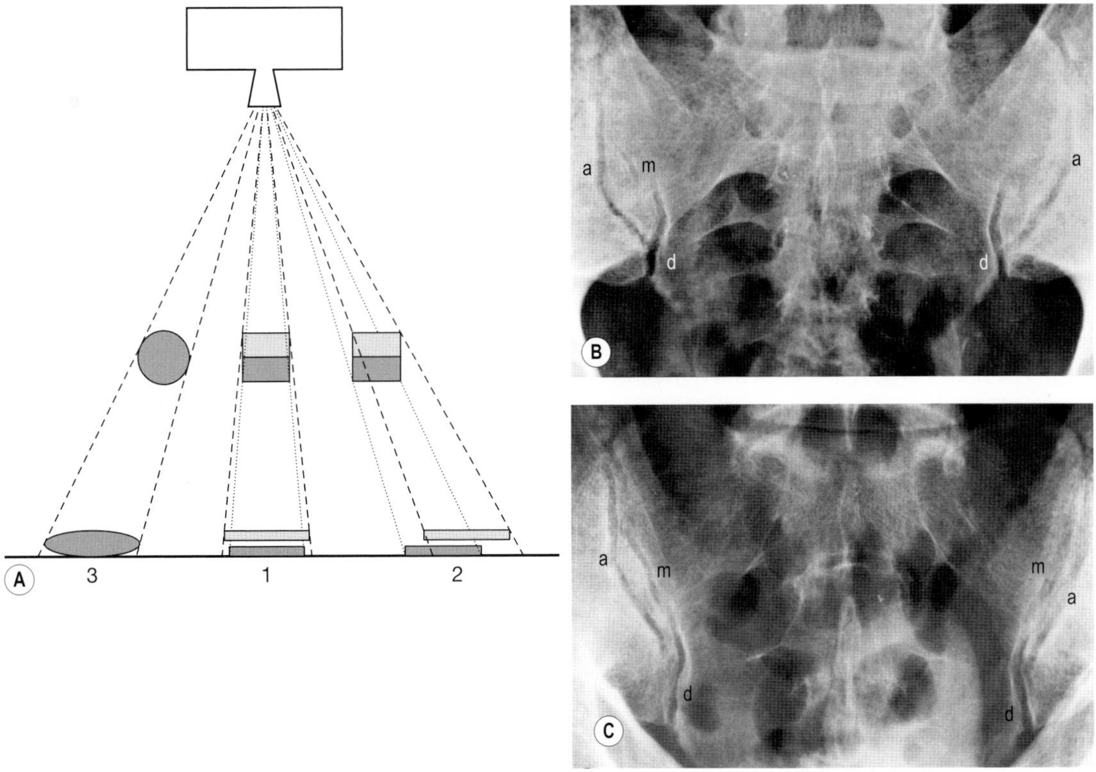

Fig. 4.28 Effects of X-ray visualization of the SI joint determined by angulation of the projected beam. (Fig. 4.28A) The place of the object in the X-ray beam determines the object's projection. In the central ray (**A1**), the top and bottom of the square are projected on top of each other, but the top is slightly larger than the bottom. At the right (**A2**), top and bottom are shifted. The sphere on the left (**A3**) is projected as an oval structure. (**Fig. 4.28B,C**) A normal sacroiliac joint (SIJ) in two anteroposterior projections: a. ventral; m. middle; d. posterior parts of the joint. (B) The caudal part of a lumbar spine view. The SIJs are seen in the same projection as the lateral square in [FIG. 4.28A]. The posterior part of S3 is more accentuated and the middle part of the joint is usually not seen. (C) Cranial angulated AP view. The SIJs are in the centre of the X-ray beam. Because the ventral and middle parts of the joint are closer to the X-ray tube, they are projected more to the lateral of the X-ray. The middle part of the joint is more easily seen. *(Courtesy of Dijkstra 2007.)*

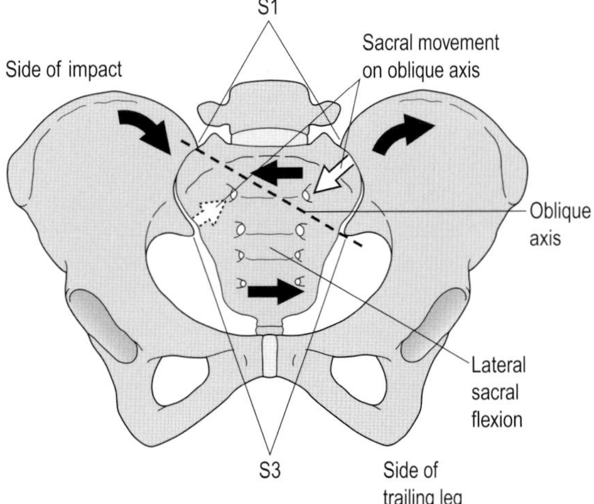

Fig. 4.29 Posterior rotation (right) and anterior rotation (left) demonstrating joint closure at S1 (right) and at S3 (left) to create an oblique axis (OA). A functional destabilization occurs at S1 (left) and S3 (right), allowing the joint to open and move on that oblique axis. *(Courtesy of DonTigny 2007, reproduced from DonTigny 2004.)*

In someone who is in alignment, X-Rays taken at right heel-strike, left toe-off during the gait cycle on one side would show 'closure' of the upper part of the right joint (S1 level) and 'closure' of the lower (S3) aspect of the left joint; in other words, the right superior, or short arm, and left inferior, or long arm, segment of the L-shape joint, respectively (Fig. 4.29). 'Jamming' together of the surfaces at these parts of the SI joint will be apparent on X-Ray; there will be relative 'opening' of the right lower and left upper segment of the joints (Figs. 4.31, 4.33). The pattern reflects the maximum movement of the pelvic bones in the gait cycle: the right and left innominate, rotating in opposite directions in the sagittal plane relative to the sacrum, which is undulating around the right and left oblique axes (Fig. 2.41). When malalignment is present, it is as though the pelvic bones have become 'stuck' in a particular part of this cycle. 'Outflare/inflare' (Figs 2.13Aiii, 4.30), 'anterior/posterior' rotation (Figs 4.31, 4.33) and 'sacral torsion', especially, result in a reorientation of the right compared to left SI joint surfaces in opposite directions relative to the plane of the film and the X-ray beam being projected. If the reorientation of these surfaces is in opposite directions, as it is particularly with 'rotational malalignment' and a 'flare', it will compound any difference that already exists in the orientation of the short and long arms of the joints relative to the vertical axis (Figs 2.2, 2.3). Therefore, on reading the film:

1. there is more evidence of 'opening' and/or 'closing' (approximation), affecting different parts of the SI joint than would be normal, also asymmetry on comparing the right to the left side, or combinations of these (Figs 2.8, 4.6, 4.24, 4.31, 4.33, see also Ch. 2)
   a. the joint may be all 'open' on one side and appear partially or fully 'closed' on the opposite side (Figs 4.6, 4.31A)
   b. some of the joint may be 'open', with the adjacent borders clearly evident but other parts of the joint hidden by overlapping of the sacral and iliac surfaces; any overlapping of roughened joint surfaces may be misinterpreted as 'sclerosis' and changes indicative of 'osteoarthritis' or other pathological conditions in a person whose SI joints are actually normal (Figs 4.34, 4.38)
2. different sections of the joint can appear 'open' and 'closed' to the beam ('ventral', 'mid- or 'posterior'; 'upper' or 'lower') on side-to-side comparison, depending on:
   a. the projection of the beam (Fig. 4.27), and
   b. reorientation of the joint surfaces in someone with malalignment (Figs 4.24, 4.28, 4.31, 4.33)

On realignment and barring any underlying pathology the same views of the pelvis and spine are now likely to show near-symmetry of the right and left SI and facet joint surfaces on exposure to X-ray beams projected at the same angle, or on a CAT scan or MRI (Figs 4.33, 4.34).

Spine

Rotation of the vertebrae occurs with the formation of cervical, thoracic and lumbar curves. Consider, for example, the typical rotation of L1–L4 into the lumbar convexity (Figs 2.42, 2.96, 4.6, 4.24, 4.33). Displacement of the spinous processes toward the concavity may also be clearly evident on anteroposterior views of the thoracic and cervical spine (Fig. 4.31B). In keeping with the clinical examination findings of a spinous process having been displaced relative to that of the vertebrae above and below, the rotational displacement of an isolated vertebra will usually be evident on X-rays:

1. If the vertebral rotation is further into the convexity, there may be an obvious accentuation of the displacement of its spinous process relative to those above and below (Fig. 4.31B).
2. If the rotation is in the direction opposite to the vertebrae above and below, there may be an obvious interruption of the curve formed by these other spinous processes (e.g. right lumbar convexity in Fig. 2.96B).

Facet joints

Malalignment also results in a reorientation of the facet joints relative to the beam, so that they will appear open on one side and narrowed or closed on the other. The rotation of L1–L4 into a left convexity, for example, 'opens' the left and 'closes' the right facet joints (Figs 2.96C, 4.33). Rotational displacement of individual vertebrae will augment or diminish this effect. The difference will be most evident on oblique films of the lumbar spine (Fig. 2.74B). Narrowing of the joint space on one side of the X-Ray may be wrongly attributed to degeneration of the surface cartilage; widening, to laxity of the capsule and the supporting ligaments.

Sacrum

A shift of the sacrum is sometimes easily apparent on X-ray. Standing anteroposterior views of the pelvis, for example, may show the following.

In the presence of 'rotational malalignment', concomitant rotation of the sacrum around one of the oblique axes will show that a line through the midline of the sacrum and coccyx runs off-centre, angled to the right or left of the vertical or Y-axis with rotation around the right or the left oblique axis, respectively (Aitken 1986; Figs 2.10, 2.21, 2.42, 2.52A, 4.31A, 4.35A). The sacrum and coccyx will realign with the Y-axis on correction of the malalignment (Fig. 4.35B).

In the presence of a pelvic obliquity attributable to either an anatomical or a functional LLD, the sacrum, as part of the pelvic unit, will usually have rotated around the sagittal axis in the coronal plane, so that the sacral base is inclined (Fig. 3.90A). Depending on the underlying cause (e.g. anatomical LLD, 'upslip', or other), the iliac crest will be higher on the right or left side. In an attempt to adapt to such a sacral base inclination to the left:

1. The L5 vertebra may side-flex to the right in an attempt to decrease any compensatory scoliosis but this change creates new stress points, may impair its normal function and, eventually, precipitate lumbosacral pain (Fig. 3.90C)
2. With time, the sacrum itself may adapt to the obliquity in an attempt to decrease the stress on the lumbosacral region and to decrease any compensatory curves of the spine. In that case, the sacral base will end up partially or completely level, even though the iliac crests still show a persistent obliquity, being high on one side (Fig. 3.90B). It is important to know whether or not such a sacral adaptation has occurred, especially when contemplating prescribing a lift for someone known to have had previous unleveling of the sacral base but:

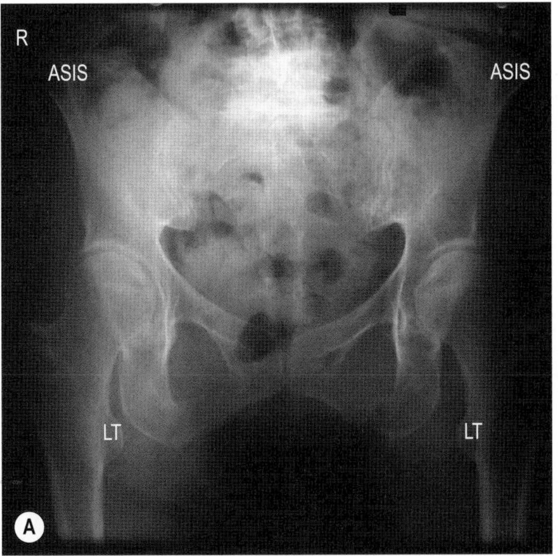

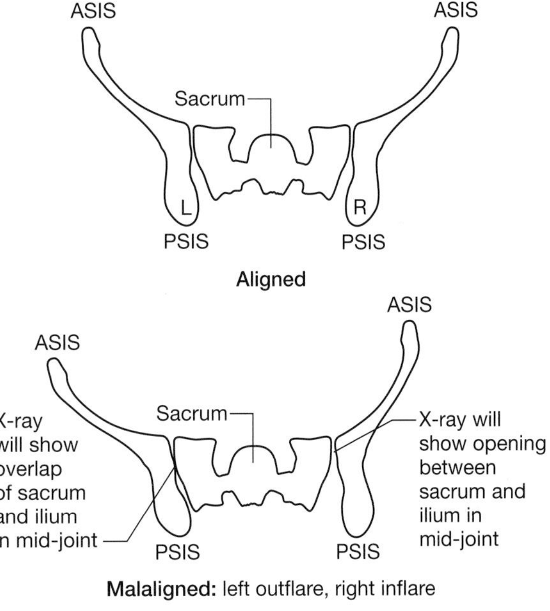

Fig. 4.30 X-ray changes with 'left outflare, right inflare'. (A) A-P projection of pelvis and hip joints. The femoral heads remain at the same level as the left acetabulum moves outward and the right inward in the transverse plane. Innominate width appears to be increased on the left and decreased on the right. The anterior superior iliac spine (ASIS) appears to be increased in overall size and broader on the 'outflare' (left) side, and smaller and narrower on the 'inflare' (right) side. The left femoral neck appears to be further away from, the right closer to, the ipsilateral inferior pubic ramus. The left lesser trochanter (LT) appears to be smaller with overlapping on external rotation, the right more obvious with internal rotation of the leg (see also Fig. 2.75). (B) Diagramatic conceptualization of A-P X-ray beam projection onto the pelvis when 'aligned' and with a 'left outflare, right inflare' present; superoinferior view (see also Figs 4.28, 4.29).

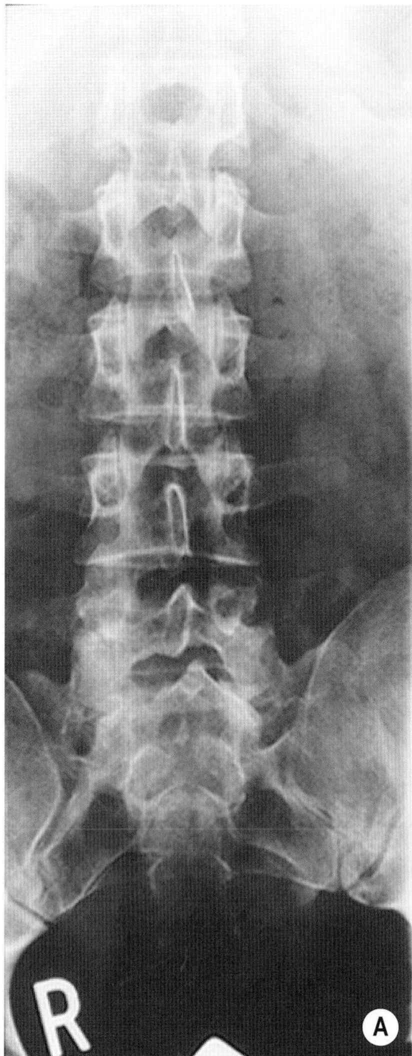

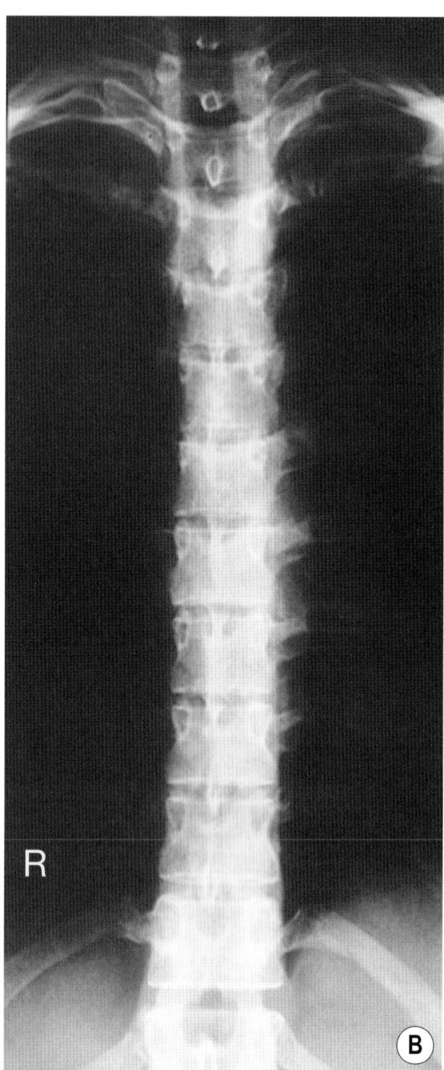

Fig. 4.31 X-ray changes reflecting a variation in orientation of the sacroiliac joint surfaces and the vertebrae to the beam as a result of 'right anterior, left posterior rotational malalignment', with the lumbar spine fairly straight and some thoracic levoscoliosis (see also Figs 2.75, 4.24). (A) Most of the right sacroiliac joint is visualized; whereas the left appears 'closed' except for the lower third. The facet joints appear variably open or closed at the different levels. (B) The mid-thoracic vertebrae (T4-T9 inclusive) have rotated into the left convexity, especially at T4-T7, suggesting vertebral rotational displacement (maximal at T6).

a. now presents with an anatomical (true) LLD and a seemingly 'short leg' side, and persistent pelvic obliquity, or
b. has failed to respond to attempts at correction of a functional LLD attributable to an 'upslip' or 'rotational malalignment' and is left with a pelvic obliquity.

If there has been accommodation with sacral base leveling, adding a lift on the seemingly 'short side', in an attempt to level any residual pelvic obliquity noted on comparison of right and left iliac crest height would unfortunately again raise the sacral base up on the side of the lift, with possible reappearance of the compensatory curves, associated stresses and previous symptoms.

Hip joints

'Anterior' innominate rotation results in an anteroinferior displacement of the superior acetabular

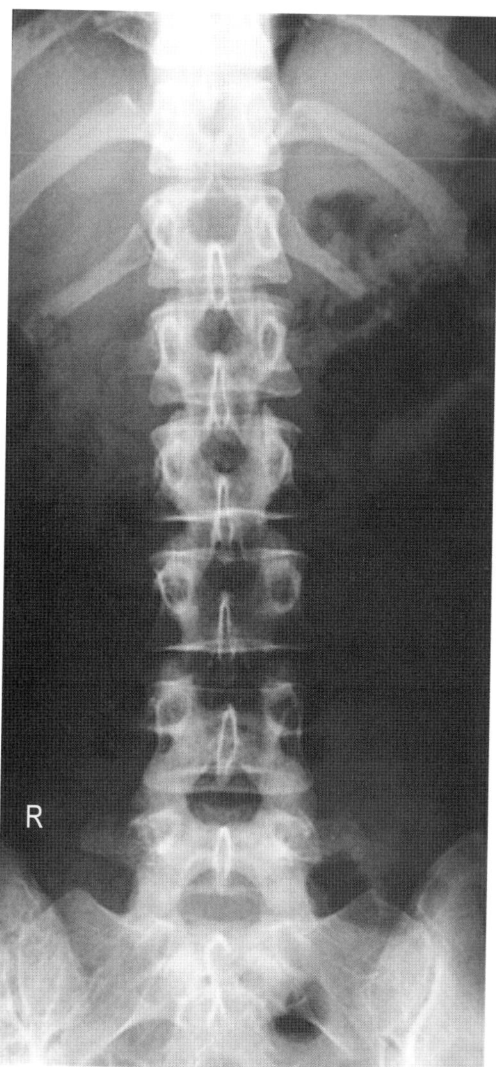

Fig. 4.32 On realignment of the person shown in Fig. 4.31, the sacroiliac and lumbar facet joints appear to be more symmetrically open and the spine relatively straight.

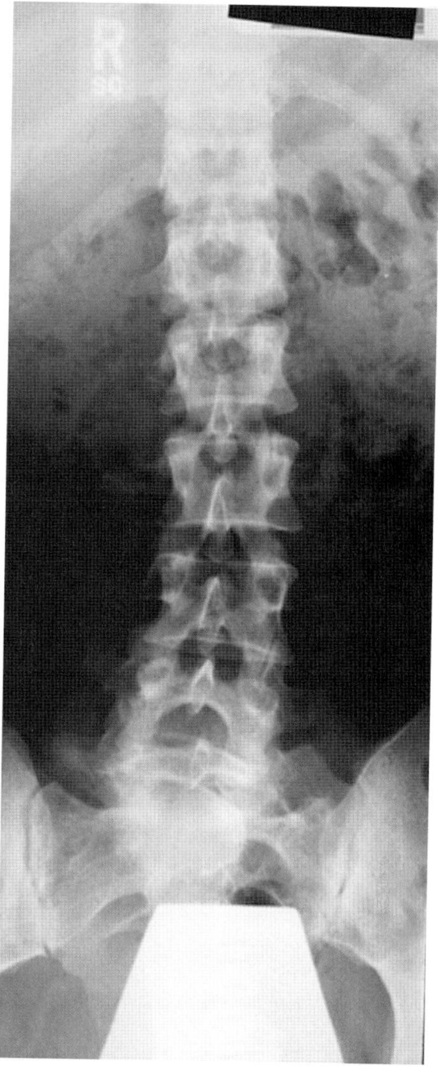

Fig. 4.33 X-ray changes with malalignment: the effect on sacroiliac and facet joint orientation to the A-P beam. L1-L4 vertebral rotation into the left convexity opens the left mid-lumbar facet joints and aggravates the closing/compression of the right facet joints that results with the simultaneous left rotation and right side-flexion. L5 is sacralized on the left.

rim, with increased overlapping of the femoral head that could be misinterpreted as a narrowing of the hip joint on an anteroposterior X-ray. 'Posterior' rotation has the opposite effect: posterosuperior displacement of the superoanterior rim can make the joint appear wider anteriorly on comparison to the opposite side (Fig. 2.75). There will also be:

1. with 'outflare/inflare':
   - a reorientation of the hip joints caused by the rotation around the vertical axis in the transverse plane, so that the acetabulum ends up facing more forward on the 'inflare' and outward on the 'outflare' side on the A-P view (Figs 2.75, 4.30, 4.35)
2. with an 'upslip':
   a. rotation of the pelvic unit around the sagittal axis in the coronal plane (Fig. 4.35) and pelvic obliquity on standing, sitting, lying A-P views

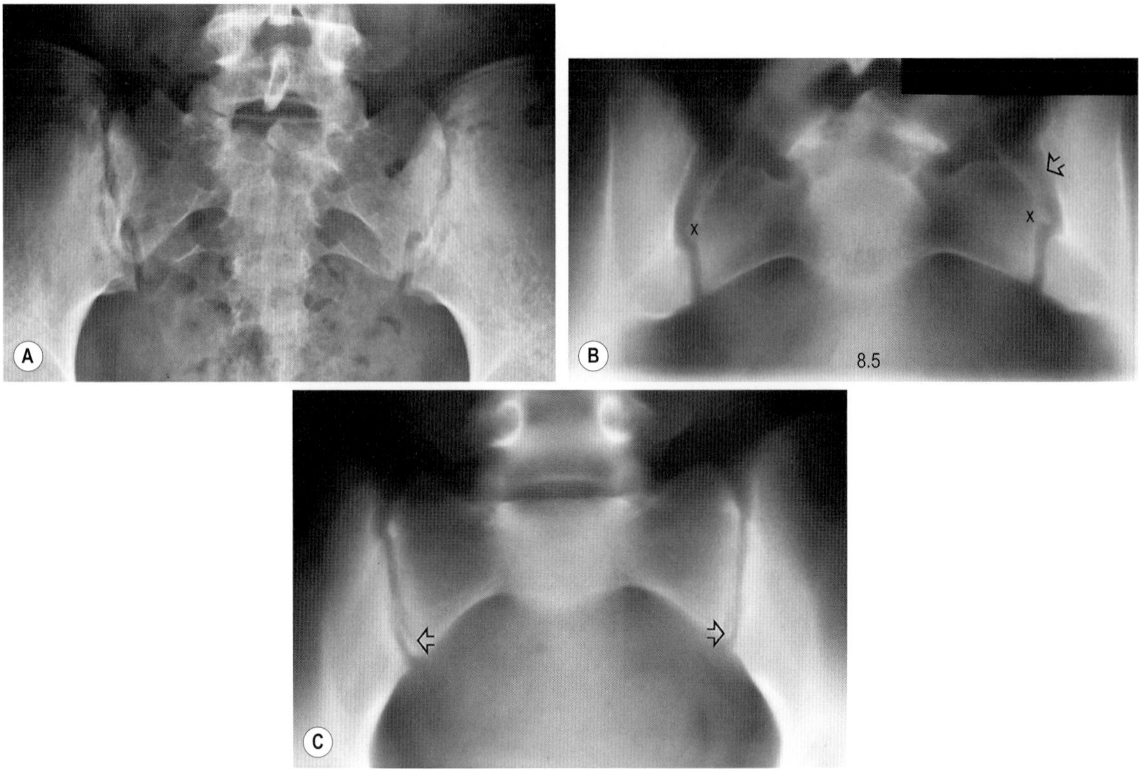

Fig. 4.34 (A) Plain X-ray of the sacroiliac joint (SIJ) in a 17-year-old boy in which parts of the joint are superimposed, giving the impression of irregularity on the left [see also Figs 4.24, 4.30, 4.31, 4.38]. The differential diagnosis was ankylosing spondylitis or closing epiphysis. Tomography revealed closing epiphyses and congenital irregularity of the joints. (B) Tomography of the posterior part of the left joint shows a hooklike (X) projection into the axial joint on both sides and a left-right asymmetry with bony exostosis (arrow) of the sacrum in the left axial joint. '8.5' depicts the distance of the slice from the table top. (C) Tomography of the ventral part of the joints. There is a slight sclerosis of the left joint, due to the closing of the epiphysis. In the caudal area, an epiphysis (arrows) is seen in the sacrum, especially on the right side. *(Courtesy of Dijkstra 2007.)*

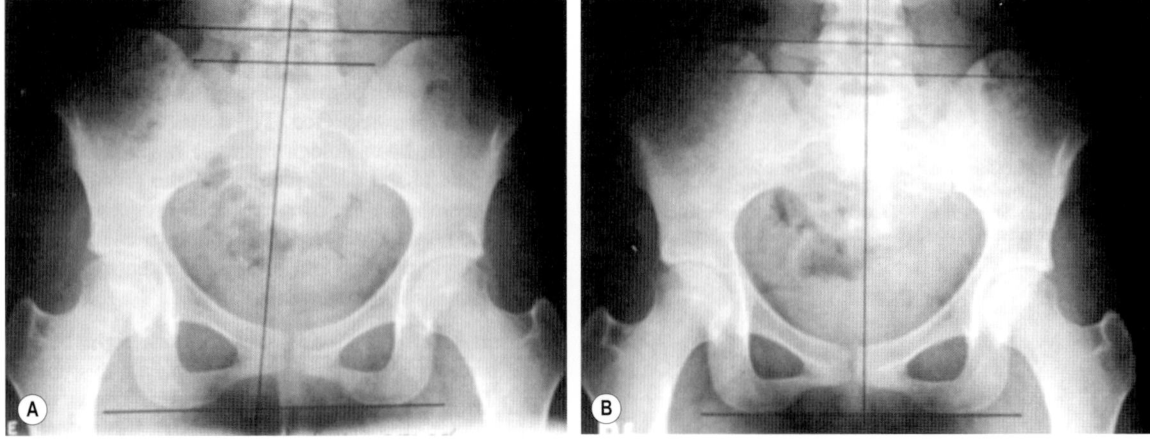

Fig. 4.35 Changes in the relationship between the lumbar spine and the pelvis on a standing anteroposterior view. (A) Before manual treatment: left axis deviation is evident. (B) After manual treatment: realigned with vertical axis. *(Courtesy of Aitken 1986.)*

b. a possible narrowing of the superior aspect of the hip joint with the upward (craniad) movement of the femur in the vertical plane
c. upward displacement of all the landmarks, including the hip joint, relative to the sacrum and the opposite (normal) side, uniformly present in standing, sitting, lying

3. with an 'upslip' and 'rotational malalignment':
   a. one lower extremity ends up rotating externally, the other internally
   b. on external rotation, the greater trochanter is pulled posterior and the femoral head forced anterior, with:
      i. stretching of the anterior capsule and ligaments (Figs 2.48, 4.3)
      ii. compression of structures of the anterior hip and subinguinal region, which may be evident on MRI (Fig. 2.104)
   c. on internal rotation, the femoral head is forcing posteriorly and stretches the posterior capsule and ligaments
4. with any of these presentations
   - an increase in tension or actual reflex spasm involving any of the surrounding hip girdle muscles will tend to pull the femoral head upward and more closely applied within the acetabulum and may result in an apparent joint space narrowing

Trochanters

Varying degrees of asymmetry occur as the proximal femurs rotate in contrary directions relative to the acetabulum and as the greater and lesser trochanters rotate into and out of view with the external and internal rotation of the lower extremities that occurs with an 'upslip' and 'rotational malalignment' (Figs 2.75, 4.3, 4.30A). A difference may also be apparent with an 'outlare/inflare' if any rotational forces are exerted on the lower extremities with the reorientation of the acetabula as the innominates rotate in the transverse plane; this is more likely to be evident on non-weight-bearing A-P views (e.g. when lying supine).

Symphysis pubis

Normally, the right and left pubic bone surfaces match and are separated by about 2-3 mm (although even 5-6 mm need not necessarily be considered abnormal if the person is asymptomatic and there is no suspected instability).

A step deformity of 2-3 mm or more at the symphysis pubis may reflect changes in the alignment of the superior pubic rami:

1. with a 'right anterior, left posterior' pattern of 'rotational malalignment', the right ramus is displaced downward relative to the left - reflecting right anteroinferior and left posterosuperior innominate rotation, respectively (Figs 2.10, 2.42, 2.75, 4.26)
2. with a 'right upslip', the right is displaced straight upward relative to the left.

These findings may be erroneously interpreted as reflecting an instability of the symphysis pubis. However, instability should not be presumed unless:

1. it has been proven radiologically using the active straight leg raising (ASLR) test or on a 'flamingo' or 'figure-4' standing stress test (Fig. 2.102A,B)
2. separation at rest exceeds 5 mm (though this does not confirm a problem of instability, especially in someone who is asymptomatic, until it has actually been proven by these tests)
3. realignment fails to correct these abnormal findings (Fig. 4.35),
4. malalignment keeps recurring if the joint is not stabilized (see Ch. 2).

Computed axial tomography (CAT scan)

A CAT scan may be able to confirm that:

1. there are indeed degenerative changes evident in one or both SI joints - it may help define their nature (Figs 4.34B,C, 4.36, 4.38B). Although that does not confirm they are causing the patient's pain or that there is any ongoing joint inflammation (see 'bone scan' below)
2. there is symmetry or asymmetry of the joint surfaces at respective levels - the latter could indicate that the person was out of alignment at the time of the scan; asymmetrical pressure on surfaces, especially if the joint is osteoarthritic and/or inflammed (Fig. 4.36), could be responsible for pain, especially if that pain decreases or actually disappears when a pressure point is shifted or abolished by realignment.
3. SI joint instability is probable, by disclosing a significant displacement of the SI joint surfaces relative to each other, which may persist despite realignment (Fig. 4.37)
4. other pathological features are present or absent (e.g. iliopectineal bursa, fracture of the acetabular

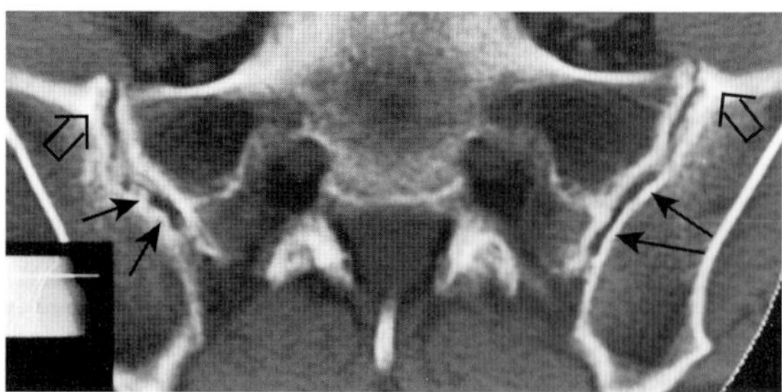

Fig. 4.36 Osteoarthritis with CT. In this patient (CT at the level of S2), severe sclerosis of the ventral sacroiliac joint (SIJ) ligaments and the joints margins was found. Even bony ankylosis (arrows) can be found. *(Courtesy of Dijkstra 2007.)*

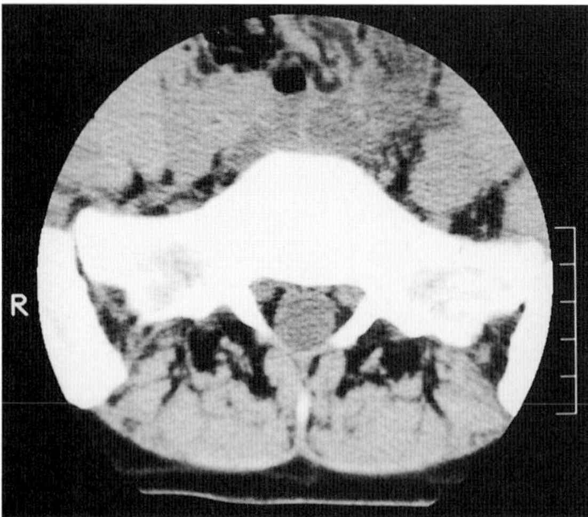

Fig. 4.37 An unstable right sacroiliac joint. The computed tomography scan shows 1 cm posterior displacement of the right innominate relative to the sacrum. A block with local anaesthetic resolved the pain.

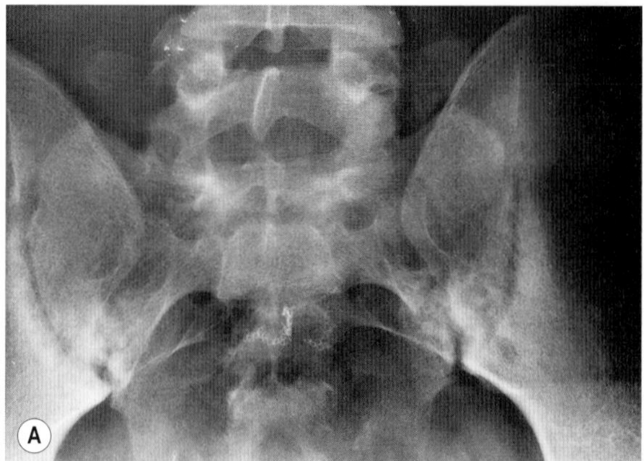

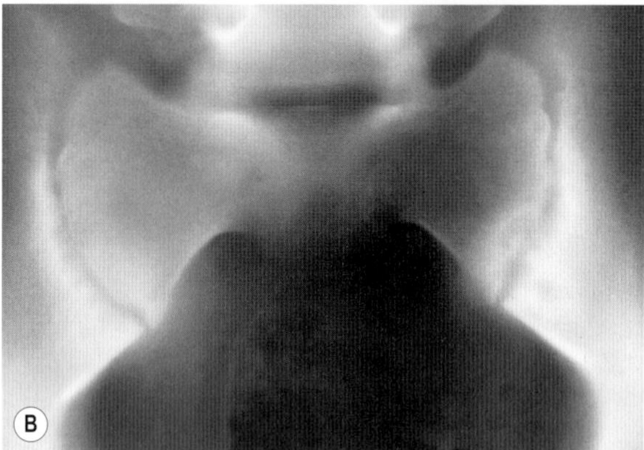

Fig. 4.38 'Ankylosing spondylitis' in a patient with Crohn's disease. (A) On X-ray, there are irregular joints with sclerotic borders and probably signs of ankysosis on the left side. (B) Tomography of the ventral part of the same sacroiliac joint (SIJ). Erosions and sclerosis are clearly seen, but no ankylosis. The 'ankylosis' seen was, in fact, a superimposition of parts of the joint. *(Courtesy of Dijkstra 2007; see also Fig. 4.34)*

rim, sacroiliitis, ankylosing spondylitis, chondrocalcinosis or other rheumatologic conditions; Fig. 4.38).

Magnetic resonance imaging (MRI)

An MRI is particularly helpful for:

1. ruling out other causes of pain originating from the spine, pelvic or hip region that may have been missed or were not clearly defined on ultrasound (e.g. a bursa, accessory piriformis) or previous CAT scan (e.g. disc protrusion, annular tear)
2. give information regarding the soft tissues that a CAT scan is unable to define (e.g. acetabular labral tear)

Findings on a CAT scan, MRI and ultrasound (Klauser et al. 2005) may be enhanced by injection of contrast material, preferably under fluoroscopy: into a joint (e.g. MRI arthrogram) or even muscle (e.g. to assess atrophy, enlargement; Fig. 4.19).

Bone scans

Patients presenting with pain localizing to the lumbosacral and/or SI joint areas often undergo bone scans to rule out or confirm problems such as facet joint osteoarthritis and sacroiliitis. In the presence of malalignment, and with no indications of a spondyloarthropathy on clinical examination, these scans:

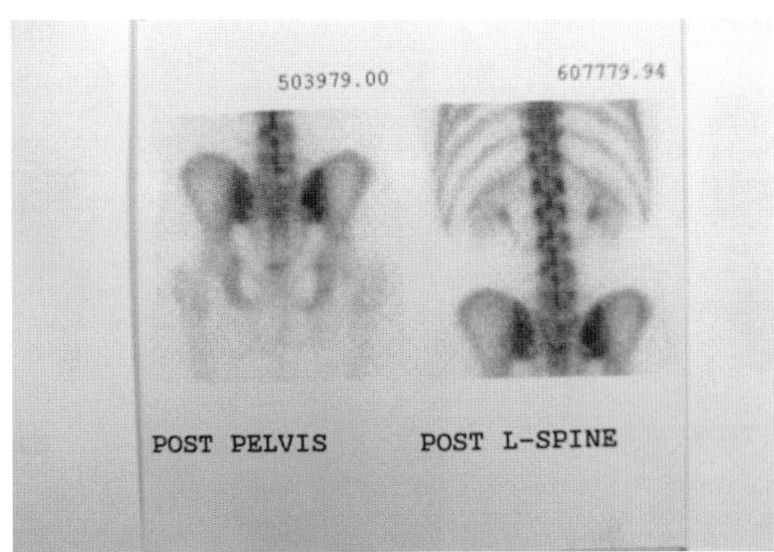

Fig. 4.39 Typical changes on a bone scan when malalignment is present: there is a variable tracer concentration, here considerably higher in the right sacroiliac area than in left, as reflected by the asymmetrical SIS ratio (right 1.37 versus left 1.17). However, the ratio was still within normal limits (less than 1.5). The spine was unremarkable. There was neither any history of remote injury nor any clinical or laboratory indications of spondyloarthropathy.

1. are usually normal
2. may reveal a suspected or unsuspected underlying problem with increased bone turnover (e.g. osteoarthritis involving the facet or hip joints)

These scans sometimes do, however, show:

1. an asymmetrical increase in overall activity in the SI joint region on one side compared to the other, albeit the activity may still be within normal limits bilaterally
2. increased activity affecting only one or more small localized areas of the surfaces of an SI joint on one or both sides (Fig. 4.39)
3. an abnormal increase in activity localizing to:
   a. the symphysis pubis, usually interpreted as representing changes consistent with 'osteitis pubis'
   b. one or more facet joints that may show osteoarthritic changes on X-ray or CAT scan and/or whose surfaces are constantly being subjected to increased pressure on account of the malalignment, stimulating cell turnover

These changes in activity may be no more than a reflection of an increase in bone turnover that has resulted from the asymmetrical stress on these joints caused by the malalignment, now that the joint surfaces no longer match, and there may be a component of instability attributable to a failure of 'form' and/or 'force' closure.

Block with local anaesthetic

Blocks can be helpful for localizing sites from which pain originates and guiding treatment, particularly when realignment fails to affect pain or resolves it only incompletely. Typical selective blocks include:

SI joint block

- to see if pain is originating from the posterior pelvic ligaments, from within the SI joint or both sites (see Fig. 7.42)

facet joint block

- to help define if the pain is originating from within the joint, its capsule/ligaments, or its nerve supply

nerve root block

1. suspected irritation or frank compression by a disc bulge or protrusion
2. query of hypersensitivity of nerve fibres or a neuroma entrapped in scar tissue formed after previous laminectomy, disc resection

epidural block

1. when a trial with any of the above blocks fails to localize the problem or bring relief
2. post-operatively (e.g. after multi-level decompression), when hypersensitive scar tissue or neuroma formation is suspected or when there is evidence of L4 or L5 instability
3. to rule out dural irritation and cauda equina pathology

The presence of malalignment can usually be diagnosed from changes evident on X-rays. Reporting these findings should be part of the regular interpretation of these films:

1. to decrease the possibility of their misinterpretation on subsequent reading by those not familiar with the entity of 'malalignment'
2. to help decide on an appropriate treatment approach and need for any follow-up investigations (e.g. bone scan, ultrasound, CAT scan or MRI) to verify pathology suggested by the X-rays

For further information regarding technique and findings specific to the SI joints and symphysis pubis, the reader is referred to Bernard & Cassidy (1991), Bjorglund et al. 1996, Dorman & Ravin (1991), Mens et al. (1997) and Ravin (2007). Also recommended are overviews of: the basic problems encountered with SI joint visualization (Dijkstra 1997, 2009); the role of CAT scans and MRIs (Jurriaans & Friedman 1997; O'Neill & Jurriaans 2007) and of ultrasound (Klauser et al. 2005; Stokes et al. 2007) when investigating these areas; the use of SI joint injection for pain referral mapping and arthroscopy (Fortin et al. 1994, 1997) and the application of radiology to clarify coccydynia (Maigne 1997).

IMPLICATIONS FOR RESPIROLOGY

Respiration is tied in closely with the function of the musculoskeletal system and the biomechanics of the trunk and spine in particular. For a more detailed description of what exactly occurs, and the implications of malalignment, the reader is referred to writings by Hodges & Cholewicki 2007, Hodges et al 2005a, Chaitow et al. 2002, Chaitow 2004, 2007, Thompson et al. 2006 and Lee 2003. A resume of their writings, and a subsequent correlation with malalignment, follow.

The respiratory cycle

Inspiration

This consists of elevation of the ribs and a lateral expansion of the rib cage, an action normally achieved by contraction of:

1. the diaphragm, to depress the central tendon and elevate the lower ribs (Fig. 4.40A)
2. pelvic floor muscles, to help support the abdominal contents as the intra-abdominal pressure is increasing; this provides the resistance needed for the diaphragm to exert its effect on the central tendon and ribs (Fig. 4.40B)
3. muscles to extend and help stabilize the spine and rib cage (e.g. latissimus dorsi, erector spinae; Cala et al. 1992).

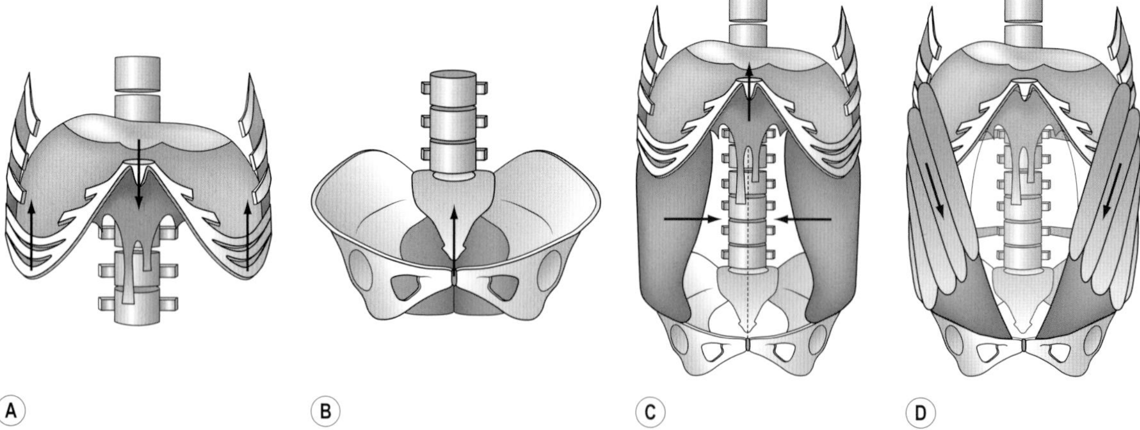

Fig. 4.40 Contribution of the muscles of the abdominal cavity to respiration. (A) Diaphragm contraction depresses the central tendon and elevates the lower ribs. (B) Pelvic floor muscle activity prevents depression of the floor when intra-abdominal pressure is increased. (C) Transversus abdominis activity narrows the waist and elevates the diaphragm via displacement of the abdominal contents. (D) The superficial abdominal muscles, including obliquus externus abdominis (shown) depresses the rib cage and increases intra-abdominal pressure. *(Courtesy of Hodges & Cholewicki 2007.)*

Expiration

While in part a passive event, with elastic recoil of the ribcage and the lungs, there is also felt to be contraction of particular muscles, namely:

1. abdominal muscles (Figs 2.30, 2.31, 4.40 C)
   a. in particular, transversus abdominis, which lets the diaphragm ascend (DeTroyer 1997; Urquhart & Hodges 2005; Hodges & Cholewicki 2007)
   b. external obliques, which apparently come into play with increased respiratory effort (Hodges et al. 2005) to help the lower ribs descend (Figs 2.32, 2.33, 4.40D)
2. probably also erector spinae (paravertebral) muscles, to counter any tendency for the spine to flex (Hodges et al. 2007)
3. a phasic increase of pelvic floor muscles contraction to support abdominal contents (Campbell & Green 1955) which is seemingly linked primarily to abdominal muscle activity and, less likely, to changes in intra-abdominal pressure with expiration (Hodges et al. 2007).

The action of respiratory muscles is obviously interlinked with that of a number of other muscles which, specifically, act together to ensure stability of the spine. In addition:

1. Respiratory muscles themselves are also important in helping stabilize the trunk just prior to or during an activity. For example, diaphragm and transversus abdominis contract:
   a. phasically, just 'prior to rapid limb movements' (Hodges & Richardson 1997)
   b. tonically, such as with repetitive movements of the arm (Hodges & Gandevia 2000a, 2000b) and walking (Saunders et al. 2004, 2005).
2. Muscles active in respiration, such as the diaphragm, are obviously interlinked with efforts to achieve stability (Hodges & Gandevia 2000a, 2000b), though their role in ensuring respiratory function seemingly (and not surprisingly!) forgoes all else.

> *When, however, a challenge occurs that makes postural stabilizing demands on the diaphragm at the same time that respiratory demands are occurring, it is the stability element that suffers.*
>
> (Chaitow 2007: 568)

3. Their role in ensuring stability of the spine can create problems.
   a. if respiratory muscles are not functioning normally:
      i. stability is likely to be impaired
      ii. it is suspected that this person is then at increased risk of developing back pain (Finkelstein 2002; Smith et al. 2006)
      iii. incontinence may occur on account of impaired pelvic floor function
   b. in someone who presents with low back pain, the action of the respiratory muscles is likely impaired secondarily and this affects breathing; similarly, recruitment of the diaphragm and pelvic floor muscles appears impaired in those with sacroiliac pain (O'Sullivan et al. 2002). Compensatory measures include an attempt to stiffen the spine, probably by:
      i. CNS mediated co-contraction of trunk muscles to 'compensate for reduced osseoligamentous stability of the spine' (Panjabi 1992a,b; van Dieën & de Looze 1999; van Dieën et al. 2003)
      ii. recruitment of the superficial 'outer' core muscles, in addition to the 'inner' core muscle activity noted above

Unfortunately, these adaptations to pain and particularly the resultant stiffening may have long-term negative mechanical and physiological effects on the spine because of the increased compressive loading (Kumar 1990).

Hodges & Cholewicki (2007) indicated that respiration will be affected in those presenting with somatic complaints. In particular, those with LBP:

1. are likely to show stiffening of the spine with increased deviation of the centre of gravity with breathing
2. less frequently prepare the trunk in anticipation of the movement that occurs during rapid arm movements, so that there results an increased trunk displacement with that arm movement (Mok et al. 2004a); there is also a reduction of counter-rotation of the shoulders and pelvis during locomotion (Lamoth et al. 2002) and decrease in intervertebral motion during trunk flexion (Kaigle et al. 1998).

Hyperventilation and emotional states

Hyperventilation has been shown to compromise spinal stability by 'increasing tendency to greater muscle tension, muscle spasm, interfering with the intra-abdominal pressure stabilization functions of the diaphragm' (Schleifer et al. 2002). Overbreathing, such as may occur intermittently with daily activities that are physically demanding, has been shown experimentally to temporarily reduce or even eliminate the postural (tonic) and phasic functions of the diaphragm and transversus abdominis. The suspected decrease in spinal stability was felt to increase the person's propensity to injury of the spine (Hodges et al. 2001; Hodges et al. 2002)

Hyperventilation has been closely linked with emotional states, such as apprehension, anxiety and fear, and somatic complaints such as LBP. Voluntary hyperventilation has in fact been able to bring on such emotional and somatic states in patients with known anxiety disorders and stress-related complaints (Chaitow 2004, 2007).

Breathing retraining aimed at re-establishing a normal breathing pattern, with particular emphasis on abdominal breathing to slow down expiration, has shown improvement of postural control, also beneficial effects as concerns the emotional states and any somatic complaints (Aust & Fischer 1997; Han et al. 1996; Mehling & Hamel 2005). Chaitow (2007: 569) stressed that:

> *'although seldom causative, BPD [breathing pattern disorders] can be seen as to potentially be a major factor in encouraging and maintaining musculoskeletal dysfunction in general, and back pain in particular...'*

> *'unless BDSS are looked for and evaluated, they are unlikely to be recognized in a manual medicine setting'*

Malalignment-related effects on the mechanics of breathing

Discussion to this point has concentrated on the role of respiratory muscles and how that interlinks with the muscles that ensure stability of the pelvis and spine, with mention of:

1. the complications resulting from impairment of respiration, in particular, and
2. the effect of emotional and some somatic complaints, such as back pain, on respiration

The biomechanical changes and pain associated with malalignment can further alter the mechanics of breathing and impair ventilation. An 'upslip' and 'rotational malalignment' typically result in pelvic obliquity and compensatory curves of the spine. Given a thoracic convexity to the left (Fig. 3.15A):

1. the ribs on the right side move closer together; whereas those on the left separate
2. after costal motion has stopped, there is some further side flexion of the vertebrae to the right (Fig. 3.15B); this causes the right ribs to rotate anteriorly and the left ribs posteriorly
3. the overall changes include:
   a. alteration in the space available for the right compared with the left lung
   b. stress on the costovertebral and costotransverse joints, also the costochondral junctions, bilaterally (Figs 2.94, 3.15, 3.16)
   c. increased tension in some soft tissue structures, in particular the thoracic diaphragm and intercostal muscles
   d. conceivably, a decrease in the minute lung volume on the right compared to the left side
   e. an increased chance of pleural irritation when coughing

With a thoracic convexity to the left, the typical finding on clinical examination of the supine-lying person is a 'forward and down' displacement of the upper segment of the ribs on the left side, relative to those on the right (Fig. 2.93B). Displacement is maximal

1. between the 1st and 2nd left rib and
2. on the left compared to right side

These differences decrease gradually, until the adjoining right and left ribs come to match up horizontally (usually at the level of the 4th, 5th or 6th ribs). Below this particular level, the ribs again come to be rotated in the opposite direction so that the right ones are now noted to lie increasingly 'forward and down' compared to the rib just above and its partner on the left side. The pattern reflects the effect of the vertebral rotation caused on the ribs above, at and below the apex of the convexity, respectively. With a convexity to the right, the opposite finding of anterior rib displacement is usually seen. Other factors, particularly rotational displacement of individual vertebrae (Fig. 2.94) or reversal of the convexity at a level below the cervicothoracic junction (Fig. 2.91) will affect the pattern described.

Breathing normally involves an elevation of the ribs and a lateral expansion of the chest cage, with a descent of the thoracic diaphragm - so-called 'lateral costal breathing' (Figs 4.40, 4.41). Joints already placed under stress by pelvic and spine

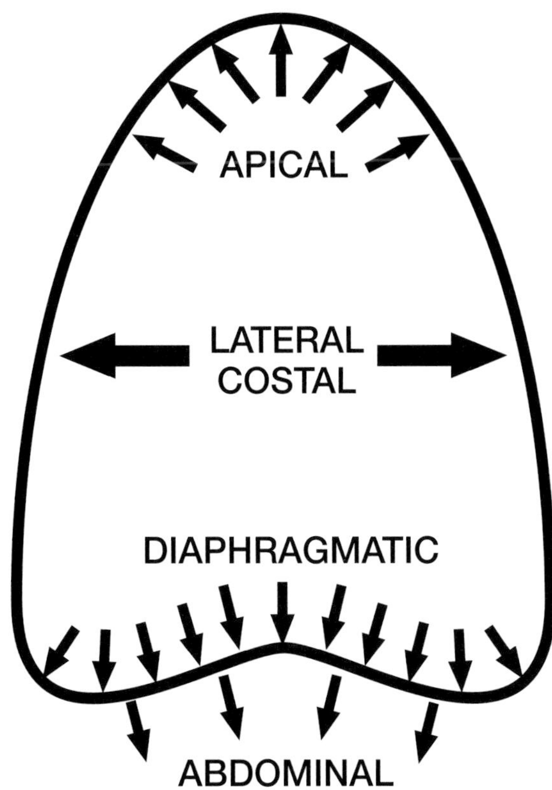

Fig. 4.41 Breathing patterns.

malalignment - sternocostal included - and especially by rotational displacement of any thoracic vertebrae (i.e. the costochondral junctions and the costotransverse and costovertebral joints) will be stressed even further by any movement of the rib cage (Figs 2.93, 2.94, 3.15, 3.16). Pain from these joints can impair normal lateral costal breathing and result in one of the following patterns.

Apical breathing

Breathing is carried out mainly using the upper parts of the lungs; the result is a shallow pattern, with a failure to ventilate the major part of the lungs.

Abdominal breathing

Movement of the ribs is impaired. To compensate, the diaphragm descends to allow the lungs to open up but the descent is limited, sometimes as a result of restriction caused by problems with the stomach, liver, spleen or bowel. Unless an effort is made to breathe in deeply, the result is often a shallow breathing pattern that may also impair normal gastric and bowel motility, resulting in a feeling of 'bloating' of the stomach.

The shallow breathing associated with the 'apical' and 'abdominal' patterns results in a compensatory increase in respiratory rate which can result in excessive blowing-off of carbon dioxide, a respiratory alkalosis and earlier fatiguing of the respiratory muscles. Weakness and early fatigue may eventually become noticeable even on attempts at retraining for lateral costal breathing. A vicious cycle can develop, with pain from the thoracic spine and rib cage limiting retraining efforts and resulting in further weakening.

Another complicating factor is the asymmetry of muscle tension and strength typical of an 'upslip' and 'rotational malalignment' superimposed on the overall increase in muscle tone that has been noted with a breathing pattern dysfunction. Muscles that are already abnormally tense on account of the respiratory problem are more likely to become symptomatic when subjected to any further increase in tension as part of the 'malalignment syndrome', albeit this increase is in an asymmetrical pattern. Certainly a number of 'inner'/'outer' core muscles and 'sling' systems are in a position to affect respiration.

IMPLICATIONS FOR RHEUMATOLOGY

The 'malalignment syndrome' *per se* is not an arthritic condition but malalignment can result in irritation and inflammation of the SI joints, symphysis pubis or any other joint put under increased mechanical stress by chronic asymmetrical overloading. The question of whether or not the stresses related to malalignment can actually lead to osteoarthritis, with accelerated joint degeneration, still needs to be answered (Figs 3.81, 3.82, 4.39).

Differentiating between malalignment and arthritis

Back pain and stiffness felt on waking that decreases or resolves with activity is typically attributable to increased irritability of soft tissues, actual inflammation, shortening or even contracture; it tends to recur temporarily on standing up from sitting or getting up after lying down during the day. However, the stiffness or aching may become more persistent as the person continues with an activity, such as a prolonged walk; this probably reflects the increased stress on joints and the supporting soft tissues as the muscles eventually start to fatigue. Morning stiffness and pain that decreases with activity is characteristically seen when there is soft tissue involvement, also with some of the seronegative spondyloarthropathies (e.g. ankylosing spondylitis). The initial stiffness and aching has been attributed to a stretching-out of the soft tissue(s) affected; in particular, the thoracodorsal fascia and posterior pelvic ligaments that tend to contract or 'gel' during a rest period (see 'Tissue types', Ch. 8). In contrast, pain attributable to mechanical factors (e.g. hip and SI joint osteoarthritis) tends to get worse on weight-bearing as the day progresses and decrease with sitting and lying.

Any back stiffness and aching seen with malalignment can have features of both types as there is usually an element of:

1. soft tissue irritation/inflammation, especially involving the posterior pelvic ligaments
2. mechanical pain, with the increased stress affecting particularly the lumbosacral (e.g. discs, facet), hip and SI joints

Tests specific for the SI joint area may provoke pain in someone presenting with malalignment, and some of the tests discussed in Chapter 2 are appropriate for this purpose. Most of these tests, however, do not differentiate between pain arising from the joint surfaces, capsule, interosseous or surrounding ligaments or even a specific site (e.g. hip versus SI joint).

Radionuclear scans sometimes detect a difference in the degree of activity in one SI joint compared with the other, though the actual degree of activity on both sides is often still within normal limits (see 'Implications for radiology and medical imaging', above; Fig. 4.39). This relative increase in uptake may just reflect early degeneration that is somewhat worse on one side. It may also, however, simply reflect an asymmetrical increase in bone turnover attributable to the asymmetrical increase in pressure on these joint surfaces and the change in weight-bearing that occurs with the malalignment. Such an increase in pressure could conceivably accelerate the degeneration of the joint cartilage, known to occur at an earlier age on the iliac than the sacral side (see Ch. 2; Cassidy 1992). Also, degeneration may not be uniform, reflecting the differences in pressure distribution on the joint surfaces caused by malalignment; e.g. long versus short arm, S1 versus S3 segmental level (Fig. 4.29)

In contrast, in the case of an inflammatory arthritis affecting the SI joints (e.g. sacroiliitis), bone scans typically delineate a generalized - and symmetrical - bilateral involvement.

'Malalignment syndrome' versus a 'chronic pain syndrome'

The 'malalignment syndrome' is frequently confused with some of the chronic pain syndromes thought to arise primarily from muscle, in particular 'myofascial pain syndrome' and 'fibromyalgia'. These three are, however, distinct entities, even though they may coexist. In addition, the chronicity of the biomechanical stresses and pain associated with malalignment can result in findings consistent with the 'myofascial pain syndrome'. There is an ongoing debate about whether malalignment can eventually lead to the development of a coexistent 'fibromyalgia syndrome'.

Myofascial pain syndrome

The key features of this syndrome are as follows:

1. It occurs more frequently in females than males (3:1).
2. The pain and tenderness usually localize to one quadrant or even just one muscle.
3. There is a trigger point - an area of acute tenderness localizing to a taut nodule or band - which is palpable within a muscle in the area of the muscle spindle (Costello 1998).
4. Transverse snapping of the taut band manually, or the insertion of a needle into the band, both may elicit a local muscle twitch response that can be seen and recorded.
5. Palpation of the trigger point may, in addition to causing localized pain, also elicit pain or altered sensation in a typical referral pattern (Travell & Simons 1992; Fig. 3.45).
6. The pain from the trigger point can be relieved by stretching or injection of a local anaesthetic.

Fibromyalgia syndrome

This pain syndrome is also referred to as 'generalized fibromyalgia' or 'fibrositis', compared to the 'myofascial pain syndrome' which is sometimes referred to as 'localized fibromyalgia' (Malyak 1997). Classical 'fibromyalgia rheumatica' is a chronic diffuse musculoskeletal pain syndrome of unknown etiology: non-inflammatory, non-autoimmune (though the incidence is increased in association with autoimmune diseases such as hypothyroidism, rheumatoid arthritis, systemic lupus erythematosus and Raynaud's disease). There are characteristic tender points. It occurs primarily between the ages of 30 and 50 years, females being affected 10 times more often than males. If the onset of similar symptoms is after age 55–60, they are usually due to a disease other than fibromyalgia (e.g. arthritis, infection, neoplasia).

Chronic, generalized, muscular aching pain involves, in particular, the shoulder and hip girdles, neck and lower back. The tender points are paired, occurring at specific sites bilaterally: the suboccipital muscle insertion, the anterior aspect of the C5-C6 intertransverse space, the midpoint of the upper border of trapezius, the origin of supraspinatus, the second rib just lateral to the costochondral junction, the lateral epicondyle, the upper outer quadrant of gluteus maximus, the posterior aspect of the greater trochanter and the medial aspect of the knee at the joint line (Fig. 4.42). The diagnosis of 'fibromyalgia syndrome' rests on a history of widespread pain and localized tenderness in at least 11 of these 18 sites.

The paired 'tender points' specific to classical 'fibromyalgia rheumatica' syndrome are distinct from 'trigger points' in that there are no palpable nodules or bands, the sites are symmetrical and their location does not change.

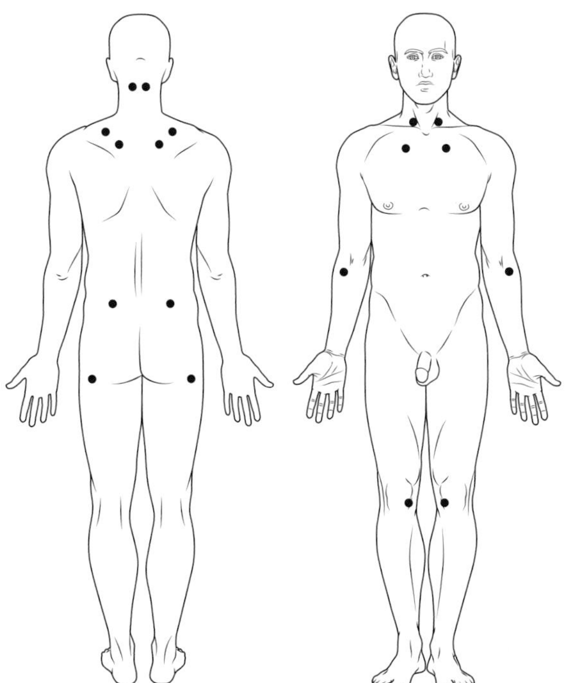

Fig. 4.42 Location of the 18 (9 pairs) specific tender points in fibromyalgia patients.

The individual suffers from generalized, chronic stiffness and fatigues easily. There is a non-restorative sleep pattern associated with:

1. a disturbance of the characteristic low-frequency (0.5–2.0 Hz) delta waves of non-rapid eye movement sleep by faster (7.5–11.0 Hz) alpha waves, leaving the person feeling tired rather than refreshed in the morning
2. muscular fatigue, aching and development of the tender points.

Differentiating: malalignment, myofascial pain syndrome and fibromyalgia

Given these distinguishing features of 'fibromyalgia' and 'myofascial pain' syndrome noted above, it should be easy to differentiate these entities from the 'malalignment syndrome', which:

1. occurs in an approximately equal number of females and males
2. may have tender sites, less frequently actual 'trigger points', associated with it; however, these occur in a seemingly 'random' distribution, involving primarily the muscles showing an increase in tension and tenderness in an asymmetrical pattern as a result of:
   a. an altered sympathetic response, with asymmetric 'facilitation'
   b. a change in the length-tension ratio
   c. a reaction to an irritating focus or pain (e.g. joint compression or distraction)
   d. an attempt to stabilize a joint
   e. a combination of these factors (see Ch. 3)
3. is characterized by musculoskeletal pain from specific structures, mainly in an asymmetrical pattern that can usually be explained on the basis of the factors noted above, and is usually attributable to the biomechanical stresses that typically occur with malalignment
4. does not feature the generalized stiffness, specific pairs of tender points or non-restorative sleep pattern seen with 'fibromyalgia rheumatica'.

According to some authors (Barral & Mercier 1988; Barral 1989; Selby 1992; Upledger & Vredevoogd 1983), the chronic increase in pelvic floor tension has been considered to be a possible cause for the decrease in vitality, or even the 'chronic fatigue syndrome', complaints that are not uncommonly noted in association with the 'malalignment syndrome'; in particular, in those with a complicating 'levator ani syndrome' or coccydynia (see below).

IMPLICATIONS FOR UROLOGY, GASTROENTEROLOGY, GYNAECOLOGY AND OBSTETRICS

In the peri-partum period, acute pain localizing to the symphysis pubis is often incorrectly attributed to a separation of the pubic bones, even though a separation may not actually be palpable or evident on ASLR or a standing 'figure-4 radiological view intended to stress the joint (Fig. 2.102A,B). In these cases, the problem is more often triggered by the additional stresses being superimposed during this time on a joint that is already under constant stress as the result of a pre-existing long-standing 'upslip', 'rotational malalignment', 'outflare/inflare' or combinations of these. The malalignment, and the associated excessive displacement and rotation of the pubic rami relative to each other, may also result from the trauma of delivery, any surgical intervention (if such occurred) and subsequent muscle spasm.

> Because of its location, pain triggered by malalignment and originating from the pelvic region can mimic gastrointestinal and genitourinary disorders.

Take, for example, pain originating from the right anterior SI joint ligaments, which are usually located immediately posterior to the appendix (Fig. 2.4A,B). This pain can localize to McBurney's point and mimic the pain of appendicitis. In addition, as discussed in detail below, all of these ligaments and other somatic structures are segmentally related to viscera that have an autonomic supply from the same segment (Barral & Mercier 1988). For example, the bowel derives autonomic supply from the same S2, S3 and S4 root that provides somatic structures such as the nearby sacrococcygeal joint and coccyx.

Norman (1968) reported on 74 patients who presented with lower abdominal, groin or rectal pain 'which, after extensive investigation ... defied the efforts of the examiners to implicate any of the organ systems to explain the protracted pain' (p. 54). 72 of the 74 patients had no complaint of back pain or sciatic radiation, and none responded to antispasmodic medications. 71 obtained relief from their pain within minutes on the injection of 3 cc 2% procaine into the ipsilateral SI joint; 52 required a second and 32 a third injection, spaced 3 days apart. By 1 month, 58 (81%) were pain-free. The various symptoms reported by some of those who were successfully treated in this way are of particular interest, as noted in Box 4.7.

BOX 4.7 Symptoms documented in Norman's study (1968)

1. an acute onset of right groin pain
2. right lower quadrant pain with radiation to the groin, treated unsuccessfully by repeated dilatation of the ureter for 'spasm of unknown origin'
3. severe right lower quadrant pain radiating to the back, with only a partial response using a ptosis corset for bilateral 'renal ptosis' noted on X-ray
4. left lower quadrant pain in a patient diagnosed as suffering from 'diverticulitis'
5. symptoms of acute right lower quadrant pain in a patient with a previous appendectomy, felt to indicate 'another attack of appendicitis'
6. severe pain and muscle spasm in the rectum with radiation down the right leg, which failed to respond to haemorrhoidectomy, improved only temporarily after a paravertebral nerve block and caudal block, and worsened on anaesthetizing the coccyx
7. severe sciatica, as well as abdominal pain on coughing
8. pain in the lower left part of the abdomen on taking long steps when walking

There is no reference to pelvic malalignment in Norman's report but the symptoms listed have all been reported in association with malalignment (see Ch. 3; also 'Thoracolumbar syndrome' above, and the descriptions below). The negative investigations, and the positive response to SI joint injection, suggest that the pain arose from stress on the joint capsule, interosseous ligaments and/or cartilage. Norman correctly identified 'sacroiliac disease and its relationship to lower abdominal pain'. The question remains of how many of his patients actually had the SI joint problem to begin with because they were out of alignment and might have responded just as dramatically to realignment.

It is not unusual for someone to experience symptoms involving the gastrointestinal or genitourinary system when they are out of alignment. The acute onset of these symptoms can coincide with the recurrence of malalignment and their abrupt cessation with successful realignment. Typical symptoms include:

1. an increased need to void (daytime frequency and nocturia), urgency and stress incontinence

2. episodic loose stools, or even diarrhoea, lasting 1–3 days and sometimes alternating with the onset of constipation on realignment
3. a build-up of gas with abdominal distension
4. a marked exacerbation of premenstrual and menstrual pain
5. unilateral vaginal wall/labial/testicular pain
6. sexual dysfunction and pain on intercourse (dyspareunia)

An awareness of the commonly encountered referral patterns involving the gastrointestinal and genitourinary systems is important when questioning a person, as they often fail to report such patterns spontaneously. Males, for example, may not volunteer a history of unilateral testicular pain. In a man presenting with malalignment who is afebrile and has no evidence of testicular tenderness or swelling, and whose investigations for infection, tumour and hernia are negative, this pain may be on the basis of referral from the ipsilateral iliolumbar ligament to the testicle (Fig. 3.46). In females, irritation of this ligament may account for dysaesthesias felt in the ipsilateral vaginal wall and/or labia. Irritation of the 'anterior' cutaneous perforating nerve branches of T12 and L1 can also cause dysaesthaesias in the ipsilateral lower abdominal wall, groin, scrotum or labia majora (Fig. 4.23A2,B2).

Effects of malalignment: somatic versus visceral?

The fact that problems involving somatic structures can result in visceral symptoms has long been recognized. In this respect, Hackett (1958) did much to clarify the visceral effects relating to ligaments, while Travell & Simons (1983, 1992) documented those associated with trigger points.

Recognition that visceral problems can result in somatic symptoms is in large part attributable to the translation in 1988 of the landmark *'Manipulations viscerales'* published by Barral & Mercier in 1983.

> Barral and Mercier's studies, and the experience of others skilled in 'visceral manipulation', have resulted in an increasing awareness that the problems related to malalignment, rather than being restricted to the musculoskeletal or somatic system, can also affect the autonomic and visceral systems.

In fact, many of those using visceral manipulation are convinced that it is more often the visceral problem that is the cause of the recurrent malalignment rather than the other way around (Barral 1989; personal communications: J.L. Cole-Morgan 1993; J.S. Gerhardt 1999; H.L. Jones 1999; J. Wells 2009). Their success in treating these cases resistant to other approaches would certainly support this contention. They speak of organs or viscera not lying in their proper place as the result of trauma, and not fully functioning because of displacement or a restriction of their mobility, much as one might talk about the rotational displacement of a vertebra or the pelvis being 'out of place' with malalignment. The liver, for example, is suspended in the abdominal cavity by six major ligaments (Fig. 4.43) and normally moves some 200 meters a day as it repeatedly ascends and descends in harmony with the movements of the diaphragm on expiration and inspiration, respectively. Tightness of any of these ligaments can result from postoperative scar formation or blunt trauma, such as a seat-belt or airbag injury, also secondary to inflammation or infection.

Tightness will impair the smooth upward and downward movement of the liver and, by impairing the glide of the fascia that envelops the liver, is also felt to interfere with the craniosacral rhythm. These restrictions can eventually interfere with the proper functioning of this organ. Dysfunction may initially be experienced as unexplained visceral symptoms attributable to biliary stasis and a decrease in hepatic metabolism. Nervous depression and a decrease in the immune response have been linked to the same mechanism (Barral & Mercier 1989).

> Patients who present with malalignment that fails to respond to other manual therapy approaches may finally respond to visceral mobilization, used either alone or in combination with one of these more 'traditional' mobilization techniques.

Ligaments and referral to viscera

Hackett (1958) was one of the first to point out that pain originating from somatic structures, namely the ligaments, could be referred to the viscera and was, therefore, capable of evoking symptoms involving the gastrointestinal and genitourinary systems. He blamed the problem on a laxity of these

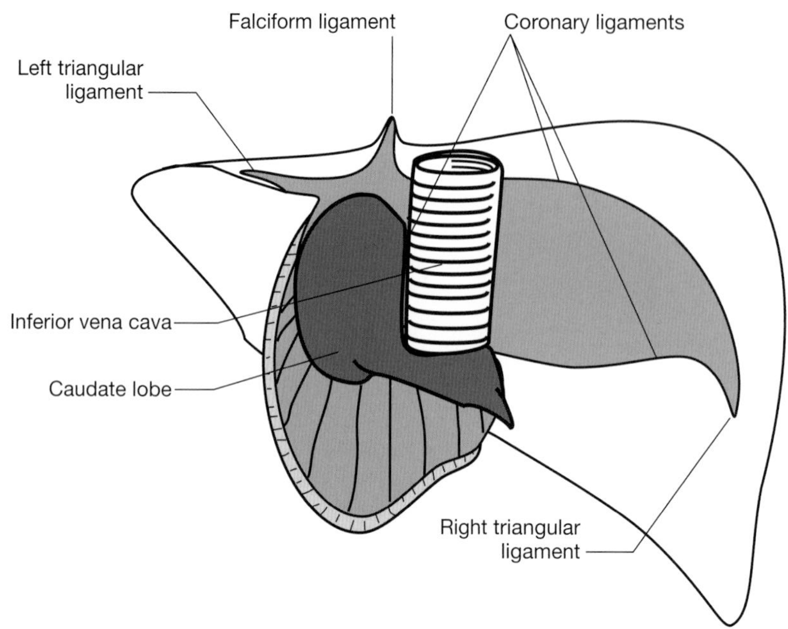

Fig. 4.43 The six ligaments supporting the liver. *(Redrawn courtesy of Grant 1980.)*

ligaments. By injecting hypertonic saline or glucose solution into specific ligaments, he was able not only to map out the patterns of referred pain into the extremities (see Chs 2, 3) but also to record consistent responses involving the viscera. Some of his findings warrant repeating here as they have been supported in numerous subsequent publications (e.g. Barral & Mercier 1988; Maigne 1997; Maigne & Chatellier, 2001; Steege et al. 1998) and, in the author's experience, have been borne out in clinical practice. Direct quotations regarding symptoms referred from specific ligaments to the viscera (Box 4.8) are taken from Hackett's 1958 monograph.

Hackett wrote that:

> *The pain in the intestine and testicle has been reproduced by needling in the dorsal 12th, lumbar articular and the iliolumbar ligaments, and the tendon attachments to the transverse processes of all the lumbar vertebrae.*
>
> (Hackett 1958: 90–91)

BOX 4.8 Visceral symptoms caused by referral from ligaments

Iliolumbar ligament (Figs 3.46, 3.63)

1. ipsilateral testicular discomfort
2. discomfort involving the penis
3. unilateral vaginal or labial pain, with or without dyspareunia
4. unilateral groin pain (capable of mimicking appendicitis)
5. nausea

Lumbosacral ligament (Fig. 3.63)

1. bladder discomfort and a frequent urge to void, which can signal a recurrence of malalignment and may not be relieved by voiding
   [Author's comment: in addition to involvement of this ligament, another mechanism to consider in the differential is a strictly mechanical one, malalignment having resulted in irritation of the bladder outlet by distorting the bladder and squeezing and/or twisting the urethra or bladder neck; see also Figs 2.56, 2.57 and 'Visceral problems and the pelvic floor' below]
2. rectal pain

Sacroiliac ligaments (Figs 3.63, 4.10)

These can refer pain to the lower abdomen, possibly 'accompanied by tenderness' in that area (Hackett, 1958: 91).

Lumbar and lumbosacral spine ligaments (Fig. 3.63)

Irritation of these ligaments has been connected to bowel disturbance; with the recurrence of malalignment:

1. some may experience an acute onset of diarrhoea that is abolished by realignment
2. in others, it is associated with a coincident episode of severe constipation, bloating and 'gas'

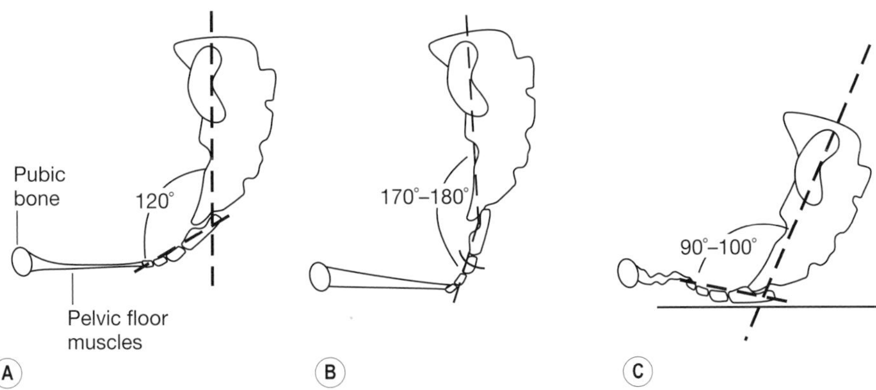

Fig. 4.44 Effect of angulation of the coccyx on the inserting ligaments and pelvic floor muscles. (A) A normal angulation of 120 degrees relative to the sacrum, with a 30 degree range of motion; there is normal pelvic floor tone. (B) Excessive 'extension angulation' resulting in hypertonus of the pelvic floor. (C) Excessive 'flexion angulation' resulting in hypotonus of the pelvic floor (e.g. passively on sitting in a 'slouched' position); however, this angulation may itself result actively with a chronic increase in tension of these muscles from whatever cause (e.g. irritation by a pelvic cyst, mass).

'Anterior' rotation of the coccyx (Fig. 4.44C) has also been associated with bowel disturbance, possibly by affecting the autonomic supply to the bowel as it exits with the S2, S3 and S4 nerve roots (Fig. 4.15) in close proximity to the anterior aspect of the sacrococcygeal articulation and the coccyx itself (Barral & Mercier 1988; Maigne & Chatellier 2001).

Problems relating to the female reproductive system

Females are sometimes reluctant to volunteer information relating to sexual function and menses, in which case questions are in order relating specifically to the following:

Dyspareunia (painful sexual intercourse)

Pain in the vaginal wall or labia on one side may manifest itself as 'introital dyspareunia'. Pain can be referred to these sites from the ipsilateral iliolumbar ligament or result from irritation of the T12/L1 anterior cutaneous branches as part of the 'thoracolumbar syndrome' (Fig. 4.23A2, B2). The following problems are more likely to result in 'deep-thrust dyspareunia':

1. tension and tenderness involving the pelvic floor muscles themselves
2. torsion of the vagina in conjunction with the bladder/uterine complex when the latter is distorted by malalignment (Fig. 2.53C)
3. a painful coccyx, which may reflect:
   a. a chronic increase in tension in the attaching muscles and ligaments (Figs 2.53, 4.44B)
   b. problems involving the sacrococcygeal junction itself, such as subluxation, rotational or torsional strain, or excessive anterior or posterior displacement (Fig. 4.44); an intercoccygeal joint, if present, may become a source of pain for similar reasons (Figs 2.3A, 3.68)

These problems are discussed in more detail under 'Coccydynia, pelvic floor dystonia and levator ani syndrome', below.

Dysmenorrhoea

Typical changes in the menstrual cycle (which tends to occur with increased frequency) include a longer and more painful premenstrual phase, increased back pain, increased abdominal and/or pelvic discomfort, a heavier flow, a longer duration and irregularity. The periods revert to the habitual pattern with realignment. Possible explanations for these phenomena include:

1. increased engorgement of the reproductive organs resulting from torsion of these organs and increased tone in the pelvic floor muscles
2. torsion resulting in increased tension in some of the ligaments that suspend the uterus and ovaries
3. an actual recurrence of the malalignment, which is more likely to happen around the time of the period, possibly as a result of:
   a. an increase in ligament laxity associated with the transient increase in the blood relaxin level known to occur around this time (and also with ovulation)

b. a transient increase in the stress level which, in turn, causes an increase in muscle tone; muscles that are at present relaxed but have previously been tense and tender, whether as a result of malalignment or some other insult, tend to be the first ones to react to an increase or recurrence of stress

'Pelvic girdle pain' or 'PGP'

Up to this point, there has been considerable discussion of sites capable of causing groin and pelvic floor pain. Some of the ones that should be considered in the differential diagnosis include:

1. iliolumbar ligament referral to the groin/testical/vagina (Figs 2.4A, 3.46)
2. the SI joint and upper posterior sacroiliac ligaments (Fig. 3.63)
3. the sacrotuberous and sacrospinous ligaments (Figs 2.4A, 2.5A, 3.64)
4. the 'thoracolumbar syndrome', with 'anterior cutaneous branch' involvement (Fig. 4.23A2,B2)
5. sometimes even trigger points in piriformis (Fig. 3.45)

Over the past two decades, there has also been extensive discussion regarding the origin of pelvic/groin pain typically encountered with pregnancy. The so-called 'pelvic girdle pain' (PGP) has been considered to result from:

1. poor control of the motion of the pelvic joints
2. disturbance of the activity and coordination of the large stabilizing muscles around the SI joints (Hungerford et al. 2003, O'Sullivan et al. 2002, O'Sullivan & Beales 2007)
3. subsequent development of pain, secondary to the increased demand on these pelvic muscles, ligaments and joint capsules

PGP is described as follows (Östgaard 2007):

1. occurs in about 20% of pregnancies, rarely after trauma or arthritis
2. a specific form of LBP, localizing 'between the posterior iliac crest and gluteal fold...in the vicinity of the SIJ'
3. can radiate into the posterior thigh, but not below the knee
4. may occur in conjunction with pain in the symphysis pubis region
5. makes it difficult and painful to turn over in bed
6. results in lower endurance for sitting, standing and walking

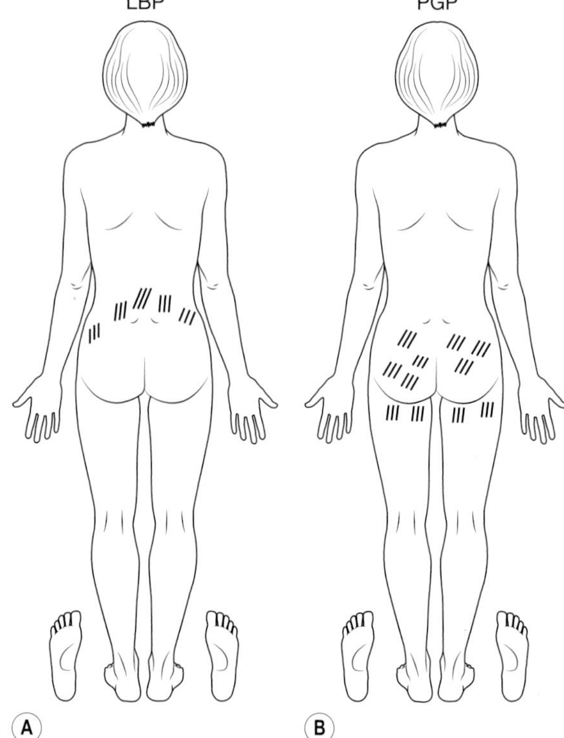

Fig. 4.45 Pain drawings of (A) lumbar back pain (LBP) and (B) pelvic girdle pain (PGP). *(Courtesy of Östgaard 2007.)*

7. may occur together with LBP but 'diagnosis of PGP can be reached only after exclusion of lumbar causes'; back pain of lumbar origin is noted to be restricted to the lumbosacral region and upward of L5 (Fig. 4.45B)
8. the 'pain and functional disturbances in relation to PGP must be reproducible by specific clinical tests' which, basically, provoke pain from one or both SI joints; the tests have been described in Ch. 2 and include: posterior pelvic pain provocation, Gaenslen's stretch (e.g. passive right hip flexion, left hip extension in supine-lying, to stress bilateral SI joints and left hip flexors), long (dorsal) sacroiliac ligament, Patrick's (or FABERs), modified Trendelenburg and active SLR tests or ASLR (Figs 2.19B, 2.107, 2.108, 2.126, 2.128, 2.129, 2.130)

The description of the post-partum period given above notes that, whereas the PGP usually disappears within 3 months after delivery, 'lumbar back pain' tends to persist. Some women with PGP seemingly develop chronic pain even after the ligaments have 'regained their normal tension'. There is no indication whether this 'normal tension' is in keeping with having regained pre-partum body weight, alignment, or other parameters. However, their recommendation is for referral to a physiotherapist for training of pelvic muscles initially, to gain control of movement of the pelvic joints, followed by training of back muscles (Dumas et al. 1995, 1995b). Retraining is noted to be 'slow, 6–12 months, and always includes periods of serious relapse' (Östgaard 2007). Some women are described as doing well immediately post-partum but can develop PGP 'months after' that may require 'several years' of rehabilitation. Östgaard (2007: 358) went on to note that:

1. 'coordination and exercise of the stabilizing muscles of the pelvic girdle, as well as a pelvic belt, help relieve pain and will eventually often cure the condition'
2. 'uncontrolled, but not unnecessarily increased motion, of the SIJs resulting in extreme positions and in tense joint capsules and ligaments, instead of well-controlled muscular dynamic stabilized joints' is likely to result in pain in the joint capsules and ligaments.
3. this pain triggers 'reflex isometric contraction of the same stabilizing muscles of the pelvic girdle': they now work in a 'static instead of dynamic' fashion and become 'painful and insufficient'; with the increased tension causing more pain, a 'vicious cycle is initiated' involving the soft tissues that are at the root of the PGP so that it 'might go on indefinitely if left untreated'.

There has been no indication of any correlation between PGP and oral contraceptives (Östgaard et al. 1991a; Bjorklund et al. 2000), hormonal and ovulatory changes resulting with post-partum breast-feeding (Östgaard & Anderson 1992) or problems with the infant/child (e.g. disability) or the delivery itself (Östgaard et al. 1991a, 1996).

Other comments in the literature of note:

1. The SI joint and posterior SI joint ligaments have been recognized as a 'known source of posterior PGP (PPGP), although the relationship between the pain and the patterning of pelvic motion remains unclear' (Fortin et al. 1994; also Vleeming et al. 2002, Hungerford & Gilleard 2007).
2. Already in 1999, Mens et al. reported increased amplitude of anterior rotation of the innominate in PPGP patients, also that there was a correlation between a positive ASLR test with posterior pelvic pain (O'Sullivan et al. 2002; Fig. 2.102).
3. Buyruk et al. 1999, Damen et al. 2001 reported that:
   a. ASLR is positive in the presence of asymmetric stiffness of the SI joint, which is:
      i. indicative of impaired load transfer between trunk and lower limb
      ii. prognostic for pain and pelvic impairment
   b. SI joint stiffness is asymmetric in subjects with PGP; whereas healthy individuals had symmetrical stiffness (Damen 2002a)

In the 'pelvic groin pain' syndrome, the pain is noted to localize to the SI joint area and 'most likely to emanate from the large, stabilizing muscles around the pelvis' (Östgaard 2007: 354); whereas any pain felt in the posterior iliac crest level and above was attributed to problems in the lumbosacral area (Fig. 4.45).

Overall, the description of the 'PPGP' repeatedly overlaps that of the 'malalignment syndrome'. Certainly malalignment can be a cause of problems during and after pregnancy, and a major part of the 'malalignment syndrome' includes the features noted to comprise the PPGP phenomenon:

1. the joint instability, reflex muscle contraction and secondary development of pain in the muscles, ligaments and joint capsules; in particular, the SI joint, interosseous and posterior SI joint - ligaments that Fortin et al. (1994) and Vleeming et al. (1992a,b) referred to in trying to explain the PGP phenomenon some time ago, and which continue to be part and parcel of the current description of this entity
2. pain typical of the PPGP is sometimes noted to come on months after delivery; this time sequence would be more in keeping with development of a 'malalignment syndrome' in someone who has delivered but:
   a. was out of alignment at the time of the delivery but never had treatment aimed at achieving realignment and has now become symptomatic
   b. went out of alignment post-partum, which is not uncommon, given the demands on the mother, and more likely to occur:
      i. as the baby gains weight
      ii. if lifting is done incorrectly (often with a torsional component)

However, there is no indication by these authors:

1. whether there was any evidence of one or more of the three common presentations - an 'upslip', 'outflare/inflare' or 'rotational malalignment' - in the expectant women who were diagnosed as having PPGP

2. if malalignment was actually noted:
   a. whether there were any obvious symptoms and signs that could be attributed to the malalignment itself (i.e. typical of a 'malalignment syndrome', with a pelvic floor dysfunction component) and, if so
   b. whether these signs and symptoms differed from those noted in:
      i. the women who were diagnosed as having a 'PPGP' and
      ii. those diagnosed as not having PPGP; e.g. those who were not pregnant and the 75-80% who were pregnant but were felt not to have a PPGP problem (but who may well have been out of alignment, given that the three common presentations together are found in 80-90% of the general population)

Coccydynia, pelvic floor dystonia and levator ani syndrome

Involvement of the coccygeal region is not uncommon in association with malalignment. The author found that 12% of those presenting with malalignment had tenderness over the coccyx (Schamberger 2002). Abnormalities of the sacrococcygeal joint, an intercoccygeal joint (if present; Figs 2.3, 3.68) and the attaching pelvic floor muscles and ligaments are now recognized as a cause of:

1. both acute and chronic pain seemingly arising from the 'spine', sometimes hard to differentiate from symptoms that originate from the lumbar region because of the overlap in the pain distribution
2. pelvic floor dystonia (both hyper- and hypotonicity)
3. visceral dysfunction
4. levator ani (spasm) syndrome
5. failure to achieve realignment of the pelvis and spine, or to maintain any correction.

The role of coccydynia and pelvic floor dystonia as a cause of ongoing problems, including chronic pelvic pain and visceral symptoms, has been receiving increasing recognition (Maigne 1997; Maigne & Chatellier 2001; Steege et al. 1998) The following is a summary of developments in this area and an approach to assessment and treatment based, in part, on a succinct account delivered by Seelby in 1992.

The coccyx and sacrococcygeal articulation

Barral & Mercier (1988: 260) stressed the importance of the sacrococcygeal articulation in stating that:

> *...It has a physiological role in copulation, defecation and micturition. It plays an integral part in lumbosacral dynamics; problems with the coccyx can contribute to lumbosacral restrictions.*

1. This diarthrosis is normally capable of up to 30 degrees of motion (Fig. 4.44A). It is reinforced by the anterior, posterior and lateral sacrococcygeal ligaments, which help to maintain the position of the coccyx and distribute forces to the coccyx and adjacent structures (Fig. 3.68). In addition, the coccyx serves as a point of attachment for almost all the other soft tissue structures of the pelvis (Barral & Mercier 1988).
2. Excessive forward angulation (= flexion), such as occurs with sacral counternutation, slouching, or as the result of a fall, can result in pelvic floor hypotonus with eventual contracture of these muscles and ligaments (Fig. 4.44C). Excessive backward angulation (= extension), as may occur with birth trauma or prolonged nutation, increases the tension and can eventually result in lengthening of these soft tissue structures (Fig. 4.44B).

The continuations of the dural tube that exit through the sacral hiatus also blend into the periosteum of the coccyx. Manipulation of the coccyx thus allows those using craniosacral treatment a direct means of acting on the spinal dura (see Chs 7, 8).

Anatomy of the pelvic floor

The pelvic floor muscles serve to anchor the low back and the hip joints, support the pelvic organs and stabilize the pelvic ring (Pool-Goudzwaard et al. 2004). The floor is made up of five layers of muscle and fascia, which attach to the pelvic bones (Fig. 2.53):

1. The anal sphincter forms the first (superficial) layer.
2. The urogenital triangle, or second layer, consists of the urogenital diaphragm and vaginal and urethral sphincters; it stretches from the ischial tuberosities posteriorly to the pubis anteriorly.
3. The pelvic diaphragm, or third layer, is made up of the three levator ani muscles (pubococcygeus, iliococcygeus and ischiococcygeus), which blend with the rectal sphincter posteriorly and the superficial perineal muscles anteriorly (Fig. 4.15). Together, they support the base and neck of the bladder (Sapsford et al. 1997, 2001, 2008). Herman (1988: 87) noted that these muscles not only:

...have the potential to decrease the urethral, vaginal and rectal canals, but they can decrease the anteroposterior relationships of the bony ring; and some authors believe that they can change the angle of the sacrum to the lumbar spine.

4. In addition, as Heardman pointed out in 1951, there are fascial connections between the levator ani muscles and the piriformis, biceps femoris, semitendinosus and obturator internus muscles, so that a change in tension in any of these muscles can affect the tone of the pelvic floor.
5. The smooth muscle diaphragm and endopelvic diaphragm complete the floor.

The pudendal nerve and vessels that supply these muscles travel within the fascial layers (Fig. 4.15), which puts them at risk of being irritated or compressed by any abnormal increase in tension and/or contracture of these myofascial tissues. Any compromise of the neurovascular supply can result in spasm, trophic changes, vasomotor effects and pain involving the pelvic floor structures (Barral & Mercier 1988; Herman 1988).

Visceral problems and the pelvic floor

Typical visceral problems that have been attributed to pelvic floor dysfunction include:

1. incontinence of bowel or bladder attributed to a lax floor (Smith et al. 2007)
2. constipation and incomplete voiding with excessive tension
3. dysmenorrhoea, dyspareunia, impotence and sexual dysfunction
4. recurrent cystitis and urinary tract infection

Pelvic malalignment distorts the ring formed by the pelvic bones and, therefore:

1. disturbs the normal relationship of the points of attachment of the pelvic floor muscles
2. can affect the tone in these muscles (Fig. 4.46)
3. puts a twist on structures that exit by traversing the pelvic floor (the urethra and distal rectum/anus) or lie in close proximity to the pelvic floor (the vagina, uterus, bladder and rectum; Figs 2.53C, 4.46, 4.47).

Twisting of the bladder and its outlet may be one explanation for the reports of urgency and frequency of voiding that sometimes disappear immediately on realignment, only to return just as quickly when malalignment recurs, a phenomenon that has also been attributed to irritation of the lumbosacral ligaments (Hackett 1958). Distortion of the vagina and uterus may account for problems of dyspareunia and dysmenorrhoea, which can also sometimes disappear promptly with realignment.

Visceral pain can also cause pelvic floor hypertonicity and spasm, which may deform the sacrococcygeal joint and lead to back pain. Alternately, a bladder infection can result in spasm of the levator ani muscles and may, in turn, be responsible for the inability to void completely and the eventual development of back pain.

> In other words, sacrococcygeal pain may cause visceral problems or may itself be the result of an underlying visceral problem.

Therefore, in the absence of a history of trauma to the sacrococcygeal region, a concerted effort must be made to exclude any underlying visceral pathology affecting the bowel, rectum or urogenital system. If preliminary tests (e.g. blood screen, urinalysis and ultrasound scan) are negative, the problem(s) may simply be related to a coexistent malalignment. In particular, distortion of the pelvic ring, L4 or L5 vertebral displacement and sacrococcygeal rotation should be sought for and addressed. Further investigations (e.g. RTUS of pelvic floor, bladder; Figs 2.56, 2.57, 2.58, 4.46) and treatment (e.g. trigger point injection, pelvic floor exercises and biofeedback; Fig. 4.47) may be in order if the symptoms fail to respond to realignment alone (see Ch. 7).

Coccydynia: relation to coccygeal positioning, mobility, displacement

Hypotonicity of the pelvic floor muscles has been attributed to anterior movement of the coccyx that may have occurred as a result of trauma or the pressure of faulty sitting. McGivney & Cleveland (1965) were able to show this anterior movement radiologically. Their studies indicated that the coccyx is normally tilted forward some 120 degrees on the sacrum (Fig. 4.44A; see also Maigne & Chatellier 2001, below). The angle of the sacrococcygeal joint tended to decrease considerably when the patient was placed in a 'slumped position' on the X-Ray table, 'indicating substantial flexion of the sacrococcygeal joint' (Fig. 4.44C).

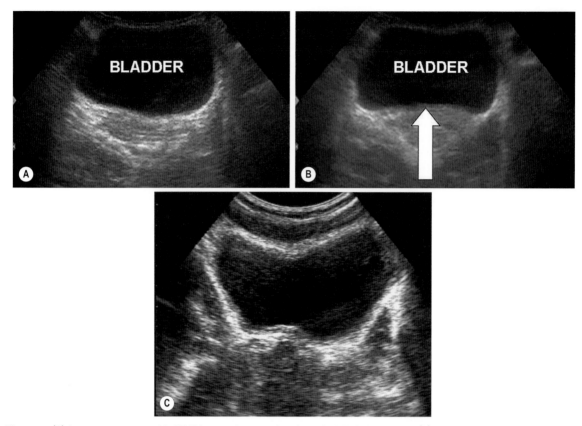

Fig. 4.46 (A) A transverse suprapubic RTUS image of a normal moderately full bladder at rest. (B) During a contraction of the pelvic floor the profile of the bladder changes and the inferior aspect of the image rises. (C) Transverse suprapubic real-time ultrasound (RTUS) image of [patient J's] bladder at rest. Note the asymmetry of the inferior border of this image compared to the normal bladder in (A). The profile of the bladder is by itself not diagnostic of any particular dysfunction. Either the endopelvic fascia on the left could be stretched or torn, or the pelvic floor muscles on the right could be hypertonic. Further tests are necessary to differentiate the cause of this asymmetry. *(Courtesy of Lee 2007b.)*

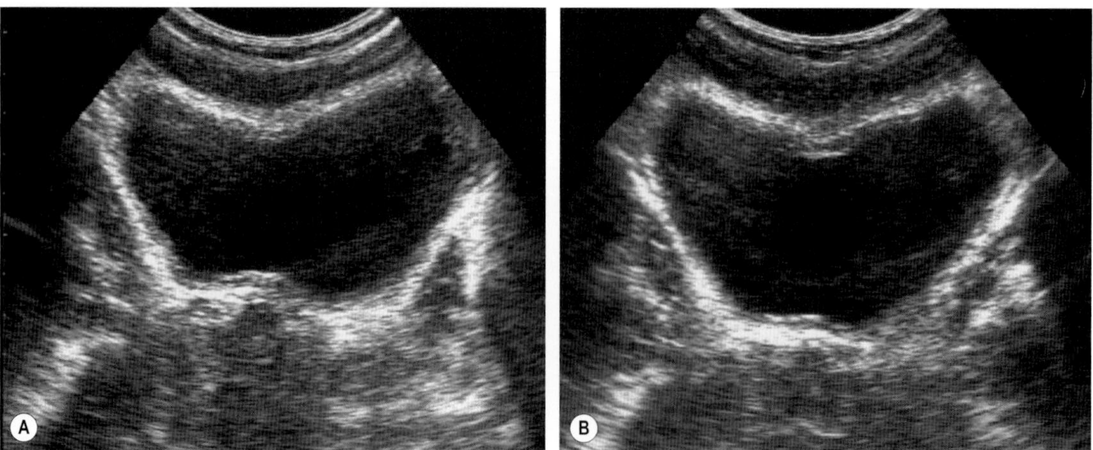

Fig. 4.47 (A) This is a transverse suprapubic RTUS image of [patient J's] resting bladder before she learned to relax the ischiococcygeus and the external rotators of the right hip. (B) RTUS image of [her] resting bladder immediately after she stopped 'butt-gripping' for comparison. Note the change in shape of the right inferior aspect of the bladder. *(Courtesy of Lee 2007b.)*

Like Thiele (1963), they stressed how:

1. a habitual poor sitting posture was common in patients with coccygeal pain
2. slumping in a chair caused the sacrum and the coccyx to press against the hard surface and produced increased flexion of the sacrococcygeal joint, and
3. the coccygeal pain was often relieved simply by sitting on a firm surface, trunk erect so that its weight was now supported by the ischial tuberosities rather than the coccyx (see Ch. 7)

Use of a coccygeal relief pillow (Fig. 7.43) has also proven helpful:

1. a central cut-out posteriorly prevents any weight-bearing on the coccyx
2. a firm lower-half foam base is covered by a piece of memory foam tapered forward; the lower-half can absorb more shock but the upper part is good at accommodating to and recovering from any indentations made by the often 'uneven' weight-bearing parts
3. tapering the foam forward cushion helps shift weight-bearing onto the right and left ischial tuberosity and posterior thighs (Fig. 7.43C)

Traumatic or habitual anterior rotation of the coccyx moves it closer to the pubic symphysis, bringing the origin and insertion of the pelvic floor muscles, ligaments and fascial sheaths closer together (Fig. 4.44C); pelvic floor muscle tone and strength are thereby decreased. When the bladder and rectum are relaxed in this way, incontinence may result (Barral & Mercier 1988).

The role of excessive or abnormal movement of the sacrococcygeal (and any intercoccygeal joints; Figs. 2.3, 3.68) in the causation of coccydynia and pelvic floor dysfunction continues to be explored using approaches like the dynamic method using radiology and coggygeal discography (Maigne and co-authors: 1994, 1996, 1997, 2001), combined with taking a lateral X-Ray in standing and when sitting on a hard surface, the back 'slightly extended...a posture in which the pain is most pronounced'. Maigne warned that it could take several minutes for pain to develop in the sitting position and that it was therefore crucial to wait before drawing any conclusions as to whether any of the findings on the X-Rays actually did play a role in the causation of the coccydynia. His studies disclosed a breakdown of these findings into the following categories:

1. 20-25% with 'sagittal (posterior) subluxation or luxation (displacement by 25% or more)'
   a. in most of them, these findings were 'reduced' on standing
   b. while about 40% of the subjects in this category were asymptomatic, there were frequent reports of an acute pain felt on changing from sitting to standing
2. 20-25% with coccygeal hypermobility in flexion; that is, flexion exceeding the 'normal' 20–25 degrees seen on standing
3. 15% with coccygeal 'spicules'
   a. described as a bony spicule on the dorsum of the tip of the coccyx that juts out under the skin; there may be a 'pit' in the overlying skin or even a pilonidal sinus
   b. found most commonly on the dorsum of a non-mobile coccyx, making pressure on the spicule worse as the coccyx cannot move 'to take evasive action'
   c. pain is felt on sitting and is localized to the tip, relieved with local anaesthetic
   d. onset of the 'coccydynia' is 'spontaneous', there is no obvious precipitating cause
4. 40% with idiopathic coccydynia - the 'dynamic' films were normal; the differential was felt to include:
   a. referred pain, possibly originating from the SI joint or lumbosacral area
   b. intradiscal inflammation
   c. chronic bursitis (e.g. presenting as pain at the tip of the coccyx, even without a spicule being present)
   d. irritation or inflammation of the sacral origin of the sacrotuberous ligament [Author's comment: also consider sacrospinous ligament origin; Fig. 3.64]
   e. psychogenic pain (hysteria); noted to be rare and characterized by permanent pain that was not increased by sitting

Levator ani syndrome and coccydynia

Levator ani syndrome, also called 'levator spasm syndrome', may result from a persistent increase in pelvic floor muscle tone. For example, acute trauma to the sacrococcygeal region, such as from a fall, direct blow or unaccustomed and prolonged pressure in a poor sitting posture, can result in reflex hypertonicity of the levator muscles. As Selby (1992: 3) pointed out, this may create further:

irritating deformation of the joint in the same anterior direction as the original traumatic insult ... This scenario can go on for years, fuelled by sitting in soft chairs and certain car seats (e.g. bucket seats). However, simple manoeuvres (e.g. direct mobilization of the sacrococcygeal joint) that break into the vicious cycle can often totally alleviate this sort of distress, both acute and chronic, in short order.

A history of trauma to the coccyx is often overlooked or hard to come by in patients who have sustained an injury many years ago. Specific questions may trigger a memory of a tobogganing accident or of a fall from a bike or down a staircase. Sexual abuse is another cause to consider. Athletes are less likely to recall specific incidents, especially if their sport is one in which falls are par for the course.

In female patients, questions repeatedly bring forth the realization that the symptoms that have now brought them to the doctor's office have, in retrospect, been present since the time of a pregnancy and delivery. Birth trauma and inadequate postpartum strengthening are very likely to result in excessive relaxation of the pelvic floor. Malalignment is almost a guaranteed aspect of any pregnancy, given:

1. its high prevalence in the general population to start with (80% plus), and
2. the increased chance of it occurring during the pregnancy itself, in part as a result of:
   a. the altered body biomechanics, with the increased lumbar lordosis to counter the weight of the fetus (Fig. 3.56),
   b. the increased lumbosacral stress, and
   c. the fetus exerting asymmetrical pressure on the 'inner' core muscles, the pelvic floor in particular, and the coccyx - initially by constantly moving about at different angles, later often by 'being stuck' in one position prior to triggering repeated spasms while negotiating and dilating the narrow birth canal at the time of the actual delivery.

Malalignment can become a major stress factor around the time of delivery, one that often is not diagnosed or treated post-partum, usually just ignored with the shift of attention: initially to any soft tissue trauma (tears, surgery) and then to the increasing demands of the newborn. However, while the soft tissues usually heal, chances are that there will be a persistent malalignment problem – if that is not diagnosed and treated right there and then, it can become responsible for symptoms of ongoing groin, back and/or coccygeal pain reported months or sometimes years later, if at all. If physiotherapy treatment is instituted, it is likely to be limited to the 'standard' approach, given that exposure to manual therapy is not usually part of the basic training course for qualification as a physiotherapist. In Canada, for example, only 20-25% have subsequently persued a structured post-graduate training course to subspecialize in the diagnosis and treatment of alignment-related disorders. The fact that symptoms can often be dated back to this period of the patient's life, yet usually still respond to realignment and a subsequent course of treatment that addresses the complications typically seen with malalignment, would be in keeping with this assumption. The subject continues to be studied extensively as part of the 'PPGP' (Mens et al. 1992; Östgaard 1998, 2007; Hungerford et al. 2007).

Coccydynia: diagnosis and treatment

Selby (1992: 4) described radiation of pain from the coccyx as follows:

spinal pain due to coccyx strain and hypertonicity of the pelvic floor is commonly felt in the mid to low sacral area referring outward toward the greater trochanter unilaterally or bilaterally (resembling trochanteric bursitis) and not infrequently down the posterior thigh

He also documented cases of chronic groin and anterior thigh pain that completely resolved following mobilization of the coccyx. Symptoms were typically provoked by sitting in soft chairs and by prolonged standing and repetitive activities such as stair-climbing that 'demand effort from the pelvic floor muscles to contract in order to stabilize the pelvis and thus are potentially provocative' (1992: 4).

In this regard, Barker & Briggs (1999: 225) pointed out that gluteus maximus has tendonous attachments to the sacrococcygeal capsule, and that if one could reproduce the pelvic floor pain with resisted hip extension (e.g. stair-climbing) it was 'indicative of coccyx dysfunction due to that relationship'.

Increased pelvic floor tension, in addition to causing localized or referred pain, must be considered as a possible cause of a general decrease in vitality or even a 'chronic fatigue syndrome' that has frequently been noted in these patients (Barral & Mercier 1988; Selby 1992; Upledger & Vredevoogd 1983).

Diagnostic and treatment approach

A simple approach to assessment proposed by Selby is as following:

1. an initial evaluation of the gross range of motion of the whole spine, of sacroiliac mobility (using the

kinetic rotational or Gillet test; Figs 2.121-2.125) and of the spinal dural system for irritability (using manoeuvres like Maitland's 'slump' test; Fig. 3.75)
2. the coccyx is then palpated to note its anterior/posterior angulation, any deviation from the midline, tenderness and thickening or hypertrophy of the soft tissue inserting into it; it may be possible to carry out the palpation and subsequent steps through the clothing [Author's comment: this decision is largely based on the individual therapist's preference and local standards of acceptability]
3. with the patient in standing or side-lying, the edges of the coccyx are then briefly massaged, noting its flexibility and end-feel while attempting to release any tension in the soft tissue and to mobilize the joint gently; alternatively, sustained pressure can be applied 'deeply' on the lateral margins of the coccyx
4. the range of motion of the back and neck is then immediately re-evaluated, as is the 'slump' test (if it was positive). [Author's comment: an initial ASLR and subsequently as part of the re-evaluation might also be appropriate]

Selby (1992: 5) also noted that:

> *coccydynia and abnormal tonicity of the pelvic floor is almost always associated with loss of lumbosacral extension, unilateral or bilateral side-bending and sometimes loss of flexion*

After rubbing the margins of the coccyx deeply, there may be a surprising resolution of these restrictions. Selby felt that mobilization of the sacrococcygeal joint and the surrounding soft tissues 'frees up sacral extension' so that the sacral base can once again tip anteriorly (which is the physiological movement of the sacrum that occurs with lumbar extension; see 'nutation', Fig. 2.18C). He postulated that these effects may come about as a result of influencing inhibitory reflexes mediated by the Golgi tendon organs, proprioceptive changes resulting from mobilization of the sacrococcygeal joint and possibly also a reflex decrease of tone in the iliopsoas and piriformis muscles (see Chs 2, 4, 8).

Other treatment approaches for coccygeal involvement include:

1. Maigne & Chatellier (2001) advocated 3 manual therapy techniques
   a. manipulation of the coccyx
      - consists of using a finger in the rectum to mobilize the joints and stretch the attached muscles and ligaments
   b. massage of the pelvic floor
      i. initially described by Thiele in 1937
      ii. primarily using a finger in the rectum to massage the levator ani and piriformis muscle (Fig. 2.53B)
   c. mild stretch of the levator ani and external sphincter, without moving the coccyx
2. Injection

   With the patient in side-lying and hips flexed, coccygeal discography is carried out under fluoroscopy at the level that showed luxation or hypermobility radiologically and/or was tender to palpation. According to Maigne, these patients responded better to the intradiscal cortisone injection than those with a normal coccyx. A spicule may be injected directly. If there is a problem of instability due to luxation or hypermobility, other injection techniques may have to be considered; e.g. prolotherapy (see Ch. 7).
3. Surgical coccygectomy (see also Bilgic et al. 2010)

   Criteria for surgery are limited:
   a. the patient fails to respond to the above treatment approaches
   b. the coccygeal problem is primarily responsible for the failure to maintain any realignment achieved

In a pre- and post-operative study by Maigne (1996: 6-7; 2001)

1. 91% were 'better' by 4 to 8 months
2. development of a 'phantom limb syndrome' was one possible complication, in keeping with the fact that the surgery was indeed an 'amputation'

SUMMARY

A recognition of the common presentations of malalignment and the 'malalignment syndrome' is important in order to allow one to differentiate these from other specific medical problems. Clearly, the symptoms arising from malalignment and these other medical entities can overlap; it is not until realignment has been achieved that the true nature of any underlying problem may finally become apparent. Malalignment must itself always be considered as a possible unifying cause of the complaints with which the patient presents, especially when:

1. the symptoms and signs are consistent with those typically associated with malalignment
2. the examination and investigations fail to reveal one of these 'well-recognized' clinical conditions.

Chapter 5

Clinical correlations in sports

CHAPTER CONTENTS

DOI: 10.1016/B978-0-443-06929-1.00005-3

Back pain and a variety of injuries are complaints common to numerous sports. They are even more likely to be a problem in those athletes who present with malalignment and who:

1. overtrain and/or compete
2. engage in sports that involve repeated:
   a. lifting, extension or forward flexion, which increase the mechanical stresses on the lumbosacral region in particular (e.g. weight-lifting, tennis)
   b. extreme torsional stresses on the trunk and pelvic ring (e.g. golf, dance routines)
   c. landing on one leg after a routine or jumping from one leg to the other (e.g. figure skating, gymnastics, running)
   d. collisions or falls (e.g. hockey, basketball)

These athletes are more at risk of injury because of the malalignment. Eventual failure of the tissues and joints to adapt to the additional stress imposed by malalignment can result in microtears in muscles and ligaments, actual sprains or strains, stress fractures and other injuries.

Malalignment itself may occur secondary to:

1. insults of this type; in particular, strains, falls and fractures, also
2. repeated asymmetrical throws and torsional stresses (e.g. lacrosse, baseball, tennis).

Malalignment alters body biomechanics and, in addition to predisposing to injury, creates stresses that may hinder the athlete's ability to progress and do well in a given sport, prolong recovery time or even prevent full recovery. This chapter takes a closer look at the detrimental effects of malalignment on athletic activities. The first part discusses the clinical correlations relating to specific biomechanical changes, the second looks at the effect of malalignment on specific sports, and the third analyzes the biomechanical changes underlying some of the recurrent injuries seen when malalignment is present. The chapter concludes with considerations regarding:

1. whether failure to advance in some sports:
   a. is primarily a 'natural' process of elimination, or
   b. may, at times, actually be determined by the restrictions and the asymmetries imposed by the presence of malalignment (especially in sports that reward symmetry and alignment) and could, therefore, be preventable
2. the effect of malalignment on the validity of research that involves investigation of biomechanical aspects of certain sports and treatment techniques.

CLINICAL CORRELATIONS: SPECIFIC BIOMECHANICAL CHANGES

Clinical correlations associated with vertebral rotational displacement and pelvic malalignment relate primarily to stress patterns that result from limitations of ranges of motion, changes in muscle and ligament tension, and alterations of weight-bearing and leg length. Irritation of joint structures, soft tissues, and the peripheral nerves and autonomic nervous system, eventually can give rise to typical pain phenomena.

VERTEBRAL ROTATIONAL DISPLACEMENT

In the thoracic region, stress resulting from a vertebral displacement is also transmitted through the costovertebral and costotransverse joints to the ribs, and anteriorly to the sternocostal and costochondral junctions (Figs 2.94, 3.15, 3.16). Further rotation into the direction of the displacement is restricted, affecting the overall movement of the spine and predisposing to injury.

> The term 'vertebral rotational displacement' refers to excessive rotation of one or more vertebrae relative to those immediately above and below (see Ch. 2), which can result in increased stresses and strains on soft tissue structures, facet joints and discs at the level(s) involved.

Vertebral levels commonly involved

The general findings on examination at an affected level have been described in Ch. 2. Rotational displacement can affect any vertebra between the occiput and the sacrum but it does involve certain levels of the spine with increased frequency (see Ch. 3). Note is here made of some of these levels.

L4, L5 or both vertebrae

Though these are involved infrequently (affecting some 5% of those with recurrent pelvic malalignment), there are three major problems that can result with rotational displacement at these levels: pain, restriction of range of motion and secondary malalignment of the sacrum and the SI joints (Figs 2.52, 2.96). Instability of the lumbosacral area may be caused by the initial injury or develop subsequently with the stress arising from recurring vertebral rotational displacement.

Pain

Usually pain is severe and of acute onset, coincident with the displacement of one or both vertebra. It may be localized to the low back region but there may also be radiation to the buttocks or even referral to the lower extremities as a result of:

1. increased tension on soft tissue structures
   - involves primarily the paravertebral muscles, interspinous, supraspinous and other intervertebral ligaments and, at the L4/5 level, also the iliolumbar ligaments (Figs 2.4, 2.5, 2.52, 3.61B, 3.68, 7.40)
2. stresses on facet joints
   a. compression on the side contralateral to the direction of vertebral rotation, and
   b. distraction (opening) ipsilaterally (e.g. clockwise trunk rotation results in approximation of the left and separation of the right joint surfaces; Fig. 2.52B)
3. torquing of the annulus and the disc

Clockwise rotation of L5, for example, increases tension in the right iliolumbar as well as the supra- and interspinous ligaments, also multifidi and rotatores muscles, primarily from the L3 to S1 level (Figs 2.29, 2.52B, 3.68). It compresses the left and separates the right L5–S1 facet surfaces. Distraction or entrapment of the facet joint capsule, ligaments and the nerve fibres supplying these joints can account for localized pain and referred symptoms to the ipsilateral buttock and lower extremity as far down as the ankle (McCall et al. 1979; Mooney & Robertson 1976; Travell & Simons 1992).

Restriction of range of motion

> Vertebral rotational displacement is usually multidirectional, involving not only rotation in the transverse plane but a combination of either forward flexion (F) or extension (E), the rotation (R) around the vertical axis and side-flexion (S): the 'FRS' or 'ERS' presentation, respectively.

The 'FRS' and 'ERS' patterns result in a restriction of further movement into the directions indicated. L1–L4, for example, would normally rotate into a convexity; therefore, rotation would be counter-clockwise into a left (Figs 2.42, 4.6, 4.26, 4.33) and clockwise into a right convexity (Fig. 2.96A). Superimposing a clockwise rotational displacement of L4 on a pre-existing right convexity will accentuate the already existing forward flexion (or extension), rotation and right side-flexion, limiting any further movement of L4 into all of these directions. Counterclockwise displacement of L4 would limit further movement into the opposite directions (Fig. 2.96B).

1. Assuming that the lumbar spine is forward flexed and L1-L4 have rotated clockwise into a right lumbar convexity (Fig. 2.96A):
   - L1-4 would be in an FRS (forward flexed, right rotated, left side-flexed) position and further movement into these directions would be limited
2. if L4 now rotated to the left, its range of rotation into the opposite (left) FRS directions may be slightly increased
3. if L4 rotated even further to the right with an excessive force, it could be literally 'jammed' into a right FRS position.

Malalignment of the SI joints

A clockwise rotation of L4 or L5 exerts a rotational force on the innominates (anterior on the left and posterior on the right) because the simultaneous rotation of the transverse process - forward on the left, backward on the right - displaces the iliolumbar ligament origins away from their insertions and increases tension in these ligaments on both sides (Fig. 2.52A). There is also the torsional effect on the sacrum transmitted through the compressed left facet joint (Fig. 2.52B) and the L5-S1 disc. Reactive spasm in the adjacent quadratus lumborum and psoas can cause a recurrent ipsilateral 'upslip' (Fig. 2.62). Always remember that in the case of recurrent 'rotational malalignment' or an 'upslip', two common causes to consider (especially when there is excessive pain, usually acute in onset) are:

1. a failure to correct L4 and/or L5 vertebral rotational displacement, and
2. an actual instability of L4/L5, L5/S1, or both levels.

Thoracolumbar junction: T11, T12 and L1

Degenerative changes at the thoracolumbar junction are common in sports that call for repeated high spinal loading, high-velocity hyperflexion and hyperextension, and rotary motion (d'Hemecourt & Micheli 1997); in particular, gymnastics, ballet, wrestling, diving, waterski-jumping, and the bowling action of cricket, with gymnastics consistently receiving most mention (Kesson & Atkins 1999).

Rotational displacement at this junction typically involves T12 and/or L1, less often T11. These vertebrae may be involved in isolation or in combination; for example, the commonly noted 'T12 right and L1 left' rotation. In addition to the increased stress on facet joints, discs and ligaments, often with reactive muscle spasm localizing to the thoracolumbar region, rotational displacement at these levels may be complicated by the presence of an 'upslip' and/or 'rotational malalignment' of the pelvis, with:

1. pelvic obliquity and the compensatory scoliosis that creates stress points at the sites of reversal: the lumbosacral, thoracolumbar and cervicothoracic junctions
2. 'facilitation' of the left quadratus lumborum muscle; this increase in tension would act directly on the upper origins of this muscle from the L1 transverse process and may help explain the frequently seen L1 left vertebral rotation
3. 'thoracolumbar syndrome' (see Ch. 4; Figs 4.20-4.23)
4. rotational stresses on the attaching rib(s) and thoracic diaphragm

A rotational displacement of T11 and/or T12 results in increased stress on their costovertebral and costotransverse articulations. The associated torquing increases the stress on the anterior articulation of the 11th rib at the costochondral junction and its continuation as the costal cartilage. Pain can usually be provoked by applying pressure anywhere along the affected rib(s), and localized by direct pressure on the tender anterior and/or posterior articulation(s). Torsion of the lower ribs can also present as discomfort and even spasm of the attaching diaphragm. Any of these structures may become symptomatic, sometimes presenting as 'chest' or 'abdominal' pain and leading to extensive investigations to rule out a cardiac, respiratory or gastrointestinal problem (see Ch 4).

The T4 and T5 level

A rotational displacement of one or both vertebrae at these levels is a frequent occurrence and may reflect the fact that:

1. reversal of the curvature of the thoracic segment, which helps to ensure that the head ends up in the midline, may start as low as T4 or T5 (Fig. 2.91B)
2. forces normally associated with upper extremity activities intersect at this level; unopposed or unequal forces predispose to displacement of one or both vertebrae through muscle action (e.g. different muscles on opposite sides that can created a torsional component when acting together; unopposed unilateral rhomboid action because of weakness of its partner or a difference in tone, with 'facilitation' on one side and 'inhibition' on the other):
    a. asymmetrical throwing; e.g. bowling, curling or track and field events that involve throwing an object with one arm (Figs 3.18, 3.51)
    b. lifting a weight with one arm at a time
    c. asymmetrical resisted manoeuvres; e.g. canoeing (Fig. 5.1)
    d. sudden rotational forces on the trunk, especially when the pelvis is fixed, as in sitting or lying; e.g. collisions with players and objects; wrestling (Fig. 5.35).

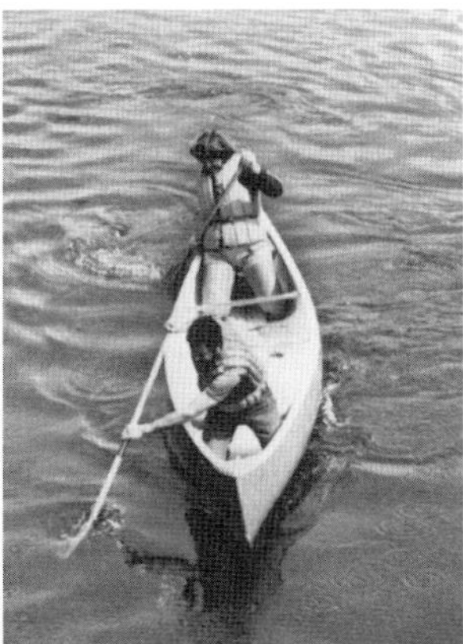

Fig. 5.1 Canoeing in the kneeling, half-squatting position: torquing through the trunk, pelvis and even legs to carry out a 'stern pry and bow cross-draw' manoeuvre. *(Courtesy of Harrison 1981.)*

> The spinous processes will deviate from the midline in a direction opposite to that of the vertebral body rotation. As a result, the otherwise uniform curve formed by the thoracic spinous processes, convex to right or left, will be interrupted at the level of the deviated spinous process.

The associated pain is commonly felt in the interscapular area and/or under one or both scapulae. Pain from these sites can also be referred directly through the thorax to the anterior chest region, simulating angina (see Ch. 4). Other referred pain patterns to the shoulder girdles were discussed in Ch. 2 (Figs 3.12, 4.8). The athlete may localize the discomfort mainly to an area of increased tension and tenderness, or actual localized spasm. These changes may be palpable within the immediately adjacent rhomboid, mid-trapezius and paravertebral musculature (sometimes just on one side), or more laterally (e.g. subscapularis, infraspinatus, teres minor). The abnormal tension may simply reflect an increase in distance between the origin and insertion of these muscles. For example, a right deviation of the T4 spinous process, away from the left scapula, will increase tension in the attaching left rhomboid and mid-trapezius muscles. Alternately, the vertebral rotation may be secondary to an increase in tension with spasm, sprain or other injury affecting right rhomboid, pulling T4 to the right. Pain from T4/T5 can also trigger a reflex contraction of adjacent muscles in an attempt to splint this site. One is usually looking at a combination of factors (see Ch. 3). The area may, however, remain asymptomatic. Just as an imbalance in muscle tension can cause rotation of a vertebra in the interscapular region, specific muscles can be harnessed to rotate that vertebra back in line (see Ch. 7: 'using rhomboid to effect realignment of T3'; Fig. 2.97).

On examination, pain may be evoked with posterior-to-anterior and/or rotatory pressure to the spinous process of the vertebra, possibly also to the one above and below. There may be discomfort with pressure applied to the soft tissues within the immediate vicinity. As in tests carried out for thoracolumbar syndrome, the findings may suggest an irritation of specific facet joints (Fig. 4.20). Trigger points are common in the muscles and ligaments at these levels and the adjacent posterior shoulder girdle regions. In addition, upper extremity ranges of motion may be restricted if they exert a rotational force on a tight, affected segment of the thoracic spine and provoke pain.

The 'T3' or 'T4' syndrome

As initially described by Maitland (1977), this refers to a symptom complex caused by the rotation of one or more vertebrae between T2 and T7, with T3 or T4 being most commonly involved. The symptoms are vague and widespread, with a report of pain and paraesthesias in the upper limbs and/or head pain (initially described as a dull aching or pressure feeling in an 'all-over' distribution). Symptoms may occur as a result of referral through the autonomic nervous system, originating from the upper thoracic region. In the series of 90 patients with T4 syndrome published by McGuckin in 1986, all had involvement of the upper extremity, either uni- or bilaterally, with a glove-like distribution of paraesthesias: fingers up to the wrist(s), or to the forearm, elbow or an even more proximal level (Fig. 4.9).

Fraser (1993) described a 'T3 syndrome' following trauma (e.g. a fall onto the shoulder or direct trauma to the anterior rib region). Symptoms may include paraesthesias, pain, vasomotor changes, a loss of sensation, the swelling of an extremity, anterior chest wall and/or axillary pain, a weakness of grip and difficulty breathing. The dramatic results achieved with manipulation to restore joint play at T3, the T3 costotransverse junction and sometimes also T2 and T4 led Fraser to propose that:

1. the correction 'affects the vaso-motor system probably via the sympathetic ganglion at T-2' (1993: 5)
2. it may be worth considering injection of local anaesthetic into this ganglion.

Examination and diagnostic techniques

Palpation of the paraspinal muscles in the vicinity of the displaced vertebra(e) may reveal tenderness and increased tension, or even muscle that has become hard and unyielding with recurrent spasm and now feels like a piece of rope running alongside the spinous processes on one or both sides. Chronicity of the problem can result in an increase in fibrous content, with the feeling of crepitus on palpation. The facet joints can be stressed:

1. non-specifically on side-flexion, back extension alone, and back extension combined with rotation to the right or left

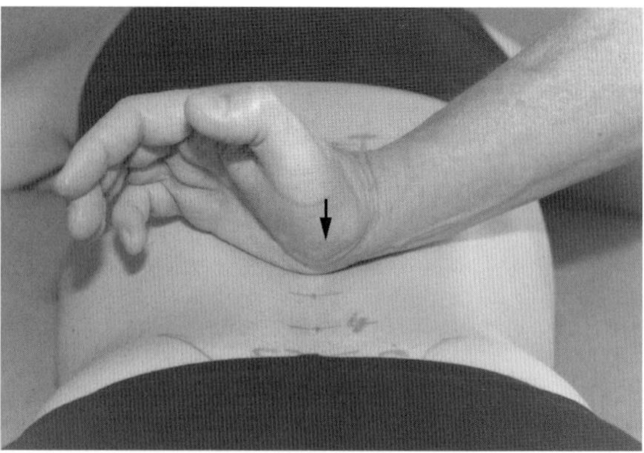

Fig. 5.2 Posteroanterior compression of individual spinous processes using the heel of the hand (pisiform bone).

2. more specifically, by applying a translatory rotational (Fig. 4.20A) or direct forces to individual spinous processes (Figs 4.20B, 5.2).

> In the case of vertebral rotational displacement, applying a further rotational force will reveal a restriction into the direction of the displacement and may provoke pain.

Posteroanterior translation or 'glide' in the sagittal plane may be similarly decreased or abolished, making the affected level(s) feel 'stiff' and unyielding. These changes are usually most easily appreciated in the region of T12–L1, where the reversal of the lumbar and thoracic curves in the sagittal and coronal planes itself already results in a restriction of joint play, even in the absence of any superimposed rotational displacement of one or both vertebrae (Fig. 3.14C). The levels adjacent to a site of such excessive rotation sometimes also lack 'give' and feel stiff; whereas hypermobility may be evident at sites immediately adjacent or some distance away, where the spine is attempting to compensate for this restriction of movement or has been stressed to the point that actual ligament laxity or joint degeneration has occurred.

Rib involvement can be assessed by examination for side-to-side asymmetry and by stressing the anterior and posterior rib attachments, either directly or by selectively springing the individual ribs along their length (Figs 2.93, 2.94). Diagnostic nerve root blocks can be helpful if involvement of posterior root or intercostal nerve fibres is suspected. Selective blocks of the rib articulations - costochondral, costotransverse and costovertebral - may also help to localize the origin of the pain (see Chs 3, 4, 7 and Figs 3.15, 3.16).

Correlation to sports: vertebral rotational displacement

Rotational displacement of a vertebra is most likely to become symptomatic with sports that require repeated flexion, extension, rotation or combined motions of the spine. These include, in particular, weight-lifting, court sports, sports involving a swinging motion (e.g. golf, baseball, lacrosse, ice hockey), rowing sports, canoeing, kayaking, throwing events and martial arts. Whether or not such a displacement actually becomes a problem depends on several factors (Box 5.1).

Sports requiring rotation of the trunk while standing

The orientation of the lumbar facet joints in a near-sagittal direction allows for little rotation of the lumbar vertebrae around the vertical axis in the transverse plane. When standing, most of the movement on trunk rotation in sports such as golf, baseball and hockey occurs through the thoracic segment and, if permitted, the cervical spine. Rotation of the trunk results in stress especially through the thoracolumbar and cervicothoracic junctions. There is some simultaneous rotation of the lower extremities possible; whereas the pelvic ring and lumbar segment rotate more or less as one unit. Stress through the lumbosacral junction is maximal once all the rotation of the thoracic segment, pelvis and lower extremities has occurred and the few degrees of rotation possible in the lumbar spine segment levels above L5 (i.e. L1-L4) have been exhausted.

Sports requiring rotation of the trunk while sitting

The pelvis is now fixed, rotation again occurring primarily through the thoracic segment and at the thoracolumbar junction. Once no further rotation is possible through these levels, the lumbar spine will start to rotate as one segment. Rotation, however, is limited and quickly results in increased stress on the lumbosacral junction. This athlete is, therefore, more likely to develop symptoms from the mid- (thoracolumbar) and low back (lumbosacral) regions with activities such as kayaking, yet may have no problem with asymmetrical paddling. For example, when canoeing in the kneeling position, the rotational stress can be distributed along the length of the spine, the pelvic region and even partly through the lower extremities (Fig. 5.1).

LIMITATION OF SPORTS PERFORMANCE BY THE COMMON PRESENTATIONS OF MALALIGNMENT

The changes associated with the three common presentations of pelvic malalignment may limit sports performance by:

1. interfering with the desired or required range of motion
    a. limiting range in a direction specifically needed for a certain sport (e.g. reaching outward and back to catch a ball; trunk rotation in kayaking, golfing; Figs 3.5, 3.49)

BOX 5.1 Factors that influence whether vertebral rotational displacement becomes a problem

1. Restrictions at the level of the spine affected are superimposed on the restrictions already caused by the normal orientation of the facet joints (thoracic more flat or horizontal, limiting flexion and extension; lumbar aligned more in the sagittal plane, limiting rotation; Fig. 3.9)
2. The degree of rotational displacement determines the degree of:
    a. excessive facet joint compression or distraction (Fig. 2.52)
    b. stress on the discs and rib joints (Fig. 2.94)
    c. stress on any soft tissues connecting these structures (Fig. 3.68)
3. The particular sport places further stresses on the level at which the displacement has occurred. Excessive rotation of a lumbar or thoracic vertebra, for example, does not necessarily pose a problem with repetitive, symmetrical flexion/extension activities such as sculling or using a rowing machine. The deciding factor here would be whether the degree of extension required is such that it causes a further approximation on the side on which the surfaces have already been brought closer together, to the point of actually provoking pain.
4. The athletic activity puts an additional rotational stress through the level(s) affected (e.g. court sports or kayaking); this is especially true for the lumbar segment, where the minimal rotation normally available may already have been reduced to a critical point on one side by the rotational displacement.

b. limiting combined trunk, pelvic and limb ranges of motion, which could create problems especially in those sports which require all parts of the body to be able to move through a full range of motion at any time, sometimes at high speed (e.g. court sports, lacrosse, white water kayaking)
2. provoking discomfort or pain
3. causing problems with muscle weakness and fatigue
4. altering weight-bearing, balance and controlled progression (ice skating, dancing/ballet)
5. disturbing symmetry, posture and style (synchronized swimming, competitive weight-lifting).

Appendix 10 notes the changes that can occur and some of the sports affected as a result.

CLINICAL CORRELATIONS: SPECIFIC SPORTS

Specific sports create specific demands, and malalignment can affect the ability to meet these demands, often in a predictable manner. We are sometimes too quick to blame hand and foot preference, muscle tightness or weakness in an attempt to explain why one athlete is unable to change his or her style and repeatedly carries out a manoeuvre in the same way, or why another athlete has suffered a specific injury (especially if it is recurrent). A knowledge of the biomechanical changes and limitations imposed by the malalignment may allow for a more rational explanation. Appendix 11 details the clinical correlations related to some specific sports and Appendix 5 lists those specific to running.

COURT, RACQUET AND STICK SPORTS

A specific sport may appear to have been singled out as carrying an increased risk for a certain type of injury but the injuries outlined below are common to a number of these sports, and the mechanisms of injury often similar. Malalignment may well be a unifying factor.

Excessive rotation into a pelvic or thoracic restriction

Typical here is the rotation of the trunk required in tennis or golf (see below). Take the example of a right-handed tennis player with 'right anterior, left posterior' innominate rotation and a lumbar segment convex to left (Fig. 2.42). When he or she attempts a right backhand with both feet fixed to the ground (Fig. 5.3), the initial left rotation is restricted:

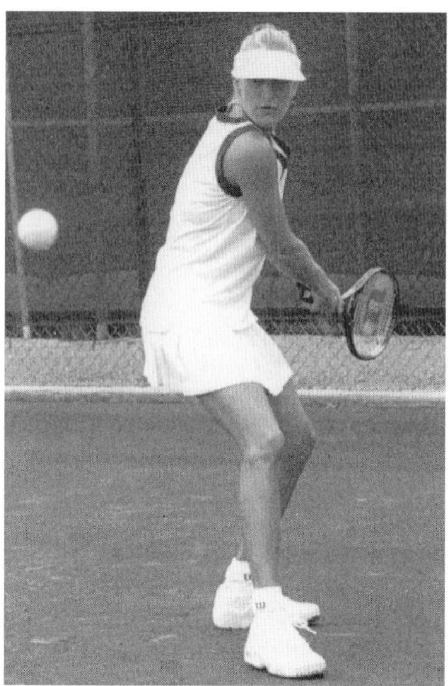

Fig. 5.3 A right backhand in tennis: the feet are relatively fixed to the ground and the trunk is rotated counterclockwise in preparation for hitting the oncoming ball. *(Courtesy of Schwartz & Dazet 1998.)*

1. through the lumbar segment, by the fact that the vertebrae have already rotated partly to the left, into the convexity (Fig. 2.42)
2. through the pelvic unit around the vertical axis in the transverse plane (Fig. 3.5C)
3. through the legs, especially by a limitation of further left internal, right external rotation, as these are already partially rotated in these directions

The combined effect is to restrict rotation through the lumbar spine and below. The rotational component has to occur, in large part, through the thoracolumbar junction and thoracic spine. Reaching backward in preparation for the backhand further increases the possibility of causing an injury to any one of these regions. This manoeuvre, which requires a counterclockwise rotation, again occurs primarily through the trunk when the feet are fixed. The player may be able to compensate by increasing rotation through the knees but is at increased risk of suffering an acute knee injury and acceleration of wear and tear because the counterclockwise rotation augments the tendency toward:

1. right pronation and knee valgus angulation
   - with internal rotation of the tibia relative to the externally-rotating femur, increased stress on the soft tissue structures (e.g. the medial collateral ligament) and increased pressure within the lateral joint compartment (Figs 3.37, 3.81B, 3.82)
2. left supination and knee varus angulation
   - with external rotation of the tibia relative to the internally-rotating femur, increased stress particularly on the lateral collateral ligament and increased pressure within the medial joint compartment.

Actually hitting the ball involves a clockwise thoracic rotation which is suddenly slowed, arrested, or even forced counterclockwise as the racquet contacts the ball. If any simultaneous clockwise rotation of the pelvis and lower extremities continues, there results a torsional stress, maximal through the already compromised thoracolumbar junction. In addition, at contact the ball may force the wrist into flexion and/or there is an acute contraction of the right wrist extensors in an attempt to counter any wrist flexion; both manoeuvres exert a jarring force on the origin that can result in a typical lateral epicondylitis or 'tennis elbow'.

A lay-up in basketball requires a maximum range of trunk and pelvic rotation. Limitations associated with malalignment may make it more difficult to approach the basket from one direction and may, in fact, be responsible for a preference to execute a lay-up from left or right, clockwise or counterclockwise. The risk of injury is increased should circumstances such as the proximity of other players or a blocking of the preferred approach force the player into choosing a different angle or rotating into an already restricted direction in order to complete the lay-up.

Excessive movement into a restricted hip range of motion

'Right anterior, left posterior' innominate rotation results in a limitation of right hip flexion and internal rotation, left hip extension and external rotation (Figs 3.71–3.75). There is, therefore, an increased risk that a quick forward movement of one leg or backward of the other may exceed the available hip flexion or extension range of motion, respectively. In the example given, there would be an increased risk in a lunge with the right leg leading and the left receding (Fig. 5.10C). Similarly, rotation of the body to the right or left over a planted, relatively 'fixed', foot may exceed, respectively, the remaining external or internal rotation available for that extremity, possibly to the point of 'engaging' the anatomical barrier and causing injury (Figs 3.78-3.80, 5.14B,C).

Thoraco-abdominal injuries

Injuries involving rectus abdominis, transversus abdominis and external and internal abdominal oblique muscles have been seen to occur more often in tennis players than in those playing handball and racquetball. Lehmann (1988) may well have been right in attributing these injuries to the increased need for overhead activity in tennis. Malalignment can, however, also increase the chance of suffering a sprain or strain of these 'inner' and 'outer' core muscles with the sudden rotational, reaching and extension movements characteristic of some of these sports (Figs 5.4A,B,C).

> Injury is especially likely if such movement occurs at a time when that muscle is already shortened by adaptive contracture and/or an increase in tone (e.g. as occurs with 'facilitation' and in reaction to pain or instability caused by the malalignment).

Athletes presenting with malalignment sometimes complain of pain in the lateral flank and abdominal region on one or both sides. Problems relating to transversus abdominis or the external or internal obliques can cause pain in these generalized areas, given the overlapping of these muscles and their role as part of the anterior abdominal slings. Tenderness may localize to their origins from the ribs, the main muscle bulk itself or the insertions onto the innominates (Figs 2.31B, 2.32, 2.33).

External abdominal obliques

Most frequently injured, uni- or bilaterally, are the external abdominal obliques (Fig. 2.32) which:

1. originate from the posterolateral aspect of the lower eight ribs and run forward and downward, to

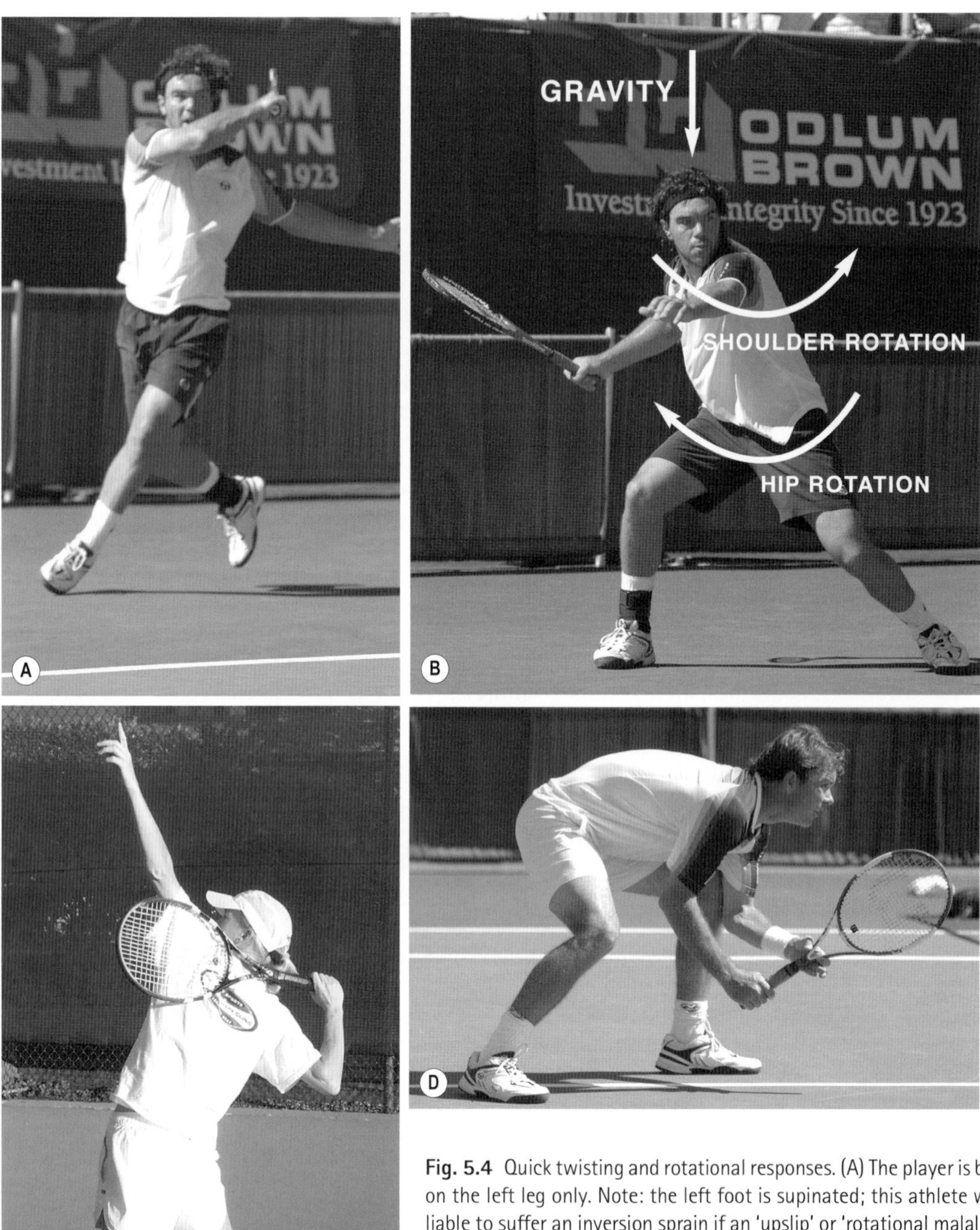

Fig. 5.4 Quick twisting and rotational responses. (A) The player is bearing weight on the left leg only. Note: the left foot is supinated; this athlete would be more liable to suffer an inversion sprain if an 'upslip' or 'rotational malalignment' were present, with the associated shift in weight-bearing toward left supination and functional weakness in left peroneus longus (see Fig. 3.37). (B) Torsional stresses increase risk of injury to soft tissues and joints in thoracic and lumbar spine regions in particular. (C) Overhead serve, a combination of back hyperextention and trunk rotation, results in torsional and 'jamming' (compressive) forces on the back. (D) The forward-flexed posture, common to tennis and a number of other competitive sports, predisposes to malalignment when combined with trunk rotation and side-flexion. *(Courtesy of Petersen & Nittinger 2006.)*

2. insert into the iliac crest and, along with the inferior segment of transversus abdominis and lateral rectus abdominis
3. also insert into the iliohypogastric and ilioinguinal region and onto the lateral aspect of the superior pubic ramus

Tension in the right external muscle is increased by 'right anterior' innominate rotation, and by clockwise trunk and counterclockwise pelvic rotation around the vertical axis, also 'left outflare/right inflare'. Tension increases simultaneously in other abdominal muscles, such as transversus abdominis and rectus abdominis, which are interlinked with the external obliques (Fig. 2.39).

Internal oblique

This muscle originates from the thoracodorsal fascia and anterior iliac crest, inserting into ribs 9-12, through the aponeurosis into the linea alba and to the superior pubic ramus and pectineal line. In the example given above for the effect of 'right anterior' rotation on the right external oblique (Fig. 2.32), tension is especially likely to increase in the contralateral (left) internal oblique (Fig. 2.33) if there is a compensatory 'posterior' rotation of the left innominate, also with a 'left outflare'.

Transversus abdominis

Tension will increase in the ipsilateral transversus abdominis (Fig. 2.31). This muscle originates from the lateral inguinal ligament, iliac crest, thoracodorsal fascia and cartilages of the lower ribs, to insert into the linea alba, the superior pubic ramus and the pectineal line.

Rectus abdominis

'Anterior' innominate rotation increases tension in the ipsilateral half of rectus abdominis by separating its origin and insertion (Fig. 2.31B). As indicated above, transversus abdominis and the external and internal obliques blend with rectus abdominis and are, therefore, also affected indirectly by tension changes in this muscle.

Tension in all four muscle groups is further increased by reaching and extension movements (e.g. serving in tennis, bowling in cricket, going up for a spike in volleyball). Injury is more likely when rotation, reaching and extension movements occur at a time when these muscles and their tendons are already under increased tension because of pre-existing malalignment (Figs 3.51, 5.4)

Low back pain

Marks et al. (1988) stated that the four strokes used in racquet sports - forehand and backhand ground strokes, the overhead serve and the volley - all put the back at risk. The overhead serve in tennis, for example, is a combined action of rotation and hyperextension of the back (Fig. 5.4B). Rotation occurs through the lower extremities, pelvis and primarily thoracic segment of the spine. Any malalignment-related restriction of movement increases the stress on sites that are already attempting to compensate.

Field hockey deserves special mention here because of the prevalence of low back pain. Part of the problem stems from the constant need to lean or actually bend forward with the trunk while handling and reaching with what, for many of the players, amounts to a relatively short stick. In addition, the trunk is repeatedly rotated clockwise and counterclockwise when attempting to hit the ball from the left or right, respectively. If this manoeuvre is carried out while moving forward, the ability of the pelvis to rotate into the side of the leading leg is at times restricted so that the legs and trunk have to compensate, further increasing the rotational stress (especially on the thoracic spine).

Players may already be aware of a mechanical restriction on wind-up or follow-through. The pelvic restriction is more likely to be to the left, partly because of:

1. restriction of further internal rotation of the left leg and
2. the associated restriction of pelvic rotation around the vertical axis in the transverse plane to that side, especially when both feet are on the ground (Fig. 3.5C).

Pelvic restriction can only increase the stress on the thoracic spine, whose ability to rotate to one side or the other may be further decreased by the rotational displacement of any individual thoracic vertebrae (Fig. 3.49B). It should be remembered that thoracolumbar dysfunction, rather than causing mid-back pain, may be felt as low back pain and also as lateral hip/buttock pain (e.g. as in the 'thoracolumbar syndrome' with cutaneous nerve involvement; Fig. 4.23A,B).

Shoulder injuries

Malalignment impairs both shoulder stability and ranges of motion (Fig. 3.17), partly as a result of the:

1. compensatory scoliosis, so the glenoid socket faces downward on the concave and upward on the convex side of the thorax (Figs 2.90, 2.120C)
2. trunk rotation around the vertical axis (increasing the tendency to shoulder protraction on one side and retraction on the other (Chs 3,6)

Those with an 'upslip' or one of the 'more common' rotational patterns typically show an increase in right external, left internal rotation of the gleno-humeral joint (Fig. 3.17A).

When a player is serving overhead or hitting an overhead volley, the shoulder is initially in a position of maximum external rotation, and the anterior capsule, ligaments and internal rotators are maximally stretched. In someone with malalignment, using the right arm to serve, the increased right external rotation range seen with the malalignment may allow the player to develop more force when serving but:

1. the increased external rotation puts these anterior tissues under even more strain, at the risk of stretching and eventual anterior gleno-humeral joint laxity (Fig. 4.7)
2. a forceful swing-through is more likely to come to an abrupt halt by the limitation of internal rotation on the right side if he or she tries to go through the full ROM (Fig. 3.17A)
3. to avoid stressing these anterior tissues, especially if there is already some discomfort, the player may avoid using the extra external rotation available on the right side and instead compensate by increasing rotation and extension of the spine to 'wind-up' for the throw, at the risk of precipitating or aggravating back pain (Fig. 3.18).

In contrast, external rotation will be decreased on the left side and may not allow the player who serves with the left arm to develop as good a force as would be possible when in alignment. Again, the player may try to compensate by increasing spine extension and/or rotation to improve arm external rotation, at the risk of precipitating or aggravating pain especially in the upper back and thoracic spine region.

Groin strain

Balduini (1988: 352) described two mechanisms that can result in groin strain in tennis players, both resulting from an attempt by the player to stop lateral progression.

1. One tends to occur on clay surfaces and involves the leading foot sliding outward. A loss of traction can result in the slide ending up as a split, in which case the adductors, and less often the iliopsoas, can be strained or the lesser trochanter avulsed (Figs 3.50, 5.21)
2. The other mechanism occurs by 'posting' the leading foot outward on a surface where the footing is secure, such as a synthetic court. In other words, lateral movement is abruptly stopped. Here 'the efforts of the adductors and hip flexors are opposed by lateral momentum, and contraction results in muscle tearing rather than the anticipated deceleration'.

The majority of those with the 'right anterior, left posterior' rotational pattern present with a restriction of both left hip adduction and abduction range (see also Ch. 6). Tension is typically increased in:

1. the left hip abductors and tensor fascia lata/iliotibial band (TFL/ITB) complex, through 'facilitation' (Figs 3.41, 3.44)
2. the iliacus component of iliopsoas (Figs 2.46B,C, 2.59, 3.42, 4.2B), especially when 'posterior' innominate rotation is present (which it is more often on the left side; see Ch. 2)
3. iliopsoas as a unit, sometimes unilaterally in an attempt to stabilize an SI joint or decrease pain
4. psoas, as a result of 'facilitation' linked to T12, L1 or L2 vertebral rotational displacement.

The combined effect of these restrictions predisposes to injury of the hip adductors, as well as pectineus and the individual components of iliopsoas (Figs 2.62, 4.2. 4.14), with either a lateral 'slide' or 'posting'. Forced adduction can cause pain by compressing these same structures, while putting a tight gluteal/TFL/ITB complex at risk of sprain or strain (Figs 3.41, 3.44Aiii, 5.17).

Reference should also be made at this point to the occurrence of a painful hemipubic bone in court sports as a result of irritation of the anterior cutaneous branches in association with T12/L1 rotational displacement and the 'thoracolumbar syndrome' (Fig. 4.23A2,B2; Appendix 9). These branches are vulnerable especially in those playing tennis or soccer (Maigne 1995). Certainly, repeated trunk hyperextension and reaching manoeuvres (e.g. serving), as well as excessive or repetitive hip extension stressing the back, will put the anterior branches under stretch while simultaneously narrowing the intervertebral foraminal outlets as the player leans backward.

Knee injury

Typical alterations of knee biomechanics relating to malalignment, and predisposing to acute injury or accelerated wear and tear, have been discussed above under 'Excessive rotation into a pelvic or thoracic restriction' and Ch. 3 (Figs 3.37, 3.81, 3.82).

Ankle sprains

The 'more common' rotational patterns and an 'upslip' predispose to various types of ankle sprain (Box 5.2 and see Ch. 3).

BOX 5.2 Malalignment predisposes to ankle sprains

In someone with an 'upslip' or one of the 'more common' patterns of 'rotational malalignment':

1. *left ankle inversion sprains*: caused by the tendency to supination and lateral weight-bearing, weakness of the peroneal muscles and pre-positioning by internal rotation of the left lower extremity
2. *right ankle inversion sprains*: occur less frequently and are probably attributable in some cases to the increase in right varus angulation observed when non-weight-bearing (Fig. 3.26); as the lateral aspect of the right foot hits the ground at this more acute angle, there is a momentary instability of the foot that, literally, can cause it to 'fall outward' (instead of rolling into eversion and forward into pronation, as would be usual)
3. *right ankle eversion sprains*: caused by the tendency to pronation and medial weight-bearing, weakness of the ankle invertors, and pre-positioning by external rotation of the right lower extremity

Collision with a fixture or opponent

As a result of a collision, parts of the body may be involuntarily rotated into one of the restrictions of range of motion imposed by the malalignment, 'jamming' a facet or SI joint or actually exceeding the anatomical barrier earlier to the point of causing soft tissue and joint injury (Fig. 2.51B).

Recurrence or aggravation of malalignment

Torsional sports are among the worst that athletes presenting with malalignment could engage in while symptomatic or undergoing treatment.

The activities are already asymmetrical, with rotational components, and often also involve repeatedly shifting weight-bearing or jumping from one leg onto the other. Carrying out manoeuvres in a flexed position increases the risk of imbalance (Figs 5.3, 5.4D). Going out of alignment only augments all these asymmetries and any imbalances. Because of the competitive element of a game, movements often occur almost reflexly as the athlete throws all caution to the wind, something which can only add to the risk of sustaining an injury or causing the recurrence or aggravation of an existing malalignment problem.

CURLING

The curler delivering the 'rock' gathers enough momentum to slide about ten meters from the 'near hack' line at the back to finally release the rock at the 'near hog' line. The position assumed for the slide is similar to a 'lunge' (Fig.7.18B). Throwing with the right arm, he or she:

1. weight-bears and slides on the left foot, with the hip and knee fully flexed
2. trails the right leg, with the hip in partial extension and the leg sliding along the top of the ice
3. leans the trunk forward some 20 to 30 degrees but keeps the head level, eyes focused on the target ahead

Basically, the player is in a 'left leg forward' lunge position. Assuming the presence of a:

1. 'right anterior, left posterior' innominate rotation
   a. right side: hip extension is increased (posteroinferior acetabular rim moved upward;

iliopsoas and rectus femoris relaxed; hamstrings 'facilitated'; pelvis would rotate easily clockwise (Fig. 3.5B)
   b. left side: hip flexion is increased (hip extensors released; anterosuperior acetabular rim moved upward)
2. 'left anterior, right posterior' rotation
   a. right side: hip extension impaired by the acetabular rim and tightening of hip flexor muscles by a change in the length-tension ratio
   b. left side: impairment of hip flexion by the acetabular rim and tightening of the extensors

Malalignment is more likely to precipitate problems on account of:

1. increasing stresses on sites that are already vulnerable because of the posture the player has to assume; namely, the lumbosacral and cervicothoracic junctions
2. repetitive torsion through these same sites on delivery of the rock, with the thorax having to counter any rotational movement of the pelvis.

At the same time, the lunge position may help correct a 'rotational malalignment' through a leverage effect on the innominate:

1. on the side of the flexed hip, the femur could exert a corrective effect on an 'anterior' rotation; whereas
2. on the side of the extended hip, the effect would be to correct a 'posterior' rotation (see Ch. 7, Figs 7.16-18)

CYCLING

The legs should move symmetrically in the sagittal plane, knees equidistant from the crossbar, in order to generate an equal amount of force. The cyclist who presents with malalignment may, however, be aware of an asymmetry of form and strength in that:

1. leg strength feels different, the leg on one side 'feeling weak' in terms of the amount of power it can generate and having a tendency to fatigue more easily
2. the legs appear to move differently, movement generally feeling not as 'spontaneous', possibly even awkward, on the weak side

Several laboratory studies have attributed these problems to a malalignment-related leg length difference (LLD). On the side of the 'short' leg, Dunn & Glymph (1999) showed:

1. a decrease in the power generated (up to 5%)
2. a loss of pedal stroke efficiency, the round and smooth 'electronic motor' type effect being replaced by a piston-like action.

Studies were carried out using a standard bicycle mounted on a CompuTrainer, which allowed for a measurement of torque applied to each crank arm at every 15 degrees of rotation, as well as of the power split percentage between the right and left legs. These studies documented that, on realignment, the cyclist:

1. regained a smoother, more rounded stroke on the previously 'short' side, more in keeping with that on the opposite side
2. could ride for a longer time-period at maximum output
3. showed a continuing improvement on repeat studies over time, which was thought to be indicative of the body's continuing adaptation to the newly aligned position.

The right leg is more likely to feel weaker than the left. Given the large percentage of those presenting with 'right anterior' rotation (around 80%), the right leg is more often the shorter leg in the sitting position (see 'Sitting-lying test' in Ch. 2; Figs 2.77-2.79).

Foran (1999: 12) pointed out that an LLD of more than 3 mm is a sign of 'spastic contracture' (perhaps caused by muscle 'facilitation') originating at an upper motor neuron level, and that:

> *The spastic musculature responsible for the functional leg insufficiency remains hypertonic, even while wearing orthotics and heel lifts. This means a torqued pelvis and microtrauma on one side while seated.*

Only realignment was thought to improve matters. In addition to the above observations regarding form and strength, the following may become obvious to the cyclist or trainer.

The knees end up a variable distance away from the crossbar

With 'right anterior' innominate rotation, the right knee comes closer to midline than the left as the foot reaches the lowest point on pushing down on the pedal (Fig. 5.5A). This inward movement reflects the increasing tendency to foot pronation and knee valgus angulation on this side, with the leg straightening but still in external rotation as 'weight-bearing' increases (Fig. 3.3). As the right pedal moves upward, the right knee very obviously moves away from the crossbar, a movement in

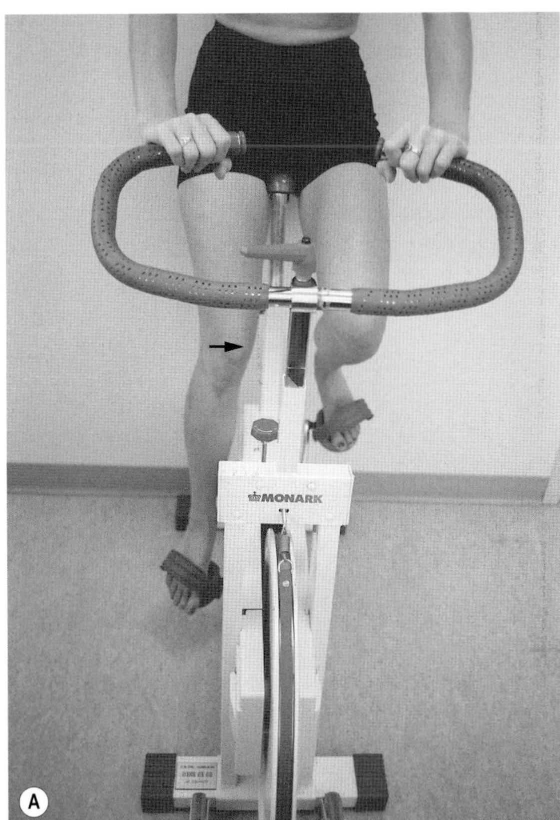

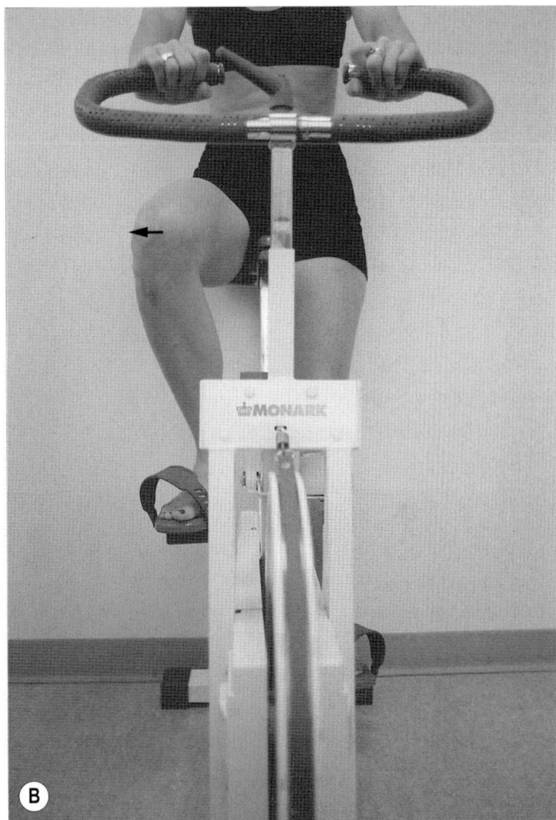

Fig. 5.5 Relationship of the knees to the midline (crossbar) in a cyclist with (i) an 'upslip' or one of the 'more common' patterns of 'rotational malalignment' and (ii) the typical rotation of the legs (right externally, left internally). (A) The right knee is moving toward midline (= medial translation along the coronal axis; see Fig. 2.9) on knee extension, with foot pronation and a tendency toward genu valgum. The left knee appears relatively neutral, travelling primarily in the sagittal plane. (B) The right knee is moving away from the midline (= lateral translation) with external rotation of the leg as the knee flexes. The left knee again maintains a relatively neutral position.

keeping with the fact that the right leg goes into exaggerated external rotation as it flexes and weight-bearing decreases (Fig. 5.5B).

Seen from the front, the right knee appears to be moving in a circle around the coronal axis in the sagittal plane, as well alternately moving in and out relative to the crossbar along the coronal axis (Fig. 2.9). In contrast, the left knee moves more straight up and down in the sagittal plane, maintaining a more consistently even distance from the bar. The overall movement of the left leg also appears to be smoother in comparison to that of the right.

The cyclist can improve matters by adding toe clips in the hope of stabilizing the feet and counteracting any tendency toward right pronation and left supination.

1. The right toe clip can be adjusted by rotating it counterclockwise so that the right foot, rather than pointing outward as the malalignment would dictate, now ends up pointing more or less straight ahead or even slightly inward at the lowest point of pushing downward. Fixing the foot in this position might be expected to counteract the tendency to external rotation of this leg, improving the mechanical advantage of the right leg and its ability to generate a force by:
   a. orienting the leg muscles more in the sagittal plane, so that they are working more in the line of progression
   b. increasing right ankle stability by decreasing the tendency to pronation

Unfortunately, the right leg has really had to be forced into this 'straight' position because, as long as malalignment is present, there will be a force trying to rotate this leg outward. If the toe clip now counteracts this tendency to external rotation as the knee extends and the foot increasingly weight-bears pushing down on the pedal, the rider may experience increased pressure or actual pain:

1. on the lateral border of the foot, as its usual movement outward with the leg is arrested by the toe-clip
2. around the right knee
   a. limiting pronation of the foot:
      i. decreases ankle and foot mobility
      ii. increases the tendency to knee valgus angulation and the twisting force between the femur and now relatively 'fixed' tibia
      iii. increases stress on soft tissue structures on the medial aspect of the knee (e.g. MCL)

On the left side, the increased tendency to internal rotation of the leg, varus angulation of the knee and supination of the foot on pushing maximally at end-of-range puts the TFL/ITB and the lateral knee structures (e.g. LCL) at risk of becoming symptomatic. A toe-clip can be adjusted medially to prevent this tendency to inward rotation and supination of the left foot. However, the cyclist may feel:

1. the toe-clip press against the medial aspect of the foot
2. discomfort from the increased stress on the lateral aspect of the knee and/or thigh.

The addition of an orthotic which has been modified to counteract any obvious tendency to pronation or supination could also be tried but the only long-term solution is realignment followed by reassessment to see if there are indeed some residual problems for which orthotic fitting might be appropriate (see Ch. 7).

Back pain with cycling

In some cyclists, riding with the trunk in a forward-flexed position (Fig. 5.6A) precipitates or worsens malalignment-related back or pelvic pain by:

1. increasing the stress on the cervicothoracic junction as the cyclist keeps the head and neck in compensatory extension throughout the ride
2. increasing the tension in already tense and tender paravertebral and extensor spinae muscles the length of the spine, to further extend the head and neck intermittently in order to see the road ahead and to counter any tendency to forward flexion of the trunk
3. putting the posterior pelvic ligaments (especially the iliolumbar, sacrotuberous and interspinous) under tension
4. putting direct pressure on tender sites such as the sacrotuberous insertions, hamstring origins and coccyx.

One alternative is to temporarily train on a stationary bicycle, sitting with the trunk upright and the arms relaxed at the sides. This minimizes tension in the muscles and ligaments of the back, sacral and coccygeal regions. Weight-bearing is more effectively shifted onto the ischial tuberosities and may, in fact, spare the coccyx completely, depending on the seat construction (see below).

An even better option may be to use a recumbent bicycle, which effectively relaxes the back muscles and ligaments by providing support, helping to maintain the lumbar lordosis and, thereby, decreasing the tension in these structures. It may also avoid putting pressure directly on tender sites, although this is not always guaranteed.

When out on the road, trunk flexion can be minimized by raising the handle bars as high as is feasible and still comfortable. Mountain bikes, ridden on a smooth surface, are preferable; shock absorption can be further increased by using a visco-elastic gel seat or similar cover over the actual bicycle seat. Accommodative seats with a mid-line groove lying directly under the coccyx and genitalia (labrum, testicles) will further decrease pressure on these structures, which are particularly vulnerable when leaning forward for extended periods of time (Fig. 5.6B,C).

Seating may be impaired

In addition to the problem of sitting on painful structures, discussed above, impaired seating can also be caused by some of the uneven weight-bearing aspects of malalignment. With a 'right anterior' rotation, for example, the left ischial tuberosity may end up lower by as much as 1 cm relative to the right (Figs 2.73C, 2.76D, 3.86C, 6.4A). The cyclist may be aware that he or she is bearing more weight on the left side and that the pelvis is shifting to accommodate; he or she may actually try to counter

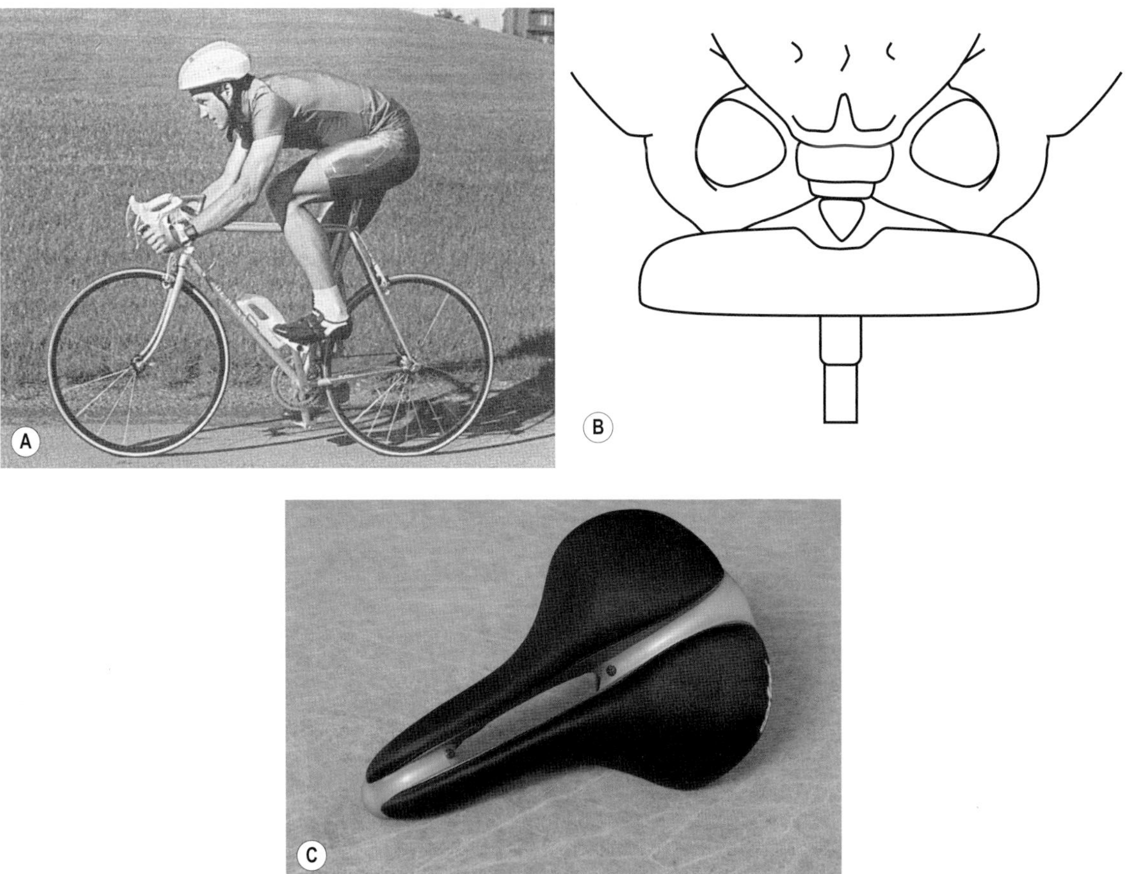

Fig. 5.6 Seating in cycling. (A) The supposedly 'good' position, with the back flat and the head up, may still cause problems when malalignment is present by stressing tense/tender structures (e.g. the paravertebral muscles and posterior pelvic ligaments). *(Courtesy of Matheny 1989.)* (B) and (C) A seat with a central depression concentrates weight-bearing on the ischial tuberosities and relieves pressure on the coccyx and genitalia (see also Fig. 7.43).

this feeling of 'imbalance' by filling the gap between the right buttock and seat with a thin pillow, or with material stuffed inside the training pants.

Toe cleats, orthotics, cleat shims and adjustments to the saddle, peddle and crankshaft to accommodate for the short leg may result in some improvement but realignment remains the only definitive treatment. If cycling repeatedly stirs up coccygeal symptoms or other musculoskeletal pains, this activity is best avoided until the problem has responded to treatment. Finally, those who are cycling and still going out of alignment must make sure that they are not doing so when getting on and off the bicycle. If that is the case, a bicycle without a crossbar is preferable (Fig. 5.7). Making use of a foot stool or the curb also cuts down the amount of asymmetrical rotation through the hip girdle and pelvis that would otherwise occur.

DANCING

Today's dancers start training at an earlier age and often train longer and harder than those in previous decades in order to excel. Chronic or overuse-type injuries are more common than acute ones, and the lower extremities are injured more often than other areas in most forms of dance. The biomechanical limitations imposed by malalignment may play a key role in causing these injuries.

Take, for example, the 'turnout' of the legs. As Adrian & Cooper (1986: 409) indicated:

> *...the amount of turnout is influenced by bony, ligamentous, and musculotendinous factors [and] optimum turnout ... will result if the dancer has adequate strength in the deep external rotators and adductor muscles of the hip joint and uses appropriate muscle activation patterns.*

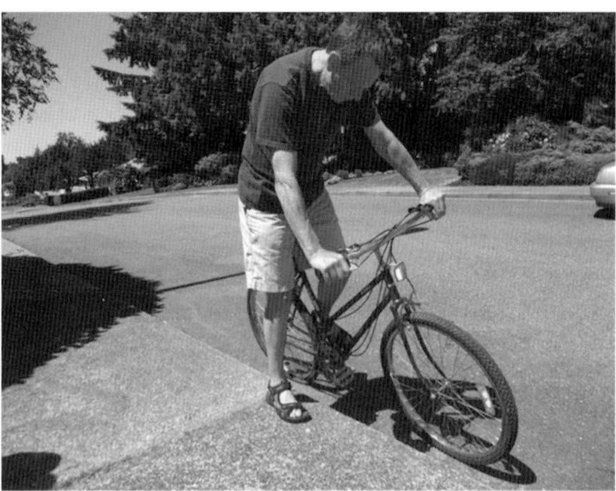

Fig. 5.7 Riding a bicycle without a crossbar and using a step-up (e.g. the curb) will decrease rotational forces through the pelvis when getting on and off, thereby decreasing the risk of recurrence of malalignment while the pelvis and spine are still relatively unstable.

This may be true for the dancers who are in alignment but those who present with malalignment are fighting needlessly imposed restrictions on ranges of motion and, in addition, limitations relating to altered strength and activation patterns. The following discussion will focus on how malalignment can affect basic ballet steps.

The five basic positions of classical dance

Dance is a flow of movements based on fundamental patterns of alignment of the head, arms, trunk, pelvis and legs. These movements repeatedly strain the available ranges of motion of these various parts of the body to their limit. The five basic positions in classical ballet, for example, involve a progressively increasing degree of difficulty in terms of their effect on the orientation of the lower extremities in relation to the rest of the body (Fig. 5.8). In all five positions:

1. the pelvis remains facing forward; that is, it is aligned in the coronal (frontal) plane
2. the trunk is usually aligned in the coronal plane but it can rotate on the pelvis with some manoeuvres (e.g. *ports de bras*)
3. the lower extremities are externally rotated (*en dehors*).

In the ***first position***, the lower extremities are externally rotated so that the feet are aligned at an angle of 45 degrees or less relative to the frontal plane, with the heels touching (Fig. 5.8A - 1st). The ***second position*** resembles the first except that the lower extremities are abducted to an equal extent in the coronal plane and are externally rotated to 90 degrees (Fig. 5.8A - 2nd). In the ***third, fourth and fifth positions,*** the lower extremities are adducted so that the legs are crossed and placed either together (Fig. 5.8A - 3 rd and 5th), or with one foot in front of the other (Fig. 5.8A - 4th; 5.8B), with the overall orientation of the feet in line with the coronal plane. The stress created in the lower extremities, pelvis and trunk by these five positions is further augmented by progressing from the *à plat* (flat) to *sur la demi-pointe* to *sur la pointe* (up on the toes) placements of the foot, combined with the various possible positions of the head and arms, and whether the dancer is supported on one or two legs.

Problems related to the basic positions

The ranges of motion specifically taxed by these positions are external rotation, abduction and adduction of the lower extremities and, to a lesser extent, pelvic and trunk rotation in the transverse plane around the vertical axis. Nixon (1983: 465) bluntly stated that:

> *The position of the leg* en dehors *(turned out) is contrary to nature. The position necessitates constant training from a very early age and laborious exercise to force it. There is little wonder ... that musculoskeletal strain becomes manifest.*

Micheli (1983: 474), on discussing the causative factors of back pain in dancers, indicated that the increased lordosis evident in a large number of dancers is usually acquired; the accompanying extension of the pelvis actually allows increased external rotation of the lower extremities and would, therefore, facilitate turnout. He also identified the following as risk factors for overuse injuries in dancers:

> *... anatomic malalignment of the lower extremity, including differences in leg length; abnormality or rotation of the hips; position of the kneecap; and bow legs, knock-knees, or flat feet*

Sammarco (1983: 487) made the point that 'children who begin classical ballet training during their juvenile years ... have the benefit of developing turnout while at the same time developing the femoral neck angle'; whereas:

> *... after the age of 11 the shape of the femoral neck can no longer be altered through the moulding process of continual pressure, such as lying on the floor with the hips abducted and externally rotated ... turnout is achieved by stretching the hip capsule.*

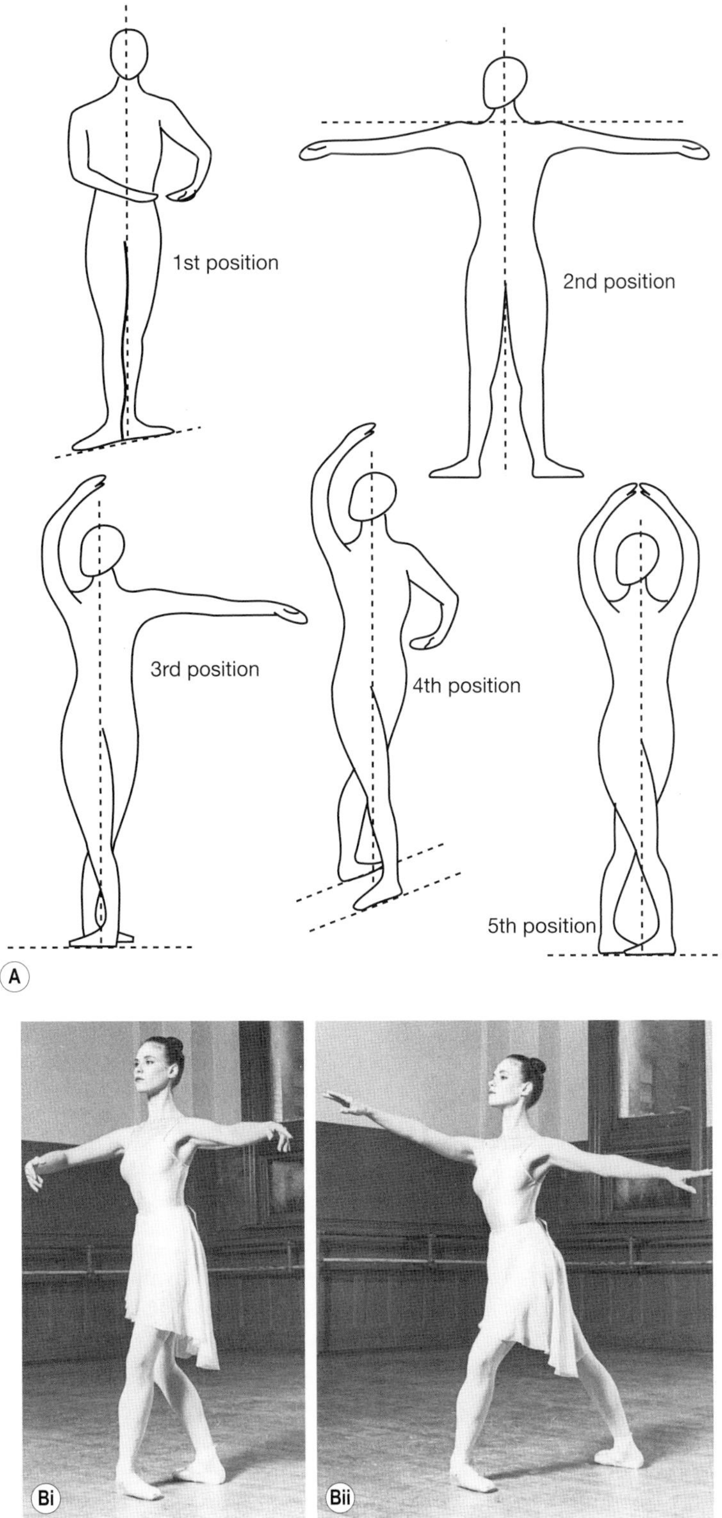

Fig. 5.8 Classical dance. (A) The five basic positions of dance. (B) Narrow and wide fourth position preparations for a *pirouette en dehors*. *(Courtesy of Laws 1984.)*

BOX 5.3 Common complications in the hip region in dancers (Sammarco 1983)

1. Prolonged forced hip abduction [*second position*] stretches the capsule, whereas strain at turnout puts the medial internal capsule under stretch and compresses the superolateral aspect of the acetabulum; there is eventual capsule scarring and calcification, with osteophyte formation on the acetabular rim and the femoral neck [Figs 2.48, 4.3]
2. Hamstring - excessive traction on the origin
3. Hamstrings – tears involving, in particular, the short head of biceps femoris
4. Strain of the adductor origins or muscle belly
5. Iliacus tendonitis and myositis, often seen bilaterally and in association with the *developpé* manoeuvre, in which: the hip and leg are brought from the first dance position outward and upward in external rotation [at which point the flexed knee is extended] and the lower extremity returned to the *first position* again
6. Greater trochanteric bursitis [especially considering the TFL/ITB strain with adduction in the 3rd - 5th position and on external rotation manoeuvres]
7. A snapping sensation as the tendon of tensor fascia lata moves across the greater trochanter, most likely to be visible [or even audible] when the dancer lands from a leap
8. Snapping in the groin region, probably of iliopsoas, when the hip is still 45 degrees flexed 'as the leg is brought from a flexed, abducted, externally rotated position with the knee extended back to the *first position*' (495) in the second half of a *developpé*
9. Traumatic sciatic neuritis from striking the buttocks against the floor when doing the splits

He pointed out the common complications that occur around the hip region (Box 5.3).

In addition to these, there are the problems related to the Achilles tendon, knee and great toe. Howse (1983: 499) stressed the importance of the 1st toe in allowing the dancer to 'maintain the correct line through the foot', thereby avoiding 'the secondary production of injuries elsewhere in the lower limbs', which could result from 'the difficulty or inability to maintain correct line and weight distribution from the foot up the leg and through the trunk'. He cited the following common problems:

1. metatarsus primus varus, resulting in secondary hallux valgus
2. a short first ray, forcing the dancer to attempt maintaining stability by weight-bearing over the second and third toes (commonly known as a Morton's toe; secondary to Point 1, the 2nd and 3 rd metatarsal heads come to lie increasingly forward of the 1st; Fig. 3.39A)
3. hallux rigidus, with pain and a progressive loss of dorsiflexion
4. injury to the capsule and ligaments of the first metatarsophalangeal joint, aggravated by a rotational twist of the toe itself.

Effect of malalignment

The above are among the more common injuries seen in dance. Some of them can be related to repetitive movements that place an abnormal stress on a specific structure.

On looking at the structures commonly involved, however, it becomes obvious that these are also, in large part, the structures that can be put under abnormal stress merely by the malalignment being present, even before superimposing the additional stresses incurred in dancing.

> The stresses inherent to the dance movements and malalignment must be regarded as being capable of augmenting each other and increasing the risk of the dancer becoming symptomatic.

The following is a consideration of how some dance manoeuvres can be affected by the specific stresses associated with malalignment.

Presentation: 'right outflare, left inflare'

The pelvic ring rotates clockwise, the left ASIS protrudes and there is reorientation of the acetabulae in the transverse plane: the right facing partly posterior, the left partly anterior. For a dancer, it results in:

1. asymmetry of the pelvic ring even when just standing
2. limitation, in this case:
   a. to rotate the pelvic ring counterclockwise when the feet are both weight-bearing (Fig. 3.5)
   b. to swing the right leg forward, the left back (see Ch. 3)

Presentation: 'upslip' and 'more common' patterns of 'rotational malalignment'

The following will be based on the assumption that the dancer is afflicted with an 'upslip' or one of the 'more common' rotational patterns ('outflare/inflare' will be mentioned as appropriate).

Turnout

The malalignment-related limitations that will interfere with the ability to achieve maximum, symmetrical turnout include:

1. a restriction of left lower extremity external rotation and abduction, right internal rotation, in part as a result of the asymmetrical orientation of the hip sockets
2. the asymmetrical increase in muscle tension around the hip joint, which involves right hamstrings and gluteus maximus, left hip abductors and TFL/ITB complex
3. contracture of soft tissues that have been put into a shortened position for prolonged periods of time

The dancer may try to force the feet past the amount of left turnout that is readily available. Adrian & Cooper (1986: 409) pointed out how the dancer may be able to:

> *assume the perfect turned-out position while the lower legs are flexed, and then straighten the legs and attempt to adjust alignment from the floor ... by pronating the feet excessively, by 'screwing (twisting) the knees' and/or by hyperextension of the back – all of which may cause a myriad of dance injuries if continued over time*

When malalignment is present, attempts at such faulty adjustments would be further compromised by:

1. an inability to pronate the left foot as much as the right or, at worst, not at all because of a tendency toward frank left supination
2. an inability to 'twist' through the left knee as easily as the right side on carrying out manoeuvres that require external rotation, with a limitation of the amount of internal rotation of the left tibia relative to the femur (Fig. 3.81)
3. any decrease in lumbar lordosis, and with it decreased flexibility of the lumbar spine segment and ability to extend, that can result in:
   a. compensatory lateral curvature (e.g. 'scoliosis')
   b. rotational displacement of individual vertebrae
   c. excessive posterior rotation of the sacral base (counternutation)
   d. coccygeal involvement, and
   e. pain from stress on the junctional regions (lumbosacral and thoracolumbar), with a reactive increase in tension in the adjacent paravertebral muscles.

Pattern of weight-bearing

The typical dance shoe offers little, if any, support. The feet are, therefore, at liberty to pronate or supinate on movement and to collapse into positions of medial or lateral weight-bearing, respectively. With malalignment:

1. on the left side
   a. the left foot tends to supinate and becomes more rigid, increasing the chance of developing metatarsalgia, plantar fasciitis, symptomatic Morton's neuroma, stress fractures and other complications caused by an impaired ability to absorb shock
   b. the risk of left ankle sprains is increased, given the shift to lateral weight-bearing and the weakness of specific ankle muscles, especially left peroneus longus
2. on the right side
   a. a relative increase in right pronation under high load, especially with the impact on landing, which results in excessive or repeated traction on the abductor hallucis longus and plantar fascia, as well as the origins of tibialis posterior, and predisposes to longitudinal arch pain and medial 'shin splints', respectively; medial shin pain may also occur from a sustained contraction of tibialis posterior as the dancer attempts to prevent excessive pronation (Kravitz 1987)
   b. increased right pronation also results in increased stress on the medial aspect of the first metatarsophalangeal joint and rotation of the great toe, increasing the chance of hallux vulgus formation and progressive degeneration
   c. accentuated internal rotation of the right tibia and increased right knee valgus angulation predispose to an excessive stress on medial knee structures (e.g. MCL) and patellofemoral compartment syndrome or 'dancer's knee' (Figs 3.37, 3.81).

These and other asymmetries affecting the lower extremities may be responsible for a dancer's disconcerting sensation of instability of one or the other ankle or extremity when pushing off or landing, more likely to involve the right leg (see Ch. 3: 'A problem with balance and recovery'; Figs 3.92, 5.19).

Asymmetry of strength, tension and range of motion
Muscular imbalance, presenting in the form of differences of strength, endurance and flexibility in opposing muscle groups, is frequently cited as a cause of pain in dancers if not corrected (Adrian & Cooper 1986; Fitt 1987). The imbalance is attributed to structural factors and to 'consistent patterns of misuse or overuse' (Adrian & Cooper 1986, p. 412). Although these factors may indeed be operative in dancers, there is also the possibility that the dancer prefers to carry out these manoeuvres in a certain pattern for the simple reason that it feels better or is easier to do that way, or that there just is no choice if the manoeuvre is to be executed at all.

> If malalignment is present, it probably plays a role in determining the easiest way to carry out a particularly difficult manoeuvre.

Most of the imbalances cited above can, in fact, be more easily explained by the asymmetries associated with malalignment rather than inherent structural changes or limitations resulting from faulty repetition. Given that malalignment is already evident in 75% graduating from elementary school (Ch. 2), it will have affected a large number of younger dancers during the 'formative' years. Certainly malalignment should be considered as possibly having played a major part in the development of any faulty patterns and even structural changes.

Failure to progress

Dancing, especially ballet, is one of the disciplines that calls for a stepwise progression to more and more demanding routines in terms of physical skill, balance and grace. The dancer is at risk of dropping out at the point at which the restrictions imposed by the malalignment make it increasingly difficult, if not impossible, to advance to the next stage (see Ch. 3).

DIVING

The asymmetries associated with malalignment will affect especially those dives which have a sagittal or vertical component by preventing perfect symmetry and increasing the splash at entry. Examples include dives incorporating vertical take-off followed by a somersault back layout or a somersault pike.

The restrictions imposed by malalignment are, however, even more likely to affect those dives incorporating a twist produced by simultaneous rotation around two or three axes. For example, a dive starting with a vertical take-off with an angular component, followed by 1.5 reverse somersaults and 1.5 twists, will incorporate rotation around all three axes (Fig. 5.9). If the diver leans

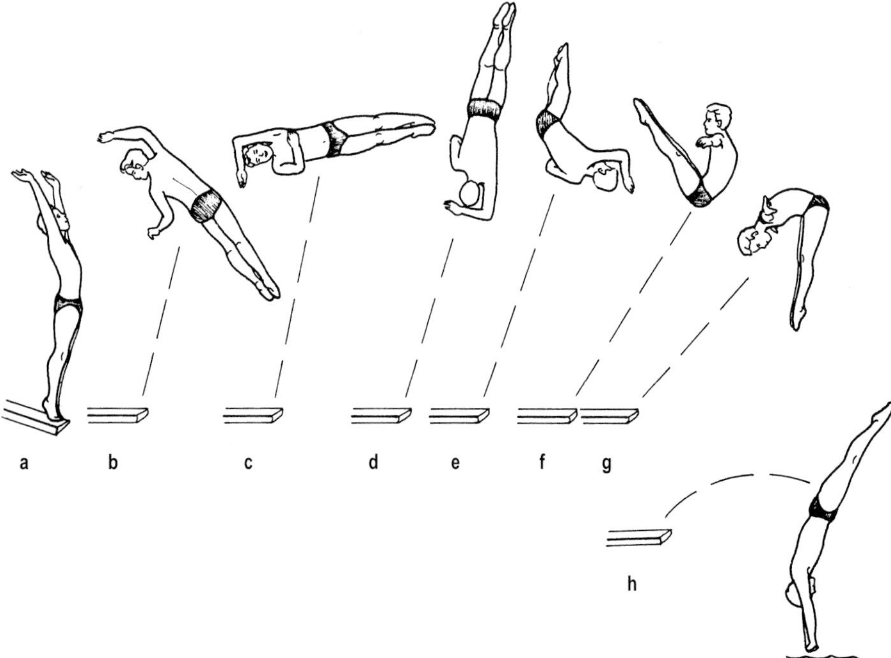

Fig. 5.9 Reverse 1½ somersault with 1½ twists from 1 m height. *(Courtesy O'Brien 1992.)*

into the twist too soon, it may be difficult to initiate the somersault. A problem of a similar nature could conceivably result because malalignment pre-sets the body in a 'twisted' position from top to bottom.

Another problem common to diving is the recurrence of malalignment, more likely with dives that incorporate a twist. Recurrences can occur either while performing the twist or on entry into the water, especially if the entry is not perfectly symmetrical and/or there is still a spinning component at the time the body hits the water. Some teams actually make sure that someone skilled in manual therapy examines the diver following each dive and, if necessary, carries out realignment immediately, in an attempt to ensure the quality of a subsequent dive and to decrease any risk of injury.

Dives from a springboard may be affected by asymmetry in the ability of the ankles to dorsiflex as the board is depressed, and to plantarflex maximally on pushing off (Figs 3.75, 3.84). A unilateral cuboid subluxation restricts range of motion in all four directions and may prove increasingly painful if stressed repeatedly in this way (Fig. 3.85A) The ability to gain lift will be affected by the asymmetry in the strength of the hip and knee extensors, also by the weakness attributable to the tendency toward excessive right pronation and genu valgum, left supination and genu varum. The diver may actually complain of one leg, usually the right, feeling weaker.

The coccyx is especially vulnerable in somersaults, 'lead-ups' and other reverse dives and training drills in which the feet enter the water first and the body leans back. On back dives from the 5 or 10 m board, for example, the body tends to overlean backward as the feet enter the water and the coccygeal area can end up taking the brunt of the blow. The amount of buttock cushioning may play a protective role here. With some dry-land drills, such as somersaults carried out at floor level or off a low box, the diver actually lands on the mat sitting on his or her buttocks with the legs in front. Always suspect the possibility that pelvic floor dysfunction may have developed and is complicating the recovery when coccygeal pain fails to respond to rest, repeated realignment and the modification of dives and dry-land drills (Figs 4.44, 4.45). Aside from temporarily discontinuing these dives, there may be need for special measures including use of a coccygeal relief pillow, possibly coccygeal/pelvic floor mobilization (Chs 3, 4, 7; Fig. 7.43). Return should be graduated, starting with dives without a torquing component from the 1 m board and gradually more difficult ones at increasing heights.

FENCING

Classical fencing is a 'unidirectional' sport requiring speed, balance, strength and timing as the body repeatedly lunges forward and retreats. The feet are placed at a right angle to each other; a right-handed fencer will have the right foot pointing straight at the opponent (Fig. 5.10A). This stance provides stability in both the coronal and sagittal directions. Stability also comes from a proper positioning of the knees:

> *the knees should be above the feet to reduce the moments of force and stress at the knee joints*
>
> (Adrian & Cooper 1986: 623)

Stability is decreased by any deviation of the knees to either side from this ideal position directly over the feet (Fig. 5.10B).

The lunge is initiated by kicking the leading foot toward the opponent and rapidly extending the knee of the back leg so that the body moves forward in as straight a line as possible (Fig. 5.10C). There is a simultaneous extension of the back arm and hand from their initial position: held overhead, with the shoulder, elbow and wrist bent to 90 degrees. The knee of the front leg stays flexed and, in order to increase the force of the lunge, is flexed even further once the lead foot has been planted securely. This knee flexion is controlled by eccentric quadriceps contraction. Forward motion and flexion of the front leg are eventually arrested by a concentric contraction of the quadriceps, hamstrings and gluteus maximus. The motion is then reversed by the combination of the front leg extending, the back leg pulling the weight of the torso backward, and the back arm resuming the flexed position overhead.

The lunge requires, of necessity, some pelvic rotation around the vertical axis in the transverse plane; bringing the hip forward augments the distance by which the foot can advance on the lunge side (as in the swing phase in walking; Fig. 2.12). In the fencer leading with the right leg, pelvic rotation will be counterclockwise. Throughout the encounter, the trunk is turned one-half to three-quarters to the front in order to minimize the chest surface area exposed to the opponent (Pitman 1988; Fig. 5.10).

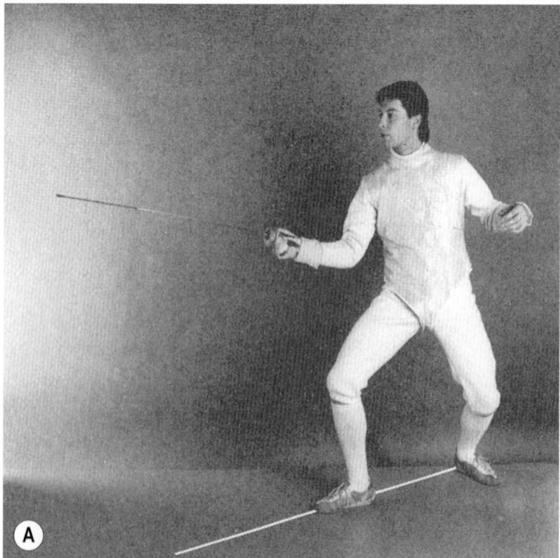

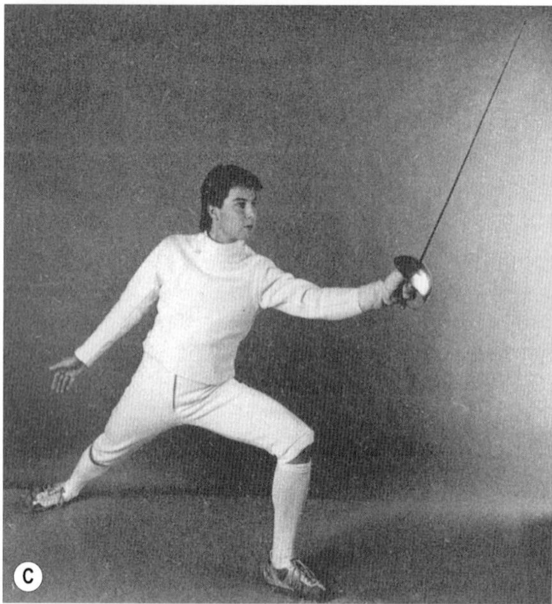

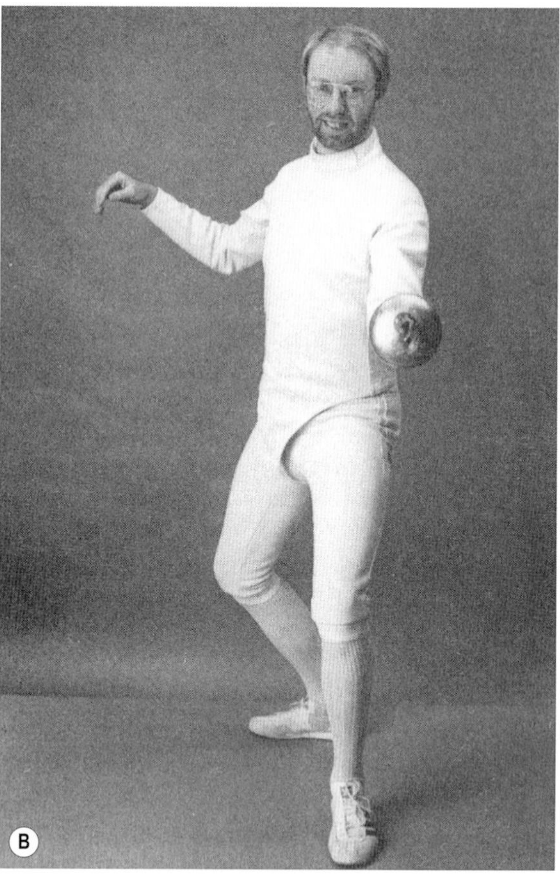

Fig. 5.10 Classical fencing: positioning for speed, strength, balance and timing. (A) Side view of a right-handed fencer in the 'on guard' position: the right foot is pointing at the opponent, the left foot is at a right angle and the trunk is turned one-half to three-quarters to the front. (B) Front view of a left-handed fencer in the 'on guard' position: the left knee is balanced directly over the foot. (C) The sabre lunge: note how the left knee is balanced over the left foot, and the feet are at a right angle. *(Courtesy of Pitman 1988.)*

Needless to say, fencing is a precision sport. Malalignment can ruin that precision, with the result that the fencer may miss the target, becomes more vulnerable and is at increased risk of injury.

The possible impact is illustrated here using the example of a fencer who leads with the right leg and presents with one of the 'more common' patterns of 'rotational malalignment', that of 'right anterior, left posterior' innominate rotation.

As indicated, stability is greatest when the feet are at right angles, which requires that both lower extremities are in a position of relative external rotation. The malalignment will limit external rotation of the left leg while increasing it on the right. If left external rotation is less than 45 degrees, the left foot may end up angled at less than 90 degrees to the sagittal plane, diminishing stability in the coronal and perhaps even sagittal planes. Compensation may be achieved by active clockwise rotation of the pelvis, to ensure the right foot points at the opponent and simultaneously increase the amount of external rotation of the left leg. This clockwise rotation of the pelvis may help improve stability in both planes, albeit at the cost of:

1. resulting in passive clockwise rotation of the trunk, with increased exposure of the vulnerable chest area
2. more compensatory manoeuvres to ensure the right arm moves in the sagittal plane if the trunk is now actively counter-rotated (i.e. counterclockwise, in this case)
3. placing the right acetabulum further backward so that it takes more time to advance from, and retreat to, this position with a lunge
4. decreasing the ability to rotate the pelvic ring counterclockwise

Forced external rotation on the left side puts the hip joint ligaments and the TFL/ITB complex under even more tension and risks precipitating pain from the left hip, greater trochanter and lateral thigh area (Fig. 3.41). Other internal rotators of the left lower extremity (e.g. gluteus medius/minimus) will also be wound up passively and put at risk.

Any 'posterior' rotation of the left innominate to compensate for the 'right anterior' rotation will restrict the counterclockwise rotation of the pelvis around the vertical axis in the transverse plane, decreasing the ability to use pelvic rotation to help advance the right leg at the time of the lunge (Fig. 3.5C). In addition, the decrease in left hip abduction range may further decrease the length and force of the right forward lunge that would otherwise be possible (see Ch. 3).

If the above limitations make it impossible to have the leading right foot point directly toward the opponent, and move forward and backward in a straight line, balance will be impaired. For maximum stability, the knees should be positioned directly over the feet at all times. The right arm is said to deviate by 2 degrees for every degree that the leading right knee deviates medially or laterally from that ideal position, increasing the chance of missing the target (M. Conyd, pers. comm. 1993, 2009). The right knee may deviate because of:

1. *a tendency of the right lower extremity toward external rotation*

   This change increases the chance for the foot to end up pointing out from midline (Figs 3.3B, 3.19B, 3.20). As the knee flexes on going into the lunge, the foot tends to pronate. The simultaneous valgus angulation of the knee predisposes to an inward deviation of the knee relative to the foot, decreasing stability, increasing tension in the medial knee structures (e.g. the medial collateral ligament) and compressing the lateral compartment (Figs 3.37, 3.81). The movement pattern, and the stresses, will be reversed on extending the knee to recover from the lunge
2. *compensatory internal rotation of the right leg*

   The fencer may try to increase the stability of the lunge by actively rotating the leg inward to bring the outward-pointing right foot back to midline and the knee more in line with the sagittal plane. As in the case of the cyclist using toe clips, however, the femur will still want to rotate externally on the fixed foot. On a right forward lunge, the knee may actually drift outward into varus, decreasing stability, increasing stress on the lateral knee structures (e.g. the lateral collateral ligament) and compressing the medial compartment.
3. *weakness of the quadriceps*

   The functional weakness of the right rectus femoris, possibly coupled with an actual wasting of the right vastus medialis, will make the eccentric contraction of the quadriceps mechanism less effective for stopping the lunge (Figs 3.57-3.60). The knee is more likely to collapse inward (valgus strain) and the patella to track outward, increasing tension across the patellar groove, compression within the patellofemoral compartment and traction on the tibial tubercle. Weakness may also affect the subsequent concentric contraction needed to extend the knee and reverse the lunge.

The knee is the most common site of injury in fencing (M. Conyd, pers. comm. 1998, 2009). Increased valgus angulation at a time when the right knee is under load, coupled with a wasting of the right vastus medialis, increases the risk of developing a knee injury (Box 5.4).

The fencer can try to overcome the restriction of stride length that results with malalignment by lifting the right leg higher but this, unfortunately, means coming down harder on the heel, increasing the chance of sustaining a heel bruise. It also increases the amount of shock transmitted upward to the knee joint, where it may accelerate the degeneration of the menisci and cartilaginous surfaces.

BOX 5.4 Common knee injuries in fencing

Patellofemoral compartment syndrome and chondromalacia patellae

If retropatellar pain is already a problem, the fencer can sometimes avoid it by forcing the knee into varus angulation. The improved patellar tracking might avoid putting pressure on tender patellar facets or femoral condyles but it comes at the cost of increased deviation of the knee from midline and decreased stability.

Joint degeneration

Varus or valgus angulation under load increases the pressure in the medial or lateral compartment, respectively, and predisposes to premature degeneration (Fig. 3.82).

Injury to the medial or lateral meniscus

1. Anything that counteracts the increased tendency toward external rotation of the right leg associated with an 'upslip' and the 'more common' patterns of 'rotational malalignment' will increase pressure on the medial compartment.
2. Medial meniscal entrapment is more likely when the foot is relatively 'fixed' and:
   a. the foot/ankle are pointing inward (i.e. stabilized in supination) and do not allow the tibia to rotate externally when the knee extends with the medial compartment closed
   b. the knee quickly moves from a position of flexion and valgus angulation (with the tibia in internal rotation) to a position of extension and neutral (or even varus) alignment with associated external rotation of the tibia.

Perhaps more significant is the fact that it also raises the centre of gravity and decreases stability even further at a moment when the fencer is already in a precarious position.

The left foot is more likely to supinate, which may increase the tendency toward:

1. the knee collapsing toward varus angulation at times when the fencer is in a more upright position
2. the foot and ankle collapsing toward inversion at push-off, increasing the risk of an inversion sprain at a time when the trailing leg is helping to accelerate the body forward when carrying out a lunge.

The fencer with the 'left anterior and locked' presentation (Figs 3.3A, 3.22B) who leads with the right foot will have:

1. *a limitation of right external rotation*

   It will be more difficult to rotate the right leg externally in order to point the right foot directly at the opponent. A counterclockwise rotation of the pelvis can compensate for this limitation. Simultaneous compensatory clockwise rotation of the trunk to allow movement of the right arm in the sagittal plane may be inevitable and will make the chest more vulnerable; compensatory active trunk rotation will result in increased rotational stresses and energy demands.

2. *problems related to supination*

   The tendency is for right foot supination and right knee varus angulation, which increases the risk of a right inversion sprain on heel-plant and weight-bearing during a lunge. The increased rigidity of the right foot results in more shock being transmitted proximally to the knee, hip, SI joint and spine.

3. *impaired left leg stability and push-off strength*

   These will result if the left foot collapses into pronation and the knee buckles into valgus at the time of the lunge.

Malalignment affects the classical fencing form in particular, decreasing versatility by limiting the repertoire of actions. It is less likely to affect the modern form, which consists, in large part, of a 'flash' combining a running motion, jump action and quick recovery. It has, however, adverse effects on both types, particularly in terms of increasing susceptibility to injury by increasing tension in certain ligaments and muscles, limiting some ranges of motion and decreasing stability.

GOLF

For the right-handed golfer, the initial action is one of winding up the spine by twisting the trunk clockwise and then unwinding to strike the ball and continuing into swing-through, effectively winding up counterclockwise. Adrian & Cooper (1986: 558) have described the golf swing as a combination of the arms moving across the body primarily in the coronal (frontal) plane while the trunk rotates around the vertical axis in the transverse plane. The shift of weight onto the right foot on the backswing, and the left foot on the swing-through to left increases the range of hip rotation. According to their analysis, at the height of the backswing 'pelvic action is seen to have rotated the pelvis almost 90 degrees and spinal rotation to have turned the upper torso more'.

The right-handed golfer with an 'upslip' or 'rotational malalignment', may present with problems relating to the following:

Asymmetrical limitation of upper extremity rotation

The increase in right external and left internal rotation at the glenohumeral joint seen with malalignment (Fig. 3.17A) is an advantage on the backswing but may be a limiting factor on right-to-left swing-through. The golfer can attempt to compensate by increasing trunk and pelvic rotation but this may not be possible if counterclockwise rotation is limited and may stress these sites inadvertently (see below; Fig. 3.5C). Limitation of right forearm supination, left pronation (Fig. 3.17C,D) are also factors to consider relating to gripping and swinging the club, especially if there are recurrent or chronic upper extremity soft tissue problems (e.g. medial epicondylitis, or 'golfer's elbow', which may also be on a referred basis when malalignment is present; see Fig. 3.12Bii).

Limitation of rotation through the thorax

Trunk rotation to one side is typically decreased (Fig. 3.49). This limitation results from a combination of factors including the direction of the thoracic convexity, an asymmetrical increase in paravertebral and shoulder girdle muscle tone, the presence of any vertebral rotational displacement and/or rib rotation (Lee 1993). Efforts to compensate through the pelvis or lower extremities may be limited by the asymmetry of available ranges of motion.

Limitation of pelvic rotation around the vertical axis in the transverse plane

'Left posterior' innominate rotation and 'left inflare' both limit pelvic rotation to the left and will affect the right-to-left swing-through (Fig. 3.5). With a 'right posterior' rotation or 'right inflare', the limitation is to the right and will affect the right backswing. To avoid compromising the backswing or swing-through, any reduction in the pelvic rotation may be compensated for by increasing rotation primarily through the thoracic segment of the spine (especially T/L junction), hip joints and lower extremities, albeit at the cost of increasing stress on these structures.

Asymmetrical limitation of lower extremity, ankle and foot ranges of motion

1. The golfer with the 'left anterior and locked' pattern of 'rotational malalignment' has a limitation of right external and left internal leg rotation, both of which could affect the right-to-left swing-through.
2. On the other hand, the golfer with an 'upslip' or one of the 'more common' rotational patterns has a restriction of right internal and left external rotation, which could create problems with an attempt at a left-to-right swing-through.
   a. On completion of the right backswing, the right leg has passively rotated internally; the right foot has moved toward neutral or frank supination and comes to weight-bear more laterally. The left leg has passively rotated externally and the foot rolled inward, toward neutral or actual pronation, and plantarflexed (to weight-bear more on the medial MT heads and lengthen the leg, respectively).
   b. On right-to-left swing through, these changes are reversed so that at the end of the 'drive', the left leg is in maximal internal rotation and the foot and ankle supinated; whereas the right leg is in maximal external rotation and the foot plantarflexed.
   c. All these changes occur to maximize the extent of the backswing and swing-through. Problems are more likely to occur if the feet move inadequately or, worse still, remain planted on the ground, increasing rotational strains through the knees and hips. Malalignment affects these movements of the lower extremities unfavourably: they become asymmetrical, with restriction of right internal rotation and plantarflexion, left external rotation and dorsiflexion.

Acute blockage of trunk rotation

When the golfer driving from right to left takes a divot the wrong way or hits a covered root or a rock in the rough, thoracic rotation to the left can be suddenly limited or even completely stopped; whereas the rotation of the pelvis and to some extent the head and neck continues. This twisting of the head and neck through the cervicothoracic junction, and of the pelvis on a fixed trunk through the thoracolumbar junction, can aggravate problems attributable to pre-existing malalignment or precipitate the onset or recurrence of malalignment.

The author is reminded of the golfer who reported going out of alignment each and every time he 'took a divot'. He solved this problem by lying down on the links in order to carry out an immediate correction using a muscle energy technique he had learned at the workshop. This allowed him to get on with the game until he 'took the next divot'. The suggestion of having someone assess his style in the hope of cutting down on the number of times he took a divot was not well received.

Using different clubs should also be considered, especially on the driving range where there is a risk of repeatedly hitting the mat. For example, unlike traditional steel clubs, titanium and graphite clubs will yield a bit on impact and absorb some of the shock.

Increased stress through the thoracolumbar junction

> Restrictions imposed by limitations of pelvic or lower extremity rotation require a compensatory increase in rotation more proximally. The resulting stress is maximal through the thoracolumbar junction and trunk but can also affect the shoulder, elbow and wrist joints.

A typical history is that of the golfer who presents fit and unaware of any problems at the start but develops back pain over the first half of the course. The pain typically increases as the game progresses, sometimes forcing him or her to abandon play. The pain is often limited to the mid-back region or may be maximal there. Other parts of the back may eventually become a problem as impaired rotation and pain result in protective muscle spasm and faulty technique. An irritation of the T12 and L1 cutaneous fibres can trigger a full-blown 'thoracolumbar syndrome' (Figs 4.20-4.23).

Posterior ligament and muscle stress

Malalignment results in increased stress on the posterior pelvic ligaments (Figs 2.5, 2.6). They are more likely to become a problem with golf, particularly when working out on a driving range. To drive the ball, the trunk is slightly flexed on the pelvis, further increasing the tension in these ligaments. Similarly, the erector spinae muscles are at increased risk as they are contracted for prolonged periods of time to control trunk flexion. Maintaining this stance while adding a twisting insult to the trunk and pelvis also repeatedly stresses the anterior and posterior oblique muscles. Eventually, it can precipitate or worsen pain from individual muscles and ligaments, with possibly distal effects, given that they are all part of the system of oblique 'slings' (see Ch. 2).

The results of treatment can be most gratifying, with repeated reports that realignment finally allowed the golfer to complete 18 holes without pain being 'par for the course'. The biggest problem in most cases is one of convincing the golfer not to play for a while to ensure that treatment attempts will be successful. Unfortunately, few are willing to stop until the season is over before making time for the 3-4 months sometimes required to get to the point of maintaining the realignment and tolerating the rotational stresses inherent to playing golf without triggering a recurrence of the malalignment. In that case, a proper course of treatment aimed at realignment and stabilization may not be possible until the off-season.

GYMNASTICS

Gymnastics may be divided into floor exercises and those carried out on apparatus. Some problems, including back and knee pain, are common to both.

Back pain

Tsai & Wredmark (1993) postulated that the increased incidence of back pain in gymnasts relates to the commonly noted hyperlordosis aggravated by repeated hyperextension manoeuvres, an increased trunk length and a low sacral inclination. Micheli (1985) identified four entities responsible for back pain in gymnasts.

1. **Pars interarticularis fracture or spondylolysis**

   These presentations can sometimes be attributed to trauma or to a single episode of hyperextension. It is, however, more often felt to be related to the increased lordosis and/or repeated and extreme degrees of hyperextension required for some routines.

Stinson (1993: 86, 519) cited studies also implicating heredity and the combination of lordotic stress on a neural arch weakened because of an inherited defect in the modelling of the cartilage. He felt, however, that the high prevalence in certain athletic disciplines (gymnastics, diving, football, weight-lifting and wrestling) makes 'spondylolysis in the athlete in some respects a unique entity'. It may occur unilaterally or bilaterally. The history is usually one of an insidious onset of low back pain with or without radiation to one or both buttocks, 'often first noted when the gymnast does a back flip or back-walkover'.

2. **Vertebral body fracture**

   Micheli (1985: 89) cited fracture of the vertebral end plates as another cause of back pain in young athletes. Fractures are detected particularly at the anterior margins and 'appear to be usually the result of repetitive microtrauma – most probably repeated flexion ... and can result in frank vertebral wedging'. He went on to say that 'in the gymnast, these fractures usually occur at the thoracolumbar junction and may involve three or more vertebral bodies, although one or two levels of involvement are more common'. These athletes may be mistakenly labelled as having Scheuermann's disease.

3. **Discogenic back pain**

   Micheli (1979) reported an increasing incidence of this condition in the athletically active adolescent population. Back pain may actually be overshadowed by unilateral or bilateral hamstring tightening or the development of a 'sciatic scoliosis'.

4. **Spondylogenic back pain**

   This is often a presumptive diagnosis based on the exclusion of the above three categories and ruling out a tumour or infectious process.

Malalignment increases the stress on both the discs and the pars interarticularis, and conceivably increases the chance of the gymnast developing any of the above complications. Gymnastic manoeuvres that call for a maximum movement of the vertebrae in all three planes are superimposed on a spine that is already moving abnormally because of the malalignment. L5 vertebral rotational displacement to the right, for example, compresses the left L5-S1 facet joint and will automatically increase the stress placed on the left pars whenever a movement involving extension, left side flexion or clockwise rotation of the trunk is superimposed (Fig. 2.52B). As stated by Ciullo & Jackson (1985: 97), the pars can fail 'when subjected to unusual repetitive forces of hyperextension, tension, torque and compression'.

Malalignment can cause or augment all of these stresses. A compensatory lumbar convexity to the left, for example, entails a rotation of L1–L4 into the convexity. The right facet joint surfaces are compressed, both by the counterclockwise rotation and right side-flexion into the concavity, increasing stress on the pars on that side, while reducing the overall flexibility of the lumbar segment (Figs 2.42, 4.6, 4.33). Pressure will be increased even further, especially on the right facet joint surfaces and pars, with:

1. the addition of a left rotational displacement of one or more individual vertebrae (see above; Fig. 2.96B)
2. any malalignment-related increase in sacral nutation that accentuates the lumbar lordosis, and
3. any increase in side-flexion from reflex contraction of right psoas, quadratus lumborum, paravertebral and/or erector spinae muscles

Micheli's observation (1985) that vertebral body fractures in gymnasts usually involve the anterior aspect of only one or two vertebrae in the thoracolumbar junction may be an indication of the stress on this site caused by the change from a lordosis to a kyphosis (a change from an 'extension' to 'flexion' stress, respectively). If, however, these anterior fractures are indeed related to increased or repetitive flexion stresses, the flexion stress caused by the kyphosis would be expected to be least at the thoracolumbar junction and maximal at the apex of the thoracic kyphosis. In addition, because of the orientation of the facet joint surfaces, most flexion and extension movement occurs in the lumbar segment, to lesser extent at the thoracolumbar junction and least in the thoracic segment itself (Fig. 3.9).

Malalignment may offer a more plausible explanation for finding vertebral fractures at the thoracolumbar junction. In addition to the shift from a lumbar lordosis to a thoracic kyphosis, there is:

1. the torsional and lateral flexion strain on the discs attributable to the reversal of the lumbar and thoracic convexities, L1 being rotated one way and usually T12 (sometimes also T11) in the opposite direction (Fig. 3.14C)
2. in addition, vertebral rotational displacement involving T12 or L1 is very common, typically occurring in conjunction with an 'upslip' and 'rotational malalignment' of the pelvis and correcting with realignment

All these changes result in a loss of the normal joint play or 'glide' so that there is, typically, increased resistance or stiffness at the level of the junction which diminishes the ability of this area to yield to stresses of any type (Fig. 5.2).

Superimposing a flexion stress more readily increases the load on the anterior disc and adjoining vertebral margins, predisposing to fracture. The fact that pain elicited by posteroanterior and side-to-side transverse pressure on the spinous processes often localizes to the thoracolumbar and lumbosacral junction areas is indicative of the increased stress on these sites that comes with malalignment (Figs 4.20, 5.2). If there are any sensory symptoms, or suggestions of referred paraesthesias, a coexistent thoracolumbar syndrome may have to be ruled out. Even though tenderness can often be elicited on palpation or stressing of either site, the athlete may be asymptomatic until something like a tear of the annulus fibrosus, an end plate fracture or pars stress fracture finally occurs and brings these areas to his or her attention.

Knee pain

A review published by Andrish (1985) indicated that knee pain in gymnasts relates primarily to patellofemoral compartment problems, ligament sprains, meniscal tears, contusions and Osgood–Schlatter's disease. The stresses on the patellofemoral region that result with malalignment must also always be kept in mind (see Ch. 3). If there is no history of direct trauma, or if the complaint is unilateral, this should raise suspicions that malalignment may be playing a role (Figs 3.37, 3.81, 3.82, 4.5).

Let us now look at the effect of malalignment on the demands of the individual gymnastic disciplines.

Apparatus: specific problems

Malalignment will primarily affect the dismount, those routines which are asymmetrical and those requiring rotation around the vertical, sagittal and/or coronal axes. Problems relate to the following changes that occur with malalignment.

Limitations of thoracic spine and pelvic rotation

These affect the ability to do somersaults and twists as part of routines carried out on the rings, parallel bars, the side-horse and balance beam, or in the course of vaulting.

A limitation of rotation of the pelvis around the vertical axis in the transverse plane into the side of a 'posterior' innominate rotation or an 'inflare' may become a problem, especially at times when the gymnast is holding on to the apparatus with both hands; for example, with manoeuvres on the pommel horse (Fig. 5.11B,C) or the rings (Fig. 5.11D). Holding on this way automatically decreases the ability to rotate through the thoracic region and, therefore, increases the rotational stresses through the thoracolumbar, lumbosacral and pelvic regions, including the hip and SI joints.

> The ability to rotate through the lower extremities is restricted in some routines by holding the legs close to each other; for example, when doing double-leg circles on the pommel horse or horizontal bars (Fig. 5.11A,B) as opposed to a scissor-action (Fig. 5.11C).

The restriction increases the rotational stresses through more proximal structures. If the pelvis and spine cannot accommodate because of a malalignment-related limitation of rotation in specific directions, the result can be awkwardness, a decreased ability – or even inability – of the gymnast to carry out these routines, and actual injury.

The ultimate test of any limitation of the hip, pelvic or thoracic range of motion must occur while carrying out high double-leg circles on the pommel horse (Fig. 5.11B). This requires rotating the closely applied legs in one direction across the top of the horse, limiting rotation through the hip girdles, while the rest of the body rotates in the opposite direction, supported by each arm alternately holding on to one of the handles.

The ability to rotate the upper trunk to either right or left while in the cross-hang (iron cross) position on the rings will be compromised, in particular by any limitations of:

1. the thoracic spine
   a. any movement of this segment is restricted or 'fixed' by having to tense most shoulder girdle and trunk muscles to maintain the 'iron cross' position, which can result in
   b. augmented tension/discomfort in muscles that are already affected unfavourably by pelvic malalignment and/or a complicating vertebral rotational displacement
2. the pelvis and legs
   a. when the trunk is 'fixed' (Point 1), added muscle contractions may be needed to counter

any tendency of the pelvis and legs to twist relative to the trunk and to each other on account of malalignment being present, in order to maintain as symmetrical a position as possible for point evaluation (Figs 3.5, 5.11D).

Asymmetry of lower extremity muscle strength, a feeling of 'instability' in one leg and a problem with balance
These may present difficulties especially on dismount and with routines carried out on the balance beam, more likely those incorporating a twist of the trunk relative to the pelvis or around the long axis of the body. Dismount stability is further compromised by the various asymmetries affecting the lower extremities, and though these asymmetries obviously affect both legs, the athlete may feel one leg in particular is 'weak' or 'unstable', to the point that his or her routine has been modified to rely on the leg 'they can trust' (see Ch. 3: 'A problem with balance…').

Floor exercises

Floor exercises require the ultimate in flexibility and balance as the gymnast carries out tumbles, springs and double and triple twists in quick succession, landing on either one or both feet or in the split position. As the difficulty of the routines increases, so does the chance that the asymmetries associated with malalignment will become a limiting factor or cause of an injury.

The athlete may be aware of stiffness, limitations of movement, asymmetries in push-off strength, possibly a feeling of insecurity or imbalance on trying to come to a controlled stop at the end of a routine. Athletes probably tailor their routines, consciously or subconsciously, in order to avoid these problems; for example, by carrying out a manoeuvre in the direction that avoids the restriction of range of motion, repeatedly landing on the more stable leg, or putting more weight on that leg when landing on both.

> This 'lop-sided' repetition predisposes to overuse problems; whereas an inadvertent deviation from these routines puts the gymnast at increased risk of injury.

HIKING AND CLIMBING

Hiking, and even more so climbing, can demand the utmost in agility and strength, as dictated by the terrain. Any weakness or restriction of range of motion puts the person at increased risk. Slopes augment any shift in weight-bearing and predispose to inversion or eversion sprains, especially when on uneven terrain in other than supportive high-tops or boots (Fig. 3.31). Asymmetrical activities increase the chance of vertebral and/or pelvic malalignment occurring or worsening (Fig. 3.36). Hiking poles, preferably adjustable ones used bilaterally, help decrease possible effects of an existing malalignment by diminishing any asymmetries on weight-bearing and decrease demands on the lumbo-pelvic-hip complex by distributing the weight between the legs and arms. The person should be on the look-out for any recurrence during the climb, or at least do a self-assessment on return to base camp or home, in order to carry out realignment as soon as possible and avoid becoming symptomatic again. In someone fit and muscular, corrective manoeuvres such as traction for an 'upslip' may require more effort in terms of the amount of traction/weight and how long it is applied (see Ch. 7).

INTERCEPTIONS IN TEAM SPORTS

Interceptions result in an unexpected turn-over of the ball or puck to the opposition; they are mentioned here because they are an important part of a number of athletic activities. They do present an unexpected opportunity to turn the game around. However, the 'lucky' opposition players usually cannot plan for the event; that is, prepare the body for any associated impact, excessive rotation or loss of stability. The response is usually spontaneous, with no time to consider the increased risk of:

1. exceeding any restrictions of range of motion
2. losing equilibrium
3. having to twist the pelvis and spine to an extreme, sometimes in opposite directions, with or without superimposed acute trunk flexion or extension.

Interceptions are, therefore, more likely to result in injury, especially in the athlete already presenting with malalignment. They must also be considered as a possible cause of initial occurrence or recurrence of malalignment.

JUMPING SPORTS

Limitations relating to malalignment affect primarily the following aspects:

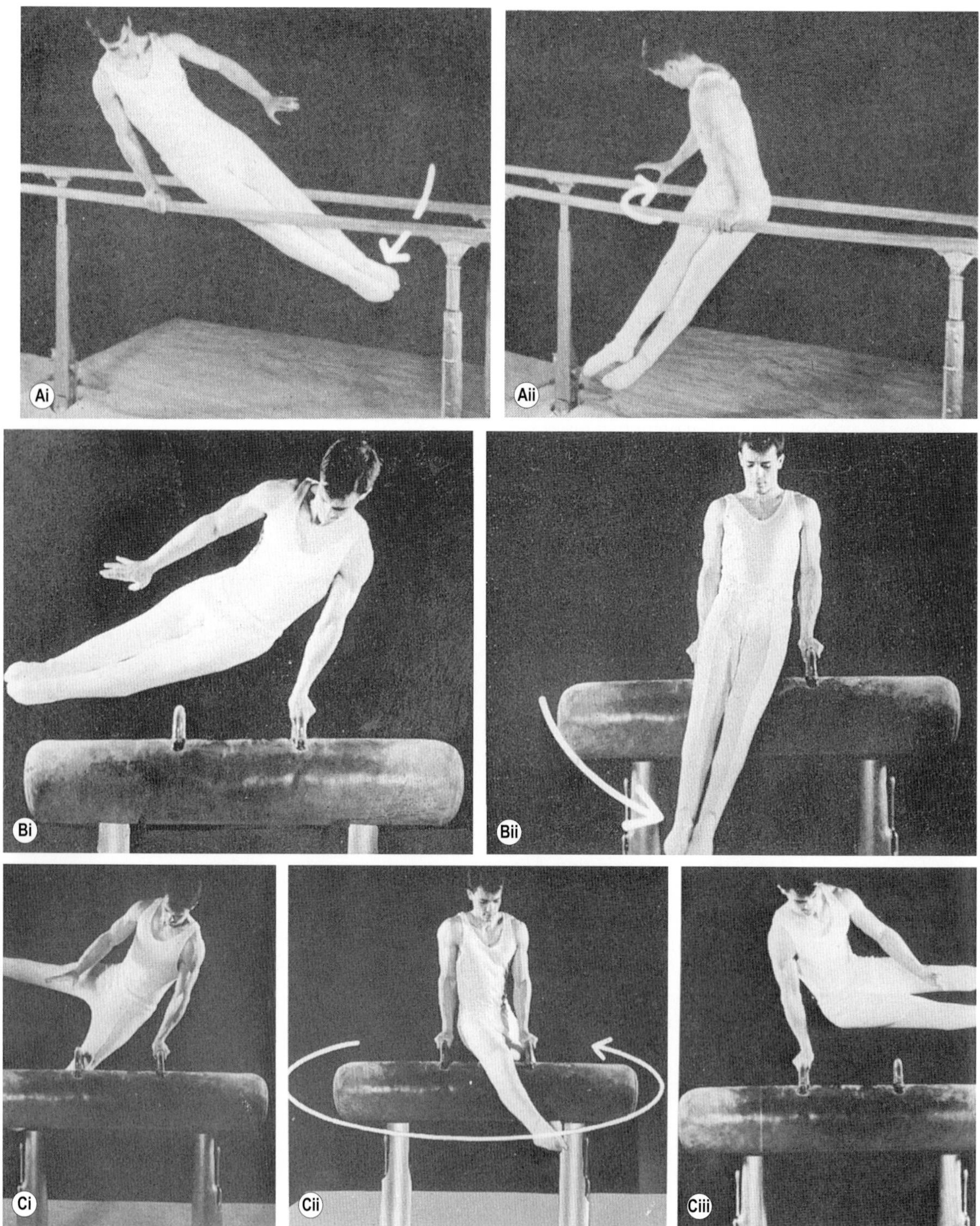

Fig. 5.11 Gymnastic manoeuvres. (A) Front support turn on the parallel bars. (B) Double-leg circle on the pommel horse. (C) Single-leg circle with scissor-action.

(Continued)

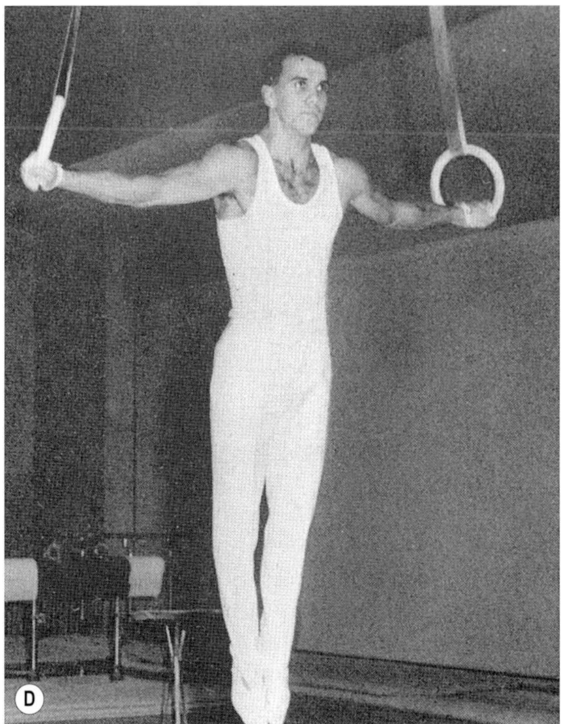

Fig. 5.11—cont'd (D) Straight-body cross-hang (iron cross) position on the rings. *(Courtesy of Loken & Willoughby 1977.)*

Rotation

Most jumps have a rotational component. For example, after the take-off in a high jump using the Fosbury flop (Fig. 5.12), or on ascending and when reaching the top in the pole vault.

Hip extension and flexion

'Right anterior, left posterior' innominate rotation restricts right hip flexion and left hip extension; the reverse occurs with the 'left anterior, right posterior' pattern of 'rotational malalignment' (Figs 3.71, 3.72). These changes will affect the stride length and hip flexion or extension required for clearance (hurdles and steeplechase), the extent of reach (the long and triple jumps) and push-off (pole vault and high jump). The final upward thrust in the vault and high jump, for example, comes from simultaneously kicking one leg up in the air (hip flexion) and extending the opposite hip and knee after initial flexion. Stride length can also be affected by an asymmetry of pelvic rotation in the transverse plane; for example, by limitation into the side of a 'posteriorly' rotated innominate or an 'inflare' (Fig. 3.5).

The jumper may be able to change style to adapt to the limitations imposed by malalignment (Figs 3.71-3.85). Leading off with the left leg in steeplechase and hurdle events might, for example, get

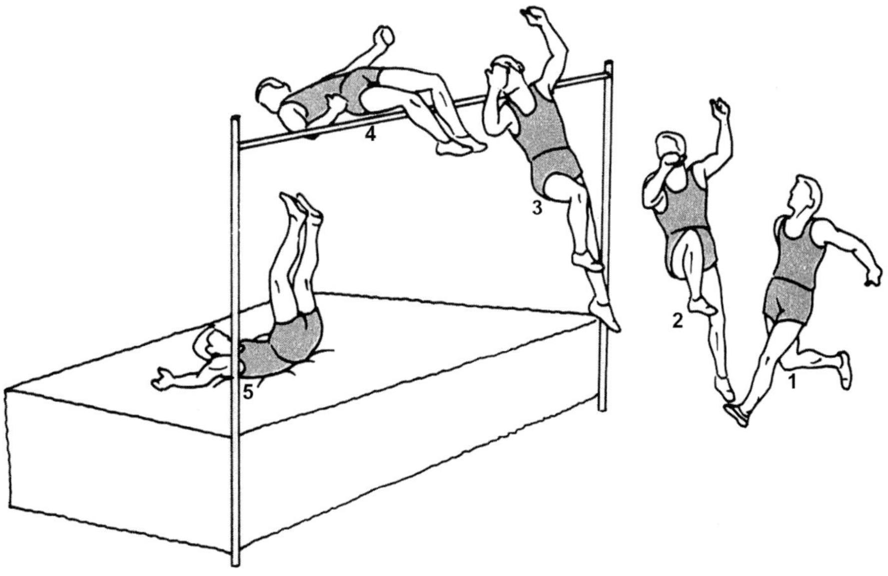

Fig. 5.12 Fosbury flop: approaching the bar from the right. *(Redrawn courtesy of Worth 1990.)*

around any restriction of right hip flexion caused by 'right anterior' rotation, 'right outflare' or increased tension in the right gluteus maximus, piriformis and/or hamstrings. For the same reason, the pole vaulter might fare better swinging up with the left leg and pushing off with the right, provided that functional weakness affecting the right quadriceps and, in a minority, also right hip extensors is not a major problem. The way in which an athlete finally executes a specific manoeuvre is probably by trial and error, in part influenced by the limitations imposed by malalignment.

High jumping

Take, for example, the high-jumper with one of the 'more common' patterns, a 'right anterior, left posterior' rotational malalignment, who intends to execute a Fosbury flop by approaching the bar in one of the following ways:

From the right side

The jumper will run toward the bar in a curved approach (Fig. 5.12-#1). After planting the left foot, lift-off is combined with simultaneous counterclockwise rotation of the pelvis and trunk, forcing the leg into internal rotation (#2). Lift-off comes through initial flexion and external rotation of the left leg and then, simultaneously, extending that leg fully while kicking the right leg (closest to the bar) up in the air (#2). Once airborne (#3), the thorax and pelvis continue to twist, in an attempt to achieve clearance of the bar with the buttocks while sailing backward with the extended back 'draped' across the bar (#4).

In other words, acceleration is converted into a vertical force by the kicking action of the right leg with simultaneous left leg extension, initiating a counterclockwise rotation of the trunk and then pelvis and, finally, back extension (Paish 1976; Worth 1990). The malalignment may affect the factors listed in Box 5.5.

From the left side

Acceleration is converted into a vertical force by simultaneously extending the flexed right leg and kicking up the left leg, with clockwise rotation of the trunk and then the pelvis initiated while weight-bearing on the right leg and continued when airborne. Effects of malalignment include the following:

1. internal rotation is decreased on the weight-bearing right leg, which is forced into that direction as the trunk rotates clockwise
2. stability of the push-off foot and strength of the right leg is decreased, given the asymmetrical functional weakness that typically affects the right hip flexors and extensors, tibialis anterior and posterior, extensor hallucis longus and other toe extensors, so that the right leg may feel weak compared to the left (Figs 3.53-3.55, 3.57-3.60)
3. a decreased ability to plantarflex the right foot on any attempt to increase leg length (Fig. 3.84)
4. a torsional strain on the spine and thoracolumbar junction (Figs 3.14, 3.49).

Depending on the type of malalignment present, and which pattern of restriction is dominant, the jumper may find that it 'feels easier' or 'more natural' to approach the bar from one side than the other,

BOX 5.5 Factors affected by malalignment in a right-side Fosbury flop approach

The most common pattern of 'rotational malalignment' ('right anterior/left posterior') would affect the attempt as follows:

1. The ability to drive the right thigh upward (hip flexion) may be limited by:
   a. the mechanical restriction of the femur that occurs with anteroinferior rotation of the anterosuperior rim of the acetabulum (Figs 3.71-3.75).
   b. tightening of the right hamstring/sacrotuberous complex by a change in the length-tension ratio and complicating 'facilitation', particularly of right biceps femoris (Figs 3.42, 3.43)
2. An increased risk of an ankle inversion sprain on the weight-bearing left side, given the functional weakness of left peroneus longus and tendency to supination on this side (Figs 3.22A, 3.53B, 5.12[1])
3. A torsional stress on the spine, especially thoracolumbar junction, if there is a restriction of counterclockwise rotation of the thorax affecting especially Phase 2 of the jump, while still weight-bearing (Figs 3.5, 3.49, 5.12[2,3])
4. Stress on the already 'ill-fitting' thoracolumbar junction - especially asymmetrical alignment of the facet joints - on hyperextension of the back (Figs 3.9, 3.14, 5.12[4])

with better results. In that respect, the malalignment may be thought of as providing a 'biomechanical' advantage to the athlete. If malalignment does indeed appear to result in improved performance in an 'established' jumper, perhaps there may be no point in attempting realignment, provided that the athlete is asymptomatic. However, there will still be an increased risk of injury, especially if that athlete participates in other sports as well (e.g. high-jump as part of a pentathlon, heptathlon or decathlon).

MARTIAL ARTS: KARATE

Karate involves fighting with the hands and feet, punching and kicking being the two most common forms of attack. The intent is to deliver as forceful a blow with as small a surface area as quickly as possible, while at the same time maintaining balance. When advancing to deliver a punch or kick, the athlete - or karateka - moves forward in a straight line in order to minimize the displacement of the centre of gravity and to shorten the time required to reach the opponent. Increased mobility occurs at the expense of stability: the 'one-and-a-half-footed' cat stance (Fig. 5.13A), for example, provides mobility but is less stable than the wide-based 'two-footed' horse stance (Fig. 5.13B) or 'back' stance (Fig. 5.13C). Increasing the distance through which an extremity moves increases the amount of force generated but this again comes at the expense of stability.

The karateka with the common 'right anterior, left posterior' pattern of 'rotational malalignment' has limitations that may decrease effectiveness and increase the risk of injury, as described below.

First, stride length is decreased as a result of a restriction of:

1. counterclockwise rotation of the pelvis
2. right hip flexion and left hip extension

This karateka is at increased risk of a sprain or strain of the tight right hip extensors and left hip flexors when advancing the right foot in front stance or lunging, especially with the 'lunge punch', a particularly deep lunge required to deliver a low blow (Fig. 5.13D). He or she can compensate for a decreased stride length by moving closer to the opponent in order to 'connect', at the increased risk of being hit and injured.

Second, the reach of the right leg is usually decreased and the high kicking action hampered, making this leg a less formidable striking weapon. Reach could be increased by plantarflexing the right foot but this ankle motion is already restricted on this side (Fig. 3.84B).

Third, the restrictions affecting counterclockwise rotation of the pelvis, and internal rotation of the right and external rotation of the left leg, may become a limiting factor for any rotational manoeuvre of the trunk carried out while supported on one or both feet. These restrictions could, for example, impair those manoeuvres in which the body quickly rotates through 180 degrees to face alternately to right and left while both feet are weight-bearing. These restrictions could also interfere with assuming a specific stance, such as:

1. the 'horse' stance, in which both feet point forward or out and the knees are then flexed, to rotate both legs externally (Fig. 5.13B)
2. the 'back' (Fig. 5.13C), 'cat' (Fig. 5.13A) and 'front' stance (Fig. 5.13D): in all of these, the feet are placed at a right angle to each other
3. the 'straddle' stance, in which the feet are rotated outward at the start, followed by simultaneous knee flexion to accentuate this external rotation (similar to Fig. 5.13B)

The force that can be generated with either leg may be decreased because of limitation of strength and/or range through which the leg can now be moved, with a reduction of the length of the possible lever arm:

1. The weakness of the right hip flexors and the decrease in right hip flexion can result in a decreased strength and range of kicks with a flexion component (e.g. the high right forward, or 'crescent', kick; Fig. 5.14Ai).
2. The weakness of left hip abductors and the decrease in left hip abduction and also extension range can result in a decreased strength and reach of any kicks with an abduction and extension component (e.g. a left 'spinning back' or 'roundhouse' kick; see Fig. 5.14B of a right one).

The ability to abduct the lower extremity is usually less on the left than the right, in part due to the increased length-tension ratio and left adductor 'facilitation' (Figs 3.43, 3.44). This could decrease the effectiveness of a left 'forward roundhouse' kick because the kick might end up being delivered low. The karateka can compensate by side-flexing to the right to elevate the left thigh further but this will be at the expense of stability as the centre of gravity is displaced to the right of midline (Fig. 5.14C).

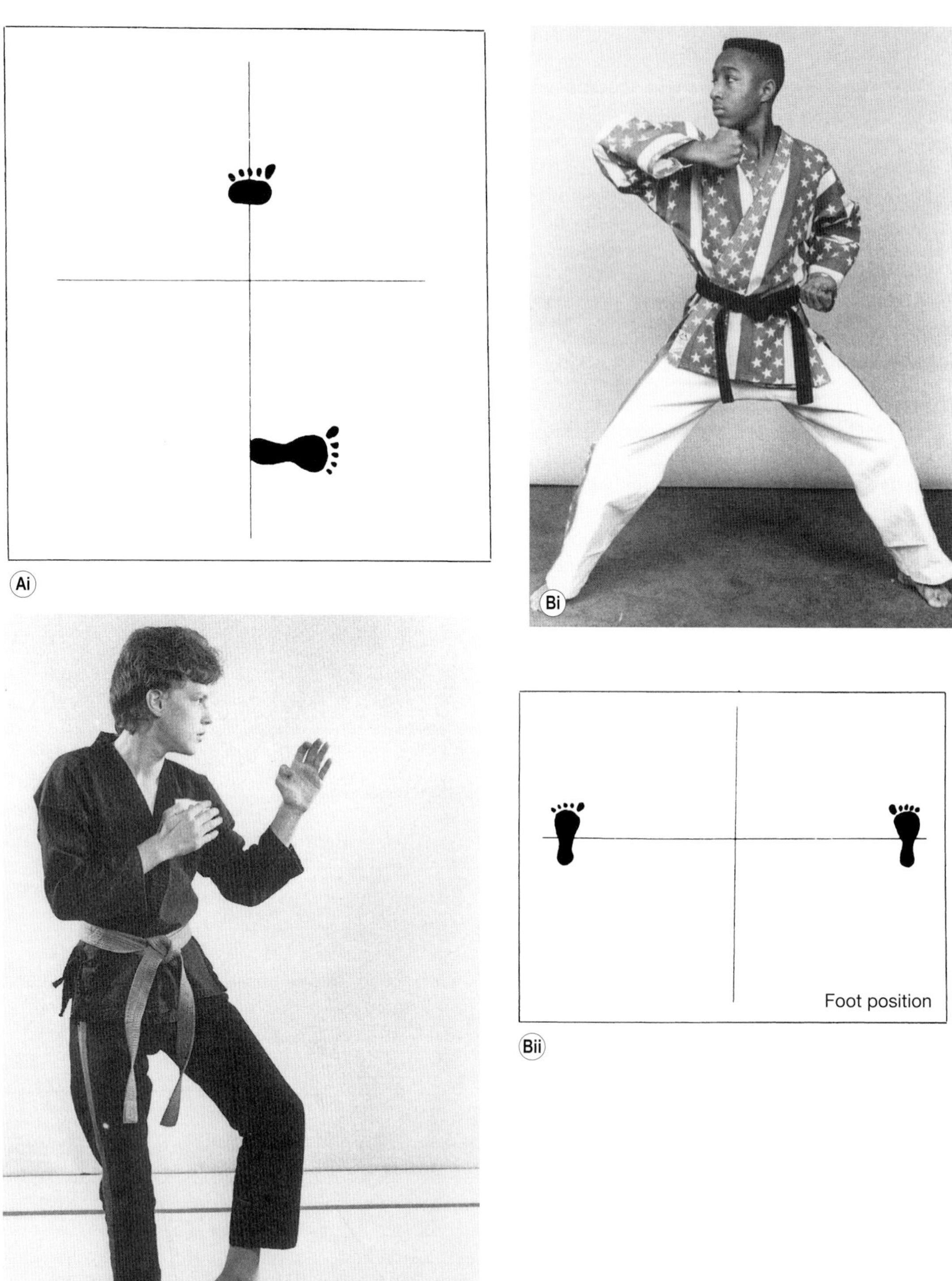

Fig. 5.13 Karate: typical positions and movements. (A) Cat stance. (B) Horse stance.

(Continued)

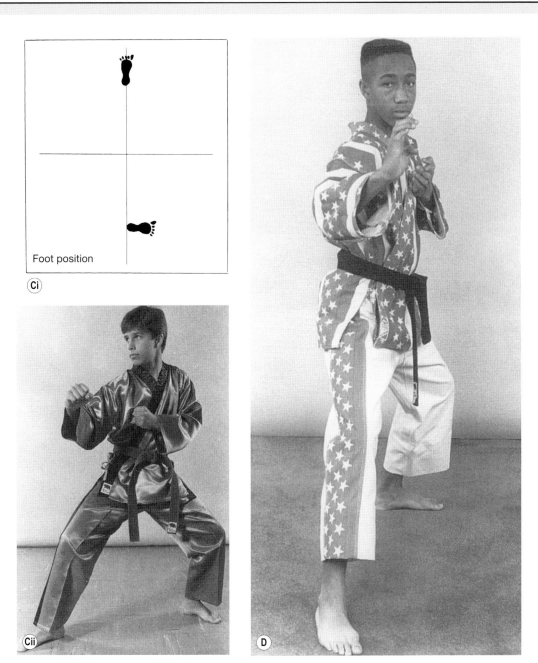

Fig. 5.13—cont'd (C) Back stance. (D) The 'lunge punch' from the front stance position. *(Courtesy of Queen 1993.)*

An impaired ability to externally rotate the left lower extremity may limit the ability to 'close the gap' properly in the right 'backward roundhouse' kick (Fig. 5.14B), which requires that the left foot rotate outward 90 degrees from its starting position (Hobusch & McClellan 1990).

Limitations of ranges of motion can decrease the effectiveness of the impact of a kick:

1. *in side-kicking*

   There may be difficulty striking the opponent with a small surface area, such as the lateral edge of the foot, because of a limitation of internal or external rotation of the leg and variations in the varus/valgus angulation of the non-weight-bearing foot (Fig. 3.26). The blow is more likely

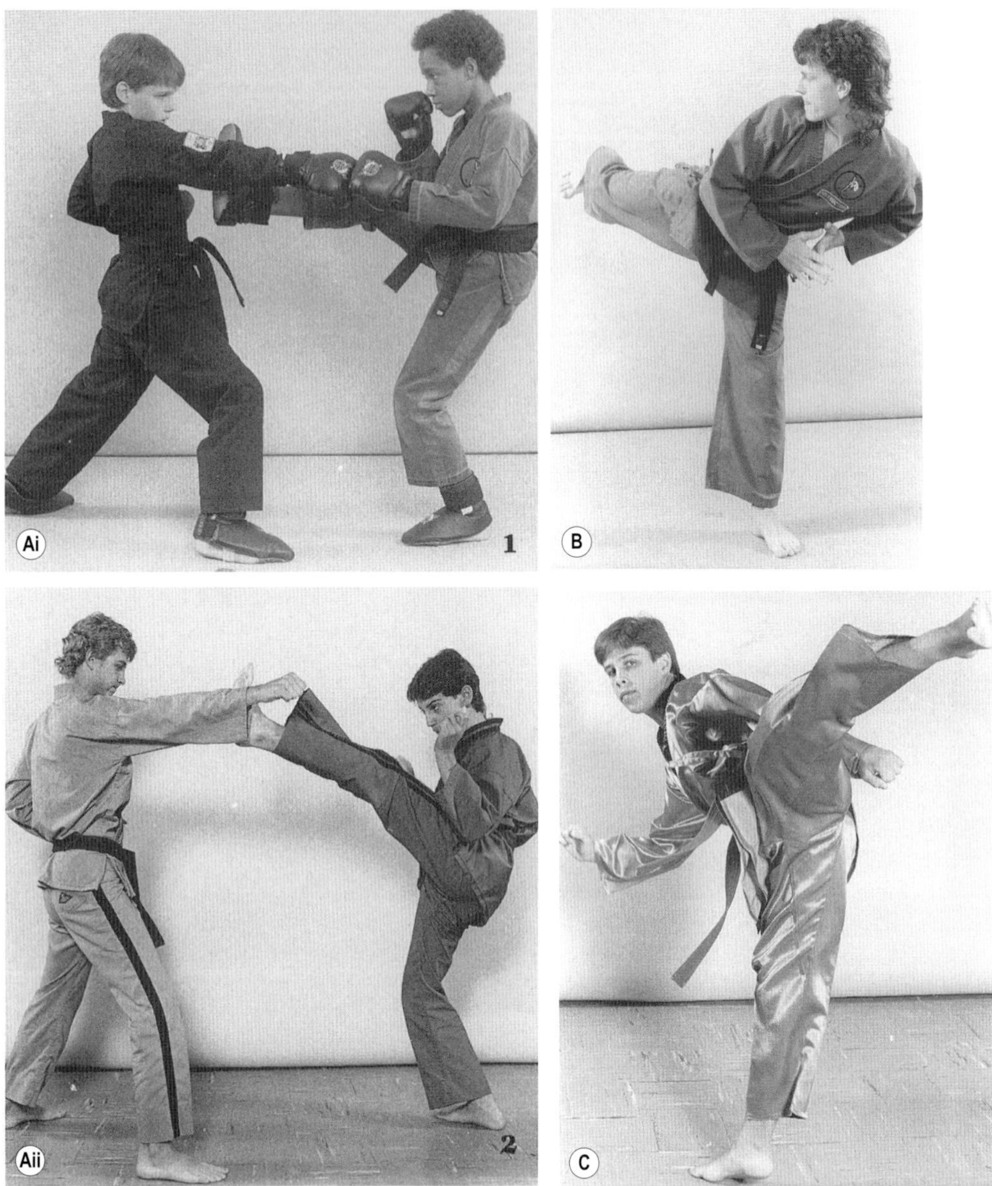

Fig. 5.14 Typical karate kicks. (A) Right (1) and left-sided (2) 'crescent' kick incorporating hip flexion (limited on the right side). (B) Right 'spinning back' or 'roundhouse' kick. (C) Left 'forward roundhouse' kick. *(Courtesy of Queen 1993.)*

to be delivered with the sole of the foot, which is less effective because the force is dissipated over a larger area. There is also an increased risk of fracturing the toes.

2. *a direct kick*

   Such a kick to the opponent's body should impact on the ball of the foot; that is, the foot is in maximal active dorsiflexion and may be passively pushed into further dorsiflexion on contact.

3. *a 'roundhouse' kick*

   Impact is with the dorsum of the foot and requires maximum active plantarflexion; the foot is forced into further plantarflexion passively on contact.

The malalignment-related limitation of plantarflexion on one side, dorsiflexion on the other (and of both dorsi- and plantarflexion on the side of a cuboid subluxation; Fig. 3.85A) may decrease the effectiveness of these kicks and increase the risk of injury by passively forcing the foot past the physiological and then anatomical barriers (Figs 3.84B, 3.85).

Instability when standing on one leg alone may be more noticeable on kicking, especially when using the *'forward'* or *'reverse' roundhouse kick*, in which the kicking action is combined with rotation to increase the force of the blow. The side of this instability may become evident with the kinetic rotational (Gillet) test or simply carrying out a one-legged partial squat (Figs 2.121, 2.122, 3.92A). Right single-leg stance is more often a problem and may relate to

1. the instability inherent to right pronation, tendency to right knee valgus, and weakness of muscles that would normally help control these
2. increased stability of the left leg, with 'locking' of the foot and ankle, more neutral alignment action of the knee joint and the muscles acting on it

The karateka requires a stable base when advancing and when delivering punches. As in fencing, advancing rapidly requires a quick forward movement of the foot and flexion of the knee on one side, combined with extension of the opposite hip and knee (Fig. 5.10). Maximum stability in the sagittal plane is achieved by having the right or left knee end up directly over the respective foot (Figs 5.10, 5.13D). Instability results with deviation of the knee to either side relative to the foot because of the:

1. inward or outward rotation of the leg, and
2. valgus or varus angulation of the knee, with a tendency toward pronation or supination, respectively.

Instability attributable to these factors is even more likely with leaping movements, both forward and backward, along the sagittal plane.

MARTIAL ARTS: JUDO

The intent is to throw the opponent off balance without losing one's own. Adrian & Cooper (1986: 629) pointed out that 'the weight is often maintained over the leading foot so that the rear foot can be quickly used for sweeping and for other attacks'. In the presence of malalignment, the stability of the lead leg will be decreased by the same factors discussed above for fencing and karate. Impaired balance is a factor to consider when weight is borne on one leg only.

In addition, the ability to use the sweeping leg effectively may be decreased by limitations of rotation. 'Right anterior' innominate rotation, for example, limits the ability of the right leg to sweep behind the opponent from right to left by:

1. decreasing the ability to internally rotate the fully extended weight-bearing right leg
2. limiting the ability of the pelvic unit to rotate counterclockwise around the vertical axis in the transverse plane, which would normally (i.e., when in alignment) allow the right hip and leg to swing forward with the pelvis on that side to gain some precious extra length for the sweep (Fig. 3.5C).

Also, the torquing forces used in judo to throw the opponent increase the chance of injury by inadvertently forcing the thorax, pelvis or legs into the direction of a restriction.

RUNNING

Problems relating to running have been discussed throughout the previous chapters, especially in regard to problems resulting from:

1. an asymmetry of weight-bearing, pronation and supination tendencies (Figs 3.22, 3.37, 3.81, 7.1)
2. contrary rotation of the legs; e.g. a whipping action of either heel, or 'clipping' of the opposite side (Fig. 3.21)
3. functional leg weakness, fatiguing and instability
4. an alteration of gait, including 'blocking' of swing-through on the side of an 'outflare' (see Ch. 3)

SCULLING, SWEEP-ROWING, KAYAKING AND CANOEING

These sports differ primarily in the amount and symmetry of trunk rotation, flexion and extension that occur from the 'catch' through the 'drive' and eventual recovery phase (Dal Monte & Komor 1989).

Sculling

The rowing action for single, double and quadruple sculls is symmetrical, and a similar action occurs when the athlete uses a rowing ergometer. The force generated by the extending legs and trunk is transferred to the arms and finally the oar. At the 'catch' - intended to put the oars into maximal working position - the trunk and legs are flexed and the arms extended; the scapulothoracic muscles, in particular serratus anterior, are maximally contracted, which helps to stabilize the scapula against the thorax. The 'drive' phase involves extension of the lower extremities, extension of the trunk and flexion of the upper extremities. Style is determined primarily by the timing and the degree of initial trunk flexion and final extension.

Malalignment will increase the possibility of restricting ranges of motion and developing back pain by:

1. increasing tension and often tenderness in thoracic (and sometimes lumbar) paravertebral muscles and posterior pelvic ligaments, thereby restricting forward flexion
2. increasing the stress on the now asymmetrical facet joints, sacrum and SI joints, restricting lumbosacral extension, flexion and pelvic tilt

Other complicating factors relating to malalignment include:

1. There is a functional inequality of leg length and strength, resulting in an unequal force through the feet on leg extension, asymmetrical strength pattern and shift in weight-bearing (right pronation, left supination)
2. Forward flexion can provoke pain by further increasing tension in other tender and/or tight muscles; e.g. the right hamstrings, which very often already show an increase in tension on account of 'facilitation' and length-tension changes with 'right anterior' rotation (Figs 3.42, 3.43).
3. Tender structures subjected to direct pressure will limit sitting time. Seat comfort varies with body proportions and seat design. Appropriate cut-outs on the seat help to avoid direct pressure on the ischial tuberosities and coccyx but may not spare a tender muscle (e.g. piriformis, gluteus maximus) or sacrotuberous ligament. The peroneal and tibial components of the sciatic nerve are also vulnerable to pressure on exiting from the greater sciatic notch, by (or through) a tense piriformis and into the posterior thigh region (Fig. 4.17)
4. Asymmetry of the ribs, rib rotation or even subluxation all increase the chances that the bellows-type effect on the chest cage will result in irritation of the costochondral junctions and costotransverse, costovertebral and clavicular joints (Figs 2.93–2.95, 3.15, 3.16).

Sweep-rowing

> The significant asymmetry involved in sweep-rowing results in specific injury patterns not seen in sculling as it involves considerable forward flexion combined with side-flexion and repetitive rotation into the side of the boat.

Complications with malalignment relate primarily to limitations of range in these directions because of tender or asymmetrically tight soft tissue structures, also an impaired rotational ability of the pelvis and the various segments of the spine, especially if there is a complicating rotational displacement of one or more vertebrae. The pelvis is relatively 'fixed' in the sitting position; the effect, therefore, is mainly on the thoracic spine and shoulder girdles. The compensatory curves and changes in muscle tension resulting with malalignment can, for example, easily limit trunk rotation into either the port or starboard side by 5–15 degrees (Fig. 3.49B).

Sweep-rowing also results in unbalanced muscle development and strength, particularly involving latissimus dorsi and quadriceps on the side of the rigger frame, an asymmetrical development which could well predispose to recurrence of malalignment after alignment appears to have been achieved.

Kayaking

In the typical recreational kayak, the double-bladed paddle allows for stroking on alternate sides in a cyclical fashion. The legs and pelvis are essentially fixed because of the low seating position and the fact that each foot may be stabilized on the hull or a foot pedal for rudder control, and the knees braced against the sides of the boat. In a flat-water kayak used for competition on lakes, there is no rudder and the knees are not braced when racing, so that the trunk is subjected to more intrinsic forces; whereas in whitewater kayaking – racing down rapids, a canyon or other natural challenge – the body is subjected to more extrinsic forces.

The cyclical paddling action in all events is primarily one of forward flexion, combined with alternate side flexion, and clockwise or counterclockwise rotation of the trunk around the vertical axis in the transverse plane. With the pelvis relatively fixed in sitting, most of this rotation occurs through the thoracic segment which, in the presence of malalignment, usually shows restriction into one side (Fig. 3.49B). The maximum stress will be through the transitional region for facet orientation: the thoracolumbar junction (Figs 3.9, 3.14). Pain is, therefore, more likely to develop in the mid-back region. Low back pain also occurs because there is some rotation of the lumbar segment as a whole once thoracic rotation reaches its limit, compounding the stress already imposed on the lumbosacral junction by the malalignment.

The increased demand for trunk rotation that is part of whitewater kayaking might be expected to precipitate back symptoms more readily than flat-water kayaking but the repetitive nature of the latter action, and the generally increased duration of ocean and river kayaking, can make these outings just as devastating. Factors that may prove complicating in any situation include:

1. the pressure exerted on tender sites (e.g. ischial tuberosities - the sacrotuberous insertion and hamstring origin - and the coccyx)
2. increased tension forces on structures that are already tender (e.g. the posterior pelvic ligaments and muscles such as piriformis and quadratus lumborum), exerted by prolonged or repetitive forward flexion and/or the repetitive trunk rotation
3. limitation of specific shoulder girdle ranges of motion is more likely to become a problem when kayaking:
    a. with a 'right anterior, left posterior' rotational malalignment, which typically involves limitation of:
        i. glenohumeral joint: left extension and right internal, left external rotation (Fig. 3.17A,B)
        ii. forearm: right supination, left pronation (Fig. 3.17C,D)
    b. movement in these directions occurs normally as part of stroking on alternate sides; problems can arise if the person needs the full range of motion to carry out a manoeuvre, in which case he or she may have to change style to prevent excessive strain on specific joints and soft tissues already compromised by the malalignment
    c. adaptive changes may include increased rotation and/or side-flexion of the trunk to make up for the asymmetry of upper extremity ranges of motion, at the cost of decreasing stroke efficiency and increasing energy expenditure

Canoeing

The positioning and combination of movements required in canoeing make the stroke the most asymmetrical of the ones described and, therefore, probably more vulnerable to the effects of malalignment.

Right-sided stroke

To carry out a stroke on the right side, the canoeist can kneel on both knees, right hip in neutral or some flexion, and weight-bearing on the left foot with the left hip slightly extended, knee flexed and foot anchored (Fig. 5.1). The stroke is initiated by reaching forward and outward, followed by a clockwise rotation of the trunk and pelvis reinforced by increasing left hip extension, and progressive extension of the trunk as the blade is driven backward. Restrictions seen with certain patterns of malalignment include:

1. a 'right anterior/left posterior' rotational pattern
    - restriction of left hip extension (and, hence, ability to extend the left leg fully) because of left posteroinferior acetabular rim impingement and increased tension in left hip flexors with the change in length-tension ratio
2. a 'right inflare'
    - restriction of further clockwise rotation of the trunk

Left-sided stroke

The canoeist will be kneeling on both knees, left hip in neutral or slight flexion, with the right hip extended, knee flexed and foot anchored. The stroke requires initial forward flexion and left side-flexion of the trunk, followed by counterclockwise rotation of the trunk and pelvis with progressive extension of the trunk and right hip, to drive the blade backward. Restrictions with malalignment include:

1. with a 'right anterior/left posterior' rotation, when driving the left blade backward:
    a. increased rotational stress on the thoracic segment because of limitation of left pelvic rotation in the transverse plane (Figs 3.5A, 3.49)
    b. increased stress on any tensed or shortened hip flexors as the trunk extends (Fig. 2.59)
2. with a 'left inflare': restriction of pelvic rotation counterclockwise

Even though sculling and kayaking may be symmetrical, these activities, along with sweep-rowing and canoeing, are all associated with an increased risk of having the athlete go out of alignment when:

1. getting in and out of the boat (Fig. 5.15A,B)
2. getting the boat into and out of the water or on and off a transport vehicle (Fig. 5.16A-D).

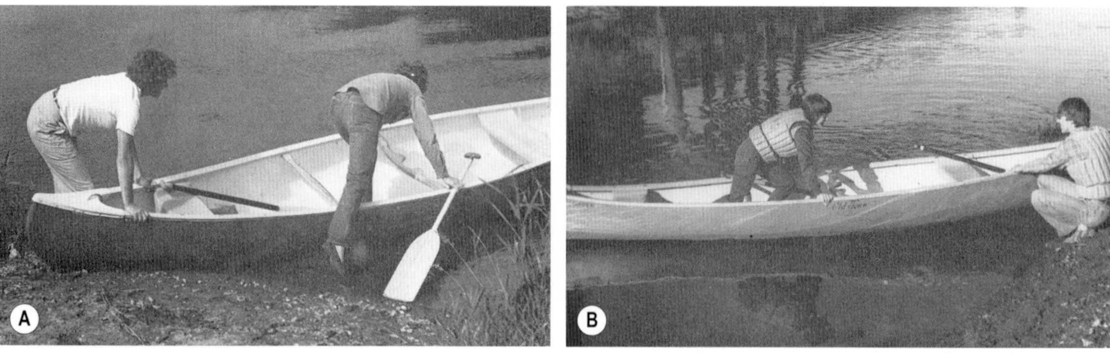

Fig. 5.15 Suggestions for steadying the boat and decreasing torsional stresses on getting (A) into or (B) out of the boat. *(Courtesy of Harrison 1981.)*

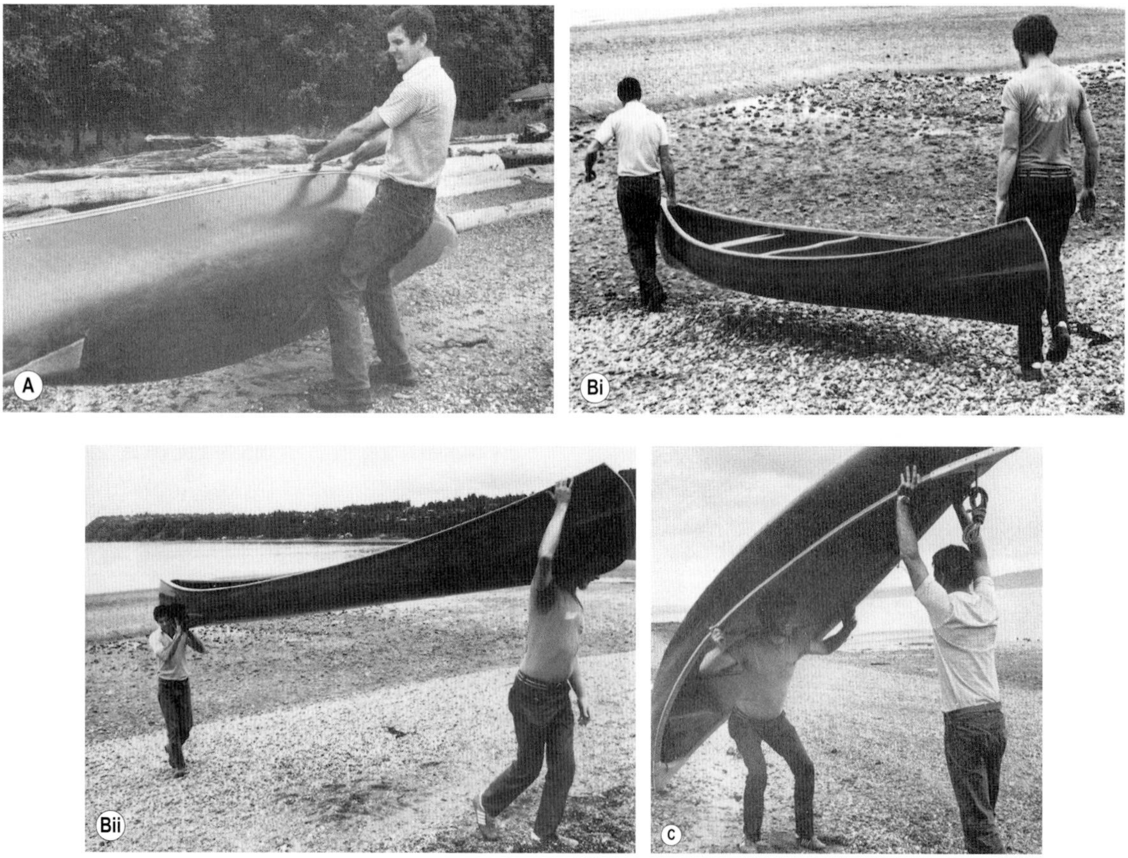

Fig. 5.16 Safe carrying and lifting techniques. (A) One-person carry over a short distance (minimal torquing). (B) Two-person (i) low and (ii) high carry (minimal torquing). (C) One-person assisted lift (no torquing).

(Continued)

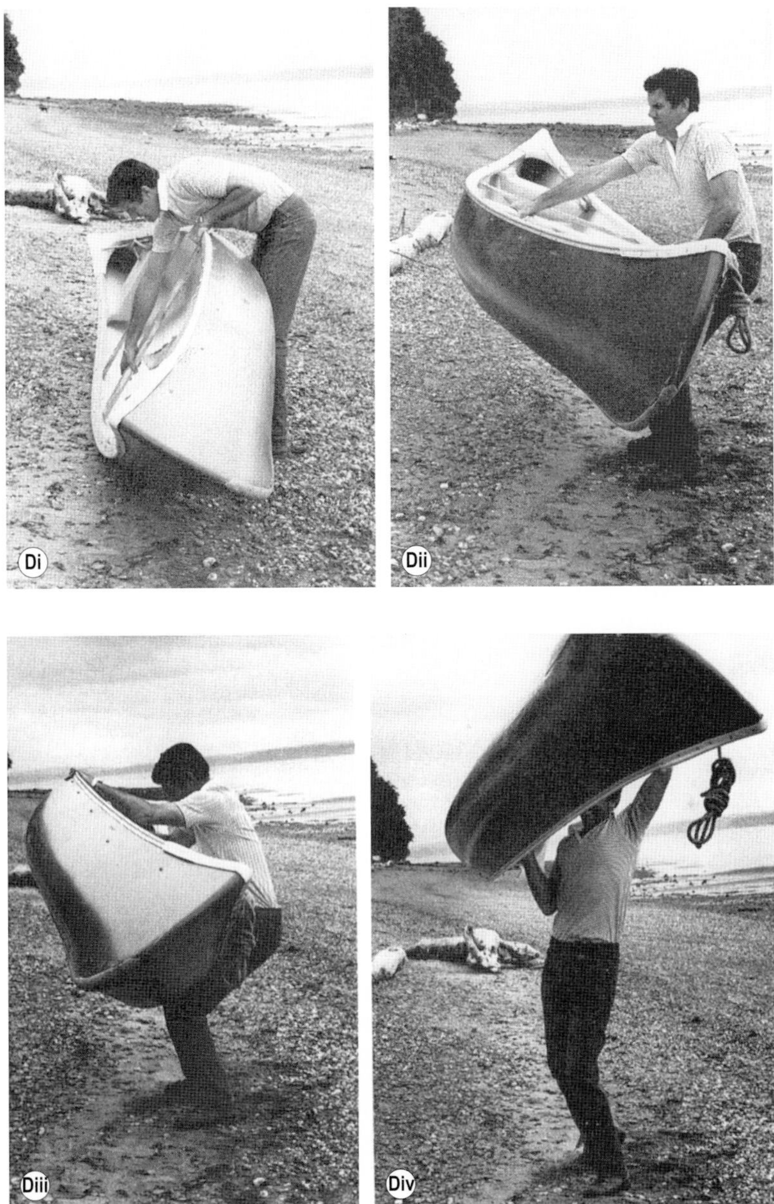

Fig. 5.16—cont'd (D) One-person unassisted lift (with considerable torquing). *(Courtesy of Harrison 1981.)*

The risk of losing alignment on these occasions can be decreased by having the athlete try to carry out the action symmetrically as much as possible (Box 5.6).

If malalignment recurs as a result of being unable to heed these precautions (usually for lack of help), or even when activity is limited to symmetrical sculling or recreational kayaking, the athlete should avoid these activities until realignment is being maintained and core strengthening has restored pelvic and spinal stability.

SKATING

The skater has to defy gravity while at the same time trying to balance the weight of the body over a thin blade. In the presence of

BOX 5.6 Techniques aimed at preserving symmetry when boating

1. Slide in and out of the boat: use the dock or side of the boat to sit on, or hang on to both sides of the boat at the same time for support while stepping in or out (Fig. 5.15A).
2. When arising from or sitting down on the seat: have someone steady the boat and hang on to both sides (Fig. 5.15B).
3. When getting into or out of the boat: if at all possible, avoid leading with one leg (which usually requires excessive hip flexion or extension, abduction, rotation or a combination of these); try, instead, to hold the legs together and move them as one unit while sitting on the dock or side of the boat (see also Fig. 9.1).
4. When alone and carrying the boat to and from the water: with the boat lying parallel to the water's edge, face the boat and pick it up with both hands as symmetrically as possible (Fig. 5.16A); preferable would be a two-person low carry (Fig. 5.16Bi).
5. When having to lift: try to get someone to help by simultaneously lifting the boat up on the other side or end in order to avoid as much torsional strain as possible (Fig. 5.16Bi,C).

malalignment, these challenges may become highly problematic.

Edges

There are basically four edges - inside and outside, forward and backward - and the skater has to be able to switch from one to the other quickly. Also, the more the lean of the body, the 'deeper' the edge and the less support is available from the blade.

These factors can make for a very insecure foot in terms of weight-bearing support and push-off stability.

> Edging is affected by any tendency to pronation or supination. The tendency to go either way is, in turn, augmented by the lack of a supporting base, any angulation and/or off-setting of the way in which the blade is fixed to the boot and the fact that the foot is elevated (and usually tilted forward) by the boot.

Falling inward or 'losing the edge' on the side of the pronating foot appears to be a more common complaint than toppling outward, probably because the neutral or frankly supinating foot is a more rigid foot, better suited for supporting the skater, for push-off and for 'holding the edge'. Any medial or lateral deviation of the knee from a position directly over the foot will further decrease stability (as in the case of fencing, judo and karate; see above and Figs 5.10B,C, 5.13D).

The combination of custom-made skates with medial or lateral reinforcement, and possibly longitudinal arch supports with or without posting, may increase the stability at the ankle and minimize such deviations of the knee. If, however, the tendency toward excessive and asymmetrical pronation or supination is attributable to malalignment, only realignment can be expected to resolve the problem completely, by:

1. putting the feet into a more secure and symmetrical position for weight-bearing
2. removing any resistance to controlled shifting onto the inner or outer edge

Executing turns

Turning is accomplished by shifting the weight onto the appropriate inner or outer edge. To make a left turn, for example, the skater can simply lean onto the left outer and/or right inner edge (Fig. 5.17). Malalignment, by affecting the ease with which the skater can shift onto a specific edge, will make it easier to make a turn into one direction. Whether this is to right or left may be predictable from the presentation of the malalignment.

Presentation: an 'upslip' or one ot the 'more common' patterns of 'rotational malalignment'

The associated tendency to supinate on the left and pronate on the right facilitates turning to the left; the skater is already predisposed to leaning onto the left outer and right inner edge. By the same token, the same skater may find it harder to execute a turn to the right because of the increased difficulty to shift weight onto the left inner and right outer edges. Biomechanically, making a left turn is like 'going with the flow'; whereas on attempting a turn to the right, he or she is 'going against the current', so to speak.

The right foot and ankle may, however, tend to feel 'sloppy', collapse inward and fatigue more readily than the left because of the functional weakness of tibialis anterior and posterior, and the

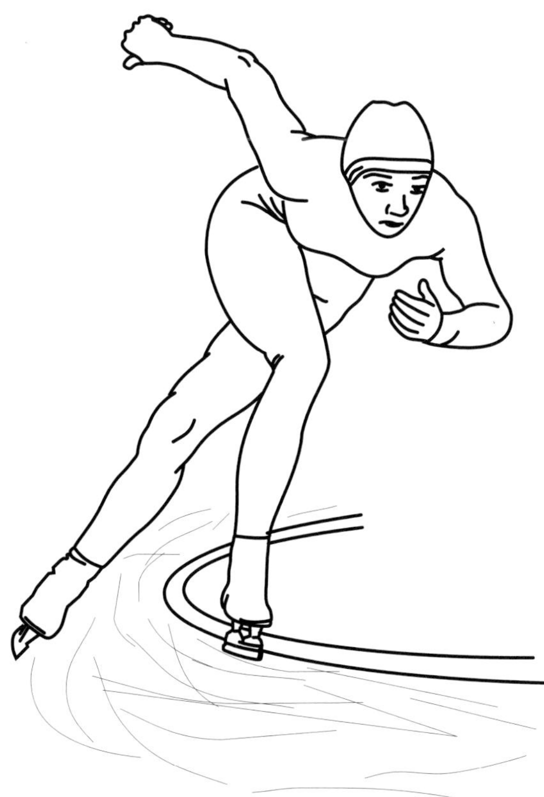

Fig. 5.17 Speed-skating: leaning inward to help push off from the right inner, glide on the left neutral or outer edge while the right and left leg are both in some adduction.

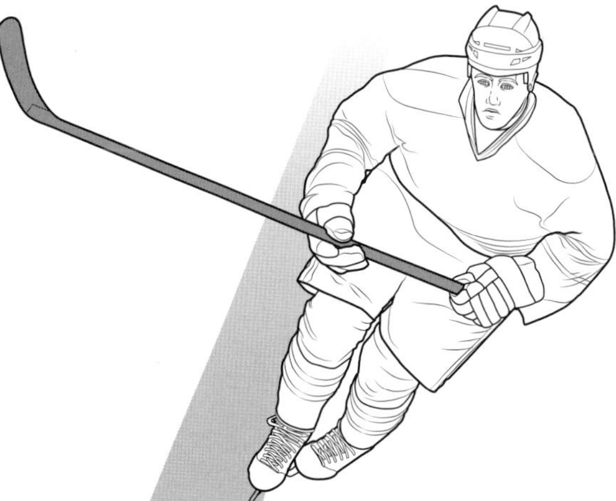

Fig. 5.18 Hockey player circling counterclockwise, leaning inward and weight-bearing on right inner, left outer edge of skate.

collapse of the medial longitudinal arch, so that the skater may prefer to put more weight on the more stable left foot and ankle.

If the same skater attempts to skate circles of a small diameter, such as in free-style figure skating or compulsory figures, the following might occur:

It will likely be easier to go counterclockwise
Counterclockwise circling requires alternately transferring the weight onto the left outer and right inner edges. The transfer from left to right is achieved by adducting the right leg to cross it in front of the left. This manoeuvre again demands getting onto what are already this particular skater's preferred edges, also for adduction of the right leg, which has a greater adduction range than the left in someone with one of these presentations of malalignment (Figs 3.44, 3.77). An 'upslip' and the 'more common' rotational patterns would also favour the speed-skater going counterclockwise around the track, especially when the right leg has to adduct across the front of the left leg while leaning to the left, into a curve (Fig. 5.17). Similarly, these same biomechanical changes would favour someone circling counterclockwise behind the goal or along the rim of a hockey rink (Fig. 5.18)

It will be relatively more difficult to go clockwise
Attempts to transfer weight to the right outer and left inner edge run counter to the tendency to 'right pronation, left supination' imposed by these patterns of malalignment. In addition, there is the restriction of left hip adduction relative to the right. The skater may try facilitating getting onto the left inner, right outer edge by leaning to the right, into the curve (i.e. toward the ice) but this comes at an increased risk of falling.

An exception to the above is an attempt to go counterclockwise supported only on the right outer edge
This is required, for example, on the 'back or backward outside eight' part of a figure-of-8 or as part of another configuration (e.g. 'camel spin'; Fig. 5.19B). Here, the skater with an 'upslip' or one of the 'more common' rotational patterns is at risk of 'losing the edge'; that is, attempts to stay on the right outer edge may eventually fail as the foot tends to fall inward. An astute 'pro' may notice that the right knee also falls inward the moment that the edge is lost. If both edges on the right skate end up contacting the ice, this constitutes a 'flat' which, in competition, results in loss of points.

Presentation: 'left anterior and locked'
This skater tends to pronate on the left and supinate on the right and may, therefore, find it easier to

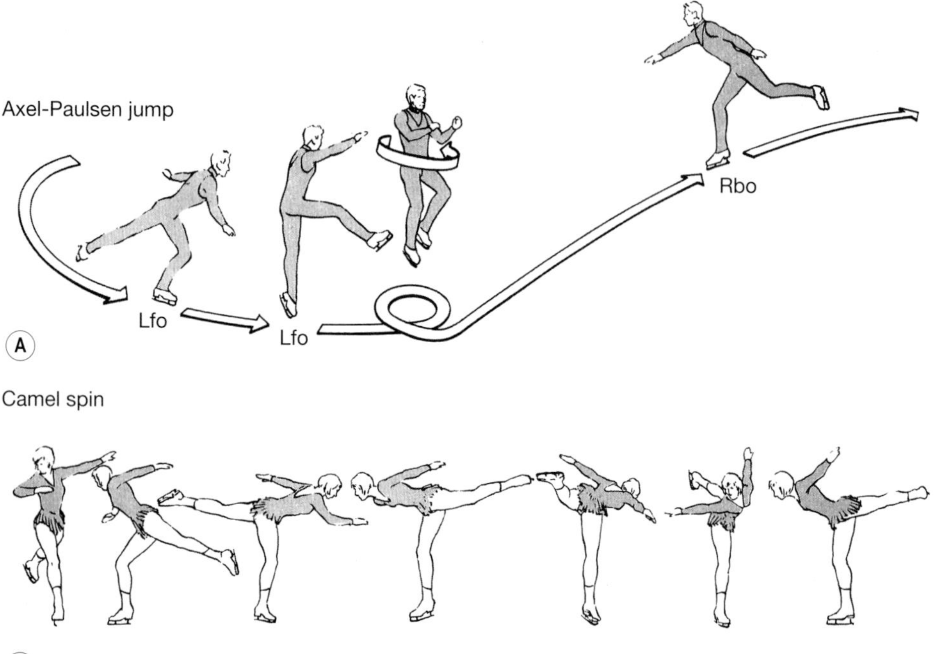

Fig. 5.19 Edging and weighting during typical ice-dancing routines. (A) Axel-Paulsen jump; note the weighting of specific edges (Lfo, left forward outside; Rbo, right backward outside) and the landing on the right leg after the jump. (B) A 'camel spin' (which incorporates the 'spiral') carried out weight-bearing on the right leg. *(Courtesy of Worth 1990.)*

execute circles clockwise rather than counterclockwise. The speed-skater with this presentation would be at a disadvantage when racing on a track in the usual counterclockwise direction.

Balance, take-off and recovery in figure skating

Figure skating has aptly been called 'a balancing act'. For those participating, progression depends, in part, on development of:

1. upper body strength, especially in males, to allow them to carry out lifts and throws
2. quadriceps strength, and
3. core strength to help maintain pelvic and trunk stability and control movement of the body in the air while carrying out any rotation(s) called for in a specific jump

The six common jumps in skating are divided into two groups:

1. toe jumps - the 'toe loop', 'flip' and 'lutz'
2. edge jumps - the 'salchow', 'loop' and 'axel'

The jumps are named for the take-off technique, since in all but the 'axel' the skater lands on the right back outside edge. For example, the 'axel' is an 'edge jump' that sees the skater launch off the front outside edge, carry out one or more loops (e.g. a double or triple axel) and land on the back outside edge of the opposite skate. Looking at one of the 'toe-jumps', the 'lutz', there is again an emphasis on edges: take-off is from a back outside edge, landing on the back outside edge of the opposite foot.

Needless to say, using the appropriate edges is one of the key determinants that allows the skater to carry out the compulsory short and long programs in figure skating.

The skater with an 'upslip' or a 'more common' rotational pattern may feel insecure when landing on one leg, more likely the right, as, for example, on completion of an Axel-Paulsen loop jump (Fig. 5.19A). The skater in the illustration takes off from the left outer edge, does a full rotation counterclockwise and lands on the right outer edge. On landing, there may be extraneous movements of the arms, trunk and left leg in an attempt to maintain balance because stability is decreased by the combination of:

1. losing the outer edge as the right foot tends to pronate
2. the right knee collapsing inward into valgus, away from its more stable position directly over the foot.

The biomechanical limitations imposed by malalignment can become blatantly obvious with some of these routines. Simply 'doing the splits' as part of a routine, legs either in abduction (= a 'horizontal split'; Fig. 5.21A) or in flexion/extension (= a 'sagittal split'; Figs 5.20, 5.21B), may become difficult because of asymmetrical limitations of ranges of motion, tense or contracted muscles and other changes attributable to the malalignment. Inability to carry out the manoeuvre without obvious effort or hesitation and to maintain symmetry and/or a specific posture can only lead to loss of points on evaluation. The 'spiral' itself calls for flexion of the trunk to horizontal, arms out to the side, gliding along supported on only one skate with the other leg extended in a horizontal position, in line with the trunk (Fig. 5.19B). The skater with 'right anterior, left posterior' innominate rotation doing the 'spiral':

1. will be able to raise the right leg further up in the air while supported on the left leg than he or she could raise the left while supported on the right leg, consistent with the increased amount of hip extension and ease of flexing the trunk to horizontal possible on the side of the 'anterior' rotation; the addition of right knee flexion may allow for a seemingly effortless performance, like the one shown in Fig. 5.20.
2. when attempting the 'spiral' supported on the right leg

   The 'left posterior' innominate rotation may interfere with the ability to bring the left leg to horizontal or higher by:

   a. the posteroinferior acetabular rim now creating a mechanical block to extension (Figs 3.71, 3.72)
   b. tightening up both left iliacus and rectus femoris by separating their origin and insertion even further (Fig. 3.42)
   c. limiting compensatory counterclockwise rotation of the pelvis around the vertical axis in the transverse plane (Fig. 3.5C)
3. will find it harder to flex the trunk to a horizontal position when supported on the right leg than on the left
   - when right weight-bearing, the pre-existing 'right anterior' rotation tightens right gluteus maximus, the hamstrings and the sacrotuberous ligament, thereby limiting forward tilting of the pelvis, so that any need for further controlled flexion now has to come more from the trunk itself

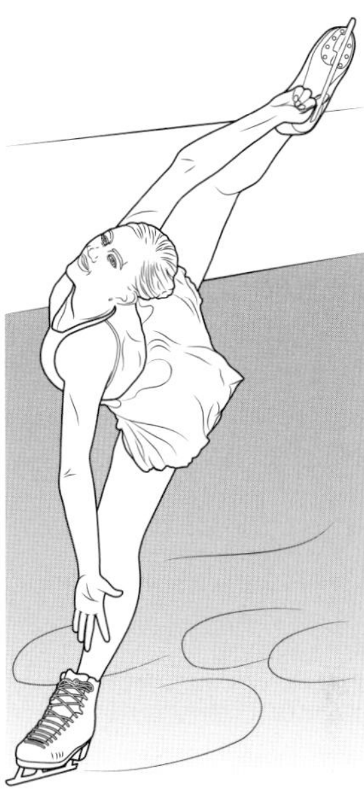

Fig. 5.20 Figure skater performing seemingly 'easy' spiral routine, which involves weight-bearing and balancing on left skate while maintaining the trunk in flexion to horizontal and right hip in full extension.

Balance is also more likely to be a problem with right single-leg support. Balance becomes progressively more precarious with routines that combine single-leg support, trunk flexion and cutting a circle. An example is the addition of a turn to the 'spiral' - known as a 'camel spin' (Fig. 5.19B) – which calls for staying on a specific edge throughout the routine. For a 'back inner edge', for example, the skater in the spiral position supported on the left leg would maintain the weight on the back part of the left inner edge.

> Because of the tendency to supination on the left, those with an 'upslip' or one of the 'more common' rotational patterns may lose that inner edge more easily and end up with what is called a 'flat', or even shift onto the outer edge of the left skate.

Losing an inner edge or going into frank supination results in a simultaneous increase in varus stress on the knee (Figs 3.37, 3.41C, 3.81). If the knee ends up no longer positioned directly over the foot, the stability of the left lower extremity will be compromised.

Malalignment, by affecting balance and edging, can only:

1. compound the difficulty of mastering the progressively more demanding routines, such as the 'triple axle' or 'quadruple toe loop', or combinations like the 'triple axle-triple toe loop'
2. increase the chance of a mishap occurring when attempting these routines, given that most require a high-speed landing on one blade – in most cases, the right back outside edge – as the body continues to rotate
3. interfere with recovery and increase the margin of error

Propulsion and speed

Because of the low coefficient of friction between the ice and the blade, propulsion in ice-skating is not possible by pushing the blade straight backward. As van Ingen Schenau et al. (1989) pointed out:

1. the blade has to be positioned at right angles to the gliding direction of the skate; this requires some external rotation of the lower extremity on the side pushing off
2. the smaller the angle between the push-off leg and the ice, the more effective the push-off; the angle is decreased by increasing the amount of abduction of that extremity.

The skater with an 'upslip' or one of the 'more common' rotational patterns, especially the speed-skater going around the track counterclockwise, may derive some benefit from the malalignment. The tendency toward right pronation, coupled with the increased ability to externally rotate and abduct the right lower extremity, should make it easier to position the right blade properly and to move onto the inner edge for push-off from this extremity. However:

1. **on the right side**
   a. The combination of pronation, functional weakness of the ankle invertors (especially tibialis anterior and posterior) and increased fatiguability of the right lower extremity may result in a feeling of weakness and instability that could affect right push-off unfavourably, especially in the longer distance events
   b. An 'anterior' innominate rotation will limit right hip flexion and hence right swing-through
2. **on the left side**
   a. The limitation of left hip external rotation, and usually also of abduction, plus an exaggeration of the tendency toward supination and the apparent weakness of peroneus longus, all combine to make it more difficult to get onto - and stay on - the inside of the left blade, diminishing the ability to push off from that side
   b. In the skater with a left 'posterior' rotation, left push-off may be further compromised by the restriction of left hip extension (i.e. in late stance phase) and the limitation of left counterclockwise rotation of the pelvis.

Increased velocity is associated with an increased forward inclination of the trunk, as seen in the tendency of speed-skaters to hold the trunk in a near-horizontal position. This is partly to counterbalance push-off but mainly to lower the centre of gravity and to reduce drag. van Ingen Schenau (1982) was able to show that the drag force increases by more than 20% with a vertical deviation of the trunk of only 20 degrees from the horizontal position. In the presence of malalignment, the ability to achieve the maximum forward inclination possible may be limited by:

1. right or left anterior innominate rotation, resulting in an ipsilateral restriction of hip flexion; e.g. 'left anterior' rotation results in decreased left hip flexion
2. an inability to tolerate any further increase in tension in posterior pelvic ligaments and the erector spinae, gluteus maximus and piriformis muscles, most of which are already under increased tension and may have become tender to palpation because of the malalignment.

Stopping

A stop is usually accomplished by digging in the opposite edges perpendicular to the line of progression. The skater with an 'upslip' or one of the 'more common' rotational patterns is already oriented to bear weight more easily on the right inside and left outside edges, which should make it easier to make a sudden stop with a quick turn to the left. Stopping by turning to the right may prove both awkward and ineffective in comparison. However, excessive right pronation and a feeling that this ankle is 'wobbly' or insecure may prevent the skater getting onto the right inside edge, a problem that is sometimes solved by:

1. using an orthotic that provides increased support under the collapsing right medial longitudinal arch
2. turning to the right instead, if that is felt to increase the stability of the right foot

The ice hockey goalie

Goalies frequently use their legs to stop the puck. Injuries are often blamed on lack of flexibility or on having had to elongate a muscle that has not yet had time to relax completely after having been activated for some other manoeuvre immediately preceding the one that caused the injury. Malalignment, by restricting some ranges of motion and increasing the tension in certain muscles and ligaments, is another cause to consider, especially if the goalie is subject to recurrent injuries. In that respect, structures especially vulnerable include the following:

Hip adductors and flexors

Quickly abducting one or both legs (e.g. doing the splits) can protect a large area of the goal crease and may block a sliding or low-flying puck but these manoeuvres risk tearing the adductors, pectineus and/or iliopsoas, and may even avulse the lesser trochanter (Figs 3.50, 5.21B). Left hip abduction is decreased and hip flexors tightened with the increase in internal rotation seen in the majority of those with malalignment, increasing the risk of injury on this side.

Iliopsoas

1. 'posterior' innominate rotation increases the tension in iliacus, 'anterior' rotation that in psoas minor, by separation of the origin and insertion of these muscles (Figs 2.59 and 2.62, respectively).
2. the tension in iliopsoas *per se* may be increased:
   a. in reaction to pain and/or an attempt by part or all of that muscle to stabilize the SI joint (Figs 2.46B,C, 2.62)
   b. through 'facilitation'
   c. by separation of the T12–L3 level transverse process muscle origin from its insertion, or
   d. passively, with internal rotation of the lower extremity

Piriformis

Tension in the right and left piriformis can be increased reflexively in a large number of those with malalignment to help stabilize the SI joint(s), also on account of trigger points (Fig. 3.45A). A tense piriformis is at risk of being sprained or strained if:

1. the muscle contracts to externally rotate the leg but that movement is suddenly blocked
2. the muscle is subjected to a further increase in tension by a manoeuvre that requires leg internal rotation, adduction, flexion or a combination of these

In a goalie with 'right anterior' innominate rotation, the ipsilateral piriformis is already put under

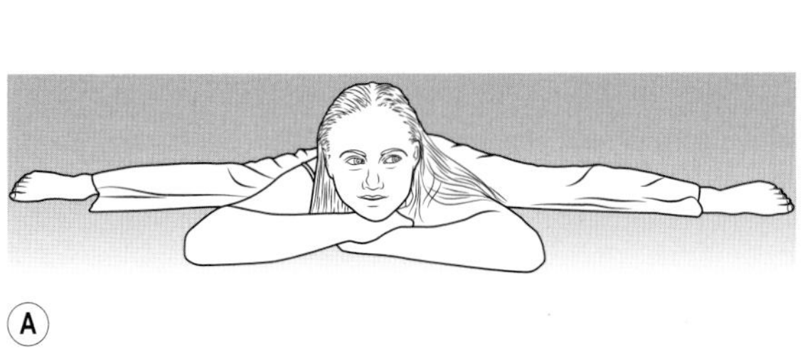

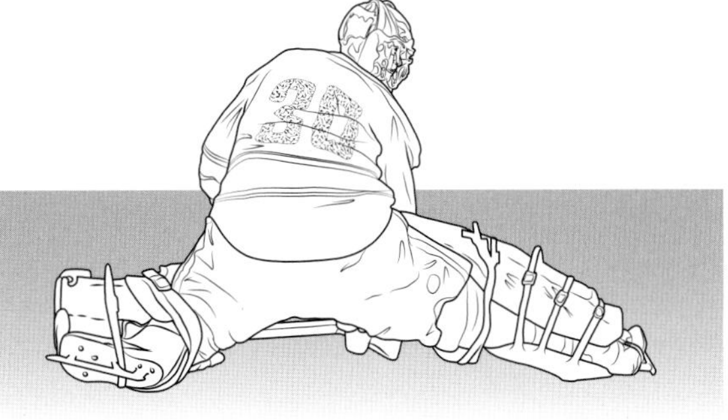

Fig. 5.21 (A) Gymnast with hips in full 180 degrees abduction in the frontal plane (= 'horizontal' split); (B) Goalie blocking low shot using a 'sagittal split'. Both positions stress the bilateral hip adductor muscles. The goalie's left thigh has been forced into internal rotation, increasing tension in the external rotator muscles, and the 'sagittal split' increases the risk of him suffering a 'rotational malalignment' with 'right posterior, left anterior' innominate rotation (see Chs 2, 3 and Fig. 5.29).

increased tension, limiting further right hip flexion, internal rotation and adduction and making that muscle more vulnerable when the leg is forced into any of these directions (Figs 3.71, 3.77 3.78B).

Hip flexors/extensors, and the sacrotuberous ligaments

Increased tension in gluteus maximus, hamstrings and the sacrotuberous ligament on the side of an 'anterior' innominate rotation puts these structures at risk in attempts to block a puck by kicking the leg straight out front or to the side, flexing the ipsilateral hip joint. The increased tension in iliacus and rectus femoris on the side of the 'posterior' rotation puts these structures at risk when kicking the left leg straight back, hyperextending that hip joint. A sagittal split would jeopardize these respective structures on both the flexed and extended side simultaneously. The ability to perform these movements would also be affected by an increase in tone that results with 'facilitation' of any of these muscles.

Pelvis, trunk, shoulders and neck

A goalie has to be extremely agile in order to move quickly from one side of the goal to the other, or to rotate to the right or left when standing, squatting or sitting in the goal crease. Any malalignment-related limitation of range of motion will interfere with this agility and increase the risk of injury. The areas listed in Box 5.7 are particularly vulnerable.

Undoubtedly, hockey players - even when in alignment - are at increased risk of having their trunk, pelvis or extremities moved passively into directions of restriction and past physiological and sometimes anatomical barriers on collision with other players, goal posts or the boards (Fig. 5.22).

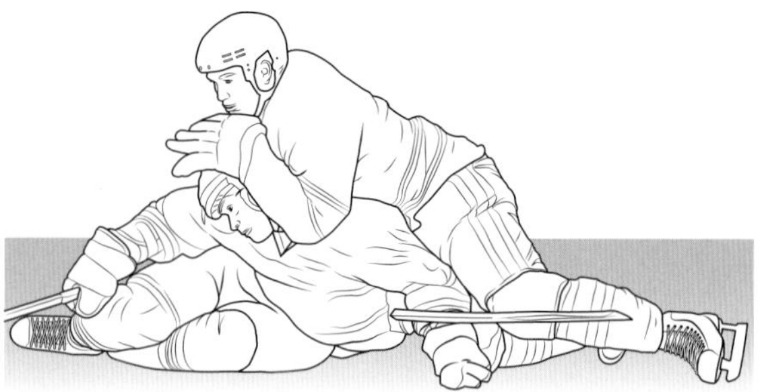

Fig. 5.22 Hockey and many other contact sports put the athlete's pelvis and spine at increased risk of being subjected to active and passive forces that can cause them to go out of alignment.

> Ice skaters and goalies, especially, are prone to suffering the complications of coccydynia and pelvic floor dysfunction from repeated falls onto the coccyx.

Also, a single incident of an SI joint shear injury, or repetitive microtrauma with repeated falls onto the buttock on the same side can result in eventual instability of that SI joint (Fig. 2.51). Given the increased potential for collisions and/or falls, skaters are also at increased risk of going out of alignment in the first place and encountering set backs in their attempts to achieve and maintain correction.

SKIING: ALPINE OR DOWNHILL

All boarding and practically all skiing events incorporate elements of asymmetry. In the aligned skier, torquing of the 'body's muscle and fascial systems [lead] to an imbalance in the length and strength

BOX 5.7 Ice-hockey goalie: body areas particularly vulnerable to injury with malalignment present

The trunk: especially on collision with a goal posts or other players, and even more so when the pelvis is fixed by sitting on the ice and trunk rotation is attempted (or forced) into a restriction (Figs 3.49C, 5.22)

The shoulders: especially on reaching attempts that require rotation into a restricted range or being passively forced into one of these directions; for example, in a goalie with an 'upslip' or one of the 'more common' rotational patterns, having the left arm forced into extension or external rotation, or the right arm into internal rotation (Fig. 3.17A,B)

The neck and back: pain may be triggered by having to assume an awkward stance for longer periods of time; for example, maintaining the hips flexed, trunk near horizontal and the head and neck extended creates a prolonged increase in stress in structures that are often already tender because of the malalignment: the paravertebral, erector spinae and other extensor muscles of trunk and pelvis, the posterior pelvic ligaments, and the sites of curve reversal and vertebral rotational displacement.

of the muscles and tendons...the soft tissues around the spine are always working dynamically in three dimensions...to protect from the forces of gravity and rotation' (Petersen 2009: 160). He goes on to say that 'few skiers make it through an entire season without experiencing some form of malalignment of the pelvis, spine and extremities, which can be an unrecognized cause of back and leg pain'. Malalignment can only increase the stresses already imposed on a skier who starts out in alignment. It also affects performance by creating unwanted stresses during the preferably symmetrical lead-in part of jumping events - ski jumps, freestyle and aerials - and the airborne phase of these and also boarding events. Difficulty making rotations and turns into one side, tending to veer off course, any increase in falls and injuries suffered should raise suspicions that an underlying problem of malalignment may be interfering with performance and enjoyment of the sport.

As described in Chapters 2 and 3, the malalignment:

1. can occur with an action that combines simultaneous side-flexion, rotation and flexion or extension of the trunk; in skiing, this could result from a seemingly simple motion (e.g. just leaning forward and side-ways to pick up the skis or a backpack) or when the system is subjected to a force (e.g. hitting a bump or taking an evasive action)
2. may result in acute pain (especially if there is an element of L4 or L5 rotational displacement) or pain that comes on gradually as inflammation increases in the injured tissues and from the stress on soft tissues and joints caused by the malalignment itself.

Alpine skiing events - Downhill, Super-G, Giant Slalom, Slalom, Super Combined - are one of the athletic activities that maximally stresses the ability of all body parts to move through the full available ranges of motion. As so aptly described by Luttgens et al. (1992: 572):

> *The movement problems encountered by the alpine skier revolve around changing directions and maintaining balance at high speeds while undergoing a variety of horizontal and vertical disturbances.*

Executing a normal turn

Turns are initiated primarily by a rotation of body parts, unweighting and transferring weight onto the appropriate edges. Almost any body part can be used to initiate a turn but the feet and arms tend to be the least effective because they are the farthest away from the centre of gravity. In addition, as indicated by Adrian & Cooper (1986: 672):

> *Arm and trunk rotations, initiated by movements at the shoulder, hip and spinal column will cause the skis to turn if the action is forceful enough. This necessity for force, acceleration, and large motions is a source of 'overturning' and loss of control.*

Rotation of the pelvis around the vertical axis in the transverse plane thus proves most effective for initiating a turn, given the proximity of the pelvis to the centre of gravity and the need for only a minimal displacement of this part of the body (Fig. 3.93).

As observed from below, the skier shown in Fig. 5.23A is initially travelling to the left and perpendicular to the fall line. He or she is gliding on the inner edge of the downhill (left) and outer edge of the uphill (right) ski, while putting more load on the downhill than the uphill ski. The edging is facilitated by leaning with the hips and knees into the mountain while the trunk is maintained in a vertical position or leans downhill, creating a right varus stress (outer soft tissues and medial patellar compartment) and left valgus stress (inner soft tissues and lateral compartment; Figs 3.37, 3.81). In order to execute a left downhill turn (Fig. 5.23B), the skier:

1. transfers weight to the inner edge of the uphill (right) and outer edge of the downhill (left) ski; this transfer is aided by leaning the body downhill, the combined effect being to:
   a. unload the downhill ski while at the same time loading the uphill one
   b. create a force toward valgus angulation of the uphill (right) and varus angulation of the downhill (left) knee
2. rotates the pelvis counterclockwise around the vertical axis in the transverse plane, which helps to initiate the turn by advancing the uphill leg and increasing the ability to weight the inside edge of that ski
3. progressively pivots through the turn, the uphill (right) leg from external to internal rotation, the downhill (left) leg from internal to external rotation; i.e. in contrary patterns

When the first half, or 90 degrees, of the turn has been completed, the skier will be facing downhill

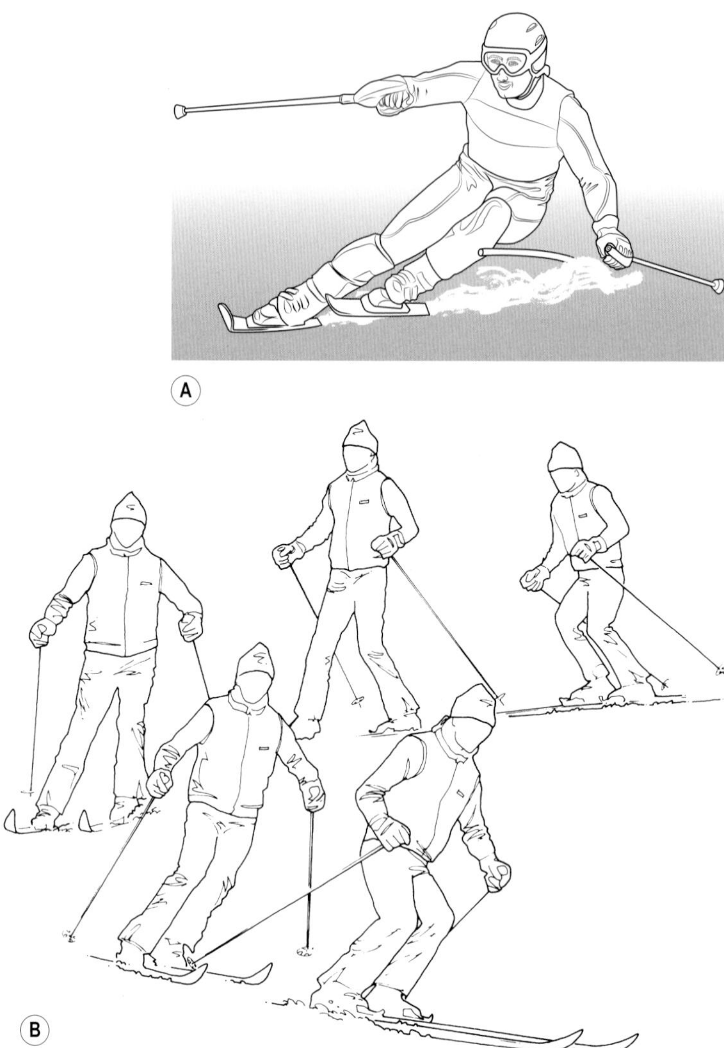

Fig. 5.23 (A) Edging is facilitated by leaning hips and knees into the hill while keeping the trunk vertical or even leaning downhill. (B) The basic 'stem turn' in skiing: proceeding initially perpendicularly to the fall line and then down the fall line and on around the turn. *(Courtesy of Parker 1988.)*

with the legs and trunk in alignment and weight equally distributed on both skis. If the skier decided at this point to head straight down the mountain, the pelvis would rotate clockwise back to neutral, facing the fall line. In order to continue the turn to a full 180 degrees, the skier has to:

1. maintain the forward rotation of the right side of the pelvis
2. help weight the inside of the right (now downhill) and outside of the left (now uphill) ski.

This weight transfer is aided by leaning the knees and hips into, and the body away from, the hill, thereby accentuating the left varus, right valgus angulation stress on the knees.

Effect of malalignment on executing a turn

Adrian & Cooper (1986: 674) rightly observed that 'human beings tend to be asymmetric; that is, they perform a turn more successfully in one direction than in the other'. They went on to state that 'leg dominance with respect to balance usually determines the preferred turning direction'. While 'leg dominance with respect to balance' may be involved, the chief determining factors in this author's experience relate to the presence of malalignment that affects:

1. rotation in/around the vertical axis in the transverse plane, with limitation into the side of a 'posterior' innominate rotation or an 'inflare' (Fig. 3.5C)
2. edging
   a. limiting the ability to get onto the right outer and left inner edge with an 'upslip' or one of the 'more common' rotational patterns
   b. the reverse limitations when the 'left anterior and locked' pattern is present.

The ease with which a turn is executed to left or right is influenced by several factors:

1. those presenting with a 'left posterior' innominate rotation will generally find it easier to turn to the right; those with a 'right posterior' rotation, to the left
2. the tendency to right or left pronation and supination on account of a shift in weight-bearing with malalignment, but this does not appear to be as influential as the limitation imposed on turning into the side of a 'posterior' rotation (Point 1)
3. limitation into the side of an 'inflare'
4. the ski boots themselves, especially rigid ones which may counter any tendency to pronation/supination, and stabilize the body on the skis
5. ability to compensate with the trunk/upper body and limbs, even though this may increase displacement of the centre of gravity and increases energy demands

Let us look at the difficulties that four different presentations of malalignment create for skiers attempting a turn.

'Right anterior, left posterior innominate rotation'

When attempting a left turn, there should be no problem unweighting the left (downhill) and weighting the right (uphill) ski, unless the skier is one of those athletes who has difficulty balancing on one leg (something that might become apparent on single-leg stance doing the kinetic rotational or Gillet test; Figs 2.121–2.125).

The weight is transferred more easily to the outside of the left and inside of the right ski, which should favour making a left turn. However, some athletes with an 'upslip' or one of the 'more common' rotational patterns report how the right foot feels 'sloppy' or 'insecure' even within the boot, how it is difficult to 'get an inner edge' on the right side and how the addition of a right medial longitudinal arch support increases the stability of that foot and ankle and allows them to dig in that edge more convincingly. A weakness of the right ankle invertors, combined with external rotation of the right leg and a tendency to right pronation, may account for this feeling of right foot and ankle instability.

Pelvic rotation around the vertical axis in the transverse plane is restricted to the left. The side-to-side difference can be appreciable: 10–25 degrees is not unusual (Fig. 3.5). In addition, the restriction of left pelvic rotation increases as the degree of 'left posterior' innominate rotation increases, and may progress to the point at which it becomes ineffective for initiating the turn. The skier may then accomplish the turn by:

1. transferring all the weight onto the left ski and literally 'hiking up' the right hip, in order to clear the right ski and allow the skier to rotate the right leg and attached ski internally by muscle action, in combination with
2. increasing left trunk rotation to compensate for the loss of left pelvic rotation, in an attempt to get onto the left outside edge

All of the above is occurring at a time when the skier is supposed to be unweighting the left ski and weighting the right. Needless to say, having to unweight the right ski to effect a left turn completely forfeits the benefits that would usually derive from transferring onto its inner edge.

Trunk rotation around the vertical axis in the transverse plane is typically restricted to the left, although restriction to the right can also occur and depends, in part, on the convexity of the thoracic segment (Fig. 3.49). Left limitation will decrease the ability to use trunk rotation to initiate or carry through a left turn, even though that would constitute poor technique.

> To compensate, the skier may resort to using the arms to help initiate and control turning; this, unfortunately, proves to be an even poorer technique in that it results in a greater displacement of the centre of gravity, further decrease in stability and an increase in energy demands.

'Left anterior, right posterior' innominate rotation; right sacroiliac joint 'locked'

The main problem with this 'more common' pattern is the restriction of clockwise rotation of the pelvis, which is likely to make it harder to use the pelvis to initiate a turn to the right and easier to initiate a turn to the left. There will also be restriction of left hip flexion, right extension which may cause problems especially with Nordic/cross-country and telemark skiing (see below).

'Left anterior and locked'

The tendency for the left foot to pronate, and the right to supinate, should be of help in digging in the appropriate edges to initiate a right turn. However, the associated limitations of left internal, right external rotation, and the decrease of clockwise rotation of the pelvis around the vertical axis in the transverse plane all become a hindrance to initiating and carrying out a right turn.

'Right outflare, left inflare'

The pelvis appears rotated clockwise, acetabulum forward on the 'inflare' side, with an increase of left swing-through and right stance phase range of the walking cycle, all of which facilitates a turn to the right. The reverse will occur with 'left outflare, right inflare'

Turning problems related to degree of malalignment

As indicated, the difficulty with turning into the side of the 'posterior' innominate rotation appears to be directly related to the degree of posterior rotation. The ability to turn in one direction can certainly worsen from one day to the next, or may even deteriorate as the day progresses, perhaps because of increasing posterior rotation and/or reactive muscle tensing. Other aggravating factors to consider include:

Tightness in muscles attaching to the innominate that are capable of exerting a rotational force

1. a posterior rotational force: e.g. from gluteus maximus and hamstrings at the back, external abdominal oblique and psoas minor at the front (Figs 2.32, 2.59, 2.62)
2. an anterior rotational force: e.g. from the rectus femoris, iliacus, TFL, quadratus lumborum and internal oblique (Figs 2.33, 2.36, 2.46, 2.59)
3. rotation in either direction may cause or aggravate an existing compensatory rotation of the contralateral innominate into the opposite direction

Unskilled turns initiated by excessive trunk rotation

Excessive trunk rotation at a time when the lower extremities are fixed can exert a rotational effect on the innominates:

1. *directly*: by way of the attachments of muscles (e.g. quadratus lumborum, latissimus dorsi and the abdominal obliques) and ligaments (e.g. the iliolumbar; Fig. 2.52A)
2. *indirectly*: by exerting a rotational force down through the lumbar spine, straining the lumbosacral junction and compressing the facet joint on one side to cause torsion of the sacrum (Fig. 2.52B).

Impact to the innominate bone

The direction of rotation that results from a direct blow to the innominate as a result of a fall or collision depends on whether the impact came from an anterior or posterior direction, and whether the force was applied above or below the inferior transverse axis or ITA (the axis of rotation of the ilia in respect to the sacrum, at the inferior aspect of the SI joint; Figs 2.50, 2.51).

Leverage effect on the innominate

A fall or collision can easily turn the lower extremities into levers capable of effecting innominate rotation: anterior with inadvertent hyperextension posterior with forced hip flexion (Fig. 2.47).

Simultaneous 'inflare' on the side of an innominate 'posterior' rotation

For example, the skier with a 'left inflare' and/or 'left posterior' rotation may note that turns to the right can be carried out with increased ease and speed, and at a more acute angle, if necessary. In contrast, turns to the left are harder to execute, tend to take more time and are less acute. At worst, the skier literally lifts the right leg and twists the body into the direction of the left turn.

Whenever these limitations become apparent, the skier should carry out a self-assessment and proceed with the appropriate self-treatment technique(s) if malalignment is indeed present (see Chs 7, 8), in the hope of allowing for an immediate return to unhindered skiing. Alternatively, a trip to the foot of the slope right there and then to see someone skilled in manual therapy might prove worthwhile. Correction will certainly make for a better day of skiing in that it should again allow turns to be carried out with equal ease, speed and ability to lean into either side, as well as decrease the risk of further injury.

Problems 'getting a good edge'

Skiers are acutely aware of side-to-side differences in the ability to fit comfortably into a boot and to dig in the inner and outer edge. Unfortunately, they often go on to make modifications by trial and error on their own.

The following comments apply also to Nordic and cross-country skiing and telemarking.

One common complaint is that of feeling a weakness of the ankle, with an inward collapse of the foot. Skiers may use terms such as 'pronation', a problem they may counter by using either a medial inside arch support or a build-up under the binding. Skiers who supinate bilaterally may feel an improved ability to get onto the inner edge by adding a lateral raise under the binding. For those with an 'upslip' or one of the 'more common' rotational patterns, the tendency toward supination may be quite obviously accentuated on the left, so that they may end up with a left lateral raise only, or one on the left that is higher than the one on the right side.

The binding on one side may be fixed facing outward in an attempt to accommodate an increased tendency toward external rotation of that leg, typically on the right side in those with an 'upslip' or a 'more common' rotational pattern (Fig. 5.24B). Provided that the amount by which the binding is rotated outward exactly matches the external rotation of the leg:

1. it may help to minimize stresses at the ankle and knee that would otherwise result from a mismatch
2. the foot, ankle and knee may not feel more stable but there may be a relief of the discomfort previously felt on the lateral aspect of the foot; this is in contrast to the cyclist who has rotated the toe clip inward in the search for increased comfort, stability and ability to generate power with that leg (see 'Cycling' above)
3. it will do little else to counter the other stresses relating to the malalignment (e.g. on the pelvis and spine).

In other words, the skier may be able to make some changes that decrease discomfort caused by the malalignment. However, failure to actually correct the malalignment leaves him or her at risk of incurring long-term unwanted biomechanical changes and injury.

If the binding is maintained in a neutral position (sagittal plane), so that the boot points straight forward (Fig. 5.24Ai), or if the amount by which the binding is offset outward fails to match the external rotation of the leg exactly, and given that movement of the foot and ankle is usually limited by the boot, any persistent tendency for the leg to rotate outward:

1. will accentuate the tendency to external rotation of the femur relative to the tibia (which is now more or less 'fixed' at the tibio-talar joint by the boot), genu valgum (with increased stress on the medial structures; e.g. MCL) and pressure on the lateral femoral joint compartment (Figs 3.37, 3.81)
2. may result in a pressure feeling along the lateral aspect of the foot, particularly the forefoot, as it tries to rotate outward but is restrained by the boot
   a. this pressure sensation may be aggravated by the addition of an orthotic made to counteract the tendency to pronation: by raising the medial longitudinal arch or adding a medial posting (especially to the forefoot section), the orthotic shifts weight-bearing laterally and encourages further external rotation of that leg, thereby increasing the pressure exerted by the boot against the lateral part of the foot
   b. provision of an orthotic with a lateral raise of the forefoot may relieve the pressure on the outside of the foot but, unfortunately, accentuates the forces tending to pronation, knee valgus and lateral tracking of the patella.

The initial temptation is often to offset both bindings outward, usually to the same degree. In someone with an 'upslip' or one of the 'more common' rotational patterns, whose left leg has actually rotated inward (sometimes to the point at which the foot now points straight ahead or may even have crossed the midline; Fig. 3.19Bii), offsetting the binding outward on the left side will create a counter-rotational force:

1. There will now be increased pressure against the medial aspect of the left forefoot as the leg tries to turn inward. This pressure may be alleviated

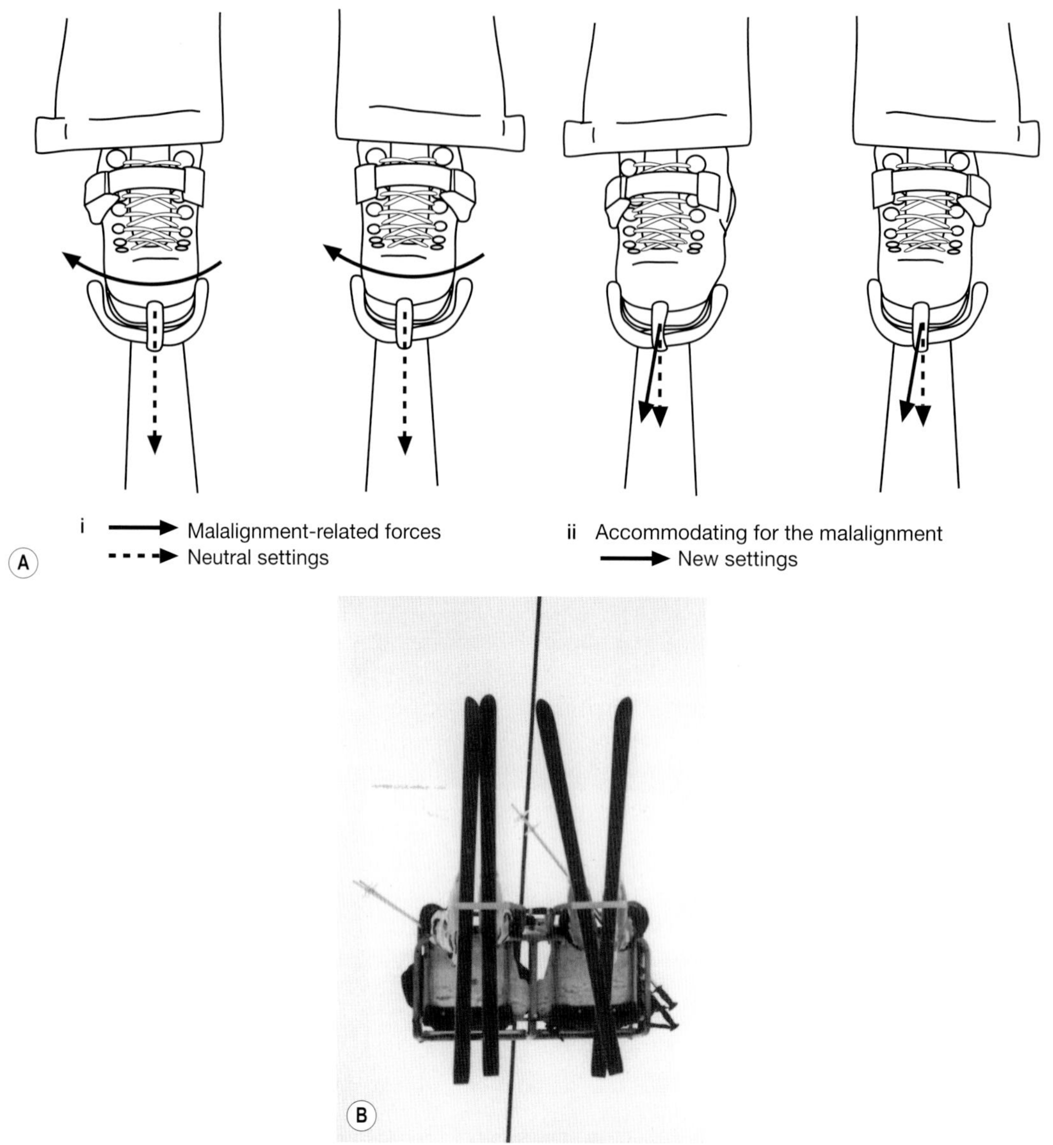

Fig. 5.24 Typical manifestations of a malalignment-related tendency to right external, left internal rotation in skiing. (A) The ski bindings have been offset outward from the midline on the right and inward on the left in (ii) to accommodate for the increased stress exerted on the right lateral and left medial foot in (i) as the legs attempt to rotate within the boot. (B) When riding the lift: malalignment is probably present in the skier sitting in the left seat (appearance from below), where right ski (leg) is turned outward relative to the left. The skier in the right seat is more likely to be in alignment, with both skis pointing in the same direction.

with an orthotic to 'counter pronation'. An orthotic that shifts weight-bearing laterally would, however, further increase the rigidity of a foot that is often already in a neutral to supinated position.

2. There will be a residual varus stress on the knee as the femur attempts to rotate inward relative to the 'fixed' tibia. The skier may complain of symptoms related to stress on lateral joint line soft tissues (e.g. LCL) and the medial femoral compartment.

The ongoing need for any modifications that have already been made to skis, orthotics, bindings or boots must be reassessed following the correction of the malalignment.

Weight-bearing and lower limb orientation may change dramatically with realignment, so that the biomechanical effect of any prior provision with orthotics or modifications to skis, bindings or boots may now:

1. be completely inappropriate if they are left in place
2. actually cause malalignment to recur

Problems relating to 'getting' a good inner or outer edge are also influenced by the inherent weight-bearing pattern (neutral, or a tendency to bilateral pronation or supination) and the alignment of the lower extremities (neutral, genu valgum with compensatory pronation, genu varum with a tendency toward supination, or external or internal rotation). Following realignment, these factors have to be reassessed and accommodated for, as indicated (Fig. 3.33). Once alignment has been achieved, a good approach is to:

1. have the person put on the boots and stand comfortably on the skis; attach bindings accordingly
2. if it seems advisable, insert off-the-shelf orthotics to provide symmetrical medial arch support; subsequently make modifications to these orthotics if these seem indicated (e.g. medial posting to counter excessive pronation, lateral forefoot posting to shift weight-bearing medially and relieve pressure on a Morton's neuroma)
3. next, consider providing custom orthotics incorporating any or all of these trial modifications, if they were deemed helpful; remember, a semi-rigid model will absorb more shock but may allow more movement within the boot than a rigid one

Knowing whether or not the skier is in alignment may be helped by observing the orientation of the skis on the next ride up on the lift: are both pointing forward or outward by the same amount, or is one rotated outward relative to the other (Fig. 5.24B). If malalignment is suspected, the first step is to confirm this; establish the type of presentation on hand, proceed with realignment and a trial of maintaining alignment for a few weeks before making any further changes to skis, bindings or orthotics.

Difficulty weight-bearing on one lower extremity

The skier may describe a feeling of weakness, insecurity or imbalance when weight-bearing on one leg alone.

Alpine, cross-country and telemark skiers often end up, unexpectedly, having to place most or all of their weight on one ski for short distances. How they fare when that happens to be the 'insecure' leg depends in part on their level of skill, the speed at which they are travelling and the difficulty of the terrain. The problem may be attributable to malalignment, in which case the effectiveness of realignment can be easily ascertained.

Preference for attempting a sudden stop

A sudden stop, which Parker (1988: 52) appropriately referred to as a 'hockey stop', entails 'a rapid two-footed twisting and resultant two-footed skid', the skis ending up parallel to the fall line but the skier still looking downhill (Fig. 5.25). In other words, the pelvis rotates with the skis; whereas the trunk continues to face the fall line to a varying degree. This rotation occurs around the vertical axis in the transverse plane, with trunk rotation primarily through the thoracic segment and in a direction opposite to pelvic rotation.

For most skiers, the combination of impaired rotation of the pelvic and thoracic segment to one or other side, difficulty getting an edge and perceived weakness on one side makes it consistently easier to accomplish such a quick stop by preferentially turning to either the right or left. The main determining factors appear to be those listed in Box 5.8.

The skier is at increased risk of injury at times when fellow skiers or the terrain prevent the quicker, and usually more stable, turn into the preferred direction for stopping. For those in competitive ski events, the combination of problems relating to turning preference and the asymmetry of turning, getting an edge and lower extremity strength and balance, assumes more significance as a potential cause of poorer performances and injuries.

The ability to squat, crouch or assume a 'lunge' position in order to reduce drag may be hampered, especially by:

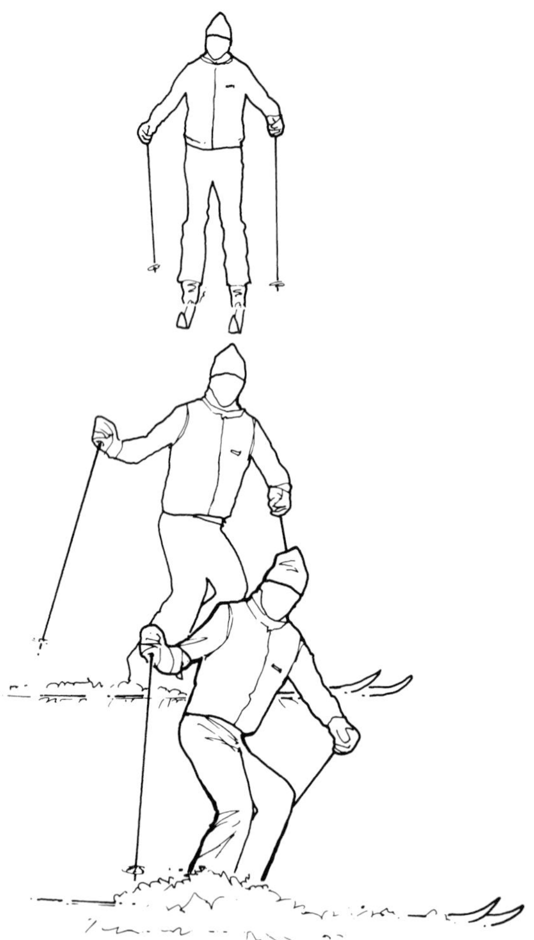

Fig. 5.25 'Hockey-stop' on skis. *(Courtesy of Parker 1988.)*

1. an inability to tolerate a sustained increase in tension on tender posterior pelvic ligaments and muscles
2. restrictions imposed by innominate rotation, especially a restriction of hip flexion with an 'anterior', hip extension with a 'posterior' rotation (Figs 3.71A, 3.72B,C, 3.76B)
3. pressure on a tender/swollen iliopsoas, pectineus, bursa or acetabular rim, with groin pain on attempted hip flexion

SKIING: NORDIC OR CROSS-COUNTRY AND TELEMARK

Differences between the various styles relate primarily to the method of achieving propulsion and making turns.

Traditional Nordic and track skiing

Propulsion is usually achieved using an alternating stride pattern, the most common being the diagonal stride, in which pole action is coupled with a backward thrust of the opposite, trailing ski. This thrust is produced by rapid hip extension with terminal plantarflexion of the foot and results in the forward gliding action of the lead ski. Speed is determined, in part, by the following.

The strength of the backward thrust

With an 'upslip' and 'right anterior/left posterior' innominate rotation, the strength of the push-off thrust could be decreased on either side as a result of:

1. any ankle weakness and instability, such as occurs on the right with an increased tendency toward right pronation and external rotation
2. a limitation of left ankle dorsiflexion (Fig. 3.84A), which has been associated with a decrease in plantar flexor peak torque (Mueller et al. 1995)
3. functional weakness and increased fatiguability of the muscles acting on the ankles and feet, in particular the left peroneal muscles, and the right tibialis anterior and posterior and extensor hallucis longus

BOX 5.8 Factors that affect the ability to carry out a 'hockey-stop' in skiing

1. The ability of the pelvis to rotate in the transverse plane is limited into the direction of a 'posterior' innominate rotation or an 'inflare' (Fig. 3.5C).
2. In some, the ability to dig in the more 'secure' edges may be a more important factor. The 'more common' rotational pattern of 'right pronation, left supination' should make it easier to dig in the right inner and left outer edges, respectively. This pattern, especially when combined with a 'left anterior' innominate rotation would allow for increased pelvic rotation counterclockwise, may make it easier to complete a left turn.
3. If, however, the pronating right ankle feels weak and insecure, the skier may prefer to get onto a more secure right outer edge and turn to the right instead; 'right anterior' rotation and also a 'right outflare' will facilitate turning in this direction.

4. cuboid subluxation, causing unilateral limitation of dorsi- and plantarflexion, calcaneal inversion and eversion
5. limitation of left hip extension by the backward displacement of the posteroinferior acetabular rim with 'left posterior' innominate rotation

Stride length

Stride length will be influenced by the asymmetry of hip and ankle ranges of motion and any limitations imposed by the innominates. On the left side, for example:

1. left hip extension is decreased by 'left posterior' rotation (Figs. 3.71, 3.72)
2. left hip flexion is impaired by 'left outflare' (obstructing left swing-through; see 'Outflare-inflare', Ch. 3)
3. the concurrent limitation of left ankle dorsiflexion seen in those with an 'upslip' or one of the 'more common' patterns of 'rotational malalignment' (Fig. 3.84A).
4. as weight is transferred to the left forefoot in preparation for push-off, further stretching of the already tight calf muscles and plantar fascia engages the 'windlass' mechanism prematurely and results in earlier, accelerated plantarflexion of that ankle

In an attempt to compensate for the limitation of left hip extension, the skier may try actively to exaggerate left plantarflexion in order to increase the leg length on push-off. Active counterclockwise rotation of the pelvis around the vertical axis in the transverse plane will also increase left leg length to help even out the stride length but this thoracic/pelvic range is already limited in those with 'left posterior' innominate rotation or a left 'inflare'. Either way of dealing with the asymmetry means more work and an increase in energy expenditure.

Problems on turning are primarily related to difficulties in getting an inside or outside edge, and restrictions of pelvic and trunk rotation, similar to those discussed above for downhill skiing.

Ski-skating: 'marathon' and 'V-skate' stride

These are two common skating strides used in cross-country skiing. The marathon skate stride is accomplished with the thrust coming from only one lower extremity while the other glides in a track (Fig. 5.26A); whereas with the V-skate the thrust comes alternately from one and then the other leg

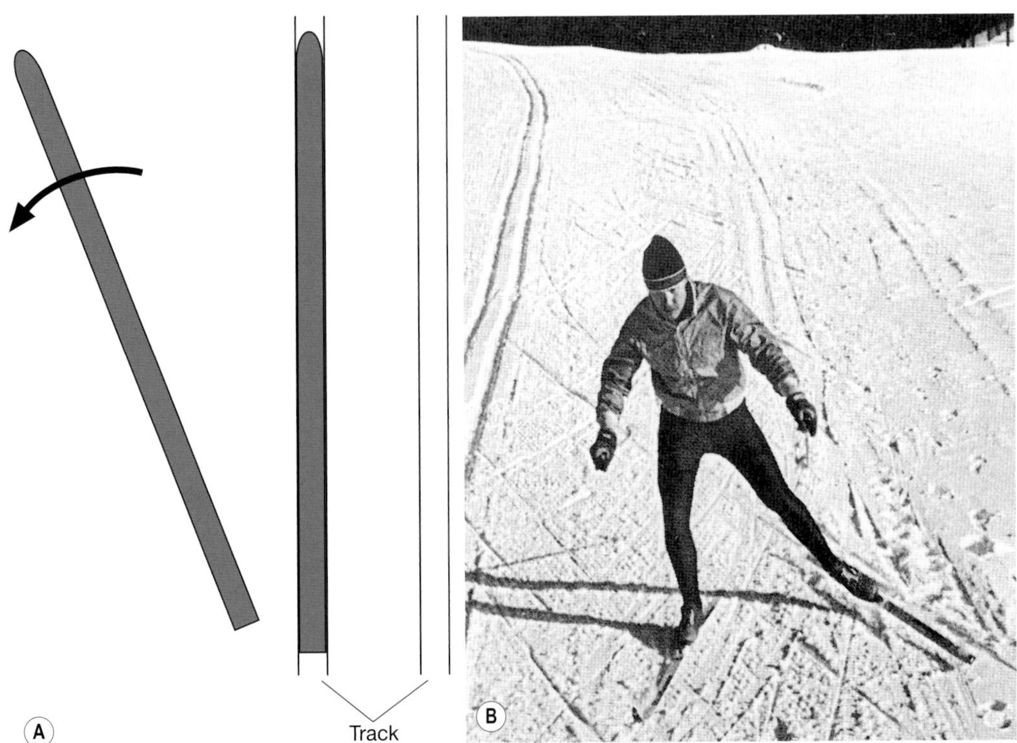

Fig. 5.26 Ski-skating: (A) Marathon skate stride; (B) V-skate stride. *(Courtesy of Matheny 1989.)*

(Fig. 5.26B). In both methods, the rear or thrust ski is angled at approximately 30 degrees to the direction of the glide (Watanabe 1989).

The skier with an 'upslip' or one of the 'more common' patterns, for example, is affected by the limitation of left hip abduction and external rotation, as well as the tendency to left supination, all of which make it more difficult to angle the left ski outward to 30 degrees and get onto the left inner edge. There is also the functional weakness of peroneus longus. As a result, the left push-off thrust may be decreased compared with the right and there is an increased risk of suffering a left calcaneal inversion sprain.

With the 'left anterior and locked' pattern, the tendency to inward collapse of the left foot and ankle (pronation), and an increased ability to rotate that extremity outward, may make it easier to get onto the left inner edge, while making these same manoeuvres more difficult on the right side.

Telemarking

A turn to the right can be initiated from the 'half-wedge' position, where the right (inside) ski points straight and the left is wedged, or pointed inward, by a slight internal rotation of the left leg (Parker 1988: 34; Fig. 5.27). Although most of the weight remains on the straight-running right ski, 'the pressure that develops on the wedged ski initiates a slight direction change'.

To make a telemark turn to the right, the left ski leads and assumes the half-wedge position, pressure being applied to the left inner edge. The right leg is 'tucked under', the hip extended and the knee flexed as the foot moves back, with pressure applied to the right outer edge. The left half-wedged ski continues to advance so that the right hip extends and the right knee flexes even further to allow the skier to sink into the telemark stance: the left foot forward and the right slightly back. The weight is primarily on the leading (left) leg at the beginning of the turn. As the turn progresses, the skier rocks back, putting increasingly more weight on the trailing (right) leg (C. Adamson, pers. comm. 1993).

Turns, therefore, require a partial squat, dorsiflexion of the foot and ankle, and partial flexion of the hip and knee on the leading half-wedged leg (which will end up being downhill at the completion of the turn); whereas the eventual 'uphill' leg is trailing, with the hip extended, knee flexed and ankle plantarflexed.

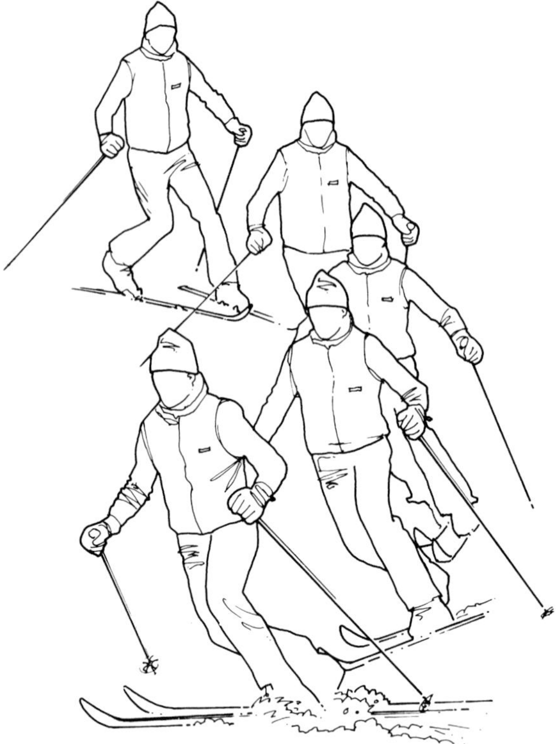

Fig. 5.27 Basic turns in telemarking. Illustrated is a right 'half-wedge turn', initiated by 'wedging' what will become the leg on the outside of the turn, by rotating the left leg and ski inward. Most of the weight remains on the straight-running right 'inside' ski; while the pressure on the inside edge of the wedged 'outside' ski is gradually increased as the turn progresses. For progression to a right 'telegarland' or telemark turn: as the 'outside' left ski is 'wedged', the left leg is simultaneously internally rotated and slid forward, the skier sinking into the 'telemark' stance by flexing the right knee further and extending the hip on that side. *(Courtesy of Parker 1988.)*

Turns will be affected by limitations of ranges of motion:

1. dorsiflexion and plantarflexion (Figs 3.75Aii, 3.84)
2. hip extension and pelvic rotation on the side of a 'posterior' innominate rotation or an 'inflare'; hip flexion on the side of the 'anterior' rotation (Figs 3.5, 3.71, 3.72)
3. trunk/pelvic rotation required for turns (Figs 3.5, 3.49)
4. the asymmetries evident on squatting (Fig. 3.76)

> A restriction of pelvic rotation will be even more of a problem than in downhill or Nordic skiing, given that the telemark skier is squatting to a variable degree, and the turns are much tighter. The tendency will be to compensate by rotating more through the trunk on executing a turn into the restricted side.

SNOWBOARDING

Snowboarding includes going downhill, riding moguls or powder, and performing 'tricks' in half- and quarter-pipes. It requires a combination of strength and balance. Quadriceps and hamstring, lower leg and ankle/foot muscle strength is vital. Core muscle strength, by helping stabilize pelvis and spine, contributes to maintaining balance. Those in the 'pipe' events also depend on an element of acute spatial perception to allow them to carry out various aerial tricks, often in quick succession. As indicated below, malalignment can affect performance both on the ground and when airborne.

Like skateboarders, snowboarders have their feet placed on the board pointing either out toward one edge of the board or rotated to a varying degree toward the front relative to a line bisecting the board (creating the so-called 'stance angle'; Fig. 5.28A). The left foot leads in a 'regular', the right in a 'goofy-foot' boarder (Fig. 5.28B). Steering is accomplished largely with the rear foot when the board is on the ground, as well as with rotation of the hips and pelvis; the trunk is angled at about 45 degrees to the fall line. In a 'regular' snowboarder, whose feet face the right edge of the board and who uses his or her right (rear) foot for steering, the effects of malalignment with an 'upslip' or 'right anterior/left posterior' innominate rotation are as follows.

The more the feet face forward, the greater the stance angle and the more the bindings are actually fixed in a way that runs counter to the abnormal tendency to 'right external, left internal' rotation of the lower extremities that results with this pattern of malalignment.

> The snowboarder may eventually feel more comfortable with adjustments, perhaps even with the bindings mounted so that the stance angle is zero degrees (Fig. 5.28Aii).

The feet will then be in better alignment relative to the tendency to right external and left internal rotation, and there may be more comfort and ease of control.

The limitation of counterclockwise rotation of the pelvis around the vertical axis in the transverse plane may interfere with the ability to rotate the pelvis to the left; this is likely to create more of a problem with 'zero stance angle' when a 'regular' boarder tries to manoeuvre the board on the ground (Fig. 3.5C). The boarder may compensate by increasing trunk - and possibly also head and neck - rotation to the left.

Limitations of ranges of motion can become a problem especially at the time of a fall or collision, not only when riding the board, but also when airborne, performing vertical 'tricks' in snowboard cross, giant slalom and halfpipe events. For example:

1. For the 'backside rodeo' (Fig. 5.28D) the 'rider' gathers speed, does a slight toe-side carve just before reaching the lip of the jump, then shifts weight onto the heels to prepare for the 'flip'. On becoming airborne, he or she throws back the head and trailing shoulder to initiate the 'backflip' while, at the same time, grabbing the edge of the board, either with the front hand on the heel side or rear hand on the toe side, to help steady the rotation. Once the flip is completed, the rider lets go of the board to initiate a final 180° spin before landing.
2. When 'riding the half-pipe', a number of torsional stresses initiated in the air continue once the rider again contacts the ground, so that trunk and pelvis are repeatedly subjected to rotation into extreme ranges of motion while the feet are relatively 'fixed' with the board now on the ground. Alternatively, the board may already be rotating in the opposite direction as the 'upper' part of the rider twists to prepare for take-off and the next trick.

The more difficulty the rider has getting onto an edge because of a malalignment-related shift in weight-bearing, functional LLD and asymmetries (particularly of ranges of motion), the more he or she depends on rotating the trunk and arms or on leaning the body toward the ground in order to carve a turn, take off or land 'cleanly'. Also, malalignment is likely to impair shock absorption by altering the ease of movement of the lower extremities, pelvis and trunk relative to each other.

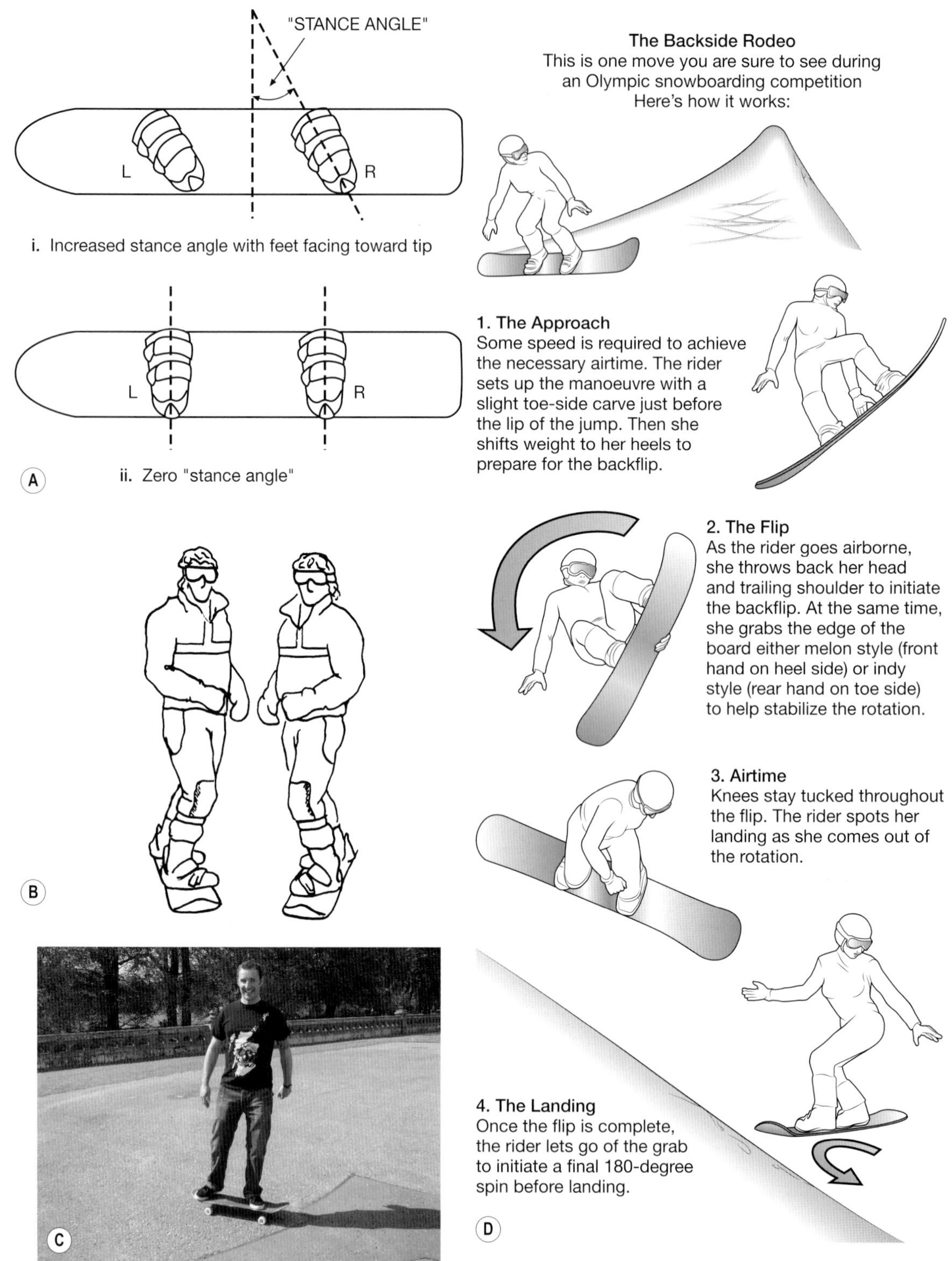

"STANCE ANGLE"
L
R
i. Increased stance angle with feet facing toward tip
L
R
A
ii. Zero "stance angle"
B
C
The Backside Rodeo
This is one move you are sure to see during an Olympic snowboarding competition Here's how it works:
1. The Approach
Some speed is required to achieve the necessary airtime. The rider sets up the manoeuvre with a slight toe-side carve just before the lip of the jump. Then she shifts weight to her heels to prepare for the backflip.
2. The Flip
As the rider goes airborne, she throws back her head and trailing shoulder to initiate the backflip. At the same time, she grabs the edge of the board either melon style (front hand on heel side) or indy style (rear hand on toe side) to help stabilize the rotation.
3. Airtime
Knees stay tucked throughout the flip. The rider spots her landing as she comes out of the rotation.
4. The Landing
Once the flip is complete, the rider lets go of the grab to initiate a final 180-degree spin before landing.
D

Fig. 5.28 Snowboarding. (A) A 'regular' foot placement relative to a line dissecting the board: (i) increased stance angle, with the feet facing toward the tip; (ii) zero stance angle. *(Redrawn courtesy of Bennett & Downey 1994.)* (B) A 'regular' snowboarder (left foot leading) and a 'goofy-foot' (right foot leading). *(Courtesy of Bennett & Downey 1994.)* (C) Skateboarder: 'normal' footing is similar to that of a 'regular' snowboarder's. (D) Snowboard 'backside rodeo' illustrating techniques described in the text: 1. approach, 2. flip. 3. airtime, 4. landing. *(Redrawn courtesy of The Vancouver Sun 2010.)*

Compared to the right, the left leg tends to be somewhat more 'rigid', given the restriction of left foot dorsiflexion, the tendency to left supination, and knee varus or neutral alignment (Figs 3.37, 3.81).

Freestyle and aerial skiing are affected similarly by factors imposed by being out of alignment.

SLEDDING: BOBSLEIGH, LUGE AND SKELETON

These competitive events involve careening downhill on an ice-covered course of straight stretches connecting curves of surprising configurations. In all three, racers may reach speeds of up to 140 km. However, the key to winning lies in an 'explosive' start: a 1/10th of a second advantage at the start is acknowledged as multiplying to a lead of 3/10th of a second at the end. The fast start calls on the following for each event:

Bobsleigh

The 'pushers' are in a 'get set' position, similar to being in blocks for a track sprint event; at the 'start', they generate the strength to get the sled moving and then attempt to build up speed as quickly as possible, before filing in - preferences are for football players for strength and sprinters for speed.

Luge

Racers depend on shoulder girdle and arm strength, initially to hold onto the starting gate handles on the side of the track to rock the sled back and forth before bursting out of the gate, then to make use of spiked gloves on the ice surface for extra acceleration before finally lying down on their back, feet stretched out in front and head back, to be as 'aerodynamic' as possible.

Skeleton

The racer crouches down in a 'get set' position as for a track sprint event, except that the pelvis and trunk are turned toward the sled

1. he or she explodes out of the blocks into the 'push phase', running side-flexed to hold on to the sled handle with one hand in order to generate as much acceleration as possible as it travels along a groove for the first 30 meters
2. at that point, springing forward and landing on the 'saddle' of the sled adds further momentum

Steering the bobsleigh depends on the driver pulling on a piece of rope and the team coordinately leaning to the right or left to help negotiate corners safely. In luge and skeleton, steering is accomplished by varying contact to the runners/steering bows by changing head, shoulder and leg position.

Effects of malalignment to consider

1. *increased risk of injury in some stages of these races*

   Trunk, pelvis and legs are especially twisted over to one side in the bobsleigh and skeleton start and would be affected by:

   a. superimposing further asymmetries and torsional strains typical of malalignment through these structures
   b. any limitation of rotation around the vertical axis into the side they are trying to twist into (e.g. a racer with a 'left inflare' or 'left posterior' innominate rotation running along on the right side, twisted and side-flexed to left, into the typical restriction of counterclockwise rotation of the pelvis; Figs 3.5, 3.49)
   c. Push-off would be affected if it has to rely on action from functionally weak and/or tight muscles (e.g. left TFL/ITB complex, peroneals and hamstrings on pushing off with the left leg in bobsleigh and skeleton, when the sled is on the athlete's right side).
2. *difficulty pushing on one side and/or vaulting over a particular side*

   By trial and error, they may have found that they perform these functions better approaching the sled from the opposite side, but malalignment and problems such as obvious limitation of left trunk/pelvic rotation should be ruled out as a possible cause for such a preference (Figs 3.5, 3.49).
3. *difficulty with control in luge and skeleton*

   For example, when the innominates rotate clockwise and the left ASIS ends up forward of the right ASIS with the 'left inflare', also with sacral torsion around the 'right-on-right' axis. This clockwise shift may be compensated for by counterclockwise rotation of the trunk. Before even making any adjustments:

   a. the skeleton racer, lying prone, is making stronger contact with the left pelvis (ASIS) and right anterior shoulder
   b. the luge racer, lying supine, contacts more firmly with the right buttock (PSIS) and left scapula

Adjustments to control the 'sleigh' have to incorporate these asymmetries; better still would be to correct the malalignment first and recheck to see if there are residual 'promontories' that can then be accommodated somehow to allow for better control of the sled.

Tobogganing, a seemingly more 'benign' sledding activity, has been discussed particularly in regard to 'coccydynia' and 'pelvic floor dysfunction' (see Chs 4, 7).

SWIMMING

Detrimental effects seen with malalignment relate primarily to asymmetrical propulsion, increased resistance and the increased energy required to correct for any torquing of the pelvis, trunk or lower extremities.

Head and neck

The frequently noted limitation of head and neck rotation to the right and of side flexion to the left (Fig. 3.10) may interfere with the ease with which breathing can be carried out on the right side when attempting alternate breathing on swimming freestyle or doing the crawl. The increase in tension found consistently in the right upper trapezius and scalenes, compounded by repeatedly straining to rotate the head and neck into the direction of the limitation, may precipitate or exacerbate neck and upper back pain. The swimmer may compensate for any limitation by increasing the clockwise rotation of the trunk but this could prove costly in terms of efficiency of style and energy expenditure.

Upper extremities

Decreased right internal and left external rotation

Asymmetry of glenohumeral internal and external rotation (Fig. 3.17A) will affect arm entry and pull-through where these are dependent on trying to achieve maximum range in the direction of the restrictions. The end result is:

1. increased soft tissue strain at the end of an increased range of motion; e.g. the right anterior and the left posterior glenohumeral capsule are susceptible to being stretched with an increase in right external and left internal rotation, respectively
2. increased soft tissue strain on trying to force past a restriction; e.g. the left anterior capsule, especially if it has undergone any shortening or even some contracture, is at increased risk of stretching with any efforts aimed at overcoming the limitation of maximal left external rotation
3. stretching the capsule/ligaments repeatedly can predispose to eventual joint laxity, subluxation/dislocation and accelerated joint degeneration (Fig. 4.7)
4. an asymmetrical contribution of the arms to propulsion and lift.

Decreased left arm extension

The butterfly swimmer who has less left than right arm extension (Fig. 3.17B) could conceivably compensate by:

1. pulling with increased force on the left side
2. torquing the body (trunk) counterclockwise, to allow the left arm to clear the water to the same extent as the right one, or limiting right arm extension to match that available on the left

Trunk and pelvis

Impaired rotation of the cervical, thoracic and pelvic region relative to each other may lead to corrective manoeuvres, including increased torquing of one part to attain more symmetry with the others.

Corrective manoeuvres that entail torquing of the trunk or pelvis may achieve symmetry of stroke strength. However, torquing of one part can result in contrary rotation of the other and often involves the cervical segment and legs as well. In other words, all four levels may be off-set relative to each other. These changes, at worst, are capable of introducing a 'wobble' that would increase energy expenditure by decreasing efficiency and increasing overall resistance.

Rotational displacement of any vertebra(e) will result in:

1. stiffness that can, for example, limit back extension in the breast stroke
2. impaired rotation to one side, calling for a compensatory increase in rotation of the adjacent vertebrae at the cost of increasing stress on these sites

Lower extremities

Propulsion using extension, adduction and internal rotation

The kick used for the breaststroke requires initial hip and knee flexion followed by forceful extension. Richardson (1986: 110) described how 'maximal valgus force is applied to the knee and the foot is maximally dorsiflexed and everted' during the flexion phase, so that 'abduction of the hips is minimized during the pushing phase'. As a result, the lower extremities go from an initial position of internal rotation, adduction and extension, to one of external rotation and flexion, and then again assuming the initial, fully extended position by the end of the kick.

> In other words, the propulsion phase consists of simultaneous hip and knee extension, leg adduction and internal rotation, ankle plantar flexion and foot eversion.

The propulsive force is created, in large part, in reaction to the water displaced by the inner aspect of the shin and the bottom of the foot.

Any asymmetry of movement will result in an asymmetrical contribution to the propulsion force. With an 'upslip' and the 'more common' rotational patterns, for example, there is more external rotation possible on the right than the left side. The sole of the right foot is, unfortunately, set in increased varus angulation compared to the left when non-weight-bearing (Fig. 3.26), decreasing the surface area that can generate a propulsive force on extension. This balance of factors may result in asymmetrical propulsive forces being generated by the right compared to the left side.

Lower extremity orientation, joint ranges of motion and strength

The efficiency of propelling the body is also affected by lower extremity side-to-side differences of orientation and asymmetries of joint ranges of motion and strength. An 'upslip' and the 'more common' rotational patterns, for example, limit right internal rotation and plantarflexion, left external rotation and dorsiflexion. These asymmetries may help to explain the predicament of the occasional swimmer who is slow to move forward, or worse, fails to move forward or even moves backward when using the flutter kick hanging on to a board, but proceeds forward without problem once back in alignment.

It helps to think of the lower extremities as acting like two propellers. Because of the malalignment, each of these propellers is set at a different angle. In addition, there are the side-to-side asymmetries in strength. Significant here is the common finding of a relative decrease in right hip flexor and extensor strength; whereas these specific muscles, which are crucial for doing the flutter kick, are usually full strength on the left side. In comparison, weakness on the left side affects primarily the hip abductors, hamstrings and ankle evertors, none of which play much of a part in this movement. The combined effect of these asymmetries appears to be that, in some swimmers, the 'propellers' actually work against each other, so that the propulsion effect is reduced, cancelled or even reversed. Correction of the malalignment serves to realign the 'propellers' and promote forward movement.

Swimming is, with exceptions such as the side-stroke, mainly a symmetrical activity. However, asymmetrical stresses imposed by malalignment increase the likelihood of specific injury occurring on one side. Frequently seen knee injuries, for example, include medial collateral ligament stress syndrome, patellofemoral compartment syndrome, medial synovitis and medial synovial plica syndrome. These are more likely to occur on the right side with an 'upslip' and one of the 'more common' rotational patterns, and on the left with the 'left anterior and locked' pattern. Ankle and foot extensor tendonitis commonly associated with the flutter and dolphin kick are more likely to occur on the side on which the extensors are tight and plantarflexion is decreased; those with a cuboid subluxation would be even more vulnerable, given that both dorsi- and plantarflexion are reduced on the side of the subluxation compared to the other.

In addition, symmetrical strokes will result in increased stress on structures that are now asymmetrical. In the butterfly, for example, back extension further compresses facet joints that are already approximated on one side by vertebral rotation, especially at the thoracolumbar junction, where this problem is compounded by the segmental curve reversal (Figs 2.52B, 3.14). Box 5.9 summarizes the overall effects of these asymmetries.

In a sport in which races may be won by one-hundredth of a second, these effects can prove costly indeed.

SYNCHRONIZED SWIMMING

Problems with malalignment relating especially to an asymmetry of lower extremity ranges of motion may be more easily evident in routines in which the body is submerged with the legs protruding from the water in specific, and usually symmetrical, patterns relative to the waterline. In a participant who is not

BOX 5.9 Effects of asymmetry on swimming

1. Speed is reduced by any decrease or asymmetry in propulsion and the lift forces generated.
2. Energy is wasted by the need for corrective action in order to 'keep an even keel' and counterbalance any asymmetry of the propulsive forces generated by the right versus the left side.
3. Asymmetry and corrective torquing forces further increase energy requirements by increasing drag.
4. Injuries, involving especially the back, hips and knees, are more likely to occur.
5. When malalignment is present, the swimmer may find it easier to carry out a stroke (e.g. crawl) facing constantly to one side rather than rotating from right to left and back again. He or she may thereby avoid any discomfort and/or impediment to propulsion and speed felt on alternate breathing or whenever facing the opposite side.

blessed with a general degree of increased mobility, malalignment may well result in difficulties.

Limitations of hip flexion and extension seen with all three presentations of malalignment will affect those positions in which one leg has to flex at the hip to 90 degrees and the other remains vertical, either completely (e.g. the 'crane'; Fig. 5.29A) or partially (e.g. the 'knight'; Fig. 5.29 C3). Restrictions of flexion or extension may also cause a problem with a 'split' in the sagittal plane (Fig. 5.29 C4), which the athlete may be able to correct by 'opening' the pelvis: rotating the pelvis around the vertical axis in the transverse plane, so that it ends up forward on the side of restricted flexion and backward on the side of restricted extension (Fig. 2.12). Similarly, with a 'right inflare' the ipsilateral innominate (i.e. acetabulum) moves forward in the transverse plane, allowing for increased right hip flexion; whereas with a 'left outflare' the innominate moves backward, allowing for more hip extension on that side. However, in those with 'left posterior' innominate rotation, the limitation of pelvic rotation counterclockwise in the transverse plane may make this manoeuvre less effective to compensate for any restriction of right flexion and left extension.

Extension can also be increased by accentuating the lumbar lordosis, at the risk of affecting style and precipitating back pain.

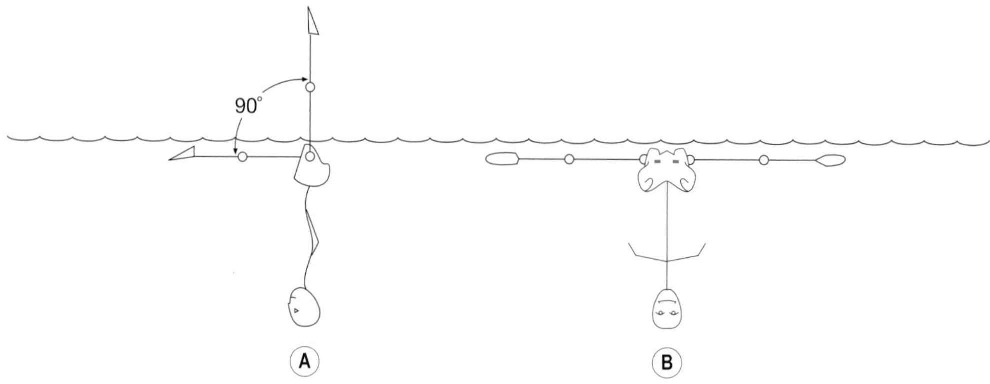

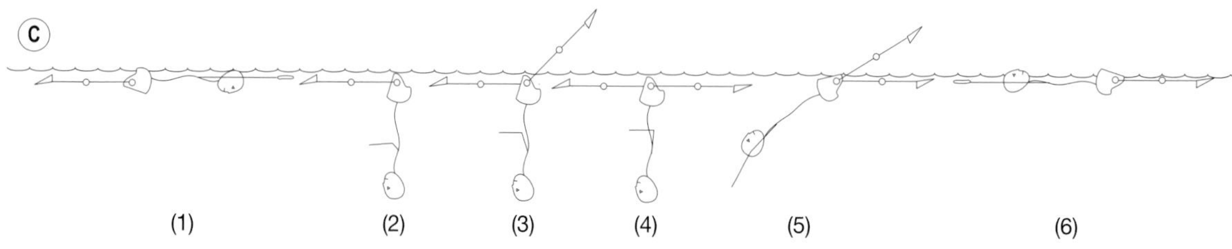

Fig. 5.29 Synchronized swimming positions. (A) 'Crane'. (B) A 'split' in the frontal plane (abduction). (C) A 'walkover front' sequence: (1) initial position and (6) finale; (2) back pike; (3) 'knight' or 'castle'; (4) 'split' in the sagittal plane (extension/flexion).

For the 'split' in the coronal plane, both legs should abduct 90 degrees to become horizontal with the water (Fig. 5.29B), but malalignment may result in an obvious limitation to one side (usually the left). Symmetry may be preserved by actively limiting abduction on the more mobile side to match that on the restricted side but then both will fall short of horizontal. Also, the asymmetry of plantarflexion may result in an obvious inability to point the foot on one side as much as on the other (Fig. 3.84B).

Any attempts to compensate are probably easier to achieve when the swimmer carries out a routine on his or her own and just floating freely than when restricted by being interlinked with a partner or a group, trying to match up to what the others are doing and to maintain the symmetry of the routine at all cost.

As in swimming, asymmetries related to malalignment may also play a role in the causation and localization of the injuries seen with synchronized swimming. Weinberg (1986: 161) pointed out the following common problems.

Back pain

Back pain has been attributed to an increased lumbar lordosis and to the hyperextension required to carry out manoeuvres such as the 'split' in the sagittal plane, the 'knight' position and the 'walkover' sequence (Fig. 5.29C); for example, going from the 'back pike' (2) into the 'knight' position (3), with one leg extended and the other vertical, into a sagittal 'split' (4), and finally bringing the trunk into horizontal alignment with the legs.

Needless to say, back pain is more likely to develop when an increased lordosis or repeated hyperextension is superimposed on the asymmetry of pelvis and spine, and the rotational stresses that result with malalignment - notably at the thoracolumbar and lumbosacral junction. Also, when confronted with someone with back pain who is seemingly in alignment, remember to check for signs of excessive rotation of the sacrum around the coronal axis:

1. a 'bilateral sacrum anterior' rotation (= excessive counternutation), with loss of the lumbar lordosis, stiffness of the lumbar segment and associated pelvic/neurological symptoms
2. a 'bilateral sacrum posterior' rotation (= excessive nutation), with an increased lumbar lordosis, a 'subtle/elastic' feel to the lumbar segment and other typical signs and symptoms (see Ch. 2).

Knee injuries

Cited as one of the common overuse injuries is chondromalacia patellae, possibly related to 'the constant emphasis on forceful extension of the knee' repeated use of the 'eggbeater' kick, as well as exaggerated Q-angles which increase the tendency to lateral tracking of the patella on knee extension (Figs 3.37, 3.81, 4.5). These knee problems are more likely to occur on the right side in those with an 'upslip' or one of the 'more common' rotational patterns, for reasons previously noted to predispose to patellofemoral compartment syndrome (see Ch. 3).

Shoulder injuries

Shoulder pain can come on with the stress inherent to extensive support 'sculling' that is part of many of the routines, inflammatory conditions (e.g. as seen with rotator cuff impingement syndrome) or actual joint degeneration. On sculling, the shoulder is 'slightly abducted and maximally rotated [externally] on the outward phase, and adducted and internally rotated on the inward phase. The major stress ... is a stretching of the anterior capsule at the point of maximal external rotation' (Weinberg 1986: 162), which predisposes to developing glenohumeral joint laxity, subluxation or even dislocation. A malalignment-related limitation of external rotation on one side and internal rotation on the other, combined with asymmetrical strength, may reduce the overall effectiveness of the sculling manoeuvre. Stress on the anterior capsule will be increased on the side on which external rotation is relatively increased (Figs 3.17A, 4.7).

THROWING SPORTS

In most sports, the execution of a throw involves the whole body rather than consisting of an isolated arm action. Most throws basically require some rotation of the pelvis, thorax and extremities in order to generate maximum velocity. The following two throws serve to illustrate these points.

Javelin

At the end of the run up, the right-handed athlete transfers weight from the right to the left foot in preparation for release. Just prior to this transfer, he or she 'winds up' for the throw by rotating the trunk clockwise, simultaneously extending the

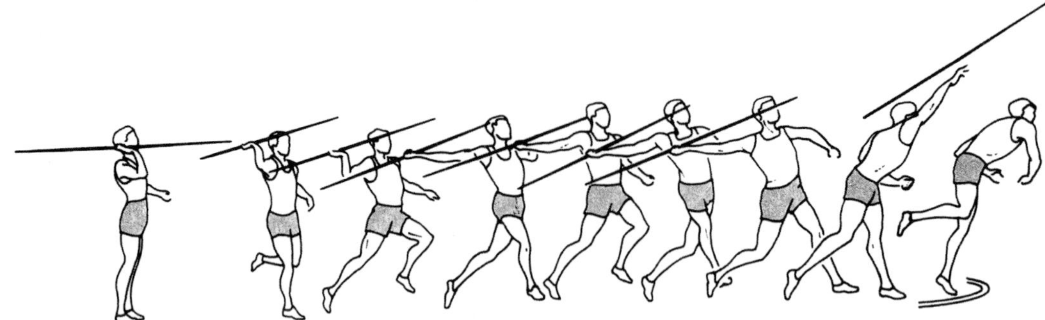

Fig. 5.30 Javelin throw: the wind-up phase leading to weight transfer onto the left leg, with passive internal rotation of that leg just prior to release. *(Courtesy of Worth 1990.)*

spine, side-flexing to the right and rotating the right arm externally (Fig. 5.30). The transfer to the left foot is accompanied by a counterclockwise rotation of the pelvis to advance the right hip and thereby add to the length of the step. The trunk then flexes and unwinds counterclockwise as the right arm rotates internally. 'The final force, added to the forward movement of the body, is derived from pelvic and spinal rotation, [and] medial rotation . . . of the humerus' (Adrian & Cooper 1986: 526), with simultaneous passive internal rotation of the weight-bearing left leg.

Pitching

The movement of the throwing arm and the trunk is much the same as the sequence after the run-up described for throwing the javelin. Looking at a right-handed pitcher throwing overhand, the initial 'wind-up' phase calls for balancing on the right leg while accentuating the passive internal rotation of that leg as the body winds up (Figs 5.31A, 3.18, 3.51). Simultaneous pelvic rotation to the right during this phase 'can be more than 90 degrees from the intended direction of flight of the projectile' (Adrian & Cooper 1986: 498). The trunk rotates along with the pelvis until it also is at a right angle to the intended direction of the throw. As the 'wind-up' proceeds, the left leg rises upward in the air, partly to counterbalance simultaneous right side flexion of the trunk and partly in preparation for stepping forward onto the left foot. During the 'forward force' phase or actual 'cocking' phase, the hands separate (the right hand moving backward), the throwing arm moves into extreme external rotation, and weight is transferred onto the left foot (Fig. 5.31B).

> *Acceleration' sees an increased weight-shift forwards onto the left foot, and a simultaneous 'unwinding', consisting of a counterclockwise rotation of the pelvis that subjects the now-supporting left leg to passive internal rotation [Fig. 5.31C]. Further rotation of the pelvis, unwinding, and forward flexion of the spine, combined with internal rotation and extension of the upper extremity, constitute the 'deceleration' phase and all aid the force of the release [Fig. 5.31D]. Control of the throw is perfected by going through the 'follow-up' phase, which also involves passive internal rotation of the left leg [Fig. 5.31E].*

Some of the restrictions imposed by malalignment are capable of affecting the 'four axes of motion' felt to be crucial for the execution of any of these throws. Limitations of joint ranges of motion, combined with asymmetries of strength and problems with balancing on one leg, impair speed and accuracy and can result in a suboptimal throw. Take the example of the pitcher with an 'upslip' or one of the 'more common' rotational patterns who pitches with either the right or left arm.

Arm rotation

In the 'wind-up' phase

In the absence of any other shoulder pathology, adding up the degrees of internal plus external rotation on each side will show the combined range of motion to be the same on the right and left sides (Fig. 3.17A). However, the limitation of either internal or external rotation will alter the rotation around the axis of the arm and affects its contribution to the throw.

1. *right-handed pitcher*

   Right external rotation is increased relative to left and unlikely to be a problem, barring excessive repeated stretching of the anterior glenohumeral capsule.

2. *left-handed pitcher*

   The limitation of external rotation on the left is more likely to be a problem that may result in:

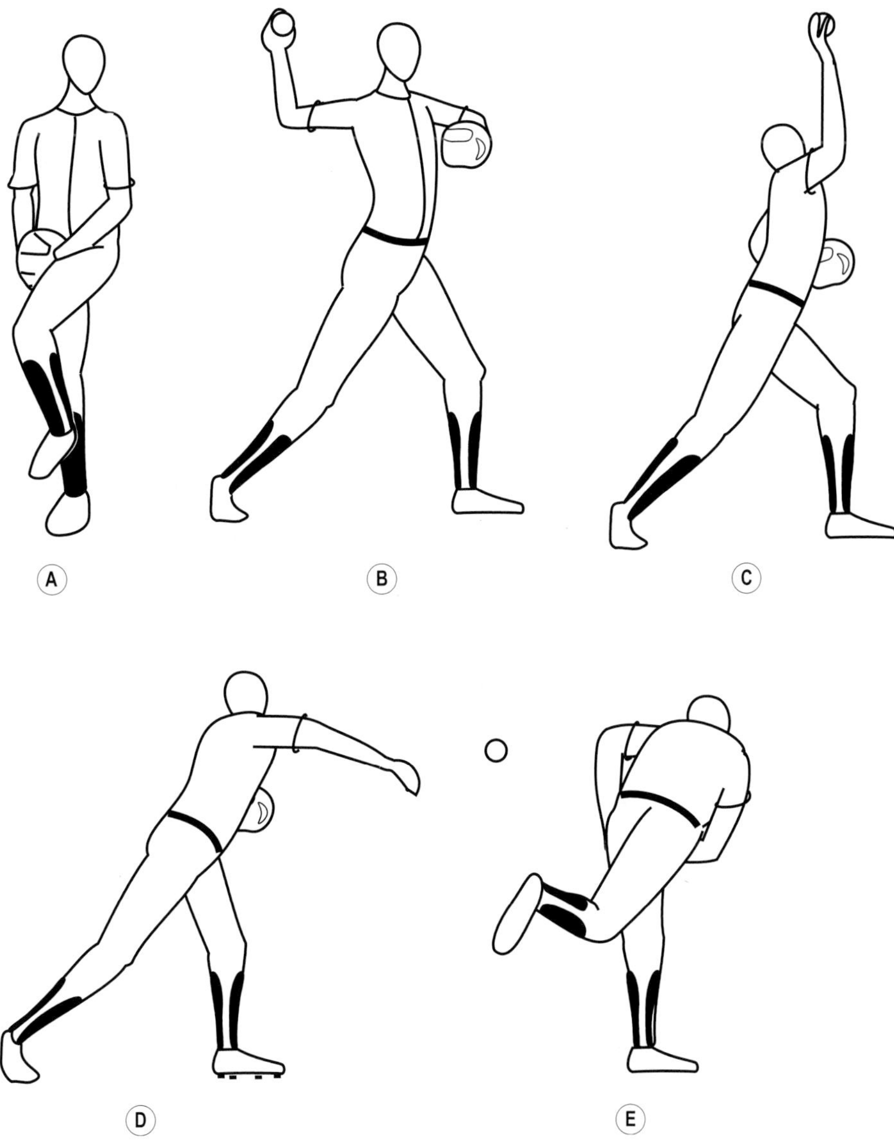

Fig. 5.31 Phases of ball throw: right-handed pitcher (see Fig. 3.51). (A) Wind-up (including 'cocking' of the left leg). (B) True 'cocking' phase. (C) Acceleration. (D) Deceleration. (E) Follow-through.

a. a compensatory increase in left elbow flexion and forearm supination, which will increase tension on the ulnar nerve and increase the chance of precipitating or aggravating nerve subluxation, irritation and inflammation, possibly an ulnar nerve palsy
b. increased valgus stress (medial elbow stress syndrome and injuries to the medial elbow ligaments and capsule)
c. increased lateral elbow joint compression (e.g. humeroradial joint).

Arm rotation in preparation for the release

The limitation of right internal rotation could conceivably present a problem in the right-handed pitcher on release if carried through to the end of range as it may increase:

1. traction forces on the right lateral elbow ligaments and capsule
2. right medial elbow joint compression forces (e.g. humeroulnar joint).

Leg, pelvic and thoracic rotation

Asymmetries affecting the pelvis and lower extremities are likely to affect the throw. In the case of the right-handed pitcher with an 'upslip' and/or one of the 'more common' patterns of 'rotational malalignment':

1. internal rotation of the right lower extremity is restricted compared with that of the left and may limit the 'wind-up'

> Once the limit of right leg internal rotation has been reached, any further movement into the right required for the 'wind-up' either cannot occur at all or has to take place through increased right side-flexion and/or increased clockwise rotation of the pelvis.

2. limitation of counterclockwise rotation in the transverse plane of the pelvis with a 'left posterior' innominate rotation may limit rotation in the 'release' phase, especially whenever weight is supported on both feet; this would also be affected by a concomitant left 'inflare'
3. any restriction of pelvic rotation to the right or left increases the torque force through the thoracic segment - especially through the thoracolumbar junction - in either the 'wind-up' or 'acceleration/deceleration' phases
   a. unilateral limitations of thoracic spine side-flexion and rotation can be seen with a compensatory curvature of this segment, rotational displacement of individual vertebrae and/or asymmetry of paravertebral and extensor spinae muscle tension
   b. these restrictions could impair normal function of the segment through these phases and decrease its ability to compensate for any shortcomings of rotation in arms, pelvis or legs

Balance

Balance may also be a problem, whether on account of a functional weakness, an alteration of proprioceptive input or additional factors. This is more likely to occur during the single-support phase on the right leg in conjunction with one of the 'more common' patterns of 'rotational malalignment' (see Ch. 3 and 'Figure skating', above).

WATERSKIING

The waterskier's success depends in large part on maintaining balance while trying to execute turns and other manoeuvres by getting onto an inner or outer edge of the ski(s).

Two skis

The ability to turn to the right or left is determined largely by the ease with which the skier can simultaneously get onto the inside edge of one and outside edge of the other ski. The skier can seemingly accomplish this simply by leaning the body to one or other side. The ease with which this shift can occur will, however, also be influenced by any facilitating or restricting effect imposed by coexistent malalignment. It will, for example, conceivably be easier to execute a turn to the left with an 'upslip' or one of the 'more common' rotational patterns as these make it easier to get onto the right inside and left outside edge of the foot.

Slalom

Malalignment will have a more pronounced effect on the ability to execute turns in this event. Most slalom skiers have the left foot mounted forward on the ski, the rear right foot steering by selectively weighting the inner or outer edge. Again, in those with an 'upslip' or one of the 'more common' rotational patterns, the associated tendency to right pronation and left supination:

1. increases the ease with which they can weight the left edge
2. may make it easier to turn and to fall to the left
3. allows a more acute lean of the body to the left before triggering a fear of falling
4. may allow them to raise a higher wall of water more easily when executing a left turn

The insecurity experienced by some on a right turn may relate, in part, to the difficulty they have with shifting onto the right edge and with an increased need to lean the trunk into the right side, toward the water, in order to do so.

As in snowboarding, the slalom skier who has the right foot mounted forward is known as a 'goofy foot' (Fig. 5.32). This may again be an indication of an underlying malalignment problem. Certainly the 'left anterior and locked' pattern increases the ease with which weight can be shifted to the inside of the left foot and the outside of the right, which should make it easier to steer with the left foot trailing and to get onto the right edge to execute a right turn.

WEIGHT-LIFTING

Some power lift competitions, such as the squat exercise or deep knee bend, are judged partly on style. A spotter on each side looks to see whether

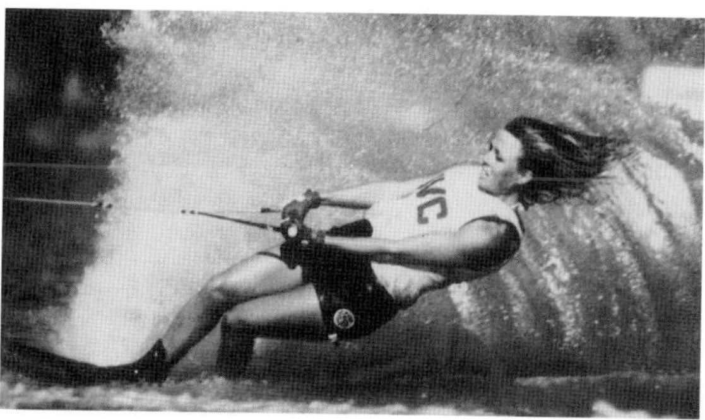

Fig. 5.32 'Goofy-foot' slalom water skier: the right foot leads, the left steers. *(Courtesy of West 1989.)*

each buttock has dropped below the level of the ipsilateral bent knee when the athlete is in the full-squat position. Points may also be deducted if the height of the buttock and knee on one side does not match that on the other side.

Factors to consider when the squat is not symmetrical:

1. Counterclockwise rotation of the pelvis in the transverse plane brings the right acetabulum forward, the left backward so that the knees no longer match: the right femur may appear longer than the left.
2. With 'right anterior, left posterior' innominate rotation
   a. the right buttock (ischial tuberosity) and iliac crest are usually noticeably elevated relative to the left (Figs 2.76B, 3.76A, 3.86A,B, 6.4).
   b. the right acetabulum has rotated downward and back so that, compared to the left, the right thigh may be noticeably lower proximally, seemingly shorter and angled upward more acutely to the knee (Fig. 3.76B).
3. the symmetry of the squat will be influenced by any limitation of innominate rotation by tight and/or tender muscles/ligaments:
   a. anterior rotation: primarily by gluteus maximus, piriformis and/or hamstrings and the sacrotuberous ligament
   b. posterior rotation: by iliacus and rectus femoris involvement

Tightness or discomfort from these structures may also create problems with the full squat required part way through:

1. the 'snatch' lift, when the weight-lifter is in the 'catch' or 'receiving' position (Fig. 5.33A3)
2. the 'clean-and-jerk' lift, when the weight-lifter is in the catch or receiving position for the 'clean' (Fig. 5.33B3).

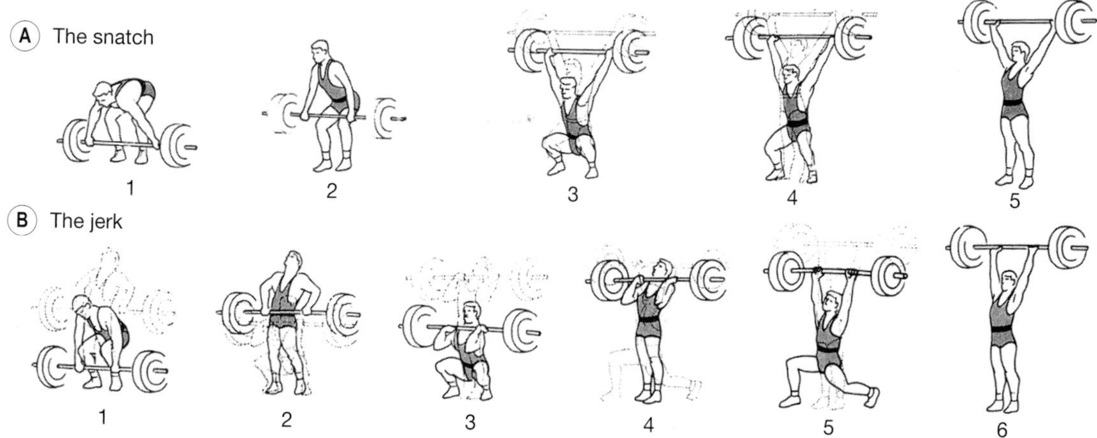

Fig. 5.33 Weight-lifting positions affected by malalignment. (A) *The snatch.* The bar is pulled upward from the ground (1, 2) to the full extent of both arms being vertical above the head (3), 'splitting' or bending the knees to a deep squat in the process (3), before proceeding to the full standing position (4, 5). (B) *The clean-and-jerk lift.* For the 'clean', the bar is brought in a single motion to the shoulders (1, 2, 3), simultaneously 'splitting' or bending the legs (squatting) into the catch or receiving position for the 'clean', which is then achieved by going on to stand (4). The arms are next brought vertically above the head, the legs at the same time being split by flexing one hip and extending the other. This manoueuvre results in the catch or receiving position for the 'jerk' (5) which is then achieved by standing up while maintaining the arms vertical (6). *(Courtesy of Worth 1990.)*

The 'clean-and-jerk' lift proceeds to the 'catch' or receiving position for the 'split' jerk, which is an asymmetrical position with one leg fully extended behind the body and the other flexed to approximately 90 degrees at the hip and knee and in the sagittal plane, as in a 'forward lunge' (see Fig. 5.10C). At the same time, the fully extended arms balance the weight directly above the head (Fig. 5.33B5).

The weight-lifter who presents with 'right anterior, left posterior' rotation or a 'right outflare, left inflare' may experience a problem with this part of the lift, when he or she is supported by the flexed right hip and knee with the left leg in extension, because of the associated limitation of right hip flexion and left hip extension. The tight right sacrotuberous ligament, gluteus maximus and hamstrings, and left iliacus and rectus femoris, are at risk of injury, given the rapidity of moving from the standing position (Fig. 5.33B4) into the 'catch' or lunge-like position (Fig. 5.33B5) and then on to the 'jerk' (standing up again; Fig. 5.33B6) with the weight lifted above the head.

Weight-lifters with an 'upslip' or one of the 'more common' rotational patterns have also reported:

1. the legs in the squatting, split or bend positions not being oriented in the same direction (as in the 'snatch', on moving from B2 to B3), often with the right knee and foot pointing more outward relative to the left (in keeping with external rotation of the right leg; Fig. 3.76Bi)
2. the right leg not feeling as strong as the left, something that disappears on correction of the malalignment, or that they may be able to correct for, in part, by actively rotating the right leg inward so that the foot now points forward.

Any exercises with weights, regardless of whether they are resting on or held above the shoulders (Fig. 5.34), increase the risk of going out of alignment, especially when:

1. the weights are excessive and, therefore, more likely to result in even a momentary aggravation of any asymmetries of balance and muscle contraction
2. there are asymmetries in the weights being handled, either individually by one hand (e.g. as for alternate right and left biceps curls) or attached to the ends of a bar
3. torsional movements are carried out with the trunk while supporting a weight in this manner; if the feet are both weight-bearing, the ability of the pelvis to rotate can be limited in certain directions (see Fig. 3.5C), increasing rotational stress through the thoracic segment

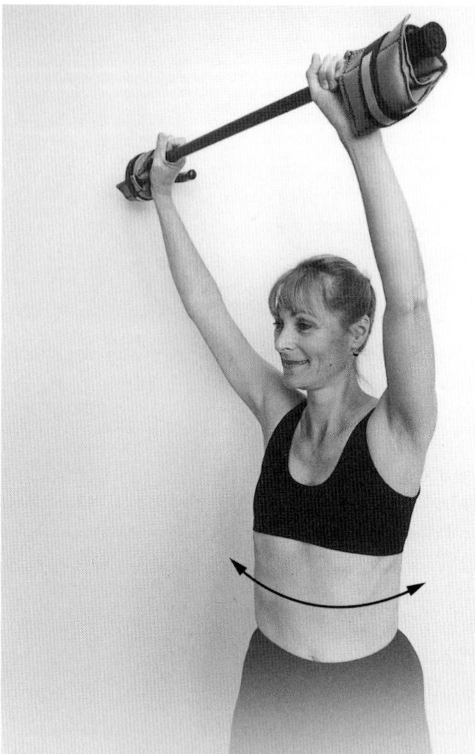

Fig. 5.34 Weight-lifting: torquing the trunk in the transverse plane (arrows) with a bar and attached weights supported above the shoulders, while the feet (and pelvis) are relatively fixed.

> Interestingly, the weight-lifter's belt is applied in exactly the same location as the sacroiliac belt and has been shown on magnetic resonance imaging studies to run across the short upper arm of the L-shaped joint.

This finding led Snijders et al. (1992) to speculate that the benefit derived by a weight-lifter from wearing a belt when in a stooped position may relate more to its ability to stabilize the SI joint than to improving back strength by increasing the intra-abdominal pressure. However, the belt not only results in compression forces to the SI joints but also complements the support provided by transversus abdominis anterolaterally. It thereby affects the 'inner' core muscle complex and helps maintain intra-abdominal pressure (Figs 2.28, 7.34-7.36). The combined effect is to stabilize the pelvis and spine, a key factor for carrying out weight-lifting routines effectively and safely.

WINDSURFING

A windsurfer needs to be able to control the board and sail it from either side, yet many will have a side preference. This sport requires, in addition to agility, flexibility and the ability to rotate the limbs, pelvis and trunk through the maximum available ranges of motion. Whereas the preference for one side may be determined, in part, by laterality and habit, a restriction of motion in directions frequently called upon to manoeuvre the board and sail probably also play a role. A problem in shifting weight onto the medial or lateral edge of a foot could affect the ability to maintain a stable position, lean to either side and to steer the board. Asymmetry in the pectoral muscles, with malalignment-related trunk rotation resulting in shoulder protraction on one and retraction on the other side, also 'facilitation' of some shoulder girdle muscles, might help to account for the observed increase in pectoral muscle ruptures (Woo 1997).

WRESTLING

Wrestling has been referred to repeatedly in discussion relating to excessive torsion of one part of the body, especially when another part is 'fixed' and unable to move. Typical examples are described in Box 5.10.

BOX 5.10 Effects of torsional stresses in wrestling

1. Torsion of the trunk into the restriction at a time when the pelvis is 'fixed', as may occur with:
   a. a contestant forming a bridge to prevent a 'fall' (Fig. 5.35A)
   b. an opponent preventing the pelvis from moving while forcing rotation of the trunk (Fig. 5.35B)
2. Torsion of the pelvis and legs into the restriction when the trunk is 'fixed' (Fig. 5.36A,B); consider:
   a. one contestant with a 'right anterior, left posterior' rotation, now lying supine with the hips and knees flexed
   b. the opponent, while pinning down the trunk, somehow forces the flexed lower extremities to the left (Fig. 5.36A,B), into the combined limitations of left pelvic rotation (Fig. 3.5C) and right internal, left external leg rotation (Figs 3.78 and 3.79, respectively).

FORETHOUGHT TO CHAPTER 6: HORSEBACK RIDING AND PLAYING POLO

The interplay of malalignment and horseback riding is covered in detail in Chapter 6. The comments here are limited but intended to precede, in part, the material in 'A 'natural' process of elimination?', below.

Failure to advance in riding

Riding may well be one of those sports in which malalignment makes the difference between whether the athlete progresses as expected, gives

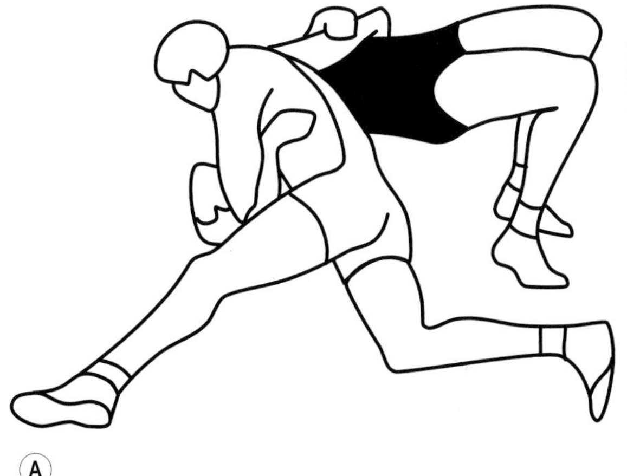

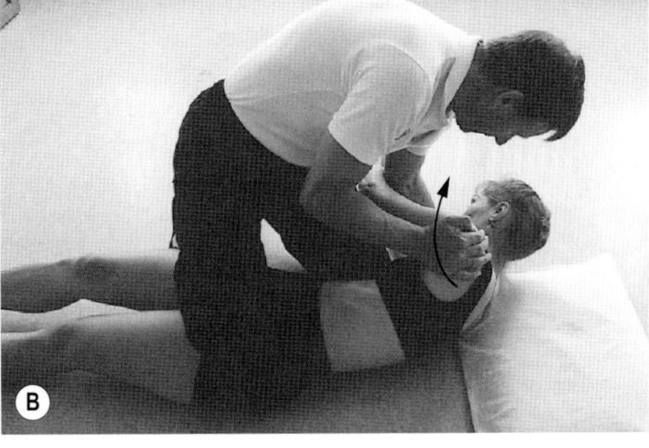

Fig. 5.35 Wrestling action in which the trunk may be forcefully rotated (actively or passively) relative to a 'fixed' pelvis. (A) Forming a bridge (black shorts) to prevent a fall, with the pelvis 'fixed' by keeping both feet anchored to the ground. (B) The opponent (white top) is rotating the trunk clockwise while pinning the pelvis down on the floor.

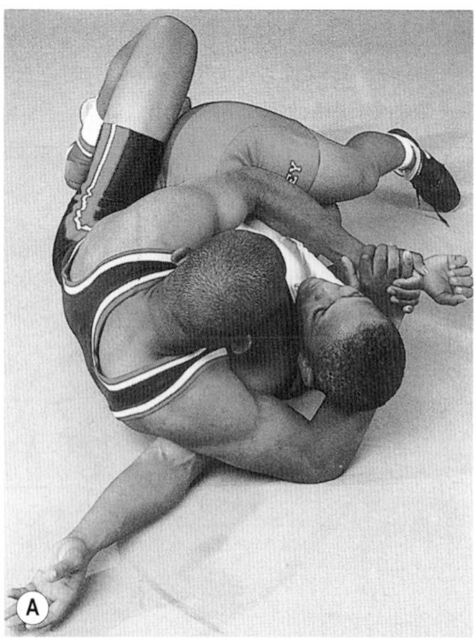

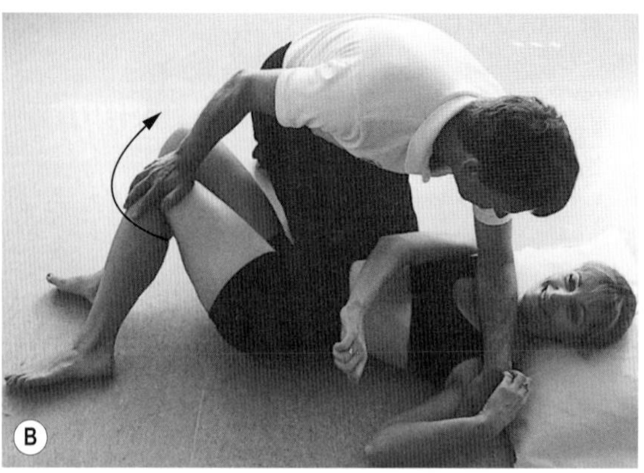

Fig. 5.36 Wrestling action in which the pelvis may be forcefully rotated (actively or passively) relative to a 'fixed' trunk. (A) A clockwise rotational force on the pelvis of the red-white [right/lower] opponent, whose shoulders (= trunk) are pinned to the mat. *(Courtesy of Savage 1996.)* (B) The flexed hips and knees are forced to the right, rotating the pelvis clockwise relative to the 'fixed' trunk.

up riding altogether or settles for less challenging equestrian pursuits. Wanless, more or less, said as much in 1989 in her lesson on 'The positioning of the body and an introduction to asymmetry'. She cited the case of 'Jan' who:

> *...had reached a stage in her riding where she was continuously depressed about her apparent inability* [to do dressage], *whilst simultaneously becoming desperate in her attempts to 'get it right'. Finally ... she decided to take up long-distance riding in the hope that 'letting herself off the hook', combined with long hours in the saddle, might somehow give her the seat and the abilities for which she longed. She is not the first person I have met who had made this transition; however, she is also not the first to have admitted that although long-distance is great fun, it is for her a substitute - and if she felt competent enough she would really prefer to do dressage.*
> (Wanless 1995: 78)

Wanless described how a rider may feel that he or she is sitting symmetrically in the saddle when, in fact, the right thigh is turned outward [=external rotation] and the left inward [=internal rotation], and how placing the rider symmetrically in the saddle makes him or her feel rotated to the left (Fig. 5.37). The description is in keeping with a rider who most probably has an 'upslip' or one of the 'more common' patterns of 'rotational malalignment', with rotation of the lower extremities: the right externally and the left internally (Figs 3.3B, 3.19B, 3.78B, 3.79). A 'left inflare, right outflare'

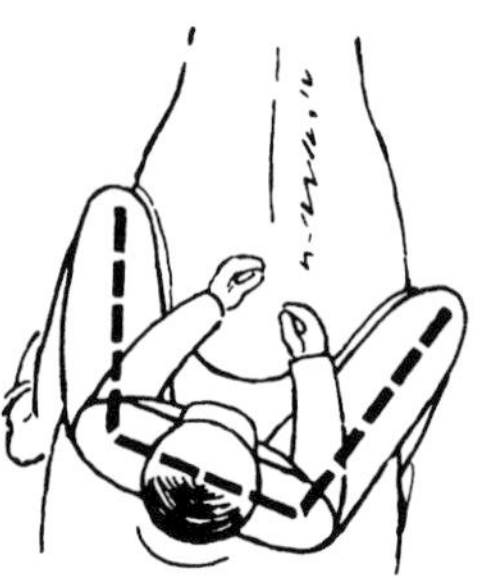

Crooked rider to the right is actually placed like this

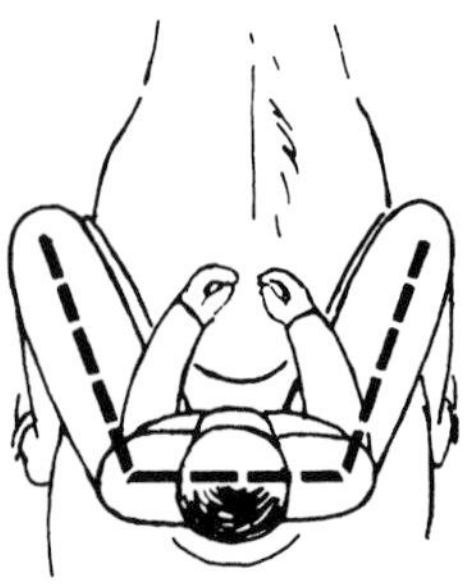

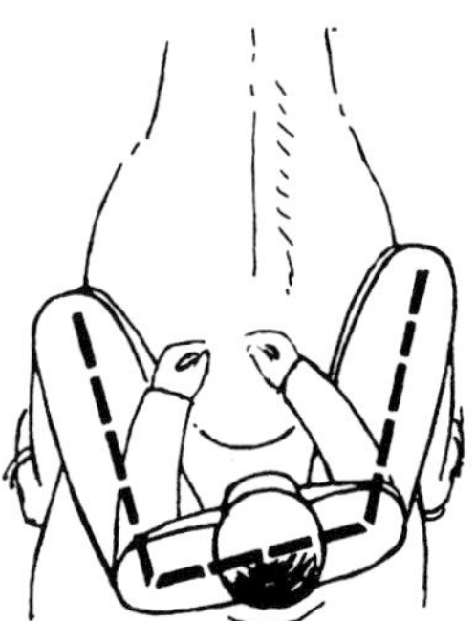

When she is actually well placed she feels like this

Fig. 5.37 With crookedness, in particular, subjective feelings are not to be trusted. When you counteract your natural asymmetry ['malalignment'], you will feel as if you have brought your outside seat-bone so far back that you are facing too much to the outside. *(Courtesy of Wanless 1995.)*

pattern would result in clockwise rotation of the pelvis around the vertical axis so that the left ASIS would come forward and the inside of the left thigh apply against the horse, with the findings reversed on the right. These changes would make it more difficult to maintain a proper seat. Loss of contact with the right thigh probably also interferes with being able to communicate properly with the horse (see Ch. 6).

Wanless then gave Jan's presentation, which was really typical of someone with an 'upslip' or one of the 'more common' rotational patterns. She went on to describe, complete with illustrations, how the right leg was turned outward and concluded with the advice to Jan that she should start the recovery process by making a conscious effort to turn the right leg inward when both riding and walking. Initiating such an effort did indeed improve Jan's posture, and seemingly the horse 'responded beautifully with this change in her carriage ... Jan could feel a distinct difference in the way she was moving' (Wanless 1995: 86). However, she did point out that:

> *This initial change can happen in a very small amount of time, but it can take years for it to become so ingrained that it feels natural and effortless. With every lapse of concentration, the rider tends to fall straight back into her old pattern - but at least she knows how to redeem herself.*
> (Wanless 1995: 87)

The temporary nature of these treatment attempts - seemingly limited to consciously effected postural adaptations - would really not be very surprising if the findings were indeed attributable to an underlying problem of malalignment.

> Unfortunately, malalignment can be corrected only in part by any conscious effort and will recur as that effort ceases, even momentarily.

Realignment of the rider, and often also of the horse, may offer the only long-term solution. Maintaining the alignment of the horse and rider may become as simple as checking regularly to detect - and reverse - any recurrence early, using mounting blocks, and getting into the habit of mounting from alternate sides (see Ch. 6 and Wagner-Chazalon 2000).

Playing polo

Polo deserves special mention here because of the extreme demands on the ability to:

1. side-flex the trunk and/or
2. combine extension and rotation to twist backward, in preparation for reaching the ball
3. rotate the trunk on the pelvis when hitting the ball and on follow-through

Whenever the player is sitting, the pelvis is relatively 'fixed', increasing any rotational stress through the thorax, especially the thoracolumbar region. Added to all this is the momentum of the action and the possibilities for close contact or collision with an opponent. The stage is set for injuries related particularly to the limitations of trunk and shoulder ranges of motion typically seen with malalignment.

CONCLUSION

Appendix 10 notes clinic correlations typical for some specific sports other than running, and Appendix 11 provides some non-specific correlations that apply to a number of sports. It is obviously not possible to mention every individual athletic activity in this book. It is, however, to be hoped that the discussion of the basic biomechanical changes in the preceding chapters, and of the application of this information to the sports mentioned above, will give those working with athletes the insight needed to make use of this material when trying to analyze problems and injuries encountered in a certain sport. Also, as indicated in 'work and hobbies' below, injuries in any of these three settings can be caused by similar biomechanical forces and the problems evolving with malalignment caused in one setting may be perpetuated by activities carried out by the person in some other setting that has so-far not been revealed or even suspected.

RECURRENT INJURIES

The following are the most common recurrent problems seen in association with 'right anterior, left posterior' innominate rotation.

1. left hip abductor and ITB sprain
2. left trochanteric bursitis

3. left ankle inversion sprain
4. right patellofemoral compartment syndrome
5. back 'sprain' or 'strain', typically localizing to the right and/or left of the lumbosacral junction, sometimes very definitely over one or both SI joints
6. referred dysaesthesias or paraesthesias in typical patterns, corresponding to the joint, nerve or soft tissue being irritated
7. 'shin splints': medial, lateral and anterior

Factors contributing to the first six conditions have been discussed throughout the text, and are indicated again in Appendix 12, but shin splints deserve further mention at this point.

'SHIN SPLINTS'

Shin splints may be medial, lateral or anterior and the etiology may include:

1. **periostalgia**
   - bone tenderness, along the origin of a muscle (e.g. medial tenderness, along the tibialis posterior origin)
2. **a stress fracture**
   - tending to result in more localized pain and often involving the junction of the mid- and distal third of the tibia
3. **compartment syndrome**
   - presenting as a feeling of 'tightness', 'swelling', with an increase in circumference, tension and tenderness confined to a specific compartment; e.g. lateral shin pain with peroneal compartment involvement
4. **asymmetrical stresses and/or referred pain with malalignment**

Similar to ligaments, pain attributable to periostalgia is typically relieved with rest and initially worse on getting up but decreased on continuing with an activity, in keeping with an increase in blood flow, stretching and 'loosening up' of the fibro-osseous junction and the muscle itself (see Chs 4, 8). In contrast, pain from a stress fracture or compartment syndrome is worsened by weight-bearing activity but may persist on non-weight-bearing and with rest. Depending on the history and examination findings, specific investigations and treatment may be in order. Discussion regarding malalignment-related shin splints follows.

Whether athletes presenting with malalignment develop medial, anterior or lateral shin splints will be determined, in part, by factors such as their inherent weight-bearing pattern, tibial torsion, genu varum and valgum and the patterns of referral triggered by the altered biomechanics.

Medial shin splints

These are usually activity-related and result from excessive traction on the medial periosteal origins of tibialis posterior. With an 'upslip' or one of the 'more common' rotational patterns, they may present just on the right side, or worse on the right than the left, because of the increased tendency toward right pronation and medial weight-bearing, aggravated by the functional weakness of tibialis posterior and the increased ease of fatiguability of the muscle on this side.

Lateral shin splints

These are usually the result of excessive traction on the lateral compartment muscles, peroneus longus and brevis. With an 'upslip' and the 'more common' rotational patterns, lateral shin splints may occur just on the left, or be worse on the left than the right, because of the increased tendency toward supination and lateral weight-bearing, compounded by the functional weakness and ease of fatiguability of these muscles on this side. Like medial shin splints, they are usually activity-related.

Pain may also be referred to the lateral shin region from the upper posterior SI joint ligaments (Fig. 3.63A,B), and to the anterolateral shin region from the structures in the anterior hip region; amongst these, the iliofemoral and pubofemoral ligaments (Hackett 1958; Fig. 3.67).

Other possible causes of 'lateral shin pain', more likely on the left side with the lateral shift in weight-bearing, include:

1. a tender ITB, vastus lateralis or biceps femoris insertion (Figs 3.37, 3.41)
2. a painful, displaced proximal tibiofibular joint (Figs 3.81Bi, 3.83)
3. irritation of the common peroneal nerve or its deep and superficial branches as they wind around the fibular head (Figs 3.37, 3.38)

Anterior shin splints

If trigger points (Travell & Simons, 1992), stress fracture, periostalgia from overuse of tibialis anterior and/or an anterior compartment syndrome have been ruled out, anterior shin splints in the presence of malalignment are usually in keeping with referred pain. Hackett (1958: 30) showed how irritation of the sciatic nerve associated with SI joint instability 'resulting from relaxation of posterior sacroiliac, sacrospinus and sacrotuberus ligaments' can result in a pain that localizes 'to either side' of the upper anterior tibia (Fig. 5.38).

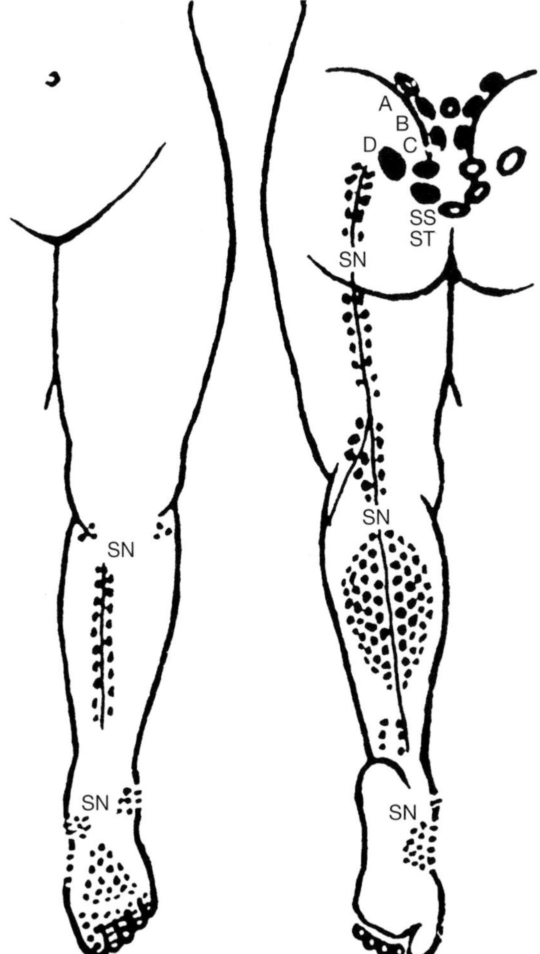

Fig. 5.38 Pattern of 'sciatica' caused by sciatic nerve (SN) irritation that can occur with sacroiliac joint instability from 'relaxation' of the posterior sacroiliac (A, B, C, D), sacrospinous (SS) and sacrotuberous (ST) ligaments. *(Courtesy of Hackett 1958.)*

In the presence of malalignment, therefore, one must always suspect that shin splints tending to localize medially, laterally or anteriorly may be occurring on the basis of referred pain, especially if:

1. the shin splints are not necessarily activity related, at times coming on even at rest
2. there may be variation in the shape or the area involved, though they consistently overlie one area (e.g. the anterior shin), change from one to another of these confined regions, or may involve two or three simultaneously, depending on which structures are being irritated that day
3. typical of referred pain, the area involved is 'non-anatomical'; i.e. not in keeping with the pain confined to the area supplied by a specific nerve
4. there is no localized soft tissue or bone tenderness to suggest overuse periostalgia or possibly a stress fracture, and the bone scan is negative
5. these 'shin splints' are relieved by realignment or by injecting a local anaesthetic into the ligaments from which they originate

Compartment syndrome

The shift in weight-bearing with an 'upslip' and 'rotational malalignment' can selectively increase stress on the medial, anterior and posterior compartments and the muscles within. It may play a role in triggering or maintaining an actual compartment syndrome. Pain and oedema localize to the compartment and/or specific nerves that have been compromised.

Always consider the malalignment-related biomechanical stresses, as these aggravating stresses can be decreased or removed with realignment and may speed up recovery when having to deal with stress fractures, shin splints or compartment syndromes.

WORK AND HOBBIES

In addition to being involved in sports activities, athletes may be working either part or full time, doing housework and possibly persuing physically demanding hobbies. If they are adhering to recommendations in respect to curtailing their athletic activities, yet have ongoing symptoms and the malalignment keeps recurring, their work or hobbies may be the culprit. Of particular concern are those activities involving:

1. asymmetrical movements, such as repeatedly having to lift, reach and twist (e.g. putting things on to high or low shelves, or into filing cabinets)
2. repeatedly getting in and out of bed or a vehicle with one leg leading, thereby exerting a torsional force through the lumbo-pelvic-hip region; similarly, getting on and off a bike or horse, down to and up from a rowing machine or any other piece of exercise equipment that sits low or actually on the floor can result in major asymmetrical strains through this region if the action is done improperly (Figs 5.15, 5.39)
3. dealing with periodic or constant stress (e.g. competitive, emotional or financial)
4. repeated squatting, especially when this is combined with rotation of the trunk and reaching with the arms to either side (e.g. gardening).

The problem may be as simple as that of the runner who had stopped running while undergoing mobilization treatments but who continued to go out of alignment. At the author's recommendation, he had discontinued running in favour of the 'symmetrical' activity of cycling. The recurrence of malalignment was attributed to the torquing of the pelvis required to swing one leg over the seat and crossbar on getting on and off the bicycle. The problem was solved by using a step-up stool or the curb to decrease the amount of torquing (Fig. 5.39).

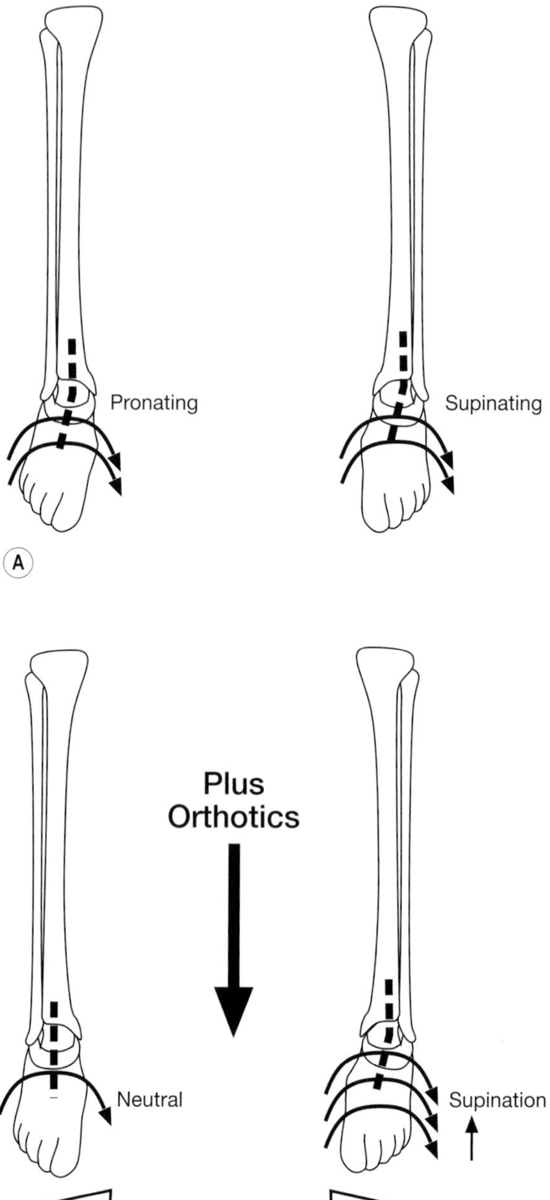

Fig. 5.39 A person with a 'right anterior, left posterior' innominate rotation. (A) Tendency to right pronation, left supination. (B) The effect of providing bilateral orthotics with a medial raise (posting): a decrease of right pronation and an accentuation of the tendency to left supination.

A 'NATURAL' PROCESS OF ELIMINATION

> Malalignment is a ubiquitous condition, yet not everyone who is out of alignment is symptomatic or has developed complications that are evident on examination.

In a study of 136 patients being seen at an intake clinic for admission to a cardiac rehabilitation programme (Schamberger 2002), 80% were out of alignment, in keeping with the percentage reported in multiple other studies (see Ch. 2). 37% of these patients were asymptomatic, other than for their cardiac problems, and on examination had no musculoskeletal findings that could be related to the malalignment; that is, no tenderness of specific muscles or ligaments, or pain with pressure over the spine or on stressing the lumbosacral region, hip or SI joints. The other 63% either had complaints and/or findings on examination that could be attributed to, or aggravated by, the malalignment. These patients were, admittedly, in an older age group (60–80 years) and had been relatively inactive, most of them for many years. There are,

BOX 5.11 Malalignment: factors that can precipitate symptoms

1. The person may become symptomatic when another insult - such as a fall or collision - is imposed on a system already subjected to the stresses inherent to being out of alignment. Athletes, depending on their sport, may be at increased risk of such a mishap occurring, particularly in contact sports (e.g. soccer, American football, hockey).
2. Another mechanism, one that also applies to athletes especially, is the sheer increase in demand placed on the musculoskeletal system. Aggravating factors include starting up or accelerating an exercise programme too quickly, or subjecting specific parts of the system to increased forces by changing equipment or terrain (e.g. suddenly adding up- and downhill to previous all-flat terrain runs). This 'overuse' increases the chances that one of the structures already under excessive stress because of the malalignment will eventually fail and become overtly painful.
3. A third mechanism sees the athlete progress to a level of difficulty at which the malalignment finally interferes with performance, to the point at which it prevents the athlete from advancing in that sport. A typical scenario is the previously cited example of the skater with one of the 'more common' patterns of 'rotational malalignment' who considered dropping out of the training programme because a malalignment-related right leg instability and inability to hold the right edge prevented her from advancing to more demanding routines (see 'Figure skating', above). It is for reasons like these that athletes may get 'eliminated' from their sport altogether, or they settle for alternate, often not as fulfilling, ways of participating in that same sport (see 'Failure to advance in riding', above).

however, definitely people who have been known to be out of alignment for some time but who have become symptomatic only recently. Some of the more common precipitating factors to consider are described in Box 5.11.

Nonetheless, a large number of those athletes who do make it to the top are also out of alignment. There are several possible reasons why they have been able to succeed despite the malalignment:

1. They have somehow been able to compensate, surmounting any limitations imposed by the malalignment. Some compensation may have been achieved through selective stretching and strengthening or the use of devices such as a lift, orthotics, ankle supports, SI joint or weight-belts.
2. They may be able to use the malalignment to their advantage. A high-jumper may, for example, adopt a certain style and side of approach in order to take advantage of the best ranges of motion available, and to avoid any of the restrictions imposed by the malalignment that would become limitations on attempting an approach from the opposite site (Fig. 5.12).
3. They are naturally hypermobile, or they have increased their mobility with stretching and relaxation to the point at which they can now attain ranges of motion which are adequate enough to make any restrictions attributable to the malalignment inconsequential when carrying out a specific manoeuvre.
4. The restrictions do not matter because of the way in which they have learned to cope with the demands of their sport; their personal 'style' or preferences, so to speak. Alternatively, the very nature of the sport may never require them to go past the point at which a limitation of range or a functional weakness will become a problem. For example, an oarsman sweep-rowing in a four or an eight:
   a. is less likely to be affected by lower extremity asymmetries
   b. may be able to compensate for any limitation of pelvic or trunk range of motion by always rowing on the same side
   c. may not have to move the trunk to the point at which:
      i. flexion might pull on posterior ligaments and/or muscles (e.g. latissimus dorsi) which typically show an increase in tension on account of the malalignment
      ii. extension might irritate a tight transversus abdominis or external/internal oblique, or compress facet joints to the point of provoking pain.

EFFECT OF MALALIGNMENT ON THE VALIDITY OF RESEARCH IN SPORTS

Malalignment affects a number of parameters that, in turn, alter the biomechanics of a person's body. The results of any research that involves body biomechanics are, therefore, suspect if the investigator has failed to take into account whether or not malalignment was present in the participants.

These parameters, for example, will affect research looking at, or influenced by, range of motion, muscle strength, muscle tension, leg length and weight-bearing patterns. The author's concerns noted in the first edition still stand: the results of any research dealing with biomechanics and the musculoskeletal system need to be questioned if they have failed to take into account the changes attributable to a coexistent malalignment.

The previously cited studies continue to serve as good illustrations. For example, note was made of studies looking at the effect of orthotics on weight-bearing and oxygen consumption. Most of these studies made no mention of whether the participants were in alignment or not; some (e.g. Delacerda & McCrory 1981) made mention of 'leg length differences' but did not specify whether these were anatomical (true) or functional LLDs.

Let us assume that a participant presents with:

1. a 'right anterior' innominate rotation, the right leg rotated externally, and an obviously pronating foot on this side
2. a 'left posterior' rotation, the left leg rotated internally, and the left foot and ankle appearing to be in neutral or actually supinating slightly on weight-bearing (Figs 3.3, 3.19C, 3.21, 3.22A, 3.23A,B).

Because we are still generally more attuned to detecting pronation, and because the pronation on the right side is often so easily discernible when the presentation of malalignment described is present, the fact that the left foot really remains in neutral or actually supinates slightly may be easily overlooked unless those carrying out the research are familiar with malalignment and specifically looking for an asymmetry of weight-bearing by:

1. doing some simple tests to determine whether malalignment is present, and what type
2. possibly looking at a pair of runners or shoes that have been worn for a few months, to help confirm that an alignment problem is likely present.

Otherwise, the participant stands a good chance of being labelled as a 'pronator' (see 'Introduction 2002'). Initial force plate studies will probably show some difference(s) between the right and left side (Fig. 3.25A,Bi). Any difference may well end up being attributed to a 'leg length difference' that was evident at some part of the examination. One iliac crest may have been observed to be higher than the other in standing, or one leg longer than the other in long-sitting or supine-lying. However, none of the studies cited mentioned whether leg length was checked in more than one position, and it is highly unlikely that the specific 'sitting-lying' test was performed with the intent to note a difference or even shift in length, changes that typically occur with an 'upslip' and 'rotational malalignment'. Simply noting that one iliac crest is higher in standing and possibly finding that there is still an obliquity of the pelvis evident on sitting would (or should) raise suspicions that this is not a simple matter of an anatomical (true) LLD. Unfortunately such comparisons are not likely to be made unless the examiner is trained in assessing alignment (Figs 2.72B, 2.73, 3.86A,B). In the presence of an 'upslip' or 'rotational malalignment', any measurement of leg length, other than by standing X-ray (Figs 2.74A, 2.75) would have been erroneous, as it would have been an assessment using landmarks that could have appeared asymmetrical purely on a functional basis.

Following the initial oxygen uptake studies, each participant was made to run without orthotics, with orthotics that were in neutral, and with different pairs of orthotics that were built-up or 'posted' to varying degrees of equal extent bilaterally on the medial aspect to counteract the supposed 'bilateral pronation'. For example, the right and left orthotics, at one stage, were posted two degrees medially, hindfoot and forefoot. Repeat testing detected a continued side-to-side difference on force plate studies, with no significant change in oxygen consumption for the same workload while wearing the different types of orthotic.

The results should hardly be surprising. What has really happened with the addition of the orthotics? On the right side, the medial posting may have decreased pronation and provided some feeling of stability by increasing support of the medial longitudinal arch. On the left, the orthotic will have increased the tendency toward supination and decreased the ability to absorb shock by decreasing movement in the subtalar joint and mid-transverse arch; the foot may feel comparatively 'stiff'. On repeat force plate studies, there is likely to be a persistence of side-to-side differences which are unlikely to decrease the workload of walking or running. The workload may actually have been increased by:

1. an accentuation of the side-to-side differences, and compensatory changes involving the limbs, pelvis and trunk
2. a loss of shock absorption that results from forcing both feet, especially the left, toward increased lateral weight-bearing

By looking at the combined results for several participants, one also runs the risk of diluting or cancelling out data if different presentations of malalignment are unknowingly included in the sample; e.g. an 'upslip', one of the 'more common' or the 'left anterior and locked' pattern of 'rotational alignment'.

The correct procedure would be to look for any malalignment initially, correct it if present and then reassess weight-bearing. In a number of the participants, any previously noted pronation may be less obvious, or the pattern may now actually be one of bilateral supination (Fig. 3.33). The posted orthotics that are then provided should be appropriate for the weight-bearing pattern now evident: medial for pronation, lateral for supination. In about 90% of cases, the leg length will be equal following realignment. An appropriate lift for the other 10% will ensure that the pelvis is level in all the subjects carrying out the subsequent tests.

The only factor being studied now will be whether oxygen consumption is affected by providing a pair of orthotics, neutral or appropriately posted to correct for any residual tendency toward pronation or supination. In addition, the weight-bearing pattern is now more likely to be symmetrical, something that will become evident on initial and repeat force plate studies.

SUMMARY: RESEARCH AND MALALIGNMENT

1. Researchers frequently appear to assume, usually incorrectly, that we are built more or less symmetrically or that 'minor' asymmetries do not matter. However, malalignment can result in several asymmetries, some or all of which may significantly affect the impact of any interventions. To ascribe side-to-side differences to discrepancies in leg length may be true in part, especially when malalignment is present. However, one must not:
   a) suggest the problem is due to an LLD, without actually identifying the cause of that LLD
   b) imply that the difference is the result of an anatomical (true) LLD, which ignores the fact that:
      (i) 80-90% of participants are likely to be out of alignment, and
      (ii) approximately 90% of these will have an equal leg length once realignment has been achieved.
2. Restrictions in range of motion are easily attributed to a tightness of capsules, ligaments or muscles when there may, in fact, be no true restrictions but merely the functional asymmetries typically seen with an increase in muscle tension and joint orientation seen in association with malalignment. Asymmetries of weight-bearing, muscle bulk and strength may be just as misleading.
3. Much of the research on biomechanics published today continues to ignore malalignment and the entity of a 'malalignment syndrome' and may, therefore, be based on erroneous assumptions. Side-to-side differences may be attributable to malalignment rather than to the effect of an intervention. Alternatively, the malalignment may have a 'cancellation' effect on some interventions, if these interventions act differently on the asymmetries on one side compared to the other (see comments regarding 'orthotic posting', above). The malalignment should, therefore, be corrected before carrying out research likely to be influenced by these asymmetries.

Research should be suspect if it:

1. involves investigation of biomechanical aspects that can be affected by malalignment
2. fails to acknowledge the presence or absence of:
   a. any of the common presentations of malalignment
   b. an underlying 'malalignment syndrome', seen with an 'upslip' and 'rotational malalignment'.

Chapter 6

Horses, saddles and riders

David Lane, DVM

Lauren Fraser

CHAPTER CONTENTS

THE EQUESTRIAN TEAM

All equestrian sports reflect a partnership between horse and rider, a partnership built on communication (Fig. 6.1A). Much of this communication is conveyed through the rider's body position (Fig. 6.2). The higher the team aims to perform, the more subtle these postural clues need to be. Hand position, tension through the reins and bit, shifts in weight along the spine and pelvis, together with a deep seat and relaxed legs, stimulate impulsion and the movement of the horse's back. Only a relaxed rider sitting correctly can apply aids (the signals by which the rider communicates with the horse) well. An effective but soft seat is dependent on the correct position of the rider's pelvis and spine.

Imbalances on the part of either horse or rider can result in 'disconnect' that may adversely affect performance. For instance, if the rider's posture has become imbalanced or asymmetrical secondary to a vertebral or pelvic malalignment, this information will unwittingly be communicated to the horse. The horse may then respond to commands that the rider is unaware he or she is making.

DOI: 10.1016/B978-0-443-06929-1.00006-5

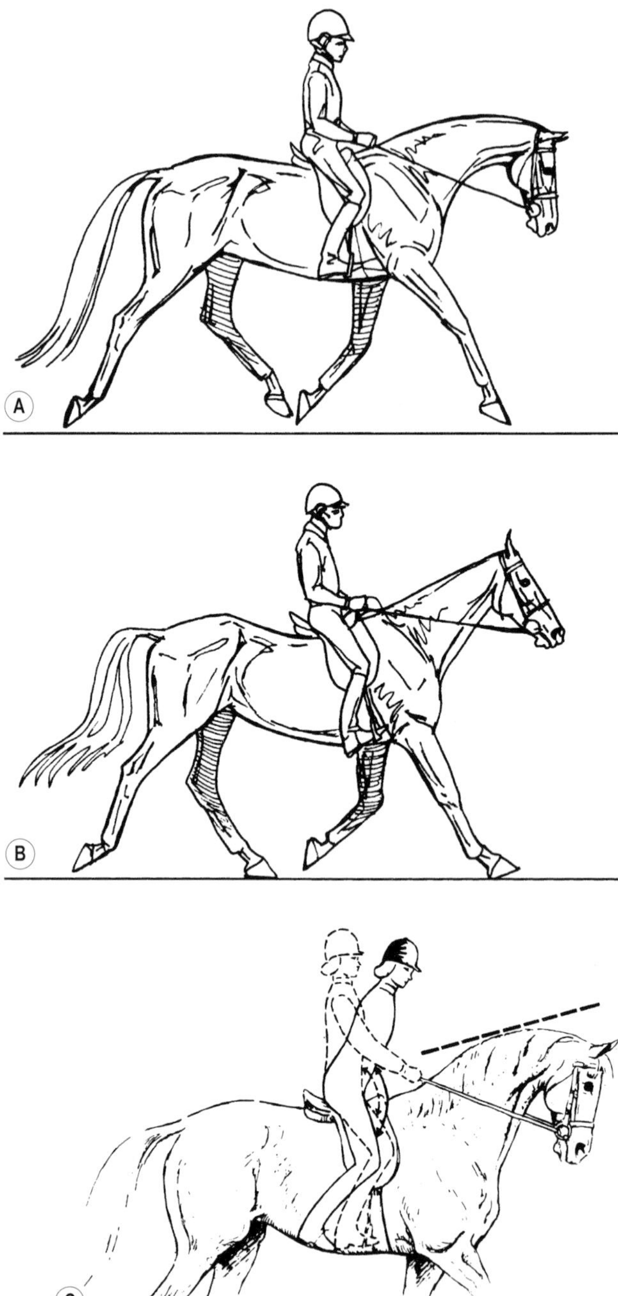

Fig. 6.1 The horse's back and neck as an indicator of problems. (A) Correct: The horse moves 'round' with the back raised. Proper movement can occur with a round, swinging back and not too much tension in the back, neck and hind legs. (B) Incorrect: The horse moves 'hollow' with the back dropped. A tense, hollow back may be caused by problems relating to the horse, the rider or an ill-fitting saddle; it results in a high head and a stiff, uncomfortable gait that prevents the horse engaging the hind legs well, responding correctly to seat aids and 'working on the bit'. (C) When the horse 'overbends', the rider's trunk tends to tip onto the 'fork', the body tilts forwards and the thigh moves too much towards the vertical, the foot tending towards plantarflexion. *(A,B, courtesy of Harris 1996; C, courtesy of Wanless 1995.)*

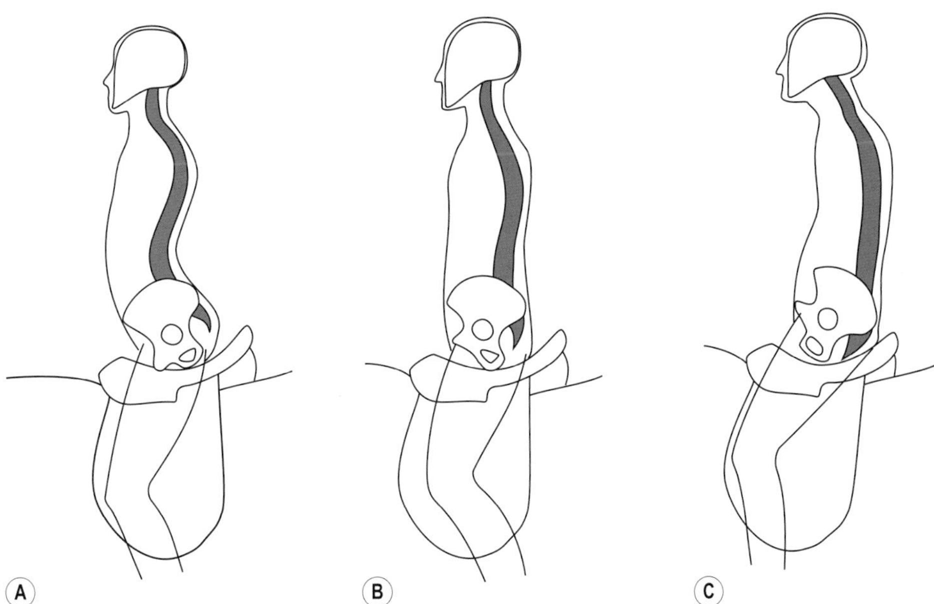

Fig. 6.2 The balance of the rider relative to the alignment of the horse. (A) The pelvis is rolled forwards (anterior rotation: an attempt to balance in the saddle when the horse's head is held high), causing an increased lumbar lordosis and rounded shoulders. (B) The pelvis is correctly balanced, resulting in the normal slight curves of the spine and a straight, strong back. (C) The pelvis is rolled backwards (posterior rotation), causing a rounded back and shoulders, a collapsed chest and a protruding head. *(Redrawn courtesy of Swift 1985.)*

Unexpected or unwanted responses (e.g. failure to turn as easily to one side as the other) frustrate the rider and can be inaccurately attributed to a behavioural, training or limb lameness issue in the horse.

Another example involves the use of aids. The intensity of a rein aid, for example, is made by slight pressure from the ring finger, by a rounding of the wrists or by using the whole arm. The intensity is sustained while increasing forward drive aids to the horse. When the horse submits, the hand relaxes and light control is maintained. An imbalance and asymmetry of the scapulae associated with pelvic malalignment will unwittingly interfere with rein tension (Figs 2.90, 2.120 C).

If the horse is afflicted with malalignment, it may not be able to perform to an expected level. Loss of collection, altered head carriage, refusing jumps or resisting the bit are just a few examples of how the horse's performance may be affected. Because malalignment often remains undiagnosed, these performance issues are frequently assumed to be behavioural in origin.

Furthermore, because malalignment often results in proprioceptive deficits and reduced muscle mass, if the horse continues to attempt feats it is no longer fit to perform, it is at an increased risk of incurring a secondary injury.

Not only can malalignment issues predispose the horse to further injury, they may also be the result of an underlying subclinical or undiagnosed limb lameness. Frequent recurrence of the same malalignment lesion should raise the suspicion of an underlying lameness.

Proper evaluation of the equestrian team must look at horse and rider, both in and out of the saddle. Consideration must also be given to the saddle itself, to determine how well it fits. An ill-fitting saddle can adversely affect both team members.

> To determine the cause of the problem, the conformation of both the horse and the rider must be evaluated, individually and as a working team.

Team evaluations require an assessment of each member individually and with the horse and rider working in tandem. Trainers frequently err by using substitute riders when evaluating the horse, which negates the opportunity to diagnose conditions resulting from the specific pairing of team members.

> Another rider, except possibly an instructor who is trained to notice these types of difficulties, may complicate the situation by bringing a new set of skills, and often new problems, to the scene.

Several questions need to be asked to determine whether the horse and rider are suited for each other:

1. Is the horse too big or small?

   A basic rule of thumb is that the combined weight of rider and tack should not exceed 20% of the horse's weight, but such rules are dependent on multiple other factors such as rider experience, saddle size, horse back length, etc.

2. Are their skill levels well suited?

   An experienced rider's vertebrae are mobile but controlled. The spine moves laterally from a convex to a concave position with ease, and the low back moves primarily forward and backward with the sway of the horse (Figs 6.1A, 6.2B, 6.3). The rider can apply a signal to the horse with the action of the spine to urge the horse forward. This mobility and control is not often seen in the novice and the senior rider. A well-trained performance horse may not understand the signals provided by an inexperienced rider's vertebral movements.

If the team is experiencing a performance issue, one first needs to determine where the problem lies. For instance, if the team veers to the left, the assessor needs to decide whether incorrect guidance from the rider is at fault, or if the problem originates from the horse. Perhaps the rider has a malalignment of the pelvis with a 'right anterior' innominate rotation. The right ischium will be found to be high (Figs 2.73 C, 3.86B, 6.4A,C); whereas the left ischial tuberosity is lower and puts pressure on the horse's left paravertebral muscles, causing a reflex increase in tension in these muscles. The rider's right shoulder and hip are too far ahead of the action, so that the rider appears to be perching on the saddle (Figs 5.37, 6.4Bii, C). The right hip ends up in extension, and the right leg goes too far behind the girth of the saddle. **Incorrect signals are communicated to the horse because the sitting position of the rider is incorrect**. Conversely, trapezius and paraspinal restrictions of the horse's mid-thoracic region could shorten the left forelimb stride length, which can also result in the team veering off course. Both conditions could exist concurrently.

In many cases, the rider complains of muscle spasm and in some cases stiffness when mounting and dismounting. Muscle spasm can be evoked in the vicinity of an injury or lesion as a protective reflex to prevent unwanted movement. This protective reflex is also operative if the pain originates from a joint. The muscles are not necessarily in

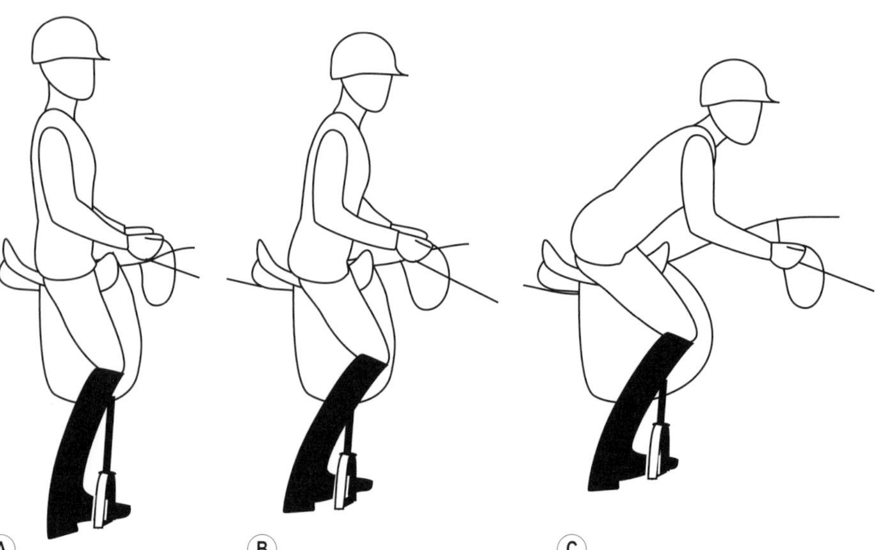

Fig. 6.3 The three main seating positions in riding. (A) Dressage seat. (B) Light seat. (C) Forward (or jumping) seat. *(Redrawn courtesy of Harris 1996.)*

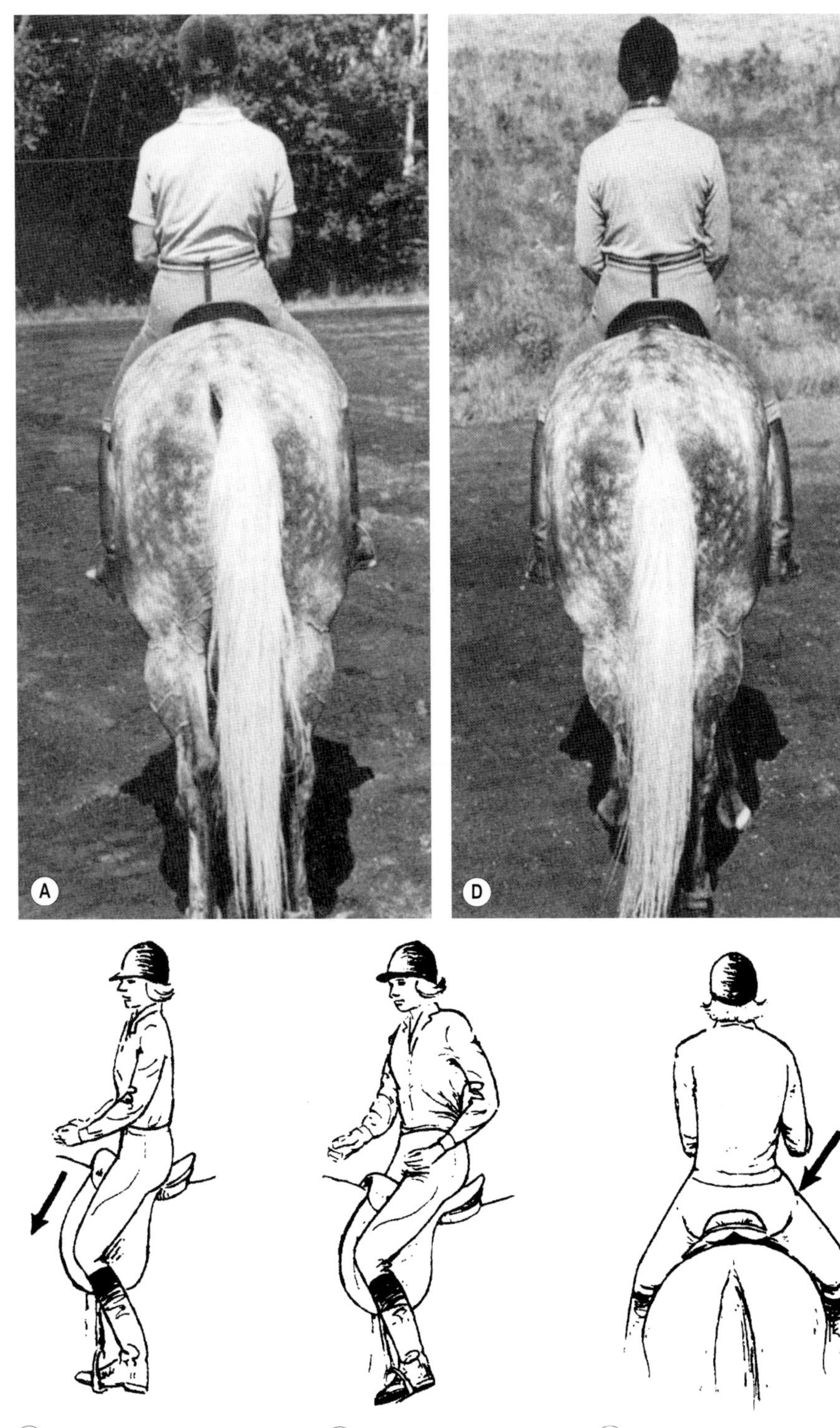

Fig. 6.4 A rider sitting 'off centre' (A) The right shoulder and pelvic (iliac) crest are obviously higher than the left, the pelvis being rotated to the left (forwards on the right). (B) The rider's 'good' (i) and 'bad' (ii) sides. As the rider collapses (i.e. goes out of alignment, with right anterior rotation), more of the chest shows, and the twist carries through to her thigh, so that it hangs away from the saddle: she clings on with just part of it. (C) The 'collapse', seen from the back. The rider's inside leg-body angle closes, whereas the outer angle opens. (D) The rider. . .is now sitting squarely in the saddle: the pelvic crests and shoulders are even and the spine straight. *(A,D, courtesy of Swift 1985; B,C, courtesy of Wanless 1995.)*

constant spasm around the injured joint, but movement beyond a critical point can trigger specific groups to contract. The observed pattern of spasm can then be interpreted to determine the type of malalignment present in the horse and/or rider. Spasm in the left quadratus lumborum, the left paraspinal muscle at L2 and L3, and/or the left latissimus dorsi can, for example, indicate pelvic malalignment with thoracic and shoulder involvement.

MALALIGNMENT IN THE RIDER

THE BALANCE AND SEATING POSITIONS OF THE RIDER

Equestrians communicate instructions to their horses through subtle changes in body and limb position. Different sports place different demands on the horse and, therefore, require a different 'seat' or riding position. Each seat is intended to guide and provide harmony of movement with the horse. Balance needs to remain centered, yet also needs to flow with the dynamics of the horse. In traditional English riding, there are three main seating positions in equitation (Fig. 6.3):

1. the dressage seat (also called the basic seat)
2. the light seat
3. the forward (or jumping) seat

Following is a description of these seats and how they may be adversely affected by malalignment of the rider.

The dressage seat

> The dressage seat is considered to be the basic seat for training a horse and rider in flat work.

To achieve this seat, the rider should assume a normal upper body position, with a vertical spine centered above the sacrum and the pelvis evenly positioned (Fig. 6.3A). By engaging and relaxing the paraspinal muscles, the rider is able to move harmoniously with the horse. The shoulders should be slightly retracted and depressed at the scapulae. Shoulders and heels should be in perfect vertical alignment.

The upper arms should be relaxed and move freely in a flexion–extension motion from the shoulder joint. The elbow is flexed, and the forearm is in a mid-position with the wrists straight, the fingers flexed and the thumbs uppermost. Relaxed shoulders, elbows and wrists ensure that the rider's body movements are not transmitted through their hands. The head is carried erect, with vision directed toward the intended direction of movement. The chin must stay in line and not push forward.

The ischia and pubic symphysis form the triangle of the seat. The thighs lie flat against the saddle, with sufficient coxo-femoral internal rotation to allow the medial surface of the knee to contact the saddle fully. The line of the rider's thigh should be as vertical as possible without taking the weight off the ischium (Figs 6.1A, 6.2B, 6.3, 6.4Bi). Having a long line to the thigh ensures a deep knee position which enables the rider to apply the lower leg to the barrel of the horse.

The rider's legs below the knee usually slope backward and downward. Depending on the length of the leg, the knee joints are typically flexed to 30 degrees. The medial surface of the calf keeps a light contact with the side of the horse.

The toes and forefoot are dorsiflexed and everted, pointing forward and slightly outward. The stirrup is positioned under the metatarsophalangeal joints and the weight of the rider normally transfers backward from the metatarsophalangeal joints to the heel. The ankle needs to flex freely with the horse's movements.

Should the rider be affected by a malalignment of the foot and ankle resulting in supination of the forefoot, the foot will plantarflex and elevate the heel. Consequently, weight can no longer be distributed backward through to the heel, the upper body is shifted forward and the hands drop. The head moves forward as well, into a 'poking chin' posture (see Fig. 6.2C).

Pelvic imbalances such as sacral torsion and/or locking of a sacroiliac joint can prevent the rider from maintaining correct positioning. For example, an 'anterior' rotation of the pelvis on one side, in which the innominate ends up rotated forward and upward (Figs 5.37, 6.4, 6.5), causes asymmetry in thigh position. If the rider attempts to compensate, the knee on the side of the 'anterior' rotation is forced either externally or internally. The former position leads to an insecure seat (Figs 5.37, 6.4Bii,C); the latter rotates the lower leg away from the horse, reducing the ability of the rider to communicate using the medial calf or heel.

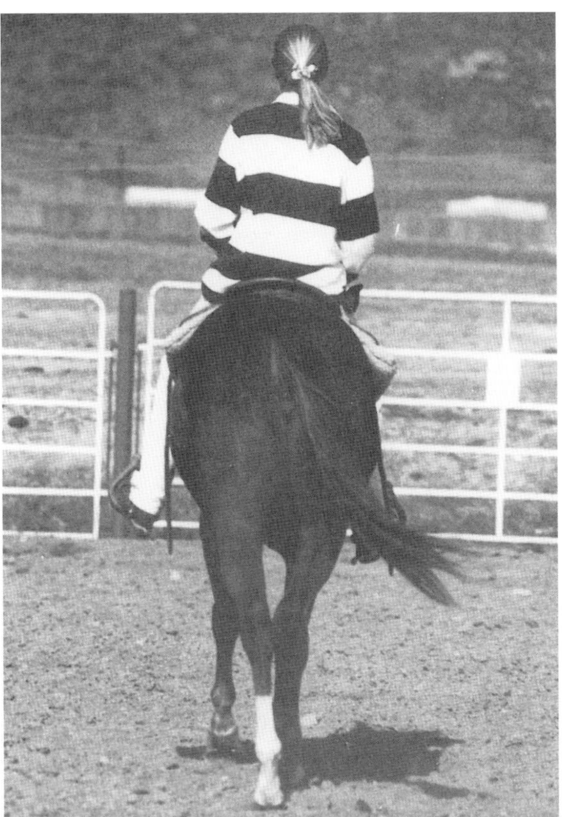

Fig. 6.5 Left anterior rotation can be one cause of an abnormal sitting position or 'crookedness'. The left ischial tuberosity is raised off the saddle, losing contact and resulting in a shift of position, with the left pelvis and shoulder in forward rotation. *(Courtesy of Hill 1992.)*

The light seat

The light seat is useful for flat work with show jumpers and when there are frequent changes between the flat work and jumping.

The light seat reduces the burden of weight on the horse's back (Fig. 6.3B). The stirrups are shortened two holes to lean the rider forward and increase flexion at the knee. This position releases some of the weight from the ischium and puts more of it through the upper leg. It also engages the hip flexors and adductors.

Pelvic malalignment results in an asymmetry of strength through the hip girdle and leg muscles (see Ch. 3, Appendix 3). This imbalance, in addition to the malpositioning of the legs, contributes to uneven weight distribution in the saddle. For the rider to achieve a true light seat, there can be no malalignment of the pelvis and spine.

The forward (jumping) seat

The purpose of the forward seat is to give freedom to the horse's back and enable the rider to follow quickly all the balance and movement changes of the horse.

The forward or jumping seat is an advanced position recommended only after acquiring a safe, balanced dressage and light seat (Fig. 6.3C). It is used for both jumping and galloping and the rider must be able to transition easily between this and the light or forward seats between jumps. Failure to execute these transitions in a balanced or symmetrical fashion can throw the horse off stride.

The stirrups are again shortened to promote knee flexion and ankle dorsiflexion, and are placed mid-metatarsal rather than at the metatarsophalangeal joints. Failure to position the stirrup correctly or maintain the forefoot in plantarflexion, rather than dorsiflexion, can result in ankle joint immobilization (see Ch. 3; Fig. 3.30)

CONFORMATION OF THE RIDER

One of the most common problems to arise in training is that the horse shows signs of stiffness or a lack of willingness to laterally flex the neck and body (Fig. 6.6).The assumption is all too frequently made that this lack of willingness comes from the temperament of the horse. Changes in equipment are made, or stronger aids are used to make the horse comply.

Failure to respond to these measures should trigger the notion that a physiological imbalance may be at the true root of the problem. If a malalignment exists, it first needs to be determined whether the problem originates with the horse or the rider. Practitioners will find that in most chronic cases, both the horse and the rider are affected and both will require treatment.

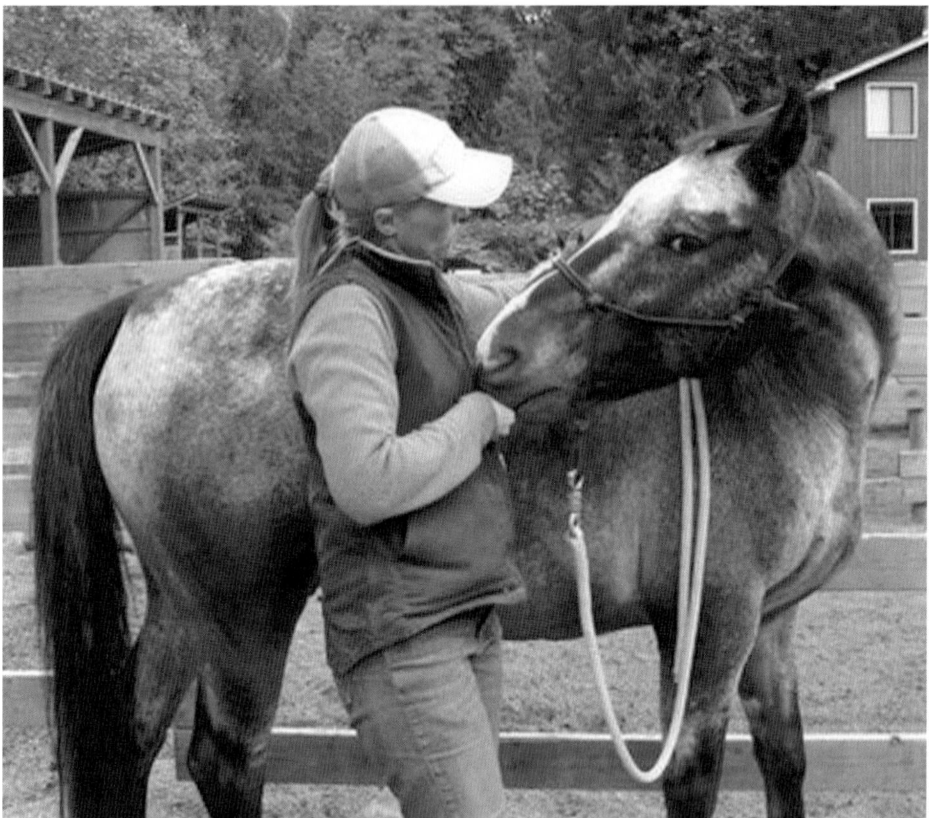

Fig. 6.6 Neck lateral flexion ROM test. A treat is offered from behind the horse, encouraging it to voluntarily stretch the neck laterally. Horses with reduced neck flexion will be unwilling or unable to hold their neck in sustained lateral flexion for more than a second, or they may externally rotate their skull in order to achieve additional reach. This horse is showing normal left lateral neck range of motion.

The following questions are useful in determining whether the problem is originating with the horse or the rider:

1. When riding, is there any pain or aching between the shoulder blades (scapulae) or on one side of the neck or shoulder?
2. Has the trainer commented that, when sitting square in the saddle, the rider has:
   a. one shoulder higher than the other (Figs 6.4A,C, 6.5) ?
   b. the pelvic crest elevated on one side (Figs 6.4A, 6.5) ?
3. Is there low back pain during or after riding?
4. Does the rider have trouble sitting deep in the saddle?

If the answer to any of these questions is 'yes', the rider's weight is not distributed evenly through the saddle, resulting in an incorrect seat. 'In balance' in the saddle means that the pelvic (iliac) crests are even (Figs 6.4D, 2.71A,B), and that each ischium sits deeply. There is no rotation in the spine (lumbar to cervical). When the horse is working 'in balance', there is a rhythmic upward thrust to the pattern of movement conveyed to the rider through the horse's back.

When riders are not in alignment, or are significantly rotated around the pelvis, their ability to control and communicate with the horse is reduced. Injury-induced asymmetries are common. Even though chronic pain may not yet be in evidence, riders often exhibit a limited range of motion that can prevent them from reaching peak performance.

The rider compensates by bringing the trunk back to vertical, rotating the pelvis forward and, thereby, increasing the lumbar lordosis (Fig. 6.2A).

As indicated above, an aid is a form of communication between the horse and rider, through the use of hands, legs and seat position. Weight transferred from the spine and pelvis, together with a deep seat and relaxed legs, stimulates impulsion and the movement of the horse's back. The rider creates and maintains the horse in a forward movement. In doing so, the rider seems to 'sit the horse on the bit'; that is, to convey a message via the reins and bit. In addition, contact with the bit via the reins to the rider's hands permits additional communication. The horse must be supple and in balance with the rider in order to take the rein aids willingly and to rebalance itself by movement of its head and neck.

The rider's seat: weight aids

Only a relaxed rider sitting correctly can apply the weight aids efficiently. An effective but soft seat is dependent on the correct position of the rider's pelvis and spine. Malalignment reduces the stability of the rider in the saddle by altering the 'correct' position and hence the distribution of the weight.

Shoulder girdle and upper extremity: rein aids

The intensity of the rein aid depends on whether it is made by slight pressure from the ring finger, by a rounding of the wrists or by using the whole arm. This rein aid is sustained while increasing forward drive aids to the horse. When the horse submits, the hand relaxes and light control is maintained. The imbalance and asymmetry of the scapulae associated with pelvic malalignment will interfere with any application of the rein aids (Figs 2.90, 2.120).

The rider's seat is the key to identifying rider-based malalignment. The pelvis must be level and symmetrical in the transverse and sagittal plane to allow the horse to be balanced and free to move (Figs 6.2B, 6.4Bi,D). An uneven pelvis compromises this balance and ability to move. 'Anterior' rotation of the left innominate results in having the left side high when sitting (Fig. 6.5) and will cause the hip and knee on that side to become raised and forward (the reverse of the situation illustrated in Fig. 6.4). These changes can prevent the horse from flexing and moving easily to the left.

Presentations of the malaligned rider

Box 6.1 outlines two common presentations of malalignment in the rider; in both, the left hip is lowered and the right ilium elevated.

Complaints of the rider

Malalignment is most likely to result in complaints involving the facet, hip or SI joints, as well as the scapular region. Pain can result from these sites being put under stress either directly or as a consequence of malalignment-related impairment of pelvic, spine or limb function resulting in abnormal or increased strain while riding.

Sacroiliac joint pain

Decreased mobility at the SI joint can alter the ability of the rider to achieve a deep seat in the saddle. When the range of movement is lost at the hips, vertebral and sacroiliac movement must increase to compensate. Pain from the SI joint usually radiates into the buttock, the groin, and/or down the leg of the affected side (Fig. 3.63). On examination, the pelvis is no longer balanced, the right ilium is probably elevated if the left hip is lowered (Fig. 6.4A,C). Tests intended to stress specific structures, such as

BOX 6.1 Two common presentations of malalignment in the rider

Presentation A: there is rotation of the lumbar vertebrae to the right into a right convexity of the lumbar spine, usually from L1 to L4 (see Fig. 2.96), the maximum rotation generally being found at L2. A mild compensatory rotation to the left occurs throughout the thoracic spine. The scapulae are uneven and the left shoulder is elevated and rotated forward. The rider complains of pain in the low back and between the scapulae.

Presentation B: there is no rotation of the lumbar spine but rotation occurs throughout the thoracic spine, beginning to the right at T10 and being maximal at T3–T5. There is also a compression and narrowing of the space between the right transverse processes of T1 and C7. Stress on the cervical spine is increased. The rider exhibits a bobbing head and reports pain between the scapulae and often numbness and tingling radiating into the right shoulder and arm.

the anterior and posterior sacroiliac ligaments, may be positive, indicating SI origin pain (see Ch. 2). In addition to realignment, the preferred treatment for sacroiliac and lumbosacral pain includes:

1. SI joint support in the form of a lumbosacral support (somewhat more extensive than an SI belt; Figs 7.34, 7.35), to be worn while riding and working with the horse
2. Electrotherapy, Interferential Current, laser; for example, IFC with Vacomed attachment or the HeNe Scan Laser with infrared beam component (2–4 J/cm^2; area 10 × 15 cm), which has been found particularly helpful.

Facet joint pain

Facet joint injury can result from:

1. prolonged or excessive compression (Fig. 2.52)
   For example, when the right innominate is rotated 'anterior' and the pelvis elevated on the right, there is usually a lumbar curve, convex to left, with subsequent vertebral rotation into the convexity of the curve (Fig. 2.42). The facet joint surfaces on the right are compressed; whereas those on the left are separated. The pain that can result in prolonged or excessive compression is often felt as a 'deep in the bone' ache, which is commonly referred from the low back to the buttock, and can also be referred down the thigh to the knee.
2. an acute sprain or strain
   With an acute right lumbar facet sprain or strain, spasm of the surrounding muscles (e.g. paravertebrals and quadratus lumborum) elevates the right pelvis, narrows the lumbar disc spaces on the right side and prevents rotation through the lumbar spine. Pain is commonly referred forward or around the iliac crest and into the pubic area (compare to Fig. 4.21).

Alterations of weight-bearing and ranges of motion

1. Leg orientation and foot posture patterns
   The therapist should look at the legs:
   a. with the feet in the stirrups, when the horse and rider are stationary, and
   b. from the front and the back, when they are moving toward and away.
   With the 'more common' presentations, right innominate rotated 'anterior' (Figs 5.37, 6.4), the right leg may be obviously externally rotated, with the knee falling outward to the point at which the right foot ends up on tiptoe with the heel elevated (plantarflexed). The left leg may, however, be internally rotated, the left knee hugging the side of the horse and the foot collapsed inward and dorsiflexed (pronated). The opposite pattern may be seen with, for example, the 'left anterior and locked' presentation (Fig. 6.5).
2. Hip ranges of motion
   These are tested to determine the ability of the rider to have the correct leg position, which is needed to communicate with the horse using pressure signals from the calf, knee and thigh. Malalignment results in an asymmetry of hip range of motion. For example, with the right pelvis elevated and rotated forward in the sagittal plane:
   a. external rotation of the right leg is increased, as is adduction and abduction; whereas right internal rotation is limited (Figs 3.44, 3.78, 3.79, 6.4 C)
   b. right hip flexion is decreased and extension is increased (Figs 3.71, 3.72, 3.76Bi).

Hip joint pain

Pain from the hip can be referred forward to the groin and goes down the anterolateral thigh to the knee (Fig. 3.67). It can radiate down the anterior aspect of the lower leg but stops proximal to the ankle joint. Hip joint pain can be assessed by determining the hip ranges of motion, both passively and on resisted movement (see Chs 2, 3). Note should be made whether

1. there is any weakness
2. pain occurs on passive and/or active movement
3. pain is experienced at a particular point of the available range.

Scapular pain

With an imbalance of the scapulae, the rider complains of pain in the paraspinal muscles between the shoulder blades. This imbalance also decreases the range of scapular abduction and retraction when the shoulder is elevated and can lead to inconsistency with rein aids. Imbalanced rein tension communicates unwanted signals to the horse. Furthermore, rigidly held reins can prevent the horse from bending or flexing correctly.

Begin the scapular examination with the rider standing, and then sitting on a stool with no back support. Note the level of the scapulae, bearing in mind that alterations of the level can indicate weakness in the trapezius muscles, serratus anterior or latissimus dorsi. To demonstrate abnormal mobility of the scapulae against the thorax, ask the rider to shrug the shoulders. Riders, especially those who engage in hunter-jumper, 2-3-day eventing and endurance activities, occasionally develop hand numbness when riding. If thoracic outlet syndrome is suspected (Figs 3.12, 3.13), have the rider elevate the scapulae and shrug the shoulders, holding this position for approximately 1 minute. Adson's manoeuvre and the 'military position' should also be tried. Pain into the arms or tingling may indicate a thoracic outlet syndrome but other tests and appropriate investigations are needed to confirm or eliminate this often elusive diagnosis.

ASSESSMENT OF THE HORSE: ANATOMY AND GAIT

ANATOMY

On a microscopic level, the equine musculoskeletal system is virtually identical to a human's. As a result, most physiological principles remain the same for both species. However, there are also fundamental anatomical differences that prevent direct extrapolation of all principles.

One key difference is that the equine spine is not a vertical column like a human's; it is aligned horizontally, like a suspension bridge.

Another difference lies in the fact horses frequently weigh more than 400 kg. Their skeletal systems must routinely endure forces that ours cannot. This creates significant limitations when treating certain equine orthopaedic conditions. Comminuted long bone fractures are fatal, even with the best surgical care at hand. Technology has yet to design an orthopaedic implant that can withstand the stresses placed on it by a large convalescing animal, and few horses convalesce well.

Like humans, horses of different builds have an affinity for different sports. Jumpers tend to be more heavily muscled with long sloping scapulae, endurance horses are typically flat muscled with smaller builds and deep chests, and western stock horses usually have short backs and short metacarpals/tarsals.

The back

The horse has 7 cervical vertebrae, 18 thoracic and either 5 or 6 lumbar (depending on the breed). A variable number of transverse spinous processes of the caudal lumbar vertebrae articulate via synovial joints. These intertransverse joints provide rotational stability while exerting the hip extensors. The 16th thoracic dorsal spinous process stands upright; everything superior to it is angled backward, and everything inferior to it is angled forward (Fig. 6.7).

Head and neck

The carriage of the head and neck and the contents of the intestines determine the position of the centre of gravity.

When standing in neutral posture, the horse is said to be 'standing square'. All four limbs are in line, with the metacarpals and metatarsals positioned vertically. The centre of gravity is approximately at the height of the sternum under the centre of the trunk, closer to the front legs or 'forehand' (Fig. 6.8).

The forelimbs

When standing square, the forelimbs carry 20% more weight than the hind limbs (60-65% and 35-40%, respectively). Equine shoulder joints are less flexible than humans', being restricted to predominantly forward and backward movements, but are more stable than their human counterparts. Figure 6.9 shows the normal forelimb skeletal anatomy and hoof conformation. Landing jumps, braking and turning are activities that increase forelimb strain.

The hind legs

The hind legs and associated musculature provide the immense power associated with equine athletic endeavours – sudden turns, big jumps and explosive starts (Fig. 6.10). Because the hind legs directly connect to the pelvis and spine, malalignment of the pelvis or the lumbosacral junction interferes with this propulsive force and subsequent performance. Subclinical tarsal inflammation or degenerative arthritis is not uncommon, and frequently leads to secondary pelvic imbalances.

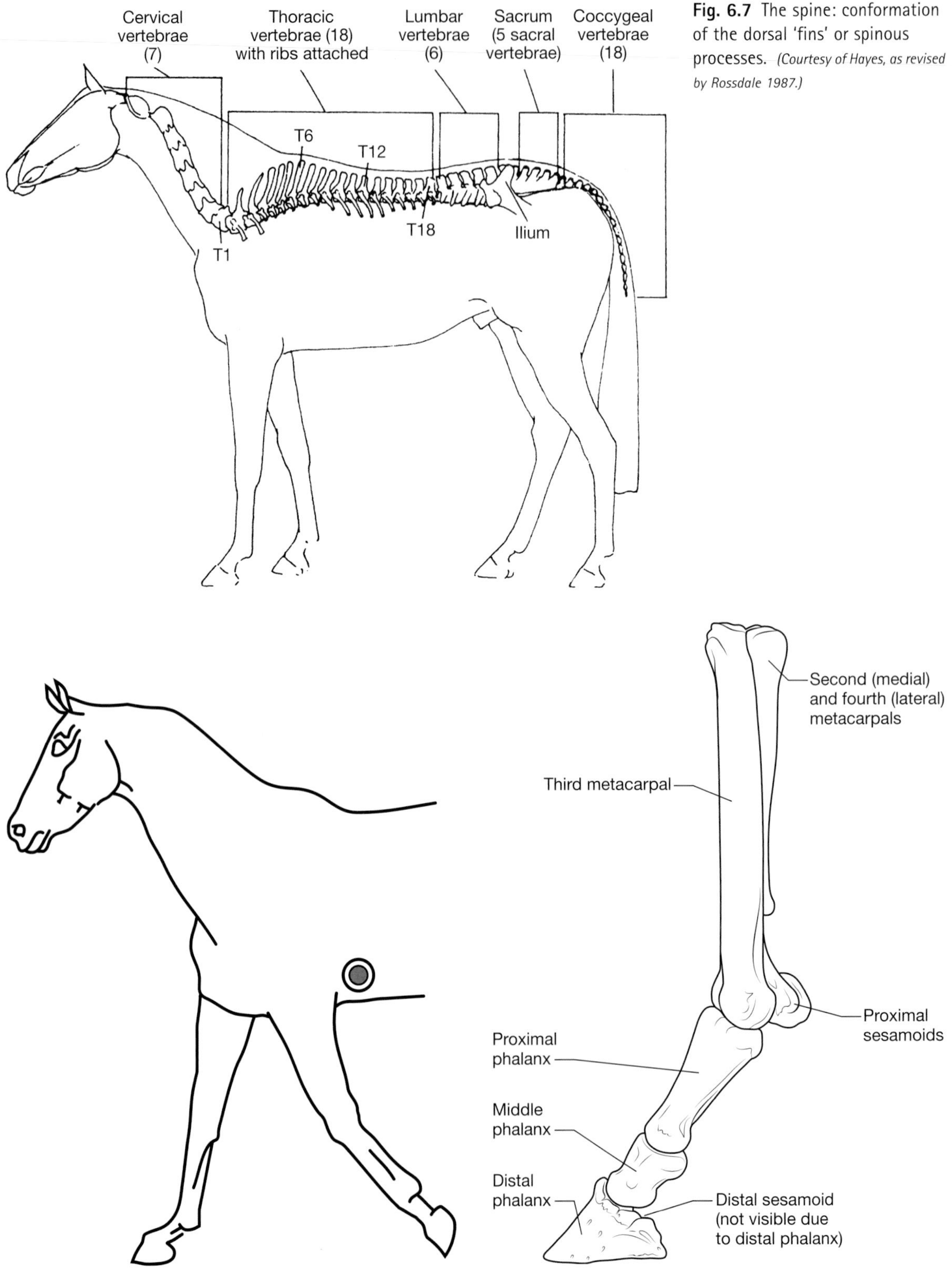

Fig. 6.7 The spine: conformation of the dorsal 'fins' or spinous processes. *(Courtesy of Hayes, as revised by Rossdale 1987.)*

Fig. 6.8 Location of the centre of gravity. *(Redrawn courtesy of Strasser & Kells 1998.)*

Fig. 6.9 Horse's 'thoracic limb' (forelimb) anatomy. *(Courtesy of T.S. Stashak, Ed., Adam's 5th edition 2002.)*

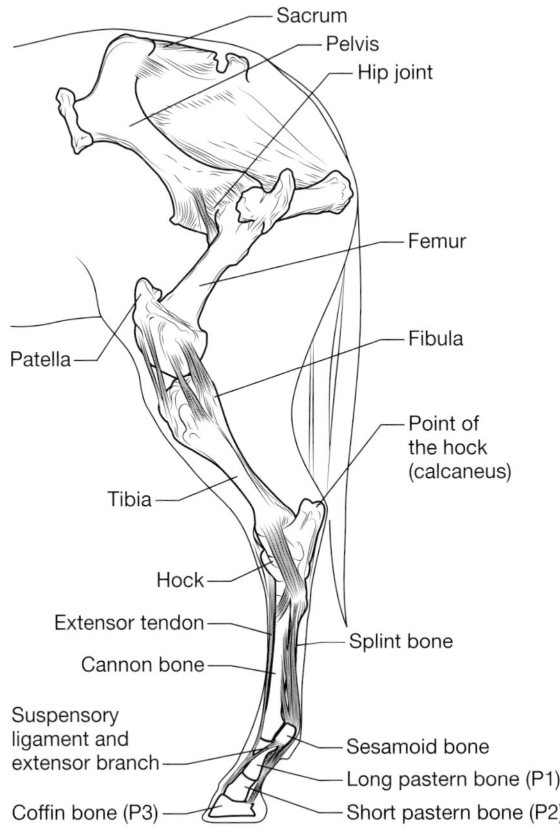

Fig. 6.10 Horse's 'pelvic limb' (hindlimb) anatomy. *(Courtesy of T.S. Stashak, Ed., Adam's 5th edition 2002.)*

GAIT

There are four typical gait patterns – the walk, trot, canter and gallop. The horse should be able to switch from one to the other easily, either spontaneously or with appropriate commands.

Walk

At the walk, the horse takes separate steps with each leg. Movement initiates with a hind leg, followed by the front leg on the same side; for example, left hind then left front, followed by the right hind and finally the right front leg (Fig. 6.11A). One foot remains on the ground at all times. Stride lengths are generally even; failure of the hind foot to fall at least partly into the footprint of the front leg on the same side may indicate a malalignment issue.

Trot

At the trot, the horse springs from one diagonal pair of legs to the other; e.g. the left hind and the right front coming to the ground together. When the horse springs off that pair of legs, there is a moment of suspension where no foot is in contact with the ground, followed by synchronous placement of the right hind and left front (Fig. 6.11B). The movement is continuous and should be rhythmic, with a two-time beat.

Canter and gallop

Both the canter and the gallop are 3-beat gaits, e.g. left hind to left diagonal, onto right hind and left foreleg; then to right foreleg, followed by a period of suspension with all four legs off the ground (Fig. 6.11C). Because these gaits require greater strength and fitness, younger horses find them more difficult to perform while carrying a rider. Consequently, the rider may overcompensate to counterbalance and could develop an increased rotation in the thorax with a shift of the pelvis, so that the opposite ischium bears more weight.

FACTORS AFFECTING MALALIGNMENT IN THE HORSE

Malalignment in the horse can cause malalignment to develop in the rider and vice versa.

Malalignment in the horse is frequently a 'chicken or the egg' situation: physiological imbalances or sports injuries frequently lead to secondary malalignment and vice versa. There are many factors that can contribute to equine vertebral kinetics, probably many more than we currently appreciate. The most commonly implicated factors are listed below:

Conformation and posture

As mentioned earlier, different horses have different conformation or body builds that lend themselves to certain tasks. Some horses have poor conformation which predisposes them to certain injuries. For example, horses with long backs and weak paraspinal musculature are more likely to suffer from back injuries. These horses frequently present with poor posture – lordosis of the thoracic vertebrae just inferior to the scapulae and a secondary elevation of the head (Fig. 6.1B). Malalignment can lead to this posture, and vice versa.

Horses that are asked to perform tasks for which they are inadequately suited, be it as a result of poor

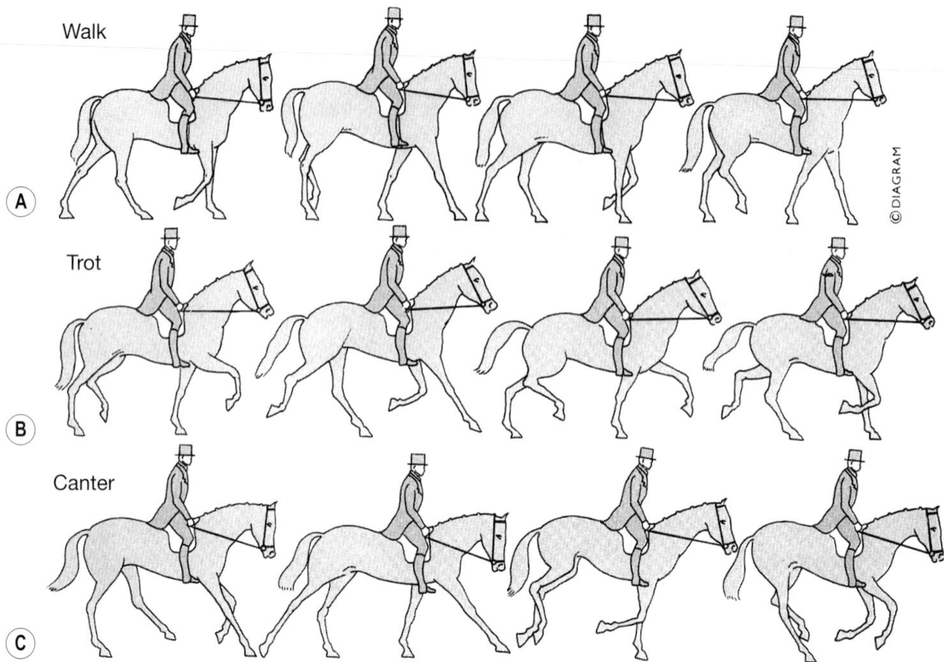

Fig. 6.11 Riding gait: the walk, trot and canter. (A) The walk: there are separate steps, one after the other (right hind, right front, then left hind and left front). There is no moment of suspension. (B) The trot: the horse jumps from one diagonal to another (right hind and left front, then left hind and right front). There is a moment of suspension with all four legs in the air. (C) The canter: a three-time pace. In the right canter, the sequence is left hind leg, left diagonal (right hind and left foreleg) and right foreleg, followed by a period of suspension. *(Courtesy of Worth 1990.)*

conformation, inadequate fitness level, subclinical disease, or unrealistic expectations on the part of the rider, are predisposed to malalignment issues. It takes experience and sound judgment to determine what a horse is truly capable of. The horse must be well suited to the rider, in size, experience and ambition.

There are many details to consider when evaluating a horse's conformation, far too many to be considered within the scope of this chapter. Multiple books have been written on this topic.

Lameness

Equine malalignment issues infrequently present as a clinical single limb lameness. Horses with an obvious limp need to be seen by a veterinarian for diagnosis. Basic information on how to detect the presence of a limp can be found within the discussion on 'Evaluation of the horse', below.

Subclinical, or difficult to detect lameness, is relatively common and often initially presents as a malalignment issue. Horses will frequently compensate for mild lamenesses by shifting their weight off the affected limb and guarding it. Such protective measures can be enough to prevent them from manifesting observable disease but can easily lead to secondary malalignment issues or injury. For example, a horse with left tarsal arthritis may mask the discomfort by throwing its weight forward on a diagonal into the right forelimb, triggering spasm of the trapezius or other muscles associated with scapular movement. This results in an abnormally shortened right forelimb stride length which, coupled with the increased weight load of a rider, could result in secondary tendonitis or thoracic malalignment issues.

Horses presenting with either a primary limb lameness, or a chronically recurring malalignment issue should receive a full lameness exam from a qualified veterinarian. Such examinations routinely include extensive gait evaluation, radiographs and regional nerve blocks.

Hoof care

Hoof pain is a leading cause of lameness in horses. Abscesses of the hoof wall, bruising of the sole, inflammation of the laminae that connect the hoof wall to the foot itself are just a few examples of common conditions. Part of any proper examination for lameness will focus on the hoof (Fig. 6.12).

Horses were designed to move constantly. Wild horses typically travel 20 to 30 miles each day. Normal grazing behaviour consists of taking a few bites of grass, walking several steps, taking another few bites, and so on. The hoof is a dynamic structure that expands and contracts with the repeated change from bearing weight to non-weight-bearing. Each footfall contributes to the circulation of blood. Many horses today are kept in unnatural conditions; confined to 12 by 12 foot square stalls and shod with metal shoes that restrict normal foot dynamics. Consequently, hoof wear of a confined horse differs significantly from that of a free range or wild horse.

Hoof conformation greatly affects how weight is distributed through the remaining structures of the limb and eventually the vertebral column. Toe length affects the 'breakover' point of the hoof and determines how much force is applied to the sensitive laminae. Poorly trimmed, shod, or otherwise cared for feet can contribute to a wealth of medical conditions and should always be considered when evaluating a horse's condition.

Roughened and irregular hoof walls, abnormal conformation, chipped or cracked hoofs, hoof walls

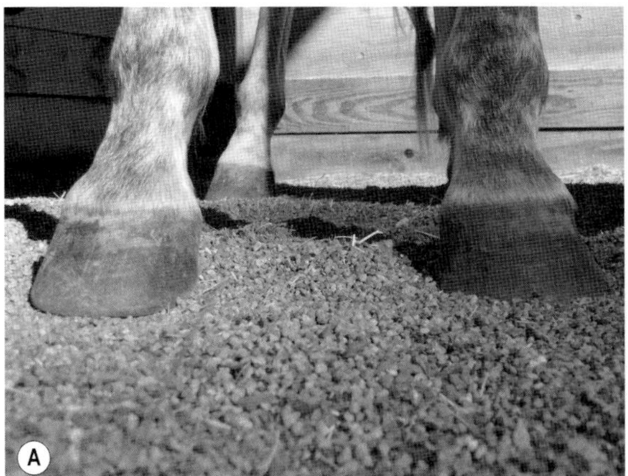

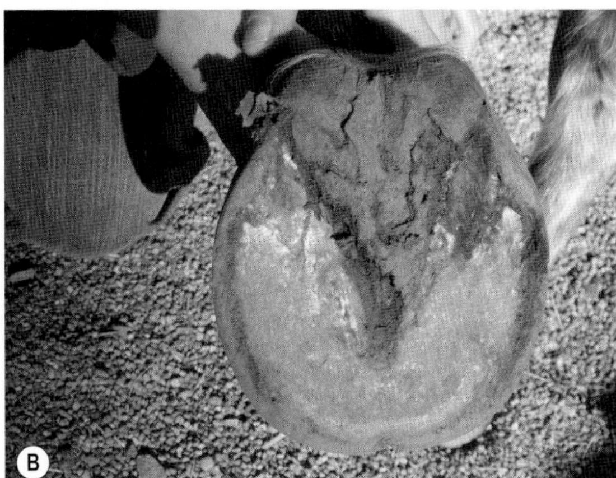

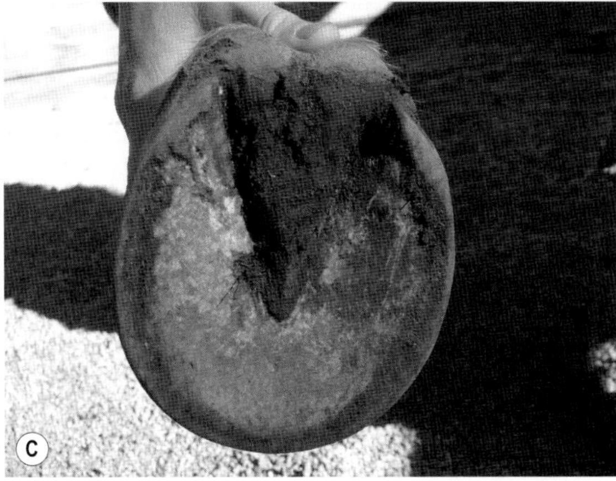

Fig. 6.12 Demonstration of the connection between hoof conformation and weight bearing of more proximal structures. This horse suffers from a chronic lower motor neuron injury to the right shoulder, causing subsequent shifting of weight from right to left. (A) Front view: note that the horse's left hoof flares at the bottom and that the right hoof is more narrow and upright with a longer heel. These differences would be even more noticeable if the horse was not being treated with frequent corrective trimming. (B) The sole of the left hoof is more flattened with loss of concavity. The frog is wider and flatter than it should be secondary to chronic increased load bearing. (C) The right hoof does less weight-bearing and consequently has greater sole concavity, a deeper sulcus and narrower frog.

that extend well past the sole, or simply a history of not having had the hooves trimmed in more than 8 weeks is enough to suggest that further hoof care may be needed.

Considerable debate exists between farriers and other hoof professionals about how to best care for a horse's feet, and no single answer can be applied to all horses. Genetic phenotype, environment, husbandry practices and intended use of the horse are all factors that need to be considered. Again, a discussion that does justice to this complex issue lies beyond the scope of this chapter and the reader is encouraged to review the vast amount of material that has already been written on this topic.

Dental care

Horses, like rodents, have continually erupting teeth. They lengthen by 3 mm each year (hence the term, 'long in the tooth'). This growth is countered by slow erosion; as horses chew grass, they grind their teeth in a circular motion. If their teeth are well aligned, the erosion is even. However, frequently it is not: secondary sharp points form, leading to discomfort and altered chewing habits. Such imbalances can be transferred through the entire stomatognathic architecture, affecting the temporomandibular joints, pharynx and proximal cervical musculature. As with people, there are a large number of proprioceptors associated with these structures (see 'Dentistry', Ch. 4).

Wild horses normally feed from the ground but domestic horses frequently feed from elevated feeders. Head position, or the degree of elevation, affects the resting occlusal position between the maxillary and mandibular dental arcades. Feeding horses from elevated troughs is thought by many to contribute to an increase in malocclusion issues.

Malalignment of dental origin can lead to compromised proprioception and reduced flexibility of the cranial cervical vertebrae. Affected horses frequently present with reduced cervical flexibility, reluctance to turn in certain directions, or 'bracing against the bit'. Severely affected animals may have altered ear carriage, irritability, decreased mentation (presumably secondary to headaches) or respond explosively when asked to perform certain tasks. Routine veterinary dental care is the best way to prevent this condition. Many performance horses receive dental examinations every 6 months. A history of tossing the head while feeding, dropping feed (sometimes called 'quidding'), or reluctance to have the cheeks palpated are all indicators that the teeth should be examined.

Saddle fit

Much like an ill-fitting running shoe, ski boot, or backpack can cause discomfort in people, the saddle is a precision piece of sports equipment that must fit both horse and rider to function well. Poorly fitted saddles are frequently associated with malalignment issues in both team members. A more detailed discussion of saddle fit follows below.

EVALUATING THE HORSE

Evaluation of the malaligned horse can be a daunting task, and one best left to appropriately trained medical professionals. Unfortunately, useful modalities for horse care are poorly regulated in many countries (including Canada), which opens the door for unqualified individuals to claim undeserved expertise. There are a myriad of do-it-yourself books or weekend courses available that teach hoof trimming, dental care, chiropractic treatment, massage, etc. but such brief educational experiences are inadequate instruction for true medical professionals. If one works with equestrian teams, one should find qualified individuals for referral purposes, as the quality of one's referrals is a reflection of one's own expertise.

Having said that, there are a number of simple ways to evaluate whether or not a problem exists:

Gait evaluation

It takes experience to read a horse's gait well, but consideration should be given to the following:

Head bob

Forelimb lameness often presents with a 'head bob'. Unsound horses will shift weight off painful limbs, creating asymmetric head movements. As the painful limb strikes the ground, the head will go up and possibly to the opposite side in an effort to shift weight away. As the sound limb assumes weight bearing, the head will drop down again. A common mnemonic for remembering which leg is affected is that: 'The head is DOWN when the SOUND foot hits the GROUND'.

Hip hike

Similarly, with hind end lameness, the horse will attempt to shift weight off the affected limb by affecting a 'hip hike', an upward tilt of the pelvis on the side of the lame limb.

Pastern sink

The pastern, or distal metacarpal/tarsal and 1st phalangeal joint (Fig. 6.10) sinks with weight-bearing. Uneven sinking of the pasterns, which can be best observed by trotting on pavement, indicates uneven weight-bearing. The pastern sinks less on the affected limb and more when weight-bearing on the opposite side. The problem manifests itself as an asymmetry of the pelvic roll (Fig. 6.13).

Footfalls

Listen to the clopping of the hoofs on a paved surface. Asymmetrically loud footfalls indicate increased weight-bearing compared to the other side.

Footprints

Stride lengths should by symmetrical on each side; the hind foot should fall, at least partly, within the print of the forefoot. Footprints should be of equal depth, left side compared to right. Having the horse walk through a smooth sand surface can help with this evaluation.

Some lameness problems will improve with exercise, some will worsen. Some are more pronounced on hard ground, some on soft. Some may appear only when circling clockwise or counterclockwise. Some only appear when the horse is under saddle. The gait may need to be tested under all these conditions in order to determine if a lameness problem exists.

Cervical range of motion

Horses with full cervical range of motion should be able to comfortably look at their own sacrum (Fig. 6.6). Horses unwilling to voluntarily do so, that

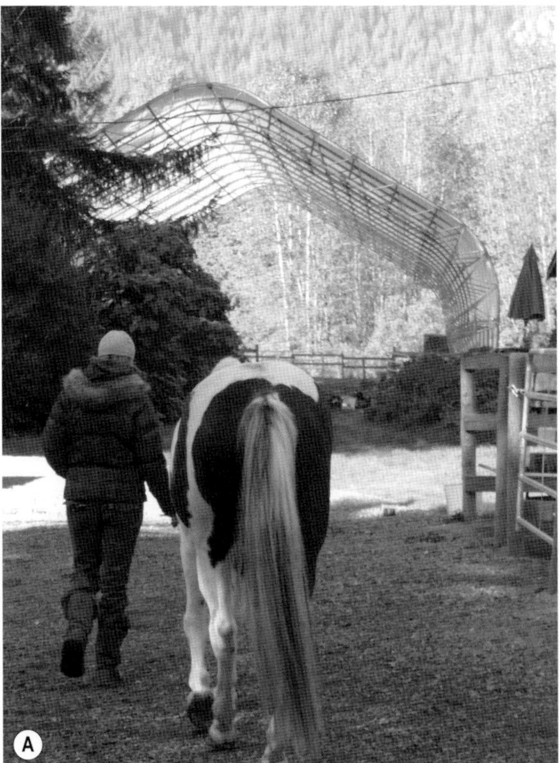

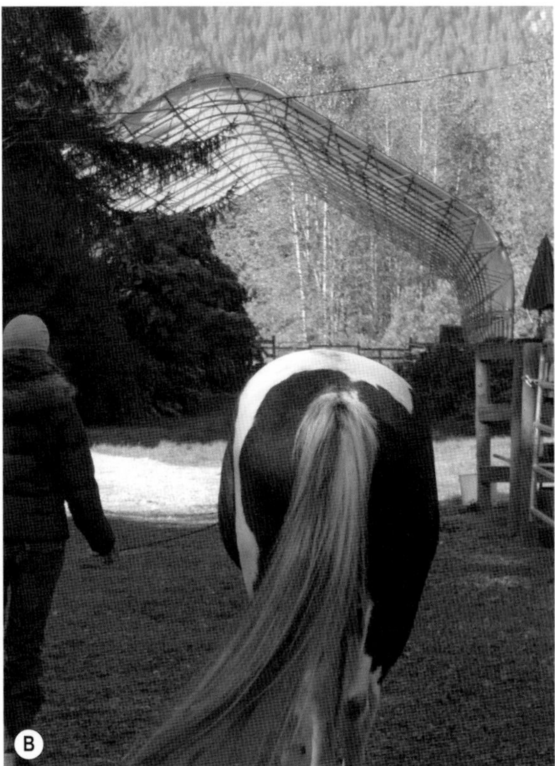

Fig. 6.13 The tuber coxae (TC) or hip bones of a horse rock from side to side. The movement should be symmetrical; asymmetrical pelvic range of motion while walking on flat, firm ground indicates asymmetrical SI joint mobility which, in turn, can reduce the horse's hind limb power. (A) Right TC elevated: this horse is bearing weight on the right hind leg, resulting in normal elevation of the right tuber coxae. (B) Right TC level: the horse's left tuber coxae is only mildly elevated above the right, despite the fact that it is fully weight-bearing on the left hind leg. Such asymmetries are clinically significant.

sink into that position only briefly before returning their head forward, or that externally rotate their head in order to increase their reach likely have some sort of vertebral kinetic or malalignment issue. Voluntary range of motion can be tested by offering grass or some other treat to the horse in such a way that they need to reach for it.

Pelvic movement

The pelvis rotates from side to side as the horse walks. If the horse is standing square and symmetric, the position of the pelvis should be even. Evaluate the horse's pelvis under both situations. Pelvic malalignment will often manifest with one tuber coxae (hip bone) higher than the other while standing, or uneven pelvic movement while walking (Fig. 6.13).

Muscle tension

Palpate the horse while it is standing square. Muscle bulk and tone should be symmetric. Imbalances likely indicate an injury or underlying asymmetrical posture (see also Figs 3.57-3.60).

Lightly palpate the paraspinals looking for evidence of flinching or guarding. Monitor to see if the horse suddenly grows alert, holds its breath, pins its ears or quickly turns toward the person examining a suspect area. These are all indicators of a potential problem. The sacrum and caudal lumbar region, as well as the thoracic just inferior to the scapulae, are areas commonly affected by malalignment issues.

Performance issues

Malalignment issues in the horse most commonly present with a history of impaired performance or altered posture. The most common complaints are listed below:

1. Altered head carriage – either vertically or laterally
2. Irritability
3. Walking on an angle
4. 'Resisting the bit'
5. Sensitivity when being groomed
6. Problems changing leads or turning in a given direction
7. Altered topline/backline posture
8. Discomfort or resistance when the cinch is tightened
9. Refusing jumps or bucking
10. Undiagnosed, mild, or shifting lameness
11. Gait abnormalities such as short striding, interfering, forging, or cross-firing: these are common terms for a variety of ways that a horse's feet might knock together during movement, an indication of abnormal or asymmetric stride lengths (see also Fig. 3.21A,B). Horses with normal gaits do not knock their feet together.
12. Non-specific decrease in performance or fitness
13. Increased stumbling
14. Loss of collection or impulsion
15. Refusal to pick up a lead
16. Difficulty flexing at the poll or atlanto-occipital joint
17. Pulling on one rein
18. Recurrent colic

SADDLE FIT

As mentioned earlier, proper saddle fit is an essential component of a performing team. Poor saddle fit is frequently implicated as a cause of malalignment issues for both horse and rider. The horse's back is dynamic and the saddle needs to move with it. Thoracic lordosis, elevated head, muscle bruising or atrophy, skin lesions, pain and reduced performance can all result from an ill-fitting saddle.

> The saddle should be checked for fit every 4-6 months.

Saddle fit should be frequently re-evaluated, every 4 to 6 months or every time the horse's body shape changes – a saddle that sits well on a horse in its prime will no longer fit if that same horse gains weight (Harman 2004).

Saddle evaluation is as much an art as it is a science, with many opinions about what constitutes the perfect saddle. It is best left to those with extensive formal training but a few basic considerations are listed below:

1. The saddle should sit level just behind the retracted scapulae. It should not interfere with normal movement of the shoulder blades. Too far forward will affect the horse's movement; too far backward will render the horse vulnerable to injury and cause the rider to rotate too far forward. No weight-bearing aspect of the saddle should extend inferior to the origin of the last rib.

Atrophy of thoracic musculature is a frequent consequence of poor saddle fit. Always evaluate saddle position while the horse is standing square on level ground.
2. With the rider on the saddle, confirm that there is clearance over all of the dorsal spinal processes – 2 or 3 fingers' worth. Saddles that are too wide will often lose this clearance.
3. There should be even pressure beneath all the panels. Panels with a wider surface area are preferred. Weight-bearing should be on regions of wide musculature, and not the scapulae or spinous processes. The wider the panel surface area, the better. Panel pressure is increased when the saddle is too narrow. Examine the sweat marks after a horse has been working – even sweat marks indicate even panel pressure.
4. Monitor the horse's response to the saddle; a guarded or irritated response should always be heeded.
5. Check the saddle for asymmetric wear; it can indicate if malalignment is present in one or other party (Fig. 6.4A,C). Horses tend to wear the underside asymmetrically; whereas the rider tends to wear the seat asymmetrically.

Ensure that the girth is not being over-tightened, tightened quickly, or tightened with the use of a commercial leverage device. One should be able to slip multiple fingers between the girth and the sternum. Reliance on an over-tight girth indicates an unbalanced rider.

Inspect the horse beneath saddle contact areas for alopecia, white hairs, muscle atrophy, tender ribs or muscles and for behavioural indicators of pain – all of which indicate current or prior poor saddle fit.

Both the rider's weight and the weight of the saddle should be evenly distributed over the thoracic spine of the horse.

Even if the saddle fits well, an imbalanced rider can mimic poor fit if one ischium is more heavily weighted than the other. For example, 'right anterior' rotation and 'right upslip' both result in unweighting on the right side. The right ischial tuberosity moves upward and increased weight now has to be borne by the left ischial tuberosity, which can easily come to lie a good centimetre lower (Figs 2.76B,D, 3.86 C, 6.4A,C, 6.5). Similarly, if the horse suffers from lumbosacral malalignment, the propulsive G-force is uneven and the centre of gravity changes (Fig. 6.8). These changes can cause a torsion in the movement of the horse's thoracic spine, which can eventually result in a breakdown in the front part of the saddle where the rider's knee grips. This breakdown can cause pain in the shoulder of the horse, and the rider may experience a drop of the thigh and pelvis on the side of the breakdown.

The rider will experience an even pattern of thrusts though the pelvis, SI joints and back when the horse moves in balance.

SUMMARY

Harmony in riding can only be achieved when the horse and the rider are both in alignment and the saddle fits properly. The following are some of the problems that result from malalignment:

Malalignment of the rider

Let us consider the rider presenting with 'right anterior, left posterior' innominate rotation.

1. The right hip and knee end up elevated and positioned forward to the point of possibly blocking the horse from right side-flexing and moving easily to the right (Figs 5.37, 6.4Bi,ii).The right shoulder and hip similarly end up too far ahead, so that the rider appears to be 'perching' in the saddle on this side.
2. The right hip ends up excessively flexed, and with time there is contracture of the right iliolumbar ligament. An effort to lengthen the right leg can eventually result in a compensatory increase in the lumbar lordosis and may create difficulties when attempting realignment.
3. The right leg ends up moving too far behind the girth of the saddle and may be obviously externally rotated (Fig. 5.37). In this case, the foot tends to go into a plantarflexed position so that the heel is higher than the forefoot, preventing proper distribution of the weight backward through the heel; the stirrup may require lengthening on this side when compared with the left. Active internal rotation of the legs normally helps the knees to act as anchor points for the pelvis, stopping the rider falling back into the 'armchair seat' with the pelvis rotated backward and the back being rounded (Figs 6.1B, 6.2C).

4. The outward rotation of the right knee with external rotation results in an insecure seat because the right thigh and the medial aspect of the knee no longer lie in full contact with the saddle (Figs 5.37, 6.4). The rider can actively rotate the right leg internally in an attempt to achieve a vertical position, at the cost of losing contact between the medial calf and the barrel of the horse.
5. The iliac crests are no longer even, the right probably being higher than the left, and weight distribution is also uneven – heavier on the left buttock and stirrup (Fig. 6.4A,C). The compensatory curves of the spine result in an imbalance of scapular position and range of motion (decreased abduction and retraction on the side of the elevated shoulder) and interscapular pain, often with referral to the shoulder or arm.
6. Insecurity of the seat with right external rotation, imbalance of leg strength and uneven weight distribution in the saddle will also stop the rider from achieving a true 'light seat' (Fig. 6.3B). The rider may notice difficulty with control and giving aids, recurrent spasm, and stiffness when mounting and dismounting, if not outright back and SI joint pain.

Malalignment of the horse

Malalignment results in muscle spasm, stiffness, pain and reduced performance. There are a number of factors predisposing horses to malalignment issues, including poor dental or hoof care, horse-rider mismatch, poor conformation or fitness for the task at hand, injury or subclinical lameness. There are a number of ways that equine malalignment will manifest but most relate to behavioural changes, compromised performance or reduced flexibility. Shifts in the horse's balance can be transferred to the rider, leading to malalignment in both parties.

Malalignment and impaired saddle fit

Saddle fit is also key. Poor saddle fit can cause compression of the thoracic spinous processes, causing compensatory lordosis in an attempt to escape pain, with secondary elevation of the head (Fig. 6.1B). The rider might subsequently develop an increased lordosis in an attempt to counteract the tendency to fall forward when the horse's head is held high (Figs 6.1B, 6.2A).

In short, the horse and rider are a team. Malalignment of one will frequently trigger malalignment of the other. In chronic situations, both parties are usually affected.

This chapter has not tried to cover all the problems relating to malalignment of horse and rider. Instead, key areas have been discussed and suggestions regarding assessment techniques given. Following an evaluation of horse, saddle and rider, the physician/therapist should list the problems and plan the treatment and the protocols to be followed to correct any malalignment.

One of the principles of a treatment programme is to facilitate healing after an injury. This is achieved by regaining a full-range of movement and muscle strength as soon as possible. In addition, the riders must be taught to recognize when they are in balance. Whenever movement balance is lost, uneven and unequal stresses are created which can result in malalignment. Although the changes may be minimal at first, failure to correct the situation can eventually result in serious worsening of the malalignment-related problems of both horse and rider.

Chapter 7

A comprehensive treatment approach

CHAPTER CONTENTS

DOI: 10.1016/B978-0-443-06929-1.00007-7

Seventy-five percent of elementary school graduates are out of alignment, 80-85% by the time they finish high school (Klein 1973; Klein & Buckley 1968). Treatment is indicated if the person's history and examination indicate that malalignment is present and, in the case of an 'upslip' or 'rotational malalignment', there is an associated 'malalignment syndrome' that:

1. may be putting him or her at increased risk of injury
2. may have precipitated the symptoms or caused an injury
3. may be perpetuating and/or aggravating the symptoms
4. may be slowing down or preventing recovery from an injury
5. may be preventing the person from advancing in their chosen line of work or sport.

This chapter first looks at the shortcomings of using standard treatment approaches for back pain caused by malalignment. It then outlines a logical and proven treatment programme. The need for the person's day-to-day participation is emphasized, in order to increase the chances of achieving the best results quickly and help maintain improvements, especially in-between formal treatment sessions. The chapter concludes with a differential diagnosis of other conditions to consider, appropriate investigations and alternate treatment options should the recommended approach fail to achieve lasting realignment and resolution of symptoms and signs. It is a lead-in to Chapter 8 which looks at alternate manual therapy techniques and complementary treatment methods currently used to increase the chances of achieving lasting relief from the problems caused by malalignment and the 'malalignment syndrome'.

FAILURE TO RESPOND TO STANDARD TREATMENT APPROACHES

The judicious use of anti-inflammatory medication and electrical modalities, combined with a graduated stretching, strengthening and range of motion programme, may well help bring a symptomatic person back to regular activities, work and play.

However, if the symptoms are in any way related to, or influenced by, the malalignment, then all these measures may amount to no more than band-aid therapy as long as the malalignment is not diagnosed and corrected.

MALALIGNMENT AND THE STANDARD TREATMENT OF LOW BACK PAIN

Low back pain (LBP) is one of the most common musculoskeletal complaints in our society. The aetiology is varied yet the treatment approach often singularly unvaried: medications to counter pain, inflammation and muscle tension, the repeated application of heat or cold, use of electrical modalities (e.g. ultrasound, laser or interferential current, TNS), instruction regarding posture and proper lifting techniques, strengthening of the back and abdominal muscles, stretching of the hip extensors and flexors, arching the back while lying prone, traction and (thrown in for good measure) the 'pelvic tilt'. Some of these 'standard' exercises are more likely to cause recurrence or aggravation of low back pain in someone who is out of alignment as well.

CASE HISTORY 7.1

A runner presented with a history of gradually increasing left lateral thigh and knee pain, coming on consistently on going into the last 10 miles of a marathon and increasing to the point of forcing him to abandon the race. The pain would settle completely with standard treatment measures and time, only to recur again in the last 10 miles of the next marathon.

Examination 1 week after his last marathon attempt revealed 'rotational malalignment' with 'anterior' rotation of the right innominate. There was increased tone and tenderness to palpation in the left hip abductor muscle mass and the length of the iliotibial band down to its insertion (Fig. 3.41). On Ober's test, passive left hip adduction was significantly restricted compared with that on the right (Fig. 3.44). Gait assessment showed that he pronated on the right and supinated on the left side. A pair of running shoes he had used for training in the preceding 6 months showed changes consistent with this weight-bearing pattern: the heel cup collapsed inward on the right and outward on the left (Fig. 7.1A).

Correction of the malalignment quickly resulted in a resolution of symptoms and signs, and allowed for an immediate return to a full training schedule. Symptoms did not recur during the next marathon 6 months later and he was able to finish the race. On reassessment shortly after, alignment had been maintained, and the left hip abductors and TFL/ITB were relaxed and non-tender. The heel cups of a new pair of running shoes of the same make still maintained a neutral (vertical), symmetrical position after a comparable 6 months of training (Fig. 7.1B).

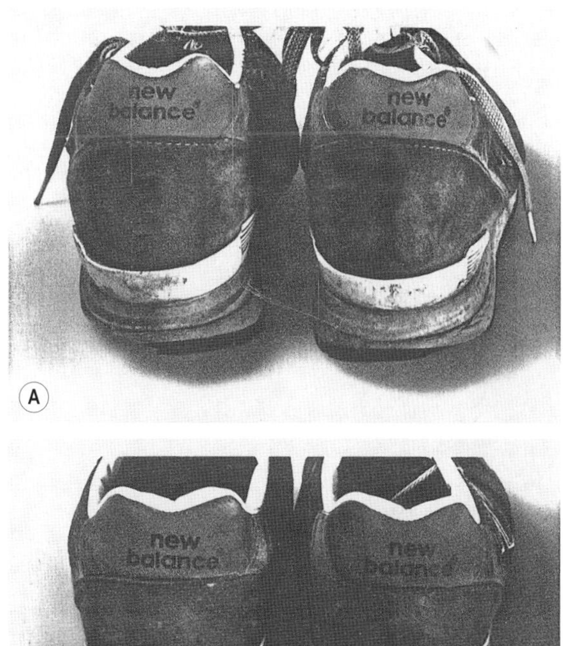

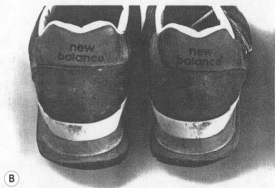

Fig. 7.1 Marathon runner's training shoes. (A) A pair used for 6 months prior to the correction of malalignment. Note the heel cup collapse (inward on the right, outward on the left) and excessive left lateral heel wear with supination. (B) A pair used for 6 months while maintaining realignment. The heel wear is even and the heel cups symmetrical, positioned in neutral (vertical).

The posterior pelvic tilt

The posterior tilt consists of actively rotating the pelvic unit posteriorly while lying supine, in order to temporarily flatten the back and decrease or eliminate the lumbar lordosis (Fig. 7.2B). In someone who presents in alignment but suffers from mechanical back pain, the tilt may be helpful in that it decreases pressure on the lumbar facet joints, opens the foramina, relieves compression pain from the posterior parts of the vertebrae, and decreases pressure within the disc and any tendency of the disc to bulge anteriorly.

In someone presenting with malalignment, however, the posterior pelvic tilt may cause more pain.

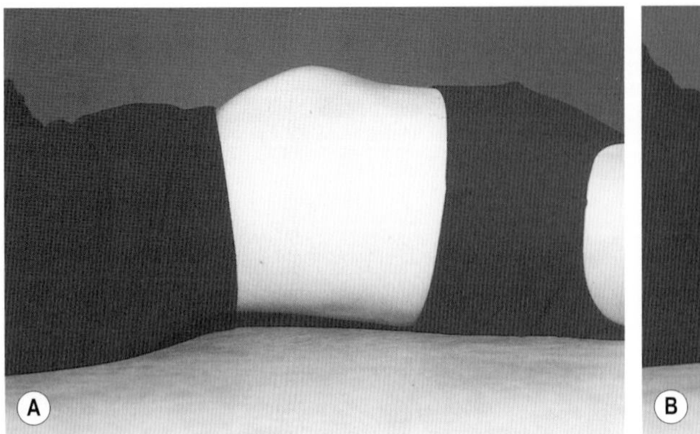

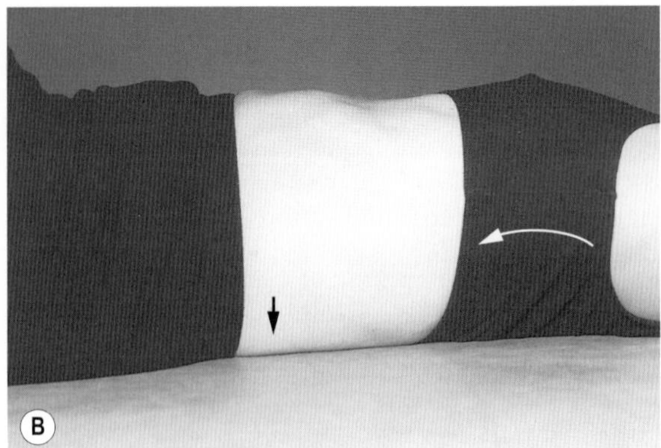

Fig. 7.2 Pelvic tilt. (A) The normal resting position showing a hollow (lumbar lordosis). (B) Active posterior rotation of the pelvis flattens the spine.

As we have seen, 'rotational malalignment' is often associated with sacral torsion, 'locking' of one or other SI joints, pelvic obliquity and a lateral lumbar convexity that reverses at the thoracolumbar junction to give rise to a thoracic curve convex in the opposite direction (Fig. 3.14). Spinal tenderness localizes primarily to the sites of increased stress: the lumbosacral and thoracolumbar junctions.

The posterior tilt aims to flatten the lumbar segment in one plane - the sagittal - in order to decrease the lordosis. This completely ignores the fact that, when malalignment is present, there will also be an accentuated lateral convexity of the lumbar segment to the right or left. In order to create that lumbar curve in the coronal (frontal) plane, the vertebrae must have undergone simultaneous axial rotation into the convexity and side-flexion into the concavity; in other words, simultaneous rotation around the vertical and sagittal axes with movement in the transverse and coronal (frontal) planes, respectively. A left lumbar convexity, for example, results from L1–L4 inclusive side-flexing to the right and rotating to the left, maximal at the apex (Figs 2.42, 4.6, 4.33). There will usually also be an element of extension, in keeping with a residual lumbar lordosis of varying degree (Fig. 3.14A). As a result, facet joint surfaces have been moved closer together on the right and separated on the left side (reverse of L5 findings shown in Fig. 2. 52B).

In someone presenting with malalignment, carrying out the posterior pelvic tilt may, therefore, actually cause more pain (Box 7.1).

Doing the posterior pelvic tilt lying supine on a hard surface also risks putting direct pressure on structures that just may not bear being pressed against that hard surface in the process of attempting the tilt:

1. tender posterior pelvic ligaments (especially those crossing the posterior SI joint (Fig. 2.5)
2. tender PSIS, ischial tuberosity (sacrotuberous insertion, biceps femoris origin; Fig. 2.6), coccyx, coccygeal spicule (see Ch. 4 and Fig. 4.44)

BOX 7.1 Factors that can cause the 'posterior tilt' to be painful

1. trying to flatten a curve in one plane (sagittal), ignoring the fact that the curve exists in two planes (sagittal and coronal) and that the individual vertebrae are rotated in three planes (sagittal, coronal and transverse)
2. further increasing stress on the points of curve reversal (thoracolumbar junction) and the twisted lumbosacral junction
3. increasing the tension on already tender posterior soft tissue structures (e.g. the supra- and interspinous ligaments, and thoracolumbar myofascia) by changing their length-tension ratio
4. stretching the tender posterior pelvic ligaments (e.g. iliolumbar)
5. aggravating the facet joint irritation that results with vertebral rotation by increasing the:
    a. joint separation already present on the convex side, further stretching joint capsules, ligaments and their nerve supply
    b. joint compression already occurring on the concave side, with a risk of entrapment of these soft tissues and nerve fibres and irritation of the innervated surfaces

3. protuberant, and particularly stiff, unyielding spinous processes of:
   a. rotationally displaced vertebrae, especially the vertebrae around the thoracolumbar junction (see Chs 4, 5; Figs 3.14 C, 5.2).
   b. the sacrum and coccyx (Figs 2.80A, 4.44B)

Traction

Traction is unlikely to straighten the curvatures of the spine if these are:

1. part of a compensatory scoliosis, with segmental vertebral rotation in opposing directions (lumbar, thoracic and cervical) attributable to an 'upslip' or 'rotational malalignment'
2. caused by the rotational displacement of one or more isolated vertebrae.

The spine, pelvis and attaching myofascia have to be regarded as a spiral structure that one may not be able to unwind just by pulling on both ends at the same time. Samorodin aptly explained this phenomenon using the analogy of the wound-up telephone cord (Schamberger 2002: 393). Traction alone may precipitate or augment pain by:

1. increasing stress on sites of curve reversal and vertebral rotational displacement
2. further increasing the tension in myofascial and ligamentous structures already tensed-up because of 'facilitation', skewing of length-tension ratios and other changes attributable to the malalignment.

However, gentle repetitive traction, aimed at relaxing in particular the paravertebral muscles (e.g. multifidi, extensor spinae), may be a useful adjunct to help achieve and maintain the correction of such a vertebral displacement. Gentle traction can certainly help if carried out immediately preceding and/or following efforts at mobilization, probably by temporarily decreasing the tension in these attaching muscles by:

1. achieving some relaxation through the 'contract–relax' mechanism (see Ch. 8)
2. opening up the spaces between the vertebrae and facet joints to relieve compression, reactive muscle tightening and any irritation of exiting nerve roots
3. minimizing or abolishing strain in muscles that have been 'facilitated'.

Extension exercises and back extensor strengthening

Extension of the back while lying prone, maximal in the 'cobra' position (Fig. 7.3), can increase the pressure on facet joint surfaces that are already approximated on one side by vertebral rotation in conjunction with malalignment (Fig. 2.52B). Back extension also causes further stress on the particularly stiff sites of curve reversal, where the adjacent vertebrae rotate in opposite directions (Fig. 3.14B,C).

This is not to say, however, that one cannot have a person do exercises for the back extensor muscles. Given the frequent involvement of these muscles (e.g. reflex spasm, tenderness, disuse weakness and wasting), a stretching and strengthening programme should be part of rehabilitation - provided a core strengthening programme is well underway to ensure pelvic and spine stability (Figs 7.25-7.29) and alignment is starting to be maintained. Any arching of the back should continue to be limited to the pain-free zone to avoid triggering reflex muscle spasm. A contraction of these muscles, done in a way that avoids excessive back extension, can be initiated in the prone position simply by:

1. extending only the head and neck (no more than 2–3 cm off the surface at first; Fig. 7.4A), progressing to also lifting the shoulders at the same time (Fig. 7.4B)
2. alternately raising the straight right and left leg 1–2 cm off the surface (Fig. 7.4C), and eventually both legs simultaneously:

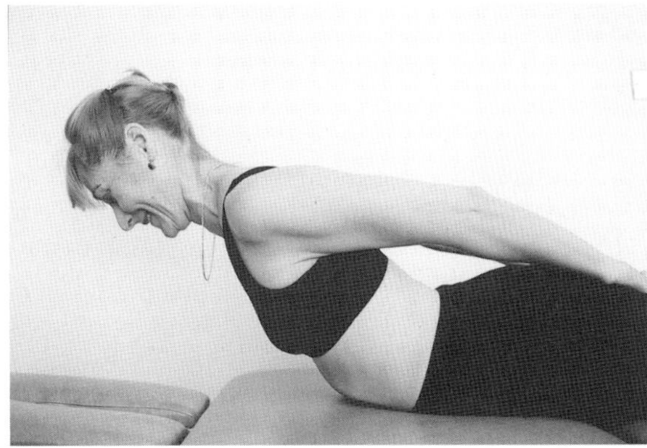

Fig. 7.3 Hyperextension of the back: the 'cobra' position.

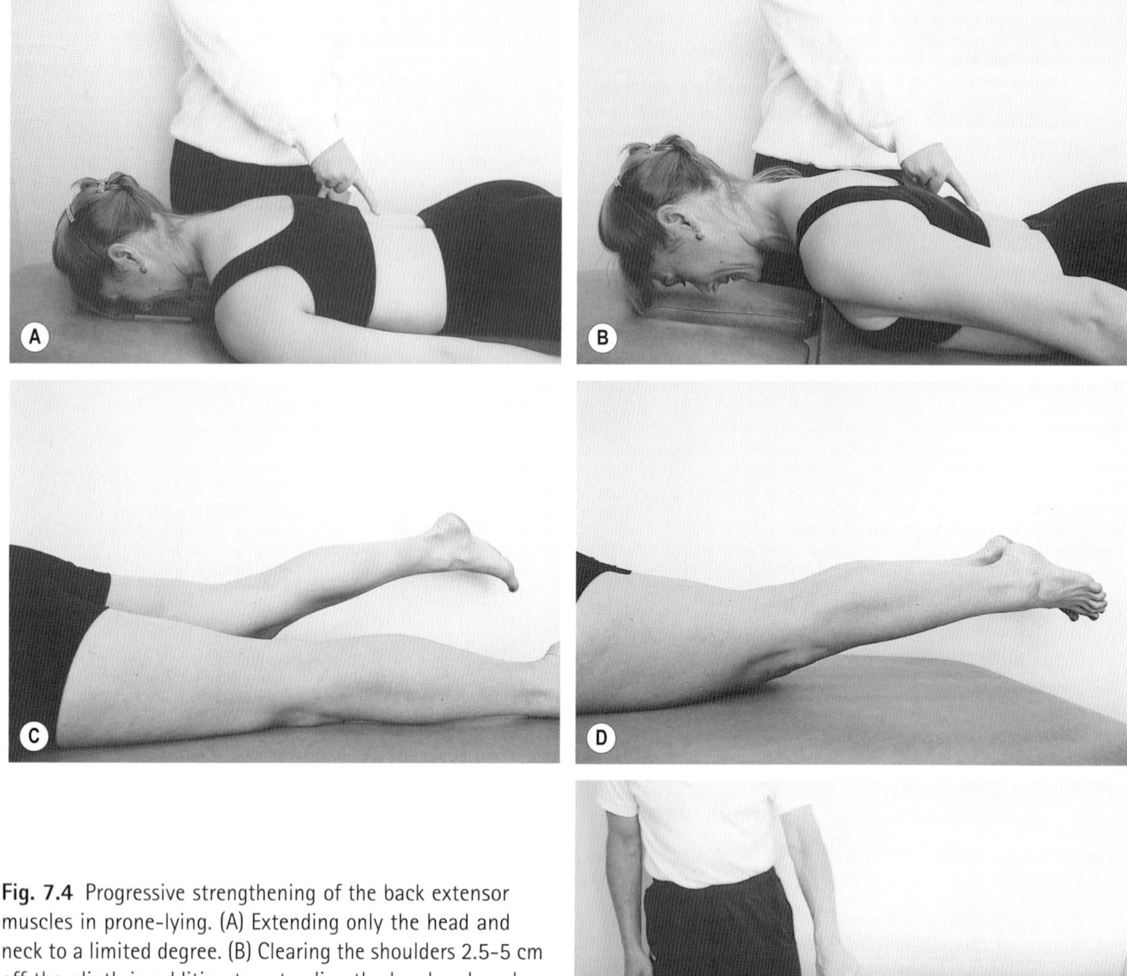

Fig. 7.4 Progressive strengthening of the back extensor muscles in prone-lying. (A) Extending only the head and neck to a limited degree. (B) Clearing the shoulders 2.5-5 cm off the plinth in addition to extending the head and neck minimally. (C) Alternately raising the right and left straight leg, knee 5–15 cm off the plinth. (D) Simultaneously raising both straight legs, knees 5–15 cm off the plinth; eventually, combining this with (B). (E) All the muscles are completely relaxed between contractions (the head and legs resting on the plinth).

initially just clearing the bed and then progressing gradually from 5 up to 10–15 cm as the pain decreases and strength increases (Fig. 7.4D).

The emphasis is on frequent repetition of contractions that are brief to start with: holding to a slow count of 1 or 2 is adequate, followed by relaxation to allow for a maximum inflow of blood and clearance of waste (Fig. 7.4E).

Initial brief repetitive muscle contractions avoid decreasing or cutting off the entry of blood and the exit of waste for too long, to avoid compounding the problem especially in those muscles along the spine which have already been subjected to the detrimental effects of a chronic increase in tension.

Once the person can do three sets of 10, the duration of each contraction is increased to a slow count of 2 but only for the first set of 10 to start. At this stage, progressively increasing the count is preferable to increasing the degree of extension. Relaxation is improved by tying the contractions in with the regular rhythm of breathing; in this case, contracting on inspiration, relaxing on expiration or vice versa, depending on whatever feels the best way. Once the person can contract to a count of 5 for 2 or 3 sets of 10 and is starting to maintain alignment, the degree of extension may now gradually be increased: first for one set, then two and so on, as tolerated. He or she should preferably be in alignment when carrying out the extension manoeuvres; a good approach is to do the self-assessment and correct any recurrence of malalignment just before the exercises. This simple progressive approach can be used for strengthening any other muscles.

Sit-ups

There seems to be some obsession in our society with doing a sit-up from supine-lying to vertical and, ultimately, perfecting the 'abdominal crunch' by touching the nose or the right and left elbow alternately to the opposite knee (Fig. 7.5). Most patients presenting with back pain, whether it be on the basis of malalignment or some other cause, are likely to run into grief with these manoeuvres. Pain often increases as the neck and trunk pass the upright (vertical) position:

1. coming up into sitting leaning slightly forward, at which point the posterior cervical and thoracic paravertebrals and erector spinae, especially, are activated to prevent the trunk from falling forward

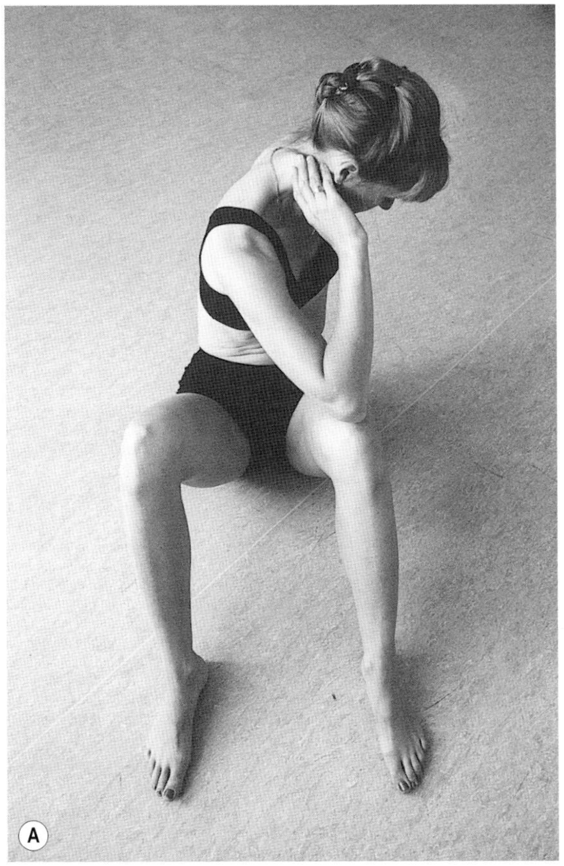

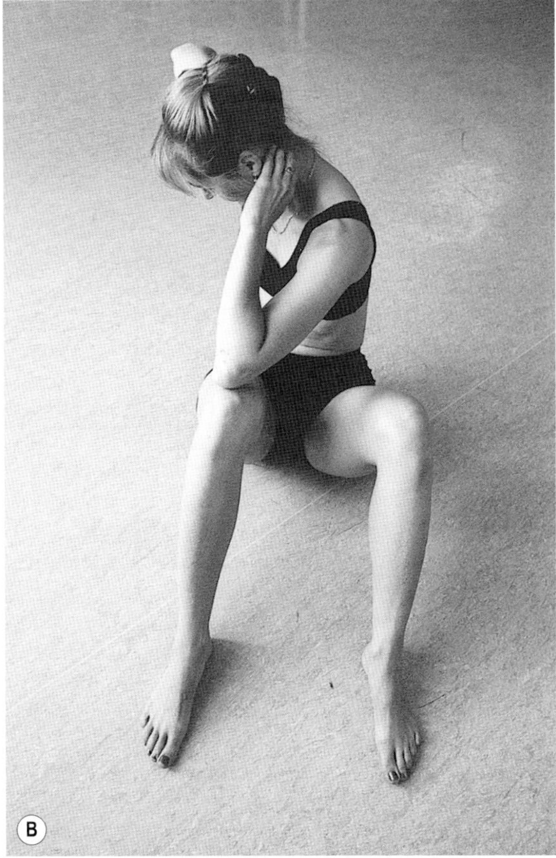

Fig. 7.5 Risking a recurrence of malalignment doing the abdominal 'crunch' with the addition of a torsional component by alternately touching (A) the right elbow to the left knee and (B) the left elbow to the right knee.

2. going back into supine-lying, at which point the anterior neck muscles (e.g. paravertebrals, scalenes and sternocleidomastoid) contract to prevent the head from falling backward.

Posterior paravertebral contraction effectively increases the pressure on both the disc and the facet joints. In someone with malalignment, the addition of twisting the trunk alternately to right and left has to be viewed as another factor capable of causing:

1. pain
    a. from attempted rotation into a restricted range on one side (Fig. 3.5 C) and further compression of the facet joints on the side opposite to the direction of rotation (Fig. 2.52)
    b. by increasing the tension on the posterior pelvic ligaments and in the thoracolumbar muscles and fascia
2. a recurrence of malalignment because of the repeated torsion of trunk and pelvis.

The intent is to strengthen the abdominal muscles, especially:

1. transversus abdominis and the obliques, which should respond to core strengthening, and
2. rectus abdominis

In someone with severe back pain, a good contraction primarily of rectus abdominis can be initiated simply by raising the head and neck while lying supine (Fig. 7.6A), then progressing to raising the shoulders just 2–3 cm off the surface (Fig. 7.6B) and possibly incorporating graduated straight-leg raises (especially if activating the neck and shoulder girdle muscles causes discomfort, as it might in someone following a 'whiplash' injury). Similar to attempts at strengthening the back extensors, the contractions should initially be of short duration, with the muscles being completely relaxed in-between contraction, carried out within the zone of comfort and avoiding triggering any discomfort or outright pain at all costs. Instructions are for an initial set of 10 contractions daily, increasing to two and then three sets as strength and endurance improve. At that point, either the duration of the contraction and/or the degree of trunk flexion can gradually be increased, following the progression outlined above for the back extensors.

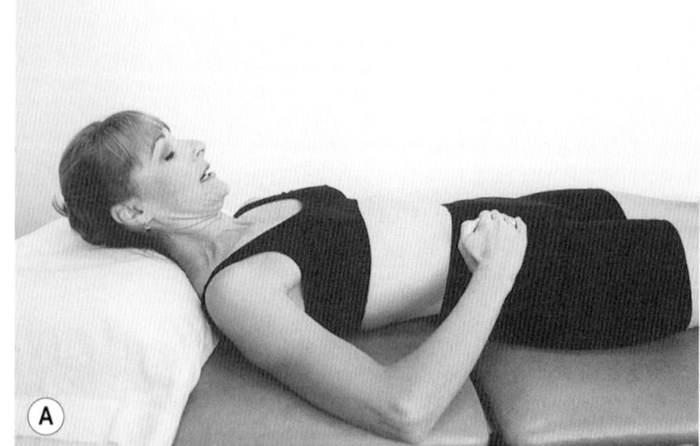

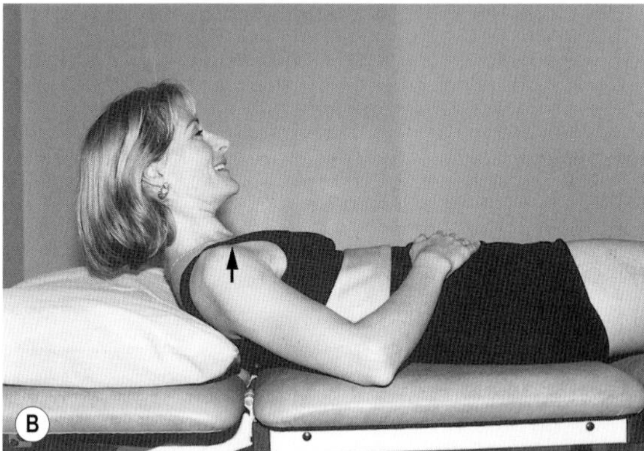

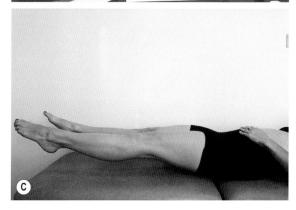

Fig. 7.6 Graduated abdominal muscle strengthening. Simultaneously drawing the umbilicus toward the plinth and tightening up the muscles around the rectum will ensure a strengthening not only of rectus abdominis, but also transversus abdominis and the pelvic floor muscles (see Figs 2.31B, 2.53). (A) Initially only the head is lifted off the plinth. (B) The shoulders clear the plinth, along with the head. (C) Both heels are just clearing the plinth (with the legs held straight).

It cannot be stressed enough that strengthening of the above muscles must be preceded by strengthening of the 'inner' and 'outer' core and by efforts at realignment, both of which are an intricate part of the overall treatment programme for the 'malalignment syndrome' and will be discussed in that context later (Figs 2.28-2.40, 7.25-7.29).

Always consider the possibility of an underlying problem of malalignment when:

1. the standard treatment measures discussed above fail to resolve the pain, or actually worsen it
2. history, examination and investigations do not disclose a disc, facet or other underlying problem.

MANIPULATION, MOBILIZATION AND MUSCLE ENERGY TECHNIQUES

The key to recovery from the 'malalignment syndrome' is to relieve the stresses and strains on the skeleton and attaching soft tissues which are attributable to the malalignment.

Realignment using an appropriate manual therapy technique should, therefore, be the first treatment measure and, in combination with core strengthening, remains a mainstay of treatment.

In approximately 80-90% of people presenting with one or more of the three common presentations of malalignment, correction can be achieved quite easily. In a small number of these, 5% at best, realignment is maintained after only one or two treatments, something that is more likely to occur in a younger person. In the majority, correction can be achieved but the malalignment keeps on recurring initially, a reflection of all the changes that the body tissues have undergone in adapting to the malalignment. Realignment is eventually maintained for longer and longer periods of time following each correction as the tissues and joints, and probably also the brain, start to adapt to the more symmetrical postures and biomechanical stresses, the 'straight' as opposed to 'crooked' you. Within 3–6 months, most of them will finally maintain alignment and require no further correction. However, that is not to say that they may not go out of alignment again at some point in the future and require further treatment, especially if they become symptomatic. Subsequent recurrence of malalignment can usually be linked to a period of increased mental and/or physical stress, excessive lifting (especially with a torsional component) or exertion (e.g. longer than usual participation in a demanding activity) or simply sitting for prolonged periods of time (e.g. when travelling).

In approximately 5-10%, correction cannot be achieved or is quickly lost following each correction. The majority of these people prove to have one or more of the following:

1. instability of one or both SI joints, the pubic symphysis and/or one or more lumbar vertebrae attributable to impaired 'form' and 'force' closure or neural control (see Ch. 2)
2. a generalized joint hypermobility (e.g. Ehler-Danlos syndrome)
3. persistently increased tension or actual spasm of muscles that are in a position to cause malalignment to recur.

In others, the recurrence may be secondary to some as yet undiagnosed problem, such as a missed central disc protrusion (see 'Asymmetries that fail to respond', below).

In addition to the muscle energy technique (MET) and traction, which are the main approaches to realignment discussed in this book, there are numerous other manual therapy techniques that find application in the treatment of malalignment - a number of these are discussed in Chapter 8. They range from the high-velocity, low-amplitude (HVLA) manipulations traditionally associated with chiropractic, the long-lever, low-velocity (LLLV) osteopathic techniques to re-establish joint play and the seemingly more gentle methods (e.g. craniosacral release, zero-balancing, NUCCA technique) which are now being embraced by many chiropractors, osteopaths, physicians and physiotherapists alike because they may be more successful in achieving long-term correction.

As suggested by Richard in 1986, the success of these more gentle techniques is possibly because they address not just the issue of the bones being out of alignment but also any persistent asymmetries of flexibility, muscle tone and strength. A failure to treat all of these aspects relating to malalignment can result in subsequent recurrence or even an inability to achieve initial correction. An HVLA manipulation, for example, may well put a rotated vertebrae or pelvic bone back into place but the malalignment may keep on recurring as long as any residual asymmetrical tension in the attaching muscles or ligaments continues to exert a rotational stress on these bones. Simultaneously treating the malalignment and any persistent asymmetries in tension is more likely to achieve long-lasting realignment and a resolution of the symptoms.

In practice, simply achieving lengthening of the tight myofascial tissue and relaxation of muscles can, at times, result in a spontaneous realignment of the bones. In other words, in some cases the problem with malalignment is primarily one of persistent asymmetrical tension and/or contracture of muscle and other soft tissues which:

1. may have led to the bones going out of alignment in the first place
2. are now the cause of recurrences of the malalignment because they continue to exert their detrimental effects, so that realignment can only be maintained temporarily

For example:

1. The myofascial tissue on the concave side of a curve in the spine is put in a relaxed position and will shorten with time (Fig. 2.60). When the curve is decreased or eliminated with realignment, excessive tension in these contracted structures will exert a unilateral force on the vertebrae that can result in a recurrence of the malalignment, unless realignment is combined with a graduated stretching programme to help them regain their normal length.
2. The persistence of a trigger point in the right quadratus lumborum after realignment may perpetuate a general increase in tension in that muscle and cause the recurrence of a 'right upslip' (Fig. 2.62).
3. Mobilization may effectively correct the malalignment of the pelvis initially caused by an L1 rotation with resultant 'facilitation' of iliopsoas on one side and 'inhibition' on the other. The pelvic malalignment is, however, more likely to recur if the L1 rotation, and any persistent asymmetry of tension in right compared with left iliopsoas, is not also attended to after realignment of the pelvis.

CASE HISTORY 7.2

This 37-year-old female runner presented with symptoms of cervicogenic brachialgia in a left C6 and C7 dermatome referral pattern and frequent headaches following a fall down a flight of stairs. On initial examination, the cervical spine range of motion was reduced in all planes of movement, the deltoid muscle weak (4/5) but the neurological screen otherwise unremarkable. In addition to a postural scoliosis, there was evidence of 'anterior' rotation of the left innominate and vertebral rotational displacement at the C2/3, C6/7 and T11/12 levels. Surface electromyography (SEMG) showed increased paravertebral muscle activity readings (the light bars in Fig. 7.7) throughout the spine, worse on the left than the right and at the levels noted to have rotated (e.g. C6/7 and T11), also the lumbosacral region. These SEMG findings were consistent with postural compensation and a reactive increase in paravertebral muscle tension throughout the back.

After three months of therapy aimed at mobilizing the pelvis and spine and relaxing the paravertebral muscles, the frequency of headaches had significantly decreased and she was otherwise asymptomatic. The neurological screen was now unremarkable. Repeat SEMG (the black bars in Fig. 7.7) still showed some higher readings, now localizing to the left C2–C4 and T7, right L1 and L3 levels, probably indicative of an ongoing attempt to compensate for the changing postural pattern. The muscle tension overall was, however, significantly reduced and more symmetrical than that recorded initially.

TECHNIQUES FOR CORRECTION OF 'ROTATIONAL MALALIGNMENT'

Some easily-learned manual therapy techniques are particularly useful for treatment of 'rotational malalignment' in a clinical setting, at home or even outdoors. It must be stressed at this point that these techniques should not be painful, if at all possible, to avoid any further increases in muscle tone.

A technique may be successful in achieving alignment but the correction is often quickly lost if the procedure has provoked or worsened pain and, with it, a reflex increase in asymmetrical muscle tone.

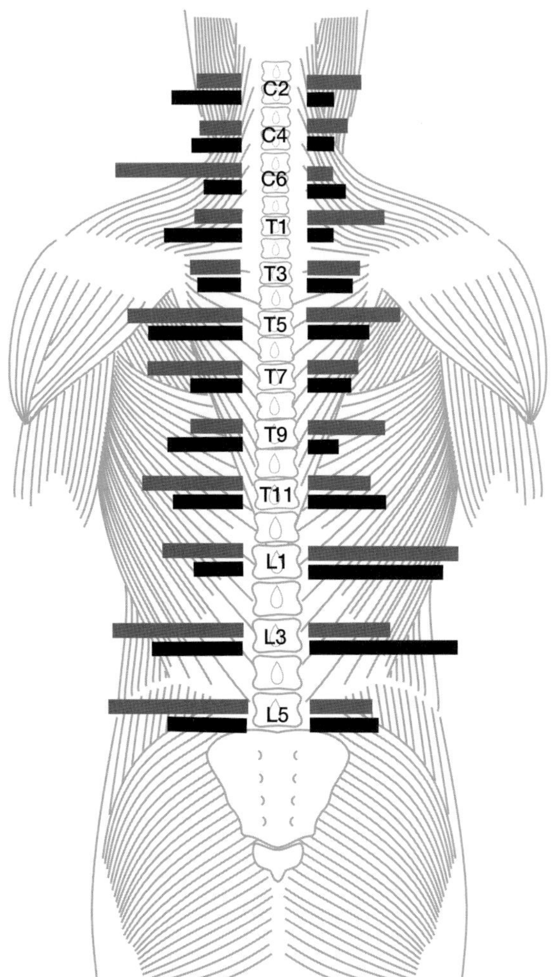

Fig. 7.7 A surface electromyograph of the paravertebral muscles to detect the tension level (see 'Case History 7.2'). The light horizontal bars indicate the findings after injury; note the asymmetry and the large number of levels showing an increase in activity. The dark horizontal bars denote the findings after 3 months of treatment, including manual therapy. The asymmetry has significantly decreased in the cervical and thoracic levels, and there are now fewer levels showing increased activity (persisting mainly in the lumbar region). *(Redrawn courtesy of D.J. McCallum, unpublished data 1999.)*

In most cases, pain can be avoided by a minor modification of the technique being used; often this amounts to no more than simply changing the position (e.g. decreasing the angle of hip and knee flexion; Figs 7.9B, 7.9Ei,ii, 7.13E,F).

Sometimes, however, a patient has such generalized discomfort and soft tissue tenderness that one just cannot use a certain approach, such as the 'muscle energy technique' (MET), during the initial stages of treatment. In that case, an even more gentle and less 'invasive' method, one that requires less effort on the part of the patient or involves working at sites distal to where pelvic and spine instability and pain are most severe, may be more appropriate (e.g. craniosacral release or the NUCCA technique; see Ch. 8). One can then try reintroducing MET, possibly in conjunction with some of the complementary methods of treatment at a later date, once the patient's condition has started to improve. However, the 'more gentle' techniques of realignment, or even just limiting initial treatment to core muscle strengthening may fail, especially if there is a problem such as soft tissue or joint inflammation and pain, or joint instability secondary to ligament laxity or joint degeneration. In that case, attempts at trying to achieve stability and realignment may have to be discontinued until the inflammation has settled down and/or the ligaments have been strengthened (see 'anti-inflammatories' and 'prolotherapy', below) to allow the patient to finally get on with a progressive core strengthening, realignment and postural retraining programme.

Muscle Energy Technique (MET)

> Muscle energy technique is one method of mobilization particularly useful for correcting a 'rotational malalignment' by harnessing the person's own muscles to generate a rotational force on a specific structure.

MET allows for correction of malalignment using the person's own muscle power to rotate a bone or bones back into their proper position. Take the example of a person presenting with an 'anterior' rotation of the right and a compensatory 'posterior' rotation of the left innominate.

Right innominate: 'anterior' rotation

A resisted active contraction of the right gluteus maximus can be harnessed to create a posterior rotational force on the right innominate in order to correct the 'anterior' rotation (Figs 2.5B, 2.36, 2.37, 7.8Ai). Essentially, gluteus maximus originates from the posterior iliac crest, along the posterior gluteal line, and inserts primarily into the greater trochanter (Figs 2.5B, 7.8Ai,ii). One of its actions is to extend the hip joint when the thigh is free to move

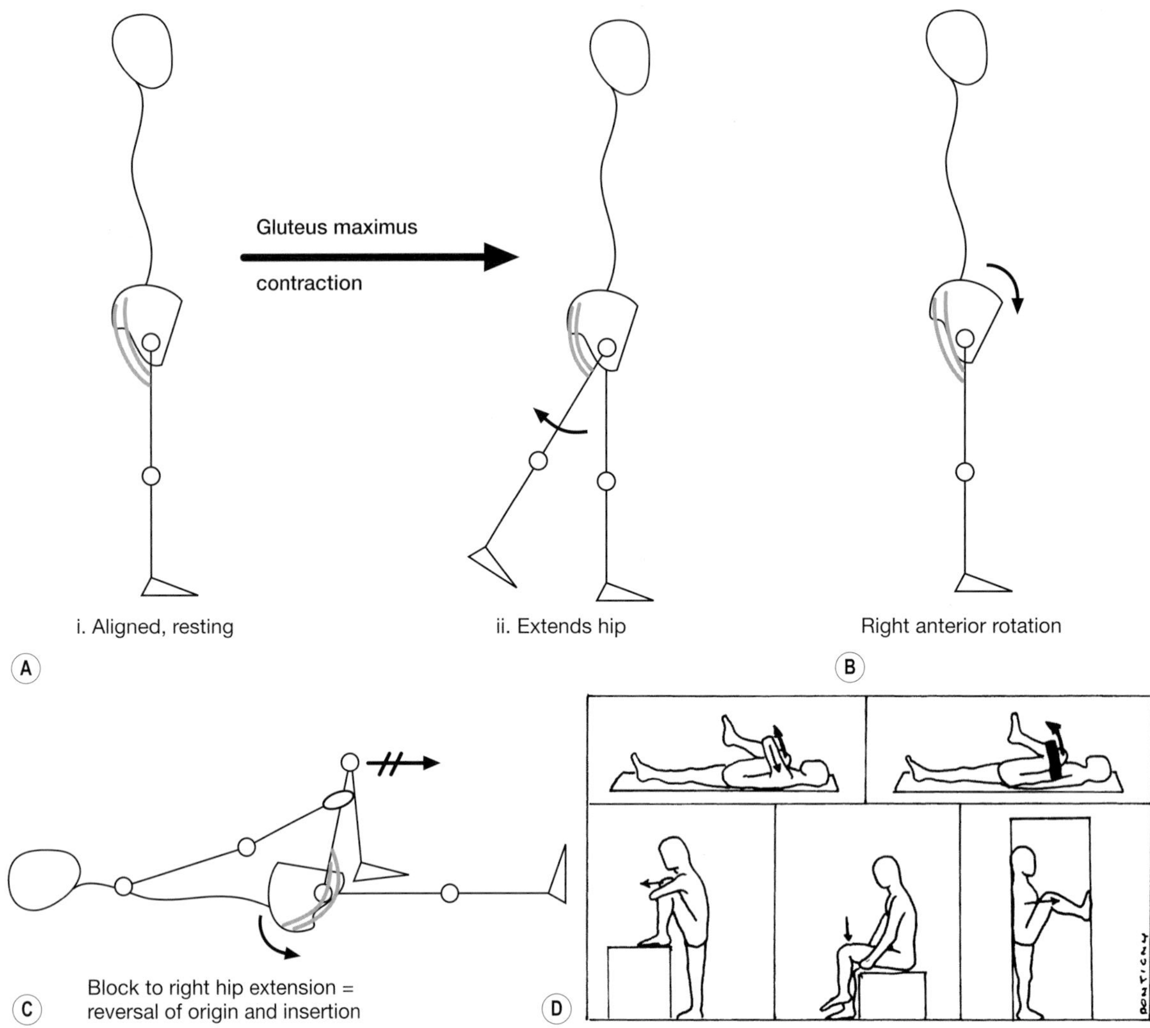

Fig. 7.8 Muscle energy technique to correct a 'rotational malalignment'. (A-C) The biomechanics of using gluteus maximus (Fig. 2.5B) to correct a right innominate 'anterior' rotation (B). (A) The muscle acts as a hip extensor when the leg is free to move. (C) Blocking right hip extension reverses the muscle origin and insertion, creating a posterior rotational force on the innominate. (D) Muscle energy techniques can be used in a variety of positions *(Courtesy of DonTigny 1997.)*

(Fig. 7.8Aiii). However, by resisting right hip extension, and hence any movement of the femur, one effectively reverses the muscle origin and insertion (Fig. 7.8C). Gluteus maximus will now exert a posterior rotational force on the right innominate, which is still free to move. The person attempts to extend the hip but this movement is prevented by having him or her:

1. hold on to the thigh or shin, with the hip and knee flexed (Figs 7.8C,D, 7.9)
2. push against another person or an object that serves to provide the resistance needed (Figs 7.8, 7.9).

Following each contraction, a muscle usually relaxes and will lengthen a bit more. In the case of gluteus maximus, one can take up the slack each time by letting the thigh drop down toward the person's chest and, if tolerated, even toward the opposite shoulder (given that gluteus maximus is oriented somewhat diagonally across the buttock) before attempting the next resisted contraction (Fig. 7.9C). The repeated contraction and relaxation of gluteus maximus in this manner will successfully correct an 'anterior' rotation in 80-90% of people. For those who have pain on knee flexion (e.g. aggravation of osteoarthritic pain;

patello-femoral syndrome), the procedure can be modified by supporting the lower leg (calf) on the assistant's shoulder or on a chair to decrease the knee flexion angle (Fig. 7.9D). Similarly, if there is hip or groin pain, one may find a position of comfort either by abducting or adducting the femur slightly or by decreasing the hip flexion angle.

Left innominate: 'posterior' rotation

Two different sets of muscles can be harnessed in order to correct a 'posterior' rotation of the left innominate.

Iliacus

Iliacus originates primarily from the anterior iliac crest and upper iliac fossa, inserting into the tendon of psoas major and directly into the lesser trochanter (Figs 2.46B,C, 4.2, 7.10A). If the thigh is free to move, the primary action of iliacus is to flex the hip joint (Fig. 7.10Aii). By resisting left hip flexion, one effectively reverses the origin and insertion and creates a force that will rotate the left innominate anteriorly (Fig. 7.10C). When sitting or lying supine, the person attempts to flex the hip, but any movement is again blocked.

One-person technique

1. the counterforce is provided by the arms/overlapping hands pushing against the anterior aspect of the left thigh (Figs 7.10C, 7.11A,B)
2. the elbows are preferably locked in extension so that, when lying supine, the force goes straight up to the shoulder girdle and through to the surface he or she is lying on
   a. there is, therefore, no need for contraction of any of the neck, shoulder girdle or arm muscles, a point to consider especially when a patient has, for example, suffered a whiplash' or a shoulder injury (Figs 7.10C, 7.11A)
   b. the only muscle working is iliacus.

Two-person technique

An assistant provides the resistance needed to prevent any movement on attempted hip flexion (Fig. 7.11B,C,F).

Rectus femoris

Rectus femoris originates from the anterior inferior iliac spine and anterior rim of the acetabulum; it inserts indirectly into the tibial tubercle by way of the patellar tendon (Figs 2.46 C, 2.59, 7.12Ai). It is the only muscle of the quadriceps complex that crosses both the hip and knee joint so that, in addition to extending the knee, it can also flex the hip joint when the knee is in full extension (Fig. 7.12Aii, Cii). This muscle can, therefore, be effectively used to create an anterior rotational force on the 'posteriorly' rotated left innominate (Fig. 7.12B) by:

1. blocking attempted extension of the left knee when that knee is flexed (Fig. 7.12Ci)
2. blocking attempted left hip flexion when that knee is straight (which actually also engages iliacus; Fig. 7.12Cii).

As illustrated, either a one or two-person technique can be used. The hip is best kept at 90 degrees of flexion or less; bringing it any closer increases the chance of using the femur on the left side like a lever and accidentally causing a recurrence of a 'posterior' innominate rotation (Figs 2.47A, 7.16-18, 7.22). The following techniques for correction of a left 'posterior' rotation are recommended:

One-person technique

The person lies supine, with the left hip flexed to about 90 degrees. He or she then resists repeated attempts at knee extension by hanging on to a towel or wide belt placed at a level between mid-shin and the ankle (Fig. 7.13A). Alternately, a sling looped around the flexed knee and secured at the other end (Fig. 7.13B) not only offers resistance to knee extension but also allows for relaxation of any sore neck, upper back and shoulder girdle muscles.

Two-person technique

When you are helping a person to use this manoeuvre, you can provide the resistance to knee extension:

1. with your hand around the left ankle (Fig. 7.13C)
   a. unfortunately, the strength in your arm is probably less compared to that of the quadriceps in most people and will, therefore, allow them to overcome your attempts to generate an adequate force even at a suboptimal level of effort on their part; the person may have to be reminded several times that when using MET they are:
      i. usually activating only one or two select muscles
      ii. never to push with a greater force than you are capable of resisting, which would run counter to the idea of harnessing the

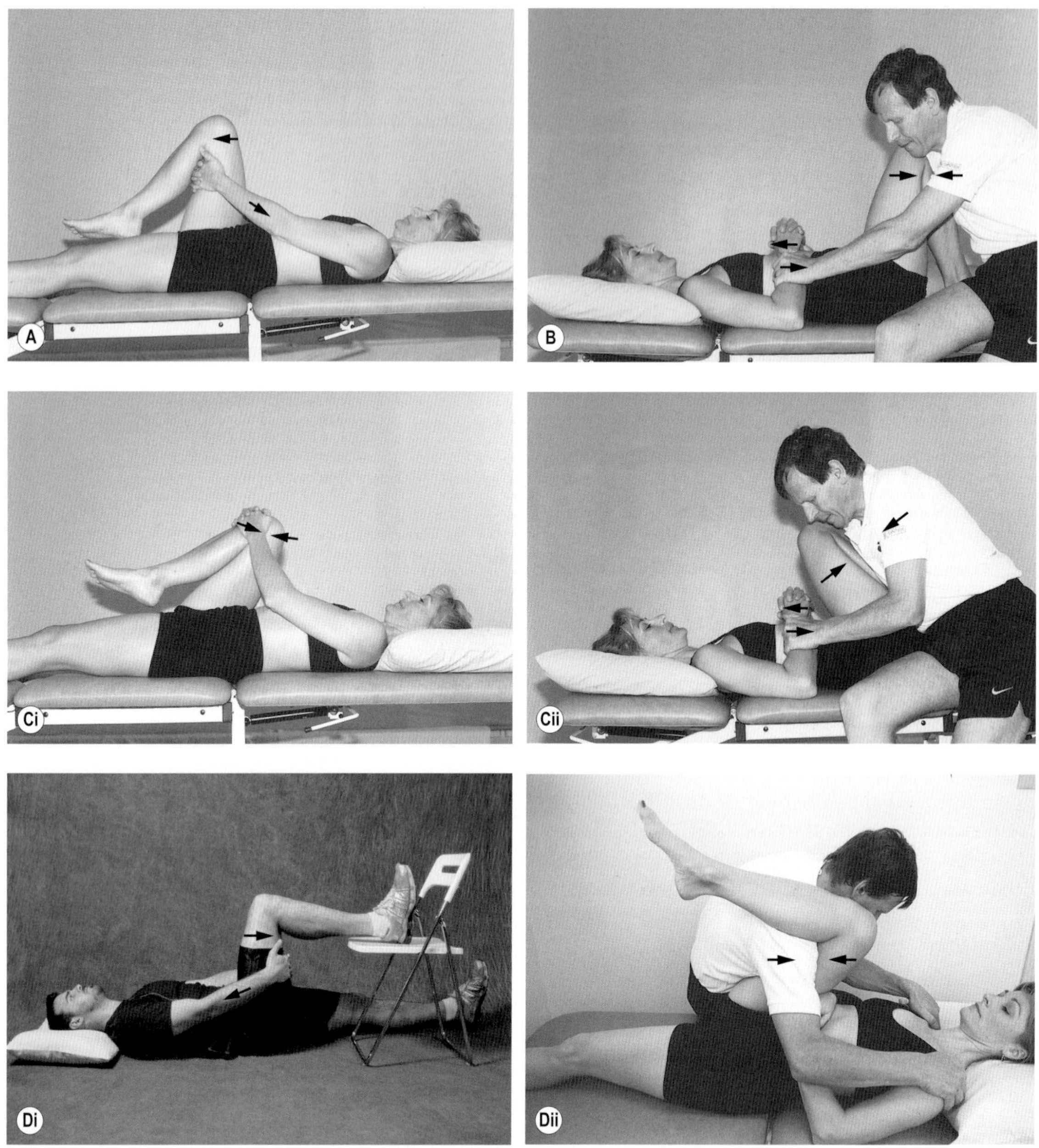

Fig. 7.9 Muscle energy technique for the correction of right innominate 'anterior' rotation: using gluteus maximus by blocking attempted right hip extension. (A) One-person technique. (B) Two-person technique. (C) To take up any slack as the hip extensors relax on repeated resisted contraction, gradually increase the hip flexion angle (compare to (A) and (B), respectively), provided that this does not cause or aggravate pain. (D) To modify the technique for a painful knee (e.g. osteoarthritis, patellofemoral compartment syndrome), decrease the knee flexion angle: (i) one-person technique - leg resting on chair; (ii) two-person technique - leg resting on assistant's shoulder.

(Continued)

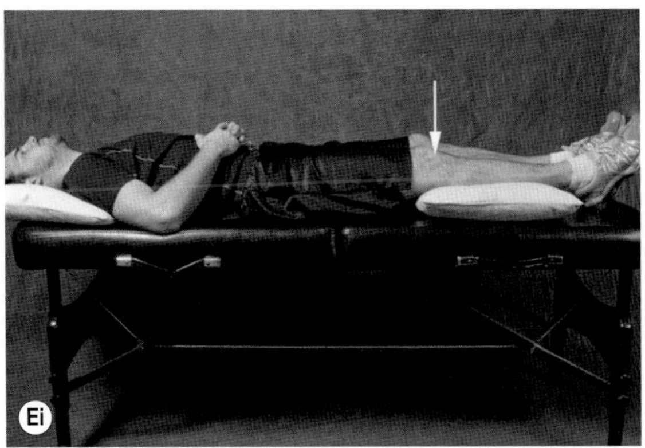

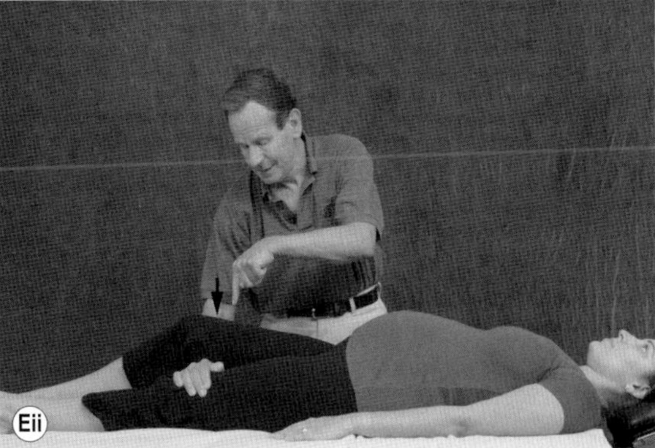

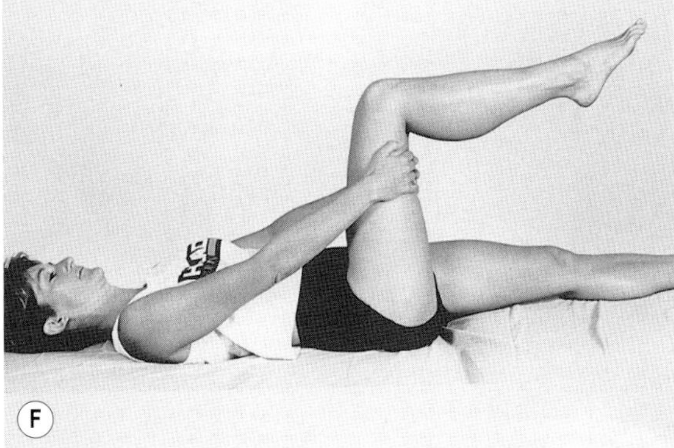

Fig. 7.9—cont'd (E) Modified technique resisting hip extension: (i) one-person (note: knee resting over pillow in some flexion, to keep hamstrings relaxed); (ii) pre- or post-partum. (F) Incorrect technique: the effectiveness of a resisted hip extensor contraction is decreased by simultaneous quadriceps contraction, seen here keeping the knee in 90 degrees flexion - the lower leg is held unsupported up in mid-air by rectus femoris which is also capable of exerting a simultaneous, counterproductive anterior rotational force on the innominate bone (see Figs 2.46 C, 2.59, 7.12).

specific muscle(s) to initiate a movement (in this case, one of 'innominate rotation', not 'knee extension')

b. if you are sitting to carry out this manoeuvre, your own pelvis is relatively 'fixed', so that your trunk is subjected to a unilateral rotational force that puts you at increased risk of going out of alignment (Fig. 2.13C)

2. with the distal part of their shin or the ankle region pushing up under your armpit (Fig. 7.13D)
   - this set-up allows you to use your own body weight to counteract their quadriceps contraction more effectively, as well as decreasing the torsional forces on your body
3. alternately, when helping someone with longer legs, the flexed knee can be rested across your shoulder and allow you to more easily, again using your body weight to advantage by hanging on to the shin to resist the attempted knee extension (Fig. 7.13E).

Application of this technique to the wrong side will obviously only make matters worse. Some facts to consider should be of help here (Box 7.2).

MET successfully corrects an 'anterior/posterior' innominate rotation in 75-85% and:

1. will usually simultaneously resolve a concomitant SI joint movement dysfunction, such as a relative decrease of movement or actual 'locking' (Fig. 2.125)
2. may also correct a coexistent vertebral rotational displacement; for example:
   a. the rotation of L1 typically seen in association with 'rotational malalignment', or
   b. L4 and/or L5 rotation (which may have caused the pelvic 'rotational malalignment' in the first place; Fig. 2.52)

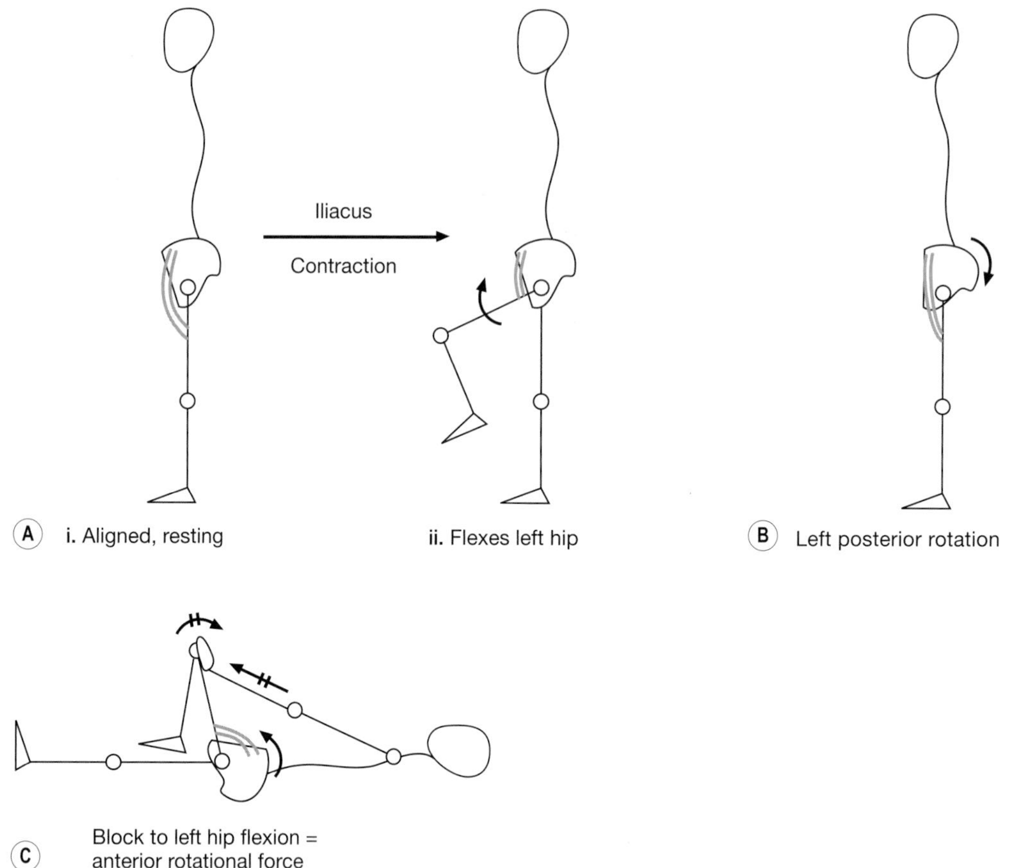

Fig. 7.10 Muscle energy technique versus innominate 'posterior' rotation (B). (A) Iliacus acts as a hip flexor when the thigh is free to move (see Fig. 2.46). (C) Blocking hip flexion reverses the muscle origin and insertion, creating an anterior rotational force.

3. corrects a concomitant sacral torsion in approximately 50%
4. may sometimes correct an 'outflare/inflare' present at the same time
5. will only rarely correct a coexistent 'upslip'.

MET can also be used to correct the rotational displacement of specific vertebrae (see 'MET for correction of vertebral rotational displacement', below).

If the person reports pain, the MET may have to be modified as follows:

Pain on correction of a 'right anterior' rotation

If the initial attempt to flex the right hip to 90 degrees, or the subsequent active extension of the right hip in the sagittal plane causes pain, try the same manoeuvre with the thigh adducted or abducted 5–10 degrees. If this makes no difference, start with the right hip flexion angle decreased to 60 degrees or even less, resistance being provided by an assistant (Figs 7.9B, 7.14A) or by lengthening the reach using a towel or wide belt (Fig. 7.14Bii). The manoeuvre can even be performed on one's own, with the right leg lying almost straight (Fig. 7.9Ei), or with the attempted right hip extension resisted by the forearm of an assistant (Fig. 7.14Ci) whose hand is secured lying across the person's opposite (left) thigh (Figs 7.9Eii, 7.14Cii). Remember, the knee should always be in some degree of flexion, to ensure the hamstrings are relaxed.

The mechanical advantage of gluteus maximus decreases as the right hip flexion angle is decreased but most people will still derive benefit with repeated contractions. In these situations especially (e.g. post-partum), the emphasis is on repetitions - rather than generating strength - in the one or two specific muscles needed to achieve the correction.

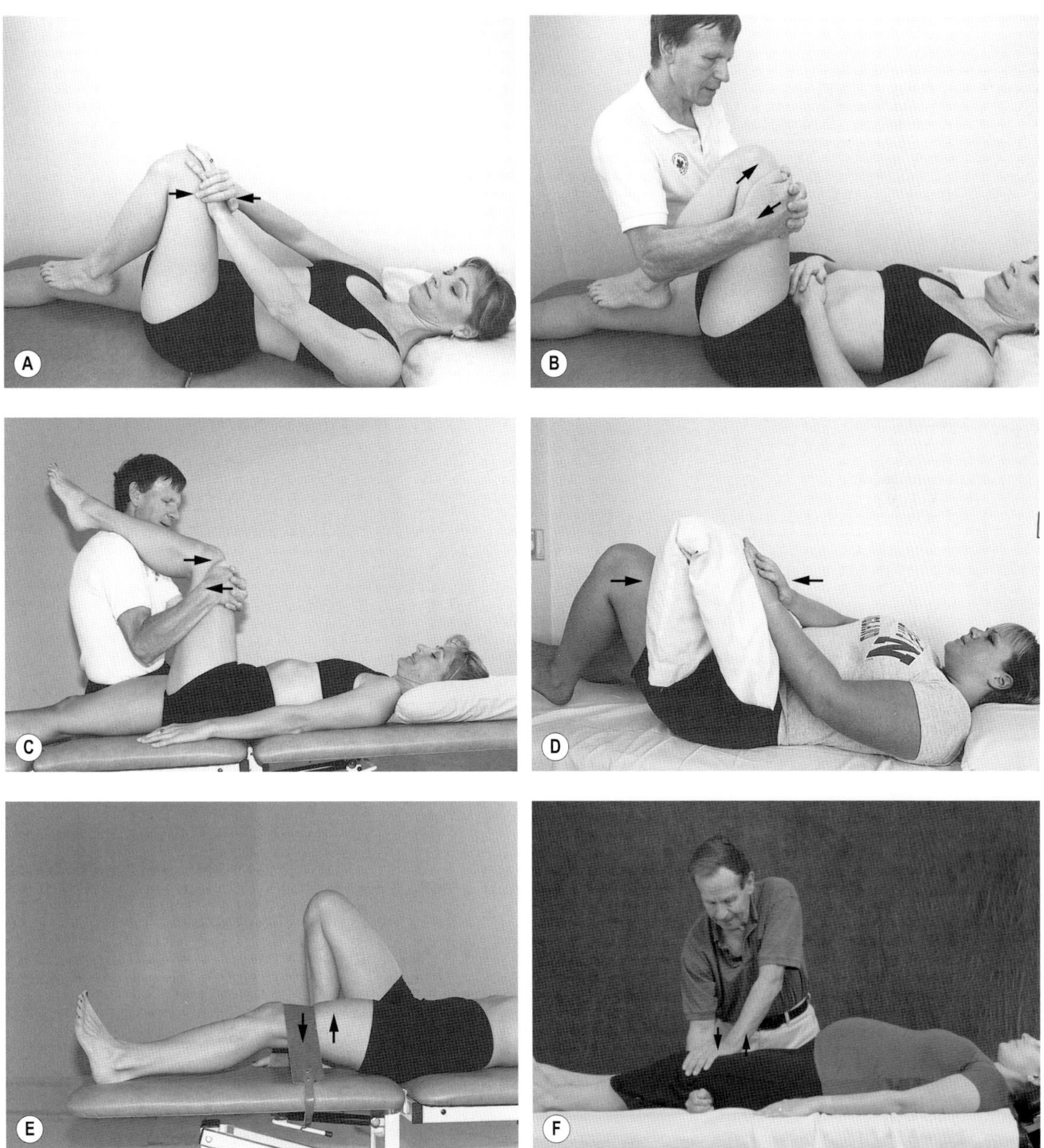

Fig. 7.11 Muscle energy technique for correcting left innominate 'posterior' rotation: using iliacus and/or rectus femoris by blocking attempted hip flexion or knee extension, respectively. (A) One-person technique. (B) Two-person technique. (C) Modification for a painful left knee; using primarily iliacus;. (D) Modification for short arms and/or an inability to flex the hip: the pillow helps to fill the gap. Note: Should it prove difficult or painful to maintain the hip at 90 degrees flexion, try decreasing the angle: (E) one-person technique - the fixed belt resists the attempted hip flexion; (F) two-person technique during pregnancy or post-partum, activating both iliacus and rectus femoris. A pillow (E) or hand-support (F) under the popliteal fossa maintains the knee in partial flexion, to ensure hamstring relaxation.

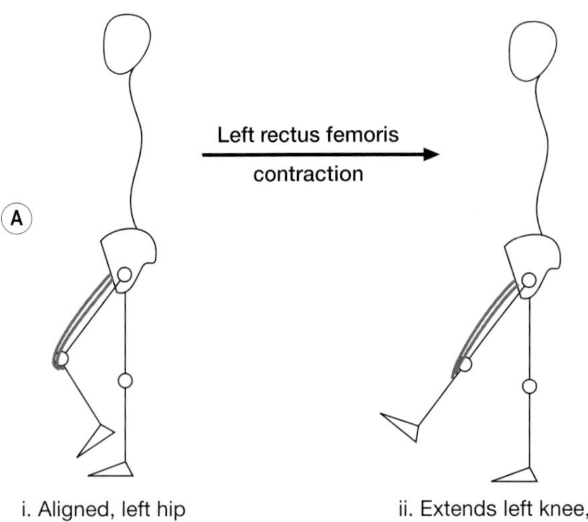

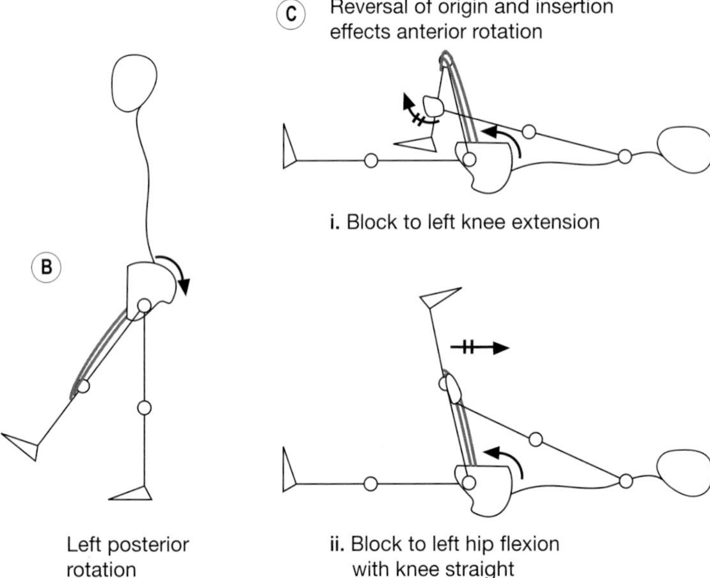

Fig. 7.12 Muscle energy technique: the biomechanics of using left rectus femoris for the correction of a left innominate 'posterior' rotation. (A) The muscle originates from the anterior inferior iliac spine on the innominate and inserts into the tibial tubercle (see Figs 2.46 C, 2.59). (B) It acts as a knee extensor when extension can occur (e.g. non-weight-bearing. (Ci) Blocking knee extension reverses the origin and insertion, creating an anterior rotational force on the innominate. (Cii) Blocking hip flexion when the knee is extended will also engage rectus femoris.

Excessive strength is usually accompanied by unwanted activation of muscles that may actually counter the rotational forces required to correct the malalignment.

If pain does occur at some point as the right hip is increasingly flexed with progressive stretching and relaxation of the gluteus maximus, simply bring the thigh back to the last position that did not prove painful. After repeating the manoeuvre a few times in that position, try it once more at an increased hip flexion angle to see whether that still provokes pain. If it does, go back to the previous pain-free position and stay there from then on. For example, if pain came on with the thigh flexed 120 degrees, do some more resisted contractions at 110 degrees and then try again at 120 degrees - if this still hurts, complete

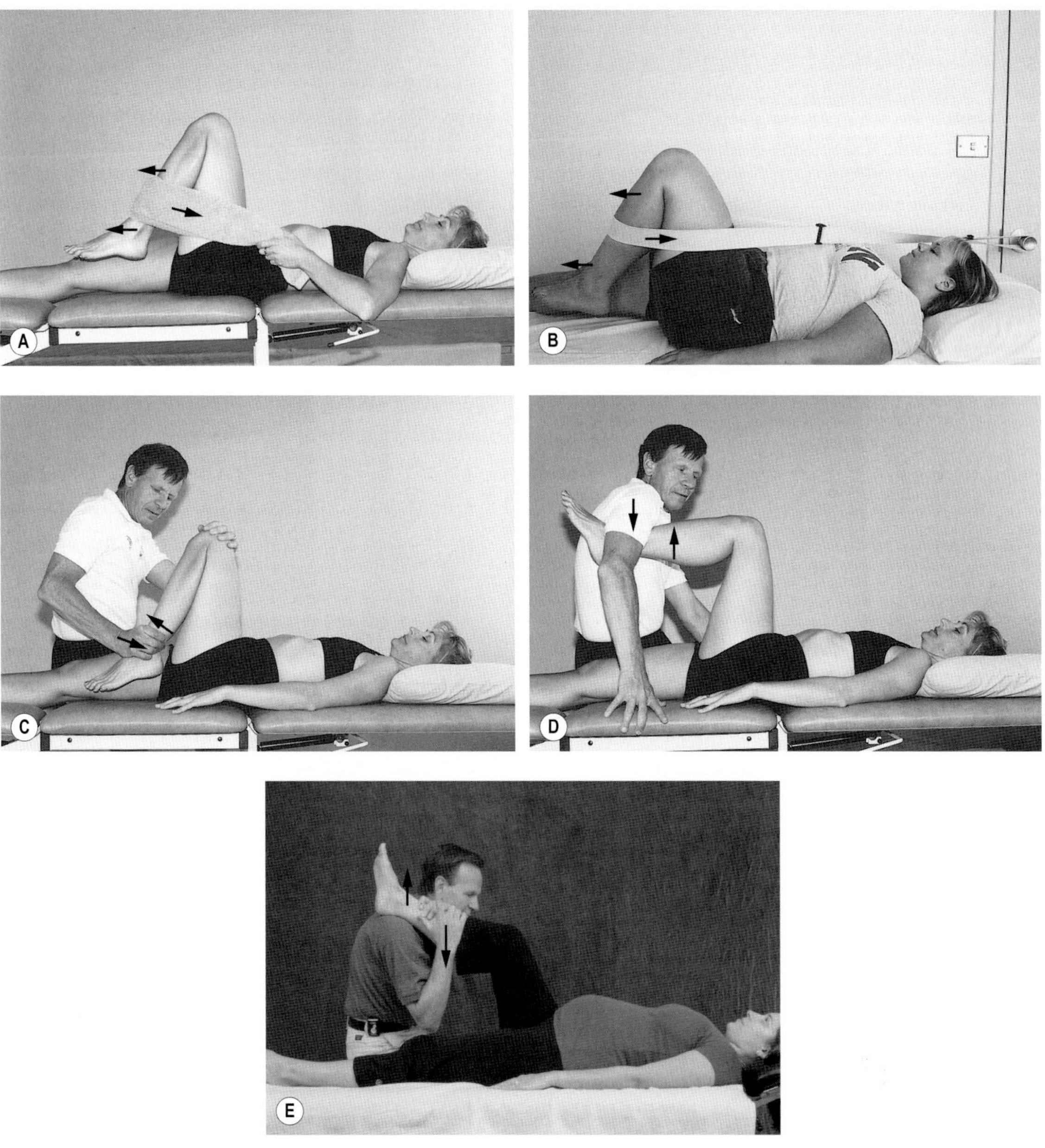

Fig. 7.13 Muscle energy technique for correcting left innominate 'posterior' rotation using rectus femoris: blocking attempted extension of the flexed left knee. (A) One-person technique (here using a towel to provide an extension for short arms, in order to avoid any posterior rotational leverage forces that can result with increasing degrees of hip flexion). (B) One-person technique using a sling: (i) as an extension for short arms, (ii) to provide resistance to knee extension at a reduced left hip flexion angle and/or (iii) as a substitute for the arms, to allow sore neck, upper back and shoulder girdle muscles to relax while using this method. (C) Two-person technique: the twisted position of the assistant's trunk increases the risk of putting himself out of alignment. (D) Improved two-person technique: any torsion is limited and the assistant can offer more counterforce using his body weight to advantage, thereby decreasing any risk to himself. (E) Leg lies on shoulder, assistant again uses his weight to advantage by hanging on to the lower leg to resist knee extension.

BOX 7.2 Determining the appropriate MET for correction of 'rotational malalignment'

1. The 'anterior' rotation is probable on the side on which the leg lengthens on going from the long-sitting to supine-lying position; asymmetry of all the pelvic landmarks verifies the presentation. These examination findings, also conditions that can result in a false test, have been discussed in Chapters 2 and 3.
2. If an 'anterior' rotation recurs, it may do so on the same side, but this is not a safe assumption and always makes a proper examination of alignment mandatory whenever treatment using MET is being considered.
3. In approximately 5-10%, a side-to-side switch from 'anterior' to 'posterior' rotation is evident from one examination to the next, a phenomenon seen particularly in those who have:
    a. generalized joint hypermobility, as the result of a natural, often time-limited, event (e.g. during a pregnancy and post-partum; Marnach et al. 2003) or congenital condition (e.g. Ehler-Danlos)
    b. suffered some recent asymmetrical (and usually torsional) stress, such as from a fall onto one side, or when carrying a heavy weight either just on one side or awkwardly across the body, with rotation into the opposite direction from usual (e.g. going down a staircase carrying a heavy suitcase on one side)
    c. laxity of one or both sacroiliac joints, or instability of L4 or L5 allowing rotation to either right or left

the corrective manoeuvre staying at 110 degrees. It may be that progressively increasing right hip flexion is causing pain by:

1. further increasing tension in already tender posterior pelvic ligaments and buttock muscles
2. compressing a tense and tender right iliopsoas muscle, pectineus or possibly an iliopectineal bursa, all of which are particularly vulnerable to an increase in hip flexion (especially when combined with adduction) where they lie within the narrow femoral triangle, sandwiched between the inguinal ligament and anterosuperior lip of the acetabulum (Fig. 4.2).

Pain on correction of 'left posterior' rotation

The person again lies supine, the left hip flexed to 90 degrees, and repeatedly resists either left hip flexion or left knee extension, about a dozen times (Figs 7.10-7.13). If either manoeuvre proves painful, he of she may have to try:

1. changing the hip-flexion angle
2. decreasing the strength of the contractions, or
3. abandoning the MET manoeuvres on this side for the time being and, instead, do more repetitions of the appropriate manoeuvres only on the opposite side if this proves less painful or, preferably, pain-free; concentrating on the correction of the 'right anterior' rotation (Figs 7.8, 7.9) will usually result in simultaneous correction of a compensatory contralateral (left) 'posterior' rotation, and vice versa.

Keep in mind that the two most common mistakes made when carrying out the MET are:

1. *generating too much force*
    a. one only needs to contract the specific muscle(s) that can act on an innominate to achieve realignment
    b. increasing force activates more and more muscles; many of these attach to the pelvic ring (e.g. transversus abdominis, external and internal obliques, pelvic floor muscles) and can interfere with achieving the desired rotation of the innominate(s)
2. *altering the respiratory rhythm*
    - recommendations are to maintain the normal rhythm as best as possible; holding one's breath or increasing/decreasing the frequency or depth of breathing in and out usually results in a generalized increase in muscle tone

The few muscles needed to achieve realignment are best:

1. relaxed in the inspiratory phase
    - during which tension in trunk muscles (many of which also attach to the pelvic ring) is increased
2. activated in the expiratory phase
    - during which the trunk muscles are relaxed

Always remind the person to relax all the muscles other than those specifically needed for a certain MET manoeuvre.

The most common mistake is to tense up the muscles in the neck and upper back region while hanging on to the towel or belt to provide the required resistance. Worse still is to actually raise the head

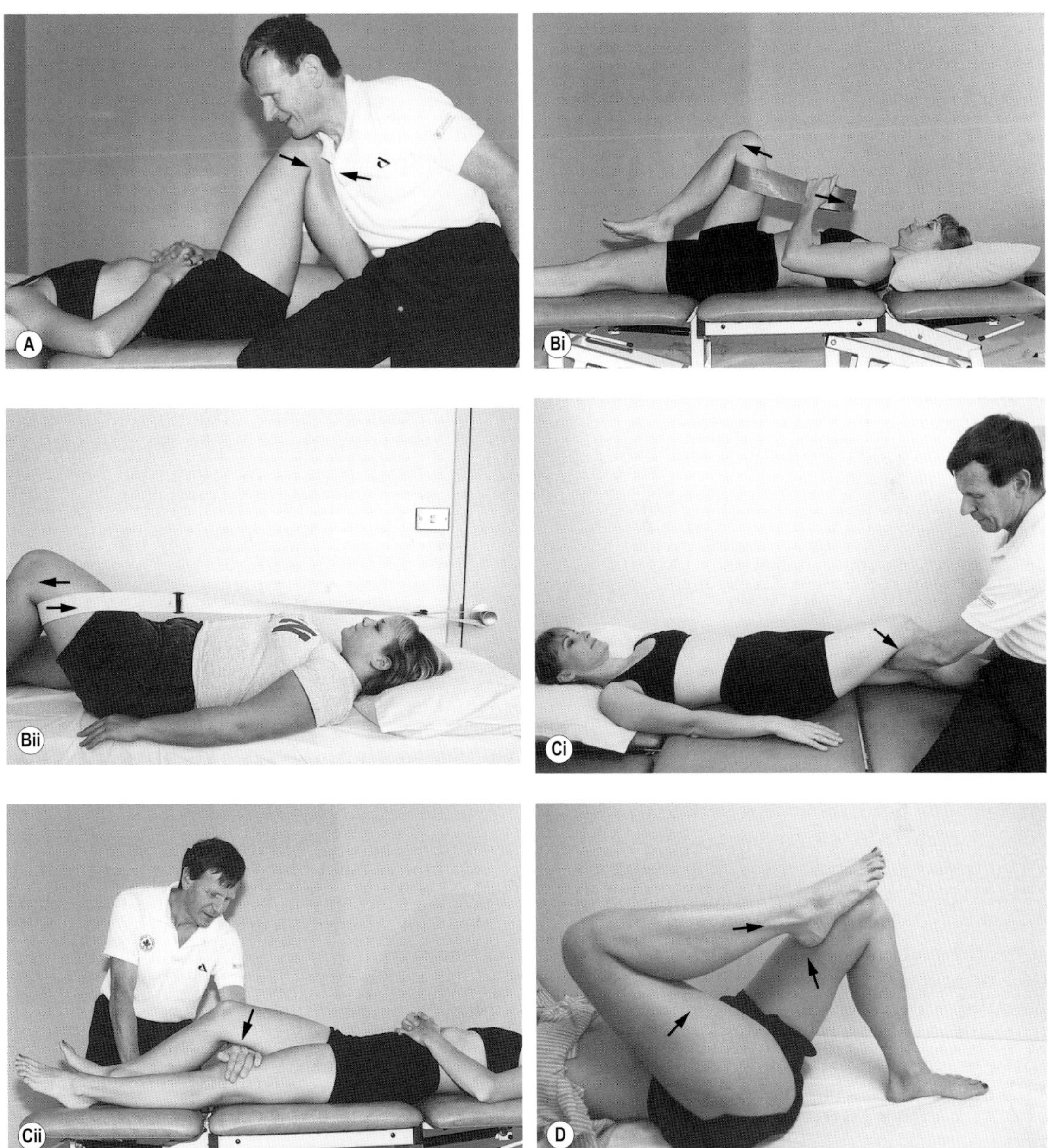

Fig. 7.14 Modifications of the muscle energy technique using resisted hip extensor contraction for the correction of 'anterior' innominate rotation. (A) Decreasing the hip flexion angle to avoid any pain noted past that point. (B) Using a towel or wide belt: (i) to serve as an extension for short arms; (ii) to allow for a decrease in the hip flexion angle and/or a relaxation of tense/painful neck/upper back muscles during the manoeuvre. (C) When the hip flexion angle needs to be markedly reduced because of obstruction (e.g. during maternity; Fig. 7.9E) or pain (e.g. postpartum or after surgery). The assistant's forearm: (i) can provide resistance; (ii) can be steadied by securing the hand on top of the opposite thigh. (D) Simultaneous resisted right hip extension (versus 'right anterior' rotation) and left hip flexion (versus 'left posterior' rotation).

and/or shoulders off the plinth. Tensing these muscles inevitably results in a domino-like involvement of anterior and posterior trunk muscles, all the way down to their attachments to the superior pubic rami, iliac crests and the thoracodorsal fascia (e.g. rectus abdominis anteriorly, erector spinae and latissimus dorsi posteriorly; Figs 2.31-2.40). A contraction of these muscles can easily interfere with the action of the one or two muscles needed to achieve rotation of the innominates in the desired direction.

Contract-Relax

The contract-relax method is one way of achieving both progressive relaxation and realignment.

> The relaxation of a muscle following an isometric contraction is usually more profound than can be achieved voluntarily.

Sometimes just achieving relaxation of any tense attaching muscles allows the bones to rotate back into proper alignment. The hold–relax method used to treat localized muscle spasm is based on the same principle. The decrease in tension following each contraction allows for the further passive movement of a body part into the direction of the restriction.

The contract–relax manoeuvre can be useful for the correction of innominate rotation, in particular the rotation and displacement that occurs anteriorly at the symphysis pubis. Realignment of the pubic bones, for example, may be achieved by alternate bilateral hip abduction and adduction against a resistance while sitting or lying supine (Fig. 7.15). The simultaneous symmetrical activation of these muscles exerts an equal pull on pelvic structures that are in an asymmetrical position to begin with, thereby allowing them to come back to the midline, or 'neutral', position. The technique is covered in some detail below under 'Self-help techniques to correct malalignment'.

When malalignment is present, there is often an increase in tone in the left hip abductors and right piriformis, which exert opposing rotational forces on the lower extremities: left internal, right external rotation, respectively. Asymmetrical tension in the piriformis also creates a sacral torsional strain by way of its origins from the anterosuperior aspect of the sacrum (Fig. 2.46A). The hip abductors and the external rotators of the thigh can be activated by resisting any movement on attempted bilateral hip abduction/external rotation while lying supine or sitting, maintaining the hips in a flexed position, the knees some 20–30 cm apart and the feet together (Fig. 7.15A,Bi,Ci). The repeated isometric contraction of these muscles may correct a sacral torsion or rotation of the lower extremities and cause them to relax to the point of re-establishing symmetry of muscle tone.

Simultaneous hip adduction against resistance, with the knees again held 20–30 cm apart, reverses the adductor origin and insertion, resulting in a symmetrical traction force on the inferior pubic rami (Fig. 7.15Bii,Cii). These forces can sometimes re-establish symmetry at the symphysis pubis; this may occur by temporarily separating the symphysis and then allowing the adjoining pubic bones to fall back into the normal, aligned position as the adductors relax. It is this separation that is felt to be responsible for the sensation sometimes reported of something having 'moved' in the region of the symphysis, often accompanied by an audible sound, much like 'popping' a knuckle. Unilateral adductor contraction, of course, can also correct an ipsilateral inflare (see 'MET for correction of 'outflare' and 'inflare', below).

Reassessment may show the partial or complete reduction of a previously-noted step deformity at the symphysis and even the correction of a 'rotational malalignment', suggesting that the manoeuvre can also exert a rotational force on the innominates by way of their attachments to the previously asymmetrical pubic bones, to bring them all back to the neutral position.

Pain experienced with this technique is primarily attributable to contracting the muscles too forcefully, too often or both.

> People easily get caught up thinking that 'more is better' but end up activating muscles other than the ones needed to carry out a specific MET; they can also develop an 'overuse' type myofascial or tendon pain. Both will interfere with the correction of the malalignment problem.

The hip adductors and abductors seem especially vulnerable, perhaps because they are not likely to be very strong muscles in comparison with the

Fig. 7.15 Contract-relax method for the correction of innominate rotation: alternating simultaneous bilateral right and left resisted hip abduction and adduction. (A) One-person technique lying supine: a belt acts to resist abduction, while a cushion between the knees helps to prevent bruising on adduction. (B) One-person technique sitting: (i) the hands (or arm rests) resist abduction; (ii) the forearm resists adduction. (C) Two-person technique lying supine: (i) resisted abduction (ii) resisted adduction.

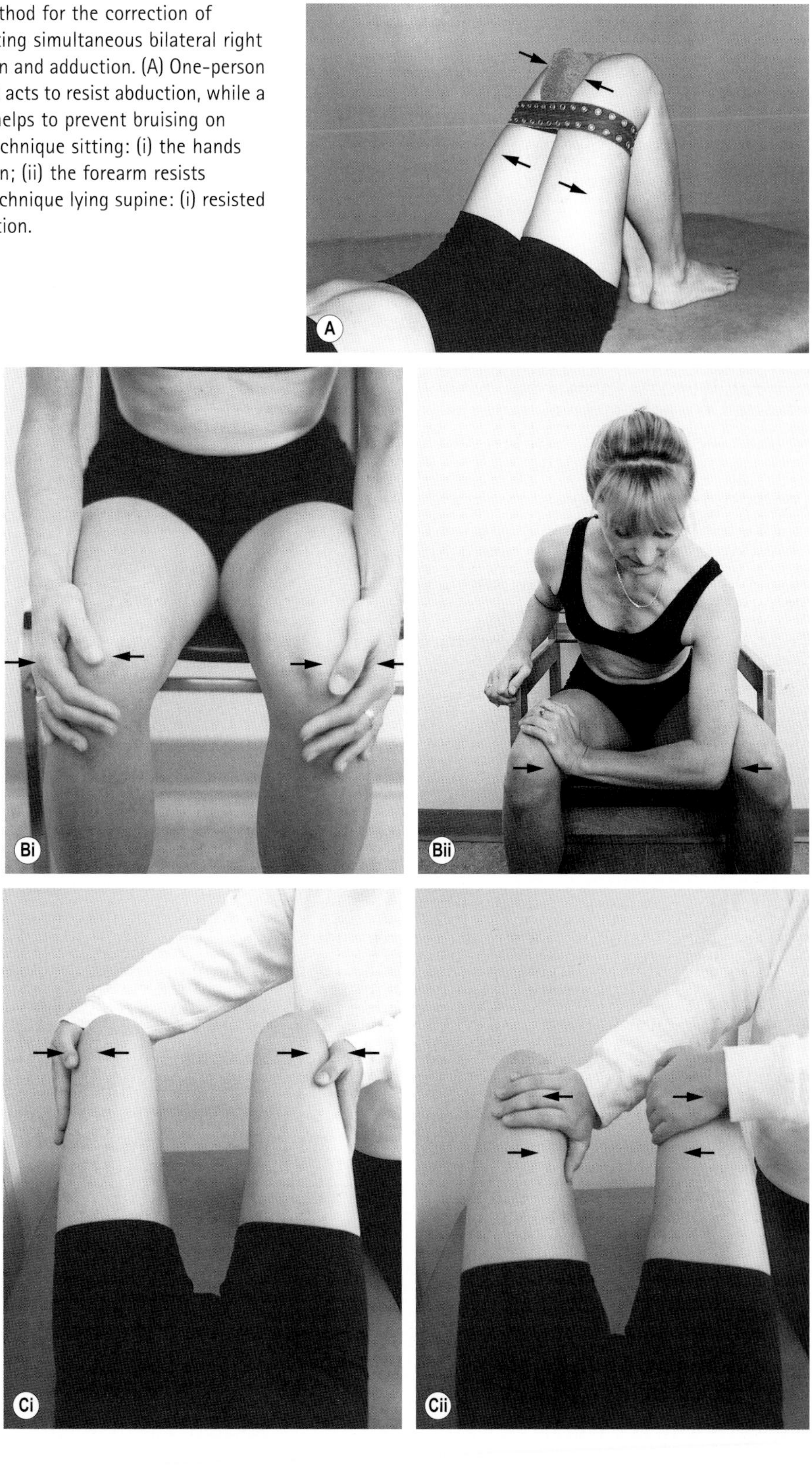

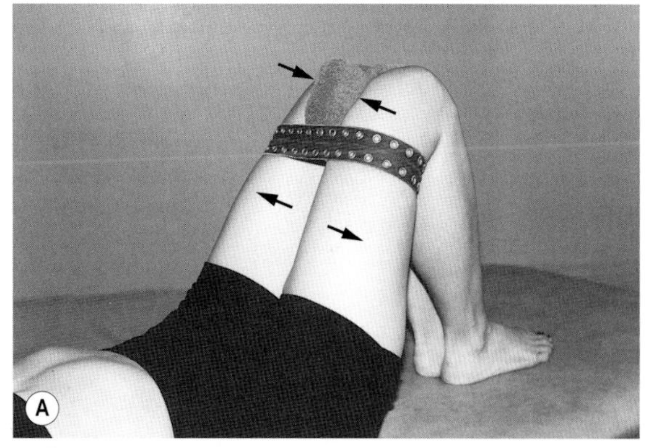

hamstrings and quadriceps, except perhaps in goalies and others who repeatedly adduct and abduct the legs as part of their work or sport (Fig. 5.21). Discomfort from overuse may not be felt for some hours after an overzealous attempt at the corrective manoeuvre described. Therefore, the following guidelines seem appropriate:

1. Limit the strength of the contraction to 50% of maximum to start with, if tolerated, in a conscientious effort to activate just the adductors or abductors and avoid triggering or increasing pain.
2. Do only five repeats to a slow count of three initially; even better, just do the contraction every time you breathe out, when the other muscles attaching to the pelvis are more likely to be relaxed. Add one more contraction every 2–3 days until you are doing a set of 10.
3. Once 10 repeats at 50% strength are easy, progressively increase either the strength or number until you can do 2 sets of 10 contractions at 100% strength of the specific muscle(s).

Leverage to effect counter-rotation

The femur can act like a lever to effect rotation of the ipsilateral innominate. Progressive hip flexion, for example, puts the posterior soft tissues under increasing tension and eventually sees the femur impinge on the anterosuperior rim of the acetabulum (Fig. 2.47A). At that point, further passive hip flexion creates a mechanical force capable of rotating the innominate posteriorly (Fig. 2.109). Progressive hip extension will eventually have the opposite effect: anterior rotation of the innominate (Figs 2.47B, 2.108A,B). This leverage effect can sometimes be used to correct a 'rotational malalignment'. For example, passive right hip flexion carried out with the person standing (Fig. 7.22A,C) or lying supine (Fig. 7.16A) may correct an 'anterior' rotation on that side. Passive left hip extension with the person standing (Fig. 7.22B) or lying prone (Fig. 7.16B) may correct a posterior rotation.

Leverage forces for the simultaneous correction of a 'right anterior, left posterior' rotation can also be achieved by:

One or two-person technique

Pushing the right thigh onto the person's chest while applying a gentle downward pressure on the left thigh (or letting it hang freely over the edge of the bed, similar to Gaenslen's test) forces the left hip into extension (Figs 2.108B, 7.16 C).

One-person techniques

Combined trunk and hip flexion (Fig. 7.17)

1. the person is standing with the right foot securely placed on a fairly high support, like a chair
2. he or she then lets the trunk bend forward as far as comfortably possible - if tolerated, the right thigh ends up alongside the chest; the head and arms simply hang down in a relaxed position, to help exaggerate the trunk and right hip flexion that creates the 'right posterior' rotational force

A modified lunge (Fig. 7.18A)

1. the standing person again starts by putting the right foot up on a high support, with the knee flexed
2. the left foot is planted on the floor behind, with the left knee in full extension - by then leaning forward with the trunk, and allowing the pelvis to gradually sink downward, he or she turns the right and left femur into levers capable of exerting a 'posterior' and 'anterior' rotational force on the respective innominates

Bouncing must be avoided at all cost when carrying out these lunges, to prevent precipitating or aggravating any pre-existing pain. Leverage manoeuvres may cause pain from stressing a degenerating hip or knee joint or an inflamed or malaligned SI joint. Pain may also arise simply from putting tense and tender structures under even more tension. For example:

1. passive hip flexion on the side of the 'anterior' rotation, especially with the knee straight, typically can precipitate pain from an involved piriformis and/or hamstring muscles, and the posterior pelvic ligaments
2. passive hip extension on the side of the 'posterior' rotation can evoke pain from a tender iliacus, rectus femoris, tensor fascia lata (TFL) or anterior SI joint ligament.

The vigour with which counter-rotation manoeuvres can be carried out should, therefore, be guided by an attempt to avoid, if at all possible, precipitating any pain and triggering reflex muscle spasm.

TECHNIQUES FOR CORRECTION OF A SACROILIAC JOINT 'UPSLIP'

As discussed, 'upslip' refers to a persistent upward shift of an innominate relative to the sacrum as the result of a vertical force (transmitted up the leg or

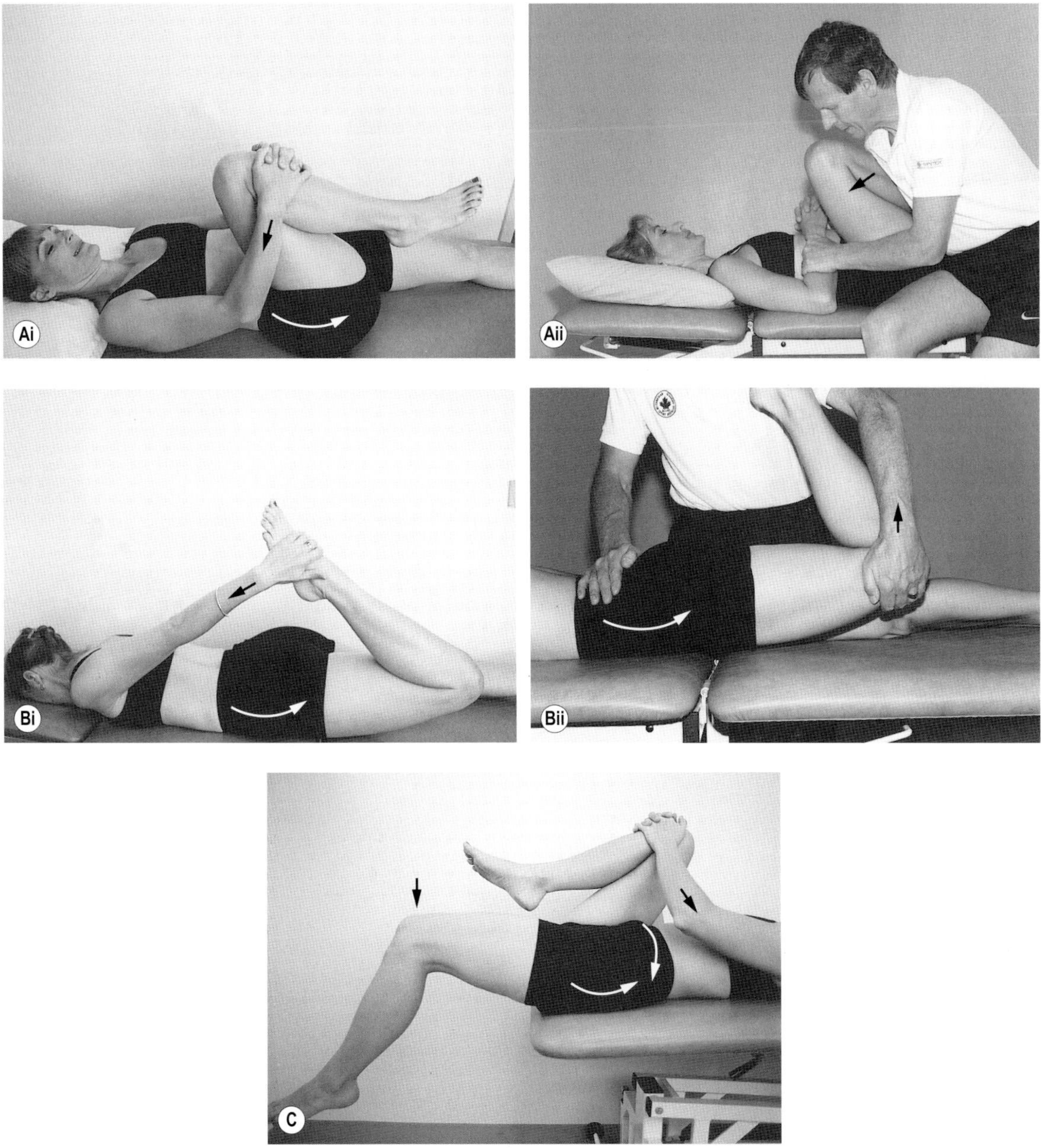

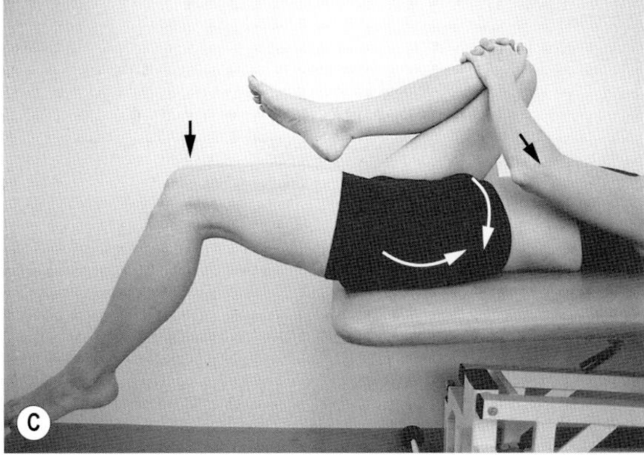

Fig. 7.16 Using a leverage effect to correct 'rotational malalignment' (see Figs 2.105, 2.108, 2.109). (A) Passive hip flexion to counteract right innominate 'anterior' rotation: (i) one-person and (ii) two-person technique. (B) Passive hip extension to counteract 'left posterior' rotation: (i) one-person and (ii) two-person technique. (C) Simultaneous correction of 'right anterior' (white arrow, down) and 'left posterior' rotation by passive right hip flexion and left hip extension, respectively.

directly onto the innominate; Fig. 2.61A) or from a persistent increase in tension in muscles that can exert a upward (craniad) force by way of their attachments to that innominate (e.g. quadratus lumborum, psoas major and minor; Fig. 2.62).

Subsequently, the 'upslip' position is often maintained on the basis of:

1. the symphysis pubis and/or SI joint surfaces being 'locked' in the abnormal ('upslip') position

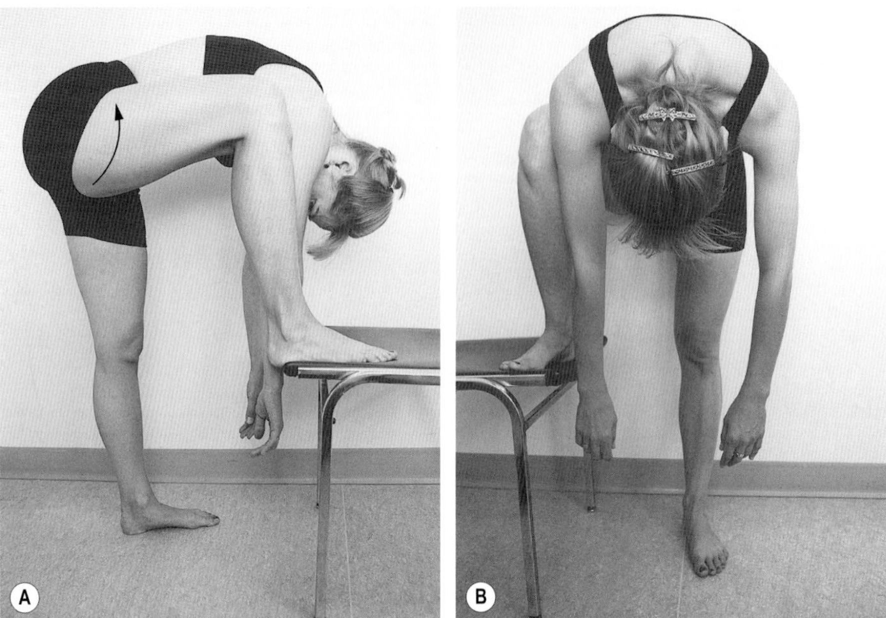

Fig. 7.17 To correct right innominate 'anterior' rotation, a right posterior leverage effect can be created with the right thigh (femur) by (A) initially resting the right foot on a high support and then (B) letting the trunk hang down in forward flexion as far as feels comfortable. Bouncing or straining while reaching down is to be avoided, as is precipitating or aggravating any pain.

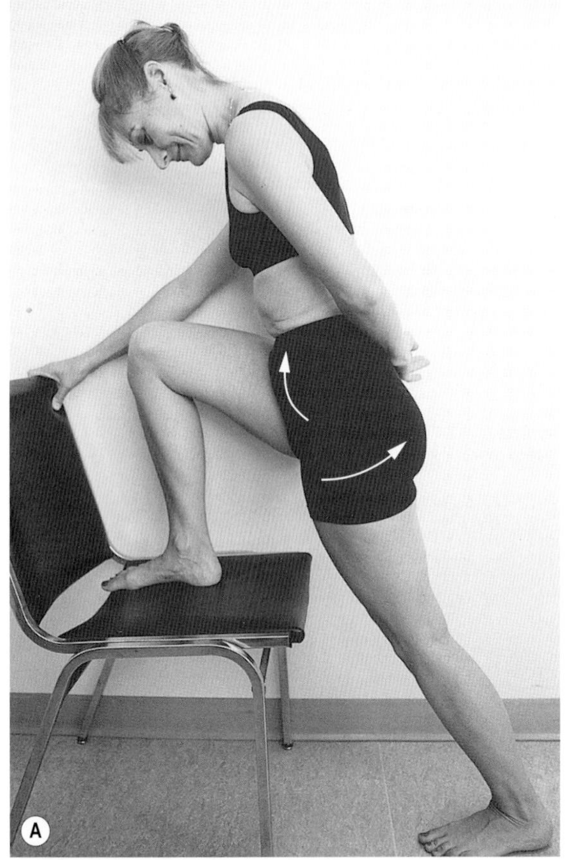

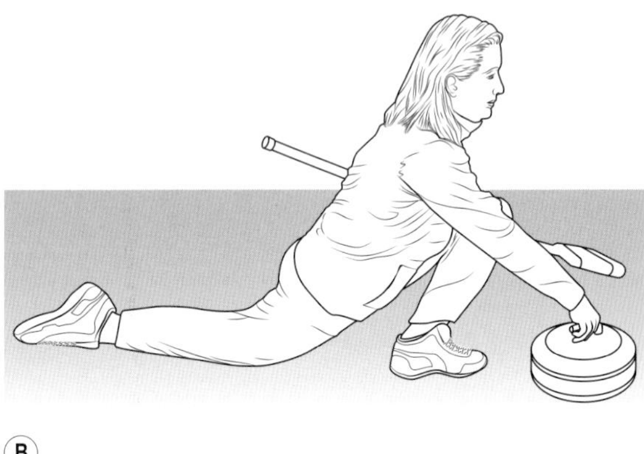

Fig. 7.18 (A). When there is a 'right anterior, left posterior' innominate rotation, this modified lunge position (right foot forward and up on a support, left leg in extension with the foot on the floor) simultaneously creates a right posterior (vertical arrow) and left anterior (lower arrow) rotational force. (B) Typical lunge position is assumed during some activities and may affect alignment favourably or unfavourably; for example, going into a lunge position for right-hand release of 'rock' in curling (i.e. left hip and knee in flexion, right in extension) could passively (1) correct a 'left anterior, right posterior' innominate rotation, (2) trigger or aggravate a 'right anterior, left posterior' rotation.

2. persistent increase in tension in muscles like quadratus lumborum, in reaction to instability and/or ongoing pain from these joints, the muscle itself or the surrounding soft tissues

Gradual relaxation of the hip girdle muscles achieved with traction may allow the innominate on that side to 'come down' and resume its normal position alongside the sacrum so that the SI joint surfaces once again match. These traction manoeuvres lend themselves to a one or two-person approach. Having someone repeatedly apply a steady downward traction force 10–12 times to the leg on the side of the 'upslip' may be adequate to resolve the problem (Fig. 7.19A). When alone, the person can try standing with a weight attached to the shin or foot of the freely suspended leg on the side of the 'upslip' (Fig. 7.19B). This approach is described in more detail under 'Self-help techniques to correct malalignment', to follow.

Manipulation, while not being encouraged as a regular corrective procedure for reasons detailed in Chs 7 and 8 may, nevertheless, be particularly helpful for correcting some types of malalignment. An SI joint 'upslip', for example, can usually be corrected with a quick downward traction on the leg. The exact position of the innominate needs, however, to be determined first, in order to establish how the manipulation should be carried out. The interested reader is referred to the literature and would need to partake in a supervised teaching programme and hands- on training before applying these techniques.

For the more gentle mobilization technique, the person is asked to lie in either the supine or the prone position. The therapist/assistant gets a firm hold of the foot and ankle on the side of the 'upslip' by having the palm of one hand rest against the Achilles insertion (the angle at the heel usually prevents it from slipping downward; Fig. 7.19A) while the other palm rests over the dorsum of the foot. There is no need for force (e.g. excessive squeezing) to maintain this hold. Next, the leg is moved into position - with the hip slightly flexed if supine, extended if prone, or in neutral, depending on the examination findings and as dictated by comfort - and then gently moved about from side-to-side or in a circle in an attempt to completely relax the hip girdle muscles. The person is distracted by conversation, and a gradually increasing traction force is exerted repeatedly about 12 times by pulling downward on the extremity, if possible in unison with the expiration phase (when the muscles attaching to the pelvis and hip girdle are likely to be most relaxed).

Successful reduction of an 'upslip' is sometimes indicated by the sensation of a joint actually having moved, similar to the feeling associated with 'popping' a knuckle, and is more likely to occur with sudden traction (manipulation).

This sensation of the joint 'slotting back into place' can often be felt by the therapist as it is transmitted through the femur and tibia down to the hands around the ankle. There is sometimes also an audible sound. The person may spontaneously report the feeling of one bone now sitting square or 'right on' with the other. It just 'feels right again', and the discomfort may immediately appear to be decreased or even abolished. If the person's anatomical (true) leg length is known to be equal, successful reduction is confirmed by finding that:

1. leg length is once again equal on the sitting-lying test
2. anterior and posterior pelvic landmarks match on side-to-side comparison (Figs 2.71, 2.72A,B)
3. hip ranges of motion are symmetrical
4. the pelvis is level in both sitting and standing
5. lower extremity muscle strength is full and symmetrical, with the possible exception of the left hip abductors and TFL/ITB complex, which usually proves stronger but sometimes takes a few days or weeks to recover full strength (see Ch. 3); easiest to test right after correction is the strength of right EHL, which should now be equal to the left - this assessment remains one of the most reliable (and quickest) to perform to ascertain whether full correction has or has not been achieved

Several attempts may be required to achieve correction; if realignment is only partial:

1. leg length may still be noticeably shorter on the sitting-lying test on the 'upslip' side, usually to a lesser extent than noted on initial assessment
2. right and left pelvic landmarks - ASIS, PSIS, pubic bones and ischial tuberosities - still do not match completely

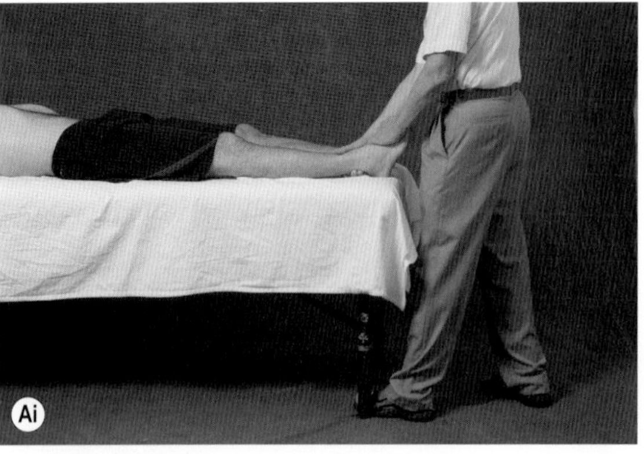

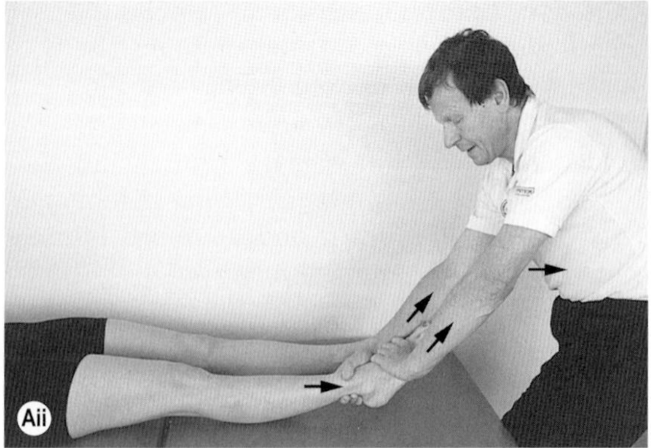

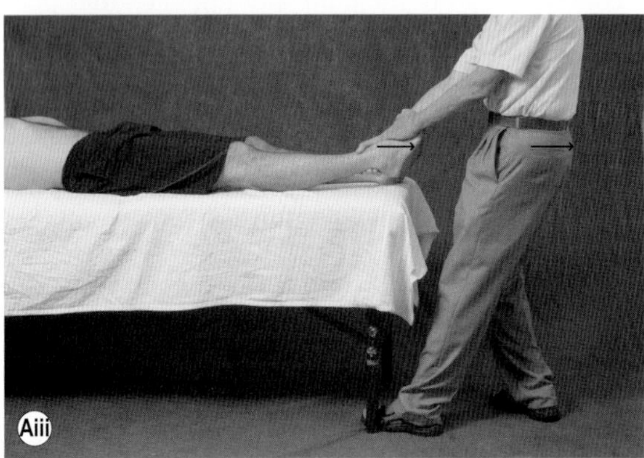

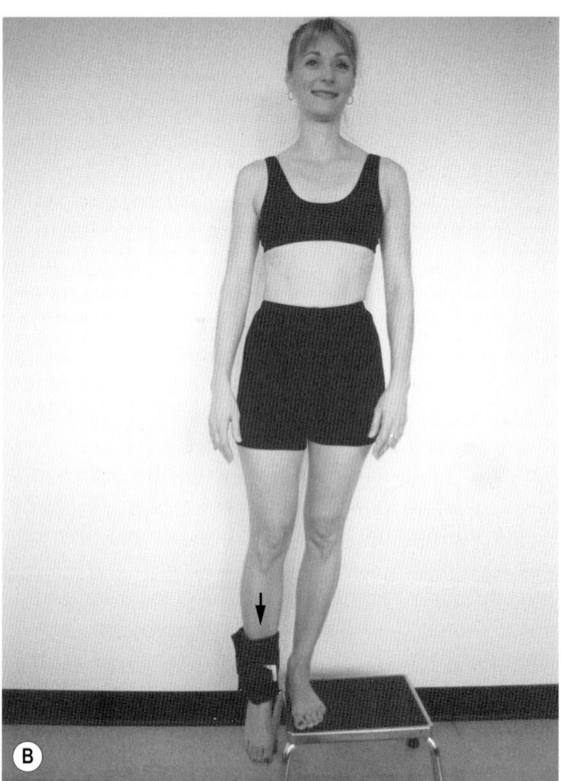

Fig. 7.19 Correction of a 'right upslip' with traction on the leg. (A) Two-person approach: (i) positioning of hands (right overlying the Achilles tendon and abutting on the calcaneus, left overlying the dorsum of the foot); (ii) direction of the forces generated with traction; (iii) the assistant maximizes use of his body weight to generate the traction forces by rocking back and forth on his feet: one is positioned posteriorly for balance/safety (Ai, iii); the legs are kept straight as the body leans back onto both heels (Aiii). Traction is applied as the subject exhales and trunk and pelvic muscles are relaxing. (B) One-person approach: using a weight attached to the suspended leg.

3. right EHL continues to give way before the left one does because of a persistant element of functional weakness

In that case, the stretch imparted by repeated downward traction has probably failed to completely relax muscles like the psoas and quadratus lumborum that are capable of exerting an ongoing upward pull on the innominate and displacing it relative to the sacrum (Fig. 2.62). It is for this reason that it may be worthwhile:

1. doing another course of about 12 traction manoeuvres immediately after the first try and rechecking alignment again right after
2. carrying out a set of tractions on a regular basis, perhaps 2 or 3 times a day, in the hope that this will relax the muscle(s) for increasingly longer

periods of time and, eventually, allow these bones to slot back into normal alignment

3. trying a manipulation, especially if repeat traction courses do not cause the person any marked increase in pain but fail to correct the 'upslip'

Underlying complications must always be ruled out, especially when the 'upslip' fails to respond to treatment as expected. These include:

1. concurrent 'rotational malalignment' or 'flare', sacral torsion, L4/L5/S1 dysfunction, or
2. other pathology that can stir up ongoing increases in muscle tension or reflex spasm and prevent the innominate sliding back into place; e.g. facet syndrome, central canal or foraminal stenosis, central or posterolateral disc bulge or protrusion, organomegaly or masses (discussed below).

MUSCLE ENERGY TECHNIQUE FOR CORRECTION OF 'OUTFLARE' AND 'INFLARE'

The pelvic movement that occurs during a normal gait cycle incorporates alternating outflaring and inflaring of the innominates, along with the upward and downward movement in the coronal plane and anterior/posterior rotation of the innominates (Figs 2.13A, 2.41). Excessive 'outflare' or 'inflare', with 'fixation' in one or the other position, can occur unilaterally, but the most common presentation is with an 'outflare' on one side and simultaneous (compensatory) 'inflare' on the other (Figs 2.13Aiii, 4.30). When an 'flare' problem is seen in conjunction with a 'rotational malalignment', correction of the 'outflare' and/or 'inflare' using MET should be carried out first because:

1. it will usually correct the 'outflare/inflare'
2. in 70-80% of those presenting with this combination, it will simultaneously correct a coexistent 'rotational malalignment'
3. in the remaining 20-30%, it may be necessary to correct the 'outflare/inflare' before the persistent 'rotational malalignment' will finally respond to attempts at correction using MET and/or other manual therapy techniques
4. although it will not correct an associated 'upslip', resolving the 'outflare/inflare' problem will at least re-establish some symmetry in the pelvic/hip girdle joint ranges of motion and muscle tone which is likely to make it easier to then resolve the 'upslip' using traction

Therefore, if an 'outflare/inflare' co-exists with a 'rotational malalignment' and 'upslip':

1. one should initially attempt correction of the 'outflare/inflare', given that it will simultaneously correct a coexistent rotational problem in 70-80%
2. use the MET for correction of those 20-30% still left with the 'rotational malalignment'
3. then apply traction for correction of the 'upslip' (which may not become obvious until the 'rotational malalignment' has been corrected)

MET for correction of a 'right outflare'

A 'right outflare' may correct with a MET that depends on resisting the contraction of the following muscles (Fig. 7.20):

Posteriorly

This involves primarily the external rotators and abductors of the right thigh (Fig. 7.21A); their posteromedial origins from the right innominate allows them to pull this part of the innominate laterally when their origins and insertions are reversed:

1. in particular, piriformis (through its origins from sacrum/greater sciatic notch area; Figs 2.46A, 7.20) and gluteus maximus (Fig. 2.5B)
2. to lesser extent
   a. the inferomedial part of the origins of gluteus minimus (from the posterior ilium; Figs 3.41, 7.20)
   b. obturator internus and externus (from the ischiopubic ramus)
   c. superior gemellus (from the outer surface of the ischial spine)
   d. inferior gemellus (from the ischial tuberosity)
   e. quadratus femoris (from the ischial tuberosity)

Anteriorly

This involves primarily right iliacus which, through its superolateral origins from the innominate, can pull it medially while external rotation is being blocked (Fig. 2.46B,C).

A person presenting with a 'right outflare, left inflare' would go through the sequence in Box 7.3.

While the technique described is correct, there are some easier ways to diagnose and to decide on how to treat the 'flare' problem at hand, as discussed next under 'Self-help techniques', below.

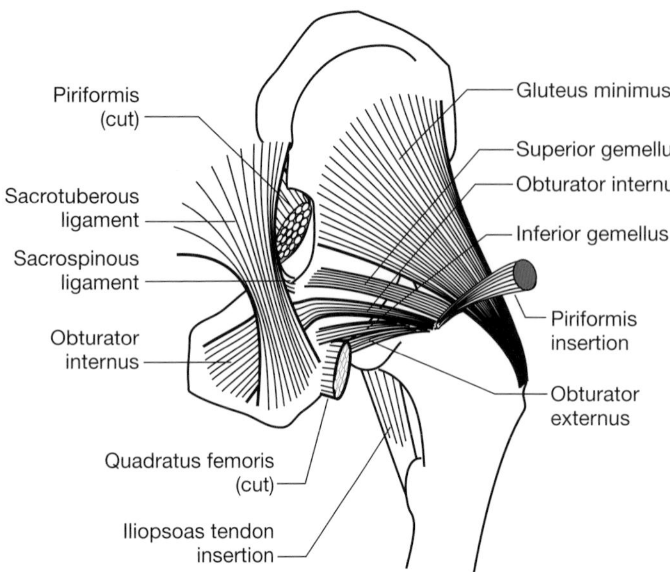

Fig. 7.20 Muscles that can be activated when using the muscle energy technique in an attempt to correct a right innominate 'outflare'. Most effective are piriformis and gluteus maximus (not shown - see Fig. 2.5B).

BOX 7.3 Technique to correct a 'right outflare, left inflare'

1. Flex the left hip and knee, leaving the left foot planted on the plinth.
2. Flex the right hip and let the right knee drop outward (= abduction and external rotation of the thigh) in order to place the lateral aspect of the right ankle against the anterior aspect of the left thigh or knee (the so-called 'figure-4' position).
3. Carry out repeated contractions against a resistance to the outside of the right knee, provided by your arms/hands, a strap/belt (fixed to something immobile or held by yourself) or an assistant (Fig. 7.21A,B)
   a. strength of the contractions is matched to the ability to resist any outward movement of that knee, keeping in mind that only a few muscles need to be activated for this manoeuvre (Fig. 7.20)
   b. if using your arms/hands to provide the resistance, try to fully extend and 'lock' the elbows to allow for transmission of forces directly to the shoulder girdle and through to the plinth, to avoid any unwanted contraction(s) involving possibly already tense and/or tender muscles in your neck, shoulder girdle and/or arm.
4. Do three sets of four resisted contractions.
5. After each set, you may be able to progressively increase
   a. passive left hip flexion (if post-contraction muscle relaxation allows for this), which could result in the left foot possibly starting to rise up a bit, off the plinth (Fig. 7.21E)
   b. a progressive increase in passive right hip flexion and adduction, to increase tension in most of the muscles activated - particularly piriformis and gluteus maximus - by taking up any slack and making the next contraction more effective.
6. Correction of the 'right outflare' is then followed by correction of the 'left inflare', if this has not already occurred spontaneously:
   a. simultaneous left hip flexion/abduction/external rotation will usually allow you to anchor the left foot by placing it against the flexed right thigh/knee
   b. on contraction, the attempt at adduction and internal rotation is resisted by pressure applied to the medial aspect of the left knee (Fig. 7.21Ci,ii; again, note the elbows 'locked' in extension).
7. Reassessment: if an 'outflare' and/or 'inflare' is still present, do one repeat of the manoeuvres outlined above.
8. Once the 'flare' is no longer evident, proceed with correction of any residual 'rotational malalignment' or 'upslip'.
9. If the 'flare' appears to have been corrected in that the major landmarks, the right and left ASIS and PSIS, now lie equidistant from the midline (Fig. 2.13Bii and Cii, respectively) but they still appear displaced in the transverse plane (e.g. left ASIS or PSIS forward compared to the right), suspect a persistent underlying problem (such as a 'sacral torsion') and see your therapist to have this assessed and treated ASAP.

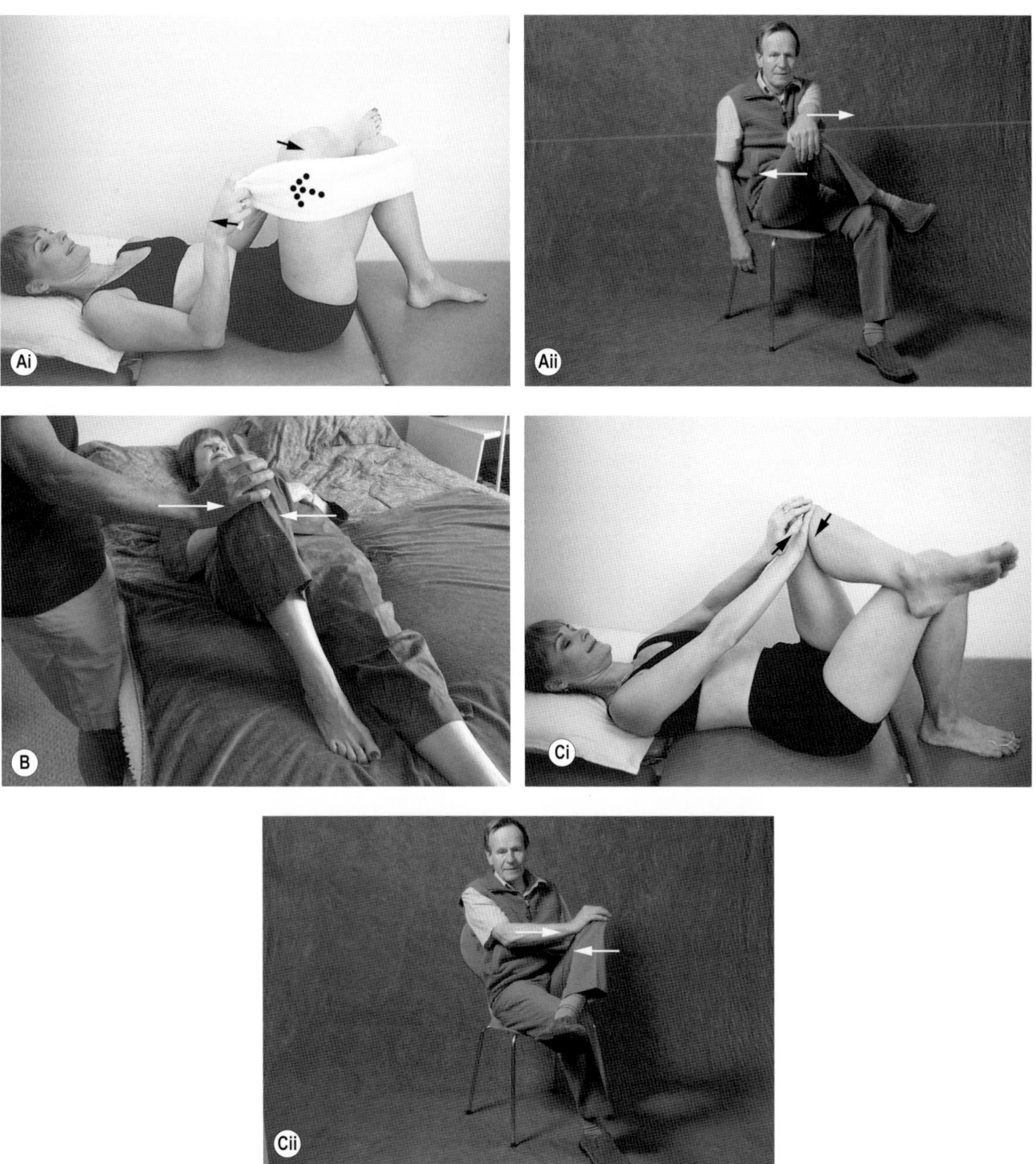

Fig. 7.21 One- and two-person muscle energy techniques. **(A,B) to correct a 'right outflare':** resist active right thigh abduction and external rotation. (A) One-person: (Ai) a towel held against the right anterolateral knee provides resistance (dotted arrow) against the outside of knee; (Aii) seated, resisting outward movement of right knee. (B) Two-person: with right foot planted on bed; not shown: assistant could also block outward movement of right knee when the person's right leg is crossed over and the foot anchored on the flexed left thigh (positioned as in Ai). **(C,D) to correct a 'left inflare':** resist active left thigh adduction and internal rotation (C) One-person: (Ci) lying supine; note: extended elbow transmits force directly through to plinth, and spares need for any muscle(s) other than left hip adductors contracting; (Cii): sitting, right forearm/hand pushing against inside of left knee.

(Continued)

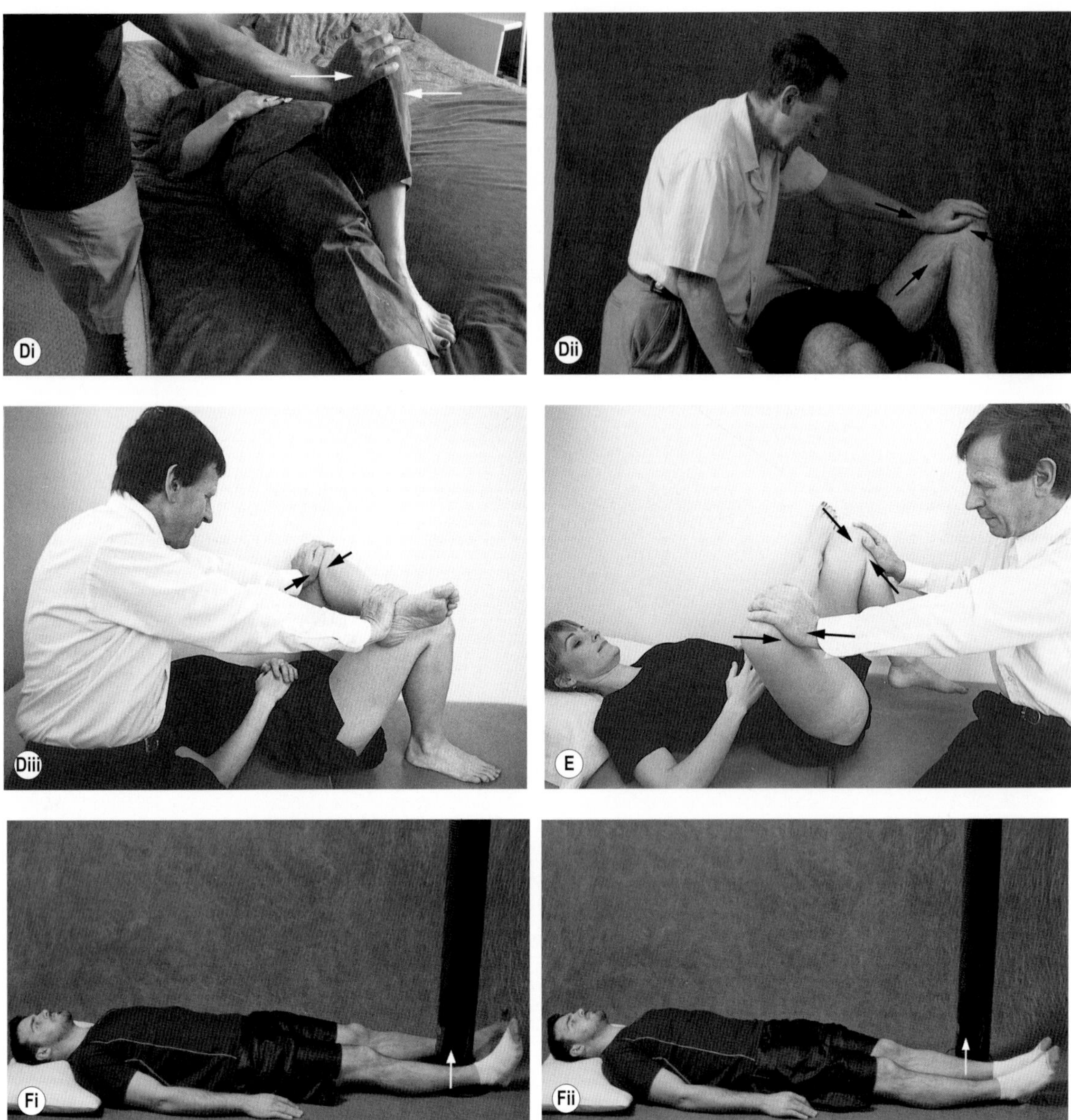

Fig. 7.21—cont'd (D). Two-person: (Di) therapist leans body into person to stop the left knee from moving inward; (Dii) adductor action pulls on medially located pubic tubercle origin to pull left innominate outward; (Diii) resistance against inside of knee of crossed-over left leg. (E) **to correct a 'right outflare, left inflare'**: the therapist can simultaneously counter attempt to move the right knee outward, left inward. **Note:** 1. The starting position can vary and is guided by comfort and circumstance (e.g. lying or seated). 2. Immobile objects (e.g. sturdy table leg) can provide the required resistance against attempted: (Fi) right hip adduction, to correct 'right inflare'; (Fii) left hip abduction, to correct left 'outflare'.

MET for a 'left inflare'

A coexistent 'left inflare' can be corrected using primarily the left adductor muscles. Both adductor longus and brevis originate from the pubic tubercle just lateral to the symphysis pubis and insert into the linea aspera of the femur; whereas adductor magnus originates from the inferior ischiopubic ramus and outer inferior ischial tuberosity (Fig. 2.40).

Given their medial origin, adductors longus and brevis are capable of pulling the left pubic bones anteriolaterally so that, when thigh adduction is blocked to reverse their origin and insertion, the effect is to make the left innominate shell rotate outward (Fig. 7.21C-E,Fi).

SUMMARY: SELF-HELP TECHNIQUES TO CORRECT MALALIGNMENT

It cannot be stressed enough that a lasting correction of the malalignment will be achieved more quickly if the person can supplement the supervised, progressive treatment programme with a regular home exercise routine that includes achieving and maintaining alignment as best as possible between the regular sessions with the therapist.

Visits to a therapist may be necessary once, twice or even three times a week initially, in an effort to achieve and maintain alignment and start on a core-strengthening programme aimed at regaining pelvic and spine stability. Time between intervals is gradually increased, depending on the person's response to treatment. However, it serves little purpose to have the therapist correct the malalignment only to have the person lose that correction within hours or days and then wait, out of alignment, until the next scheduled session in 1–2 weeks or so. Any recurrence of malalignment between treatments is a step backward because it:

1. keeps subjecting the pelvis, spine, limbs and attaching soft tissues to the same stresses and strains that have interfered with their proper function over the past months or years
2. delays attempts to decrease pain, to counter excessive muscle tension or spasm, and to increase pelvic and spine stability
3. interferes with the gradual adaptation that myofascial tissue, capsules and ligaments have to undergo in order to eventually readjust completely to the 'aligned body' position
4. stalls progressing on to postural retraining, strengthening of peripheral muscles, and a cardiovascular programme to improve overall fitness and endurance

If recurrence of malalignment during these intervals between the formal treatment sessions can be minimized or prevented altogether, the overall treatment process can be expected to take less time to complete and to be much more effective in allowing the person to return to full activities.

Correction of 'rotational malalignment'

If recurrent 'rotational malalignment' is one of the problems, a home programme with the following components is recommended.

Muscle energy technique to correct the 'rotational malalignment'

The technique, as described above (Figs 7.8-7.14), can achieve several things.

First, it can usually correct any recurrence(s) of 'rotational malalignment' between the formal treatment sessions with the therapist.

Second, even though it may fail to achieve 100% correction, it can usually decrease the degree of rotation and will, in doing so, often decrease discomfort.

Third, in those who repeatedly go out of alignment in the same pattern, it can also play an important part in helping to maintain correction because it results in a strengthening specifically of those muscles which help to counteract the 'anterior' rotation on one side (e.g. gluteus maximus) and 'posterior' rotation on the other (e.g. rectus femoris and iliacus).

Fourth, it lends itself to being helpful in many settings; e.g. at home, work or a sports event.

Significantly, a self-assessment allows the person to then carry out the appropriate self-correction manoeuvre, whenever and wherever the malalignment recurs. This is particularly important when formal help is not immediately available.

A typical example is that of the skier who has taken a fall and afterwards notices difficulty executing turns to the left because the recurrence of a 'left posterior' innominate rotation is restricting counterclockwise rotation of the pelvis/trunk around the vertical axis in the transverse plane, amongst other biomechanical changes (Figs 3.5 C, 3.49 and see 'Skiing', Ch. 5). Successful self-correction of the 'rotational malalignment' using the MET outlined above, right there and then on the side of the slope, a nearby bench or in a shelter, is likely to allow for immediate return to unhindered skiing provided there are no other restraining injuries. It will also prevent, or at least help to minimize, the chance of any recurrence of the symptoms that result with the increased stress on skeletal and soft tissue structures attributable to malalignment, a phenomenon that is definitely time-contingent: the longer the skier stays out of alignment, the more he or she is likely to experience a return of symptoms.

The person is instructed to:

1. start on the side of the 'anterior' rotation (Figs 7.8, 7.9) by resisting hip extension 12 times, taking up any slack in the gluteus maximus following each contraction (by letting the knee drop toward the chest if the muscle has lengthened a bit)
2. next, switch to the side of the 'posterior' rotation and proceed by resisting hip flexion and/or knee extension, 12 times each (Figs 7.10-7.13)
3. recheck to see whether realignment has been achieved; if not, repeat the manoeuvre and then do another reassessment
4. if the 'rotational malalignment' persists, follow up with a doctor and/or therapist to:
   a. make sure that there is not another, concomitant alignment problem, such as sacral torsion or an L4 and/or L5 instability
   b. rule out any underlying problem that can result in recurrent malalignment (e.g. facet syndrome, central or posterolateral disc protrusion, organomegaly or a mass)

If there is any pain on attempting correction of the 'anterior' rotation, the person can often avoid this simply by trying resisted hip extension with the knee moved further away, in order to decrease the hip flexion angle. The thigh may, however, end up so far away that it is out of reach. In this case, he or she can usually compensate by using a towel or wide belt, wrapped either around the back of the thigh or over the upper part of the shin (Fig. 7.14B). Another option is to rest the knee across a pillow, slightly flexed to ensure the hamstrings are relaxed, and then push the thigh down onto the pillow (Fig. 7.9Ei); this technique may be particularly helpful in the peri-partum period, when the amount of hip flexion available is usually limited (Fig. 9Eii).

Contract–relax of hip abductors and adductors

The person can do this manoeuvre alone in a number of ways.

1. **Lying supine** (hips and knees flexed to 90 degrees, feet planted; Fig. 7.15A)
   a. *abduction phase*

      Resistance to abduction is best achieved using a broad belt or other material that cannot be stretched. The loop is slipped directly around the distal part of the thighs, just proximal to the popliteal space, or over the flexed knees, 5–10 cm below the patellae (Fig. 7.15A). The knees should be able to separate about 20–30 cm and are restrained from moving past this point on attempted abduction.

   b. *adduction phase*

      A cushion or firm ball placed between the knees protects the inside of the knees from bruising and prevents any movement on attempted adduction.
2. **Sitting**
   a. *abduction phase*

      The person can push with the hands against the outside of the knees to resist repeated attempts at abducting both thighs simultaneously (Fig. 7.15Bi). Alternatively, the arm rests of a chair (e.g. on a plane) or a narrow doorway or other arrangement can serve to stop abduction.

   b. *adduction phase*

      Adduction can easily be resisted by wedging a forearm between the knees, the elbow flexed to 90 degree, wrist extended and palm against the inside of the knee (Fig. 7.15Bii). The knee on one side ends up pushing against the arm just above the olecranon, the other against the palm.

Leverage techniques

The leverage principle can also be incorporated into some effective self-help manoeuvres that attempt to correct both an 'anterior' and 'posterior' rotation simultaneously:

1. The foot on the side of the 'anterior' rotation is placed on a fairly high support (Fig. 7.17A). The trunk is then allowed to hang forward and down so that the right thigh ends up alongside the chest (Fig. 7.17B). This manoeuvre, which results in acute flexion of the thigh, is often lauded as being probably more effective (and certainly easier to do) than techniques outlined in Points 2 and 3.
2. The person sits over the edge of the bed or plinth, then lies back supine and starts to gradually pull the thigh on the side of the 'anterior' rotation onto the chest. At the same time, the thigh on the side of the 'posterior' rotation passively extends as it hangs over the edge (Figs 2.108B, 7.16 C).
3. The person can put the foot on the side of the 'anterior' rotation up on a raised support (Fig. 7.18A). The other foot remains on the ground, with the hip and knee on that side in extension. The body is then allowed to lean forward into the 'sprint start' or 'lunge' position in order to slowly hyperflex the hip on the side of the 'anterior' rotation while at the same time hyperextending the hip on the side of the 'posterior' rotation. Emphasis should be on avoiding any bouncing but, instead, sinking down gradually, holding that position for 30–60 seconds (like a stretch), and following up with four or five repeats.

These manoeuvres are simple; technique #1 and #3 have the advantage in that the person does not have to lie down. They can, therefore, be carried out anywhere: in the home or office, on the side of the playing field or a bench, and while travelling. At the very least, they will usually afford some temporary relief.

Correction of a sacroiliac joint 'upslip'

If the problem is one of an 'upslip' that fails to correct or that keeps recurring, the person should be instructed to carry out a daily home traction programme. For example, for those with a recurrent 'right upslip', the following one or two-person technique is recommended:

One-person technique

The person can stand with the left leg up on a stool, chair or staircase while ensuring balance with a hand resting on a railing or other support. He or she hangs the affected right leg down over the side with a weight attached (Fig. 7.19B). The initial weight to use depends, in part, on factors such as the person's build and the severity of muscle spasm. Wearing a runner or shoe will give a basic weight of about 1 kg to start, a hiking or ski boot approximately 2–3 kg. Shoes and boots protect the skin and allow for the gradual addition of further weight in 0.5-1 kg increments every 2, 3 or 4 days, as tolerated. This progressive increase in weight can be achieved, for example, with wrap-around weights or simply by hanging a small bucket containing an increasing amount of water or sand, or a bag gradually filled with hand-weights or cans of food, from the boot.

Two-person technique

One approach has the person lying either supine or prone while someone exerts a steady downward pull on the right leg as the person is breathing out; he or she should concentrate on relaxing completely throughout the procedure (Fig. 7.19A). A recheck should be done after a cycle of 12 traction-relaxation manoeuvres to decide if this needs to be repeated. The respiratory phases are usually quite obvious, with the increase in chest girth on inspiration, decrease on expiration; if not, ask the person to indicate the expiratory phase by blowing the air out through pursed lips in order to make a sound.

Traction is initially carried out for 10–15 minutes once or twice a day and gradually increased by 5 minutes every 2nd or 3 rd day. Eventually, 5–7 kg held for about 20 to 30 minutes usually suffices to achieve reduction. However, there may be exceptions, requiring less or more. The author recalls 2 rock climbers who repeatedly had recurrence of an 'upslip' during a climb and found that, on returning home, each could achieve correction by doing the one-person technique using 10 kg for 20 minutes.

While the weight is attached, the person is encouraged to move the right leg gently through a limited range of motion at the hip joint (e.g. circular motion through no more than 5–10 degrees). This movement, combined with the traction, helps to gradually relax the muscles and stretch out any tight structures in the hip girdle and pelvic region in order to allow for a reduction of the 'upslip'.

Recurrences of the 'upslip' may be decreased in frequency, or prevented altogether, by carrying out traction manoeuvres on a regular basis, best done as soon as possible after any activity likely to precipitate a recurrence. The quickest way to ascertain if 100% successful reduction has been achieved is to see if relative leg length remains the same in sitting and lying and whether right EHL strength is now equal to that on the left; also, pelvic landmarks should match and the pelvis be level in standing and sitting. If there is any doubt, repeat traction another dozen times. If, on recheck:

1. right EHL strength has returned and is now full and equal to that on the left but the right leg is still a bit short compared to the left
   a. there may be an anatomical (true) LLD, right leg short; if the difference is 5 mm or more, an initial heel raise of 5 mm may help maintain realignment, with subsequent increases in the height and shape of the lift, as indicated (see 'orthotics', below)
   b. there may still be tight muscles around the right hip girdle, which often relax just by maintaining alignment or with further treatment (e.g. traction, massage, acupuncture), in which case the person may actually present with equal leg length on reassessment a few weeks later and have no further need for the lift
   c. there may be other underlying pathology that can affect leg length (e.g. right hip or knee OA)
2. if the pelvic ring is still not symmetrical in some way, then other alignment problems should be considered; for example, both with a 'right outflare/left inflare', also 'sacral rotation' around the right oblique ('right-on-right') axis, there will be some clockwise pelvic rotation in the transverse plane so that the left ASIS protrudes forward while the right recedes (Figs 2.14, 2.50, 2.52).

Correction of 'outflare' and 'inflare'

It is easy to get confused by the terms 'outflare' and 'inflare', and how to diagnose them so that the correct MET technique can be used to treat them. Given the problem at hand (a 'right outflare/left inflare'), the corrective procedure outlined in Box 3 is logical but may be difficult to envision, especially if the illustrations are not available. The confusion can easily be eliminated by following the steps outlined below. Again, presume that the person has a 'right outflare, left inflare'.

As indicated previously (Chs 2, 3), the major asymmetries relate to the fact that the right innominate has moved 'outward and back', the left 'inward and forward' (as if the pelvic unit appeared to have rotated clockwise around the vertical axis in the transverse plane). Looking at the anterior aspect of the pelvic ring:

1. on side-to-side comparison, the shift in the position of the right compared to left ASIS:
   a. will be most obvious with the person lying supine: the right ASIS will appear lower, the left higher from the surface the person is lying on (Fig. 2.64A,B)
   b. in standing (with both heels against the wall) and sitting (the back pressed firmly into the back of the seat): the right ASIS appears to have moved backward, the left forward
2. assuming the umbilicus is a reliable centre marker (i.e. there has been no shift to right or left of midline on account of surgery, organomegaly or other cause):
   a. the right ASIS has moved away from the umbilicus, outward from centre (=outflare)
   b. the left ASIS has moved toward the umbilicus, inward to centre (=inflare)
   c. this shift from midline will again be most evident on lying supine (Fig. 2.13Bi) but is usually also readily apparent when standing and sitting.

Diagnosis and treatment can, therefore, be simplified by using the rule of the:

4 'O's for 'Outflare'

= THE SIDE ON WHICH THE ASIS IS LOW AND HAS MOVED OUTWARD FROM MIDLINE IS THE 'OUTFLARE' SIDE, CORRECTED BY BLOCKING ATTEMPTS TO PUSH THAT KNEE OUTWARD

4 'I's for 'Inflare'

= THE SIDE ON WHICH THE ASIS IS HIGH AND HAS MOVED INWARD TOWARD MIDLINE IS THE 'INFLARE' SIDE, CORRECTED BY BLOCKING ATTEMPTS TO PUSH THAT KNEE INWARD

The MET manoeuvres described above for the correction of these presentations can be carried out with the person first doing the self-assessment to confirm the diagnosis and then proceeding with the appropriate MET. In the case of a 'right outflare', for example, resistance to provide the force required to prevent the right knee from moving outward can be generated with one's hands, a towel or sheet applied across the right anterolateral knee region or simply by pushing against an immobile object (Fig. 7.21A,B,Fii).

MET FOR CORRECTION OF VERTEBRAL ROTATIONAL DISPLACEMENT

MET lends itself to generating the forces necessary for rotating vertebrae back into alignment. For example, mention has been made of harnessing one of the rhomboids to act on the vertebrae in the interscapular region (Fig. 2.97). The rhomboids originate from the T2-T8 spinous processes and insert along the medial scapular border. For correction of the T3 vertebral rotation to the left (spinous process off to the right), contraction in left rhomboid may be initiated:

In prone-lying

The arm can be draped over the side of the plinth or examiner's thigh. One or two fingers applied just proximal to the olecranon are usually adequate to provide the force needed to counter an attempt to bring the elbow straight up toward the ceiling (Fig. 2.97Fi). Contraction is limited to the left rhomboid and there is no scapular movement medially because of the reversal of origin and insertion using this MET. Excessive force will trigger contraction of the right rhomboid and other shoulder girdle muscles that can counter the efforts to pull T3 spinous process to the left, back into midline.

In sitting

The person is asked to try to bring the left scapula inward, toward the spine but any actual movement is prevented by applying pressure with the thumb and thenar eminence against the medial edge of the scapula (Fig. 2.97Fii).

INSTRUCTION IN SELF-ASSESSMENT AND MOBILIZATION

Those presenting with the 'malalignment syndrome' who will benefit from doing mobilization exercises at home are given a handout describing how to carry out the self-assessment to determine whether or not they are out of alignment in the first place and, if so, whether there is an 'upslip', a 'rotational malalignment', 'outflare' and/or 'inflare' or combinations of these. The handout instructs them how to carry out the appropriate MET, traction or other manoeuvre, either on their own or with someone's help, once they have established whether or not one or more of the three common presentations of malalignment is evident. They receive the handout after having been taught how to do the exercises by their therapist as part of the treatment sessions and, by the author, at the time of the initial consultation and on reassessment.

They are also asked to attend a 3-hour workshop offered once a month in order to:

1. give them a better understanding of the changes and problems that constitute the 'malalignment syndrome', in order to make it easier to recognize whether or not they are out of alignment
2. review the contents of the handout
3. do a demonstration of the self-assessment and self-treatment techniques for the three common presentations, followed by a 'hands-on' session to help them go through the diagnostic steps with a partner and then carrying out appropriate treatment techniques with that partner, under supervision
4. warn them that the type of presentation of malalignment that occurs can change from day-to-day or even on the same day, especially during the early treatment phase, and stress that they must never presume a certain pattern of malalignment has recurred without having first gone through the basic self-assessment steps each time
5. stress avoidance of inappropriate activities, especially those which are asymmetrical and/or have a torsional component
6. discuss the additional treatment options (e.g. orthotics, use of an SI belt, the role of ligament injections; see below)
7. make them aware of the educational material available, including: the author's DVD on recognition and treatment of 'The malalignment syndrome'; the complementary one on 'Alignment' by Boyd (2005) that deals primarily with the correct way to do core strengthening and exercises appropriate/inappropriate for someone just starting to achieve and maintain alignment; and others (e.g. Lee 1998; Lee 2004b)
8. advise them of a complementary workshop to review pelvic malalignment and focus on core strengthening techniques and problems of the trunk and spine (e.g. loss of specific ranges of motion, vertebral rotational displacement) that lend themselves to treatment using contract-relax and MET

> People are reminded that self-help techniques are no substitute for a supervised, progressive treatment programme but are intended to supplement it.
> Their efforts should be regarded as helping to maintain day-by-day correction; whereas the therapist does the 'fine tuning', so to speak.

In addition, it must be emphasized that the self-help manoeuvres should not provoke pain, which may trigger reflex spasm, could result in a loss of any correction that has been achieved and may discourage someone from continuing with this approach. It is always wise to have the person demonstrate on a subsequent visit how he or she has been carrying out the self-assessment and self-treatment manoeuvres, in order to ensure that these are being done correctly. If there appears to be a problem with the technique taught, they may do well to consider:

1. attending another workshop, preferably with a partner who can help them at home
2. obtaining one or both DVDs or other educational material as appropriate for their needs, so they can re-check any time a question comes up

THE POST-REDUCTION SYNDROME

Following a successful correction of vertebral rotational displacement or pelvic malalignment, some individuals experience discomfort from areas that were previously asymptomatic. A typical example is that of the person with an 'upslip' or one of the 'more common' patterns of 'rotational malalignment' who has been complaining of discomfort from a tense and tender left TFL/ITB complex. Following realignment, he or she is suddenly bothered with similar symptoms from the same complex, but on the right side. This phenomenon may be simply on the basis of:

1. **contracture of soft tissues**

   Some tissues were put into a relaxed and shortened position throughout the time that malalignment was present. In the example, the tendency to right medial weight-bearing decreased the length-tension ratio in the right TFL/ITB complex and eventually caused it to shorten. In contrast, the tendency to left lateral weight-bearing increased tension in the left TFL/ITB so that it could have lengthened with time (Figs 3.37, 3.41, 3.44, 4.1, 4.4).
2. **the redistribution of stresses that occurs with realignment**

   In the example given, tension in the shortened right TFL/ITB complex will increase as weight-bearing on the right side shifts from being medial to becoming more neutral or even lateral on realignment (Fig. 3.33).
   As tension increases in the right TFL/ITB, it may become symptomatic, especially where it is strung over, or actually snaps across, a bony protuberance (e.g. greater trochanter, lateral femoral condyle; Fig. 3.41).

Symptoms may occur in the form of localized discomfort and/or referred pain or paraesthesias originating from the affected structure(s). These symptoms usually disappear within 2–4 weeks, in keeping with the natural tissue adaptation that occurs as alignment is starting to be maintained, supplemented with appropriate stretching.

EXERCISE

During the initial stage of treatment, emphasis should be on symmetrical routines and on strengthening the thoracic and pelvic core muscles, in order to increase stability and decrease the chance of recurrence of malalignment. Asymmetric muscle activation may be specified by the therapist, and may be intended to:

1. strengthen a unilaterally atrophied muscle (e.g. often involving multifidi, rectus abdominis, quadriceps; Figs 3.57-3.60)
2. re-activate an apparently 'inactive' or 'unresponsive' muscle
3. activate a muscle in proper sequence (e.g. latissimus dorsi acting through the T/L fascia on gluteus maximus, then biceps femoris and peroneus longus; Fig. 2.37)

Graduated increases are advised to allow for progressive improvement and to minimize the chance of precipitating pain and reflex increase in muscle tension or even triggering spasm.

CONTRAINDICATED ACTIVITIES

Malalignment presents primarily as a musculoskeletal problem but the definitive treatment is realignment. Standard treatment approaches to musculoskeletal problems emphasize stretching, strengthening and flexibility routines. In the face of malalignment, some of these standard approaches and certain sports activities are contraindicated because they are more likely to cause recurrence of malalignment and/or put a person at increased risk of injury.

Contraindicated stretches

As indicated in Chapter 3, malalignment results in an increase in tension in certain muscles. This increase may be the result of a mechanical separation of origin and insertion, a response to pain or instability, or 'facilitation', with an autonomic change in the setting of the muscle spindle effected at a spinal segmental or possibly even cortical level. A chronic increase in tension can eventually result in tenderness to palpation of these muscles, their tendons and points of attachment. Discomfort from these sites perpetuates the increase in tension and initiates a vicious cycle.

It is important to note that some of the standard treatment approaches for muscles that are tight and tender are unlikely to be helpful and may in fact cause further harm.

> Stretching a tight muscle may fail if the increase in tension is occurring on the basis of malalignment and/or in reaction to a joint instability or chronic source of pain. Stretching attempted under these conditions, in fact, increases the chance of perpetuating the problem, by temporarily causing a further impediment to the inflow and exit of blood, increasing tension on the points of attachment and precipitating more pain.

This is not to preclude the gentle stretching that is often carried out:

1. to relax muscles just prior to attempts at mobilization
2. to decrease any residual increase in tension noted in specific muscles after realignment has been achieved and, thereby, decrease the chance of these tight muscles predisposing to a subsequent recurrence of the malalignment
3. to correct an 'upslip', using repetitive traction to the tight hip girdle muscles

All muscles that show an increase in tone and tenderness should be included in the routine. Stretching sessions should be short and carried out frequently, to capitalize on the nature of the contractile elements and decrease chances of provoking pain (see Ch. 8). Graduated stretching, about 4 to 6 repeats done while breathing out, should be carried out three or four, if possible even five or six times a day initially. Stretching a muscle-tendon unit only once or twice a day is more likely to be overdone and lets the tensile structures creep back to their shortened state in the 12-24-hour interval, thereby slowing the rate of recovery.

The person, unless otherwise instructed, is asked to carry out only symmetrical stretches initially. Unilateral stretches that exert a rotational force on an innominate in the wrong direction are frequently the cause of a recurrence of malalignment. Hence, there should be an emphasis on symmetrical stretching, avoiding any twisting of the trunk, pelvis or extremities until he or she:

1. is competent in deciding whether malalignment is present, and what type
2. understands how some unilateral stretches may be used to turn the femur into a lever arm to correct 'rotational malalignment'

If symmetrical stretching is not possible, the person must be cautioned to avoid stretching in any way that inadvertently creates a torquing effect on the pelvis and/or turns the femur into a lever arm that acts on an innominate to force it into the wrong direction. Consider, for example, the following stretches carried out by someone who suffers fairly consistently from recurrence of 'right anterior, left posterior' innominate rotation:

1. A left hamstring stretch while standing with the left leg up on a fence rail or other support (Fig. 7.22A): as the trunk leans progressively forward, the increasing tension in gluteus maximus and the hamstrings, in addition to the lever effect of the femur, come to exert an unwanted 'posterior' rotational force on the left innominate.
2. A right quadriceps muscle stretch in prone-lying or standing (Figs 3.42, 7.22B): as the hip is progressively extended, the increasing tension in rectus femoris and iliacus, and the lever effect of the femur, all come to exert an unwanted 'anterior' rotational force on the right innominate.

Unilateral stretches carried out on the appropriate side can be used effectively to correct a rotation but initially that should only be attempted under the express guidance of a therapist. Also, intensive stretching on one side, in an effort to achieve the same range of motion in a given direction as is possible on the opposite side, may lead to grief. In the presence of malalignment, a muscle may not be able to respond to such a stretch for completely different reasons than simply having developed myofascial tightness or undergone actual 'contracture'. Inability to stretch the hamstrings, for example, may be caused by the following:

Standing hamstring stretch

The person with a 'right anterior, left posterior' innominate rotation may find that, in standing with the right leg propped up on a support, there is a

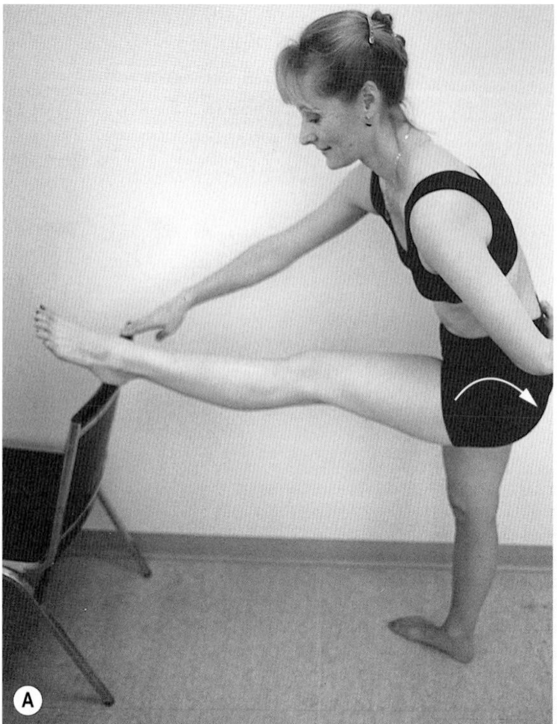

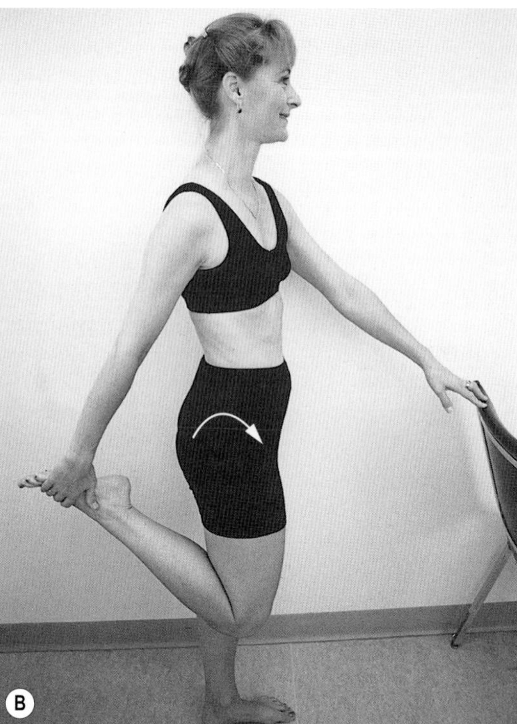

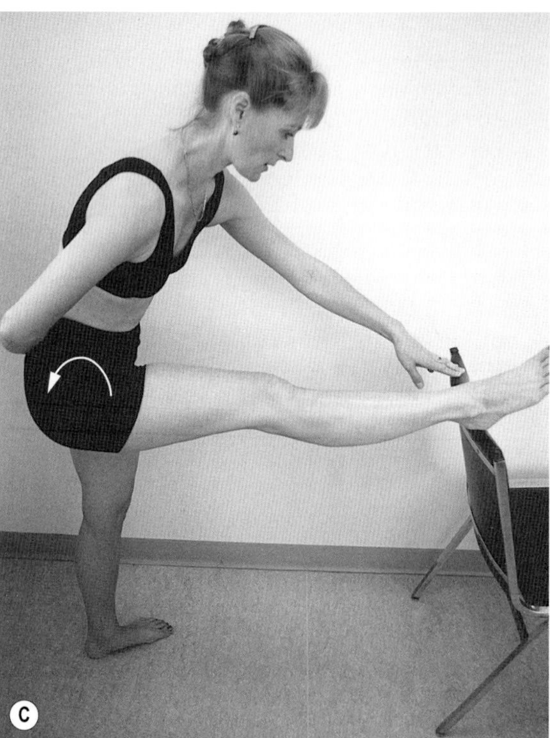

Fig. 7.22 Unilateral stretches that result in a rotational force on the ipsilateral inominate. (A) left hamstring: posterior rotation (B) right quadriceps: anterior rotation (C) right hamstring: posterior rotation.

limitation when attempting a right hamstring stretch by bending the trunk forward toward the right leg compared to carrying out the same stretch on the left side (Fig. 7.22C). The right limitation comes from the fact that:

1. tension has been increased by a separation of right hamstring origin and insertion (Fig. 3.42) and probably also by an autonomic increase ('facilitation') in muscle tone on this side
2. the anterior rotation of the anterosuperior acetabular lip of the right innominate creates a mechanical block to right hip flexion (Figs 3.71Ai, 3.72B).

Sitting hamstring stretch

When the same person attempts a hamstring stretch sitting on the floor, the legs outstretched in front and abducted, there will be a limitation of trunk flexion to the left compared to the right (Figs 3.74, 3.75). This finding is often wrongly attributed to left 'hamstring tightness'. The left limitation is actually noted in all those presenting with a right or left 'upslip' or one of the 'more common' rotational patterns, regardless of whether it is the right or left iliac crest that is elevated. In other words, the particular presentation of malalignment, other than being an 'upslip' or 'rotational malalignment', makes no difference. Possible causes to consider include:

1. unlike in the standing position, where the innominates are still free to rotate in the sagittal plane, the pelvis is now relatively stabilized by the floor in sitting

   With 'jamming' of the right in 'anterior', the left in 'posterior' rotation (the most common presentation; see Ch. 2), forward 'tilting' (flexion) of the trunk and reaching to the left is literally blocked by the posteriorly rotated left innominate. In contrast, the fact that the right innnominate is already in an anteriorly rotated position allows for more trunk flexion to that side. However, as indicated, the left restriction is also seen with other patterns of 'rotational malalignment' and an 'upslip'.
2. increased tension involving one or more muscles of a sling; e.g. 'facilitation' or reactive contraction of right latissimus dorsi in the posterior oblique system (Fig. 2.35), limiting left forward flexion
3. it cannot simply be attributed to a problem of 'hamstring tightness':
   - the right is consistently 'facilitated' and tension would further increase with the separation of origin and insertion caused by 'anterior' rotation of the right innominate, yet the limitation is consistently to the left side where contributing factors include a tightness of the left gastroc-soleus, with malalignment-related 'facilitation' of the left calf muscles, and a noticeable restriction of dorsiflexion both actively (Fig. 3.75Aii) and passively (e.g. on the 'slump' test (Fig. 3.84).

On attempts at stretching in these various positions, this person may feel increased 'tightness' of the hamstrings and calf muscles on one side as compared to the other. He or she may increase efforts to 'stretch out' these tight groups at all costs, unaware that the true reason for the muscle tightness may simply be a 'functional' increase in tone, in which case stretching may not only be futile but also dangerous as the muscle-tendon units involved are at increased risk of suffering a sprain or strain by being forcefully stretched. Following realignment, stretching for any residual muscle tightness would then be appropriate.

Contraindicated strengthening exercises

The bulk of a weak muscle can usually be improved by increasing the size of the individual muscle fibres with selective strengthening of that muscle. However, weakness of individual muscles seen in association with malalignment may not reverse with simple strengthening routines. Factors involved include:

1. The asymmetric biomechanical stresses can cause a muscle on one side to waste as a result of 'functional' disuse; whereas its partner on the opposite side may actually increase in bulk. The example of vastus medialis has been previously noted. This muscle wastes on the side of the externally rotated lower extremity, seemingly as a result of the change in biomechanical stresses and orientation (Figs 3.57-3.60). It is more likely to respond to efforts at strengthening if one first re-establishes the symmetry and normal biomechanics of the lower limbs with correction of the malalignment. The muscle is then once again subjected to normal stresses and may recover bulk just with routine use during daily activities. Recovery can be helped with the addition of appropriate

selective strengthening routines for the muscle affected (e.g. right vastus medialis).

2. The pattern of asymmetric weakness noted with malalignment disappears on realignment. Selective strengthening is unlikely to have an effect on this 'functional' weakness as long as malalignment is present, other than possibly to help prevent or slow down the development of any component of disuse wasting while the muscle is not working normally and activity may be limited as well. Once realignment has been achieved, strengthening efforts may help speed up regaining normal muscle bulk.
3. The weakness may relate to:
   a. muscle atrophy resulting from no longer incorporating the muscle in the patterns of contraction that it is normally part of, sometimes to the point that it may fail to activate at all
   b. failure to contract the muscle fully; this problem may actually relate to an inability to activate the 'inner/outer' core muscles needed to first stabilize the pelvis and spine prior to contracting a specific, seemingly 'weak' muscle
   c. failure to activate the muscle in the right sequence (see Ch. 3)

The asymmetrical pattern of 'functional' weakness seen so consistently in the lower extremities is determined primarily by factors other than lack of muscle bulk and usually disappears immediately on correction of the malalignment (see Figs 3.53-3.55).

Contraindicated flexibility exercises

There comes a point at which a further limitation of range of motion (ROM) is not a matter of lack of flexibility but one of a mechanical limitation imposed by the malalignment, a limitation that is unlikely to respond to any flexibility exercises other than to maintain the ROM that still remains. Reference is made to the asymmetrical limitation of both axial and appendicular joint ranges of motion seen with malalignment (Figs 3.5 C, 3.10, 3.17, 3.71–3.80, 3.84). Of interest is the fact that, following realignment, not only has the previously limited ROM increased so that it now matches that on the 'good' side but there is often also an immediate 5–10 degree increase in the ROM possible bilaterally compared to what was evident on the 'good' side before realignment (Fig. 3.49 C).

Specific contraindicated activities

The following activities are contraindicated on the basis that they carry an especially high risk of causing malalignment to recur. They involve, in general, actions that have a rotational component or that create asymmetrical stresses on isolated body segments. Though examples of these activities can more easily be found in specific sports, it should always be kept in mind that they are, nevertheless, also a component of many of the 'activities of daily living' (and often work routines) and that they may be responsible for the failure of a person to respond to the recommended course of treatment.

1. Caution is advised when carrying out movements involving torquing of the trunk in standing, when both the trunk and pelvis are free to move; these include:
   a. reaching to right or left, especially when this also involves lifting something up or down (e.g. stocking a shelf; Fig. 2.44)
   b. golf and court sports (e.g. tennis; Figs 5.3, 5.4).
2. Then there are those which cause rotation of the trunk relative to a fixed pelvis:
   a. twisting the trunk from one side to the other while standing and supporting a weight on or above the shoulders (Fig. 5.34)
   b. trunk rotation to reach alternately toward the right and left leg while seated on the floor with the legs apart (Fig. 3.74); gymnastic routines with an asymmetrical and/or torquing component (Fig. 5.11); canoeing in the sitting or half-kneeling position (Fig. 5.1); and wrestling moves forcing rotation of the trunk when the pelvis is pinned to the floor (Fig. 5.35).
3. Also to be avoided are activities leading to rotation of the pelvis relative to a fixed trunk; for example:
   a. wrestling moves that force rotation of the pelvis when the trunk is pinned to the floor (Fig. 5.36)
   b. lying supine, hips and knees flexed and alternately allowing both knees to drop outward and down to the right and left side;

while this may be a good way to strengthen the adductors and external and internal obliques, this exercise should be done with caution and through a limited range until the pelvis and spine are starting to stabilize (Fig. 7.23).

Activities that can turn a lower extremity into a lever arm capable of causing 'anterior' or 'posterior' rotation of an innominate are also, obviously, contraindicated if performed on the wrong side. Examples include:

1. lunges that can act like levers, mistakenly carried out in a way that accentuates or causes recurrence of an 'anterior' rotation on one and 'posterior' rotation on the opposite side (Figs 5.10, 7.18)
2. attempting to stretch a hamstring by pulling the extended leg toward the chest on the side of a recurrent 'posterior' rotation (Fig. 7.12Cii).

Unless there is a need to stretch a specific structure on just one side, the emphasis is on doing symmetrical stretches. These are possible for most lower extremity muscles and other soft tissues:

Hamstrings

1. sit with both legs extended on the floor directly ahead or abducted to some degree; flex the trunk, each hand moving along the top of the ipsilateral leg simultaneously or moving forward together on the floor, maintaining symmetry (Fig. 3.74A)
2. lie supine with knees extended; pull both legs upward and toward the chest but not to the point where the pelvic unit actually starts to tilt backward (Fig.7.24A)

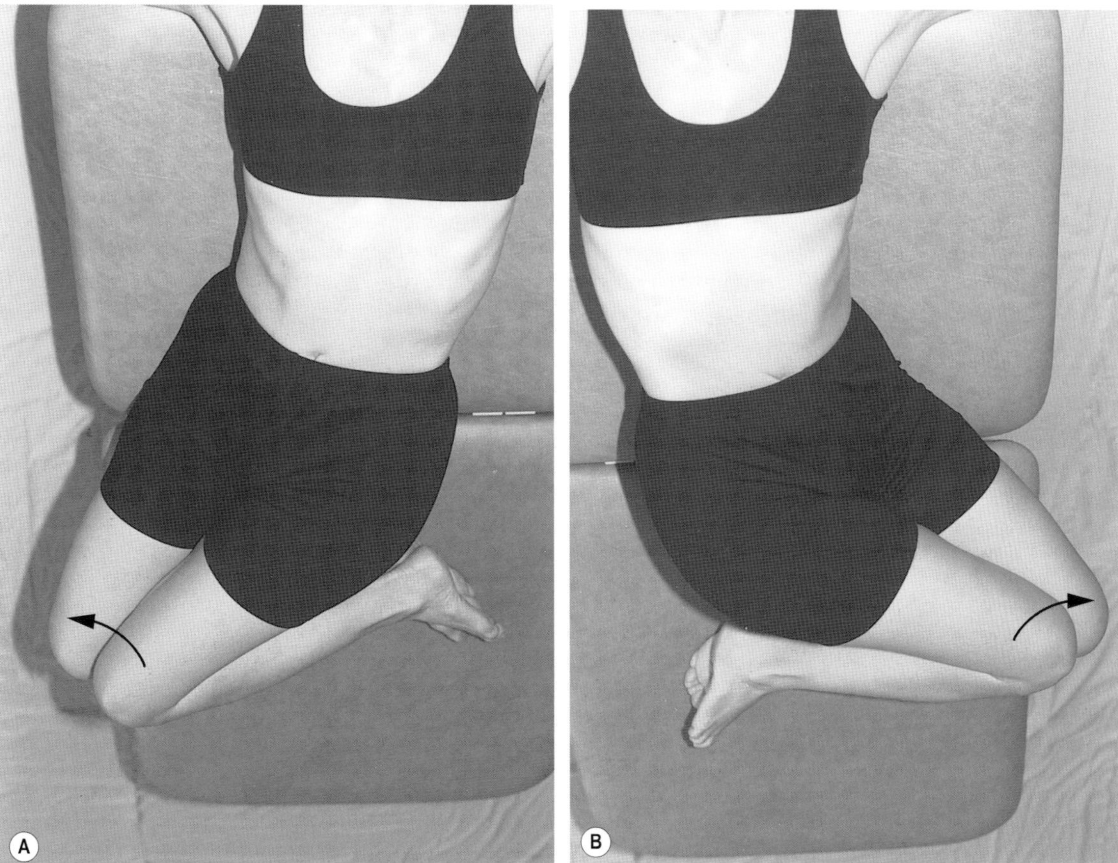

Fig. 7.23 Pelvis torquing on the relatively 'fixed' trunk: person lying supine, alternately letting the flexed hips and knees drop down to the right (A) and left side (B).

Gluteus maximus and piriformis

Lying supine, pull the knees down onto the chest as far as is comfortable, relax, and repeat the procedure to capitalize on any resultant increase in muscle length after the preceding contraction (Fig. 7.24B).

Quadriceps

Kneel, if necessary with the feet over the edge of the bed or on a pillow, to decrease pressure on the dorsum of the foot; gently lean backward with the trunk, something that may be made easier by hanging on to another person, a belt or other support (Fig. 7.24C).

Gastrocnemius and soleus complex

1. for stretch of these individual muscles bilaterally
   - with the forefoot supported on a step, simultaneously drop the heels down over the edge; stretches gastrocnemius with knees straight, soleus with knees partly flexed
2. alternately:
   a. for bilateral gastrocnemius:
      - start with the arms straight, supported by the wall or table, feet on the ground and knees in extension; drop the body progressively forward by gradually flexing the elbows but keep the knees straight (Fig. 7.24Di)

   b. for bilateral soleus:
      - initial position as for gastrocnemius, then gradually lean forward but this time with the knees flexed 10–20 degrees throughout so that gastrocnemius is relaxed (Fig. 7.24Dii)

Ankle plantarflexion range

The quadriceps stretch (described above) can also be used to increase ankle plantarflexion by stretching the dorsal ligaments and inserting tendons (e.g. tibialis anterior and posterior).

Ankle dorsiflexion range

The gastroc-soleus stretches (described above) can also be used to increase ankle dorsiflexion; e.g. by stretching the Achilles tendon, peroneal muscles and plantar fascia.

Jumping alternately from one leg to the other increases the forces transmitted through the SI joint on the weight-bearing side, as occurs in running, high-impact aerobics and some gymnastic and 'aquacise' routines. Repeated medial and lateral translation with sudden stopping and pushing off occurs in court sports and those requiring a cutting or crossing action (e.g. American football, soccer and hockey), so these activities are contraindicated for at least 2–3 months, depending on the person's response to attempts at realignment and stabilization. Repetitive actions with or without a twisting component, such as occur in certain work situations and sports, are also temporarily contraindicated (e.g. construction, roofing, cross-country running).

Low-impact aerobics may be a problem, especially if it includes a lot of asymmetrical stretches and alternating right/left weight-bearing. Sometimes even aerobic classes carried out in water may be too much, especially if the person gets carried away by the gyrations of a fit (and often younger) instructor and the natural (albeit possibly detrimental, in this situation) instinct to keep up with the rest of the group, all of which may result in temporarily forgetting the increased risk of causing malalignment to recur.

All the asymmetrical activities outlined above should be avoided until stability and balance have been regained and alignment is being maintained. Persistence with asymmetrical exercises and activities of the type listed above frequently results in a recurrence of malalignment following correction and accounts for a large number of so-called 'failures of treatment'. Keep in mind that while some people may have stopped a certain sports activity completely for the time being, they may still fail to respond to treatment because they have continued with certain demanding parts of their job or a hobby that incorporate some of these contraindicated movements. Gardening, for example, is often passed off as being only a short-lived 'seasonal activity', yet it usually involves unwanted bending, reaching and torquing while carrying out supposedly simple activities like planting or weeding, even while seemingly sitting 'safely' on a stool. In that case, there is sometimes no choice but to ask them to stop work and/or these other activities for at least 2–3 months to give their body a chance to finally respond to treatment efforts.

RECOMMENDED EXERCISES AND SPORTS

Unless otherwise indicated, the emphasis is again on symmetry during the early period of realignment, especially for those in whom malalignment keeps recurring. Training should include the types of exercise outlined below and in the DVD 'Alignment').

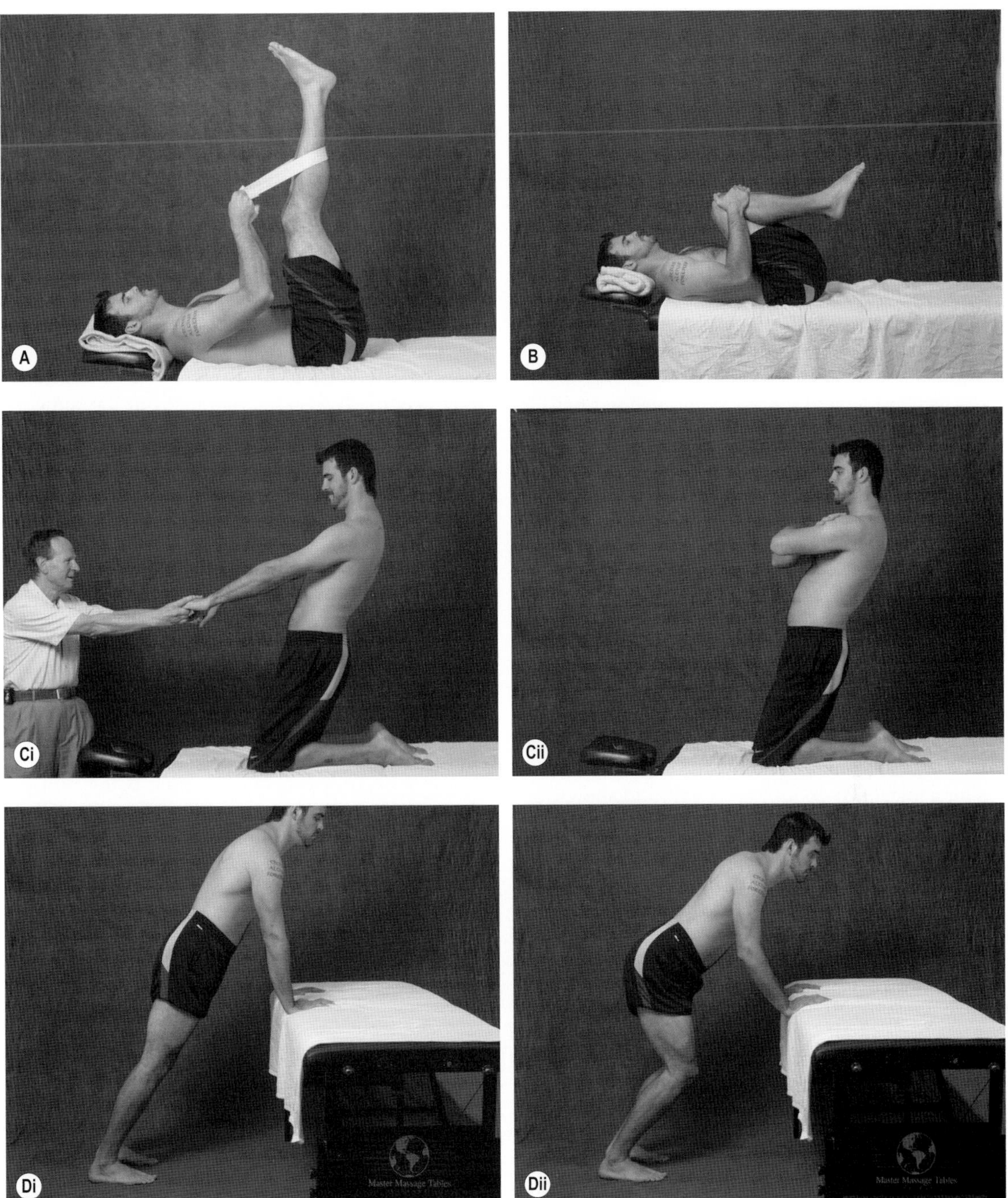

Fig. 7.24 Symmetrical stretches of lower extremity muscles to avoid causing recurrence of malalignment. (A) hamstrings (see also Fig. 3.74A); (B) applies some stretch to G. max and piriformis; (C) quadriceps: (i) with and (ii) without assist; (Di) gastrocnemius: knees are straight; stretch increases as elbows flex to allow body to lean progressively forward; (Dii) soleus: knees flex and feet dorsiflex.

Cardiovascular (endurance) training

Many of those presenting with malalignment will have lost cardiovascular (CV) fitness on account of having had to cut back or even discontinue participation in any aerobic training. Regaining CV fitness is a crucial part of their course of recovery as it:

1. increases overall axial and appendicular muscle strength (Type I aerobic fibres)
2. increases maximal oxygen uptake and allows them to do higher workloads for longer periods of time before having to resort to time-limited anaerobic means (with increased production of lactic acid and other waste products)
3. cuts down the amount of oxygen needed for working out at sub-optimal workloads; i.e. getting on with carrying out the same exercise at a certain suboptimal level but needing less oxygen to do so as overall fitness improves
4. delays onset of fatigue

Emphasis is on symmetrical CV exercises for short periods of time; initially, five minutes may be all the person can tolerate before having to rest. As the time is gradually increased, it may be best to split the session, if possible. For example, if he or she has difficulty doing a 20 minute walk, the recommendation would be for two separate 10 minute walks; this makes it easier to eventually reach 15 minutes on one or both outings for a total or 25–30 minutes a day, and allows for further step-wise increases. Walking on an elliptical trainer or outside on level ground (leaving the dog at home initially!) is a good way to start but these recommendations for a supervised progressive increase in time and/or demand apply to any of the exercises discussed. The following workouts are also appropriate in that they entail fairly symmetrical types of aerobic activity.

Swimming

Swimming is one of the best exercises for improving and maintaining CV fitness because weight-bearing is avoided and the buoyancy and warmth of the water has a relaxing effect on the muscles while the water itself offers some resistance to effort. Certain strokes are more demanding and have a torsional component; consider starting with the basically symmetrical elementary backstroke. If the person finds all strokes impossible or just can't swim, walking in progressively deeper water for longer periods of time has advantages over walking outside of the pool: walking against the resistance of the water is more demanding while the buoyancy decreases the impact on weight-bearing. Alternating short work sessions in the pool with rest periods in a shallow, and possibly warmer, side-pool to help relax muscles is more likely to allow for a gradual increase in the overall length of the work sessions.

Rowing

Rowing sports that require a symmetrical action (e.g. sculling) are suitable as long as the person takes care not to twist the trunk and pelvis getting in and out of the boat and is excused from helping to lift the boat in and out of the water or on and off a transport vehicle (Figs 5.15, 5.16). River and ocean kayaking may eventually also be tolerated but the same precautions apply. Rowing machines are best up on a platform for ease of access.

Cycling

Leaning forward to hold on to the handle bars may provoke pain by increasing tension in posterior pelvic and spine ligaments (Figs 2.5, 3.68) and in the muscles that contract to counter trunk flexion. Erector spinae are especially vulnerable as they contract to control forward movement of the pelvic unit and trunk, also to intermittently extend the head and neck to allow the rider to look at the road ahead (Fig. 5.6A). A mountain bike is, therefore, preferable to one with dropped handle bars. Better still is to start on a reclining bicycle or, if that is not available, a stationary bicycle, sitting upright initially with the arms relaxed at the side or resting on the handlebars, back straight and the legs doing all the work.

Direct pressure on a tender structure (e.g. the sacrotuberous ligament insertion, hamstring origin or the coccyx) may necessitate additional padding using a pillow or visco-elastic gel seat cover. Also now available are a variety of seats that have padded elevations to increase the weight-bearing on the ischial tuberosities, while the groove in-between decreases the pressure exerted on the coccyx and the male/female genitalia (Fig. 5.6B.C).

Stairmaster and stairs

When using a Stairmaster, the emphasis should be on frequent repetitions initially at a low resistance, preferably using a step differential of no more than 8–12 cm initially to minimize the amount of any pelvic torquing and tilting to alternate sides. If weight-bearing results in pain on one side, lead with the opposite leg, then bring the leg on the painful side up alongside. For the same reason, the person should be advised to start by going up a flight of stairs one step at a time and, initially, to limit themselves to the lowest height (i.e. first step) of the increasingly popular step-up stations used in circuit training.

It should also be stressed that the Stairmaster and treadmills are intended for a workout of the legs; the arms should be used mainly for balance. Some persons hang on to the central hand support or side-rails so fiercely that they not only do a large part of the work with the arms but also limit movement of the trunk and, thereby, introduce a major component of twisting of the pelvis on the relatively fixed trunk with every step, increasing the risk of recurrence of malalignment. The eccentric trainer, or similar models designed to have both legs weight-bearing simultaneously, may be more suitable as they make for better balance and allow free movement of the arms with minimal trunk and pelvic torsion.

Strength training

Unless otherwise specified, strengthening exercises (Box 7.4) should also be carried out symmetrically. Any weight training is preferably done lifting balanced weights using both arms and/or legs simultaneously. If for some reason strengthening is to be limited to a muscle or muscles on just one lower limb:

1. make sure that the pelvis, spine and resting limb are stabilized (e.g. sitting with the back supported)
2. avoid moving the exercising limb to the point at which it turns into a lever arm capable of rotating an innominate or vertebra.

A typical example is hip abductor strengthening carried out in side-lying. The tendency is to bring the uppermost leg toward the ceiling as far as possible, at the risk of torquing that side of the pelvis through the hip and SI joint (Fig. 7.30A). The risk of this occurring can be avoided by limiting abduction to horizontal (Fig. 7.30B). Attention must also be paid to avoid:

1. excessive forward bending of the trunk but, instead, flexing at the hips and knees at the same time; that is, squatting when lifting (Fig. 5.33)
2. actions requiring reaching or incorporating simultaneous lifting and twisting (Fig. 2.44).

Pilates exercise

Once the person has regained stability and is starting to maintain alignment to some extent, there should be an increasing emphasis on trying to regain normal movement patterns, balance and posture. The Pilates technique is one popular method used with this in mind. Joseph H. Pilates developed a dynamic form of exercise that has been very effective for those trying to regain 'form and function' and to maintain realignment. Suffering from asthma, rickets and rheumatic fever during most of his childhood in Germany, Pilates was greatly

BOX 7.4 Strengthening exercises

1. Back extensor and abdominal muscles, to improve back mechanics and strength (Figs 7.4, 7.6)
2. Pelvic 'core' muscles (Figs 7.25-7.29): exercises aimed at strengthening specifically the elements of:
   a. the 'inner' core muscles initially (Figs 2.28, 2.29, 2.53)
   -to re-establish stability of the pelvis and lumbar spine segment (i.e. multifidi, transversus abdominis, diaphragm, pelvic floor muscles and some others, such as obturators, gemelli and pectineus)
   b. the 'outer' core muscles (Figs 2.31-2.40)
   -starting with individual muscles (e.g. iliopsoas, piriformis and gluteus maximus), then those muscles integrated into the posterior and anterior oblique, deep longitudinal and lateral systems
3. The quadriceps, hamstrings and other muscles that attach to the pelvic bones, particularly those which can affect the SI joint (Fig. 2.59), with the emphasis nowadays being on:
   a. strengthening the muscles, while
   b. simultaneously re-establishing normal sequences of contraction (e.g. posterior oblique system: latissimus dorsi, through the thoracodorsal fascia to the gluteus maximus, biceps femoris and finally peroneus longus; Figs 2.35-2.38)
4. Alternating isometric contractions of the hip adductors and abductors to effect realignment of the pubic bones and, at the same time, a symmetrical strengthening of these muscles (see Figs 7.15, 7.29 and 'Self-help techniques' above)

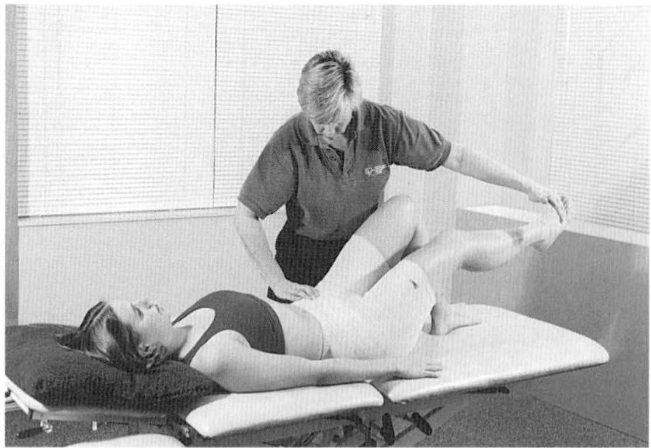

Fig. 7.25 Exercises: one leg extension with co-contraction of the inner pelvic muscle unit. *(Courtesy of Lee 1999.)*

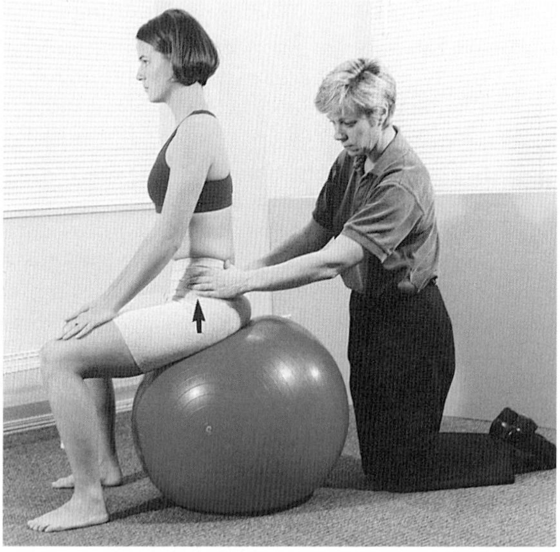

Fig. 7.26 Rise and sit with co-contraction of the inner pelvic muscle unit. *(Courtesy of Lee 1999.)*

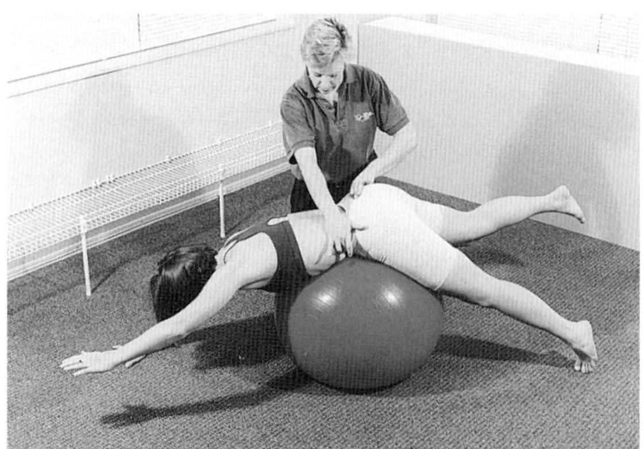

Fig. 7.27 Exercises: prone over a ball; one leg, one arm extension with co-contraction of the inner pelvic muscle unit (for the posterior obliques). *(Courtesy of Lee 1999.)*

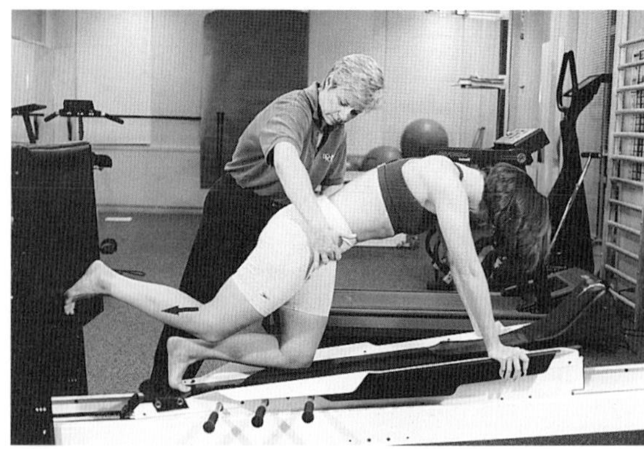

Fig. 7.28 Strengthening of one leg extensor in four-point kneeling with a balance challenge on a shuttle MVP. *(Courtesy of Lee 1999.)*

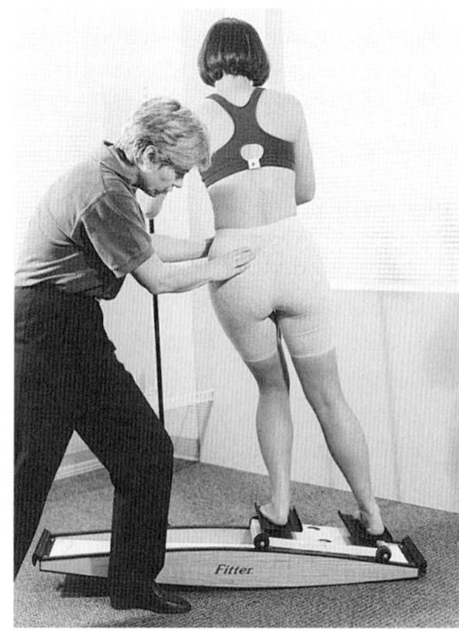

Fig. 7.29 Strengthening of the lateral system with co-contraction of the inner unit on a FITTER. *(Courtesy of Lee 1999.)*

influenced by holistic medicine and learned to use it to heal himself. While interned in England during World War I and training to become a nurse, he developed 'Pilates' mat work and also a form of resistance training that used springs attached to the hospital bed, in order to facilitate the rehabilitation of immobilized patients. He moved to New York in 1926, and over the next 60 years refined his method by developing over 500 exercises on 10 different pieces of apparatus. The technique is based on his 'Six principles of Pilates exercise', outlined in Ch. 8 (Box 8.4), and originally relied primarily on working out with springs, which can elongate

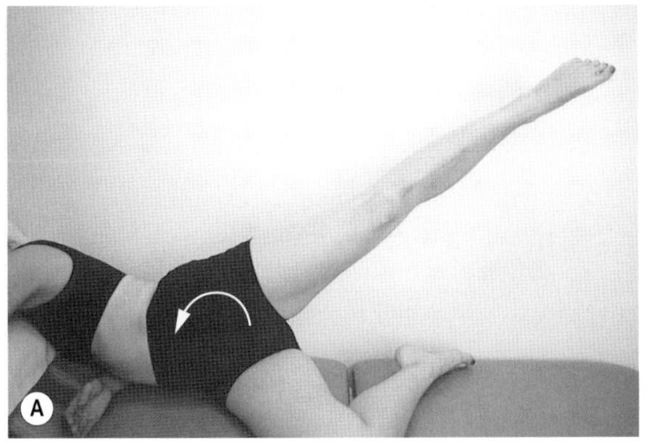

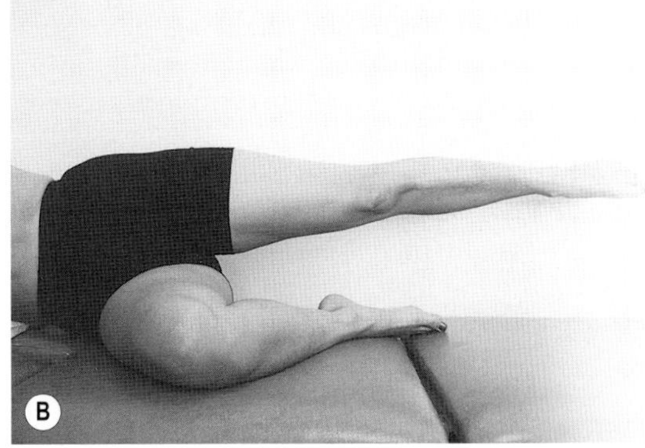

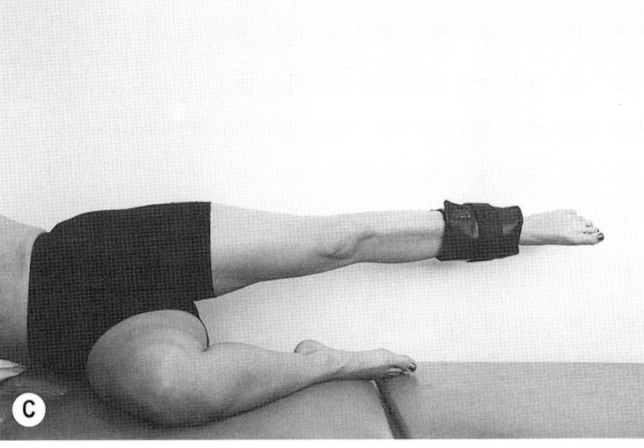

Fig. 7.30 Hip abductor strengthening. (A) Excessive abduction, creating a torsional stress on the left innominate and through the left sacroiliac joint and symphysis pubis. (B) Abduction limited to horizontal to minimize any torsional strains. (C) Subsequent progression, with addition of a 0.5-1 kg ankle weight initially while still limiting abduction to horizontal.

and contract, similar to muscles (Pilates 1934; Menezes 2000). This is in contrast to weight training, which relies on generating a resistance to gravity.

Pilates found the method proved successful in helping patients, athletes and, in particular, ballet dancers. Nowadays, it has gained recognition in helping patients progress on their road of recovery from malalignment, probably because it:

1. uses muscles synergistically rather than in isolation
2. stretches muscles and increases joint range of motion while, at the same time, also strengthening these muscles
3. improves postural alignment and increases coordination, getting the muscles to work efficiently in an effortless and graceful movement
4. takes care to work on the deeper, smaller muscle groups intrinsic to joint stability, thereby strengthening the core of the body
5. looks at the function and strength of the whole body and tries to improve on this in a graduated manner.

The Pilates treatment method will be discussed in more detail in Ch. 8.

RETURN TO REGULAR ACTIVITIES, WORK AND SPORTS

Unless otherwise instructed by their therapist, people should restrict themselves to symmetrical routines initially, until they have maintained alignment for at least 2 or 3 months. If malalignment recurs on return to work or resumption of regular sports activities, the programme needs to be re-evaluated to see whether any one component of the work or exercise routine is responsible for the recurrence. All that may be needed is to change or eliminate that component temporarily while continuing with the modified approach.

If an athlete absolutely insists on running early on, while malalignment is still recurring, he or she should first try running in water: initially, suspended with a life jacket or belt to completely avoid weight-bearing, progressing to having the toes just touching the pool floor, and eventually running in more shallow water in preparation for a return to dry land. Gradually increasing the time element is great for improving the CV component.

SHOES

Weight-bearing problems related to malalignment can be compounded by wearing shoes built to accommodate, or even counter, a specific weight-bearing pattern: pronation or supination. Over the past decades, the main features of running shoes made for a 'pronator' and 'supinator' have characteristically included:

Shoes for a pronator (Figs 3.32B, 3.35AB-'right')

1. a wedge of higher density material in the mid-section of the mid-sole, tapering from medial to lateral (the so-called 'double density' midsole)
2. a 'straight-last', to decrease any tendency toward medial (longitudinal) arch collapse and to improve stability of the mid-foot and transverse arch
3. medial reinforcement of the heel-cup to counter inward collapse
4. usually some reinforcement of the medial aspect of the midsole and upper

Shoes for a supinator (Fig. 3.35AB-'left')

1. reinforcement of the lateral aspect of the midsole and upper
2. uniform thickness and density of the midsole (the so-called 'single density' midsole)
3. a 'curved last' to allow the mid-foot to collapse inward more easily to increase movement of the mid-foot and transverse arch, thereby improving shock absorption
4. lateral reinforcement of the heel-cup, to counter outward collapse

People who presents with an 'upslip' or one of the 'more common' patterns of 'rotational malalignment' have an associated shift in weight-bearing toward right pronation and left supination (see Ch. 3). If they come to wear a pair of the typical 'double-density' shoes intended for a pronator:

1. the features of the right shoe will help decrease the tendency toward right pronation, but
2. the left will work against them by:
   a. increasing the tendency toward left supination, because of the 'straight last' and medial reinforcement of the midsole
   b. resulting in even less ability to dissipate shock at the level of the left foot and ankle because of:
      i. the fact that these are now even more rigid by having been forced into further supination (Fig. 3.30Bii)
      ii. the higher density medial wedge

Wearing such a pair of 'double-density' shoes made for a pronator has been identified as one cause of new or ongoing problems in someone presenting with malalignment. The double-density tapered midsole accentuates the left lateral weight-bearing and tendency to supinate, further increasing tension on the left TFL/ITB, lateral collateral ligament, peroneal nerve at the fibular head and the lateral ankle ligaments (Figs 3.37, 3.38). Complaints caused by irritation of these structures are common (see 'Case History 7.1'). It is interesting to speculate whether a 'pronator' shoe used in these circumstances might not also increase the chance of suffering ankle inversion sprains and stress fractures on the supinating side.

Unfortunately, there has been a preoccupation with making shoes specifically for pronators, dating back to the 1970s with the introduction of the first 'double density' runner by Brooks. Even today, there is a disproportionate number of shoes made for pronators, although the combined number of people with a neutral or supination pattern of weight-bearing is almost equal to that of the ones who pronate (see Ch. 3: 'Asymmetry of foot alignment...- a final observation on weight-bearing').

> Even now, almost 40 years later, those dealing with athletes and the public are generally more adept at recognizing a 'pronator' than a 'supinator'.

Unfortunately, someone presenting with an 'upslip' or one of the 'more common' rotational patterns is, therefore, much more likely to be labelled a 'pronator' although pronation is occurring just on one side, or happens to be worse on the right than the left; whereas the tendency toward neutral weight-bearing or even frank supination on the opposite side may go unnoticed. The sometimes very obvious tendency to right pronation probably draws attention away from actually taking the time to look properly at the action of the opposite foot and can easily lead to a quick decision biased toward a general 'pronation problem'. This person stands a good chance of being prescribed shoes intended for a pronator and, therefore, risks being subjected to the complications noted above.

In a few cases, the supination on one side may be so blatantly obvious that the person is labelled a 'supinator' and prescribed 'single-density' shoes with a curved last to allow for collapse of the longitudinal arch. This, unfortunately, would have the effect of accentuating any tendency toward pronation on the opposite side.

Common features of today's selection of runners, including the addition of a reinforcement of the medial transverse arch, medial buttressing, reinforcement around the heel and elevation of the sole under the heel are known to decrease rearfoot motion. Lately, there have been concerns that these measures:

1. make it difficult for the foot to move in a 'normal' pattern (i.e. as it would when running barefoot)
2. concentrate too much on dealing with heel-strike impact, when it appears that the forefoot is more adept at dissipating shock and that about one-third of us actually land on the forefoot (Lieberman 2008; Lieberman et al. 2010); in their case' elevating the heels may interfere with the way the feet normally deal with shock
3. affect structures proximally by interfering with the lower limb rotation

Perhaps shoes in the near future may try to allow the foot more freedom of movement and alleviate some of the above factors. Note the recent marketing of a new line of shoes that supposedly allows the foot to move more as it would when running barefoot. However, no matter what these changes may be, the shoes cannot be expected to compensate for the altered biomechanics attributable to malalignment.

FOOT ORTHOTICS

A trial with longitudinal arch supports should be considered when malalignment keeps recurring, in the hope that the orthotics will increase the chances of maintaining alignment. The person may actually report a feeling of increased pelvic stability when wearing orthotics. In addition, a previously weak and 'sloppy' foot and ankle may feel stronger and more stable on weight-bearing, at push-off and when executing turns.

ORTHOTICS: WHEN, WHAT AND WHAT NOT

The past versus present attempts

Unfortunately, a great number of those presenting with malalignment have already been provided with orthotics, often custom-made and at exorbitant prices. On further investigation, it becomes obvious that:

1. they were made from a cast of the feet taken while non-weight-bearing (e.g. sitting, lying; Fig. 3.26Aii,B)
2. even if the cast was taken when weight-bearing, the person was very likely out of alignment at the time, unless malalignment was specifically ruled out or corrected prior to the casting (Fig. 3.25Ai,Bi)

Therefore, all old custom-made orthotics should be suspect, especially if there is an obvious difficulty maintaining realignment when they are being worn. They were probably cast at a time when the person was still out of alignment and could now be setting up unwanted asymmetrical forces at the foot level. These orthotics increase the risk of recurrence of malalignment by disturbing the balance of weight-bearing that has finally been achieved with realignment (Fig. 3.26Ai). The best advice is for them to be thrown away and get on with the following recommendations.

Off-the-shelf arch supports

If orthotics are considered necessary, an initial trial with off-the-shelf arch supports is recommended when starting treatment. They can be helpful in that they:

1. are readily available 'off the shelf'
2. are guaranteed to be symmetrical (unlike the custom ones the person may have been wearing)
3. allow for a quick assessment of whether or not orthotics would really make a difference in the first place, at a price most people can afford (approximately one-tenth or even less of the cost of custom-made ones)
4. also allow for a trial of modifications to see whether any of these would be worthwhile incorporating directly into subsequent

custom-made orthotics, should these eventually be considered necessary; for example:

a. a right medial and/or left lateral raise, to counter persistent symptoms from soft tissues and joints that have usually been stressed for a long time by excessive pronation and supination, respectively, and continue to be symptomatic even though realignment is now being achieved
b. a right lateral forefoot raise to effect:
   i. a counterclockwise torquing force on an externally rotated right leg and
   ii. a more neutral/stable foot position
c. a left medial forefoot raise to effect:
   i. a counterclockwise torquing force on an internally rotated left leg and
   ii. more foot flexibility and shock absorption
d. a heel raise to make up for an anatomical 'true' LLD, if present

The changes to the orthotics noted in Points 4b and 4c, in combination, could conceivably minimize, correct or even prevent recurrence of one of the 'more common' patterns of 'rotational malalignment', possibly even an 'upslip', and the associated tendency to right external rotation/pronation and left internal rotation/supination. However, if realignment is achieved using this approach, then the situation needs to be reassessed as the orthotics may no longer be required or should be modified to accommodate the 'true' weight-bearing pattern that is revealed on correction (see 'Risks associated with orthotics', below; Fig. 7.31).

One can quickly find out if any one modification benefits or aggravates existing symptoms. If the former, one can then proceed with subsequent progressive changes as indicated; for example, gradually increasing a medial or lateral raise, up to the point that seems to give the best result.

Off-the-shelf orthotics:

1. tend to be wider than custom-made ones

   It may, therefore, be difficult to fit them into day shoes, which are usually narrower than running shoes. Currently, there are an increasing number of narrow ones available, some even intended for high-heeled shoes, so width is no longer such an issue.
2. are usually a temporary measure that may lead to:
   a. discontinuation of the orthotics altogether once alignment is being maintained and they no longer seem to be indicated
   b. a rational decision whether or not to provide custom-made orthotics, with addition of any modifications that were found to be helpful when tried on the off-the-shelf ones.

Custom-made orthotics

If the decision is to use custom orthotics, casting should be carried out with the person weight-bearing and in alignment. The malalignment-related asymmetry affects the static and dynamic attitude of the feet, the passive and active ranges of motion possible at the foot and ankle, and hence the eventual shape and fit of the orthotics (Figs 3.20, 3.25 – 3.27, 3.75, 3.84).

> Asymmetrical orthotics worn by a person who is now in alignment can result in asymmetrical proprioceptive signals from the sole and exert asymmetrical torquing forces on the lower extremities, all the way up to the pelvis. Through these and other effects, these inappropriate orthotics can, in fact, cause a recurrence of malalignment.

To prevent this complication, the person's alignment should be checked just prior to casting. If necessary, realignment is carried out first, preferably there and then, to increase chances it will be maintained during the actual casting procedure.

RISKS ASSOCIATED WITH PREVIOUSLY PROVIDED ORTHOTICS

The person presenting with an 'upslip' or one of the 'more common' rotational patterns is at risk of further aggravation of symptoms with the provision of orthotics that are posted (Fig. 5.40). For example, the tendency is to provide an increasing raise of the right medial heel, forefoot or both, in an attempt to counteract the pronation that is sometimes so blatantly obvious on the side of the externally rotated lower extremity. Aggressive medial posting of the forefoot in particular (e.g. 4 degrees, or approximately 4 mm) actually results in further torquing of the lower extremity by augmenting, at foot level, the forces already tending toward external rotation of that leg and may do little to correct the tendency to pronation, as this is a feature inherent to these two presentations of malalignment.

As indicated, the medial posting is often automatically carried out on the opposite side as well, seemingly on the assumption that if pronation is happening on one side, it must also be a problem on the other. Unfortunately, medial posting throws the left foot into further supination. Similarly, aggressive lateral posting limited to the forefoot section increases the forces promoting internal rotation of that lower extremity and can, thereby, augment the tendency to supination, especially in someone who may already be rotating internally toward neutral or even across the midline (Fig. 3.19Bii).

The problem amounts to more than just augmenting or perpetuating an abnormal weight-bearing pattern. Increasing the forces responsible for the pathological internal and external rotation of the lower extremities augments the rotational forces acting on the hip and SI joint region. In other words, incorrect posting can perpetuate the malalignment. The corollary is that malalignment can sometimes be corrected with judicious posting that sets up a torquing force to counteract an unwanted tendency toward internal or external rotation (Fig. 7.31). Malalignment can be corrected from the ground up, so to speak. A combination of appropriate postings, usually setting up contrary forces, may result in the correction of a 'rotational malalignment':

1. a lateral posting of the forefoot on the side of the externally rotated lower extremity would set up a torquing force toward internal rotation
2. a medial posting of the forefoot on the side of the internally rotated extremity would have the opposite effect, creating a force tending to external rotation

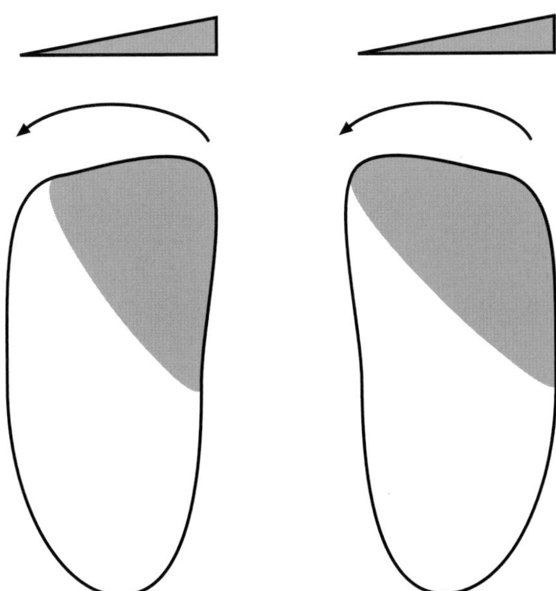

Fig. 7.31 An example of a simple approach using a forefoot posting of the orthotics to correct malalignment by counteracting rotation of the lower extremities: right laterally (to counteract external rotation of the right leg) and left medially (to counteract internal rotation of the left one).

If the person presenting with an 'upslip' or 'rotational malalignment' has been mistakenly labelled a 'pronator' because pronation or the inward collapse of a heel cup is so blatantly obvious on one side, the subsequent provision of orthotics having a medial raise bilaterally in the forefoot section will serve only to increase the forces promoting supination that are, in fact, already present on the opposite side (Fig. 5.40). On the pronating side, they may improve medial support to counteract pronation, but they could also result in a further, unwanted, external rotation of that lower extremity. The person may present with aggravation of previous symptoms (Fig. 3.37). For example:

1. *on the supinating side*
   - increased pain from the lateral structures (e.g. TFL/ITB complex), which are now put under even greater stress
2. *on the pronating side*
   - problems relating to increased external rotation, knee valgus angulation and stress on medial knee, ankle and foot soft tissue structures

> It must also be remembered that the weight-bearing pattern may change significantly once the malalignment has been corrected.

This change is most dramatically evident in children, who are usually referred for assessment because they have been noted to pronate excessively and/or display marked 'in-toeing' or 'out-toeing'. Again, these changes are often actually unilateral, or worse on one side than the other, and may be in keeping with the presence of malalignment. On realignment, the tendency toward pronation will usually be markedly decreased or may no longer be discernible: the pattern has become one of neutral weight-bearing or may have completely reversed to become one of symmetrical supination. In fact, a surprising 5–10% of adults who were seemingly pronating on one or both sides when out of alignment end up with a neutral to slight supination pattern following correction (Fig. 3.33). Reorientation of the lower extremities may also reduce any in-toeing or out-toeing.

It is, therefore, very important to reassess the gait, along with a new pair of shoes worn regularly for 2–3 months once maintaining alignment, and to recommend appropriate changes to the orthotics and footwear if the weight-bearing pattern has changed. For example, should the person now have a neutral to supination pattern:

1. remove any medial posting, especially if there are ongoing signs or symptoms consistent with lateral traction forces
2. consider the addition of a lateral raise if lateral traction signs or symptoms have failed to settle completely
3. replace rigid or semi-rigid orthotics with a soft-shell type and recommend shoes with a curved last and 15–20 mm single-density midsole cushion to improve shock absorption at the foot level.

WHEN MALALIGNMENT CANNOT BE CORRECTED

Orthotics may still play a role when realignment just cannot be achieved or maintained. They may provide an unexplained sensation of increased pelvic stability, an improvement felt sometimes even though the person is still out of alignment. More easily explained is the ability of the orthotics to decrease some of the biomechanical stresses attributable to the persistent malalignment itself.

Minimizing stresses caused by functional leg length difference

When malalignment cannot be corrected, it would seem appropriate to provide a lift on the side of the apparent, or functional, 'short' leg when standing. This will decrease stress, especially on the lumbosacral region and the spine, by decreasing the pelvic obliquity and the compensatory curvatures of the spine. It should, however, be remembered that sacral rotation, with partial or complete levelling of the sacral base, can compensate for up to 5 mm of LLD. It is, therefore, more important that a lift be used to correct any residual obliquity of the sacral base rather than an obliquity of the pelvis *per se*.

The lie of the sacrum is preferably assessed on a standing anteroposterior X-ray view of the pelvis. If the sacral base is level, no lift is indicated, even though there may be persistent obliquity of the pelvis (Fig. 3.90). If no X-ray is available, a trial with a lift may be worthwhile. The functional LLD should be measured while standing, from the iliac crest, ASIS or other pelvic landmark down to the floor. A safe rule is to limit correction to a simple heel lift of no more than 5 mm initially (Fig. 7.32A). On reassessment 4 weeks later, there are two possible outcomes to consider:

1. the 5 mm lift is well tolerated

   In this case, if the total functional LLD is greater than 5 mm, consider increasing the lift by 2–3 mm every 1–2 months as tolerated, or until the pelvis is level. It usually takes that long for soft tissue adaptations to occur. If the total difference is 1 cm, a heel lift or a simple partial or full-length insole, 10 mm high at the heel and tapering down to 5 mm at the forefoot, may suffice (Fig. 7.32B). Any further correction required usually consists of a uniform addition externally, to the bottom of the shoe. 2–3 mm layers, running the length of the heel to the front of the sole, are progressively added, as determined by any remaining discrepancy and the person's tolerance and seeming benefit following each increase.

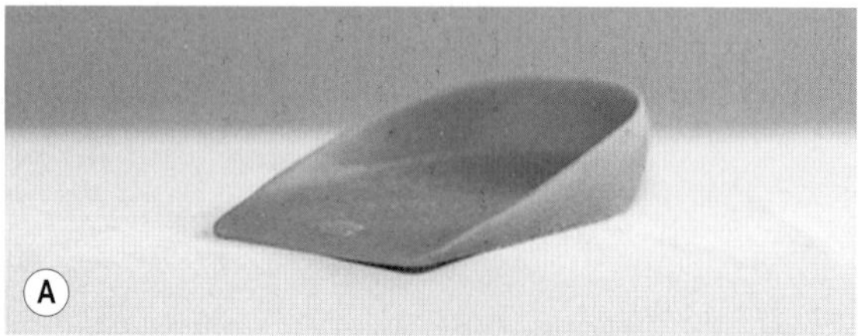

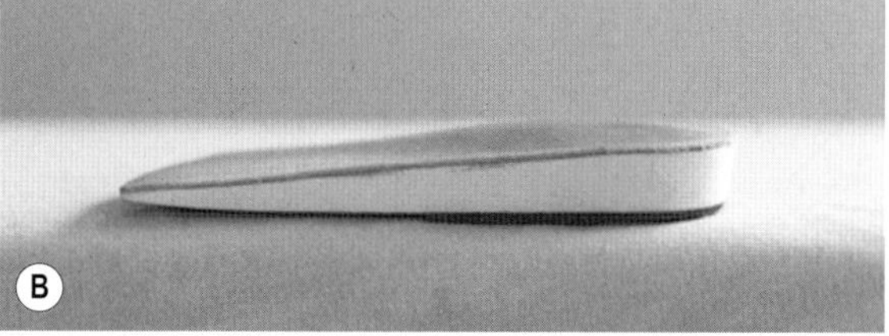

Fig. 7.32 Progressive heel lifts. (A) A simple 5 mm heel lift, used for the initial correction of a difference of 5 mm or more. (B) A 'three-quarter' length lift: 10 mm in the heel, tapering to 5 mm in the forefoot.

2. the lift is not being tolerated

   The soft tissues may have changed so much over the years as a result of the functional LLD (and, in about 10%, a coexistent 'true' LLD) that they can no longer adapt to the biomechanical changes now imposed by the lift. Alternately, a compensatory sacral base levelling may already have occurred, and the addition of the lift now creates unwanted stresses by again unlevelling the base; this may have to be confirmed radiologically in not evident on examination.

Medial or lateral posting of an orthotic or shoe

Posting should be guided by ongoing signs and symptoms that can be related to the altered pattern of movement and weight-bearing. The intent is to decrease the tension on structures that are tender as a result of being put under increased stress from persistent malalignment. This may call for:

1. medial posting on one side, to counteract stress from pronation and to stabilize the medial and transverse arch
2. lateral posting on the opposite side, to counteract lateral traction attributable to a neutral or supination weight-bearing pattern and to increase movement and shock absorption in the mid- and forefoot regions by unlocking the tibio-talar, subtalar and anterior transverse arch joints

It is best to start with a posting of no more than 2 degrees (approximately 2–3 mm) and evaluate its effectiveness 3–4 weeks later. Further increases should be guided by the response to temporary additional posting using moleskin or adhesive felt which the person can add on, one or two layers at a time at 2–4 day intervals, to the point where they seem to feel maximum benefit.

> Always be aware that the posting may exert a torquing effect on the lower extremity.

As an alternative, or in addition to posting, consider reinforcing the heel cup of the shoe medially or laterally to counteract excessive pronation or supination forces, respectively (Schamberger 1983).

WHY DO ORTHOTICS HELP TO MAINTAIN ALIGNMENT?

Some of the possible mechanisms to consider include the following:

1. An orthotic increases the stability at foot level by providing contact for weight-bearing across a larger part of the sole. Pressure is, therefore, distributed more evenly across the entire area provided by the orthotics (Fig. 7.33A). Contrast this with the kidney-shaped imprint of a bare foot in sand: weight-bearing is primarily at the heel, lateral sole and ball of the foot (Fig. 7.33B,C).
2. Orthotics can be used to decrease any persistent tendency of the feet to roll inward into pronation, or outward into supination, once the person is in alignment. They may, thereby, decrease any torquing forces on the legs that could cause a recurrence of the 'rotational malalignment', especially if these forces are in any way asymmetrical.
3. In the case of someone with a fallen anterior transverse arch, incorporation of a metatarsal button to redistribute weight-bearing to the 1st and 5th metatarsal head (where it should be), makes the forefoot more flexible and adept at absorbing shock (Fig. 4.16).
4. By providing support over the major part of the sole of the foot, the orthotics increase both the amount and the symmetry of the sensory input from the surface of the sole. Stimulation of the cutaneous proprioceptive receptors was postulated to result in pain control in three neurophysiological mechanisms proposed earlier and which are still incorporated to varying extent in some of the more recent theories in vogue (Box 7.5).

There are several end results of these mechanisms, as affected by the increased cutaneous input from the larger weight-bearing area and more uniform pressure distribution on the orthotic, including the following:

1. A decreased perception of pain results in a reflex relaxation of the muscles. This could decrease the recurrence of malalignment by decreasing or actually eliminating any asymmetry in muscle tension.
2. The barrage of proprioceptive signals could also decrease excitatory input to the muscle spindle, again resulting in a reflex relaxation of the muscles in the immediate area.

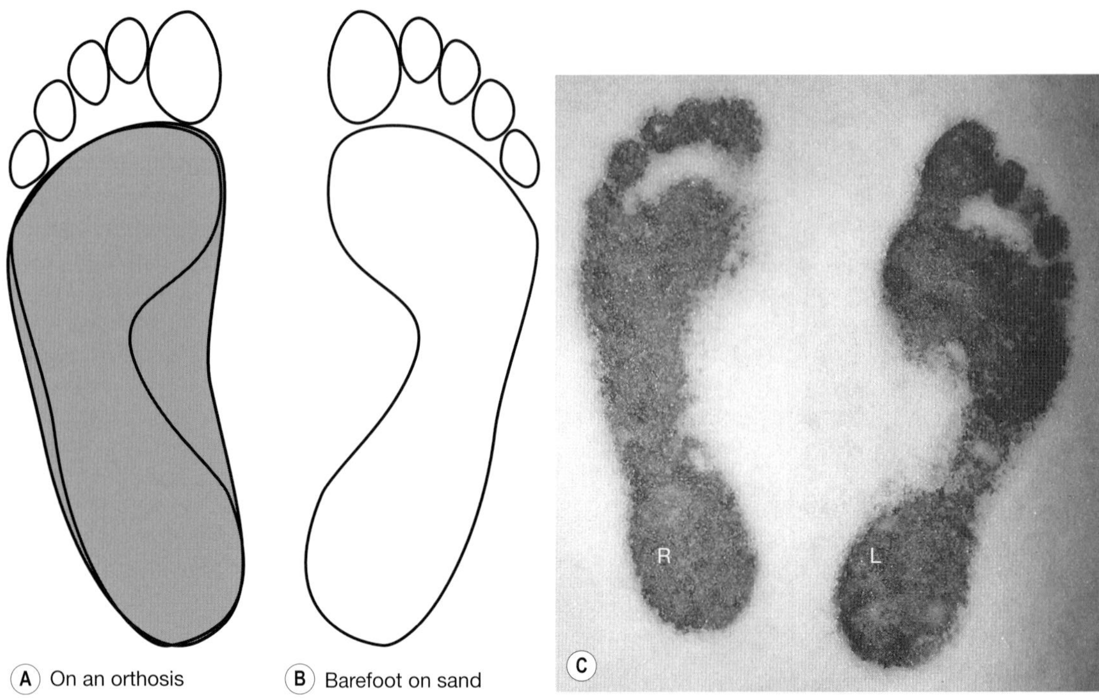

Fig. 7.33 Foot contact surface. (A) On an orthotic versus (B) barefoot on sand. (C) Barefoot weight-bearing pattern seen from below, reflecting the malalignment-related shift: medially on the right - noticeably increasing foot surface contact in the midfoot region; laterally on the left - decreasing surface contact especially along the inner (longitudinal) arch (see also Fig. 3.25A,B).

BOX 7.5 Theories of pain modulation

The gate theory of Melzack & Wall (1965)

Pain signals travel along the small-diameter, unmyelinated and slow-conducting C-fibres. Proprioceptive signals, in contrast, travel along large-diameter, myelinated and fast-conducting A-fibres. Signals from both pass through the substantia gelatinosa in the dorsal horn of the spinal cord before ascending to the brain. A barrage of proprioceptive signals arriving by way of the A-fibres may cause the substantia gelatinosa to block the signals arriving through the C-fibres. This effectively 'closes the gate', preventing pain signals from ascending further in the spinal cord and reaching the brain.

The central biasing mechanism (Mayer & Liebeskind 1974; Melzak 1981, 2001)

Pain signals ascending in the spinal cord can be prevented from reaching the brain if their transmission is subjected to the powerful inhibitory influence of the raphe nucleus in the brain stem. Cutaneous stimulation is one mechanism known to trigger activity in this nucleus, which, in turn, 'closes the gate' to pain signals ascending any further.

Release of endorphins (Pomeranz 1975)

The stimulation of cutaneous touch and pressure receptors results in the release of endorphins from the anterior pituitary gland.

3. The proprioceptive signals are ultimately transmitted to the sensory cortex where they may:
   a. effectively decrease excitatory signals to the muscles, signals that would otherwise 'facilitate' these muscles (with a resultant increase in tone)
   b. result in a more symmetrical output from the motor cortex which would, in turn, decrease any tendency to torquing attributable to an asymmetry of motor output and, hence, of muscle tone.

SACROILIAC BELTS AND COMPRESSION SHORTS

The application of a compressive force across the SI joints and symphysis pubis can afford relief from pain in these areas by decreasing the likelihood of displacement of these joints and recurrence of malalignment.

THE SACROILIAC BELT

The sacroiliac belt, also known as an intertrochanteric belt, typically fits into the space just below the ASIS and above the symphysis pubis anteriorly, and just above the greater trochanter laterally (Fig. 7.34A). It runs across the lower third of the sacrum posteriorly; if applied too low over the sacrum, or the sacro-coccygeal junction, it will exert a rotational force into counternutation (Figs 2.11, 7.34B).

The belt was developed to enhance the stability of the SI joints and symphysis pubis and can prove effective in reducing pain from these sites (Walheim 1984; Damen et al 2002b). There have been spontaneous reports of a decrease in pelvic pain, increase in comfort sitting, a tendency for the back to be straighter when sitting, and a feeling of increased pelvic girdle strength and stability on first trying on the belt. Once correction has been achieved, the belt may also prove effective in decreasing the frequency of recurrence of malalignment, if not helping to prevent it altogether in the occasional patient.

How the belt works

Possible mechanisms by which the belt exerts its effects include:

1. It brings the adjoining sacral and iliac surfaces of the SI joint closer together. As confirmed on cadaver studies, the result is an increase in the friction coefficient of the joint, decreasing the ease with which one surface can slide over the other (Vleeming et al. 1990b).
2. It enhances the 'self-bracing' mechanism (Snijders et al. 1992a) that normally ensures stability of the SI joint and allows for a transfer of the lumbosacral load to the legs while minimizing any shear between the iliac and sacral surfaces (see Ch. 2; Figs 2.25, 2.26).
3. It decreases the amount of 'anterior' rotation of the innominates and posterior tilting of the lower part of the sacrum by exerting a direct pressure against these structures (Fig. 7.34A).

Cadaver studies suggest that the belt can increase the friction coefficient and, hence, the stability of the SI joint, by bringing the apparently matching depressions and elevations on the sacral and iliac surfaces closer together (Vleeming et al. 1990b). It is, however, hard to conceive of a belt that is applied just snugly enough to prevent it from slipping up or down actually being capable of mechanically decreasing or stopping any movement of the pelvic bones relative to each other. In addition, in some patients a corset or tube-top has had equally dramatic results in helping to maintain pelvic alignment, even though these would exert only minimal pressure on the skin.

In the cadaver studies mentioned above (Vleeming et al. 1990b), doubling the tension on a belt from 50 N to 100 N decreased the amount of rotation possible at the SI joint only from 18.8% to 18.5%. Conway & Herzog (1991) hypothesized that if the SI belt did indeed stabilize the SI joint by restricting joint mobility, ground reaction forces measured in patients with SI joint problems should differ depending on whether or not they were wearing the belt; however, the authors were unable to detect any statistically significant differences.

Other mechanisms need to be considered when trying to explain the effectiveness of the belt.

First, does it favourably influence the orthokinetic reflex?

Abnormal tension in the ligaments that stabilize a joint results in a change of strength in the muscles acting on that joint. By helping to maintain the SI joint surfaces in closer to normal apposition, the belt may help even out the tension in the ligaments and, thereby, the strength in the surrounding muscles.

Second, could some of the effects of the belt be exerted by way of the proprioceptive system?

The belt applies pressure symmetrically to a large surface area. By stimulating cutaneous pressure receptors, it could flood the system with input along the fast conducting A-alpha proprioceptive fibres. In other words, the belt may be able to decrease pain by 'closing the gate' (Melzack & Wall 1965; see above). Decreasing the pain would allow for a relaxation of the muscles in which tone has increased on account of 'facilitation' or, reflexively, in response to pain and/or instability of the pubic symphysis or SI joints. If relaxation evened out tension in muscles on the right and left sides, it would decrease any tendency toward SI joint torquing.

Third, is the fact that the belt applies even pressure against the hip abductor and buttock muscles relevant?

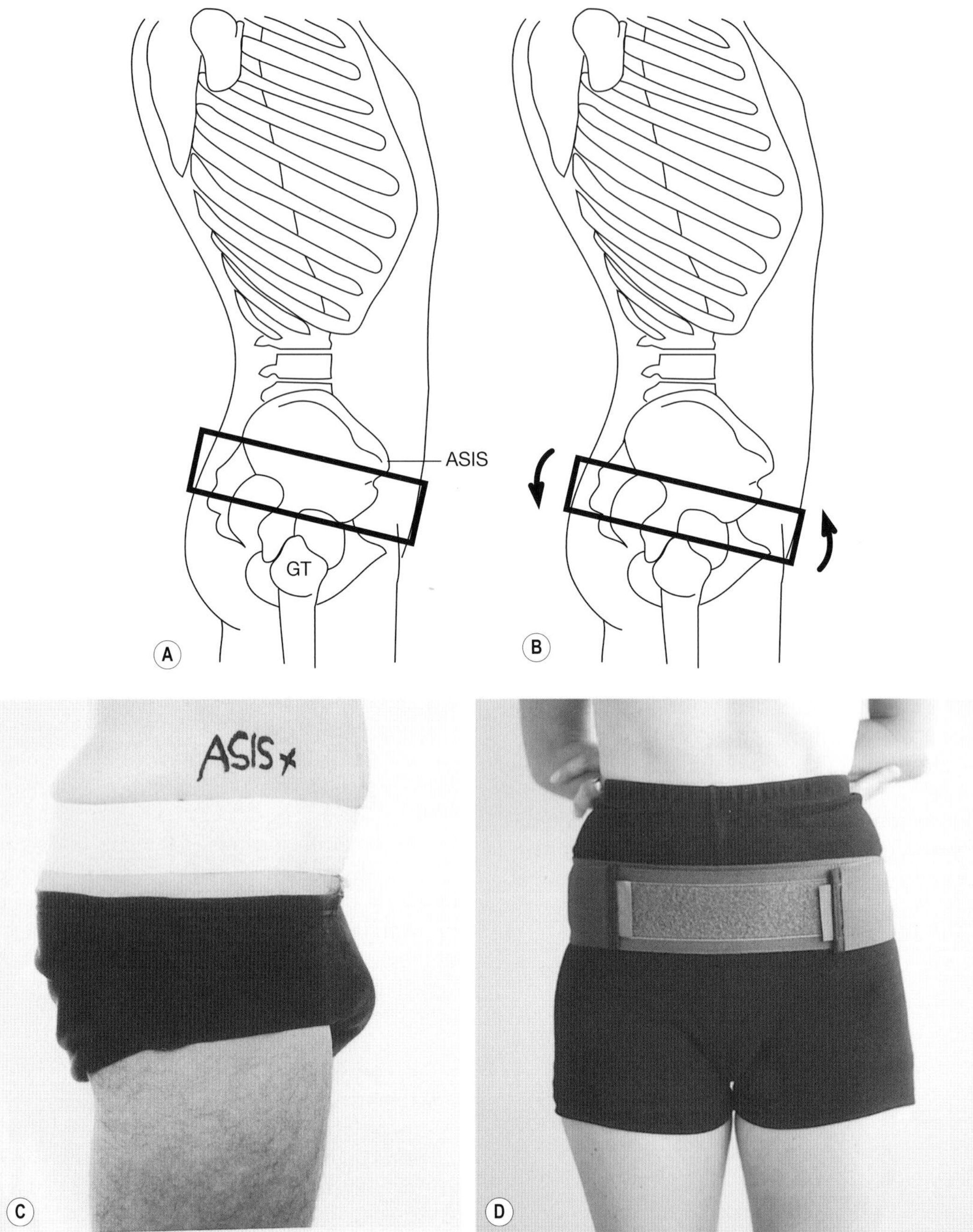

Fig. 7.34 Placement of a sacroiliac belt. (A) Correct: anteriorly below the anterior superior iliac spine (ASIS) and overlying or just above the symphysis pubis, laterally above the greater trochanter (GT) and posteriorly across the lower one-third of the sacroiliac joint; see also (C). (B) Incorrect: too low over sacrum, creating a rotational force into counternutation. (C) Sacroiliac belt: correct location. (D) Sacroiliac belt worn over clothing (Serola model). See also Figs 2.130, 7.35, 7.37 for other belt placements/effects as discussed in text.

Some of these muscles are consistently tense and tender, especially the left hip abductors and right piriformis. Applying gentle pressure may have the same effect as applying a forearm band to dimple the wrist extensor muscles in the treatment of a 'tennis elbow': the band decreases the strength of the maximum contraction that these muscles can generate and changes the torsion and traction forces in a way so that less force is exerted on the inflamed and tender muscle origins and insertions.

Finally, the belt may favourably influence posture.

One patient, for example, felt that the belt served as a reminder and 'trained her to take more care' to avoid the movements and activities that would put her at risk of going out of alignment. Another felt that a pad incorporated into the belt over the sacrum caused her back to straighten when sitting, increasing the lumbar lordosis to the point at which she no longer needed to use a back support with a lumbar roll.

As mentioned in the discussion on the active straight leg raising (ASLR) tests, re-enforcement achieved by applying medial forces to the innominates may result in improvement, presumably by counteracting SI joint instability; e.g. secondary to ligament laxity or osteoarthritis, muscle weakness or a combination of these (Figs 2.128B, 2.129B, 2.130B). More recently, it has become obvious that similar effects of improving joint stability and/or decreasing pain in the pelvic region may be achieved by application of pressure to isolated points in the pelvic region. For example, pressure on the right ASIS and the unilateral or contralateral PSIS may improve performance on the ASLR test (Fig. 2.130A). If that is the case, more consistent (and sometimes dramatic) results are achieved by:

1. reinforcing the belt with tape, pads or straps that apply pressure to a specific point or points, which could mean
2. putting the belt on in a position other than the time-honoured horizontal way, to ensure these sites are being stimulated (e.g. in the diagonal; Fig. 7.37C).

The 'Compressor™' is one of the earlier models of such a reinforced, pressure-specific SI belt (Fig. 7.35). The underlying belt is secured around the pelvic girdle. A compression strap is then attached to apply pressure over a specific point and the ASLR test repeated to see if that strap has made any difference or needs to be repositioned a bit or reinforced with a second strap. If needed, straps can be applied to overlie other points, with repeat tests to assess their effectiveness (Lee 2004a).

Indications and contraindications

The belt is used primarily for a problem of:

1. hypermobility of either SI joint or of the symphysis pubis

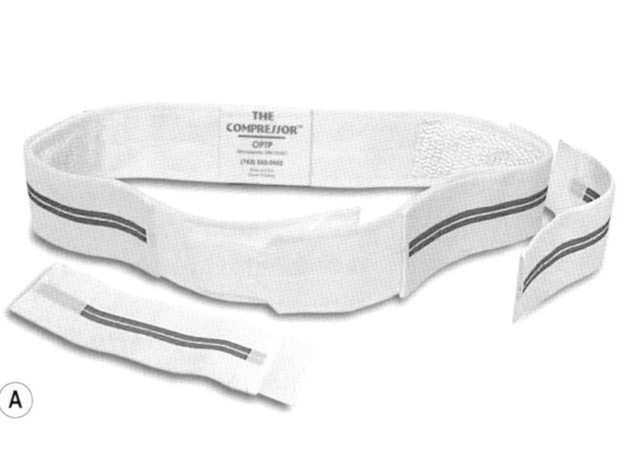

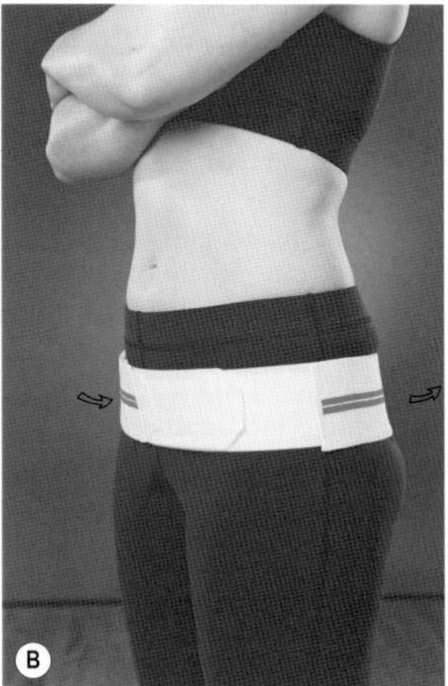

Fig. 7.35 (A) The Com-Pressor™, a patented belt that allows compression to be applied specifically to different aspects of the pelvic girdle (Lee DG 2002). (B) The Com-Pressor™ belt applied with a compression strap supporting the right anterior and left posterior aspect of the pelvis. The location of the straps is determined by the results of the ASLR test [see Ch. 2; Figs 2.128, 2.129] *(Courtesy of Lee 2011.)*

2. pain originating from any of these joints or specific sites noted on examination
3. a feeling of pelvic instability, and/or
4. recurrent malalignment

The belt is more likely to be helpful if:

1. stressing the joint(s) in the anterior-posterior or craniocaudal directions provokes the person's pain (Figs 2.98-2.101)
2. the straight leg raising test is positive; that is, passive compression of the SI joints allows the person to extend or flex the hip joint on one or both sides further and/or more easily on an ASLR test (Figs 2.128, 2.129).

The belt is likely to provide similar passive reinforcement to a symphysis pubis or SI joint(s) rendered unstable by ligament laxity or osteoarthritic degeneration (Figs 2.42, 2.102A, 4.38).

The belt is unlikely to be helpful if manoeuvres that compress the SI joints or the symphysis pubis provoke pain. The belt itself has the effect of bringing the anterior SI joint lines and superior pubic rami closer together and may, therefore, aggravate pain from these sites. If that is the case, Lee (1993b) advised resting the joint(s) by using a cane or crutches initially. One should not try an SI belt again until it no longer provokes pain, if it still seems to be indicated at that point.

Problems

Problems encountered with the SI belt include the following:

The belt is too wide and moves up and down too easily.

This becomes a nuisance, particularly when sitting down. A belt 5 cm wide is probably adequate for most people whose height is 180 cm or less; whereas those who are taller do better with one 7.5 cm in width.

The belt is applied too tightly.

Excessive pressure from the belt, buckles or stitching can irritate and even macerate the skin. The belt should be applied snugly and is best worn over the top of clothing, inside or out, especially if wearing it against the skin proves uncomfortable (Figs 7.34D, 7.35B, 7.36, 7.37A).

The belt is not worn in the proper position.

Initially, the belt could be tried lying between the ASIS and the greater trochanter. Snijders et al. (1992b) postulated that, in this position, the belt is able to exert its maximum effect to counteract any tendency of the ilium to rotate on the sacrum, as well as to enhance the 'self-bracing' of the SI joint referred to above. Of interest here is their hypothesis that the belt worn by weight-lifters, rather than acting to give extra support to the back by increasing intra-abdominal pressure, actually works by enhancing this 'self-bracing' of the SI joint in the stooped position and squat. Snijders et al. were able to show on magnetic resonance imaging (MRI) studies that the weight-lifter's belt, which is applied using exactly the same landmarks, was level with the craniad (upper) part of the SI joints. The belt was, therefore, in an optimal position to stabilize the joint by narrowing the joint space. These authors felt that if the belt were applied too far craniad, it could be useless or even detrimental, in that it would open up the caudal (lower) aspect of the joint posteriorly and decrease its overall stability.

The belt increases pain from the SI joint.

It may do so by:

1. compressing the inflamed anterior joint surfaces
2. gapping the joint posteriorly, and/or
3. stressing tender interosseous and posterior SI joint ligamentous structures

The belt interferes with efforts at elimination.

This problem is easily resolved by wearing the belt over the lower part of a T-shirt and then pulling the panties/underpants over the belt and underlying T-shirt. There is, therefore, no need to loosen or remove the belt when going to the washroom.

The belt material evokes an allergic reaction.

This is best avoided by wearing the belt over clothing, a habit already adopted by many for the sake of comfort.

The belt presses on a painful structure.

The belt may not be tolerated because it exerts direct pressure on one of the structures that has become tender because of the malalignment. Commonly involved are the piriformis (usually the right) and/or left gluteus medius/minimus. However, always rule out that the pain is not resulting from some unrelated problem, such as pressure inadvertently being applied to an underlying lipoma or neurofibroma.

Instructions for use

The belt should be worn when the person is up and about and, preferably, in alignment.

However, it may still provide some comfort even when the person is not in alignment, possibly by increasing the general stability of the SI joints and symphysis pubis and the other possible mechanisms discussed above. The occasional person derives benefit from wearing the belt at night as well, perhaps by decreasing any tendency to lose alignment when lying or turning in bed, by easing tension in some tender structure, or decreasing torquing of the pelvis. In some, malalignment is noted to recur readily on standing, in which case the belt is best applied while still lying supine, and then getting up. For a pregnant woman, there are SI belts that, in addition, provide support for the abdomen and can be let out to accommodate the progressive increase in girth (Fig. 7.36). Some belts also incorporate a triangular posterior support that overlies the sacrum.

COMPRESSION SHORTS

These shorts, commonly used in football and other sports after a 'groin injury', have also been successfully advocated for pain originating from the SI joints or symphysis pubis as a result of instability

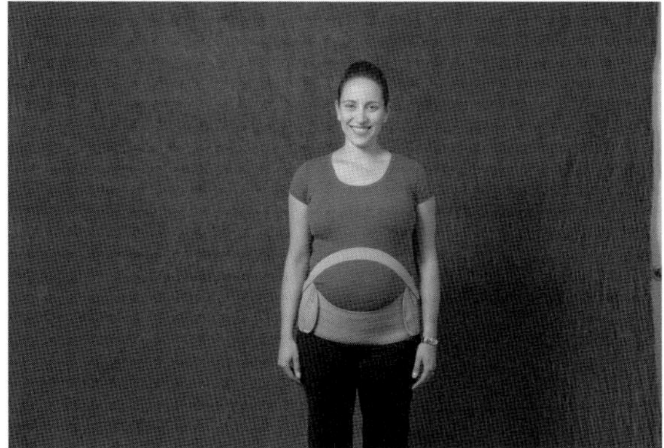

Fig. 7.36 The 'maternity mate' belt allows for progressive adjustment. By providing support for the fetus/abdomen, it helps to stabilize the lumbosacral region.

or inflammation, often in combination with a belt (e.g. Serola, *Compressor*™). They are usually made with neoprene and non-elastic materials in a way that minimizes any restriction of range of motion (Fig. 7.37A,B). Their supposed beneficial effects are noted in Box 7.6.

The shorts, in combination with the belt, have helped many patients to finally achieve some stability and comfort when the belt alone has failed. At the same time, there has been an emphasis more recently on trying to gradually start weaning the patient off the belt and/or shorts by about 4–6 weeks, in an attempt to prevent:

1. developing a false sense of 'security', and also an over-reliance on the belt/shorts
2. having the belt decrease the resting tension of a specific muscle and possibly also the strength of a voluntary contraction, at the risk of weakening and wasting of that muscle
3. reinforcing a patient's feeling that 'something is dreadfully wrong' and that they must be 'handled with care', an attitude that can actually interfere with them getting on with a progressive core-strengthening and CV programme (see Ch. 4: 'Implications for psychiatry and psychology')

COMPLEMENTARY FORMS OF TREATMENT

The aim of treatment is to achieve and maintain alignment, recover stability of pelvis and spine, decrease or abolish pain, and re-establish normal posture, muscle tension/strength and patterns of activation and movement.

In the process of trying to achieve realignment, complementary methods of treatment may be helpful, especially those that are able to temporarily reduce pain and muscle tension or spasm to improve the length of time the realignment can be maintained.

To this end, treatment by a physiotherapist who is recognized for having trained in manual therapy would be a good start as it offers the combination

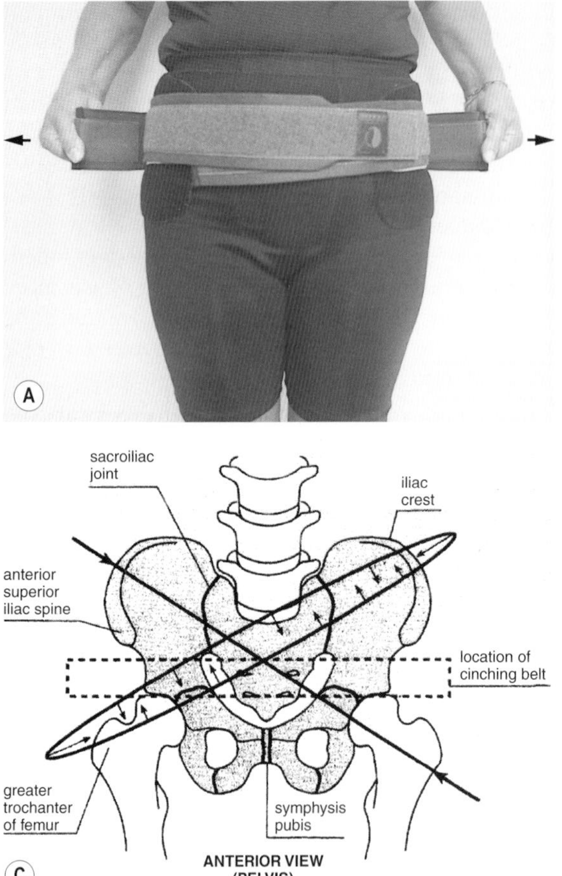

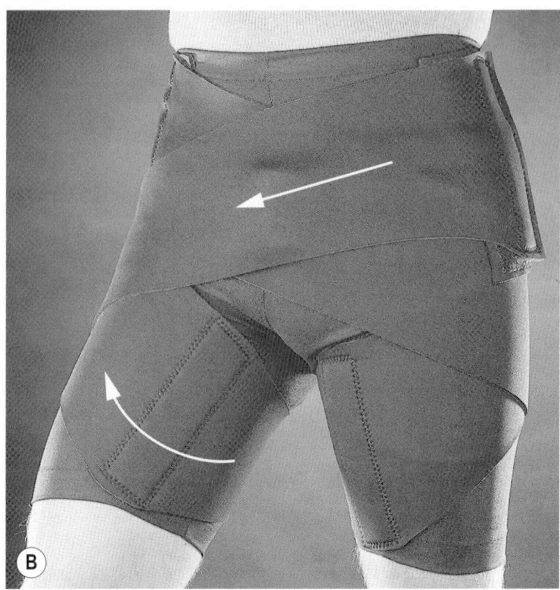

Fig. 7.37 Compression pants. (A) Incorporating a sacroiliac belt (Serola model - note the elastic side-straps stretched out sideways to be secured with Velcro anteriorly to reinforce the support). (B) With cross-straps secured to leggings and wrapped upward around the trunk (figure-of-eight). (C) Diagonal stabilizing forces created across the sacroiliac joints by the cross-straps. *(Courtesy of Active Orthopaedics Inc. 1999.)*

BOX 7.6 Beneficial effects of compression shorts

Heat retention

This may be particularly helpful when there has been injury to groin tissue and will also help to relax muscles that are tense and tender as a result of malalignment.

Compressive forces

1. These forces are spread over a larger surface area and may, therefore, be more easily tolerated by the patient.
2. Some shorts incorporate an SI belt for an additional compressive force to help to 'immobilize' these joints; the belt also helps to keep the shorts in place (Fig. 7.37A).

The addition of 'figure-of-8' hip and thigh straps provide adjustable compressive forces (Fig. 7.37B)

One strap, for example, may be anchored to the inside of the groin, wrapped anteriorly around the thigh and then across the buttocks, before being anchored anteriorly to a strap originating from the opposite thigh. The result is a diagonal compression force across both SI joints (Fig. 7.37C). A strap may apply pressure to a specific tender point to decrease pain, possibly improve perfomance on an ASLR test (see above; Fig. 2.130).

of working together with someone trained to carry out an initial comprehensive neuromusculoskeletal examination, skilled in dealing with the malalignment, usually able to simultaneously use conventional physiotherapy methods (e.g. ROM, exercise routines, electrical modalities) and capable of deciding if and when one or more of the complementary techniques may be indicated (especially to help resolve any residual problems noted once realignment has been achieved). In Canada, the Canadian Association of Manual Therapists (CAMT) governs training of physiotherapy graduates as they progress through several stages which, on completion, leads to them being designated as a 'Fellow of the CAMT', or 'FCAMT'.

Sometimes treatment aimed at the malalignment using mobilization or manipulation techniques may have been successful but proved helpful only temporarily as it failed to address the residual problems - core muscle weakness with instability of the pelvis and spine, persistent muscle spasm, trigger points - and leading to recurrence of the malalignment. Also, most patients will already have tried one or more courses of treatment with what are here considered to be 'complementary' treatment methods: massage, acupuncture, intramuscular stimulation (IMS), biofeedback, Pilates, cortisone and/or prolotherapy injections and any of a number of other treatment options available. The person's history too often indicates that therapy in the past has been limited to one or a combination of these methods (see Ch. 8), usually instituted at the time of a recurrence or worsening of symptoms. However, these methods usually fail to correct the underlying cause of their problem: the malalignment and, at best, provide only a temporary change for the better as far as concerns the muscle tension, paraesthesias, dysaesthesias and any other symptoms that have developed secondary to the malalignment (e.g. the 'malalignment syndrome', seen with an 'upslip' or 'rotational malalignment'). Usually the person will have had repeated treatment with whatever method or combination they found most consistently helpful (e.g. acupuncture, manipulation) whenever the pain returned or worsened. Unfortunately, this history keeps repeating itself again and again whenever they return to the clinic because:

1. The malalignment itself has never been addressed, or only in part, by these treatment methods.
2. Even if realignment is somehow achieved (e.g. by relaxing muscles enough to allow bones to slip back into their proper place), residual problems are never attended to and can cause malalignment to recur.
3. The patient has never been taught self-assessment, self-treatment techniques and what activities to avoid in order to help maintain realignment between treatment sessions and decrease putting him or her at risk.

Use of one or more of the complementary methods certainly may assist the manual therapist in making realignment easier to achieve and subsequently more likely to be maintained between treatment sessions. None of these methods is, however, likely to bring any more than temporary relief if used in isolation, while neglecting a simultaneous attempt at achieving and maintaining realignment.

MEDICATIONS AND ELECTROSTIMULATION

Analgesics, anti-inflammatory medication and muscle relaxants may be helpful, certainly during the initial stages of treatment. They may prove more effective when taken on a preventative basis at regular intervals around the clock. Malalignment may cause pain, or aggravate existing pain. Taking these medications in measured amounts on a regular basis (e.g. every 4 or 6 or 8 hours) during the early stages of treatment may 'head off' the development of pain, or decrease its severity, especially whenever malalignment does recur. Medications are less likely to have an effect when taken on an 'as needed' basis and certainly when one is dealing with an acute flare-up (e.g. acute muscle spasm triggered by an L4/L5 rotation relative to S1), at which time stronger medications such as percocet, oxycodone or even injections of morphine for pain or valium for muscle spasm may be indicated until the flare-up settles down.

Transcutaneous electrical nerve stimulation (TENS) is worth trying as it will decrease pain and relax the muscles in a number of patients. A unit can usually be readily supplied by the therapist for a 1 to 2 week trial. If it helps, rental or purchase of a unit should be considered. This modality is, again, more likely to be helpful when used by the patient on an ongoing basis, rather than just whenever symptoms recur or worsen. The unit is strapped to the belt and can stimulate 2 or more tender or tense sites simultaneously. It can be left on constantly or be programmed, for example, to turn on 3, 4 or more times a day for 20–30 minute intervals, whatever seems most helpful, at a setting felt to be appropriate by the therapist. The intent is to increase the overall feeling of comfort, relax muscles and, hopefully, help maintain realignment for longer periods of time.

Magnetic devices in the form or insoles or pads applied to the skin may bring relief by improving the circulation to localized sites of tender muscle or connective tissue (e.g. ligaments and fascia). More generalized effects may be achieved with the use of magnetic pillows and mattresses.

Laser stimulation is often part of an attempt to relieve pain and tension in muscle and connective tissue at deeper sites. Methods such as extracorporeal shock wave therapy (ECST) and pulsed signal therapy (PST) may be worthwhile trying in an attempt to resolve residual painful areas localizing to deep musculoskeletal tissue, especially sites that have become a chronic source of pain as a result of the insults to which they have been subjected by the malalignment and which have failed to respond to other treatment measures, even though temporary realignment is now being attained. Unfortunately, they are often one of the 'desperation measures' that were tried previously, usually at considerable expense, long before malalignment was ever diagnosed and appropriate manual therapy instituted. Hence, the patient may have to be convinced that they are worth another try, in the hope of eradicating any factors that are still capable of causing recurrence of the malalignment.

INJECTIONS

Injection is a treatment option for those presenting with:

1. recurrent malalignment caused by ligament laxity
2. ongoing pain despite correction of the malalignment, which may arise from:
   a. inflamed and/or weakened ligaments and tendons
   b. trigger points within ligaments, tendons and muscles
   c. inflamed symphysis pubis, facet, vertebral or SI joints

The stability of any joint depends on the fit of the joint surfaces and the proper function of the supporting structures: the tightness of its ligaments and capsule, and the strength and tension in the muscles acting on that joint - either directly or indirectly (see Ch. 2). Malalignment, whether it involves vertebral rotational displacement or a shift of the lumbo-pelvic-hip complex, increases tension in some soft tissue structures while relaxing others.

> Any joint connective tissue structure (i.e. capsule, ligaments) put under tension by persistent or recurring malalignment will eventually lengthen and, with time, the joint may become hypermobile because of failure of these supportive tissues.

On examination, even the SI joint that is 'locked' or hypomobile in one or both planes may actually turn out to be hypermobile on realignment and 'unlocking' of that joint. The hypermobility may be due to:

1. lengthening that has occurred in the supporting ligaments and joint capsule because of the stress imposed by the malalignment and/or joint degeneration (impaired 'form' closure)
2. release of ongoing reflex muscle spasm caused by pain and/or joint instability subsequent to a previous injury, such as a shear and partial tear
3. an element of weakening of muscles that now fail to properly support the joint (inadequate 'force' closure)
4. impaired muscle contraction, sequencing or neural control

Hypermobility of a joint can also develop because its supporting structures are being put under increased stress by the restriction of movement in a nearby or distant joint. 'Locking' of the right SI joint, for example, increases the stress on the left SI joint; decreased movement of a hip joint increases stress on the ipsilateral SI joint, the lumbosacral junction and contralateral hip joint; decreased movement of a vertebral complex increases the stress on the levels immediately above and below. All of these restrictions may also affect more distant joints and accelerate joint degeneration. Realignment may put the joint surfaces back into proper position but malalignment or vertebral displacement may now keep recurring because of failure of the supporting structures.

Sometimes the instability and/or the pain arising from the ligaments or the joint have progressed to the point where attempts at realignment prove futile - the patient may not even be able to do simple core strengthening exercises without malalignment recurring. The therapist simply cannot progress with the intended treatment regime. In that situation, strengthening and attempts at realignment have to wait until the ligaments can once again provide the needed support. When there is such an obvious problem of laxity evident, then an injection technique known as 'prolotherapy' may be indicated to increase the strength of capsules, ligaments and tendons.

Cortisone temporarily weakens connective tissue structures and is, therefore, more appropriate for the injection of persistently tender and inflamed ligaments in those cases in which alignment is being maintained, as well as for injection directly into an inflamed pubic symphysis, facet or SI joint space in the hope of settling down any inflammation within the joint (see below).

PROLOTHERAPY INJECTIONS

The word 'prolotherapy', presumably, is based on the Latin 'proles = to stimulate growth' and is a contraction of 'proliferation therapy' coined by Hackett, who pioneered research in this area and published the first monograph on prolotherapy in 1956. Based on his clinical experience and the results of animal studies, Hackett (1958) proposed the theoretical model outlined in Box 7.7.

Hackett felt that the ideal treatment would be to strengthen the fibro-osseous junction by stimulating the proliferation of fibrous tissue in this region. Solutions to induce such proliferation were readily available as they already enjoyed popularity in the treatment of venous and oesophageal varices, hernias and haemorrhoids, a treatment method commonly referred to as 'sclerotherapy' (Hirschberg 1985).

Hackett (1958) thought the term 'prolotherapy', or 'proliferant therapy', was more appropriate, given that it did indeed result in a proliferation of normal tissue. Usage of the word in this context would get away from the concept of 'scarring', which was commonly held to be the basis of the beneficial effect of these so-called 'sclerosing' injections when, in fact, injection of the solution into a vein, for example, also resulted in stimulating a proliferant reaction with collagen formation in the vessel wall, with eventual 'closing off', or sclerosing, of the vein.

Prolotherapy is based on the premises that:

1. following injury, the inadequate repair of fibrous tissue can result in chronic pain from musculoskeletal tissue (e.g. the fibro-osseous junction or 'enthesis')
2. the healing of injured ligaments and tendons may be compromised by their limited blood supply

BOX 7.7 Hackett's model of prolotherapy (also known as 'Regenerative Injection Treatment' or RIT)

1. The 'relaxation' or lengthening of the ligaments that span the joints of the spine and pelvis is a major cause of chronic low back pain.
2. The relaxation of a ligament or tendon can result from:
   a. inadequate healing following trauma (e.g. major trauma, such as a sprain or strain, or repetitive microtrauma resulting from chronic or recurrent activity or related to malalignment)
   b. congenital laxity
   c. ligament laxity associated with pregnancy
3. Relaxation of the ligaments and tendons can be the cause of pain from the 'fibro-osseous' junction, the site where the ligaments and tendons insert onto the bone.
4. Because of this increased laxity, these structures must now be considered incompetent in terms of providing adequate support to the bones and joints.
5. Pain arises as a result of:
   a. irritation of the relatively inelastic sensory nerves that lie within the ligaments and tendons
      i. even relatively normal tension forces will cause stretching of the now incompetent elastic components; whereas the relatively inelastic sensory fibres fail to stretch to an equal extent
      ii. this results in irritation of the sensory fibres, with localized and/or referred pain
   b. increased wear and tear of the now excessively mobile joints
6. Pain, ligament laxity and 'loose joints' lead to a vicious cycle of further ligament relaxation and decalcification of bone in the region of the fibro-osseous junction. Either one can induce the other: bone strength is dependent on stress imparted to the bone by the attaching ligaments or tendons, just as ligament strength is favourably affected by the stress imparted to the ligament through its connections to the bone and myofascia.

3. a lack of cells, in particular of the fibroblasts that produce collagen, may be another factor to account for the slow healing, or even failure to heal at all, of injured ligaments and tendons
4. irritant solutions can be injected to stimulate fibroblasts to proliferate, produce collagen and growth hormone and thereby promote healing

Prolotherapy injections have proven helpful in treating the problems of persistent ligament/tendon (enthetic) pain and weakness - usually maximal at the fibro-osseous junction - and also the laxity of any supporting tissues that has resulted in joint hypermobility and recurrence of malalignment. The technique aims to strengthen the connective tissue when the natural healing process:

1. has been too slow or has proven inadequate
2. has failed altogether to repair an insufficient collagen matrix that has resulted from:
    a. a single major traumatic disruption of these tissues (e.g. a shear injury to the SI joint or actual joint dislocation; Fig. 2.51)
    b. a repeated and/or chronic stretching and lengthening (e.g. recurrent malalignment, joint hyperextension or subluxation)

How prolotherapy works

Prolotherapy can help ligaments, capsules and tendons to heal by stimulating fibroblasts to produce collagen. It may do so by:

1. initiating a localized inflammatory reaction which, in turn, triggers the natural connective tissue 'healing cascade'
2. acting as a chemical irritant and initiating a chemotactic response
3. generating release of growth factors that can act directly on fibroblasts to stimulate collagen formation

Inflammation and the 'healing cascade'

A sprain, strain or other injury to a ligament, capsule or tendon triggers the 'healing cascade' of events, as follows:

1. there is an immediate release of mediators (e.g. cytokines) from damaged tissues which results in blood vessel dilatation and increased permeability, increased blood flow to the injured area, increased warmth and the development of oedema (Fig. 7. 38)
2. an initial infiltration of granulocytes is followed by monocytes, macrophages and other scavenger cells intent on the removal of necrotic tissue
3. 3-4 days after injury marks the onset of the 'inflammatory' phase, during which the release of growth factors (e.g. growth hormone) and other derivatives from platelets, macrophages, lymphocytes and similar cells stimulate fibroblasts to migrate to this area; within 2-3 days, these activated fibroblasts are already synthesizing an immature collagen
4. over the next 2 weeks, the 'inflammatory' phase gradually gives way to the 'early reparative' phase, also called the 'proliferative' phase because of ongoing fibroblast proliferation (Fig. 7.39A); the process of immature collagen formation continues for another 3-4 weeks and then decreases gradually as the number of activated fibroblasts declines to pre-injury levels by the end of the second month post-injury
5. during the weeks and months that follow, known as the 'remodelling' or 'maturation' phase, collagen fibrils become thicker, more variable in length (with some 'contracture'), more 'close-packed' through cross-linkage and orientation along the lines of stress, with a gradual increase in tensile strength (Fig. 7.39B)

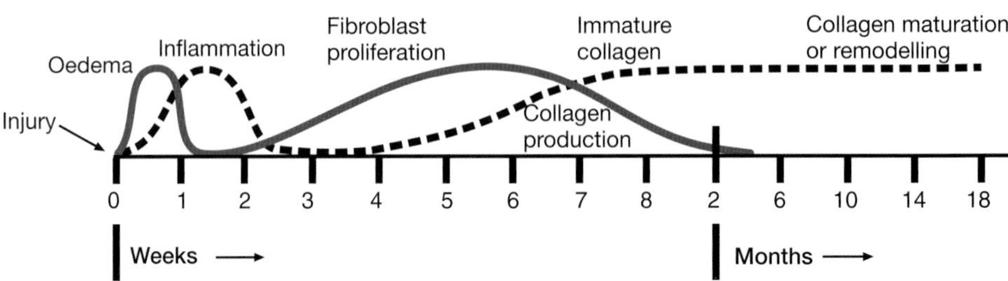

Fig. 7.38 Phases of natural connective tissue repair following sprain or strain (immature collagen = thin, short, randomly oriented fibres; mature collagen = thick, long, cross-linked fibres, oriented along lines of stress).

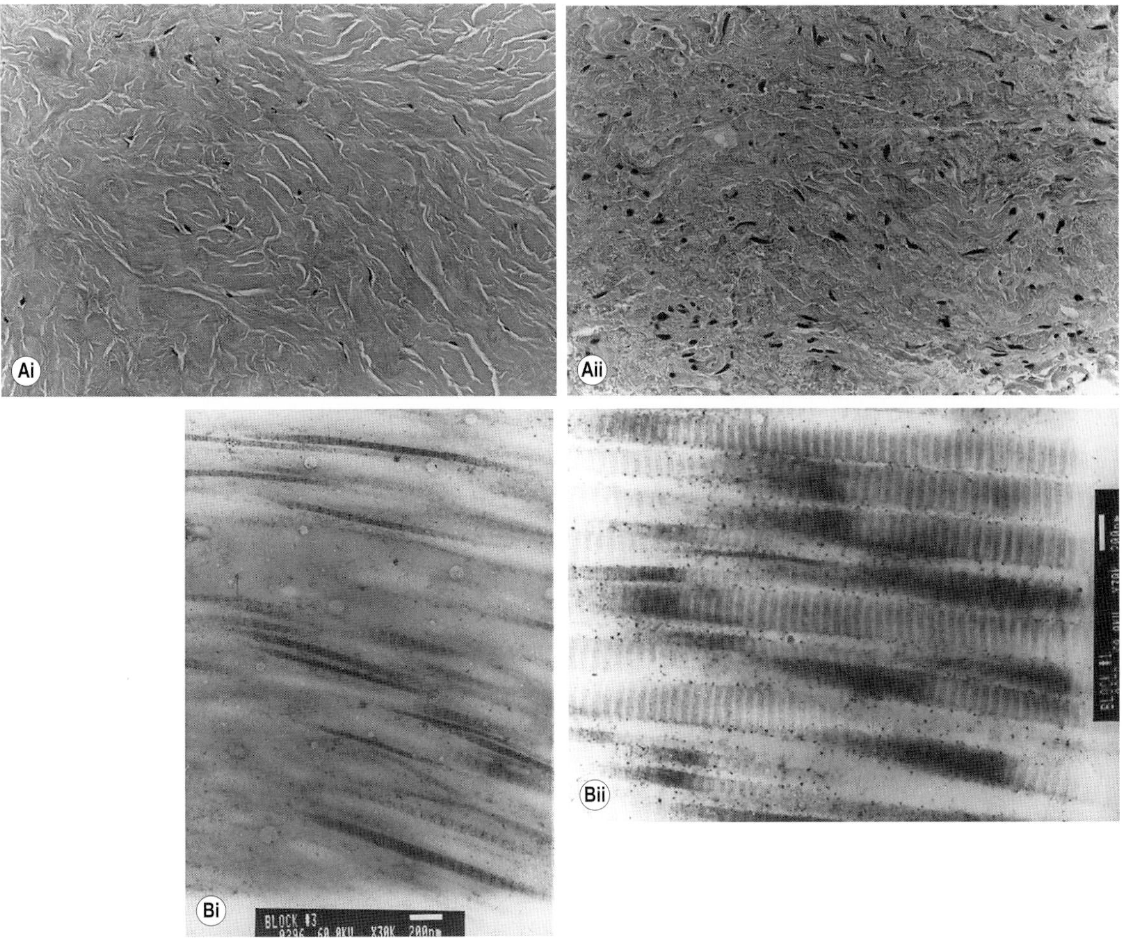

Fig. 7.39 Biopsy of the posterior pelvic ligaments before and then 3 months after a course of 6 weekly prolotherapy injections; note the fibroblastic hyperplasia, with a 60% increase in average fibre diameter. (A) Black and white haematoxylin and eosin representative slides of ligament histology (i) before and (ii) after prolotherapy. Note the increased waviness representing collagen and the increased number of fibroblast nuclei. Of significance is the absence of inflammation or disease. (B) Electron microscopy longitudinal cuts of ligament tissue (i) before and (ii) after prolotherapy. Note the increase in size of the collagen fibres as well as the increase in variation of the size of these fibres. *(Courtesy of Dorman 1997.)*

6. the process of maturation continues for some time: it may take up to 12–18 months before the tissue reaches its maximum post-injury tensile strength (which is unlikely to equal its strength prior to the injury).

When this natural process fails to take place during the first 6 months post-injury, one is usually left with a weakened, and often painful, ligament no longer capable of healing spontaneously. For example, with an injury to the SI joint ligaments:

1. failure to heal may occur because:
   a. the trauma resulted in a partial or complete disruption of ligaments (Fig. 2.51B)
   b. poor blood supply has delayed the onset of healing
   c. the nutritional status and/or immune response is inadequate
   d. mechanical factors repeatedly subject any newly-formed collagen fibres to an excessive elongation stress, either:
      i. constantly, because of persistent malalignment with separation of the joint surfaces and/or separation of a ligament's origin and insertion
      ii. with repeated recurrence of malalignment because of a lack of adequate stabilizing support from the ligaments and/or muscles

2. the pain can arise from:
   a. excessive tension on the nerve fibres, which:
      i. cannot elongate as much as the elastic tissue when subjected to increased tension
      ii. may have become entrapped in scar tissue
      iii. are most abundant in the fibro-osseous junction, which is likely to be weakened and under increased tension as a result of the malalignment
      iv. may have become hypersensitive with time because of these factors
   b. the development of trigger points in ligaments, tendons and muscles
   c. the ligaments, capsule or joint having become a site of localized or referred pain

> Prolotherapy may become the treatment of choice in that it can decrease the pain at the same time as it increases the tensile strength of the tissue by promoting collagen formation.

Prolotherapy to induce an inflammatory response

One technique relies on the injection of a solution that causes damage and incites an inflammatory response in the connective tissue, similar to what occurs with an injury, and tricks the body into initiating the natural 'healing cascade' outlined above: inflammation triggering the migration of fibroblasts to the area, with production of immature collagen fibres for the first two months and subsequent maturation of these fibres over the next 12–18 months (Figs 7.38, 7.39). In other words, someone competent in prolotherapy artificially induces the 'healing cascade' while at the same time continuing attempts to maintain alignment so that the immature collagen is not subjected to abnormal tensile stresses and has a chance to mature. In addition to recovery of strength, the ligament also regains elasticity - the ability to store elastic energy - with improvement of motion in the joint. If the intent was to get the patient back to the therapist as soon as possible to commence a progressive treatment schedule, this point is usually reached within 4–8 weeks of starting the injections. During this time, the patient is encouraged to move about as much as possible, perhaps just walking in a warm pool initially, in order to maintain residual strength and mobility. If tolerated, ongoing attempts to reverse any recurrences of malalignment using very gentle techniques (e.g. craniosacral; see Ch. 8) are also worthwhile but sometimes even this is not possible until recovery of ligament strength finally allows for resumption of the attempts at realignment and core strengthening routines.

Injections used to induce collagen formation

1. Irritants intended to induce inflammation

Hyperosmolar dextrose solution

This is one of the most commonly used 'proliferants' and probably also the safest. Dextrose solution - usually diluted to about 12.5-20% with a local anaesthetic and sterile water - draws cell fluid out of the surrounding connective tissue to such a degree that it causes cell breakdown and incites inflammation, setting the 'healing cascade' into motion. The inflammatory response subsides within 1–2 weeks as the dextrose becomes diluted again by the fluid drawn out of the cells (Banks 1991).

Concentrations of dextrose:

1. ranging between 12.5% and 20% are adequate
2. of 25% or more should be avoided, for fear of causing actual tissue necrosis, but are used for injection directly into a joint
3. of 10% do not induce an inflammation but can stimulate growth factor release

Chemotactic substances

These are capable of chemotactically attracting inflammatory mediators; i.e., inciting an immune response. They include sodium morrhuate, an extract of cod liver oil that is frequently used in small amounts in combination with hypertonic glucose.

Cellular irritants

Typical of these is 'Ongley's solution', a combination of phenol, glycerine and glucose, which both damages the cells and incites an immune response.

2. Growth factor

Dextrose, sodium morrhuate and a number of other substances not only induce an inflammatory response and the 'healing cascade' but eventually also result in an increase in growth factors that cause the division and proliferation of:

a. fibroblasts, which produce collagen for the repair of capsules, ligaments and tendons
b. chondrocytes, for the repair of cartilage

Growth factors can be injected into ligaments directly, either in isolation or combination, to stimulate growth and a healing response (Letson & Dahners 1994). The following act chemotactically (attracting fibroblasts and other cells), increase the number of fibroblasts available to replicate and produce collagen for repair, and probably have other properties that could advance healing:

a. growth factor beta type 1
b. platelet-derived growth factor (PDGF)
c. insulin-type growth factor type 1

3. Platelet Rich Plasma (PRP)

PRP is made by spinning a sample of the person's own blood in a centrifuge. The concentrate can be injected into a site such as a ligament, to benefit from the platelet's capability to:

a. bring WBCs to the injured area for clean-up of residual injured and dead cells, and
b. release of growth factors that stimulate tissue regeneration (Crane & Everts 2008)

Barring allergic reactions, xylocaine is probably the ideal local anaesthetic in that it is less likely to produce pain on intradermal and subcutaneous injection (Morris et al. 1987) and has a rapid onset of action (5–10 minutes). These advantages may, however, be offset by its short duration of action (1–2 hours). If the ligament pain does indeed stem from the irritation of hypersensitive nerve fibres at the fibro-osseous junction, longer-acting anaesthetics, such as marcaine 0.25% or procaine 2%, may be more effective for actually 'desensitizing' these nerve endings at the same time.

Experimental evidence

Early studies into the effects of proliferant solutions by Rice & Mattson (1936), Maniol (1938) and Harris et al. (1938) had already confirmed that the injection of a chemical irritant into tissue such as muscle, tendon or ligament caused an inflammatory response, then a proliferant phase and, subsequently, maturation of the collagen produced. Rice (1937) reported how the conversion to adult fibrous tissue was essentially complete in approximately 7 weeks. Hackett became a prime advocate of prolotherapy when he noted that injection of an irritant solution into a fibro-osseous junction during hernia repair resulted in 'profuse proliferation of new tissue at this union' (1956).

Hackett & Henderson (1955), reporting on the effect of injecting a proliferant solution into the Achilles tendon of rabbits, documented a progressive increase in both fibrous tissue and bone in the region of the fibro-osseous junction at 3 months. By 9 months, the diameter of the injected tendons had increased 40% and tensile strength 100% compared with control tendons. The authors remarked on the increase of continuous fibrous tissue that extended from the tendon, through the periosteum and into the bone and thereby increased the strength of the 'weld' at the junction. They also felt that:

> *...the increase of bone is significant because it results in a strong fibro-osseous union where sprains, tears and relaxation of the ligament chiefly take place and where sensory nerves are abundant.*
>
> (Hackett & Henderson 1955: 972)

Several studies have clearly validated the theories put forth by Hackett and proved the effectiveness of prolotherapy injections into the ligaments of the human pelvis and spine. Naeim et al. (1982) carried out a single-blind study that indicated that a combination of lidocaine and dextrose was more effective in treating chronic iliolumbar syndrome than was the use of lidocaine alone. Ongley et al. (1987) published the first double-blind controlled study on human subjects that proved the effectiveness of prolotherapy in the treatment of chronic low back pain.

Klein et al. (1989) presented the first histological documentation of ligament proliferation in three human subjects involved in a double-blind study into the effectiveness of prolotherapy for the treatment of chronic low back pain of at least 2 years duration (Fig. 7.39). Biopsies of the posterior sacroiliac ligaments carried out 3 months after the completion of a course of 6 weekly injections of a proliferant solution showed fibroblastic hyperplasia and a 60% increase in average fibre diameter. The three patients also demonstrated a statistically significant improvement in the range of motion in the three major axes of lumbar movement, and improved visual analogue pain and disability scores, compared with 20 controls.

Proulx (1990), injecting with a solution of lidocaine mixed with either hypertonic dextrose (12.5%) or the corticosteroid triamcinolone (10 mg), commented that, on follow-up at 8 months, the results suggested that:

1. compared with steroid therapy, prolotherapy was more beneficial the more chronic the fibrous tissue ailments
2. symptoms of prolonged immobility ('theatre cocktail party' syndrome, night pain and

morning stiffness) were good predictors of a favourable response only for the prolotherapy group
3. the SI joint dysfunction tests and ligament stress tests were of no value as predictors of outcome in either group
4. the study proved that dextrose is an 'active medication'

Klein et al. (1993: 23) reported on a randomized, double-blind clinical trial of xylocaine/hypertonic glucose (prolotherapy) versus xylocaine/saline injections into the posterior pelvic ligaments, fascia and joint capsules of 79 patients with chronic low back pain resistant to previous conservative treatment. The prolotherapy group showed greater improvement on visual analogue, disability and pain grid scores. Of interest was the finding that MRI and computed axial tomography (CAT) scans 'showed significant abnormalities in both groups but these did not correlate with subjective complaints and were not predictive of response to treatment' (p. 23), a finding that has been echoed in a number of other reports (e.g. Jensen et al. 1994; Kieffer et al. 1984; Magora & Schwartz 1976; Weishaupt et al. 1998).

More recent research has concentrated on:

1. the method of action and the analgesic and healing effects of:
   a. the concentrates typically used in prolotherapy solutions
   b. the newer injectables, including:
      i. the various growth factors mentioned above (Hauser 2004; Hauser & Hauser 2009)
      ii. autologous Platelet Rich Plasma or PRP (Barrett 2003, Crane & Everts 2008)
2. the effectiveness of prolotherapy for treatment of:
   a. an array of specific joints to stimulate cartilage and ligament repair, to strengthen the capsule, ligaments and tendons acting on the joint, and to decrease pain; e.g. prolotherapy to counter TMJ dysfunction (Ch. 4), finger and knee arthritis (Reeves et al. 2000), ACL laxity (Reeves et al. 2003; Hauser 1998, 2004)
   b. some rheumatological conditions; e.g. severe fibromyalgia (Reeves 1994)

Indications for injection

Prolotherapy may be the treatment of choice in the following situations:

1. if the malalignment has been corrected but the ligaments continue to be an ongoing source of pain, which may relate to:
   a. the severity of the injury
   b. the length of time the malalignment has been present
   c. the development of chronic inflammation
   d. the development of a hypersensitivity of the sensory endings that has failed to respond to the normalization of tension and/or a trial of repeated injections of a local anaesthetic
2. if the malalignment keeps recurring, and ligament laxity is evident or suspected
   - remember that muscles, in particular iliopsoas, gluteus maximus, piriformis and the coccygeal muscle group (Fig. 2.53), may be chronically contracted in an attempt to stabilize what may actually prove to be an SI joint that is unstable because of laxity of the supporting ligaments

Scheduling of injections

There is no consensus in the literature on how often one should inject and at what intervals. Suggestions range anywhere from one injection a week for 6 weeks, to one injection every 4 weeks for a total of three or four injections. Fibroblastic activity subsides within 6 to 8 weeks following a single injection (Fig. 7.38). Common practice is to give repeat injections within 1–2 weeks or, at the most, some 4–5 weeks later, in order to stimulate an ongoing inflammatory response and boost the changes already initiated by the preceding injection(s). In addition, given that the response rate for partial or complete relief is about 60-70% following 3–6 injections (Klein et al. 1989, Ongley et al. 1987), it seems wise to try an initial course of 4–6 injections, spaced about 2 weeks apart or as tolerated, in order to spare the majority of patients either inadequate or unnecessary injections. Those who respond only partially, or not at all, to this initial course may benefit from a further set of 4–6 weekly or bi-weekly injections.

The author's preference is to see the patient within 6 weeks after the first course of six bi-weekly injections, when the fibroblast count can be expected to have started to drop but not yet reached the pre-injection level. The response to this first set of injections is assessed in terms of pain relief and improved stability, with feedback from a therapist, if at all possible. If this response appears to be inadequate, a repeat full course is initiated. If response is only partial, a course of booster injections may suffice. These boosters are spaced further apart, starting with three boosters at monthly intervals. There follows a further reassessment 1.5-2 months after the last one and, if necessary, further boosters, with ongoing feedback to ascertain whether stability is being achieved and further prolotherapy injections are no longer felt to be necessary.

The treatment protocol obviously needs to be tailored to each person. He or she (and those involved in their care) must be made aware that:

1. improvement occurring during the course of injections to some extent reflects the effect of the local anaesthetic on painful structures (including hypersensitive nerve fibres) and temporary muscle relaxation, both of which will help the person to get on with other treatment efforts
2. the actual process of connective tissue tightening and strengthening depends on the maturation of the newly formed collagen, a process that continues over several months; that is, any treatment effects attributable to ligament strengthening using prolotherapy may not be apparent for several months
3. approximately 60-70% of cases will show some improvement at the time of the reassessment 1.5-2 months after completion of the first course (i.e. about 4–5 months after the first injection, going by the above protocol); a repeat course of injections may have to be considered in those whose response to that first set of injections proved inadequate, or a course of boosters if there was only a partial response
4. if at all possible, efforts to achieve and maintain alignment should continue during the course of injections and while waiting for the completion of the maturation process, in order to minimize any chance of either contracture or unwanted lengthening of the immature collagen fibres that are being formed (Fig. 2.60)

Throughout the course of injections, there is an emphasis on achieving and maintaining realignment and carrying on with a supervised progressive treatment course in those patients capable of doing so.

Unfortunately, there is a trend nowadays to subject patients to an ongoing course of prolotherapy injections, sometimes weekly, without attention to correction of a coexistent malalignment problem. The injections may strengthen the structure being injected and eventually abolish pain completely. However, without simultaneous attention to alignment, mobility, posture and other factors that are a key to permanent recovery:

1. any improvement with prolotherapy is likely to take longer to achieve
2. the patient is at risk of having a recurrence of symptoms and signs that are attributable to the malalignment, especially with any increase in stresses on soft tissues and joints, such as occurs on return to regular activities

Injection technique

For information, the reader is referred to Dorman & Ravin (1991), adaptations and expansions of Hackett's original 1956 monograph by Mirman (1989) and Hackett et al. (1991), and the informative books by Hauser (1998, 2004) and Hauser & Hauser (2009). Workshops with hands-on teaching for prolotherapy injection techniques are offered on a regular basis by both the American and Canadian Association of Orthopaedic Medicine and other organizations; also, there is now the 'Journal of Prolotherapy' and web site: www.getprolo.com available.

The choice of which connective tissues to inject is determined by the patient's specific problem (Fig. 7.40). If alignment is being maintained, injections may be limited to those ligaments and tendons which are persistently tender. When the SI joint is involved, injection may be restricted to specific ligaments, depending on the presentation at hand (Box 7.8; Figs 2.4, 2.5, 3.62–3.68).

To stabilize any segment of the spine (Fig. 3.68), injection must include the supra- and interspinous ligaments and the facet joint ligaments and capsules one or two levels above and below the affected vertebra(e). In the thoracic segment, injection should include the costochondral junction as well as the costotransverse and costovertebral joints at the affected levels (Figs 2.94, 3.15, 3.16). Remember that injections for instability of the atlantoaxial and atlanto-occipital region and L4/L5/S1 vertebral levels should be done by someone with the expertise to work in these areas, preferably with ultrasound guidance or under fluoroscopy. Involvement of these sites is common and must be considered as a possible trigger for recurrence of pelvic malalignment.

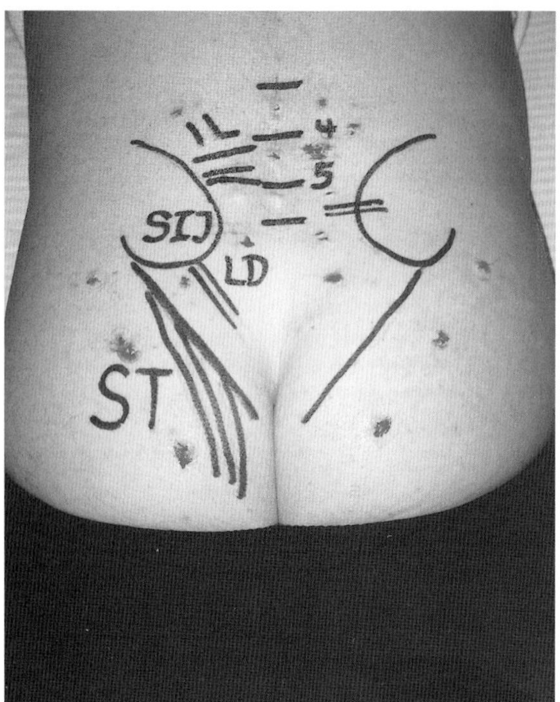

Fig. 7.40 Typical ligaments injected: IL, iliolumbar; SIJ, posterior sacroiliac joint; LD, long dorsal sacroiliac; ST, sacrotuberous; L4/L5/S1, lumbosacral level ligaments (facet joint, inter- and supraspinous ligaments). Injection at the sites demarcated by the black dots will allow one to reach the superficial and deep posterior pelvic ligaments with a 50 mm needle in most (see also Figs 2.4–2.6).

If the injection of tender superficial iliolumbar ligament insertions fails to bring relief, the pain may indicate involvement of the deep insertions (Fig. 2.4A). These, like the SI joints proper, are best injected under fluoroscopic visualization using a 7.5 cm needle or longer.

The coccyx tends to be the most tender site to inject. With recurrent coccygeal malalignment or instability, the ligaments inserting along the lateral borders, those running from the tip to the rectum and those crossing the posterior aspect of the sacrococcygeal and 1st inter-coccygeal joint should all be included (Figs 2.53A, 3.68)

The injections are usually well tolerated and can be carried out in a clinical setting. Some clinicians still like to carry out the procedure under intravenous sedation, perhaps just for the 1st injection to test the patient's response. Others proceed directly to injecting a small amount (about 0.2 cc) into multiple points of the fibro-osseous junction or the ligament itself. The author prefers to:

1. start with subcutaneous injections of a minute amount of 1% xylocaine at proposed entry points that overlie the length of the ligament, fibro-osseous junction or joint, to ease the discomfort that would otherwise be felt on the subsequent deeper injections; a 30 mm 25-gauge needle, though perhaps somewhat more uncomfortable than a 'pop gun' (Figs 7.40, 7.41), has been found to be much more effective

BOX 7.8 Injection for SI joint and symphysis pubis involvement

1. *Recurrent 'right inflare' in isolation*: right posterior SI joint, sacrotuberous, sacrospinous and long dorsal sacroiliac ligaments (Fig. 2.5A); adductor muscle origin from pubic tubercle
2. *Recurrent 'right outflare' in isolation*: iliolumbar, inguinal and anterior SI joint ligaments; also anterior symphysis pubis (SP) fibrocartilage and ligaments (Fig. 3.66)
3. *For right 'anteroposterior' rotational instability*: the above ligaments, also the interosseous, and ideally the anterior SI joint ligaments and capsule may be added by injection directly into the right SI joint (Figs 2.4, 7.42A)
4. *For a recurrent right SI joint 'upslip'* : right short/long dorsal sacroiliac and right lower posterior sacroiliac ligaments, biceps femoris origin (joined to sacrotuberous ligament in 75%; Fig. 2.6), SP
5. *For right 'craniocaudal' instability*: SP and anterior/posterior SI joint; iliaolumbar, sacrospinous, sacrotuberous and long/short dorsal sacroiliac ligaments
6. *For recurrent 'rotational malalignment' and/or 'upslip'* : injection can be limited to one side if there is evidence of unilateral SI joint laxity; however, if laxity is found bilaterally, if the 'anterior/posterior' rotation and/or 'upslip' keeps switching from one side to the other, or if there is the usually compensatory rotation of the contralateral innominate in the opposite direction, one should include the posterior pelvic ligaments bilaterally

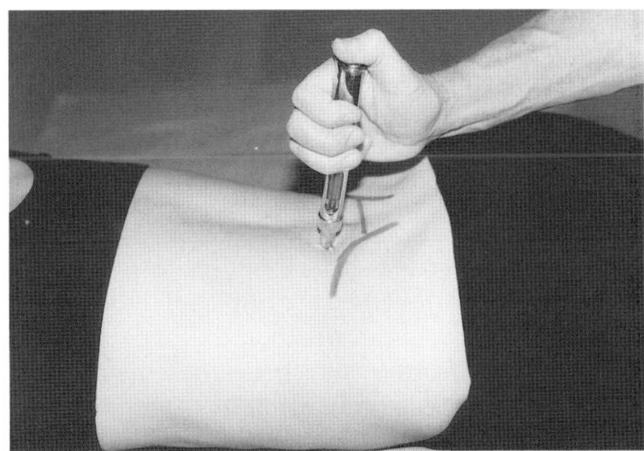

Fig. 7.41 'Pop' gun dermal anaesthetization of the needle entry sites, possibly supplemented with the injection of local anaesthetic into the deep subcutaneous tissue using a 25 mm 30-gauge needle, in order to minimize discomfort from the subsequent prolotherapy injection.

2. in 5–10 minutes, re-enter each of these sites, now to the full length of the needle, to make further injections of small amounts of xylocaine in a circular pattern with about a 2–2.5 cm diameter into the deep subcutaneous tissue overlying the ligament
3. give the injection with the proliferant solution 5–10 minutes later, using a needle suitable for reaching the site being injected (50 mm 25-gauge will do for most); the needle is advanced until it touches the bone/fibro-osseous junction, then withdrawn 1–2 mm and about 0.2 cc of the solution deposited - the procedure is repeated at the fibro-osseous junction and multiple points along the ligament itself
4. limit the 1st of the six injections to hypertonic glucose and xylocaine; if this is well tolerated, sodium morrhuate (the chemical irritant), is usually added to the subsequent injections

The time in-between the 3 steps outlined can be used for follow-up questions, writing notes, establishing if malalignment has recurred and, if so, performing a manual therapy technique (e.g. MET) to correct it.

Allergies and level of sensitivity will determine the exact components used. For example, some may require only 0.5%, others 1.5 or 2% xylocaine in the injection. The rare patient with a lower pain threshold or excessive pain is advised to take demerol 50 mg and gravol 50 mg one hour beforehand.

Following the injections, recommendations are to:

1. repeatedly apply ice for 10–20 minutes at a time, as needed, during the first day following an injection, to alleviate any immediate pain and swelling
2. keep active by walking about, in order to speed up the absorption and dispersion of the injected fluids and to prevent getting stiff
3. avoid planning any strenuous activity for the rest of the day
4. avoid using a bathtub or public swimming pool until the welts from the needle sites have healed over (usually within 2 or 3 days)
5. avoid any further irritation of the injected ligaments during the course of the injections by staying away from strenuous or jarring activities and those that put an excessive or prolonged stretch on these ligaments (e.g. deep squats, gardening, weight-lifting or simply lifting anything heavy or repeatedly)
6. avoid all anti-inflammatory medications during the course of injections, and for at least 2 weeks following the more widely spaced booster injections, given the persistence of the inflammatory phase for approximately 10–14 days after each injection (see above)
7. continue with exercises that 'work' the ligaments being injected in a reasonable manner along the natural lines of force, avoiding stretching or provoking pain; for example, following an injection of the lumbosacral and posterior pelvic ligaments, the patient is advised to do repeated easy sets of trunk flexion and extension to a comfortable end-of-range while standing, initially one set of 10, working up to 5 sets or a total of 50 repetitions each day

Short periods of gentle exercise, with frequent rests, seem to work best for most. Problems are often caused by overdoing things and suffering the consequences. Patients are frequently misled by the feeling of improvement that may follow an injection, which is most likely attributable to the time-limited effect of the local anaesthetic, with temporary muscle relaxation and decrease in discomfort.

Common sense and moderation are the key!

Reassessment for the effectiveness of a course of injections

Reassessment is carried out about 1.5-2 months after the last injection, by which time the reaction in the tissues, with formation of the immature collagen, will have largely subsided. As indicated above, by that time (some 4–5 months after the 1st injection) 60-70% will already show improved stability; this group breaks up into:

1. 20-30% in whom the ligament tenderness will have disappeared
2. 30-40% who now show only localized areas of ligament tenderness, rather than the more generalized involvement that was evident on initial examination (involving especially the posterior pelvic ligaments); for these patients, booster injections may be appropriate in an effort to eliminate any residual tenderness, instability or recurrence of malalignment, should that still be a problem
3. 30-40% who show only a partial or no improvement of the recurring malalignment, previously noted instability and tenderness.

People often expect a result from the prolotherapy injections within weeks and definitely by the time of this first reassessment. They usually need to be reminded that:

1. prolotherapy incites a process of collagen formation and subsequent maturation that goes on for over a year
2. they may not be aware of improved stability and strength for some months and maximal results may take 12–18 months to achieve
3. a clinician or therapist is more likely to be able to perceive any improvements, such as an increase in joint stability, before the person does and will tailor their course of treatment accordingly
4. significant improvement that occurs early on may be attributable to the effect of the local anaesthetic in decreasing pain, relaxing muscles, breaking muscle spasm, and possibly desensitizing nerves

> Prolotherapy initiates a course of tissue healing. However, improvements in strength and stability may not be evident for several months and people need to be encouraged by being reminded of this aspect of the treatment.

In 20-30% of those who have undergone a full course of injections, there will also be persistence of the previously-noted generalized ligament tenderness. They may report some temporary beneficial effect which often does not occur until several days after the injection, some time after the local anaesthetic has actually worn off. In these cases, it may be worthwhile initiating a second course of six injections spaced 2 weeks apart, or proceeding directly to 3 boosters spaced a month apart, followed by another reassessment within 2 months after the last injection. By this time, feedback from the therapists may indicate whether they have noticed any increase in stability of a previously unstable SI joint or vertebral complex. This feedback is helpful in deciding whether the patient might derive benefit from further boosters limited to the site of residual instability, combined with ongoing attempts to maintain alignment. Typical is a recurrent rotation of T12/L1, the mid-thoracic or any of the lower lumbar vertebra(e) that irritates musculoskeletal tissue and can also result in recurrence of pelvic malalignment.

Some patients return for a few 'booster' injection several months or a year or more after the previous course of injections. They have seemingly had a good result that lasted some time but now appears to be 'wearing off'. This problem is sometimes attributable to a recurrence of the malalignment. However, these patients may actually be in alignment now, with just some residual tenderness of the posterior pelvic ligaments. These 'repeaters' usually respond well to another short course of three injections, only to return again some time in the future for yet another possible 'booster'. Others seem to do well with 1, 2 or 3 boosters on a regular basis, spaced 4–6 months apart, similar to a 'maintenance dose'. If there is a physiological aspect to their ongoing problem, possibilities to consider include:

1. their ligaments contain inadequate collagen so that they tend to be generally weaker, but they do respond symptomatically to intermittent prolotherapy injections, perhaps by increasing collagen production and boosting strength for a few weeks or months
2. they have a congenital collagen disease and joint hypermobility; Ehler-Danlos would be an extreme presentation
3. the healing response in their ligaments is either inadequate or has been interfered with by intermittent excessive demands imposed on the ligaments

Side-effects and complications

The most common side-effect is the temporary increase in pain caused by the injection. This usually lasts no more than 1 or 2 days but in some can go on for a week, in which case one might consider increasing the interval between the injections to 2 or 3 weeks if that seems to be in the patient's best interest. Other, less frequently encountered problems include:

1. fainting, usually because of transient hypotension and bradycardia triggered by stimulation of a vasovagal attack
2. allergy to the local anaesthetic, cod liver oil or other component (including one case that seemingly narrowed down to the hyperosmolar 'glucose'; see below)
3. bleeding and bruising from the puncture of a subcutaneous vessel
4. referred pain from the transiently damaged and distended tissue
5. infection of the injection site
6. pneumothorax following injection in the thoracic region.

In a survey carried out by Dorman (1993), a total of 66 'minor' and 14 'major' complications were reported by 95 practitioners on a patient pool of 494,845 treated with prolotherapy. 'Major' was defined either as requiring hospitalization or having transient or permanent nerve damage. The conclusion was that the risk-to-benefit analysis for prolotherapy indicated a low complication rate. Allergy to cod liver oil can be established by having the patient take two or three B12 or Omega-3 capsules on a day sometime prior to starting the injections. In the author's practice, the one apparent reaction to the 'hyperosmolar glucose' solution most likely involved a preservative (although the pharmacist insisted there were none used).

Other applications for prolotherapy

Prolotherapy injections are appropriate for the treatment of any accessible ligament, capsule or tendon that is a problem on account of laxity, pain, or chronic inflammation. Prolotherapy has, for example, proved effective in:

1. increasing the stability of:
   a. subluxing or repeatedly dislocating shoulder joint(s), especially when surgery is no longer an option, or there is chronic shoulder pain (Hauser & Hauser 2009)
   b. ankles prone to recurrent sprains, when ligament laxity is evident
   c. wrists (e.g. the ligaments of a subluxing carpal bone)
2. strengthening lax cruciate or collateral knee ligaments in patients who are not candidates for surgery (Ongley et al. 1988, Hauser 2004)
3. the treatment of:
   a. chronically inflamed ligaments and tendons, especially when a trial with oral anti-inflammatories and 2 or 3 spaced peripheral cortisone injections has failed
   b. enthesopathies, such as chronic 'tennis elbow'
4. subluxing acromioclavicular or sternoclavicular joint, symphysis pubis or rib (e.g. costochondral junction), especially if these are symptomatic and/or getting worse

CASE HISTORY 7.3

A woman, 7 months post-partum, suffered a shear injury of her left sacroiliac joint in a motor vehicle accident in which her car was rear-ended and subsequently pushed into the car ahead. Her feet were braced on the floor in anticipation of both impacts. A failure to respond to ongoing attempts at realignment and strengthening of the 'inner' and 'outer' pelvic units was eventually attributed to persistent ligament laxity, maximal in the craniocaudal (vertical) plane.

Active left straight leg raising (using the method current at that time) was restricted to 50 degrees compared to 70 on the right (Figs 2.128, 2.129). 'Form' closure augmented by compression of the SI joints with pressure on the sides of the innominates increased her ability to transfer forces through the hip girdle so that left straight leg raising came to match the 70 degrees on the right. An attempt to increase 'force' closure by recruiting the right anterior oblique system (right external and internal abdominal obliques connected to the left adductors by way of the anterior abdominal fascia) was effected with pressure against her right shoulder to resist her attempt to do an oblique sit-up. This manoeuvre decreased her left straight leg raising to 40 degrees, possibly by decreasing or shutting off contraction in the 'inner' unit.

The findings were consistent with a lack of 'form' closure caused by ligament disruption; this could not be overcome by an attempt at augmenting force closure.

Recommendations were for:

1. having her use a cane in the right hand to decrease weight-bearing through the left SI joint
2. prolotherapy injections to strengthen the left ligaments that control vertical joint displacement
3. a decreased emphasis on exercises aimed at augmenting 'force' closure until 'form' closure had been improved with prolotherapy.

INJECTION OF CONNECTIVE TISSUE: CORTISONE VERSUS PROLOTHERAPY

Ligaments, especially the posterior pelvic ligaments, may continue to be acutely tender even though realignment has been successfully maintained. This ongoing tenderness relates, in part, to:

1. the severity of the ligament injury: typical of these is a sprain or strain seen in association with a shear injury of the SI joint (Fig 2.51B)
2. the amount of movement and weight-transfer through the area involved
3. the length of time that the malalignment has been present

In those patients who present with malalignment and a history of pain of recent onset (e.g. within the past 2–3 months), the ligament tenderness almost always disappears spontaneously within a matter of days or weeks following realignment. When malalignment has been present for years (e.g. with onset of symptoms sometimes relating back to a fall or to a complicated delivery some years or even decades ago) it may take up to 1 or 2 years for the ligaments to heal and the pain to finally settle down.

It is sometimes a low-grade inflammatory response that is the main cause of the ongoing ligament pain, in which case a course of oral anti-inflammatory medication may be worth trying initially. If that fails, and as long as the person is maintaining alignment, a trial with cortisone injections is warranted. In these cases:

1. if there is no improvement after one or two injections of cortisone spaced 2–3 weeks apart
   - the author prefers to proceed with a course of prolotherapy injections, which can both decrease the pain and strengthen these structures
2. if there is some improvement with one or two cortisone injections, repeat injections are carried out, but these are limited to any remaining sites of tenderness still evident at the time of each reassessment (spaced about 2–3 weeks apart)
3. once the area of tenderness noted on initial examination has been reduced to about 10-20%:
   a. any residual tenderness will usually resolve on its own
   b. in most, this goal is achieved after four or five visits, at most
4. if alignment is still being maintained on reassessment 3 months after the last cortisone injection, and overall there has been a further improvement but the person is still symptomatic and there is evidence of areas of localized tenderness
   - it should be safe by then to initiate another short course of 1 to 3 cortisone injections, limited to these persistently tender sites (the sacrotuberous origin and coccygeal ligaments are the most likely to be involved)

OTHER TYPES OF INJECTION

Pain arising from any structure can predispose to a recurrence of malalignment if it creates asymmetrical torquing forces by altering movement patterns, or precipitates an asymmetrical reflex contraction of muscles in the immediate vicinity in an attempt to decrease movement at the site of origin. Therefore, every effort should be made to assuage the painful site. The following are some other injection treatments to consider.

Injection of trigger points

Settling down the trigger point(s) with a local anaesthetic may achieve temporary relaxation of the muscle(s) to allow for a more productive treatment session and possible realignment when carried out during the 2–3 hours following the injection.

Injection of tender tendons, capsules and fascia

Cortisone may quickly settle inflammation. The fact that it also weakens connective tissue structures by disrupting the cross-linking of collagen fibres precludes injection directly into a tendon for fear of rupture. This same feature, however, makes it useful for injection into tight and tender fascia and scar tissue, to help loosen up these sites in conjunction with deep massage and stretching. If pain persists or recurs after one or two cortisone injections around a tendon or into a capsule, consider initiating a course of prolotherapy injections instead.

Injection of tense or tender muscle

Temporarily decreasing muscle tension or breaking up muscle spasm with an injection of a short-acting local anaesthetic into the motor point(s), multiple points in the muscle mass itself, or around the nerve supplying that muscle may interrupt the vicious cycle that can occur with any increase in tension or actual spasm causing more pain and perpetuating the abnormal increase in tone. Arrangements should be made so that the injections are followed by deep massage and stretching within the next 1 or 2 hours, while the anaesthetic is still active.

Botulinum-A toxin injection into the muscle affects its nerve supply and causes the muscle to relax (Childers et al. 2006). Unfortunately, the muscle may play a crucial role, directly in helping maintain the function of a joint or joints, or indirectly as part of a sling and/or a sequential contraction of muscles that, by acting together, ensure joint stability (see Ch. 2; Figs 2.35-2.40). Following the injection, the painful, hypertonic muscle can end up hypotonic and 'weak' for some weeks, making it temporarily unsuitable to function in this role.

Injection of the sacroiliac joint(s)

If injection of the posterior pelvic ligaments brings only partial or no relief, if SI joint stress tests are positive, and especially if there is a history of a shear injury, consider injecting the SI joint(s) proper (Fig. 7.42A). One may not be able to pinpoint the painful structure on examination because it is hard to stress the joint surfaces without simultaneously irritating the ligaments and capsule, or even the nearby hip joint (see Ch. 2; Figs 2.103-2.112). A bone scan may help to narrow the differential by showing increased activity limited to the SI joint (e.g. osteoarthritis, sacroiliitis) and may prove abnormal for several months to a year following injury to bone.

If the first injection dramatically reduces or eliminates the pain but only temporarily, the block may have to be repeated two or three times for an adequate trial of therapy. Common approaches to SI joint injection being used (Adrian 2009; Aprill 1992; Bernard & Cassidy 1991; Derby 1986; Haldeman & Soto-Hall 1983) include:

1. *direct joint injection, with contrast* (Fig. 7.42A)
   - this should decrease or eliminate pain from all joint structures because it will also anaesthetize the branches of the lumbosacral plexus from L3 to S2 that innervate the anterior joint capsule

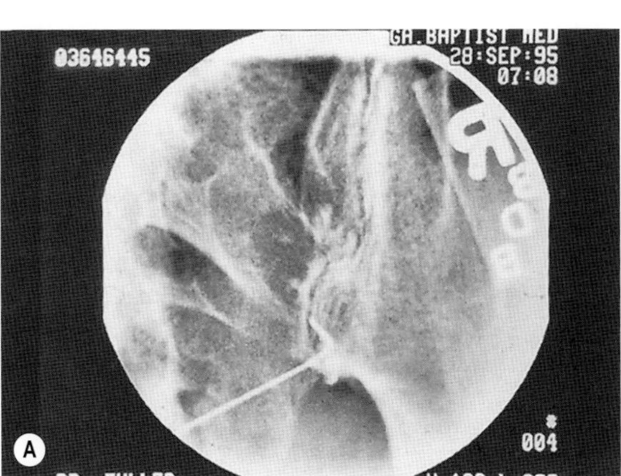

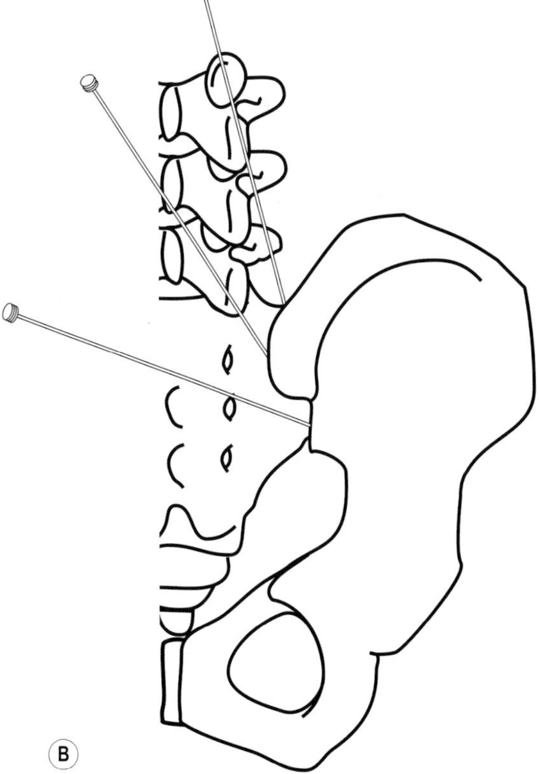

Fig. 7.42 Injection of the sacroiliac joint. (A) Direct joint injection: the position of a needle in the nexus of the ilium and sacrum is verified on fluoroscopy in preparation for sacroiliac joint arthrogram or arthrodesis (B) Needle placement for blocking the posterior primary rami that innervate the sacroiliac joint. *(Courtesy of Keating et al. 1997a.)*

2. *blocking of the posterior primary rami* (Fig. 7.42B)
   - these supply the posterior ligamentous portion of the joint; the block will not anaesthetize the anterior joint capsule

Blocks of any other sites of localized pain

Disc bulging or protrusion, foraminal stenosis and facet joint degenerative changes are some of the sites that may be suspected of causing asymmetric muscle tension and irritation or actual inflammation of nerve roots. Blocks of such specific sites can help sort out which of these, if any, actually present a problem.

Neural therapy

This technique is aimed at the chronic pain from nerve irritation which, unfortunately, is often a part of the 'malalignment syndrome', especially when the problems caused by the malalignment and/or additional insults (e.g. previous trauma or surgery) have been present for some time. Pain is reduced by injecting local anaesthetic into autonomic ganglia, peripheral nerves, scars, glands, acupuncture points and trigger points, as well as directly into tender tissues. With the decrease in pain, there is often an immediate improvement in the range of motion and ability to use and strengthen muscles, something that may increase the chance of achieving and maintaining realignment.

TREATMENT OF INTERNAL STRUCTURES

Recurrent pelvic malalignment and ongoing pain can be the result of malalignment of the sacrococcygeal joint and/or pelvic floor dysfunction, with chronic tension and, at times, trigger point formation in the pelvic floor musculature and internal ligaments. Especially likely to be involved are the levator ani muscle complex and the sacrospinous and sacrococcygeal ligaments (Figs 2.19, 2.53, 3.64, 3.65, 3.68, 4.15, 4.44). Tenderness is easily confirmed by palpation of these structures per rectum or vagina. Treatment consists of:

1. realignment of the sacrococcygeal joint and any intercoccygeal joint(s) involved
2. external massage and stretching of the tender soft tissue structures immediately alongside the coccyx (see Ch. 4)
3. internal massage of the coccygeal structures and gentle, repetitive stretching of the tense and tender pelvic floor musculature and ligaments (using a rectal or vaginal approach; Fig. 2.53B) for persistent tightness and/or tenderness
4. biofeedback, using: sensors in the rectum, vagina or both (to teach pelvic floor strengthening and relaxation routines); awareness of inspiration/expiration rhythms; information obtained on Real-Time US or RTUS; surface sensory EMG pads, or simply touch
5. ongoing efforts at correcting pelvic and spine malalignment
6. the possible addition of visceral manipulation

> The treatment of pelvic floor dysfunction often reveals that there is an associated problem involving the internal viscera.

Typical of these is a tightness, adhesion or scarring of visceral ligaments that interfere with the proper function of the bowel and can precipitate viscerosomatic reflexes (see Ch. 4; Fig. 4.43). In addition to tackling the malalignment and pelvic floor dysfunction, visceral manipulation may be required in order to finally resolve the problems typically associated with involvement of these internal structures: episodic diarrhoea, urinary frequency, urgency, nocturia, coccydynia, vaginal wall pain, dyspareunia and stress incontinence.

The discussion that follows focuses on the diagnosis and treatment of pelvic floor dysfunction, reference being made to Barral (1989, 1993) and Barral & Mercier (1988) regarding visceral manipulation, as well as to the discussion in Ch. 4.

DIAGNOSTIC AND TREATMENT AIDS FOR PELVIC FLOOR DYSFUNCTION

Kegel (1948) advocated a 'physiological' treatment for poor tone and function of the genital muscles and for urinary stress incontinence. He developed a set of exercises aimed at improving the tone of the pelvic floor muscles, especially pubococcygeus (Fig. 2.53).

In an attempt to obtain an objective measure of pelvic floor tension, Kegel invented the 'perineometer', which is basically a rectal/vaginal probe linked to a manometer. It proved helpful for giving patients feedback on how to contract these muscles appropriately and for allowing them to document any improvement in strength. Perry modified this with the addition of an electromyography (EMG) monitor to give simultaneous objective pressure measurements and an EMG read-out. This unit, the PerryMeter, has been used successfully for biofeedback (Craig 1992; Perry et al. 1988; Selby 1990). Using this device, patients are trained to appreciate when the pelvic floor muscles are over- or underactive and what they need to do to relax or contract them, respectively. Perry & Hullett (1990) also reported a high success rate in the treatment of stress incontinence using the PerryMeter in conjunction with Kegel's pelvic exercises.

Wallace (1994) advocated a combined approach to pelvic floor dysfunction in patients that included simultaneous correction of any SI joint malalignment and pelvic floor strengthening exercises using Femina cones of gradually increasing weight. 'Accommodators' of variable size will have a similar effect and allow for treatment of primary and secondary vulvovestibulodynia by increasing the ability of the vagina to accept and retain objects of increasing size without triggering painful reflex contraction of pelvic floor muscles. The tendency of a vaginal cone to slip out with the pull of gravity provides the patient with immediate feedback on which muscles to contract in order to retain the cone and thereby helps to strengthen the appropriate pelvic floor muscles. Cones may be more helpful for someone living in a rural area, where other feedback options may not be available. Possible drawbacks include that the patient may inadvertently use a cone of the wrong size or the cone comes to lie sideways, causing more irritation and tensing of muscles.

Emphasis at present is on:

1. retraining to relax the pelvic floor muscles
   a. the phase includes sensing any increase in tension, especially recurrence of spasm
   b. it may call on learning to generating a partial to full (30-100%) voluntary contraction against a probe, with feedback from an internal surface EMG sensor (or external surface-EMG pads, if an internal one is not tolerated)
2. strengthening routines, aimed at all muscle fibres, by generation of:
   a. a fast contraction, aimed at engaging fast-twitch fibres to develop speed
   b. a gradually increasing contraction, held for a longer period and aimed at activating slow-twitch fibres, to develop endurance
3. retraining of the memory patterns needed for muscle contraction and relaxation
   - this can be achieved using feedback with simultaneous surface-EMG and may be significantly improved by providing the patient with a printout of the EMG to use for home training and to learn to recognize any improvements (Wells 2009).

The use of RTUS for diagnostic purposes and feedback has been discussed in Ch. 4 (Figs 4.46, 4.47).

Treatment: non-invasive techniques

Non-invasive approaches include the frictioning and deep pressure release advocated by Selby (1990), the correction of any pelvic and spine malalignment, acupressure, myofascial release of the soft tissues inserting into the lateral aspect of the sacrum and coccyx, deep psoas and piriformis release, and the use of electrical modalities (e.g. laser, ultrasound, transcutaneous electrical nerve stimulation or TENS) over the coccyx and adjacent soft tissue structures. Kegel exercises, biofeedback approaches and use of cones or accommodators all help to ensure that the patient is actually contracting the pelvic floor muscles (rather than the intra-abdominal muscles, by mistake). Acupuncture and deep needling in the area of piriformis and the greater sciatic foramen, while 'invasive', are best mentioned in this connection.

Non-invasive techniques must also include the following:

Instruction regarding proper sitting postures

The emphasis is on shifting weight-bearing onto the ischial tuberosities by restoring the lumbar lordosis (sitting upright with use of a lumbar roll, Obus form or other supportive seating; Fig. 3.69). Weight-bearing on the sacrum or coccyx must be minimized by not slouching and not sitting for prolonged periods on hard or soft furniture or in bucket seats.

Instruction regarding proper clothing

Tight underwear, thongs and clothing material that will not stretch readily (e.g. jeans), also seamed clothing, are best avoided to decrease any direct pressure on the coccygeal and genital (vulvovestibular, testicular) regions to avoid needless irritation which could trigger a reflex increase in pelvic floor tone, if not outright discomfort or pain.

Coccygeal relief cushion

Doughnut cushions should be avoided:

1. while the ischial tuberosities may now be bearing weight as intended, they do end up on top of a rounded surface and can, therefore, shift off to the inside or outside more easily, at risk of decreasing seating stability
2. they let the sacrum and coccyx sag down into the centre hole, which increases tension on the muscles and ligaments of the pelvic floor that attach to these structures, some of which are often already tender; at worst, the coccyx may end up:
   a. actually bearing some weight directly, or
   b. being submitted to pressure posteriorly or from one or both sides by chafing against the inner aspect of the cushion, something that is more likely to occur if the coccyx is fixed in excessive 'extension angulation' (Fig. 4.44B)

Preferable would be a cushion that prevents any weight-bearing on the coccyx but instead bears it all on the ischial tuberosities and posterior thighs. An appropriate coccygeal pillow is usually made out of firm foam about 5 to 10 cm thick. It has a cut-out in the centre of the posterior edge, either square (approximately 10 cm along each edge), rectangular or triangular in shape (Fig. 7.43A). The cut-out accommodates the coccyx; it may be left open (which invites inward collapse of the edges), simply be filled with a piece of soft foam or the foam that was cut out and shredded to re-use for this purpose. The firm part of the pillow to either side provides

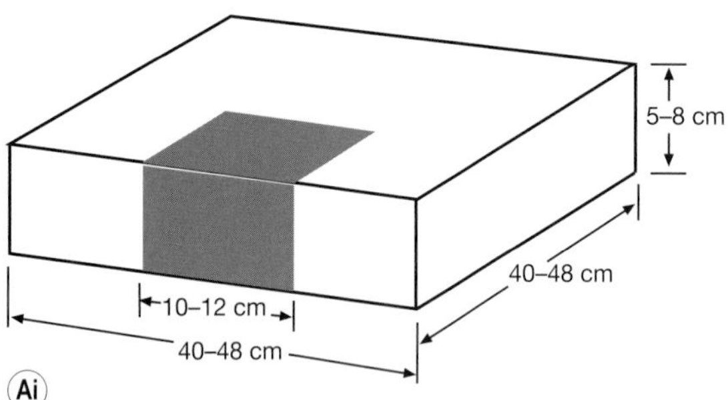

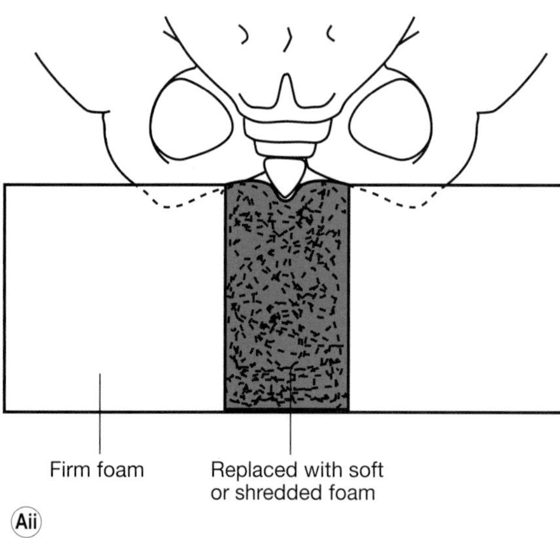

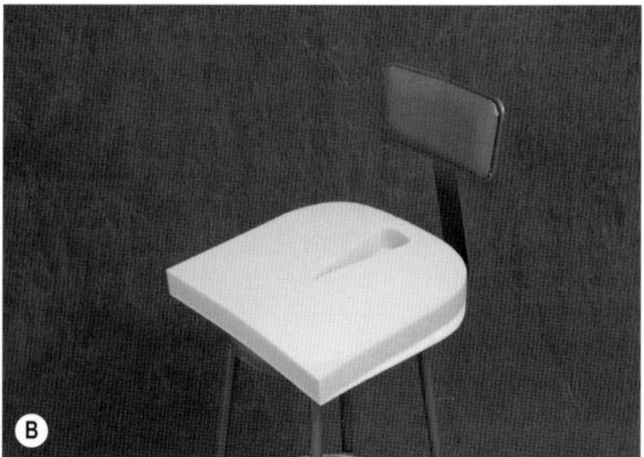

Fig. 7.43 Coccygeal relief pillow designs (see also Fig. 5.6B,C). (A). Drawing of uniform piece of foam with square cut-out; (i) posterolateral and (ii) posterior views. (B) Photo: base of firm, tapered foam (to shift weight-bearing forward from the coccyx, onto the ischial tuberosities and thighs), covered with a thick piece of memory foam (Boydhealthworks™.)

support for the ischial tuberosities, where weight-bearing should occur. A more functional design by Jan Boyd PT uses a square piece of firm foam as a base (Fig. 7.43B). On top lies a piece of memory foam, which can recover more quickly and completely after having been deformed on bearing weight. The piece of firm foam is also tapered toward the front, causing the pelvis to gently lean forward in order to shift weight-bearing away from the coccyx and more onto the ischial tuberosities and posterior aspect of the thighs. The coccygeal relief cut-out, while running through both sections, is completely surrounded by foam around its perimeter to help counter any collapse of the edges.

A home exercise programme

In addition to getting involved in a self-assessment and self-treatment regimen and, if possible, use of home biofeedback techniques to help relearn contraction/relaxation of pelvic floor muscle, exercises appropriate for the problem at hand are another vital key to recovery:

1. pelvic floor laxity
   - traditional Kegel exercises to strengthen the pelvic floor muscles, supplemented with biofeedback and other methods (e.g. intravaginal cones), can be used
2. pelvic floor hypertonicity
   - the emphasis is on relaxation exercises, including deep rhythmic abdominal breathing and visualization; muscle tightening is used only to 'get in touch' with how it feels to hold tension and to learn how to release this tension
3. pelvic instability
   - pelvic core strengthening exercises are prescribed

Treatment: invasive techniques

> The results using the non-invasive techniques may, unfortunately, be only temporary. It is sometimes not until one resorts to an invasive technique that one can finally achieve mobilization of the sacrococcygeal articulation and/or resolution of the pelvic floor dystonia, with resultant improvement.

Subsequent reintroduction of the non-invasive techniques may then help to ensure that the gains established with the invasive techniques will be maintained and that the malalignment will not keep on recurring.

Invasive techniques can reach the pelvic floor structures, also the symphysis pubis, sacrococcygeal and anterior SI joint, by way of either the rectum or the vagina. The rectal approach is sometimes not feasible because of personal preference, marked and/or painful spasm of the anal sphincter, anal fissures or other pathology. The vaginal approach has been felt to be superior by some (Barral & Mercier 1988; Selby 1990; Craig 1992; Barral 1993). It is usually more comfortable and allows the therapist to reach more of the pelvic floor musculature than would be possible using the rectal approach (Fig. 2.53B). Unfortunately, issues relating to professional ethics and medicolegal considerations may prohibit using this approach.

SURGERY

Surgery does play an important role in the treatment of problems caused by malalignment. However, more often the diagnosis of malalignment has, unfortunately, been missed, and unwarranted surgery undertaken in an attempt to rid the patient of symptoms that might well have responded simply to realignment.

SURGICAL FUSION

Patients with recurrent malalignment who fail to respond to the conservative course of treatment outlined above may be candidates for immobilization in a final attempt to gain relief from chronic pain attributable to an unstable vertebral complex or recurrent malalignment involving the SI joints and/or symphysis pubis. They are often those with generalized joint hypermobility or who have developed instability and ongoing pain as a result of ligament laxity or development of SI joint osteoarthritis. Before considering surgical immobilization, one must be absolutely certain of several factors (Box 7.9).

The very nature of the surgery may mean that a worker cannot return to a physically demanding job, or an athlete to his or her sport, for at least 6–12 months to allow for complete healing without complications.

Immobilization of a vertebral complex

Immobilization of a vertebral complex puts increased stress on the disc and facet joints immediately above and below the level(s) of fusion and

BOX 7.9 Factors to assess before contemplating surgery

The pain definitely arises from the structure considered for fusion

In the case of the sacroiliac joint, for example, there should be a dramatic temporary decrease or abolition of the pain following the injection of local anaesthetic into the joint. In addition to joint blocks, some surgeons have also had their patient undergo a 2-week trial with an external 'fixator' device (Fig. 7.44) in an attempt to establish whether or not fusion would really be helpful (Sturesson et al. 1999).

The patient has complied fully with all recommendations and the conservative approach has definitely failed

Unfortunately, patients who have 'failed' the conservative course of treatment are frequently also those who have compromised the results of that approach. Their inability to comply with the treatment programme to date only increases the chance that they are likely to compromise the outcome of a surgical procedure as well. These are typically the patients who:

1. prematurely attempt a return to work or some sport that repeatedly loads the SI joints asymmetrically (e.g. jogging), results in a torsional stress or an excessive load transfer through the lumbo-pelvic-hip region and, hence, the site considered for fusion
2. repeatedly exceed the amount of exercise that they are able to tolerate without precipitating pain, a reflex tightening of the muscles and recurrence of the malalignment

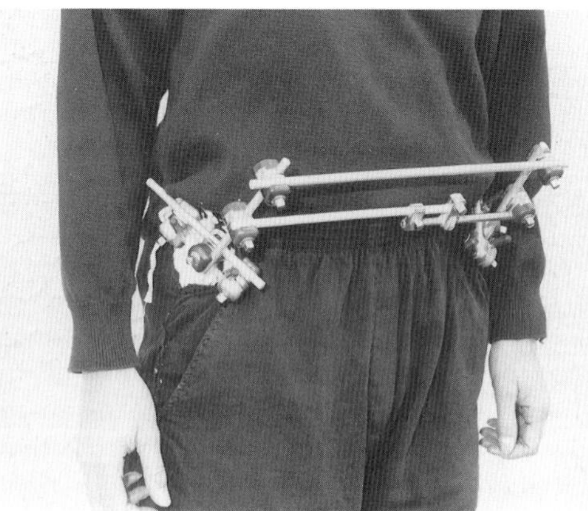

Fig. 7.44 An external 'fixator device' that has been used preoperatively to determine whether subsequent sacroiliac joint fusion is likely to relieve the pain, and postoperatively to increase chances that fusion will occur.

predisposes them to earlier development of degenerative change. These factors may preclude return to a job or sport that repeatedly loads the spine, especially if loading is accompanied by torsional stresses (e.g. lifting combined with reaching and bending).

Immobilization of the sacroiliac joints

The immobilization of one or both SI joints impairs the normal reciprocal movement that occurs in these joints during the gait cycle, with a loss of the normal shearing motion that facilitates weight transfer and helps to dissipate any residual shock from the ground forces transmitted up through the legs and hips. The hip joint, lumbosacral junction and lower lumbar spine are subjected to increased stresses because they now have to accommodate for the loss of movement at the fused SI joint(s).

For these reasons, SI joint immobilization may preclude a return to a job or sport in which an impairment of stride length, shock absorption and the ability to deal with torsional stresses can easily result in acute or long-term detrimental effects (e.g. construction, plumbing, jogging, high-impact aerobics, gymnastics).

Immobilization of the symphysis pubis

Immobilization of the symphysis pubis will also impair the reciprocal movement of the SI joints. Bone grafting with the introduction of a bone plug is likely to lead to new problems, especially when malalignment already affects all three joints of the pelvic ring. By separating the pubic bones at the symphysis, the plug causes an outflaring of both innominates with an anterior opening of the SI joints and stretching of the anterior capsule, and a posterior closing with compression of the posterior joint margins. The overall effect is to increase stress on the SI joints and to impair their movement and weight-transfer function. These stresses may eventually aggravate pre-existing pain or cause pain in SI joints that were previously asymptomatic. Fusing the symphysis pubis while it is in a displaced position because of an 'upslip' or a 'rotational malalignment' being present will defeat any attempts to correct the malalignment subsequently (Figs 2.42, 2.75, 2.76 C, 2.102A, 3.65, 3.86D)

SI JOINT ARTHRODESIS AND FUSION

SI joint arthrodesis combined with fusion, rather than fusion alone, has been advocated for patients who have failed conservative treatment. The majority have SI joint dysfunction attributed to postpartum instability, previous trauma or transitional SI joint instability following solid lumbosacral fusion (Kurica 1995). Percutaneous posterior screw fixation is carried out as an outpatient procedure in some clinics. Lippitt (1995) has been a long-time advocate of a technique that not only involves immobilization by combining arthrodesis with fusion bilaterally but also tries to avoid the detrimental effects of malalignment. He made the following observations regarding:

Unilateral 1-screw fixation

Patients who had previously undergone a unilateral one-screw fixation frequently presented with a recurrence of the pain after a year or so (Fig. 7.45A); the history and clinical examination usually indicated that ongoing rotatory/torsional effects had resulted in laxity or even fracture of that screw.

Unilateral 2-screw fixation

This procedure was also found unacceptable as it still resulted in increased asymmetrical mechanical stresses on these screws as well as on the opposite, still mobile SI joint.

Therefore, recommendations from his clinic have been for:

Bilateral 2-screw fixation to complement a lumbosacral fusion

This operation is intended for patients who had previously undergone a lumbosacral fusion and, as a consequence suffered increased stresses through the hip and SI joints bilaterally (Fig. 7.45B).

Combined bilateral SI joint arthrodesis and bony fusion

1. This is now the preferred approach.
2. The bone plugs are usually harvested from the posterior iliac crest(s) and inserted at the lumbosacral junction (i.e. sacral sulcus) to complement the arthrodesis (bilateral 2-screw fixation) with fusion of the upper SI joint.
3. To ensure the results of the surgery, there is constant monitoring during and after the procedure with:
   a. ***simultaneous monitoring of neurological function***

      This consists primarily of ongoing nerve conduction studies, with side-to-side comparison, usually using transmission of somatosensory evoked potentials (SSEPs)

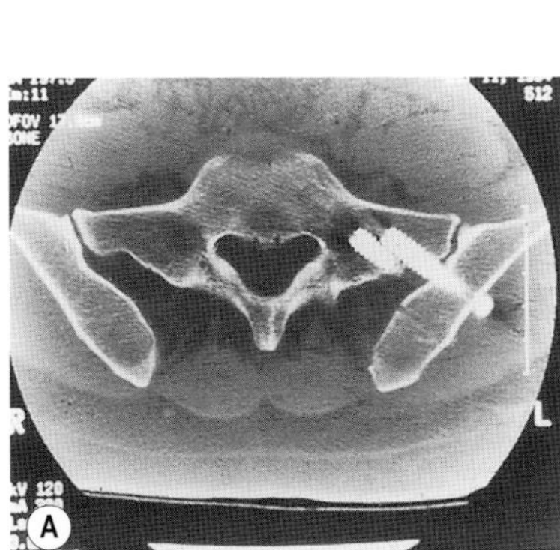

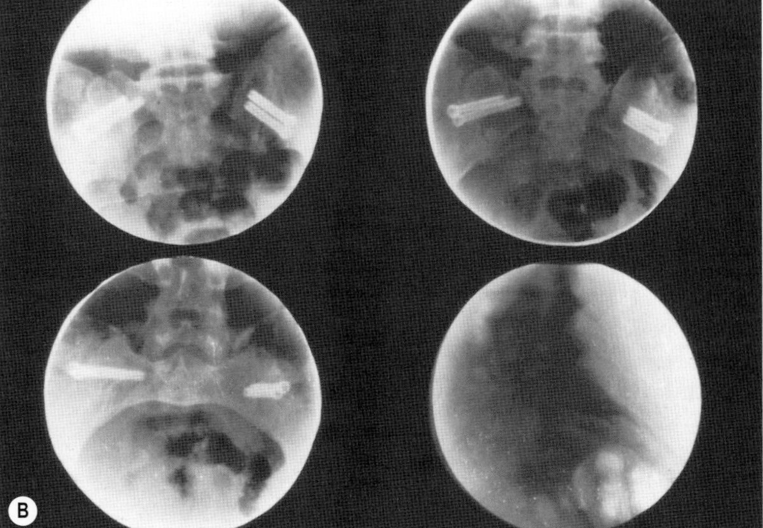

Figure 7.45 Surgical fixation of the sacroiliac joint. (A) Unilateral screw arthrodesis: postoperative computed tomography scan checking screw placement. (B) Bilateral screw fixation (with two screws bilaterally). *(Courtesy of Keating et al. 1997b.)*

from the lower extremities. These are transmitted through the lumbosacral plexus, up the spinal cord to the cerebral cortex; comparison side-to-side and to normal latencies allows for early detection of any compromise of the lumbopelvic plexus, individual peripheral nerves and/or their blood supply.

b. ***repeated assessment of the patient's pelvic alignment***
A physiotherapist skilled in manual therapy is present to ensure the patient is in alignment to start and to carry out immediate correction of any intra-operative recurrence. This measure is to avoid the situation where the patient underwent a successful SI joint immobilization but ended up having been fused with the pelvis and spine out of alignment so that, post-operatively, the legs, hips and spine continue to be subjected to the abnormal biomechanical stresses resulting with both the fusion and the malalignment, indefinitely (see 'Immobilization of symphysis pubis', above).

Post-operative course

The patient's activities are severely restricted for the first three months, with no weight-bearing, use of a wheelchair, and assisted transfers. Regular assessments are in order to rule out and correct a post-operative occurrence of an 'outflare' and/or 'inflare' or even 'rotational malalignment', all of which are possible until fusion is actually taking place. X-rays at three months may not show any evidence of healing, in which case a CAT and bone scan may be helpful to see if there is any indication of new bone formation. If early healing is evident, graduation to a walker and return to minimal physiotherapy sessions and a pool may be possible. Otherwise, the above restrictions continue to apply until repeat medical imaging at 6, 9 or 12 months finally shows that healing with fusion is taking place.

Failure of healing or return of the previous instability may occur as a result of laxity of one or more screws, failure of bony fusion, muscle spasm triggered by pain, or instability of L4/L5 or the pelvis, occasionally with recurrence of malalignment. In that case, conservative attempts to regain stability may again be tried initially: return to using a wheelchair and/or 4-wheel walker to off-load the opperative site, use of an SI belt, and/or a further one or two courses of prolotherapy injections to strengthen the surrounding ligaments. If these measures fail, or there is a definite indication of failure of bone fusion and/or instability of one or more screws, the surgical procedure may have to be repeated on the side(s) involved (see 'Case History 7.4').

CASE HISTORY 7.4

In 2000, a 40 year-old store manager slipped off a small step ladder while reaching to stock shelves. She landed straight on the left foot and then rolled and fell onto her left side. Acute left hip girdle and groin pain evolved into a chronic problem of right and/or left lumbosacral pain, radiating intermittently to the posterior thigh and occasionally also to a patch on the calf or down to the ankle. This variable pattern was in keeping with referral from the sacrotuberous and sacrospinous ligaments (Fig. 4.10). Symptoms and examination findings were in keeping with recurrent malalignment: sometimes an 'upslip', 'outflare/inflare', 'rotational malalignment', or various combinations of these. She responded to physiotherapy measures including realignment, also two courses of prolotherapy, with gradually increasing stability, strength and endurance and significant decrease in pain. Unfortunately, despite the fact that symptoms had not yet resolved completely, the employer and Workers' Compensation Board pressured her into returning to an 'office-type job', primarily desk work. Within weeks, lack of staff for health and maternity reasons saw her back stocking shelves. 3–4 months later, previous pain patterns became more intense and the pelvis more unstable, with frequent L4/L5 rotational displacement triggering muscle spasm and recurrence of pelvic malalignment. She failed to respond to a year of conservative treatment, with instability noted primarily in the left SI joint. Bilateral two-screw SI joint fixation and ilio-sacral bone-plug fusion early in 2004 were successful on the left side. However, within 6 months there was recurrence of 'right outflare' and eventually also 'right anterior' rotation. Repeat right CAT and MRI studies at 9 months showed no evidence of healing. She underwent a repeat surgical prodecure on that side which healed without complication. She went through a successful rehabilitation programme and was able to return to her former activities within a year.

UNWARRANTED SURGICAL INTERVENTIONS

Following are examples of some problems that end up being treated surgically because of a failure to realize that malalignment, rather than the condition that has been diagnosed, is the primary cause of the symptoms and signs.

Disc problems: bulging, protrusion and herniation

Disc bulging, protrusion and even frank herniation are not infrequently noted on imaging of symptomatic and asymptomatic populations alike (Kieffer et al. 1984; Klein et al. 1993; Jensen et al. 1994; Magora & Schwarz 1976; Weishaupt et al. 1998). This finding is likely to take on more significance if there are also:

1. referred sensory symptoms, some of which appear to fall within the dermatome pattern of the suspected compressed root (Figs 3.12, 3.46, 3.62, 3.63, 3.67, 4.10, 5.38)
2. weak muscles, some of which lie within the anterior myotome of that root (Figs 3.53-3.55).

A right lateral disc bulge or protrusion at L4–L5, for example, is going to take on much more significance when there is:

1. a report of paraesthesias or dysaesthesias on the lateral aspect of the right calf or dorsum of the foot or toes, or possibly even a report of altered pinprick or touch appreciation on testing in these areas
2. weakness in the right extensor hallucis longus (L5), extensor digitorum brevis (L5), tibialis anterior (L4/5) and posterior (L5/S1)
3. a 'positive' test for root irritation: a limitation of right straight leg raising; a report of back pain on straight leg raising, bowstring and/or Lasègue's test; acute back pain on the Maitland's 'slump' test; or the precipitation or aggravation of paraesthesias or dysaesthesias, with radiation to the buttock or leg in what seemingly could be a root distribution.

All the above symptoms and signs are, however, also frequently noted in association with malalignment alone. In the presence of malalignment with 'anterior' rotation of the right innominate, for example, the following may be seen:

1. There usually will be weakness ranging from 3+ to 4+/5 in right extensor hallucis longus, extensor digitorum brevis and tibialis anterior and posterior muscles; whereas their left counterparts remain strong (see Ch. 3). The fact that strength is full in the right medial hamstrings and peroneus longus/brevis (innervated by L5 but also S1) may be mistakenly rationalized as being due to the S1 nerve root contribution to these muscles still being 'intact' and, possibly, predominant compared to L5.
2. Paraesthesias or dysaesthesias lying within this 'L5 dermatome' pattern are not unusual. Hackett (1958) and others documented how these abnormal sensations associated with lumbosacral and/or SI joint instability can be referred in what seems the typical L5 distribution: from the upper half of the posterior sacroiliac ligaments to the lateral calf region (Fig. 3.63), and from the ligaments around the hip joint to the anterolateral calf and the dorsum of the foot (Fig. 3.67).

> Root stretch tests put tension not only on nerve roots but also on other soft tissue structures and their nerve supply.

These include the sacrotuberous ligament, which is tender in over 50% of those presenting with malalignment and capable of referring paraesthesias, with no indication of any symptoms localizing to the back or buttock regions (see 'Introduction 2002'). This ligament will be put under increased stretch by straight leg raising and, if it happens to be continuous with biceps femoris, also by the bowstring, Lasègue's and 'slump' tests, and any other manoeuvres that further increase tension in the hamstrings. Irritation of this ligament can precipitate or aggravate the referral of pain and paraesthesias to the lower extremity, something that can easily be misinterpreted as an indication of increased irritability of a nerve root or the sciatic nerve. Malalignment-related piriformis 'facilitation' or spasm may irritate the sciatic nerve, especially the peroneal component, directly when tension in piriformis is increased even further, especially on resisted active contraction and with tests that passively increase hip flexion, adduction and internal rotation (Fig. 4.17).

A radiculopathy typically results in a distinct pattern of unilateral sensory, motor and reflex changes. Signs on examination are fairly consistent and symptoms likely to be constantly present, though perhaps position-dependent and varying in intensity. Pain and paraesthesias are limited to a distinct distribution, and the muscles involved are all part of the myotome supplied by the specific root on that side.

In addition to the fact that bilateral reflexes remain intact, the following findings should trigger suspicions that the problem is likely to be caused by something other than a root irritation or actual radiculopathy.

Patchiness of the paraesthesias and dysaesthesias

These may, for example, involve the lateral calf region or the dorsum of the foot, not necessarily both sites at once (as would be more likely in the case of an L5 root lesion). In addition, the sites are often clearly separated from one another. In the example cited above, the person may distinguish a patch overlying the lateral calf region and another, distinctly separate, patch overlying the dorsum of the foot at times when both sites are symptomatic.

Variability of the sensations

The location and intensity of the abnormal sensations may vary. For example, there may be pain and/or paraesthesias restricted to the lateral calf region or to the dorsum of the foot at one time and both sites or neither at other times. They may also affect areas, not necessarily the same ones, on the opposite side (or even the upper limbs) simultaneously or at a different time.

Unilateral asymmetry of muscle strength

The asymmetry involves muscles from more than one myotome on the 'affected' right side; whereas other muscles in these same myotomes have retained full strength. On the right side, a typical finding on manual testing is that of a weak iliopsoas (L2/L3) but strong quadriceps (L2/L3/L4), and weak hip extensors (L5/S1) but strong ankle evertors and hip abductors (also L5/S1 innervated).

Asymmetrical weakness of muscles in the opposite limb

On comparison of the right and left side, the supposedly 'good' left side shows weakness in different muscles but involving the same myotome(s) as on the 'affected' right side. For example, on comparing muscles in the L5 and S1 myotome:

1. the right ankle evertors (L5/S1) are full strength; whereas their counterparts on the left are comparatively weaker
2. in 5-10%, the right hip extensors (e.g. gluteus maximus - also L5/S1 supplied) give way on manual testing; whereas the left ones show full strength

Ligamentous discomfort

Discomfort arises from specific ligaments, usually lateralizing to the ipsilateral right or left lumbosacral region or buttock area, overlying the region of the SI joint (rather than being central, as in a disc or root problem). Of concern are the ligaments that are put under stretch by straight leg raising: the sacrotuberous, posterior SI joint, sacrococcygeal and sacrospinous. Discomfort caused by increasing tension in these ligaments is usually reported as being off-centre, as described (Fig. 3.62).

> With a disc protrusion, the pain is more likely to localize to the centre or just to the side of the spine at the level involved, whenever the cord and roots are subjected to increased tension or compression.

Sometimes pain from the central low back region can also arise from tender interspinous, supraspinous and coccygeal ligaments put under stretch (Fig. 3.68). Low back pain reported in association with malalignment is, however, more likely to be to the right or left lumbosacral region (e.g. SI joint area). If it is in the midline, check for pain from the high-stress lumbosacral area or tenderness localizing to the inter- and supraspinous ligaments and, above all, rule out an L4 or L5 rotational displacement which can present as acute-onset pain from the central lumbosacral area.

In the presence of malalignment, the failure to find a well-defined neurological deficit on clinical examination takes on even more significance if:

1. imaging fails to show any diminution or loss of fat around the root
2. there is no evidence of root displacement or contact between the disc and root, or of any other pathological features (e.g. foraminal or central canal stenosis, central disc protrusion)
3. nerve conduction studies and EMG have ruled out radiculopathy

If there is any doubt about the diagnosis, the first step should not be disc surgery but a correction of the malalignment in conjunction with core strengthening and other appropriate exercises to see whether that will resolve some or all of the symptoms.

After achieving realignment and stabilization in the patient described above, the disappearance of any sensory and motor changes that were attributable to the malalignment may now reveal a clear-cut underlying problem, such as definite symptoms and signs in keeping with a unilateral radiculopathy. For example, if one were now to find residual weakness which is limited to the right L5 myotome, a persistence of sensory changes and dysaesthesias confined to the right L5 dermatome region, unilaterally positive root stretch test(s) and perhaps a questionable L5 reflex response, that would certainly strengthen the argument that the problem stemmed from right L5 root irritation or compression (see 'Case History 3.1'). Further investigations, including a possible root block, discogram, EMG and NCS should then be considered, if they have not already been carried out, to help decide on an appropriate treatment approach.

However, these steps are often not taken, and a discectomy may be carried out on the basis of an unfortunate coincidence of symptoms and signs suggesting the irritation or compression of a nerve root, with a disc bulge or even protrusion on the MRI or CAT scan sometimes evident at the level at which it is the most likely to catch that root. In this regard, the following observations by Kieffer et al. (1984) should be kept in mind:

1. the incidence of disc bulging increases with age after the third decade
2. a bulging disc is usually not associated with nerve root compression

MRI and CAT scanning has in the past led to an overdiagnosis of a disc protrusion being the cause of a patient's back pain. More recent studies using these imaging techniques indicate that anywhere from 10%-30% of asymptomatic subjects may show evidence of disc protrusion. As observed by Klein et al. (1993: 23), MRI and CAT scans:

> *... showed significant abnormalities ... but these did not correlate with subjective complaints and were not predictive of response to treatment*

Jensen et al. (1994: 69), using MRI, found a disc bulge on at least one level in 52%, a protrusion in 27% and an extrusion in 1% of 98 asymptomatic subjects. The findings suggested that 'the discovery by MRI of bulges or protrusions in people with low back pain may frequently be coincidental'.

The author has repeatedly had to deal with patients who had undergone futile disc resection, or even went on to fusion of one or more levels 'because the resection failed', only to have the pain finally disappear with subsequent correction of the real cause: a coexistent malalignment. The pain typically does decrease, or sometimes even disappears for a few days or weeks, following the surgery. In retrospect, patients often volunteer that this 'interlude' was probably the result of a combination of post-operative inactivity and an increased intake of analgesic medication, or the use of stronger analgesics, intended to counteract the pain caused by the surgery itself.

Aggravation of persistent symptoms or the recurrence of their previous pain often coincides with their first attempts to become more active. The pain tends to be worse than before; this may relate to the imposed rest, with a loss of overall fitness and of muscle and ligament strength. Extensive investigations may be repeated but are usually negative or inconclusive. In the absence of definite pathology relating to the disc, there is now the risk that one of the following scenarios will evolve:

1. Ongoing symptoms are attributed to scar tissue formation and/or adhesions around the nerve root that are probably the result of chronic irritation and inflammation caused by the previous disc protrusion and/or the surgical intervention. The patient is told to 'live with it', often without the benefit of instruction on how to do so. Nerve blocks or epidurals may provide temporary relief and have sometimes already been repeated to counter a flare-up. However, ongoing symptoms are likely to be, in part, the result of an underlying 'malalignment syndrome' that has so far been missed.
2. Symptoms are attributed to 'segmental instability' caused by the previous disc resection. The recommendation for a one or two-level fusion of the 'unstable' segment or segments may follow, even though flexion and extension views of the spine either fail to show definitive anteroposterior movement of 3 mm or more in either direction, or fail to do so conclusively.

The decision may be mistakenly 'strengthened' by coincidental evidence of degenerative disc changes at the level(s) in question, although such changes are not uncommon on routine imaging and, in a large number, unlikely to be the cause of their symptoms (Jensen et al. 1994; Magora & Schwarz 1976; Weishaupt et al. 1998).

Assuming that a fusion of L5–S1 or L4–L5–S1 is carried out, it is unlikely to relieve any pain that stems from malalignment of the pelvis *per se*. However, fusion at these levels is more likely to be helpful when the underlying problem is a recurrent rotational displacement of L4 or L5 that has actually been precipitating the pelvic malalignment (Fig. 2.52). Care must be taken that alignment is being maintained during the surgery. Following such a vertebral fusion, it is still possible for malalignment of the pelvic ring to occur (see 'Case History 7.4'). Realignment will hopefully effect a resolution of residual symptoms caused by such a recurrence, provided that secondary changes relating to the chronicity of the pain and the two surgeries have not progressed to the point of having become irreversible.

Either way, fusion of the segment(s) results in stresses that can increase (and eventually accelerate degeneration) of the disc spaces immediately above and below, as well as increasing stress on the SI joints and hips. The end result is a superimposed mechanical back pain, sometimes leading to surgical fusion of yet another level for advancing disc and/or facet joint degeneration.

This is a sad scenario indeed but one that is, unfortunately, all too familiar to those working with problems caused by malalignment. It is, therefore, the author's heartfelt conviction that patients in whom there is any question of whether their symptoms are caused by a disc protrusion should be seen in consultation by someone familiar with the diagnosis and treatment of malalignment-related problems. Hackett said as much (1958: 49) when he advised that:

> *Every surgeon who operates on the spine should have a conferee that is competent to diagnose the case for him unless he fully understands ligament disability.*

He was referring here to the importance of recognizing that 'sciatica' can result from causes other than disc protrusion, including a 'relaxation' of the ligaments that support the lower portion of the sacrum (Figs 3.63, 4.10, 5.38). Nowadays, if there is any doubt regarding a root or nerve involvement, recommendations would be for assessment:

1. if at all possible, by someone practising orthopaedic medicine and familiar with issues relating to malalignment
2. at an EMG clinic which, in the author's experience, continues to be one site likely to see a fair number of patients referred for a suspected 'radiculopathy' or 'peripheral nerve compression' but whose neurological exam and electrodiagnostic studies turn out normal and whose symptoms and signs are in keeping with the malalignment that was noted on the clinical examination
3. at least at a musculoskeletal clinic (e.g. sports medicine clinic), where chances are increased that one or more clinician or therapist is familiar with malalignment or, at least, more likely to know someone able to carry out an appropriate assessment and treatment for this type of problem

Other surgeries encountered in association with malalignment

Surgical 'derotation' of the tibia

At an international sports medicine meeting, a surgeon reported on the case of a female athlete who presented with obvious outward rotation of the right 'foot', which he attributed to right 'tibia varum'. He proceeded to cut through the tibia and fibula in order to rotate the distal part of these bones, and with it the ankle and foot, counter-clockwise until the toes were more or less pointing straight ahead, like those on the left side. There was no mention of any pre-operative attempt to look for evidence of malalignment. In fact, on being questioned, it became obvious that this surgeon was unaware that such an entity even existed.

As indicated throughout this text, an 'upslip' and the 'more common' patterns of 'rotational malalignment' are associated with increased tendency to 'right external, left internal' rotation of the lower extremity, and that was exactly what was evident on a pre-operative standing view of this athlete. An outward rotation of as much as 45 degrees from the midline, the other foot possibly pointing straight ahead or even across midline, would not be an unusual finding prior to realignment and no indicator of what the ultimate orientation of the lower extremities will be once alignment has been achieved (Figs 3.3, 3.19, 3.78, 3.79).

'Trochanteric bursitis' and/or iliotibial band 'tendonitis'

Several patients who have failed to respond to repeated injections of cortisone for left 'trochanteric bursitis' and/or attempts at decreasing pain arising from the tense and tender ITB have undergone resection of the left greater trochanter, the ITB or both. The other possible causes of pain in this area often were neither considered nor explored, including malalignment, trigger points, and irritation of neurological structures (Figs 3.41, 3.46, 3.63, 4.23A3B3). Typical of the latter is referral from the iliolumbar ligament to a sclerotome: the greater trochanter region. Involvement of the LFCN may have to be ruled out (Fig. 4.13). In the case of the 'thoracolumbar syndrome', there can be hypersensitivity of the skin overlying the trochanter, from irritation of the lateral perforating cutaneous branch from T12 and L1 (Fig. 4.23A3, B3). All of these causes can exist in isolation or be secondary to malalignment.

Needless to say, in these cases the resections have failed to bring relief. The long scar subsequently increases tension in the skin overlying the lateral thigh and the underlying muscles, causing them to become tender with time. Correction of the malalignment, combined with stretching and strengthening, may resolve the pain but the unsightly scar remains, and the biomechanical advantages attributable to the trochanter and the TFL/ITB complex are lost forever.

MALALIGNMENT THAT FAILS TO RESPOND TO TREATMENT

In the patient who may or may not derive temporary relief from realignment but fails to maintain that correction, the vertebral rotational displacement and/or pelvic malalignment may itself be one manifestation of an underlying problem that has so far escaped detection (see Appendix 13). In addition, it should also be borne in mind that malalignment can mimic a number of other conditions (see Ch. 4). It is, therefore, extremely important to avoid falling into the trap of attributing all symptoms to the malalignment and failing to rule out any underlying pathology by doing a thorough clinical examination and appropriate investigations, especially if there is any suspicion of abnormality that cannot be explained simply on the basis of the malalignment.

The following are examples of conditions that can result in possible overlap of symptoms and signs, and may also be responsible for the recurrence of malalignment.

Unilateral vertebral lumbarization or sacralization

The fact that the vertebral complex is fixed on one side and free to move on the other introduces a torquing effect every time the person bends forward or backward (Figs 4.25, 4.26). This torquing results in direct asymmetrical forces on the spine and the sacrum. It also exerts indirect asymmetrical forces on the innominates by way of the superior and deep iliolumbar ligament attachments to the iliac crest, especially on the side that is still mobile (Figs 2.4A, 2.52).

Unilateral pseudo-arthrosis or pseudo-joint

This usually involves a large L5 transverse process abutting the sacral ala, with definite or suggestive evidence of a joint space and sclerotic margins (Figs 4.24, 4.26). An impingement of the transverse process on only one side results in a torquing effect with any flexion, extension or rotational forces through the lumbosacral region. The pseudo-arthrosis can also become an ongoing source of pain. However, the pain may manifest itself only when malalignment is present and puts further stress on the pseudo-joint; in that case, symptoms will resolve with realignment (see 'idiopathic scoliosis', Ch. 4).

Disc protrusion or herniation

Pain from the disc itself or from irritation of the dura and/or nerve roots can result in asymmetrical muscle tension that predisposes to recurrent malalignment.

> Central disc protrusions are more likely to be missed because of a lack of findings on clinical examination. They should be suspected if there is a report of acute central low or midback pain, or even neck pain, attributable to stretching and irritation of the dura on Maitland's 'slump' test.

Symptoms commonly occur when the head is brought down on the flexed trunk and/or the ankle dorsiflexed on carrying out this test (Fig. 3.75). Central protrusion must be excluded by an MRI or CAT scan in those whose examination otherwise reveals no obvious cause for their failure to maintain alignment.

Facet joint pathology

Facet joints can be a cause of both localized and referred pain, as well as of reflex, asymmetrical muscle splinting as the result of osteoarthritic changes, ligament laxity and pain from joint surfaces or irritation of the nerves supplying these surfaces, the capsule and ligaments. Pain can be elicited on direct palpation (Fig. 4.20) or stressing the joint, bilaterally on trunk extension and contralaterally on right or left rotation.

Abdominal and pelvic masses

Masses, including uterine fibroids and ovarian cysts, can exert direct pressure on the iliopsoas and piriformis, and trigger spasm in these muscles. Iliopsoas, of course, crosses both the hip and the SI joint, and can exert rotational effects by way of its attachments to the spine, ilium, sacrum and femur (Figs 2.46, 2.62, 3.42, 4.2, 4.13). Piriformis can exert a rotational effect on the sacrum and femur (Figs 2.46, 7.20). Masses can also cause pain and asymmetrical muscle tension by exerting direct pressure on the anterior lumbosacral plexus and/or the pelvic floor on one side, or more on one side than the other (Figs 2.53, 4.15).

Visceral pathology

Pathology can occur in the form of:

1. adhesions, scar tissue or tightness of structures such as suspending ligaments, all of which can restrict the mobility of organs and viscera
2. a malpositioning of the organs and viscera (e.g. upward/downward or medial/lateral displacement; excessive rotation).

These have all been implicated as either causative or perpetuating factors for malalignment (Barral 1989, 1993; Barral & Mercier 1988). Visceral manipulation may finally allow for a prolonged correction of malalignment and bring lasting relief where other manual therapy approaches aimed primarily at realignment of the pelvis/spine have failed.

Lipomas

Tender lipomas, especially those which lie directly over the posterior SI joint margins and posterior pelvic ligaments, can mimic pain arising from the SI joint region and give one the mistaken impression that it is the joint or a ligament that is at fault. When subjected to pressure, such as from seat backs, belts or objects carried in a back pocket (e.g. a wallet), a lipoma itself may trigger pain from an underlying structure, such as the iliolumbar ligament, gluteus maximus and piriformis which can, in turn, trigger an increase in muscle tension and recurrence of malalignment. Sacroiliac belts sometimes cannot be tolerated for the same reason.

Some of the manoeuvres carried out as part of the back examination can cause pain by entrapping a lipoma. They are commonly found in the right and left lumbosacral region, often bilateral, which makes them vulnerable to compression on back extension, or even more so on simultaneous extension, side flexion and rotation to one side. This pain may be confused with a facet or SI joint problem.

Scar tissue

Nerve fibres entrapped in scar tissue can become a source of chronic localized or referred pain capable of triggering a reflex, asymmetrical increase in muscle tension. Those who practise neural therapy preach that all scars should be suspect until proven otherwise, something that can easily be done by injecting the scar with a short-acting local anaesthetic. If pain or paraesthesias disappear locally or in distal sites of referral, the scar may be suitable for treatment with a set of desensitization injections.

Referred pain

Pain referred to the lower extremities can result from a number of causes other than malalignment. These include trigger points, a degenerating or protruding disc, sciatic nerve irritation, facet joint and SI joint degeneration or compression, and increased tension or inflammation affecting the pelvic ligaments. Intrapelvic lesions (e.g. adhesions, post-surgical scars, endometriosis, fibroids and cysts) are other causes of referred pain to consider.

In such cases, investigations have to be guided by the clinical presentation and availability of diagnostic equipment. In most centres, these will include:

1. a blood screen (e.g. anti-nuclear antibody, complement factor C4 level and erythrocyte sedimentation rate for underlying connective tissue disease, HLA-B27 typing for possible ankylosing spondylitis, rheumatoid factor, B12, TSH, glucose level(s) and as otherwise indicated)
2. a bone scan to check for an inflammatory arthropathy
3. X-rays of the lumbosacral spine and SI joints
4. a CAT scan or MRI to rule out disc bulging or protrusion, scar tissue or other pathology affecting the spinal cord and nerve roots
5. ultrasound of the abdomen and pelvis looking, in particular, for organomegaly, aneurysms and masses.

A local anaesthetic block of a facet joint, pseudo-arthrosis, nerve root, scar tissue or lipoma can quickly establish whether or not that structure is the cause of some or all of the patient's pain. If the block provides temporary partial or complete relief, it should be repeated with the addition of cortisone, in the hope of obtaining long-term relief. Lipomas sometimes fail to respond to anything other than excision. Fusion of a facet joint or pseudo-arthrosis may be necessary for a permanent cure. There is, unfortunately, still a rotational element following a unilateral fusion, just as there is with a unilateral sacralization, lumbarization or SI joint fusion. Therefore, simultaneous fusion of the same structure on the opposite side is advised to prevent the recurrence of pain or of malalignment in these situations. Sensitive scar tissue may respond to attempts at desensitization with repeated injections of local anaesthetic; a course of 5–10 weekly injections usually suffices. The actual number needs to be governed by the response and repeat courses may be necessary if symptoms recur.

X-ray correlation with the presence or absence of malalignment has been, in large part, ignored. Malalignment is usually evident on films on a side-to-side comparison of major pelvic landmarks or joints (see Ch. 4; Figs 2.75, 2.102, 3.82, 4.6, 4.24, 4.30, 4.31, 4.33). For example, an 'upslip' and a 'rotational malalignment' both create a step deformity of the superior and inferior aspect of the symphysis pubis. A rotation of the lower extremities in opposite directions results in an apparent difference in the size of the lesser trochanters, which may look larger on one side by having rotated into view, and looks comparatively smaller on the opposite side because of increasing angulation to the beam and overlap with the shaft of the femur (Figs 2.74, 2.75, 4.30). Different aspects of the SI joint space will be prominent on the right compared with the left side because the surfaces are angulated differently to the beam. Especially with 'rotational malalignment', one part of the L-shape joint - ventral, middle or posterior; upper or lower - will often be more clearly defined on one side, another part on the opposite side (Figs 4.24, 4.29, 4.30-4.32). Aitken (1986) clearly showed how sacral torsion around one of the oblique axes becomes evident on an X-ray, in terms of the changes in sacral alignment relative to the vertical axis, before and after correction of the malalignment (Fig. 4.35). The fact that there can be obvious changes is not, however, to advocate the use of X-rays to establish or confirm whether malalignment is present or whether realignment has been achieved. A proper clinical examination will give more precise and useful information. However, an X-ray taken for whatever reason can help raise suspicions of an alignment problem that should be confirmed and dealt with, especially when the films show no other abnormalities. In addition, one must caution against relying on the use of X-rays taken with the person lying supine when assessing pelvic obliquity, curvatures of the spine and weight-bearing joints (especially the hip and knee joints; Fig. 3.82). Sitting views allow more accurate assessment of changes attributable to malalignment, LLD, sacral base tilt and status of these joints (Fig. 3.90); they may also help detect a sacro- or intercoccygeal joint problem (Ch. 4).

UNNECESSARY INVESTIGATIONS AND TREATMENT

It is unethical and financially unjustifiable to embark on, or persist with, standard physiotherapy treatment if an underlying problem of malalignment is not being addressed at the same time. A typical example is that of the person with an 'upslip' or one of the 'more common' rotational patterns who suffers recurrent left ankle sprains.

> Limiting care to the treatment of symptoms and signs - pain, oedema, inflammation, weakness and tightness - while failing to treat the underlying predisposing condition (the malalignment of the pelvis and spine) may, in fact, be responsible for the failure to improve and/or recurrence of an ankle sprain.

Similarly, it is unjustifiable to persist with a manipulation or mobilization technique indefinitely. If a trial of one technique over a 3- 6-month period fails to achieve lasting realignment, a trial of another technique, or a combination of techniques, should be considered. Failure to get the patient involved in the effort to regain or maintain realignment, by using self-assessment and self-treatment techniques, will also prolong recovery time or even prevent achieving complete recovery altogether.

The diagnosis of problems attributable to malalignment starts with an index of suspicion from the history. Attention has to be paid especially to the possible mechanism of injury and the presenting complaint(s) that implicate structures typically put under increased stress by the malalignment. It is the conglomeration of symptoms and signs, rather than any one specific test, that establishes the diagnosis of a 'malalignment syndrome'.

Malalignment can obviously coexist with other conditions involving the pelvis, spine, limbs, viscera or soft tissues. If there is any doubt as to whether it is the malalignment or another condition that is the cause of the problems, the first step should be to correct the malalignment to see if that makes any difference. To write the problems off as being caused by one of these other conditions, or worse still, to proceed with surgery when the diagnosis is still only part of a differential diagnosis and the possibility of malalignment has not even been entertained, is to do these patients a great disservice and invites medicolegal repercussions.

Injured athletes are usually driven by an intense desire to get back to their sport as quickly as possible. As a result, they are probably more aware of, and more willing to try out, alternate treatment approaches than other people. They are swift to register that a given treatment has failed and another one succeeded. If their problem does indeed arise from malalignment, they will have no difficulty eventually realizing that they underwent needless investigations and received improper, futile or aggravating treatment initially because the correct diagnosis had been missed.

TREATMENT IS A LONG-TERM COMMITMENT

Failure of treatment is more likely to arise from the person's failure to participate in a consistent programme aimed at regaining alignment and stability of the pelvis and spine, rather than from a failure to diagnose and treat one of the 'underlying problems' listed above. He or she will sometimes give up on the manual therapy and exercise programme after 1 or 2 months because there have been no obvious dramatic results. In some countries, the length of treatment may be governed by the number of therapy sessions covered by an insurance plan. Unfortunately, not everyone can be expected to respond fully in the time span of 12 therapy sessions or whatever limit is set by a certain policy.

When it comes to malalignment-related problems, the best results are achieved with a younger population, those in their teens to late twenties. This includes a considerable number of those who have gone through the major biomechanical changes that constitute a part of every pregnancy, yet who consistently do amazingly well in terms of achieving realignment using simple MET and maintaining that alignment while their other 'wounds' just incurred with a natural or surgical delivery are still healing (see 'Implications for… gynaecology and obstetrics', Ch. 4).

Whereas most people respond to realignment procedures within 3 to 4 months, this is not always the case. They must, therefore, be advised early on that treatment may be a long-term proposition, which requires a full commitment on their part: 1 or 2 years may be needed to undo the detrimental effects that malalignment has had on their body, often for years or even decades.

Malalignment results in long-term problems primarily related to connective tissue structures. Tendons, ligaments, capsules and myofascial structures that have either contracted or become lax over the years take time to regain their normal length and strength as they adapt to realignment. The healing response may be compromised by the poor blood supply of connective tissues. Any recurrence of the malalignment serves only to slow down the recovery process, and any interruption of the treatment programme, for whatever reason, can only have the same detrimental effect.

People often tend to settle for short-term results and may not be willing to participate in long-term treatment and a regular home exercise programme, preferring instead to return for treatment whenever their symptoms flare up. It is for this reason that right at the start all those presenting with the 'malalignment syndrome' must be made aware how malalignment puts them at risk of recurrence of symptoms and injuries, and how they can play a major part in their own recovery process.

> Treatment should not be a sporadic event, limited to time spent with the therapist at weekly or bi-weekly intervals or at the time of a flare-up but should become a day-by-day process that requires the person's involvement right from the start.

All those presenting with malalignment must be advised that they have to be willing to forego some activities for a while in order to increase their chances of regaining and maintaining alignment, and to allow injured tissues to heal. The aim is to get them to return eventually to all their activities. Thereafter, regular self-assessment and self-treatment play a vital role in the early detection and treatment of any recurrence, to prevent redeveloping symptoms or even suffering an injury on account of the malalignment. If a person fails to heed this advice and fails to play an active part in their recovery process, he or she is merely compromising the chances of ever making a complete recovery and, in the case of athletes, reaching their full potential.

Chapter 8

Treatment: Manual therapy modes

Sarah Stevens
Karina Steinberg

CHAPTER CONTENTS

DOI: 10.1016/B978-0-443-06929-1.00008-9

INTRODUCTION

This chapter provides an introduction to the body tissues typically affected by the 'malalignment syndrome' and a selection of manual treatment approaches available to correct any abnormal biomechanical forces and help these tissues recover. The best treatment approach should be based on the structure primarily contributing to the problem, the individual's expectations, philosophy and interests, as well as the availability of manual therapists in your area. It is the authors' opinion that the connection of the patient with the therapist can be as important as the type of treatment chosen, thus we encourage trying different practitioners or approaches to find the right match.

Manual therapy can be practised by numerous specialists such as physiatrists, osteopaths, physiotherapists, chiropractors, massage therapists, naturopathic doctors and athletic trainers. The techniques described in this chapter can be applied by some or all of these practitioners depending on their education and training (see Ch. 7 regarding the Canadian programme for post-graduate training of physiotherapists in the theory and practice of manual therapy, leading to designation as a 'Fellow of the Canadian Association of Manual Therapists' or 'FCAMT'). Patients should not hesitate to ask their local practitioners what post-graduate training they have had in manual therapy!

The previous chapters describe muscle energy techniques for treatment in particular of pelvic malalignment. When the pelvis is out of alignment, tissues around the pelvis must compensate, altering the optimal biomechanics and tissue length-tension relationships. There are four main systems recognized to influence pelvic dysfunction: articular, neural, visceral and myofascial (Lee 2007c, 2011). These tissues are discussed as to their anatomy, biomechanics, and the manual therapy techniques that can directly affect them.

Manual therapy is an all-encompassing term for 'hands-on' therapeutic interventions performed by various health practitioners to alleviate ailments and treat specific etiologies. The definition of manual therapy varies among health professionals and seems to be influenced by their scope of practice and how their techniques have evolved. This chapter will not attempt to review all treatment techniques available but to highlight some of the most common approaches used today. Each therapy will be introduced with a brief summary of its history and its originator(s), the physiology or biomechanics of how it functions, and a generalized description of the patient experience. The information provided is only a short description of each technique; references for further reading and resources are provided for those who want to pursue learning more about the individual techniques.

TISSUE TYPES

CONNECTIVE TISSUE

Connective tissue usually refers to fascia, ligaments, and tendons, which are primarily composed of collagen and/or elastin.

Collagen makes up about 25-35% of our entire body's protein content. This long fibrous structure contributes to the tensile strength of fascia, cartilage, ligaments, tendons, bone and skin and is a major component of the extracellular matrix supporting most of our tissues.

Elastin, unlike collagen, can stretch easily and has almost perfect recoil. With age, it loses some of its elasticity and may even calcify. The fibres are composed of protein elastin fibrils which branch and rejoin loosely. Elastin is not as organized as collagen and is usually thinner and less abundant.

Fascia

Fascia is made up of collagen, elastin and a polysaccharide gel complex forming a three-dimensional cobweb covering the body's tissues (Fig. 8.1). It has three continuous layers: (1) a superficial layer under the skin, (2) a deeper, 'ensheathing' layer which covers muscles, bone, nerves, blood vessels, and organs right down to the cellular level, and (3) the deepest layer, which connects with the dura of the central nervous system. The muscle is intimately connected with fascia, hence the term 'myofascia'. Fascia functions to support our body, absorb shock, enhance cellular respiration and metabolism, and assist with fluid and lymphatic flow.

Malfunction of the fascial system can occur from poor or prolonged postures causing asymmetrical loading, trauma, and repetitive strain. Changes in fascial mobility occur when the fascia is bound down or restricted in areas. Due to its continuous nature it causes a global effect by pulling on the body at points distal to the primary site of dysfunction (see Chs 2, 3). This stimulates nociceptors, causing pain, and reduces the body's ability to absorb and distribute forces that may be incurred with

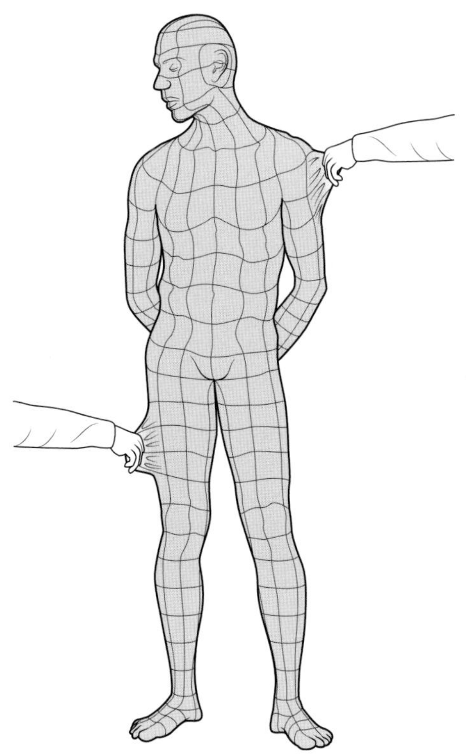

Fig. 8.1 The fascial 'cobweb' is made up of collagen, elastin and a polysaccharide gel.

sudden trauma or repetitive loading. It can also alter an individual's biomechanics and influence his or her posture and dynamic balance. Injuries to the fascial system do not result in typical nerve root or trigger point referral patterns and standard imaging tests (i.e. X-rays, CT scans, MRI, etc.) will not pick up fascial dysfunction, so typically these malfunctions usually go undiagnosed.

Therapeutic interventions can alter our fascia by: stretching its elastic component, shearing the cross-links that may have developed, changing the viscosity of the ground substance by increasing the production of hyaluronic acid, and increasing its mobility and fluid flow. Techniques which have a direct affect on fascia include myofascial release, visceral manipulation, cranial osteopathy, craniosacral therapy, Bowen therapy, acupuncture and IMS.

Ligaments

Ligaments consist of fibrous collagen tissue that connects one bone to another. Ligaments differ from other connective tissues in that their fibrils are organized in a predominantly parallel fashion. They are vascularized, have C nerve fibres which transmit pain signals, and contain mechanoreceptors. They are built to share load so that no single ligament in a joint takes the entire load at any one time. Since ligaments have elastic properties only under tension, the amount of load a ligament can adapt to depends on the speed of load application. The lengthening of a ligament up to its 'yield point' is reversible. Stretching a ligament beyond the yield point will cause tearing and irreversible lengthening.

When ligaments heal, fibrous scar tissue forms. This fills in the tear and creates a longer, weaker and less extensible structure. Ligaments respond to joint mobilization and deep transverse frictions as these help with the alignment of the collagen fibres, break up fibrous tissue deposited in the wrong direction (cross-links), stimulate a release of endogenous opioids for pain relief, and increase inter-fibre lubrication as the proteoglycans bind with water.

Tendons

Tendons are bands of fibrous connective tissue that connect muscle to bone. They are mostly made up of collagen but also have some elastin (~2%) which gives them the ability to store and recover energy in movements, similar to a spring (Järvinen et al. 1997). Their primary function is to work with muscles to exert a pulling force causing bone movement.

Tendon length will vary among individuals; there seems to be a genetical predisposition. It does not tend to lengthen or shorten in response to injury or environmental demands, thus body imbalances are believed to be due to changes in other structures such as muscles and fascia (Curwin 1994; Kvist 2002).

CONTRACTILE TISSUE

Muscles are comprised of bundles of fasciculi that, in turn, are made up of bundles of muscle fibres (Fig. 8.2; the latter) themselves are formed from bundles of myofilaments (myofibrils) composed of two main proteins, actin and myosin: the contractile elements of the muscle. Each layer of a bundle is separated by fascial tissue that helps transmit forces from muscle to tendon and bone.

Muscles are always in some degree of contraction known as 'muscle tone'. The tone of a muscle is determined by impulses coming from the spinal cord which depend on the amount of alpha activity in nerves. This activity is influenced by one's psychological state, neurochemistry, and

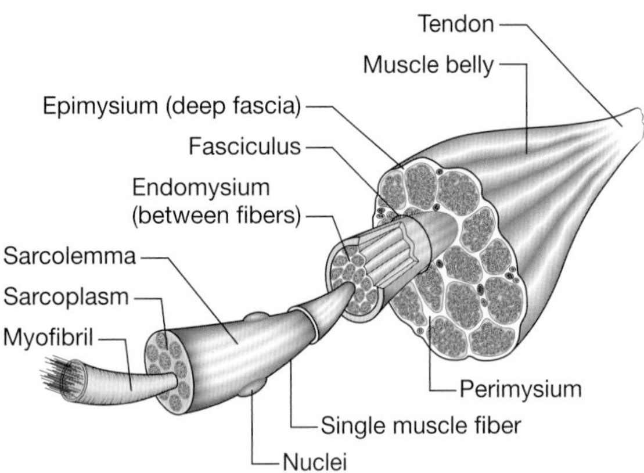

Fig. 8.2 Muscle belly split into its various component parts.

feedback from receptors within the muscles. There are two types of muscle receptors:

1. the muscle spindle, which provides feedback regarding the length of the extrafusal fibres, and
2. the Golgi tendon organ, which is located in the tendomuscular junction and gives information about muscle tension.

These muscle receptor mechanisms work in opposite ways to help control muscle tone. Muscle spindles use a positive feedback cycle to continuously monitor muscle length and rate of length change by stimulating the anterior horn cells in the spinal cord which, in turn, provides the stimuli for increasing muscle tone. Conversely, Golgi tendon organs use a negative feedback system to protect the muscle from sudden forces and tearing. They excite an inhibitory interneuron in the spinal cord to suppress the alpha motor neuron and allow the muscle to relax. This is believed to be the mechanism behind trigger point and acupressure release techniques.

When joint receptors are damaged by injury, the damage will alter the body's position sense - or proprioception - and also affects muscle tone. When the antagonist muscles are unable to relax or are pathologically shortened, the normal range of motion is restricted which will again influence muscle tone. Certain muscles are over-active and tend to shorten, while others are underactive and tend to lengthening or atrophy. These are factors that contribute to the 'malalignment syndrome', where the pattern of muscular 'facilitation'/'inhibition' and strength is noted to be asymmetrical with an 'upslip' and 'rotational malalignment' (see Boxes 8.1, 8.2 for an example of muscles which become shortened or lengthened).

BOX 8.1 Muscles that commonly become overactive and shorten

Biceps
Hamstrings
Short hip adductors
Iliopsoas
Rectus femoris
Tensor fascia lata
Piriformis
Quadratus lumborum
Upper lumbar extensors
Pectoralis major and minor
Upper trapezius
Sternocleidomastoid

BOX 8.2 Muscles that are commonly 'underactive' and lengthen

Vastus medialis
Transversus abdominis
Oblique abdominals
Middle and lower trapezius
Serratus anterior
Gluteus medius and minimus
Longus capitus
Tibialis posterior

With muscle imbalances or the 'malalignment syndrome' there is a higher tendency for injury as there is less flexibility, strength and endurance in certain structures. Treatment techniques that affect muscle tone in particular include joint mobilization, muscle energy techniques, myofascial release, and counter-strain technique (discussed below).

NEURAL TISSUE

The nervous system is a continuous network of specialized cells that communicates information from the body to the brain and vice versa (Fig. 8.3). These messages or electrical signals, including perception and movement, are responsible for interaction with the environment. The nervous system is composed of neurons and glial cells which together generate electrical impulses that travel between our central nervous system (CNS) and peripheral nervous system (PNS). Generally, our CNS processes information in our spinal cord and brain and then sends signals back to our PNS where sensory, motor, and autonomic nerves leave the spinal cord to

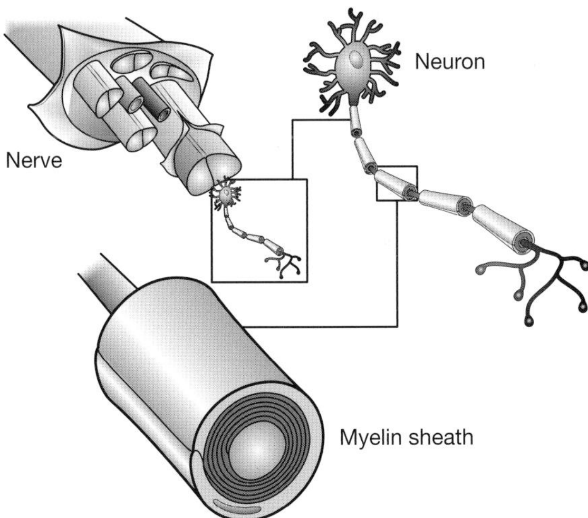

Fig. 8.3 The nervous system is continuous from the CNS to the peripheral nerves.

innervate our muscles, articular structures, organs, and glands. The neurons communicate with each other via electrochemical signals or neurotransmitters to transmit impulses from one neuron to the next.

The nervous system is continuous from the CNS to the peripheral nerves. Stress placed on one part of the system can be transmitted to other parts during movement (Breig 1978). In normal conditions, pain does not occur with movement or normal compression. However, the neural tissue can produce adverse symptoms with even minor stimuli if irritation due to a mechanical (compression or tension) and/or chemical (inflammation or ischemia) cause is present. Dahlin & Mclean (1986) showed that:

1. lack of oxygen secondary to compression will cause increased intraneural pressure that can take several weeks to reverse
2. separation of nerve fibres occurs with sustained pressure

Common sites of injury include soft tissue, osseous tunnels (i.e. a spinal nerve exiting through an intervertebral foramen), nerve branches, and tension points (C6, T6, L4, posterior knee, and anterior elbow) where nervous tissues are relatively fixed.

Neural tissue has some elastic properties and can tolerate up to 20% elongation. If compression and traction occur together, only 15% elongation is required to stimulate the nociceptors and produce pain (Sunderland 1978). In addition, neural tension can cause venous stasis and stop intraneural blood flow at approximately 15% elongation (Ogata & Naito 1986; Rydevik et al. 1981). If the nerve's distal axon shows evidence of degeneration or is injured, it will be more susceptible to mechanical and chemical irritants. Both compression and elongation contribute to the body's physiological response by causing inflammation (Dahlin & Mclean, 1986) and/or ischemia (Rydevik et al. 1981).

Treatment of the nervous system is geared to restoring proper neural mobility, reducing chemical irritation, and minimizing any mechanical pressure or tension. David Butler (2000) advocated that mobilization of the nervous system can have a mechanical effect on the vascular system by dispersing intraneural oedema. Altering the mechanical restraints on the axoplasm and improving circulation will increase the energy available for axonal transport. Mobilization may also help the axons to regenerate by allowing better contact guidance (Lundborg 1988), and causing micro-trauma that may stimulate neurite promoting factors (Heumann et al. 1987). When there is rapid improvement of the nerve, it may be due to increased blood supply or changes in availability of CSF as nerves and nerve roots get at least half their metabolic requirements from these fluids.

ARTICULAR STRUCTURES

The main components of the articular structures (the body's joints) are bones, cartilage, synovial fluid, and joint receptors. While these components are predominantly responsible for allowing movement, they have a direct influence on posture and muscle length-tension relationships which can lead to malalignment and development of the 'malalignment syndrome'.

Bone

Bone is a mineralized connective tissue that is highly vascularized and constantly adapting to external stress. It is composed of osteoblasts, cells responsible for synthesizing collagen to produce more bone, osteocytes for transporting nutritional materials and maintaining its architecture, and osteoclasts that use lysosomal enzymes to reabsorb and break down bone. In addition, bone has an intracellular matrix of collagen bundles, ground substance, water, salts and minerals. The inorganic matter gives bone its rigidity, while water provides its pliability and distortion tolerance.

Cartilage

Cartilage is mostly composed of bands of collagen fibers, proteoglycans and water. Its strong bonds with water provide elasticity, resistance to compression, and lubrication through chemical properties. The smooth nature of cartilage can also reduce friction.

There are three types: (1) hyaline, (2) fibrocartilage, and (3) elastin cartilage. Hyaline cartilage is the most abundant, found in cavities or ends of long bones and ribs; it allows for structure and flexibility in areas such as the nose, larynx and bronchial tubes. Fibrocartilage has chondrocytes scattered throughout its bundles and provides the strength and rigidity in the spinal discs, symphysis pubis, and sacroiliac joints. Elastin cartilage also has chondrocytes but they are organized in a thread-like network of fibres which provides strength to help maintain the shape of certain organs.

Cartilage has a low capacity for regeneration and therapeutic interventions mostly influence hyaline cartilage nutrition, which is provided by diffusion through synovial fluid. Thus, joint mobilization enhances joint lubrication and cartilage nutrition, and can move joint inclusions such as meniscoids or loose bodies resulting with cartilage fibrillation and degeneration.

Synovial fluid

Synovial fluid is a clear, viscous fluid found within most skeletal joints. It provides lubrication, shock absorption, heat dissipation, and nutrition for the articular cartilage, discs, and menisci. It contains phagocytic cells that aid in the removal of metabolic wastes and carbon dioxide. With movement, as the temperature or rate of shear through a joint increases, the viscosity of this fluid will decrease. Thus, with slow movement the weight-bearing capacity is maximal; whereas with fast movement the resistance to movement decreases. With injury, a post-traumatic synovitis or hemorrhagic event can occur which will cause the viscosity of the synovial fluid to decrease, thereby decreasing the ability of the joint to heal and to absorb shock.

Joint receptors

Joint receptors are mechanoreceptors which send signals to the body about injury and positional sense. According to Wyke's classification of articular receptors, there are four types, all of which differ in structural compositions and how they influence the body.

Type 1 receptors are found in the superficial layers of a capsule with a greater density in the proximal joints. They are stimulated by proprioception, vibration, and discrimination of touch, and can sense static positions, pressure changes, velocity and the direction of a person's movement. Because they have a low threshold, are slow to adapt, and fire almost continuously, they can be clinically influenced by changes of posture and positioning.

Type 2 receptors are found in the deep layers of the capsules and fat pads with a greater density in the distal joints. They are also stimulated by proprioception, vibration, and discrimination of touch. However, they only sense dynamic changes in position, such as occur with acceleration/deceleration, and are inactive at rest. Because Type 2 receptors have a low threshold and are quick to adapt, they are clinically influenced by movement such as exercise and joint mobilizations and manipulations.

Type 3 receptors are found in ligaments near bony attachments but not in the longitudinal ligaments of the spine (Fig. 3.68). These receptors are stimulated by extremes of dynamic movement when the ligaments are stressed. They are dynamic receptors that are inactive at rest, have a high threshold and are slow to adapt. Clinically, these receptors can be stimulated by providing a strong, prolonged distraction on a joint to help reduce tone in the surrounding muscles.

Type 4 receptors are a plexus of free nerve endings found in fibrous capsules, articular fat pads, ligaments, the periosteum, and the walls of blood vessels. They are pain receptors and are stimulated by mechanical and chemical factors. While they have a high threshold, they are a protective mechanism and are, thus, non-adapting and inactive at rest. Stimulation of Type 4 receptors will produce a gamma withdrawal reflex in an attempt to remove the joint from possible or further injury.

VISCERAL TISSUE

Visceral tissue is specialized tissue unique to each organ/viscera in the body, all of which are encapsulated in a fascial covering. With the support of fascia and specialized ligaments, viscera and organs are suspended in the body, decreasing gravitational strain on these important structures (Fig. 4.43). Posture, alignment of the bones and muscle balance all play a role in ensuring the proper force through the fascia required to maintain the position of the organs and viscera. When the 'malalignment syndrome' is present, fascial pull through the body can affect organ position and cause stress to affect its function. A detailed explanation of viscera and organ tissue is beyond the scope of this book. It is suggested the reader refer to more specialized anatomy and physiology texts.

MANUAL THERAPY TREATMENT TECHNIQUES

JOINT MOBILIZATION

Joint mobilization is a therapeutic technique which applies a manual force to a specific joint and causes the surfaces of joints to glide parallel to each other or gap perpendicularly. This can be done passively or with the help of the patient to reduce muscular restriction and produce movement into the joint's capsular barrier. The mechanisms of mobilization are still being investigated; however, there are several proposed mechanical and neurophysiological effects which are felt to act by influencing:

1. connective tissue length and alignment
2. neural tissue transmission (and modification) of pain signals, and
3. the function of articular structures

Connective tissue is influenced by cellular modulation. Mobilization causes the release of enzymes to break down cross-links in collagen, increasing inter-fibre distance. It stimulates fibroblast synthesis of collagen proteoglycans which bind with water and increase inter-fibre lubrication. In addition, it creates a piezoelectric current which aids in the alignment of new fibres and realignment of old ones.

Neural tissues are influenced in a way which decreases pain perception. Joint mobilization stimulates Type 1 and 2 mechanoreceptors, inhibiting nociceptive impulses and altering the afferent input to trigger efferent output or gamma bias, thereby relaxing the muscle (Sterling et al. 2000). Mobilization can also stimulate the release of endorphins and enkephalins, natural pain relievers produced by the body.

Articular structures can be mobilized to increase joint mobility by changing capsular elasticity. A 'fixated' or 'locked' joint can be corrected by moving a joint inclusion, such as a meniscoid or loose body, that is restricting the mobility. In addition, movement of the joint improves the articular cartilage nutrition and circulation which, in turn, can increase the supply of materials required for healing and aid in the removal of chemical irritants. It also alters joint lubrication; the resulting change is more significant with higher grades of mobilization.

JOINT MANIPULATION

Manipulation is a 'skilled' and highly specific joint mobilization technique that uses a 'high velocity, low amplitude' thrust technique to move a joint beyond its active range of motion but within its anatomical integrity. It is associated with an audible 'popping' noise and can be used on both spinal and peripheral joints, although spinal manipulations will have a greater influence on the neurophysiological response. Indications for manipulation include capsular and muscular adhesions, joint fixations or compressed joints, meniscoid or loose body entrapments, and segmental muscle 'facilitation'. While manipulation can be an effective treatment approach, it is a more aggressive technique with associated risks and contraindications that must always be considered. One concern is that it is difficult to control the end-point of the manipulation and that it can occasionally exceed the 'yield point' of the ligamentous supports. If minor tears were to occur repeatedly, then ligament laxity and joint instability could certainly result eventually. Though there is no convincing research evidence to support these assumptions, clinical experience suggests they are a definite possibility. Certainly, if the manipulations are being carried out on a repetitive basis (e.g. such as a weekly, bi-weekly or monthly fixed schedule), or every time symptoms recur or become intolerable, then clearly the manipulations alone are failing to address the underlying cause(s) for the problem at hand.

Mechanically, manipulation has been shown to increase the passive range of motion of a joint (Nilsson et al. 1996), by stretching the joint capsule and segmental muscles and breaking adhesions that could be found in the capsule, ligament or surrounding muscle. It can also reduce joint fixation by altering muscle tone around the joint, releasing synovial folds or meniscoid entrapments, and shifting a disc fragment. By restoring the proper joint biomechanics, a manipulation can help remove direct pressure on nervous system structures.

Neurophysiological effects include inhibition of segmental muscle 'facilitation' and pain modulation. The altered segmental muscle activity is caused by stimulation of the articular mechanoreceptors and stretch receptors – specifically, the muscle spindles and Golgi tendon organs - which cause an inhibitory reflex to the segmental muscles (Thabe 1986; Murphy et al. 1995). Pain relief is achieved using the 'gating theory' mechanism (increasing proprioceptive input to block pain signals), stimulation of mechanorecptors, relief of any mechanical irritation of the nervous system, and stimulation of the sympathetic nervous system causing an excitatory response (pilomotor response, increased sweating, flushing) to increase the individual's pain threshold. Spinal manipulation of the cervical joints has also been shown to alter sensorimotor integration; specifically, central corticomotor facilitatory and inhibitory neural processing and cortical motor control (Taylor & Murphy 2006). These findings may suggest an alternate mechanism to the 'gating theory' to explain pain relief. The manipulative technique has direct influence on the articular, neurological and myofascial systems.

Manipulations are most commonly provided by doctors, chiropractors, osteopaths and physiotherapists. In a number of countries, spinal manipulation is a restricted activity, limited to specifically designated professionals who have proven the necessary competence.

MUSCLE ENERGY TECHNIQUE

Muscle energy technique (MET) employs the patient's own muscle force in order to provide the energy required to correct tissue impairment. This technique was originally developed by an osteopathic physician, Dr. Fred L. Mitchell Sr., in the early 1950s. It has continued to evolve since then with important developments by Dr. Fred Mitchell Jr. This technique has direct influences on the myofascial, neurological and articular systems.

MET is a system of diagnosis and treatment of movement and structural dysfunction that is thought to work through neurological, mechanical, circulatory and rheologic mechanisms. As indicated by Dr. P. Kai Mitchell (2009a):

> *The majority of MET procedures use light to moderate force isometric contractions in order to relax a target muscle and make it physiologically more amenable to passive stretching and lengthening. The isometric procedures also result in concurrent micro-stretching of connective tissue, decongestion of swollen tissue, and reprogramming the nerve supply of the target muscle(s). Types of muscle contraction include: 1. Isometric contraction of varying force in order to treat one or more joints for motion impairment and/or to test muscle strength; 2. maxium force isotonic contractions to treat spasm of an antagonist muscle; 3. vibratory isolytic contractions to treat motion restriction due to fibrotic contracture; 4. concentric isokinetic contractions to treat articular hypermobility due to muscular weakness.*

A study by Lenehan et al. (2003) reported significant increases in range of motion of the thorax with one muscle energy treatment session, compared to untreated controls.

The technique requires the active participation of the patient. With the patient in a relaxed position, the practitioner positions the muscle into the feather edge of the barrier to movement. The limb is then held in place while the patient alternately contracts and relaxes the muscle, repeating this until the desired outcome is reached. MET is performed with tissue neutral tension, using an isometric contraction, and does not provoke pain. Indications for MET include: malalignment of the pelvis ('inflare', 'outflare' or 'rotation'), spine or rib dysfunction, core muscle activation and reintegration, impaired circulatory and lymphatic movement, proprioceptive nerve dysfunction (e.g. swallowing dyskinesia), and a need for bone remolding through mechanical loading using the intrinsic muscle force (P. K. Mitchell pers. comm. 2009b).

Muscle energy techniques are primarily used by osteopaths but an increasing number of physiotherapists, massage therapists, and medical doctors have sought training for this technique. MET has been found by the authors to be highly effective in treating malalignment of the pelvis and spine and the secondary 'malalignment syndrome'.

> More information on MET can be found throughout this book, as well as the website:
> www.muscleenergytechnique.com or
> www.TheMitchellInstitute.com

CRANIAL OSTEOPATHY AND CRANIOSACRAL THERAPY

Cranial osteopathy

Cranial osteopathy is a theoretical approach which primarily targets the region of the head. This approach uses light pressure or induction of pressure into the membranes around the skull to facilitate the release of stored tension within these membranes. Cranial osteopathy is one component of an osteopathic treatment, in which the whole body is assessed along with the cranium. Cranial osteopathy and CranioSacral therapy can have a direct effect on the neural, myofascial and visceral systems.

An osteopath, William G. Sutherland, was the first to theorize that the skull bones have some form of mobility throughout life, and that this is susceptible to dysfunction. In the early 1900s, he postulated that the bevelled surface of the skull bones could facilitate the rhythmic palpable sensation found within the cranium, which he called the 'primary respiratory mechanism' (PRM). The sensation of a PRM is palpable in all body tissues according to osteopathy and practitioners of craniosacral therapy.

Using the attachment of the membranes to the skull bones, the therapist may be able to affect their tension and mobility. 'The meninges or reciprocal tension membranes [Dura] . . . are the agencies for articular mobility of the cranial and craniosacral mechanism, securing balance in all diameters; aiding, controlling, and limiting motion.' (Magoun 1951: 17) It has been found that there is a small amount of mobility available within the sutures of the skull (Kostopoulos & Keramidas 1992) and that there are rhythmic flow patterns to the cerebral spinal fluid (Li et al. 1996).

CranioSacral therapy

CranioSacral therapy was developed by John Upledger, an American osteopathic physician. During a brain surgery proceedure, he was holding the dura of the patient when he noted a fluid pulse within the membranes of the skull. While working as a clinical researcher at Michigan State University from 1975-1983, Upledger experimented with techniques which can affect this pulse. As a result, he developed a series of techniques with which to test and treat the cranium, pelvis, and viscera. Upledger has since developed courses in CranioSacral Therapy, SomatoEmotional Release and Visceral Techniques (Upledger & Larni 1990).

A cranial osteopathic treatment starts with the practitioner's hands placed over specific sites around the skull, in order to feel for the strength and rate of the cranial sacral rhythm, or PRM (Fig. 8.4). The bones of the skull are assessed for movement and for position relative to the paired bone on the opposite side. The practitioner then assesses the sacrum to determine the rhythm and strength of the PRM, as

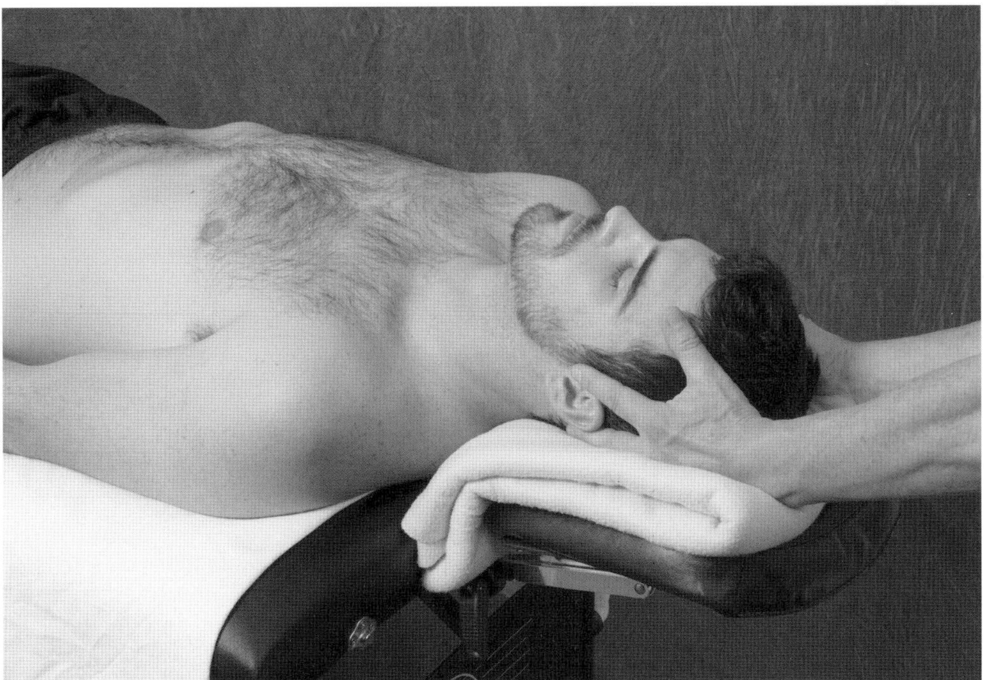

Fig. 8.4 Cranial osteopathy assessment: hand placement.

well as the bone's position and mobility within the SI joints. A treatment continues with a full body assessment of the tissues' health and mobility. Myofascial techniques may be used to treat dysfunctional tissue.

Craniosacral therapy should be considered for those presenting with malalignment, especially when other treatments have not completely resolved the patient's symptoms. For example, the technique may be effective for treating malalignment of the pelvis in patients who have failed to respond (or stabilize only temporarily) to treatment with pelvic MET, realignment of displaced vertebrae or a trial with the NUCCA approach for an apparent C1/C2 problem.

It is the authors' opinion that a high level of training is needed in order to competently assess restrictions within and around the skull. Those interested in learning craniosacral therapy should seek out practitioners who have both the extensive training and practical experience essential for teaching the technique.

CranioSacral therapy training can be sought through privately-run seminars, and osteopathy schools: www.open-source-cranio.com/sacral-training/cranio-sacral-therapy-schools. To find a practitioner from the Upledger Institute, see the website: www.iahp.com

MYOFASCIAL RELEASE

Myofascial release is a 'System of diagnosis and treatment first described by Andrew Taylor Still and his early students, which engages continual palpatory feedback to achieve release of myofascial tissues' (Binkerd et al. 2002: 1241). Myofascial release has been used in a broad sense to describe many soft tissue release techniques but this chapter will use the term to describe only those techniques in which the therapist 'listens' for tissue feedback. Myofascia is a term which describes the intimacy between the fascia covering the muscle and the fascia covering all other structures of the body. It is very hard to separate the fascial attachment to the muscle from that covering these other structures. Myofascial release is defined as a three-dimensional release technique which uses gentle traction or pressure to affect the fluid matrix contained within the fascial structure. It has a direct influence on both the myofascial and neural systems.

The technique aims to release restrictions and restore fluidity to the myofascial tissue. This process increases the mobility of fluids within the matrix of the fascial tissue, which holds components of the immune and anti-inflammatory system. Myofascial release can use mechanical traction or pressure to achieve this result. In a study conducted by Pohl (2007), high frequency ultrasound was used to measure the effects of manual treatment on the connective tissue of the skin; the changes found after treatment included a more even distribution and density of collagen.

Myofascial release uses feedback from the tissue in order to guide the treatment. As the technique is applied, the practitioner or patient may feel heat, pulling, or a wave-like sensation. The treatment is complete when the tissue resumes a normal fluctuation or 'rhythm' referred to as the PMR, or respiration of the tissue. This technique is gentle and appropriate for all ages and body types. It can be applied:

1. in an indirect fashion, where the tissue is taken into its ease of movement (such as for 'unwinding' – see Ch. 7)
2. in a direct fashion, into the tissue traction or stretch (such as with scar release)
3. into the midpoint of tension, where the tissue is half way between its ease and restriction.

Myofascial release is practised by osteopaths, some massage therapists, and others with the appropriate post-graduate training. It is highly effective in releasing accumulated tensions within the fascia of the body after injury, with faulty posture, or from chronic malalignment of the pelvis.

For information on myofascial release, to find a practitioner or to take a course, see the website by John Barnes: www.myofascialrelease.com or by D. Lee: www.discoverphysio.ca/courses

STRAIN-COUNTERSTRAIN TECHNIQUE

Strain-Counterstrain treatment involves the assessment and detection of small pea-sized tender points within a muscle's fibres. These tender points can help identify the dysfunctional proprioceptors and, therefore, guide the treatment. This technique, developed in 1955 by Lawrence H. Jones (1981) an American osteopathic physician, has direct influences on the neurological and myofascial systems.

Strain-Counterstrain is based on the idea that muscles in dysfunction have a changed neural input. Irwin Korr showed that a dysfunctional muscle spindle (proprioceptor) releases an increased neurological discharge which maintains the muscle in this dysfunction state (1986). This neurological signal is produced by the stretch receptors (muscle spindles) in response to the muscle suffering a quick stretch which, in turn, causes a constant low-level hypertonicity in the muscle. To intervene in the pattern of an inappropriately increased neural signal being produced by the stretch receptors, Strain-Counterstrain technique is used to place the muscle in a shortened position for 90 seconds. Dardzinski et al. (2000) found significant pain reduction using Strain-Counterstrain in the treatment of subjects with myofascial pain syndromes.

Treatment is passive. The tender point is localized in the dysfunctional muscle. The muscle is then moved into the appropriate position of ease by the therapist, and held for 90 seconds (or, in the case of rib dysfunctions, for 2 minutes).

> An osteopath or medical doctor may be found to provide this treatment.

VISCERAL MANIPULATION

Visceral manipulation uses gentle pressure on, or induction of movement to, the ligaments and fascia which hold the organs and viscera in place. Visceral manipulation has been used throughout history in various massage techniques. A.T. Still, an osteopath, first formally documented these techniques in a textbook in 1902. Jean-Pierre Barral (1983, 1988, 1993), a French physiotherapist and osteopath, has since developed further visceral manipulation techniques that are taught all over the world (see Chs 4, 7).

The visceral system relies on the interconnected synchronicity between the motions of all the organs and structures of the body. At optimal health, this harmonious relationship remains stable despite the body's endless variations in motion. When one organ cannot move in harmony with the surrounding abdominal structures due to abnormal tone, adhesions or displacement, it works against the body's other organs and also the muscular, membranous, fascial and osseous structures. This disharmony creates fixed, abnormal points of tension that the body is forced to move around and the resultant chronic irritation can cause postural distortion, neuromuscular dysfunction, and disease processes (Dawn Langnes, personal communication, 2009).

Visceral lesions can be caused by various traumas, resulting in dysfunctions such as ptosis (drooping), sprain of the supporting ligaments, scar formation, malpositioning or kinking, and cell damage. Visceral manipulation can help resolve these dysfunctions in the organs and viscera through:

1. resetting tone in the parenchymae, walls and supporting ligaments
2. repositioning
3. modification of scar density, and
4. restoration of nervous impulses and blood flow

A visceral manipulation treatment is done with the patient lying down or in a sitting position. The techniques are gentle and usually painless. Using light pressure, the practitioner palpates the organ location while assessing its position, mobility and primary respiratory mechanism (PRM). Techniques used to treat a dysfunction are chosen depending on the severity and type of the lesion. Other approaches used include 'fluidic' and 'energetic' techniques which are beyond the scope of this chapter.

Visceral/organ malposition or malfunction can directly effect pelvic malalignment, owing to the attachments through fascia to the posterior wall of the spine and pelvis. When repetitive treatment of malalignment through osteoarticular techniques is not effective, the visceral and fascial system should be assessed and treated.

> Courses in visceral manipulation can be found at: www.barralinstitute.com or the International Alliance of Healthcare Educators: www.iahp.com

NUCCA, GROSTIC, 'HOLE-IN-ONE' CHIROPRACTIC

B.J. Palmer, a chiropractor, strongly believed that the first two cervical vertebrae (C1/2) were the primary cause of all disease; hence, the theory of treatment he named 'hole-in-one'. In 1943, Grostic, another chiropractor, developed instruments to measure the misalignment of C1 and the cervical spine in three planes of movement. He was the first to x-ray C1 post-treatment to evaluate the degree of correction made by the adjustment/ manipulation. In 1966, Gregory founded the National Upper Cervical Chiropractic Association (NUCCA) in order to expand research and education on upper cervical spine chiropractic techniques. This treatment can have direct effects on the myofascial, neural and articular system.

An assessment by a NUCCA chiropractor includes an X-ray analysis of the first two vertebrae in the neck, as well as assessments of the symmetry of the cranium, shoulders, pelvis and leg length. With the patient in side lying, the involved vertebra is positioned so as to allow the proper force vector to be applied with a constant and firm pressure through the side of the wrist (pisiform) until the vertebra is felt to be corrected (Foran 1999a,b).

Currently, only chiropractors can be taught, and subsequently perform, the NUCCA technique. It is the authors' opinion that the findings in the cervical (C1/2) and lumbar spine regions can be adaptive or secondary to lesions within the pelvis, thorax and cranium and that these lesions should, therefore, be treated first.

Information on NUCCA, Grostic or 'Hole-In-One' techniques can be found at: www.nucca.org

ACTIVE RELEASE TECHNIQUES

Active release techniques (ART) use manual contacts combined with specific movement patterns to affect scar tissue within muscle, tendon, ligament, nerve and fascia. A chiropractor, P.M. Leahy, began developing this form of therapy in 1985 when he found he needed techniques to address the build-up of scar tissue in myofascial tissue. ART affects the myofascial and neural system.

Leahy found that overuse in muscles can cause scar tissue to build up in three ways: as the result of acute injury, micro-trauma and hypoxia (lack of oxygen). The scar tissue can restrict the free movement of neighbouring tissues and can cause tissue pain, limitation in range of movement, and reduction of strength. It is proposed that the treatment results in a mechanical release of scar tissue which then allows the particular structure to perform as intended. The decrease in scar tissue also improves blood/oxygen perfusion of the tissue. George et al. (2006) found an increase in hamstring flexibility with one ART treatment in healthy male subjects.

During an ART treatment, the practitioner manually assesses the texture of the muscle affected. This tissue is treated using a protocol specifically designed to normalize the muscle/tendon/ligament/nerve/fascia. In order to break up the scar tissue, ART uses a sufficient amount of mechanical tension, created by hand contraction to effect gradual lengthening of the structure being treated.

For more information on the ART technique, please see: www.activerelease.com

BOWEN THERAPY

Bowen therapy positions the muscle at rest, and then induces a gentle stimulus to the superficial fascia. It was developed by an Australian, Thomas A. Bowen (1916-1982), who trained with an osteopath, as well as working as a 'strapper', or therapist, on a football team which allowed him to practice and refine his technique. A number of therapists worked closely with Bowen, and each has since taught a different interpretation of his technique. Bowen approaches are variously known as: Bowen Technique, Neurostructural Integration Technique, Smart Bowen, Fascial Kinetics, Emmette Technique, Bowenfirst and BowenBridge.

Bowen therapy is a technique directed at a patient's superficial fascia while at rest. The practitioner gently rolls his/her finger(s) on the fascia, applying some minimal pressure across specific spots. The response is said to involve releasing adhesions in the collagen fibers, allowing the tissues to rehydrate, and resetting myofascial postural tone at an appropriate level. The Bowen technique has been found to be successful in enhancing flexibility in hamstring muscles (Marr 2007).

The technique is applied with the patient fully clothed. The tissue is then typically allowed to rest for two minutes or longer, in order for the nervous system to integrate the applied mechanical stimulus. Bowen therapy is gentle, and is suitable for all ages and body types.

To find out more about Bowen therapy, see: www.bowendirectory.com

OTHER COMPLEMENTARY TREATMENT TECHNIQUES

FELDENKRAIS TECHNIQUE

Feldenkrais is a movement-based technique in which the participant re-educates (neuro-) muscular patterns through repetition. The technique was created by a Ukrainian nuclear physicist, Moshe Feldenkrais (1904-1984), who had a PhD in mechanical engineering and high energy physics from the Sorbonne University in Paris, as well as a black belt in judo. He developed knee pain, and medicine at the time gave him a 50-50 chance of recovery with surgery. He decided that there must be a better way to resolve his injury.

Feldenkrais immersed himself in extensive studies of anatomy, physiology, anthropology and Zen Buddhism. His focus was on 'the human body as a cybernetic, or feedback system' (Jensen 1985: 429). He began teaching his technique in the 1950s. In order for the forces of gravity to be reduced through the body and its muscles, movements are initiated while lying on the floor, allowing the person to scrutinize habitual actions and to develop new and more efficient patterns. Therapists can also use Feldenkrais techniques through functional integration. These are one-on-one sessions, in which the individual's dysfunctional movements are assessed, and light touch or directed pressure is introduced into the area to release the restrictions.

During a Feldenkrais 'awareness-through-movement' session, the participant follows through a series of movements progressing from lying down, to rolling, then crawling and finally to standing. During all of these movements, the participant is asked to pay attention to micro-movements experienced at the joint and identify any restrictions in its motion.

Practitioners from varied backgrounds may be found using this technique. More information is available at: www.feldenkrais.com

ALEXANDER TECHNIQUE

Alexander technique allows re-patterning of dysfunctional postural muscle tone and movements within the body. F.M. Alexander (1869-1955) thought that disease has origins within a person's posture and use of muscles. Alexander was an Australian-born actor and orator. He developed problems with his voice and was unable to continue his work as an actor. He sought medical advice but found that nothing helped. He then began to seek his own solution. He practised speaking in front of a mirror and found there were peculiarities in the use of his muscles when he was speaking. He theorized that to change a muscle's control, a person must let go of the unconscious poor movement patterns which are causing problems, and to redefine new movement approaches. Alexander did not trust his own body as these abnormal movement patterns felt normal to him, and so he developed the principle of 'non-doing'. For example, instead of directing himself to stand up straight, he asked the body to 'let the head go forward and up'. Using this approach, he resolved the problem with his voice.

The Alexander technique teaches people to learn how to recognize habitual movement patterns and how to change these patterns. It essentially teaches them to break away from habitual postures and to let the body reorganize itself in the most efficient way possible. The goal is to reset postural tone and to coordinate muscle through practise of directed movement and the tactile cueing provided by the practitioner. Usually six or more sessions are required for successful motor learning to take place in postural muscles and to have a therapeutic effect on the lower back (Little et al. 2008).

In this technique, the practitioner is the coach, and no orthopaedic assessment is required. The steps are always the same, as the pattern of muscle recruitment is reorganized from the head down. The patient may first be asked to lie down and to focus on the words 'let the neck be free' and 'let the head go forward and up'. He or she may be asked not to let any intentions guide the treatment, but to find the 'path of non-doing'.

Practitioners come from varied backgrounds. To find out more about the technique: www.alexandertechnique.com

ACUPUNCTURE

There are currently two approaches to acupuncture: the Classical method or 'Traditional Chinese Medicine' (TCM), and the newer 'Western' approach known as 'Anatomical Acupuncture'. Both use the insertion of fine needles into specific points; however, the clinical reasoning and philosophy behind these methods varies.

Classical acupuncture

Classical acupuncture is a complete system for diagnosing and treating disease. It dates back over 2000 years and comes from a collection of knowledge compiled over centuries. The basic philosophy is based on Taoism: equal and opposite forces, Yin and Yang, coexist in the universe and illness is caused by an imbalance of these forces. Needling points are chosen based on comprehensive subjective and physical exams, including pulse and tongue diagnosis. They facilitate a normalization effect by adding or decreasing the amount of energy or 'Qi' flowing (Liboff 1997).

Anatomical acupuncture

Anatomical acupuncture is used as a treatment modality rather than a complete system. It combines traditional acupuncture – specifically, the predetermined points - with 'Western' anatomy, physiology and pathophysiology. Typically, practitioners will make a 'Western' diagnosis and use needling points based on the traditional 'map' or they choose their points based on anatomical position or effects on physiology.

Electro-acupuncture

Electro-acupuncture is used by both kinds of practitioners and is chosen if a stronger stimulation is desired. Needles are inserted into points and attached to a device that delivers an electrical current. The intensity and frequency can be adjusted. While there is little research supporting the specific parameters for stimulation, frequencies between 2-4 Hz are commonly used for nociceptive pain conditions and 80-100 Hz for neuropathic pain.

Proposed mechanisms of action

Acupuncture is used to control pain, decrease inflammation, stimulate regeneration, reset the autonomic nervous system and restore normal function. It influences our physiology and neurophysiology by stimulating neurotransmitters which send impulses to the spinal cord, activating centres in the spinal cord, midbrain, and pituitary/hypothalamus.

Pain modulation

As a pain-relief modality, acupuncture releases endogenous morphines known as endorphins (Pomeranz & Chiu 1976; Sjolund et al. 1977). At the spinal cord, enkephalins and dynorphin are released which cause segmental effects. At the mid-brain, enkephalins released via the dorsolateral tract in turn release monoamines (serotonin and norepinephrine) which influence our 'flight or fight response' through our sympathetic nervous system. This increase in our natural opioid or endorphin levels can be extremely beneficial for chronic pain patients. They have been shown to have low levels of endorphins in the cerebrospinal fluid (CSF), and these levels rise with electro-acupuncture (Sjolund et al. 1977).

Anti-inflammatory action

The levels of cortisol, an anti-inflammatory, significantly increase with electro-acupuncture (Cheng et al. 1980). This is a corticosteroid hormone produced by the adrenal cortex that helps reduce immune responses. Acupuncture also stimulates production of the pituitary hormone beta-lipotropin (Facchinetti et al. 1981), which also accounts for anti-inflammatory effects. It is released into the blood and CSF via the pituitary-hypothalamic complex. While the main function of beta-lipotropin is to stimulate melanocytes to produce melanin, it also performs lipid-mobilizing functions such as lipolysis and steroidogenesis. The latter includes production of steroids such as androgens, testosterone, and corticoids that aid in reducing inflammation and facilitating the healing process.

Acupuncture is performed by practitioners of Traditional Chinese Medicine, naturopathic doctors, and specifically trained medical doctors, physiotherapists, chiropractors, dentist and nurses.

DRY-NEEDLING TECHNIQUE

'Dry-needling' uses acupuncture needles to desensitize tender points and treat myofascial pain and other diseases or impairments. There are several dry-needling techniques. The two most recognized in North America are based on:

1. the 'trigger point model' developed by Dr. Travell in the 1940s, and
2. the 'radiculopathy model' developed by Dr. Gunn in 1973, known as Intramuscular Stimulation (Gunn IMS).

Trigger point model

The trigger point model specifically targets myofascial trigger points: tight knots in a muscle (thought to be due to excessive release of acetylcholine (ACh) from select motor end plates) which can affect muscle activity, range of motion, and autonomic functions. The clinician will determine which points need treatment by looking for the tight bands with spot tenderness, a jump sign, and pain. He/she may then treat these points with either a deep or superficial needling technique.

Deep needling

This approach mechanically stimulates or deforms the trigger point and can cause a 'local twitch response'. This is an involuntary spinal cord reflex contraction of the affected muscle fibres in the taut band, and is essential for achieving the therapeutic effects. The twitch response can normalize the chemical environment and diminish the endplate noise associated with trigger points (Chen et al. 2001). It is also believed that mechanical stimulation of the trigger point by the needle initiates the therapeutic effect by damaging motor endplates and causing distal axon denervation (Simons et al. 1999). The damage could trigger muscle regeneration by simulating the cholinesterase and ACh receptors in the endplates. The needle may also cause a localized stretch to the contracted structures which could help the sacromeres resume resting length. Studies by Langevin et al. (2002, 2006) provided evidence that the 'needle grasp' is not due to muscle contraction but, instead, due to changes in the surrounding connective tissue. These effects are increased by needle rotation, which causes pulling of the collagen fibres toward the needle and initiates changes in fibroblasts.

Superficial needling

This method is used to stimulate connective tissue above the motor point and indirectly affect the point without penetrating the muscle fibre with the needle. In 1980, Baldry developed a superficial needling technique to minimize risks associated with deeper penetration. A needle is inserted 5-10 mm directly over a trigger point and left in for 30 seconds. If there is still increased sensitivity, the needle is re-inserted for another 2-3 minutes. Baldry (2005) found this technique would abolish exquisite tenderness at the myofascial trigger point and eliminate spontaneous pain.

Intramuscular stimulation (Gunn IMS)

IMS is a complete system for diagnosing and treating musculoskeletal (MSK) injuries and chronic pain. It uses a deep needling technique to release shortened muscles and take pressure off nerves, allowing the body to restore the 'hard-wiring' of its MSK system. It is based on a 'radiculopathy' model that assumes chronic pain is due to compromised neural fibres (Gunn 1978, 1996).

The general principle behind the 'radiculopathy' model is that neural input to muscles becomes compromised if the nerve is squeezed by surrounding muscles or bone. This often occurs at the spine as postural adaptations (e.g. those noted with malalignment; see Chs 3, 4) and repetitive movements cause an imbalance in muscular tissues that, in turn, leads to compression in the back or neck. The compressing structures squeeze the nerves exiting the spinal column and reduce input to the muscles they innervate. Often autonomic changes (pilomotor, pseudomotor, and vasomotor signs) are noted before sensory or motor changes because the autonomic nerve fibres have the greatest diameter and will be affected first with compression of the spinal nerve. When normal neural input to a muscle is reduced, less ACh is released into the muscle and the muscle produces extra receptor sites for ACh. Since this chemical is what causes the muscle to contract, less ACh is now required to produce a contraction. Eventually, with prolonged muscle imbalances and compromised neural input to the muscle, there will be enough ACh receptors sites to respond to just the resting level of ACh stored in the muscle and the muscle will remain contracted. This is known as a 'supersensitive' structure and is explained through Cannon & Rosenblueth's 'Law of Denervation' (1949).

IMS treatment consists of needling shortened muscles in their 'ropey' and tender point, stimulating an electrical response by targeting the stretch receptor organs. This causes a quick muscle contraction, or twitch, which lets the muscle reset into a longer resting position. Not only can this increase range of motion but the lengthened muscle is also less likely to exert pressure on the nerves that innervate and/or pass through it. Pain will also be decreased because the lengthened muscle exerts less pressure on its nociceptors. In addition:

1. the increased tone noted in muscles hypersensitive to ACh decreases the physical 'holes' that normally serve as 'ports of entry', so to speak, for the Ach
2. the needles, by causing micro-injuries to the muscle, create direct channels that allow for an inflow of Ach into the muscle; with more ACh now available, the muscle becomes desensitized to ACh and decreases the number of its receptors.

After an IMS treatment, a person may feel soreness similar to a generalized muscle ache for a period of time that can last up to a few days. The aching occurs because the body has undergone a 'mini-workout', as each muscle twitch with the needle insertion is an actual muscle contraction. In addition, there may be bruising because the needles are causing micro-trauma to the tissue and can disturb the vascular supply.

Only doctors and highly trained physiotherapists are allowed to be trained in IMS and all practitioners are required to do their training out of the Institute for the Study and Treatment of Pain (iSTOP) in Vancouver, British Columbia, Canada. IMS practitioners can be found on the institute's website: www.istop.org

HORSE-BASED THERAPY

Both therapeutic riding and hippotherapy use a horse as a means of treatment for physical dysfunction. The main difference is that therapeutic riding has a goal of developing the rider's technique; whereas hippotherapy uses the horse's motion to help mobilize the rider's pelvis in different directions.

Therapeutic riding

Therapeutic riding participants are taught horseback riding in a group setting. Each horse is led by a volunteer. The rider's balance and muscle tone are developed by varying the speed of the horse. Motor planning and co-ordination of the muscles are developed while riding, and postural control is optimized in the head and trunk. Therapeutic riding is also used for its positive effects on the self-esteem of the rider.

Hippotherapy

Hippotherapy originated in 1952, when Liz Hartel of Denmark, who was previously afflicted with polio, won a dressage event at the Olympic games. It was realized that horse riding may help others with muscular dysfunction.

Hippotherapy is now an accepted medical treatment that uses the movement of a specially trained horse to facilitate changes in those with movement disorders associated, for example, with cerebral palsy, developmental delay, multiple sclerosis, autism, stroke or head injury. Common clinical impairments that can be treated with hippotherapy are abnormal muscle tone, impaired balance and/or coordination, postural control, abnormal reflexes and impaired sensorimotor function.

The key to hippotherapy is the movement that transfers from the pelvis of the horse to the pelvis and the spine of the person sitting or lying astride the horse - the actual position is determined by what particular movement the therapist is trying to facilitate in the pelvis (e.g. anterior/posterior tilt, lateral tilt, rotation in the transverse plane) or the spine. This makes it ideal for treatment of malalignment, when movements in one or more planes are usually impaired. For example, sitting sideways on the horse mobilizes the rider's pelvis in the coronal plane (see cover illustration of 1st edition!). An instructor leads the horse through a course that includes circles, diagonals and hills in order to influence the pelvic muscles and the posture of the rider. For optimal treatment, the horse's movement must be symmetrical and rhythmical. Instruction in hippotherapy is usually conducted by a physiotherapist, occupational therapist or speech therapist but can be completed by anyone with the necessary training.

To find a 'Therapeutic Riding' instructor in your area you can go to the Therapeutic Riding for the Disabled website: www.frdi.net

ROLFING

Rolfing is a form of myofascial deep tissue work and movement re-education which seeks to balance the body within the gravitational field to improve function. The Rolfing technique was created in the mid 1940s by an American biochemist, Dr. Ida Rolf (1896-1979), who had studied mathematics, physics, homeopathy, osteopathy, chiropractic and yoga. She developed an approach to treating the fascia of the body which she called 'structural integration'. Rolfing can have a direct effect on the myofascial, articular and neural systems.

Rolfing uses many deep tissue techniques to separate and allow for rehydration of adherent, dry and shortened fascia so that muscles and joints can move with more freedom. Fascia can become restrictive over time due to many factors, including poor movement strategies, malalignment, injury, and emotional 'holding' within the tissues. Rolfing technique acts to treat the whole body through release of restrictions in the fascial web. Concurrent movement re-education helps to change poor postural habits so that fascial restrictions do not recur.

A Rolfing session starts with an assessment, noting any fascial restrictions and how the person moves and holds himself/herself. Practitioners use manual pressure in tissue techniques that can sometimes be quite painful. The sessions usually follow a 10-step approach, as outlined in Box 8.3.

BOX 8.3 Rolfing sessions: the 10-step approach

The Rolfing 'ten series' can be viewed as a basic recipe which all Rolfers follow to achieve their common goal of balancing the client's body within the gravitational field. However, individual Rolfers work in different ways and also recognize that each client is unique and so adapt the recipe to suit their client's needs. The following briefly describe each of the steps (adapted from Keith Graham).

SESSION ONE- Freedom to breathe
SESSION TWO - Finding support
SESSION THREE - Creating your space, owning your place
SESSION FOUR - Finding your core, connecting earth to sky
SESSION FIVE - The next step for humankind, walking with grace and ease
SESSION SIX- Freeing the spine
SESSION SEVEN - Getting the head on straight!
SESSION EIGHT - Putting it all back together
SESSION NINE - Integration
SESSION TEN - Closure

YOGA

Yoga practice uses specific poses in order to stimulate muscle stretch and strength, facilitate focus and concentration, also to aid breathing and digestion. Yoga has been found to have roots dating back to 3000 BC. It started as a practice for spiritual growth and meditation, and is mentioned in the Bhagavad-Gita, a Hindu religious text which originated around 500 B.C. Yoga evolved into an individualized practice where the person looks inward to the breathing pattern and to the body's vitality.

Hatha yoga

The most common type currently practised is Hatha yoga, the postural form of yoga that is physically demanding. It uses postural muscles in order to hold different poses in an attempt to achieve mental and physical health. Yoga practice can affect the myofascial, neural and visceral systems. Hatha yoga may use poses in which balance on a single leg is needed, which may exacerbate malalignment-related symptoms; therefore, these poses should be modified to meet the individual's needs.

Iyengar yoga

A type of Hatha yoga called 'Iyengar yoga' emphasizes the use of precise alignment of the body while performing yoga poses, as well as using numerous props in its practice. The intent is to modify yoga poses in order to make them more comfortable for the participant. The use of props in this yoga style is key: blocks, towels, straps, the wall or even another practitioner are used in order to support the body. Each pose is fine-tuned to find the individual's most comfortable position. These poses may be held for up to 3-5 minutes or longer. Iyengar yoga may be more beneficial to patients with 'malalignment syndrome', because the poses can be more readily modified to meet the expectations of the practitioner. Small group classes maximize the instructor's ability to observe and correct the individual's position.

To find a teacher of restorative yoga, see: www.restorativeyogateachers.com

PILATES AS THERAPY

Pilates uses movement, with body weight as resistance, to strengthen and tone the body's muscles while maintaining awareness of alignment and breathing technique. It was developed by a German-born fitness instructor, Joseph H. Pilates (1880-1967). After suffering a sickly childhood, he became interested in yoga, martial arts and other athletic pursuits. He originated his program of exercises during the war, where he used slings and springs from hospital beds in order to give bedridden patients the ability to exercise. Later, in New York, with the assistance of his wife, he opened a studio which primarily catered to ballet dancers.

The Pilates technique can have a direct effect on the myofascial and neurological systems. J.H. Pilates himself used eccentric training to create long strong muscles without bulkiness (Menezes 2000, Pilates 1934). His focus was on alignment of the spine, diaphragmatic breathing, as well as maintaining core

BOX 8.4 The 'Six Principles of Pilates Exercise'

1. Breathing

Is the most important of the six principles - proper diaphragmatic breathing increases the effectiveness of the exercise program. Full inhalations/exhalations allow the breath to mobilize the ribs, massage the internal organs, enhance muscle activation and to oxygenate the tissues.

2. Concentration

As directed energy - to be mindful and pay attention to the activation of muscle groups required to perform a specific movement. Nuances and muscle patterns can be identified and thereby changed or modified.

3. Control

With concentration - learn where every part of your body is. The body teaches the brain how to interact which develops improved body responses in reactive movements.

4. Centering

Addresses the importance of spinal and pelvic stability/mobility by strengthening the abdominals. Start with a strong center and radiate out.

5. Flowing Movement

Move with the rhythm of the breath with ease and efficiency. Muscles work in systems and their job is to move the bones through a varied and wide range of movements.

6. Precision

Joe Pilates said 'Concentrate on right movements each time you exercise or else you will do them improperly and lose their value'

Working smarter with a few repetitions in an exacting manner to develop awareness, efficient form and posture.

Adapted from Karen Angelucci, Rehab Pilates instructor

muscle strength throughout by using prescribed movements (Herrington et al. 2005) and following the 'Six Principles of Pilates Exercise' (Box 8.4).

Pilates exercises use the body weight itself as resistance, and work to progressively increase the sophistication in movement with training. Pilates is usually conducted in group settings where individual assessments are not always carried out. A repertoire of exercises is used in a predetermined order which everyone follows. This type of class may use exercises which are too difficult or the sequence may advance too quickly for someone with the 'malalignment syndrome' to adapt to.

Rehabilitation Pilates

A patient with 'malalignment syndrome' is recommended to start Rehab Pilates training with one-on-one instruction following an assessment to identify the alignment discrepancies and weakness in any muscles. Specific exercises are then selected, based on the individual's specific needs. Rehab Pilates uses one-on-one or small group classes which allow individuals to control the class pace and receive individual feedback. La Touche et al. (2008) found that Pilates therapy helped maintain a significant decrease in disability in patients with chronic low back pain.

Patients with 'malalignment syndrome' are taught to identify muscle weakness and malalignment and have exercise sessions specifically designed for each individual's body needs.

To find out more about Pilates, please see: www.internationalpilates.org

ZERO BALANCING

Zero balancing was developed in the 1970s by Fritz Smith, an American MD and osteopath. The technique uses aspects of his training in osteopathy and acupuncture to create hands-on body work which facilitates energy channels within the body; in effect, using energy movement to integrate Western medical science with Eastern healing traditions. It relieves symptoms caused by an energetic or somatic imbalance and, by aligning energy with structure, enhances the natural healing process and supports ongoing optimum health. Zero balancing works in conjunction with medical therapy and is not a substitute for it.

This approach does not claim to manipulate joints. Nonetheless, release of malaligned or restricted areas is often found to have occurred in the course of a treatment session. By its very nature, in zero balancing there is an integrative theme: somatic changes tend toward integration with other somatic changes as well as with emotional and spiritual changes, and thus tend to be sustained, assuming the tissue is strong enough to hold.

The main intentions of zero balancing are to:

1. relieve pain and distress
2. improve health, vitality and wellness, and
3. help people to experience health, well-being and a higher level of consciousness

Whereas Feldenkrais treatment is often characterized as 'awareness through movement', zero balancing might be better described as 'transformation through stillness'. In contrast with most other manual therapy approaches, the person is not moved around into different positions, required to exert forces against resistance, breathe a certain way, or have body parts moved forcibly about. Rather, the fully-clothed individual lies supine and the body is handled gently and respectfully, with clear force at key sites, and briefly held in stillness, which usually induces a deeply relaxed, altered state of consciousness somewhat akin to meditation or mindfulness. These engagements are termed 'fulcrums'. In terms of tissue, all structure is, ultimately, energy. Zero balancing, therefore, focuses on bone which, as the densest structure in the body, is considered to house the deepest-held energies and restrictions. The fulcrums are generally directed at what are termed 'foundation' or 'semi-foundation' joints. These are joints that have little or no intrinsic musculature, such as the sacroiliac or tarsal joint; at these sites, the body cannot readily achieve any correction by muscular effort. Hence, even a tiny loss of range of motion can have great ramifications throughout the body in terms of alignment, freedom of movement, and compensatory efforts. It is surprising and gratifying that many joint constrictions resolve themselves readily through these simple, enjoyable interventions, while at the same time nourishing mind and spirit.

For further information on Zero Balancing, see: www.zerobalancing.com

FINDING A MANUAL THERAPY PRACTITIONER

Throughout this chapter there are references to web sites and associations which list practitioners who have taken approved therapy courses. In most countries, there is very little regulation as to the educational background of manual therapists, so it is best to ask each practitioner for their qualifications to perform a particular technique.

As indicated, manual therapy can be practised by numerous specialists including physiatrists, osteopaths, physiotherapists, chiropractors, massage therapists, naturopathic doctors and athletic trainers. The techniques described in this chapter can be applied by these practitioners, depending on their education and training. When looking for a manual therapist, one also has to consider the emotions individuals may re-live, vulnerability of being subjected to hands-on work, and the cost of treatment. Therefore, once the type of treatment has been decided on, the person may benefit from a trial of a few treatments with a couple of different practitioners to 'find the right fit', so to speak, and optimize their chances of regaining maximal body function.

CONCLUSION

Chronic pain occurs in as many as 1 in 5 of all individuals, affecting women more than men, and increasing with an aging population (Millar 1996). This is a growing financial burden on our health care system. Health care practitioners are well aware of this problem and the difficulty of finding the appropriate treatment approach.

When mainstream investigation fails to provide a diagnosis that can be corrected with medication or surgical intervention, a hands-on manual therapy approach may be needed to initiate or augment the healing process. Most research encourages a multimodal approach for maximal results but quite often the integral issue is finding the correct combination of therapeutic interventions to meet specific needs. Effective management of the 'malalignment syndrome' is no exception; it requires time and dedication by the individual to the treatment approach and prescribed exercises, the goal being a biomechanically balanced physique and ability to perform the activities of daily living without pain.

This chapter has been an attempt to describe the tissues affected by the malalignment, to explain how they are influenced, and to outline a resource list of interventions with a view toward a successful match being made between individuals and appropriate therapists. Hopefully, the ideas presented will encourage further investigation into the complementary techniques available and help individuals find solutions and management strategies for the persistent pain characteristically noted with malalignment and the 'malalignment syndrome'.

Chapter 9

Conclusion

CHAPTER CONTENTS

Malalignment of the pelvis and spine is present in 80-90% of the population. Approximately 30% of these are symptomatic; another 20-30% have evidence of discomfort when soft tissues and joints are stressed on examination. There are specific biomechanical changes that can help diagnose the three common presentations: 'outflare/inflare', 'rotational malalignment' and 'upslip'; the 'malalignment syndrome' is associated with only the last two. In addition to the distortion of the pelvis and spine, the syndrome is characterized by asymmetries from head to toe: the changes in weight-bearing, leg length, joint ranges of motion and muscle-tendon unit tone and strength are easily detectable in most people, especially in the lower extremities, and help to establish the diagnosis.

The altered biomechanical stresses predispose to restrictions and injuries. Typically, right pronation increases tension in medial soft tissues of that extremity, tendency to knee valgus and stress on the lateral tibiofemoral compartment; left supination stresses are in the opposite pattern and predispose to left knee varus and ankle inversion sprain (Fig. 3.37). A person may find these asymmetries result in an advantage or a hindrance when carrying out some activities. For example, a secondary increase in right rotation of the pelvis and trunk could improve a golfer's backswing; whereas the decrease to the left could limit follow-through (Ch. 5; Fig. 3.5)

Specific muscles show asymmetries of tension and strength. However, over the past decade, there has been an increasing emphasis on the fact that muscles act less in isolation but more as part of a system of 'inner' and 'outer' core slings (Figs 2.28-2.40).

DOI: 10.1016/B978-0-443-06929-1.00009-0

Surface electromyography (EMG), Real-Time Ultrasound and MRI are used increasingly to help:

1. detect atrophy, excessive or decreased tone, patterns of abnormal sequencing of contraction, and failure/inability to activate muscles within these slings
2. provide feedback for the patient (Figs 4.46, 4.47).

The asymmetries noted with malalignment eventually result in soft tissue changes that can predispose to recurrence:

1. contracture: involving tissues that end up in a shortened position (e.g. structures on the concave side of a curve; muscles that are 'facilitated' and/or chronically contracted reflexively to counter pain or instability)
2. lengthening: in tissues put under tension (e.g. structures on the convex side of a curve); in muscles showing decreased tone as a result of being 'inhibited'

The respective limitation of motion and joint instability makes it more and more difficult to achieve and maintain alignment the longer malalignment has been present. However, these structures usually can gradually regain their normal length with ongoing efforts. Treatment should, therefore, include teaching the person:

1. self-assessment: carried out on a day-to-day basis, to detect recurrences and correct these as quickly as possible
2. how to use self-treatment techniques (Ch. 7) or, at least, to seek help before a recurrence becomes symptomatic
3. to value symmetry as much as possible, in an attempt to decrease any torsional stresses on the pelvic unit and spine; examples include carrying out some daily activities, such as getting in and out of the bed or a car, with the legs held together and moving as one unit as best as possible (Fig. 9.1)

Total reliance on compensatory treatment methods (e.g. acupuncture, massage) and failure to recognize the symptoms and signs attributable to an underlying malalignment problem can only contribute to persistence of the malalignment. While a number of these methods may result in temporary improvement, realignment of the pelvis and spine and strengthening core muscles to recover stability remain the keys to recovery.

ONGOING CONCERNS

It has been encouraging that since the publication of the 1st edition in 2002, there has been:

1. an increasing recognition of malalignment as a cause of localized and referred pain and, in particular, of pelvic and back pain
2. a shift from focusing on the SI joint but, rather, looking at the patterns of static and dynamic action involving the core muscles and slings, and their effect on the body as a whole
3. an encouraging increase of publications in the medical literature itself, documenting results of research studies in this field

However, there are ongoing concerns that need to be considered. They relate mainly to the failure to appreciate the predominance and manifestations of malalignment in our society and how best to diagnose and treat this condition.

1. Abnormal biomechanics is still not a part of the curriculum for medical students or of the training for a number of professionals in specialties or careers that typically sees them subsequently confronted with having to deal with neuromusculoskeletal problems which may actually be caused by malalignment: in particular, orthopaedic surgeons, neurologists, rheumatologists, physiotherapists, kinesiologists and athletic trainers.
2. Medicine still fails to recognize that malalignment is a common problem that needs to be treated, and that the 'malalignment syndrome' is a common complication of malalignment and can easily lead to misdiagnosis. It also fails to appreciate the risk of needless and, sometimes, actually harmful surgery being carried out by those who have acted on the results of an incomplete examination and questionable findings on investigation because they are completely ignorant of the malalignment entity and how it can present as a seeming disc, facet or nerve root problem.
3. Ongoing prejudice regarding the diagnostic and treatment skills of osteopaths, chiropractors and physiotherapist practicing manual therapy prevents learning from these professionals and applying new skills to medical practice.

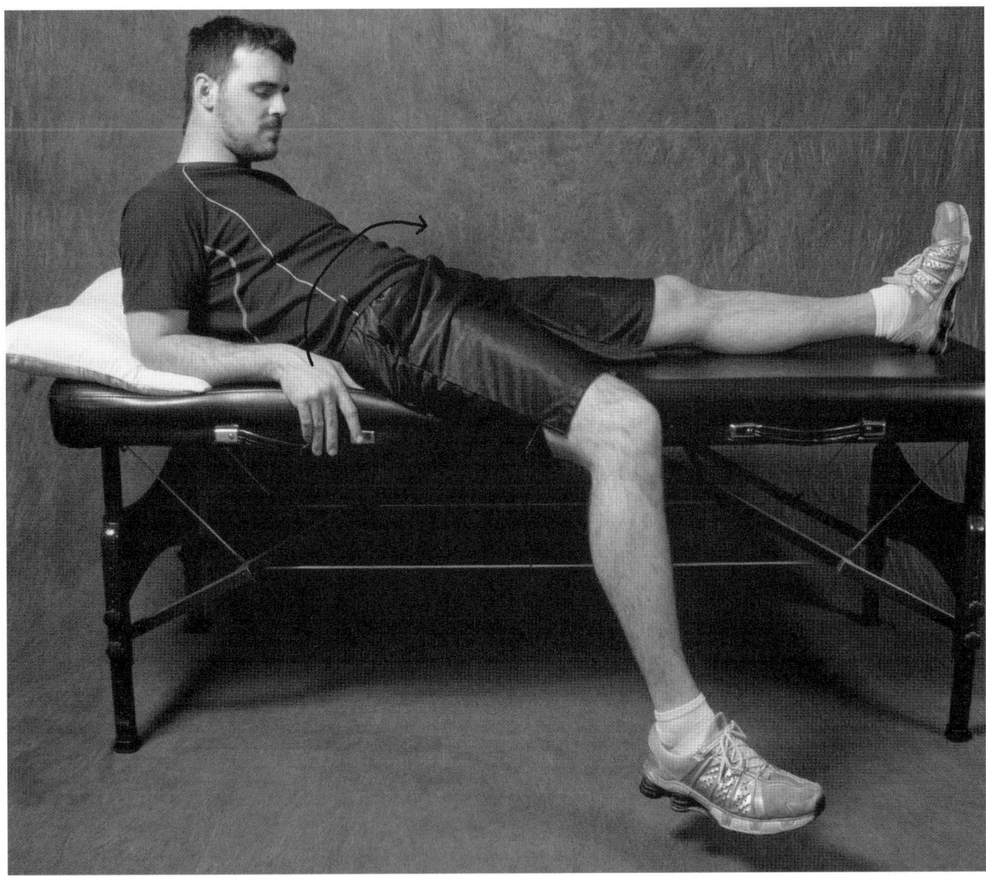

Fig. 9.1 A common mistake that results in unwanted torsional stresses on the pelvic unit: getting on and off the plinth (or into or out of the bed or a car) with one leg leading. The right thigh (femur) is in extension relative to the left and can act as a lever on the right innominate, forcing it into anterior rotation (see also Fig. 2.47).

4. If pelvic/spine alignment problems fail to resolve with efforts at realignment and core muscle strengthening to regain stability, ensure investigations have been or are about to be carried out to rule out possible underlying problems (e.g. central disc protrusions, fibroids, ovarian cysts, visceral adhesions/scars, masses).
5. Failure to recognize/accept malalignment as a distinct medical entity that can be diagnosed and treated often results in a patient being 'labeled' erroneously (e.g. 'fibromyalgia', 'chronic pain syndrome'), a 'diagnostic label' that may become engrained in the patient's mind to the point that it tends to persist even though the actual cause of the problem that had so far escaped diagnosis – the malalignment and complicating 'malalignment syndrome' – was finally treated and the signs and symptoms related to these have actually resolved.
6. There is a tendency to diagnose and treat one cause, when that cause is possibly coexistent with malalignment and one may aggravate the other. An example is 'myofacial pain' of radiculopathic origin; treatment may be limited to intramuscular stimulation (IMS) which may well relieve pressure on a root temporarily but which ignores a coexistent malalignment and secondary 'myofascial syndrome' that can continue to irritate the root and perpetuate the pain and stress.
7. Ongoing reliance on compensatory treatment methods often leads to treatment being limited to one or two modalities (e.g. acupuncture,

massage) at a time, usually followed some time later by another trial of the same or some other modality (e.g. IMS, muscle relaxants, prolotherapy). All of these are unlikely to bring long-term relief of pain and muscle spasm if they fail to correct an underlying problem of malalignment that is responsible for the increase in muscle tone and joint/soft tissue pain in the first place.

8. There is a current trend to subject the person presenting with malalignment to treatment limited to prolotherapy injections of multiple pelvic and spine ligaments to counter pain and promote collagen formation (even though there may not be a problem of ligament laxity but rather one of muscle weakness and/or joint degeneration). Even when there is an indication to use prolotherapy to decrease actual ligament laxity, failure to address an underlying problem of malalignment may result in the pelvis/spine ending up 'stabilized' but in an 'out of alignment' position that makes it harder to respond to any subsequent realignment attempts.
9. Orthotic posting is often carried out bilaterally for pronation, ignoring the fact that the pronation is more readily apparent on one side compared to the other (which may actually tend to neutral or even frank supination as a result of the shift in weight-bearing that occurs with some presentations of malalignment). Similarly, the person may be provided with shoes intended for a pronator, worsening any tendency to supinate on the opposite side. Also, providing orthotics that have been cast while non-weight-bearing will incorporate the functional shift in weight-bearing, leg length difference and other asymmetries that could have been corrected simply by first carrying out realignment and then casting while bearing weight.
10. Failure to pursue a progressive, supervised course of treatment is likely to compromise the outcome. Some may require up to 1-2 years to develop the core strength and stability, cardiovascular fitness and normal movement patterns which will ensure that symptoms finally resolve completely and their chance of maintaining alignment is again on par with that of the general population.

The signs and symptoms that develop secondary to malalignment and that comprise the 'malalignment syndrome' are attributable, in large part, to the asymmetrical stresses on joints and soft tissues, irritation of nerves and contracture of some structures and lengthening of others. Realignment in some people may allow the 'malalignment syndrome' to resolve completely and eliminate any stress it may have placed on a coexisting chronic problem, such as osteoarthritis, joint displacement and idiopathic scoliosis. In others, it may reveal an underlying problem that, up to this time, had been hidden by the signs and symptoms attributable to the malalignment and allow the clinician to finally focus investigations and treatment on that particular problem. Common examples include fibroids, ovarian cysts, abdominal masses and isolated nerve root compression that have so far evaded detection.

The field dealing with problems relating to malalignment and the treatment possibilities is indeed vast. However, one has to start somewhere, with an approach that has been well documented and stood up to testing clinically. This book has tried to present a way of diagnosing and treating the three common presentations of malalignment seen in 80-90% of those who are out of alignment. The emphasis has been on providing an easy way of detecting the biomechanical changes characteristic of each of these presentations, creating an awareness of the secondary signs and symptoms that comprise the 'malalignment syndrome' and getting the person involved in a supervised, progressive programme that includes education and encourages their participation in the treatment process.

Appendices

'The malalignment syndrome'- 2nd Edition

APPENDIX 1 SACROILIAC JOINT 'ROTATIONAL MALALIGNMENT'

EXAMINATION FINDINGS WITH THE 'MOST COMMON' ROTATIONAL PATTERNS

1. 'Anterior' rotation of the right innominate, 'posterior' rotation of the left is the configuration seen most often
2. Dysfunction of movement: usually 'locking' of the right sacroiliac (SI) joint
3. Weight-bearing: right foot pronating, left supinating
4. Gait: right leg turned outward, left inward (external and internal rotation, respectively)

STANDING

1. Compensatory, reversing lumbar, thoracic and cervical curves
2. Pelvic obliquity: most often right side higher (inclined to right)
3. Bony landmarks: the right anterior superior iliac spine (ASIS) has rotated downward, the right posterior superior iliac spine (PSIS) upward; the reverse has occurred on the left side
4. Pelvic rotation (transverse plane): decreased to the left (into the side of the left 'posterior' innominate rotation)

SITTING ON A HARD SURFACE

1. Pelvic obliquity present (most often: right side higher)
2. Trunk rotation: usually decreased to left
3. Right iliac crest and ischial tuberosity higher than left (left relatively downward and bearing more weight)

SUPINE-LYING

1. Right ASIS and pubic ramus caudad (down) compared to those on the left
2. Right leg turned outward relative to the left; right inner thigh appears to face more anterior compared to the left

PRONE-LYING

The right PSIS lies cephalad (up) compared with the left

CHANGING POSITION FROM LONG-SITTING TO SUPINE-LYING

1. The apparent leg length difference changes (shifts), the most frequent presentation being: right leg shorter in long-sitting, longer in supine-lying
2. Rule of the 5 'L's: 'Leg Lengthens Lying, Landmarks Lower' on side of 'anterior' rotation

SQUATTING

Right thigh usually higher distally and 'longer' compared to left one.

APPENDIX 2 SACROILIAC JOINT 'UPSLIP' (RIGHT SIDE)

STANDING

1. Pelvic obliquity: right side high
2. Bony landmarks: all elevated on right side
3. Compensatory, contrasting lumbar, thoracic and cervical curves
4. Pelvic rotation (transverse plane): usually right = left

SITTING ON A HARD SURFACE

Pelvic obliquity persists: usually right side higher (inclined to right)

SUPINE AND PRONE-LYING

1. Right leg shorter than left to same extent in both positions
2. Bony landmarks: right ASIS, PSIS, pubic ramus, ischial tuberosity all cephalad (up) relative to left ones

CHANGING POSITION FROM LONG-SITTING TO SUPINE-LYING

1. Right medial malleolus lies cephalad in both positions; i.e. right leg short by some amount
2. However, the actual difference between the two legs remains the same despite the change in position

TESTS FOR SACROILIAC JOINT 'LOCKING'

Negative

OTHER OBSERVATIONS

1. Suspect an 'upslip' when: hip extension/flexion are symmetrical but other ranges of motion (ROM) are still asymmetrical, all landmarks on one side are elevated, pelvic obliquity persists on sitting, and an LLD does not change on going from long-sitting to supine-lying
2. A downward force on the right leg may correct the 'upslip'
3. Findings are similar for 'downslip' of the left innominate but would fail to correct with traction on the right leg.

APPENDIX 3 ASYMMETRY OF LOWER EXTREMITY RANGES OF MOTION

ROM typical of those associated with the 'more common' patterns of 'rotational malalignment' (here presenting with 'right anterior, left posterior' innominate rotation).

	Right (degrees)		Left (degrees)	
Hip joints				
Abduction	Increased	e.g. 45	Decreased	e.g. 35
Adduction	Increased	e.g. 45	Decreased	e.g. 35
Rotation:				
external	Increased	e.g. 50	Decreased	e.g. 40
internal	Decreased	e.g. 20	Increased	e.g. 30
Total:		**e.g. 70**		**e.g. 70**
Flexion*	Decreased	e.g. 45	Increased	e.g. 60
Extension*	Increased	e.g. 20	Decreased	e.g. 5
Total:		**e.g. 65**		**e.g. 65**

*i.e. 'right anterior' innominate rotation restricts right hip flexion, 'left posterior' rotation restricts left hip extension.

Tibiotalar joints

Flexion - angle compared with neutral plantigrade foot; knee straight:

	Right		Left	
Dorsal	Increased	e.g. 25	Decreased	e.g. 20
Plantar	Decreased	e.g. 25	Increased	e.g. 30
Total:		**e.g. 50**		**e.g. 50**

Subtalar joints

	Right		Left	
Inversion	Increased	e.g. 25	Decreased	e.g. 15
Eversion	Decreased	e.g. 5	Increased	e.g. 15
Total:		**e.g. 30**		**e.g. 30**

APPENDIX 4 ASYMMETRY OF LOWER EXTREMITY MUSCLE STRENGTH

Manual assessment with SI joint 'rotational malalignment' or an 'upslip'

	Right	Left
Hip joint		
Flexors	Weak	Strong
Extensors	Weak	Strong
Abductors	Strong	Weak
Adductors	Weak	Strong

Rotators:		
internal	See text	See text
external	See text	See text
Knee		
Flexors:		
hamstrings	Strong	Weak
Extensors:		
quadriceps	*	*
Ankle		
Invertors:		
tibialis anterior	Weak	Strong
tibialis posterior	Weak	Strong
Evertors:		
peroneus longus	Strong	Weak
gastrocnemius/soleus	*	*

*minimal weakness may be hard to detect in these muscles but evident on mechanical testing; e.g. Cybex.

APPENDIX 5 CLINICAL CORRELATIONS SPECIFIC TO RUNNING

Athlete with one of the 'more common' patterns of 'rotational malalignment' or an 'upslip'

PROBLEMS RELATED TO A TENDENCY TO RIGHT PRONATION

1. Increased right hallux valgus and first metatarsophalangeal bunion
2. Right 'pump bump', or right one larger than left
3. Right plantar fasciitis, Achilles tendonitis
4. Increased tension on right medial structures: medial knee (collateral) and ankle ligaments, medial plica, tendon origins and insertions (hip adductors, pes anserinus, tibialis posterior) and periosteum (medial 'shin splints'); posterior tibial and saphenous nerve
5. Increased right knee Q-angle and knee flexion: lateral compartment pressure, patellofemoral syndrome, patellar off-tracking/subluxation, patellar tendonitis, Osgood-Schlatter's traction epiphysitis

PROBLEMS RELATED TO A TENDENCY TO LEFT SUPINATION

1. Painful left 4th and 5th metatarsal shafts and toes; possibility of causing formation and/or aggravation of a Morton's neuroma
2. Increased tension on left lateral structures: lateral knee and ankle ligaments, hip abductor muscles, iliotibial band, lateral compartment muscles/ tendons, and peroneal and sural nerve
3. Recurrent left ankle inversion sprains

PROBLEMS RELATED TO LOWER EXTREMITY WEAKNESS AND CONTRARY ROTATION

1. Right external rotation: the right heel hitting the left foot or calf on swing-through; left internal rotation: the left toes clipping the right foot or calf on swing-through
2. Ankle muscle 'functional weakness': a fish-tailing of either foot/heel, especially when weight-bearing on the toes - right inward, left outward

APPENDIX 6 CLINICAL FINDINGS: ANATOMICAL (TRUE) LONG RIGHT LEG

STANDING POSITION

1. Pelvic obliquity: right side higher (pelvis inclined to right)
2. Bony landmarks all elevated on right: ASIS, PSIS, pubic bone, iliac crest and ischial tuberosity
3. Compensatory curvatures of lumbar and thoracic spine: lumbar convexity may be to the left or right, usually with the thoracic convexity in the opposite direction and a further reversal in the upper thoracic spine or at the cervicothoracic junction
4. Right shoulder/scapula depressed if the thoracic convexity is to the left
5. Pelvic rotation (transverse plane): right = left

SITTING ON A HARD SURFACE

1. Pelvis level: the effect of the lower extremities is eliminated and the weight is now borne symmetrically on the ischial tuberosities
2. Compensatory curvatures: decreased or eliminated

SUPINE AND PRONE-LYING

1. Pelvic landmarks and greater trochanters: all level
2. Right medial malleolus lies caudad compared to the left one

CHANGING POSITION FROM SUPINE-LYING TO LONG-SITTING

1. Right medial malleolus caudad in both positions
2. The actual difference between the malleoli does not change

TESTS FOR SACROILIAC JOINT 'LOCKING'

1. Negative; on the standing sacral flexion test, the right PSIS is higher by the difference in leg length - this difference does not change on forward flexion and extension of the trunk

SQUATTING

1. If the right femur is longer: thighs equal height, right knee ahead of left; if the LLD involves mainly the tibia: right distal thigh (knee) higher

APPENDIX 7 COMBINATION OF ASYMMETRIES (1st CASE PRESENTATION)

Presentation: a person with a 'right anterior, left posterior' innominate rotation, 'locked' right SI joint, 'right upslip' and an anatomical (true) leg length difference (right longer).

FINDINGS ON INITIAL EXAMINATION

1. Stand and sit: pelvic obliquity - right iliac crest higher
2. Right ASIS caudad (down) and PSIS cephalad (up) compared to left
3. Sacral flexion, kinetic rotational test: positive on right
4. Asymmetrical lower extremity ROM as for 'more common' patterns of 'rotational malalignment' (Appendix 1)
5. Asymmetry of strength in keeping with the 'rotational malalignment'
6. Long-sitting to supine-lying: right leg lengthens, left shortens; anterior right landmarks rotated downward compared to left

EXAMINATION AFTER CORRECTION OF THE 'ROTATIONAL MALALIGNMENT'

1. Sacral flexion, kinetic rotational test: now negative
2. Standing: persistence of pelvic obliquity (pelvic landmarks and greater trochanter now *all* higher on the right)
3. Long-sitting to supine-lying: no shift ocurs now; right leg may be shorter, longer or equal to left depending on the amount of the 'true' leg length difference (LLD)

INTERPRETATION: THE FOLLOWING INDICATE PERSISTENT RIGHT 'UPSLIP'

1. The pelvic obliquity persists in sitting and lying
2. Persistent asymmetrical muscle strength/tension and joint ROM

AFTER CORRECTION OF THE 'UPSLIP', FINDINGS CONSISTENT WITH A RESIDUAL ANATOMICAL LLD INCLUDE:

1. Symmetrical landmarks (sitting, lying), strength/tension, and ROM
2. Long-sitting to supine-lying: right leg consistently longer to equal extent by the 'true' LLD

APPENDIX 8 COMBINATION OF ASYMMETRIES (2nd CASE PRESENTATION)

Presentation: a person with 'left anterior, right posterior' innominate rotation, 'locked' right SI joint, left 'upslip' and anatomical (true) long left leg

FINDINGS ON INITIAL EXAMINATION

1. Standing and sitting: pelvic obliquity, left or right iliac crest higher
2. Left ASIS caudad (down), left PSIS cephalad (up) compared to right
3. Sacral flexion, kinetic rotational test: positive on right
4. Asymmetry of lower extremity muscle strength/tension, joint ROM
5. Long-sitting to supine-lying: left leg lengthens relative to right

EXAMINTATION AFTER CORRECTION OF THE 'ROTATIONAL MALALIGNMENT'

1. Sacral flexion, kinetic rotational test: now negative
2. Standing and sitting: pelvic obliquity in both positions (direction of inclination may be reverse of that seen initially, or may change on going from standing to sitting; definitely all left innominate landmarks higher in sitting)
3. Long-sitting to supine-lying: no change in the apparent right and left leg length; in supine-lying, leg length may or may not be different depending on how the anatomical long left leg affects the left leg 'shortening' caused by the left 'upslip'
4. Persistence of asymmetrical strength/tension and joint ROM

INTERPRETATION: THE FOLLOWING INDICATE PERSISTENT LEFT 'UPSLIP'

All left landmarks elevated, pelvic obliquity in sitting, asymmetrical strength/tension and ROM

AFTER CORRECTION OF THE 'UPSLIP', THE ONLY FINDINGS REMAINING ARE CONSISTENT WITH A TRUE LLD, LEFT LEG LONG

1. Standing: bony landmarks all higher on the left side
2. Sitting and lying (prone/supine): level iliac crests, ASIS and PSIS
3. Long-sitting to supine-lying: left leg longer to an equal extent in both positions

APPENDIX 9 'THE THORACOLUMBAR SYNDROME'

DIAGNOSTIC SIGNS

1. The 'iliac crest point' sign: pain and deep tenderness localizing to the site on the iliac crest where the posterior sensory branches become cutaneous
2. Skin-rolling test: the skin and subcutaneous tissue in an area supplied by the specific cutaneous branch feels thickened and appears hypersensitive when rolled
    a. anterior branch: lower lateral abdomen and groin
    b. lateral perforating branch: lateral hip (crest to greater trochanter)
    c. posterior branch: iliac crest and buttock area
3. Pain localizing to the thoracolumbar region with pressure: creating a rotatory force on each vertebra by applying pressure to the spinous processes from the right and left elicits a pain response from involved segment(s), usually unilaterally
4. Facet joint pain: deep, vertical pressure applied 1 cm lateral to each spinous process elicits pain at the level of involved facet joint(s)
5. Diagnostic block with local anaesthetic: 2 ml local anaesthetic solution (xylocaine or procaine) is infiltrated around the painful facet joint(s); a positive block temporarily decreases or abolishes the above signs

TREATMENT

1. Correct any vertebral rotational displacement evident
2. Infiltrate corticosteroids around the facet joint(s); if 2-3 injections spaced apart fail to bring relief and there is some facet joint laxity, consider a course of prolotherapy injections
3. If the pain persists: consider surgical denervation of the facet joint(s) or percutaneous posterior rhizotomy

APPENDIX 10 CLINICAL CORRELATIONS TO NON-SPECIFIC SPORTS

SPORTS THAT CAN BE AFFECTED BY:

1. Limitation of trunk rotation in the transverse plane: golf, baseball, cricket, rowing, hockey, kayaking, court sports, baseball, gymnastics, wrestling, ice hockey, field hockey
2. Limitation of pelvic rotation (transverse plane): skiing, golf, gymnastics, wrestling, baseball, canoeing
3. Limitation of limb ranges of motion:
    a. 'anterior' innominate rotation predisposing to hamstring tears: jumping competitions (long, triple, high); running (leaving the blocks,

hurdles, steeplechase, cross-country); martial arts; soccer, football, rugby
   b. asymmetrical arm extension: swimming (e.g. butterfly; synchronized swimming)
   c. restriction of right leg internal rotation, left adduction and external rotation: ice-skating, ski-skating, horseback riding
4. Combinations of limitations in trunk, pelvis, and limbs: fencing, court sports, balance beam, martial arts, gymnastics, wrestling, soccer, windsurfing, snow-boarding, high jump, throwing events (hammer, discus, shot and javelin)

SPORTS IN WHICH SYMMETRY AND/OR STYLE IS REWARDED:

Synchronized swimming, gymnastics, ice-skating (figures competition), ballet and other classical dance routines, diving and weight-lifting

SPORTS IN WHICH SYMMETRY OF LEG STRENGTH IS IMPORTANT:

Cycling, running, swimming, skiing, skating, gymnastics, weight-lifting, body-building and power-lifting

APPENDIX 11 CLINICAL CORRELATIONS TO SPECIFIC SPORTS

An athlete with an 'upslip' or one of the 'more common' patterns of 'rotational malalignment' ('right anterior, left posterior' innominate).

CYCLING

1. Awareness of asymmetry of form (e.g. right knee moves further away from the crossbar = knee in flexion, thigh abducted and externally rotated; moves inward when extended = foot/ankle pronation; leg external rotation and knee valgus stress)
2. Awareness of asymmetry of strength (e.g. feeling that the right leg cannot generate as much power as the left, fatigues earlier)
3. Right pronation: right foot feels 'weak' and 'falls inward'

GOLF

Restrictions of trunk or pelvic rotation to the right or left; gradually increasing back pain as the game progresses

SKATING

1. Tendency to 'right pronation, left supination' would:
   a. facilitate getting onto the right inner, left outer edge and turning to the left
   b. decrease the ease of getting onto the right outer, left inner edge and turning to the right
2. Right ankle may feel 'weak', 'sloppy' and actually 'collapse inward' on account of the tendency to pronation, the functional weakness affecting right tibialis anterior/posterior and/or a feeling of instability when the foot and ankle are pronated and dorsiflexed

SKIING

1. Problem initiating or carrying out turns to one side
   - the key determinant is likely to be the limitation imposed by any restriction of pelvic rotation in the transverse plane (e.g. into the side of a 'posterior rotation' or an 'inflare')
   - tendency to 'right pronation, left supination' may facilitate getting a good right inner, left outer edge and making a turn to the left
   - functional weakness (e.g. left peroneus longus, right tibialis anterior/posterior), a problem 'getting a good inner edge' on the right and/or a sensation of right ankle/foot instability may result in the skier feeling more 'stable' or 'secure' on making a turn to the right instead

SWIMMING

1. Detrimental effects of asymmetries on the execution of strokes (e.g. asymmetrical ranges of motion: head/neck and trunk rotation, shoulder extension and rotation); compensatory torquing requires more energy
2. Contrary effect of one leg rotating internally, the other externally

APPENDIX 12 FACTORS CONTRIBUTING TO RECURRENCE OF INJURIES

Person with an 'upslip' or one of the 'more common' patterns of 'rotational malalignment'

LEFT HIP ABDUCTOR AND TENSOR FASCIA LATA/ILIOTIBIAL BAND (TFL/ITB) COMPLEX SPRAIN/STRAIN

1. Tendency to supination on the left side
2. Increased muscle tension (e.g. 'facilitation' of left hip abductors; change in length-tension ratio)
3. Functional weakness of the complex

LEFT ANKLE INVERSION SPRAINS/STRAINS

1. Tendency to supination on the left side
2. 'Functional weakness' of left peroneus longus and brevis
3. Fitting with orthotics intended for a pronator (e.g. medial raise)
4. Wearing double-density, straight-last shoes intended for a pronator

RIGHT PATELLOFEMORAL COMPARTMENT SYNDROME

1. Tendency to pronation on the right side, knee valgus strain
2. Increased right Q-angle and outward tracking of the patella
3. Tendency for the relatively 'longer' right leg to flex when standing (to lower the high right iliac crest?): increases tension in the quadriceps muscle and across the patellofemoral compartment

BACK 'STRAINS'

1. Stresses from compensatory movements required because of limitations of trunk, pelvic and limb ranges of motion in certain directions; for example, increased left trunk rotation to compensate for the limitation of left pelvic rotation whenever the left innominate is rotated posteriorly and/or 'inflared'
2. Minor insults (e.g. repetitive lifting, bending and squatting) superimposed on tissue already tender from chronic compression, distraction and/or torsional forces
3. Pelvic obliquity with compensatory scoliosis: segmental limitation of movement and increased stress at sites of curve reversal

APPENDIX 13 CAUSES OF RECURRENT MALALIGNMENT

1. Unilateral lumbarization, sacralization and pseudo-joint formation
   - creates a rotational moment on trunk flexion and extension
2. Degeneration affecting structures capable of producing 'deep', poorly defined, or referred pain*
   - hip joints, facet joints and discs
3. Disc protrusion or herniation
   - central disc protrusion may irritate the dura and spare the nerve roots or sleeves; reflex increase in tone or muscle spasm secondary to irritation of dura, root(s)
4. Spinal stenosis, arachnoiditis, root sleeve fibrosis, intra- or extradural tumours
5. Unsuspected underlying arthritic condition*
   - ankylosing spondylitis, Reiter's syndrome, gout, ulcerative colitis and Crohn's disease (regional ileitis)
6. Abdominal or pelvic masses; e.g. aneurysm, uterine fibroid, ovarian cyst, tumour
   - these may be capable of irritating muscles (e.g. iliopsoas, pelvic floor) which can, in turn, exert rotational forces on the vertebrae, the pelvic bones and/or the lower extremities
7. Pre-menstrual relaxin hormone release, causing a transient increase in ligament laxity; stress associated with menses

*NB. Bone scans may show an increased uptake in the sacroiliac joint(s) and/or symphysis pubis, leading to a diagnosis of 'sacroiliitis' and 'osteitis pubis'. Laboratory tests for inflammatory arthropathy are usually negative, and symptoms often settle with realignment of the sacroiliac joints and pubic bones.

Glossary

abduction: moving a part of the body away from the midline or, in the case of the hands/fingers and feet/toes, away from the axial line of the limbs

adduction: moving a part of the body toward the median plane or, in the case of the hands/fingers and feet/toes, toward the axial line of the limb

Adson's manoeuvre: a test for compromise of the nerves and blood vessels to the arms at the site where they run through the thoracic outlet (the narrow space between the collar bone and the underlying 1st rib) – Fig. 3.13

afferent: carrying toward a center (e.g. a nerve fibre sending signals toward the spinal cord or brain)

'aids': the signals by which the rider communicates with the horse

AIIS: Anterior Inferior Iliac Spine, a protruberant landmark on the lower part at the front of each pelvic bone; serves as attachment point for the origin of the rectus femoris part of the quadriceps muscle – Fig. 2.46C

amphiarthrodial joint: a joint that allows for little motion, the apposed bony surfaces being connected by fibrocartilage (e.g. symphysis pubis)

ankylosis: immobilization and consolidation of a joint as a result of disease, injury, or surgical procedure

anterior: on the front or forward part; referring to the front (i.e. chest, abdomen, leg) surface of the body

aponeurosis: a white, flattened or ribbon-like tendinous expansion, serving mainly to connect a muscle with the parts that it moves (e.g. the conjoint tendons of the extenal oblique and transverse muscles on the abdomen that connects them to the superior pubic bone – Figs 2.31B, 2.32)

appendicular skeleton: referring to the bones in the arms and legs (the parts that are suspended from the axial skeleton)

apprehension test: a test to check for evidence of increased irritability/tenderness at the back surfaces of the knee cap or the underlying groove that it tracks up and down on as the knee straightens and bends, respectively

arthrodesis: a surgical fixation of the joint that promotes proliferation of bone cells to achieve eventual fusion of the joint surfaces

arthrodial: referring to a joint with flat opposing surfaces (e.g. SI joint)

ASIS: Anterior Superior Iliac Spine, a protruberant landmark on the upper part of the front of the pelvic bone that serves as origin for the TFL muscle and the inguinal ligament – Figs 2.4A, 2.59, 3.42

autonomic nervous system: the part of the nervous system that regulates the activity of cardiac muscle, smooth muscle and glands; composed of the sympathetic (thoracolumbar) and parasympathetic (craniosacral) nervous system

axial rotation: rotation of the axial bones relative to an axis drawn through the axial skeleton – Figs 2.9, 2.21, 2.50

axial skeleton: referring to the bones of the head, spine, ribs, sternum (breast bone), trunk/pelvis

axon: in the peripheral nervous system, the nerve fibre that carries impulses from the neuron (nerve cell body) to its terminal branches, at which point the impulses are transmitted to another nerve cell or to cells of the organ that it acts on

bowstring test: test for irritability of the nerve roots and spinal cord; to stretch these structures, the knee is straightened (extended) when the hip is maximally flexed

brachialgia: pain in the arm(s)

bursa: a sac filled with a viscous fluid, situated at places where friction between structures would otherwise develop; e.g. iliopectineal bursa between the iliopsoas tendon and the iliopectineal eminence (a diffuse enlargement on the anterior aspect of the acetabulum or hip socket – Fig. 4.2); trochanteric bursa between the greater trochanter and the overlying hip abductor–ITB complex – Fig. 3.41

calcaneus: heel bone

caudad: directed down, toward the coccyx (tail bone)

cellulalgia: pain arising from cells

cephalad: directed up, toward the head

cervicogenic: originating from the neck region

chymopapaine 'discectomy': a treatment method for disc protrusion popular in the 1980s consisting of the injection of chymopapaine (an enzyme capable of breaking down the mucopolysaccharide–protein complexes in the protruded disc); unfortunately, the long-term effect was to accelerate development of osteoarthritis at the level injected, with complicating mechanical back pain

CNS: central nervous system

coccydynia: pain originating from the tailbone

coccyx: the tailbone

conjoint muscle: a muscle that has several components, each of which is capable of a specific action but all of which can also act together (e.g. iliopsoas made up of psoas major and minor and the iliacus – Fig. 2.62)

contralateral: located on, pertaining to, or influencing the opposite side (vs. ipsilateral)

'core' muscles: muscles that act to stabilize the SI joints and spine, consisting of an 'inner' (Fig. 2.28) and 'outer' (Figs 2.31B–2.40) unit

counternutation: backward movement of the sacral base relative to the adjacent iliac bone(s) (Fig. 2.11B)

cranio-caudal: running from head to tail

craniosacral rhythm: an alternating increase in tension of muscle and fascia, produced by the rhythmic fluctuation in the flow of the cerebrospinal fluid (CSF) from the brain down to the tailbone (see Ch. 8)

crepitus: the sensation of dry surfaces of muscle when rubbed between the fingers, indicative of chronic spasm and replacement with fibrotic tissue (increased connective tissue content)

curved last: referring to the sole of a shoe (= the last) which has an indentation on the inner border to promote inward collapse (pronation) of the foot – Fig. 3.35B

dermatome: the area of the skin supplied by one nerve root

dextroscoliosis: vertebrae turning to the right along the length of a curved segment of the spine (e.g. lumbar vertebrae will turn clockwise, into a curve that is convex to the right – Figs 2.96A, 4.24)

dorsiflexion: bending the foot upward (decreasing the angle at the ankle)

double blind study: a research study in which neither the subject nor the person administering the treatment knows which treatment any particular participant is receiving

double-density midsole: a midsole that is reinforced with more dense material on the inside (underneath the arch of the foot primarily), to counter any tendency to pronation – Fig. 3.35A

downslip: downward displacement of a pelvic bone relative to the sacrum, with apparent 'lengthening' of the leg on that side

dura: the outermost covering of the spinal cord and brain stem, continuous with the meninges

dysmenorrhoea: painful menstruation

dyspareunia: painful sexual intercourse

dysaesthesias: impaired sensation, or abnormal unpleasant sensations provoked by normal stimuli

efferent: carrying away from a center (e.g. a nerve transmitting signals from the brain or spinal cord)

enthesis: the site where a ligament, tendon, or muscle attaches to bone

enthetic pain: pain arising from an enthesis

epiphysis: the expanded articular end of a long bone (e.g. humerus at the elbow, articulating with the radius and ulna), developed from a secondary ossification centre which, during its period of growth, is either entirely cartilagenous or is separated from the shaft by the epiphyseal cartilage

eversion: a turning or tipping outward (e.g. as of the ankle in an 'eversion sprain')

evertors: muscles that act to turn a body part outward (e.g. peroneus longus everts the foot – Figs 3.37, 3.53)

facilitation: the increase in tension in a muscle resulting from an increased efficiency of transmission of nerve impulses and/or an increased number of impulses traveling in the nerve supplying that muscle

fascia: a sheet or band (Fig. 8.1) of fibrous connective tissue (e.g. thoracodorsal fascia lying deep to the skin and surrounding the muscles of this complex – Fig. 2.31A; anterior abdominal fascia surrounding the rectus abdominis muscles and serving as an anchor point for transversus abdominis – Figs 2.31B, 2.33)

femur: thigh bone

fibrosis: replacement with excessive amounts of fibrous connective tissue

fibro-osseous junction: where ligament, muscle, tendon, or capsule inserts into bone

fins: the spinous processes of a horse

foramen: a natural opening, in particular one into or through bone (e.g. at the base of the skull: foramen magnum for exit of the brainstem/spinal cord; hypoglossal foramen for exit of the 12th cranial nerve to the tongue; the foramina for the exit of nerve roots from either side of each vertebra and from the sacrum)

'forehand': the front legs of a horse

frontal (coronal) plane: any plane which passes longitudinally through the body (from side to side, at right angles to the median plane), dividing the body into front and back parts; one of these planes roughly parallels the frontal suture, another the coronal suture of the skull (Fig. 2.9)

Gaenslen's test: a test to stress the hip–SI joint–lumbosacral region by having the person flex one thigh onto the chest while achieving hyperextension on the opposite side by applying downward pressure on that thigh as it hangs over the edge of the table; pain that occurs does not define the specific site(s) affected (hip, SI joint and/or lumbosacral) – Fig. 2.108B

genu valgum: inward collapse of the knee joint

genu varum: outward collapse of the knee joint

Gillet test: kinetic rotational test – see below (Figs 2.121–2.125)

Golgi tendon organs: a mechanoreceptor found in tendons, arranged in series with the muscle and therefore sensitive to the mechanical distortion that results with passive stretch of the tendon or an isometric muscle contraction and capable of signalling changes in muscle tension; it is the receptor responsible for the 'lengthening' or 'clasp-knife' reflex, whereby stimulation of the tendon (= Golgi receptor) result in relaxation of the muscle–tendon complex which may prevent tearing but results in giving-way of the joint (e.g. knee joint giving way on sudden relaxation of the quadriceps muscle induced by activation of the tendon organs with excessive stretching of the tendon)

greater trochanter: a bony process protruding outward below the neck of the femur (Figs 2.5A, 3.41)

Grostic or NUCCA: a chiropractic technique that limits adjustments to C1 and C2 vertebrae (see Ch. 8)

hallux rigidus: painful limitation of movement of the joints of the first toe, which may be associated with flexion deformity

hallux valgus: angulation of the big toe away from the midline, possibly to the point of riding over or under the 2nd and even 3 rd toes

hypertonia: abnormal increase in tension in a muscle–tendon complex

hypotonia: abnormal decrease in tension in a muscle–tendon complex

inhibition: a decrease in muscle tension resulting from a decreased efficiency in the transmission of nerve impulses and/or a decreased number of impulses in the nerve supplying that muscle

innominate: the pelvic bone on either side of the sacrum, each made up of an iliac, ischial and pubic bone (Figs 2.4–2.6)

inversion: a turning or tipping inward (e.g. as of the calcaneal bone with an inversion sprain of the ankle)

invertor: a muscle that acts to turn a body part inward (e.g. tibialis anterior and posterior invert the foot – Figs 3.37, 3.54)

ipsilateral: located on, pertaining to, or influencing the same side (vs contralateral)

ischial tuberosities: the bones on the lower aspect of each pelvic bone which become the weight-bearing part on sitting (Figs 2.5, 2.6)

isometric contraction: muscle contraction maintained without any movement of the joint that the muscle acts on

isotonic contraction: movement of a joint carried out while maintaining uniform tension in the muscle acting on the joint

kinetic rotational test (Gillet test): test for intrapelvic torsion (ability for the pelvis to twist) and the ability to transfer weight through the pelvis when standing on one leg (Figs 2.121–2.125)

lateral: on the outside, away from the median plane or midline

Lasègue's or 'bowstring' test: pain elicited on flexing the hip when the knee is extended (i.e. straight leg raising) but abolished with the knee flexed is likely to result from irritation of the sciatic nerve, a nerve root, or the spinal cord rather than originating from the back (e.g. disc degeneration or protrusion)

LCL: Lateral Collateral Ligament, running across the outside of the knee from its attachments to the femur above and the head of the fibula below (Fig. 3.37)

lesser trochanter: a bony process that protrudes inward below the neck of the femur and serves as the insertion for the iliopsoas muscle (Figs 2.62, 3.50)

levator ani syndrome: pelvic floor muscle hypo or hypertonia/reactive spasm, with resulting pelvic floor dysfunction syndrome and recurrent malalignment (Fig. 2.53)

levoscoliosis: vertebrae turning to the left along the length of a curved segment of the spine (e.g. lumbar vertebrae will turn counterclockwise, into a curve that is convex to the left – Figs 2.42, 4.26)

linea alba: on the anterior abdomen, a white line in the midline between the rectus abdominus muscles, formed by the fascia/connective tissue that surrounds and binds these muscles together (Figs 2.39A, 2.127B)

lumbarization: partial or complete separation of the first segment of the sacrum (S1) from the second; when complete, the new vertebral segment is usually designated 'L6' (see 'sacralization' and Figs 4.24–4.26)

Maitland's slump test: a test for nerve root/spinal cord irritability such as occurs with disc protrusion; the test involves putting the roots and cord under progressively more stretch by first having the person sit with the hip flexed and knee extended and then, in succession, flex the trunk and head before the examiner passively dorsiflexes the foot

MCL: Medial Collateral Ligament, running across the inside of the knee from its attachments to the femur above and tibia below (Fig. 3.37)

medial: on the inside, or toward the median plane or midline

meniscus: a 'spacer' or pad of fibrocartilage or dense connective tissue found in a number of joints (e.g. the crescent shaped medial and lateral menisci in the knee joint)

micturition: referring to the act of voiding

'more common' rotational patterns: the possible patterns of 'rotational malalignment' other than the 'left anterior and locked' pattern

Morton's neuroma: a benign thickening of a nerve in the foot that results from repeated irritation of a natural nerve enlargement formed by the junction of branches contributed by the medial and lateral plantar nerves, usually located between the 3rd and 4th metatarsal heads (Fig. 4.16)

Morton's toe: for various reasons the 2nd and sometimes also 3 rd toe end up longer than the 1st (e.g. developmental, hallux valgus); this results in a shift of weight-bearing from the 1st to the 2nd/3rd metatarsal heads and may result in pain on weight-bearing and excessive callus formation

myelinated nerve fibre: an insulated nerve fibre, which can conduct signals more quickly than an unmyelinated fibre

myofascial: referring to tissue consisting of muscle and its fascia

myositis: inflammation of muscle

myotome: all the muscles supplied by one nerve root

neuralgia: paroxysmal pain in the course of a nerve that occurs without stimulation of a nociceptor

neurovascular bundle: a bundle of nerves and blood vessels that supplies a specific part of the body (e.g. femoral bundle to the leg – Fig. 4.14; cervicobrachial to the arm – Fig. 3.13)

nociceptor: a pain receptor cell

nutation: forward movement of the sacral base relative to the adjacent iliac bone(s) – Fig. 2.11A

Ober's test: a test of the hip abductor–ITB complex for detecting an increase in tension or evidence of contracture – Fig. 3.44

oedema: accumulation of excessive amounts of fluid in the spaces between cells of tissues, most easily evident within the subcutaneous tissue lying immediately below the skin

olecranon: the tip of the elbow

Osgood–Schlatter's disease: affects the tuberosity of the tibia (the bump or ephysisis that serves as an attachment point for the tendon of the knee cap); initially there is inflammation and degeneration (osteochondrosis) of the growth centre of the epiphysis, followed by regeneration and recalcification – by the time growth has been completed, the tuberosity often ends up enlarged and protruberant to the point that it may get in the way (e.g. when attempting to kneel)

osteoarthritis: noninflammatory degenerative disease of joints, characterized by degeneration of the joint cartilage, protruding bone growths along the margins (osteophytes), and thickening of the synovial lining on the inside of the capsule which may or may not cause pain; joints are likely to be painful with activity and to stiffen with rest

osteoarthrosis: chronic noninflammatory arthritis

parasympathetic nervous system: that part of the autonomic nervous system consisting of a cranial (ocular, bulbar part of the brainstem) and sacral division; in general, stimulation of this system has a calming effect (e.g. lowering of the heart rate and blood pressure)

paravertebral: running alongside the spine (e.g. the paravertebral muscles lying on either side of the vertebral spinous processes; Fig. 2.29)

patella: kneecap

patellar facets: the medial (inside) and lateral (outside) surface on the back of the knee cap

patellofemoral compartment syndrome: tender inflamed joint surfaces, involving the back of the kneecap (facet surfaces) and the underlying groove that the knee cap tracks up and down in on knee extension and flexion, respectively; pain is most likely to be felt with activities that load the knee joint in flexion, increasing the pressure exerted by the kneecap against the femur – going up and down stairs, rowing, cycling, jumping, squatting

pathognomonic: distinctive or characteristic of a disease or pathological condition, or a sign (finding on examination) or symptom (complaint) on which a diagnosis can be made (e.g. jaundice is pathognomonic of a probable disease process involving the liver or gallbladder)

periosteal: referring to the periosteum, a specialized connective tissue that covers the bones of the body and has the potential to form bone

PIIS: Posterior Inferior Iliac Spine, a landmark on the inferior aspect of the back of the ilium just below the PSIS; serves as iliac attachment point for the lower 'short' sacroiliac and the lateral (long 'dorsal') part of the sacrotuberous ligament (Figs 2.5A, 2.19B)

Pilates: a dynamic form of symmetrical exercises that aims at a graduated recovery of strength and mobility/movement patterns, particularly suited for those presenting with problems relating to malalignment (see Chs 7,8)

planar joint: a joint with flat adjoining surfaces (e.g. symphysis pubis; SI joint early in life)

plantarflexion: pointing the foot downward (increasing the angle at the ankle)

pleura: the membrane that lines the thoracic cavity (chest cage) and surrounds the lung on each side, enclosing a potential space known as the pleural cavity

plica: a ridge or fold of connective tissue that may be noted as a thickening (e.g. the medial plica of the knee that results from an 'infolding' of the inner knee capsule; it may become tender and painful, particularly when put under increased tension by being strung across the underlying enlarged end of the thigh bone, such as occurs with increased inward collapse of the knee joint as a result of pronation – Fig. 3.37)

posting: a raise added to build up the inside or outside of an orthotic – Figs 5.39B, 7.31

pneumothorax: an accumulation of air or gas in the pleural space; a needle that accidentally pierces the pleura can result in formation of a 'tension pneumothorax' when tissues surrounding the opening into the pleural cavity act like a one-way valve that allows air to enter, but not escape, the cavity – the patient experiences shortness of breath that worsens as the increasing positive pressure pushes the lung to the opposite side

posterior: referring to the back or 'dorsal' surface of the body, or to a part 'located in the back of' or 'the back part of' a structure

prolotherapy: a treatment method that involves injection of an irritant to promote proliferation of collagen, with the aim of strengthening a ligament, tendon, or capsule (see Ch. 7)

pronation: a rolling-inward of the weight-bearing foot, with simultaneous forefoot abduction, calcaneal (heel bone) eversion and ankle dorsiflexion – Figs 3.22, 3.37, 5.39B

prone: lying on the stomach

proprioception: the part of the nervous system concerned with providing information regarding movements and the position of the body, information that is provided by sensory nerve terminals located primarily in the muscles, tendons and the labyrinth of the ear

PSIS: Posterior Superior Iliac Spine, a landmark on the back of each pelvic bone (ilium) that serves as origin for both the long 'dorsal' sacroiliac and long dorsal sacrotuberous ligaments – Figs 2.5A, 2.6, 2,13Aii, 2.19

pudendal nerve: the nerve that comes off the sacral plexus (S2–S4) and supplies the muscles, ligaments, skin and erectile tissue of the pelvic floor

raphe: a 'seam' formed by the joining of tissues, usually in the midline (e.g. linea alba of the abdomen)

relaxin hormone: a hormone secreted in increasing amounts toward the later part of a pregnancy, to help relax the connective tissue (ligaments, joint capsules etc.) in the pelvis to facilitate delivery at term; some increase in blood levels is also noted with breast feeding and at the time of ovulation and menstruation

reticular activating system – RAS: the 'net' of cells of the reticular formation of the medulla oblongata, which is part of the brainstem – with the brain above and the spinal cord below – and contains ascending and descending tracts as well as important collections of nerve cells that deal with vital functions, such as respiration, circulation, and special senses; the RAS receives collaterals from the sensory ascending pathways and projects to higher centres of the brainstem and brain to control the overall degree of central nervous system activity (including attentiveness, wakefulness and sleep)

rotational displacement: in this text, referring to abnormal and/or excessive rotation of one or more vertebrae, with or without the simultaneous presence of malalignment of the pelvis (Fig. 2.96B)

sacralization: incorporation of the 5th lumbar vertebra into the sacral base by the formation of bone that partially or fully joins the transverse process of L5 to the sacrum – Figs 4.24–4.26

sacrococcygeal joint: the joint between the tailbone (coccyx) and the sacrum – Figs 2.3, 2.14, 2.18, 3.68, 4.44

sagittal plane: any vertical plane that runs through the body parallel to the median plane/sagittal suture and therefore divides the body into a right and left portion – Fig. 2.9

sagittal split: in synchronized swimming, this refers to separating the legs by full extension of one and flexion of the other leg; that is, separation in the sagittal plane

scapula: shoulder blade

scapulothoracic (joint): referring to the shoulder blade and the underlying rib cage (= the joint between the two)

Scheuermann's disease: osteochondrosis of the vertebrae, which can result in premature (juvenile) kyphosis or excessive forward angulation of the thoracic spine with collapse of the anterior part of one or more vertebral epiphyses

sclerotherapy: injection of an irritant into connective tissue or vessels, with the intent of producing scarring (e.g. injection for the treatment of varicose veins)

sclerotome: all the parts of bone supplied by one nerve root

serratus anterior muscle: originates from the outer surface of ribs 1-8 and inserts primarily into the inner border and lower angle of the shoulder blade; it rotates the blade and will draw it forward while keeping it applied to the chest cage when reaching or pushing against a resistance (e.g. an object, wall) with the arm straight out in front

sesamoids: 2 small bones of the foot, located underneath the big toe within the tendon that bends that toe downward (flexor hallucis longus; Fig. 4.16)

single blind study: a study in which the researcher is aware of the treatment being administered, but the participant is not

single-density midsole: midsole of uniform density to improve cushioning, useful for supinators

somatovisceral reflexes: inhibition or stimulation of visceral (intestinal) functions initiated by signals from the musculoskeletal system

somatic: referring to the musculoskeletal system (as opposed to the viscera)

spondylolisthesis: forward or backward displacement of one vertebra relative to another or to the sacrum; L4 or L5 are frequently involved because developmental separation or fracture of the pars interarticularis (see 'spondylolysis') allows L4 to move forward relative to L5, or L5 relative to the sacral base

spondylolysis: developmental or traumatic dissolution of the vertebral complex, which includes separation of the pars interarticularis (connects the vertebral body to the bony part that surrounds the spinal cord), such as can occur as a result of stress fractures through the pars with repeated back extension (e.g. gymnastics)

sprain: injury to muscle, tendon, ligament, or capsule that has resulted in rupture of some of the fibres, but the continuity of the structure(s) affected remains intact

straight last: the pattern of the sole of the shoe (last) that has the area under the inner arch of the foot filled in to provide more support – Fig. 3.35B

strain: injury to muscle, tendon, ligament or capsule that results in complete disruption (tearing) of the structure(s) involved

subtalar joint: the joint between the talus (that the tibia or shin bone sits on at the ankle) and the calcaneus (the heel bone that sits underneath)

sulcus: a groove or trench

supination: a rolling outward of the weight-bearing foot, with simultaneous forefoot adduction, calcaneal (heel bone) inversion and ankle plantarflexion – Figs 3.22, 3.37, 5.39A

supine: lying on the back

sympathetic nervous system: the part of the autonomic nervous system originating from the thoracolumbar region; in general, stimulation has an excitatory effect (increased heart rate and blood pressure, spasm of blood vessels, formation of goose flesh)

synostosis: a fusion between bones that are usually distinct, as a result of calcification of connecting cartilage or fibrous tissue

thoracic outlet syndrome: irritation or actual compression of the cervicobrachial neurovascular bundle (Fig. 3.13) from narrowing of the thoracic outlet (the space between the 1st rib and collar bone) as seen in association with drooping of the shoulder girdle or continual hyperabduction, abnormal 1st rib, cervical rib or large C7 (rarely C6) transverse process, fibrous band, tight anterior scalene muscle edge; presents with arm pain, arm/finger paraesthesias, vasomotor changes (e.g. oedema, cyanosis, pallor), weakness and wasting (with C8 and T1 fibres most vulnerable)

tibia: shin bone

upslip: upward displacement of one or other pelvic bone relative to the sacrum, with apparent 'shortening' of the leg on that side (Fig. 2.62)

urethra: the outlet from the bladder (Fig. 2.53)

uterine fibroid: a fibrous mass (fibroma) within or attached to the wall of the uterus

valgus: leaning or bent/twisted outward, angulating away from midline (right leg in Figs 3.31B, 3.36)

varus: leaning or bent/twisted inward, angulating toward midline (left leg in Figs 3.31B, 3.36)

vasovagal attack: a reaction that can be triggered by emotional stress, fear, or pain; the response involves the circulatory and neurological systems and is characterized by nausea, pallor, slowing of the heart rate and a fall in blood pressure which can lead to loss of consciousness

viscera: referring to the contents in the three great cavities of the body (e.g. lungs, bowels and organs)

visceral manipulation: a form of manual therapy that concerns itself with the viscera (e.g. freeing up adhesions, repositioning organs)

viscerosomatic reflex: a reflex effect on the musculoskeletal system triggered by stimulation of some part of the visceral system

vulvodynia: pain at vaginal entrance (vulva or labia) or vaginal wall; may be unilateral on basis of referral from iliolumbar ligament or T12 anterior cutaneous perforating branch (Fig. 4.23A2B2) irritation and a cause of dyspareunia (Box 4.8)

whiplash: excessive movement of the head and neck, typically hyperextension followed by hyperflexion in the case of a rear-end collision

Yeoman's test: a test to stress the hip–SI joint–lumbosacral region by passively hyperextending the thigh on one side while the person is lying prone; pain occurs on the affected side(s) but, as with Gaenslen's test, it fails to define the specific site(s) of the problem (hip, SI joint and/or lumbosacral?) – Fig. 2.108A

References and Further Reading

Adam's Lameness in Horses. See: Stashak, T.S. (Ed.).

Adams, M.A., Bogduk, N., Burton, B., et al., 2006. The biomechanics of back pain, second ed. Churchill Livingstone, Edinburgh.

Adamson, C., 1993. Biomechanics of a telemark turn. Personal communication.

Adrian, M., 2009. Sacroiliac joint block, with contrast dye, carried out under fluoroscopy. Personal communication.

Adrian, M.J., Cooper, J.M., 1986. Biomechanics of human movement. Benchmark Press, Indianapolis, IN.

Aitken, G.S., 1986. Syndromes of lumbo-pelvic dysfunction. In: Grieve, G.P. (Ed.), Modern manual therapy of the vertebral column. Churchill Livingstone, Edinburgh, pp. 473–478.

Albee, F.H., 1909. A study of the anatomy and the clinical importance of the sacroiliac joint. JAMA 53, 1273.

Al-khayer, A., Grevitt, M.J., 2007. The sacroiliac joint: an underestimated cause of low back pain. J. Back Musculoskel. Rehabie. 20(4), 135–141.

Andrish, J.T., 1985. Knee injuries in gymnasts. Clin. Sports Med. 4, 111–121.

Aprill, C.N., 1992. The role of anatomically specific injections into the sacroiliac joint. In: Vleeming, A., Mooney, V., Snijders, C. et al. (Eds.), Low back pain and its relation to the sacroiliac joint. European Conference Organizers, Rotterdam, pp. 373–380.

Armour, P.C., Scott, J.H., 1981. Equalization of limb length. J. Bone Joint Surg. 63B, 587–592.

Ashmore, E., 1915. Osteopathic mechanics. Journal Printing, Kirksville, MO.

Aspden, R., 1987. Intra-abdominal pressure and its role in spinal mechanics. Clin. Biomech. 2, 168–174.

Aust, G., Fischer, K., 1997. Changes in body equilibrium response caused by breathing. A posturographic study with visual feedback. Laryngorhinootologie 76, 577–582.

Avramov, A.I., Cavanaugh, J.M., Ozaktay, C.A., et al., 1992. The effect of mechanical loading on group-II, III, and IV afferent units from the facet joint and surrounding tissue. An in vitro study. J. Bone Joint Surg. Am. 74, 1464–1471.

Baker, P.K., 1998. Musculoskeletal problems. In: Steege, J.F., Metzger, D.A., Levy, B.S. (Eds.), Chronic pelvic pain: an integrated approach. WB Saunders, Philadelphia, pp. 216–240.

Baldry, P.E., 2005. Acupuncture, trigger points and musculoskeletal pain. Churchill Livingstone, Edinburgh.

Balduini, F.C., 1988. Abdominal and groin injuries in tennis. Clin. Sports Med. 7, 349–357.

Banks, A.R., 1991. A rationale for prolotherapy. J. Orthop. Med. 13, 54–59.

Barker, P.J., Briggs, C.A., 1998. Attachments of the posterior layer of the lumbar spine. Clin. Biomech. 13, 377–385.

Barker, P.J., Briggs, C.A., 1999. Attachments of the posterior layer of lumbar fascia. Spine 24, 1757–1764.

Barker, P.J., Briggs, C.A., 2004. Tensile transmission across the lumbar fascia in unembalmed cadavers: effects of tension to various muscular attachments. Spine 29, 129–138.

Barker, P.J., Briggs, C.A., 2007. Anatomy and biomechanics of the lumbar fascia: implications for lumbopelvic control and clinical practice. In: Vleeming, A., Mooney, V., Stoeckart, R. (Eds.), Movement, stability & lumbopelvic pain: integration of research and therapy. Churchill Livingstone, Edinburgh, pp. 63–73.

Barker, P.J., Guggenheimer, K.T., Grkovic, I., et al., 2006. Effects of tensioning the lumbar fascia on segmental stiffness during flexion and extension. Spine 31(4), 397–405.

Barral, J.-P., 1989. Visceral manipulation II. Eastland Press, Seattle, WA.

Barral, J.-P., 1993. Urogenital manipulation. Eastland Press, Seattle, WA.

Barral, J.-P., Croibier, A., 2007. Manual therapy for the peripheral nerves. Churchill Livingstone, New York.

Barral, J.-P., Mercier, P., 1988. Visceral manipulation. Eastland Press, Seattle, WA.

Barral, J.-P., Mercier, P., 1983. Manipulations viscerales. Maloine, Paris.

Barrett, S.L., 2003. A new approach to using growth factors in wound healing. Podiatry Today Oct.

Basmajian, J.V., Deluca, C.J., 1985. Muscles alive: their functions revealed by electromyography. Williams & Wilkins, Baltimore.

Beal, M.C., 1982. The sacroiliac problem: review of anatomy, mechanics and diagnosis. J. Am. Osteopath. Assoc. 81, 667–679.

Beatty, R.A., 1994. The piriformis muscle syndrome: a simple diagnostic maneuver. Neurosurgery 34, 512–514.

Bednar, D.A., Orr, F.W., Simon, G.T., 1995. Observations on the pathomorphology of the thoracolumbar fascia in chronical mechanical back pain. A microscopic study. Spine 20, 1161–1164.

Beighton, P.H., Grahame, R., Bird, H., 1999. Hypermobility of joints, third ed. Springer-Verlag, London.

Bellamy, N., Park, W., Rooney, P.J., 1983. What do we know about the sacroiliac joint? Semin. Arthritis. Rheum. 12, 282–312.

Bennett, J., Downey, S., 1994. The complete snowboarder. Ragged Mountain Press, New York.

Berg, W.P., Strang, A.J., 2011. The role of electromyography (EMG) in the study of anticipatory postural adjustments. In: Steele, C. (Ed.), Applications of EMG in Clinical and Sports Medicine. Intech Pub., Rijeka, Croatia.

Bergmark, A., 1989. Stability of the lumbar spine. A study in mechanical engineering. Acta Orthop. Scand. 230, 1–54.

Bernard, Jr., T.N., Cassidy, J.D., 1991. The sacroiliac joint syndrome: pathophysiology, diagnosis and management. In: Frymoyer, J.W. (Ed.), The adult spine: principles and practice. Raven Press, New York, pp. 2107–2131.

Bernard, T.M., Kirkaldy-Willis, W.H., 1987. Recognizing specific characteristics of nonspecific low back pain. Clin. Orthop. Relat. Res. 217, 266–280.

Berthelot, J.M., Labat, J.J., Le Goff, B., et al., 2006. Provocative sacroiliac joint maneuvers and sacroiliac block are unreliable for diagnosing sacroiliac joint pain. J Bone Spine 73(1), 17–23.

Bilgic, S., Kurklu, M., Yurttaş, Y., et al., 2010. Coccygectomy with or without periosteal resection. Int. Orthop. 34, 537–541.

Binkerd, J., Ward, R.C., Hroby, R.J., 2002. Glossary of osteopathic terminology. p. 1241. Available: www.interlinea.org/glossary/aoa_glossary.pdf.

Bjorglund, K., Bergstroem, S., Lindgren, P.G., et al., 1996. Ultrasonographic measurement of the symphysis pubis: a potential method of studying symphyseolysis in pregnancy. Gynecol. Obstet. Invest. 42, 151–153.

Bjorklund, K., Nordstrom, M.L., Odlind, V., 2000. Combined oral contraceptives do not increase the risk of back and pelvic pain during pregnancy or after delivery. Acta Obstet. Gynecol. Scand. 79, 979–983.

Blum, C.L., 2004a. Chiropractic and dentistry in the 21st century: guest editorial. Cranio 22, 1–4.

Blum, C.L., 2004b. The relationship between the spine, cranium and TMJ. Sacro Occipital Technique Organization, Sparta, NC.

Bogduk, N.L.T., 1997. Common anatomy of the lumbar spine and sacrum, third ed. Churchill Livingstone, New York.

Bo, K., Lilleas, F., Talseth, T., et al., 2001. Dynamic MRI of the pelvic floor muscles in an upright sitting position. Neurourol. Urodyn. 20, 167.

Boos, N., Reider, R., Schade, V., et al., 1995. The diagnostic accuracy of magnetic resonance imaging, work perception, and psychosocial factors in identifying symptomatic disc herniations. Spine 20, 2613–2625.

Bowen, V., Cassidy, J.D., 1981. Macroscopic and microscopic anatomy of the sacroiliac joint from embryonic life until the eighth decade. Spine 6, 620–628.

Boyd, J., 2005. Alignment: the missing piece of the pelvic puzzle. DVD available at: www.backhealthworks.ca.

Boyling, J.D., Jull, G.A. (Eds.), 2005. Grieve's Modern manual therapy: the vertebral column. Churchill Livingstone, Edinburgh.

Bray, H., Moseley, G.L., 2011. Disrupted working body schema of the trunk in people with back pain. Br. J. Sports Med. 45(3), 168–173.

Breig, A., 1978. Adverse mechanical tension in the central nervous system: An analysis of cause and effect: relief by functional neurosurgery. Almqvist & Wiksell International, Stockholm.

Brendstrup, T., Midttun, A., 1998. The sacrotuberous ligament pain syndrome. Danish Workmedicine.

Brooke, R., 1924. The sacro-iliac joint. J. Anat. 58, 299–305.

Butler, D., 2000. The sensitive nervous system. NOI Group Publications, Adelaide, Australia.

Butler, D., Moseley, G.L., 2003. Explain pain. Orthopedic Physical Therapy Products, Adelaide, Australia.

Buyruk, H.M., Stam, H.J., Snijders, C.J., et al., 1995a. The use of color Doppler imaging for the assessment of sacroiliac joint stiffness: a study on embalmed human pelvises. Eur. J. Radiol. 21, 112–116.

Buyruk, H.M., Snijders, C.J., Vleeming, A., et al., 1995b. The measurements of sacroiliac joint stiffness with colour Doppler imaging: a study on healthy subjects. Eur. J. Radiol. 21, 117–121.

Buyruk, H.M., Stam, H.J., Snijders, C.J., et al., 1997. Measurement of sacroiliac joint stiffness with color Doppler imaging and the importance of asymmetric stiffness in sacroiliac pathology. In: Vleeming, A., Mooney, V., Dorman, T.A. et al. (Eds.), Movement, stability & low back pain. The essential role of the pelvis. Churchill Livingstone, Edinburgh.

Buyruk, H.M., Stam, H.J., Snijders, C.J., et al., 1999. Measurement of sacroiliac joint stiffness in peripartum pelvic pain patients with Doppler imaging of vibrations (DIV). Eur. J. Obstet. Gynecol. Reprod. Biol. 83(2), 159–163.

Cala, S.J., Edyvean, J., Engel, L.A., 1992. Chest wall and trunk muscle activity during respiratory loading. J. Appl. Physiol. 73, 2373–2381.

Campbell, E.M., Green, J.H., 1955. The behavior of the abdominal muscles and the intra-abdominal pressure during quiet breathing and increased pulmonary ventilation. J. Physiol. (London) 127, 423–426.

Campbell-Smith, S., 1964. Long-leg arthropathy. Ann. Rheum. Dis. 28, 359–365.

Cannon, W.B., Rosenblueth, A., 1949. The supersensitivity of denervated structures; A law of denervation. MacMillan, New York.

Cassidy, J.D., 1992. The pathoan atomy and clinical significance of the sacroiliac joints. J. Manipulative Physiol. Ther. 15, 41–42.

Cavanaugh, J.M., 1997. Neural mechanisms of idiopathic low back pain: Inventory profiles in patients with chronic low back pain. Spine 22, 72–75.

Cavanaugh, J.M., Ozaktay, A.C., Yamashita, H.T., et al., 1996. Lumbar facet pain: Biomechanics, neuroanatomy and neurophysiology. J. Biomech. 29(9), 1117–1129.

Chaitow, L., 2004. Breathing pattern disorders, motor control, and low back pain. J. Osteo. Med. 7, 34–41.

Chaitow, L., 2007. Muscle energy techniques, third ed. Churchill Livingstone, Edinburgh.

Chaitow, L., Bradley, D., Gilbert, C., 2002. Multidisciplinary approaches to breathing pattern disorders. Churchill Livingstone, Edinburgh.

Chang, C.W., Shieh, S.F., Li, C.M., et al., 2006. Measurement of motor nerve conduction velocity of the sciatic nerve in patients with piriformis syndrome. Arch. Phys. Med. Rehabil. 87, 1371–1375.

Chen, J.T., Chung, K.C., Hou, C.R., et al., 2001. Inhibitory effect of dry needling on the spontaneous electrical activity recorded from myofascial trigger spots of rabbit skeletal muscle. Am. J. Phys. Med. Rehabil. 80, 729–735.

Cheng, R., McKibbin, L., Roy, B., et al., 1980. Electroacupuncture elevates blood cortisol levels in naïve horses: sham treatment has no effect. Int. J. Neurosci. 10(2-3), 95–97.

Childers, M.K., Wilson, D.J., Gnatz, S.M., et al., 2006. Botulinum toxin type A use in piriformis muscle syndrome. Ann. Acad. Med. 52, 243–245.

Cibulka, M.T., Rose, S.J., Delitto, A., et al., 1986. Hamstring muscle strain treated by mobilizing the sacroiliac joint. Phys. Ther. 66, 1220–1223.

Ciullo, J.V., Jackson, D.W., 1985. Pars interarticularis stress reaction, spondylolysis, and spondylolisthesis in gymnasts. Clin. Sports Med. 4, 95–110.

Colachis, S.C., Worden, R.E., Bechtal, C.O., et al., 1963. Movement of the sacroiliac joint in the adult male: a preliminary report. Arch. Phys. Med. Rehabil. 44, 490–498.

Conway, P.J.W., Herzog, W., 1991. Changes in walking mechanics associated with wearing an intertrochanteric support belt. J. Manipulative Physiol. Ther. 14, 185–188.

Conyd, M., 1993, 1998, 2009. Basics of fencing. Personal communications.

Costello, K., 1998. Myofascial syndromes. In: Steege, J.F., Metzger, D.A., Levy, B.S. (Eds.), Chronic pelvic pain: an integrated approach. WB Saunders, Philadelphia, pp. 251–266.

Cox, M., Gould, D., 1988. Swedish way to tennis success, fifth ed. A&C Black, London.

Craig, C., 1992. Notes for a workshop on pelvic floor dysfunction: examination techniques and treatment. West Vancouver, Canada.

Crane, D., Everts, P., 2008. Platelet rich plasma (PRP) matrix grafts: PRP application in musculoskeletal medicine. Pract. Pain Manage Jan/Feb.

Curwin, S., 1984. The aetiology and treatment of tendinitis. In: Harris, M., Williams, C., Stanish, W.D., et al. (Eds.), Oxford Textbook of Sports Medicine. Oxford University Press, Oxford.

d'Hemecourt, P., Micheli, L., 1997. Acute and chronic adolescent thoracolumbar spine injuries. Sports Med. Arthrosc. 5, 164–171.

Dahlin, L.B., McLean, W.G., 1986. Effects of graded experimental compression on slow and fast axonal transport in rabbit vagus nerve. J. Neurol. Sci. 72, 19–30.

Dal Monte, A., Komor, A., 1989. Rowing and sculling mechanics. In: Vaughan, C.L. (Ed.), Biomechanics of sport. CRC Press, Boca Raton, FL, pp. 53–119.

Damen, L., Buyruk, H.M., Güler-Uysal, F., et al., 2001. Pelvic pain during pregnancy is associated with asymmetric laxity of the sacroiliac joints. Acta Obstet. Gynecol. Scand. 80, 1019–1024.

Damen, L., Buyruk, H.M., Güler-Uysal, F., et al., 2002a. Prognostic value of asymmetric laxity of the sacroiliac joints in pregnancy-related pelvic pain. Spine 27(24), 2820–2824.

Damen, L., Spoor, C.W., Stam, H.J., 2002b. Does a pelvic belt influence sacroiliac joint laxity. Clin. Biomech. 17(7), 495.

Dardzinski, J.A., Ostrov, B.E., Hamann, L.S., 2000. Myofascial pain unresponsive to standard treatment: successful use of a strain and counterstrain technique with physical therapy. J. Clin. Ther. 6(4), 169–174.

Delacerda, F.G., McCrory, M.L., 1981. A case report: effect of leg length differential on oxygen consumption. J. Orthop. Sports Phys. Ther. 3(1), 17–20.

DeLancey, J.O.L., Kearney, R., Chou, Q., et al., 2003. The appearance of levator ani muscle abnormalities in magnetic resonance imaging after vaginal delivery. Obstet. Gynecol. 101(1), 46–53.

DeLancey, J.O.L., Morgan, D.M., Fenner, D.E., et al., 2007. Comparison of levator ani defects and function in women with and without pelvic organ prolapse. Obstet. Gynecol. 109(2), 295–302.

Derby, R., 1986. Diagnostic block procedures: use in pain location. Spine: State of the Art Reviews 1, 47–65.

DeRosa, C., Porterfield, J.A., 2007. Anatomical linkages and muscle slings of the lumbopelvic region. In: Vleeming, A., Mooney, V., Stoeckart, R. (Eds.), Movement, stability & lumbopelvic pain. Integration of research and therapy. second ed. Churchill Livingstone/ Elsevier, Edinburgh.

De Troyer, A., 1997. Mechanics of the chest wall muscles. In: Miller, A., Blanchi, A., Bishop, B. (Eds.), Neural control of the respiratory muscles. CRC Press, Boca Raton, FL, pp. 59–76.

Dihlmann, W., 1967. Roentgendiagnostik der Iliosakralgelenke und Ihrer Nahen Umgebung. George Thieme, Stuttgart.

Dijkstra, P.F., 1997. Basic problems in the visualization of the sacroiliac joint. In: Vleeming, A., Mooney, V., Dorman, T.A. et al. (Eds.), Movement, stability & low back pain. The essential role of the pelvis. Churchill Livingstone, Edinburgh, p. 333.

Dijkstra, P.F., 2007. Basic problems in the visualization of the sacroiliac joint. In: Vleeming, A., Mooney, V., Stoeckart, R. (Eds.), Movement, stability & lumbopelvic pain. Integration of research and therapy. second ed. Churchill Livingstone/ Elsevier, Edinburgh, pp. 299–310.

Dixon, A.S., Campbell-Smith, S., 1964. Long leg arthropathy. Ann. Rheum. Dis. 28, 359–365.

DonTigny, R.L., 1985. Function and pathomechanics of the sacroiliac joint. A review. Phys. Ther. 65, 35–44.

DonTigny, R.L., 1990. Anterior dysfunction of the sacroiliac joint as a major factor in the etiology of idiopathic low back pain syndrome. Phys. Ther. 70, 250–265.

DonTigny, R.L., 1992. Sacroiliac dysfunction: recognition and treatment. In: Vleeming, A., Mooney, V., Snijders, C. et al. (Eds.), Low back pain and its relation to the sacroiliac joint. European Conference Organizers, Rotterdam, pp. 481–499.

DonTigny, R.L., 1997. Mechanics and treatment of the sacroiliac joint. In: Vleeming, A., Mooney, V., Dorman, T.A. et al. (Eds.), Movement, stability & low back pain. The essential role of the pelvis. Churchill Livingstone, Edinburgh, pp. 461–476.

DonTigny, R.L., 2004. Pelvic dynamics and the S3 subluxation of the sacroiliac joint. CD-ROM from DonTigny, Havre, MT.

DonTigny, R.L., 2005. Critical analysis of the functional dynamics of the sacroiliac joint as they pertain to normal gait. J. Orthop. Med. 27, 3–10.

DonTigny, R.L., 2007. A detailed and critical biomechanical analysis of the sacroiliac joints and relevant kinesiology: the implications for lumbopelvic function and dysfunction. In: Vleeming, A., Mooney, V., Stoeckart, R. (Eds.), Movement, stability & lumbopelvic pain. Integration of research and therapy. second ed. Churchill Livingstone/Elsevier, Edinburgh, pp. 265–278.

Dorman, T.A., 1993. Prolotherapy: a survey. J. Orthop. Med. 15, 2–3.

Dorman, T.A., 1994. Failure of self-bracing at the sacroiliac joint: the slipping clutch syndrome. J. Orthop. Med. 16, 49–51.

Dorman, T.A., 1995. Failure of self-bracing at the sacroiliac joints: the slipping clutch syndrome. In: Vleeming, A., Mooney, V., Dorman, T.A. et al. (Eds.), Second Interdisciplinary World Congress on back pain. San Diego, CA. 9–11 November, pp. 653–656.

Dorman, T.A., 1997. Pelvic mechanics and prolotherapy. In: Vleeming, A., Mooney, V., Dorman, T.A. et al. (Eds.), Movement, stability & low back pain. The essential role of the pelvis. Churchill Livingstone, Edinburgh, pp. 501–522.

Dorman, T.A., 2001a. Pelvic mechanics and prolotherapy. Townsend Letter: The examiner of alternate medicine 213, 68–72.

Dorman, T.A., 2001b. Pelvic mechanics and prolotherapy. Townsend Letter: The examiner of alternate medicine 215, 90–93.

Dorman, T.A., Brierly, S., Fray, J., et al., 1995. Muscles and pelvic gears: hip abductor inhibition in anterior rotation of the ilium. J. Orthop. Med. 17, 96–100.

Dorman, T.A., Brierly, S., Fray, J., et al., 1998. Muscles and pelvic clutch; hip abductor inhibition in anterior rotation of the ilium. In: Vleeming, A., Mooney, V., Tischler, H. et al. (Eds.), Proceedings of the Third Interdisciplinary World congress on low back and pelvic pain. Vienna, 19–21 November, pp. 140–148.

Dorman, T.A., Ravin, T.H., 1991. Diagnosis and injection techniques

in orthopedic medicine. Williams & Wilkins, Baltimore.
Dumas, C., Reid, J.G., Wolfe, L.A., et al., 1995. Exercise, posture and back pain during pregnancy. a. Exercise and posture; b. Exercise and back pain. Clin. Biomech. 10, 104–109.
Dunn, J., Glymph, I.D., 1999. Investigating the effect of upper cervical adjustment on cycling performance. Vector 2(4), 6.
Egund, N., Olsson, T.H., Schmid, H., et al., 1978. Movement of the sacroiliac joint demonstrated with roentgen stereophotogrammetry. Acta Radiol. Diagn. 19, 833–846.
Facchinetti, F., Nappi, G., Savoldi, F., et al., 1981. Primary headaches: reduced circulating beta-lipotropin and beta-endorphin levels with impaired reactivity to acupuncture. Cephalalgia 1(4), 195–201.
Fadiman, J., Frayer, R., 1976. Personality and personal growth. Harper and Row, New York.
Faflia, C.P., Prassopoulos, P.K., Daskalogiannaki, M.E., et al., 1998. Variations in the appearance of the normal sacroiliac joint on pelvic CT. Clin. Radiol. 53, 742–746.
Farfan, H.F., 1973. Mechanical disorders of the back. Lea & Febiger, Philadelphia. PA.
Finkelstein, M.M., 2002. Medical conditions, medications and urinary incontinence. Analysis of a population-based survey. Can. Fam. Phys. 48, 96–101.
Fishman, L.M., Zybert, P.A., 1992. Electrophysiologic evidence of piriformis syndrome. Arch. Phys. Med. Rehabil. 73, 359–364.
Fishman, L.M., Dombi, G.W., Michaelsen, C., et al., 2002. Piriformis syndrome: diagnosis, treatment, and outcome – a 10-year study. Arch. Phys. Med. Rehabil. 83, 295–305.
Fitt, S.S., 1987. Corrective exercises for two muscular imbalances: tight hip flexors and pectoralis minor syndrome. J. Health Phys. Educ. Recreation 58, 45–48.
Foran, P., 1999a. NUCCA technique. Can. Chiropract. 4, 6–8.
Foran, P., 1999b. Upper cervical adjustment's impact on athletic performance. Can. Chiropract. 10–12.
Fortin, J.D., Pier, J., Falco, F., 1997. Sacroiliac joint injection: pain referral mapping and arthrographic findings. In: Vleeming, A., Mooney, V., Dorman, T.A. et al. (Eds.), Movement, stability & low back pain. The essential role of the pelvis. Churchill Livingstone, Edinburgh, pp. 271–285.
Fortin, J., Dwyer, A., West, S., et al., 1994. Sacroiliac joint referred patterns upon application of a new injection/arthrography technique. I: Asymptomatic volunteers. Spine 19(13), 1475–1482.
Fowler, C., 1986. Muscle energy techniques for pelvic dysfunction. In: Grieve, G.P. (Ed.), Modern manual therapy of the vertebral column. Churchill Livingstone, Edinburgh, pp. 805–814.
Fraser, D.M., 1993. T-3 revisited. J. Orthop. Med. 13, 5–6.
Freeman, M.A.R., Dean, M.R.E., Hanham, I.W.F., 1965. The etiology and prevention of functional instability of the foot. J. Bone Joint Surg. 47B, 678–685.
Frigerio, N.A., Stowe, R.R., Howe, J.W., 1974. Movement of the sacro-iliac joint. Clin. Orthop. Relat. Res. 100, 370–377.
Fryette, H.H., 1954. Principles of osteopathic technique. Academy of Applied Osteopathy, Carmel, CA.
Garn, S.N., Newton, R.A., 1988. Kinesthetic awareness in subjects with multiple ankle sprains. Phys. Ther. 68, 1667–1671.
George, J., Tunstall, A., Tepe, R., et al., 2006. The effects of active release technique on hamstring flexibility: A pilot study. J. Manipulative Physiol. Ther. 29(3), 224–227.
Gibbons, S., 2002. The caudomedial part of the gluteus maximus and its relation to the sacrotuberous ligament. In: Proceedings of the Fifth Interdisciplinary World Congress on low back pain, Melbourne, Australia.
Gilmore, K.L., 1986. Biomechanics of the lumbar motion segment. In: Grieve, G.P. (Ed.), Modern manual therapy of the vertebral column. Churchill Livingstone, Edinburgh, pp. 103–111.
Glencross, D., Thornton, E., 1981. Position sense following joint injury. J. Sports Med. Phys. Fitness 21, 23–27.
Gottschalk, F., Kourosh, S., Leveau, B., 1989. The functional anatomy of tensor fasciae latae and gluteus medius and minimus. J. Anat. 166, 179–189.
Gracovetsky, S., 1990. Musculoskeletal function of the spine. In: Winters, J. M., Woo, S.L. (Eds.), Multiple muscle systems: biomechanics and movement organization. Springer Verlag, New York.
Gracovetsky, S., 1997. Linking the spinal engine with the legs: a theory of human gait. In: Vleeming, A., Mooney, V., Dorman, T.A. et al. (Eds.), Movement, stability & low back pain. The essential role of the pelvis. Churchill Livingstone, Edinburgh, pp. 243–251.
Gracovetsky, S., 2007. Stability or controlled instability. In: Vleeming, A., Mooney, V., Stoeckart, R. (Eds.), Movement, stability & lumbopelvic pain. Integration of research and therapy. second ed. Churchill Livingstone/ Elsevier, Edinburgh, pp. 279–294.
Gracovetsky, S., Farfan, H.F., 1986. The optimum spine. Spine 11, 543–573.
Granata, K.P., Orishimo, K.F., Sanford, A.H., 2001. Trunk muscle coactivation in preparation for sudden load. J Electromyo Kinesiol 11, 247–254.
Grant, D., 2000. 'Asymmetric proprioception' - a possible cause of 'functional' weakness? Personal communication.
Grant, J.C.B., 1962. The relationship of the sciatic nerve to piriformis. In: An atlas of anatomy. fifth ed. Williams & Wilkins, Baltimore, MD.

Grant, J.C.B., Anderson, J.E., 1980. Grant's atlas of anatomy, eighth ed. Williams & Wilkins, Baltimore, MD.

Greenman, P.E., 1992. Clinical aspects of sacroiliac function in human walking. In: Vleeming, V., Mooney, V., Snijders, C. et al. (Eds.), First Interdisciplinary World Congress on low back pain and its relation to the sacroiliac joint. San Diego, CA, pp. 353–359.

Greenman, P.E., 1997. Clinical aspects of sacroiliac joint in walking. In: Vleeming, A., Mooney, V., Dorman, T.A. et al. (Eds.), Movements, stability and low back pain. Churchill Livingstone, Edinburgh, pp. 235–242.

Grieve, G.P., 1976. The sacro-iliac joint. Physiotherapy 62, 384–400.

Grieve, G.P., 1983. Treating backache – a topical comment. Physiotherapy 69, 316.

Grieve, G.P., 1986a. Movements of the thoracic spine. In: Grieve, G.P. (Ed.), Modern manual therapy of the vertebral column. Churchill Livingstone, Edinburgh, pp. 86–102.

Grieve, G.P., 1986b. Thoracic joint problems and simulated visceral disease. In: Grieve, G.P. (Ed.), Modern manual therapy of the vertebral column. Churchill Livingstone, Edinburgh, p. 377.

Grieve, G.P., 1988. Common vertebral joint problems. Churchill Livingstone, Edinburgh.

Gunn, C., 1978. Transcutaneous neural stimulation, acupuncture and the current of injury. Am. J. Acupunct. 6, 191–196.

Gunn, C.C., 1996. The Gunn approach to the treatment of chronic pain. Intramuscular stimulation for myofascial pain of radiculopathic origin. Churchill Livingstone, New York.

Guymer, A.J., 1986. Proprioceptive neuromuscular facilitation for vertebral joint conditions. In: Grieve, G.P. (Ed.), Modern manual therapy of the vertebral column. Churchill Livingstone, Edinburgh, pp. 622–639.

Hackett, G.S., 1958. Ligament and tendon relaxation (skeletal disability) treated by prolotherapy (fibro-osseous proliferation), third ed. Charles C. Thomas, Springfield, IL.

Hackett, G.S., Henderson, D.G., 1955. Joint stabilization. An experimental, histological study with comments on the clinical application in ligament proliferation. Am. J. Surg. 89, 968–973.

Hackett, G.S., Hemwall, G.A., Montgomery, G.A., 1991. Ligament and tendon relaxation treated by prolotherapy, fifth ed. Gustav A Hemwall, Oak Park, IL (1st edn 1956, Charles C. Thomas, Springfield, IL.).

Hackett, G.S., Huang, T.C., 1961. Prolotherapy for sciatica from weak pelvic ligaments and bone dystrophy. Clin. Med. 8, 2301–2316.

Haldeman, K.O., Soto-Hall, R., 1983. The diagnosis and treatment of sacro-iliac conditions by the injection of procaine (Novocain). J. Bone Joint Surg. 20, 675–685.

Han, J., Stegen, K., De Valck, C., et al., 1996. Influence of breathing therapy on complaints, anxiety and breathing pattern in patients with hyperventilation syndrome and anxiety disorders. J. Psych. Res. 42, 481–493.

Harman, J., 2004. The horse's pain-free back and saddle-fit book. Trafalgar Square Books, London.

Harris, S.E., 1996. Horse gaits, balance and movement: The natural mechanics of movement common to all breeds. Howell Book House, New York.

Harris, F.I., White, A.S., Biskind, G.R., 1938. Observations on solutions used for injection treatment of hernia. Am. J. Surg. 39, 112–119.

Harrison, D., 1981. Sports illustrated canoeing. Harper & Row, London.

Hauser, R.A., 1998. Prolo your pain away! Curing chronic pain with prolotherapy. Beulah Land Press, Oak Park, IL.

Hauser, R.A., 2004. Prolotherapy: An alternative to knee surgery. Beulah Land Press.

Hauser, R.A., Hauser, M.A., 2009. Dextrose prolotherapy for unresolved low back pain: a retrospective case series study. J. Prolother. 3, 145–155.

Hayes, H.M., 1987. Veterinary notes for horse owners. Random House, London revised edn. PD Rossdale; London: Stanley Paul.

Heardman, H., 1951. Physiotherapy in obstetrics and gynecology. E&S Livingstone, Edinburgh.

Hedge, J., Wagoner, D., 1999. Horse conformation – structure, soundness and performance. Lyons Press, Guilford, CT.

Hedge, J., Wagoner, D., 2004. Horse conformation – structure, soundness and performance. Lyons Press, Guilford, CT.

Herman, H., 1988. Urogenital dysfunction. In: Wilder, E. (Ed.), Obstetric and gynecologic physical therapy. Churchill Livingstone, New York, pp. 83–111.

Herrington, L., Davies, R., 2005. The influence of Pilates training in the ability to contract the Transversus Abdominis muscle in asymptomatic individuals. J. Body Move. Ther. 9, 52–57.

Hershler, C., 1989. Unpublished personal communications

Herzog, W., Nigg, B.M., Read, L.J., 1988. Quantifying the effects of spinal manipulation on gait using patients with low back pain. J. Manipulative Physiol. Ther. 11, 151–157.

Hesch, J., Aisenbrey, J.A., Guarino, J., 1992. Manual therapy evaluation of the pelvic joints using palpatory and articular spring tests. In: Vleeming, A., Mooney, V., Snijders, C. et al. (Eds.), Low back pain and its relation to the sacroiliac joint. European Conference Organizers, Rotterdam, pp. 435–459.

Heumann, R., Korsching, S., Bandtlow, C., et al., 1987. Changes of nerve growth factor synthesis in non-neuronal cells in response to sciatic nerve transection. J. Cell Biol. 104(6), 1623–1631.

Hides, J.A., Stokes, M.J., Saide, M., et al., 1994. Evidence of lumbar multifidus muscles wasting ipsilateral to symptoms in patients with acute/subacute low back pain. Spine 19(2), 165.

Hides, J.A., Belavy, D.L., Wilson, S.J., et al., 2007. MRI assessment of trunk muscles during prolonged bed rest. Spine 32, 1687–1692.

Hides, J.A., Gilmore, C., Stanton, W., et al., 2008. Multifidus size and symmetry among chronic lower back pain and healthy symptomatic subjects. Man. Ther. 13(1), 43–49.

Hides, J.A., Belavy, D.L., Cassar, L., et al., 2009. Altered response of the anterolateral abdominal muscles to simulated weight-bearing in subjects with low back pain. Eur Spine J 18(3), 410–418.

Hill, C., 1992. Making, not breaking: the first year under saddle. Breakthrough, Ossining, NY.

Hirschberg, G.G., 1985. Sclerosant solution in low back pain. West. J. Med. 143, 682–683.

Hobusch, F.L., McClellan, T., 1990. Sports performance series: The karate roundhouse kick. J. Strength Cond. Res. 12, 6–9.

Hodges, P.W., 1997. Feedforward contraction of transversus abdominis is not influenced by the direction of arm movement. Exp. Brain Res. 114, 362–370.

Hodges, P.W., 2003. Core stability exercise in chronic low back pain. Orthop. Clin. North Am. 34, 245–254.

Hodges, P.W., Cholewicki, J., 2007. Functional control of the spine. In: Vleeming, A., Mooney, V., Stoeckart, R. (Eds.), Movement, stability & lumbopelvic pain: integration of research and therapy. second ed. Churchill Livingstone, Edinburgh, pp. 489–512.

Hodges, P.W., Erikkson, A.E., Shirley, D., et al., 2005a. Intra-abdominal pressure increases stiffness in the lumbar spine. J. Biomech. 38(9), 1873–1880.

Hodges, P.W., Gandevia, S.C., 2000a. Activation of the human diaphragm during a repetitive postural task. J. Physiol. 522(1), 165–175.

Hodges, P.W., Gandevia, S.C., 2000b. Changes in intra-abdominal pressure during postural and respiratory activation of the human diaphragm. J. Appl. Physiol. 89, 967–976.

Hodges, P.W., Moseley, G.L., 2003. Pain and motor control of the lumbopelvic region: effect and possible mechanisms. J. Electromyogr. Kinesiol. 13, 361–370.

Hodges, P.W., Richardson, C.A., 1996. Inefficient muscular stabilization of the lumbar spine associated with low back pain. A motor control evaluation of transversus abdominis. Spine 21(22), 2640–2650.

Hodges, P.W., Richardson, C.A., 1997. Contraction of the abdominal muscles associated with movement of the lower limb. Phys. Ther. 77, 132–144.

Hodges, P.W., Cresswell, A.G., Thorstensson, A., 1999. Preparatory trunk motion accompanies rapid upper limb movement. Exp. Brain Res. 124, 69–79.

Hodges, P.W., Heijnen, I., Gandevia, S. C., 2001. Postural activity of the diaphragm is reduced in humans when respiratory demand is increased. J. Physiol. 537(3), 999–1008.

Hodges, P.W., Gurfinkel, V.S., Brumagne, S., et al., 2002. Coexistence of stability and mobility in postural control: evidence from postural compensation for respiration. Exp. Brain Res. 144, 293–302.

Hodges, P.W., Moseley, G.L., Gabrielsson, A.H., et al., 2003. Acute experimental pain changes postural recruitment of the trunk muscles in pain-free humans. Exp. Brain Res. 151, 262–271.

Hodges, P.W., Smith, M., Grigornko, A., et al., 2005b. Trunk muscle response to support surface translation in sitting: Normal control of effects of respiration. International Society for Posture and Gait, Marseille, France. In: Vleeming, A., Mooney, V., Stoeckart, R. (Eds.), 2007a. Movement, stability & lumbopelvic pain. Churchill Livingstone/Elsevier, Edinburgh, pp. 490–512.

Hodges, P.W., Sapsford, R., Pengel, L. M.H., 2007. Postural and respiratory functions of the pelvic floor muscles. Neurourol. Urodynam. 26, 362–371.

Hollinshead, W.H., 1962. Textbook of anatomy. Harper and Row, New York.

Holstege, G., Bandler, R., Saper, C.B., 1996. The emotional motor system. Elsevier Science, Amsterdam.

Howse, J., 1983. Disorders of the great toe in dancers. Clin. Sports Med. 2, 499–505.

Hungerford, B.A., 2002. Patterns of intra-pelvic motion and muscle recruitment for pelvic instability. PhD Thesis. University of Sydney, Australia.

Hungerford, B.A., Gilleard, W., Lee, D., 2001. Alterations of sacroiliac joint motion patterns in subjects with pelvic motion asymmetry. In: Proceedings from the fourth world interdisciplinary congress on low back and pelvic pain. Montreal, Canada.

Hungerford, B.A., Gilleard, W., Hodges, P., 2003. Evidence of altered lumbo-pelvic muscle recruitment in the presence of sacroiliac joint pain. Spine 28(14), 1593–1600.

Hungerford, B.A., Gilleard, W., Lee, D., 2004. Altered patterns of pelvic bone motion determined in subjects with posterior pelvic pain using skin markers. Clin. Biomech. 19, 456–464.

Hungerford, B.A., Gilleard, W., Moran, M., et al., 2007. Evaluation of the ability of physical therapists to palpate intrapelvic motion with the Stork Test on the support side. Phys. Ther. 87, 879–887.

Hungerford, B.A., Gilleard, W., 2007. The pattern of intrapelvic motion and lumbopelvic muscle recruitment alters in the presence of pelvic girdle pain. In: Vleeming, A., Mooney, V., Stoeckart, R. (Eds.), Movement, stability & lumbopelvic pain: integration of research and therapy. second ed. Churchill Livingstone, Edinburgh, pp. 361–376.

Jacob, H.A.C., Kissling, R.O., 1995. The mobility of the sacroiliac joints in healthy volunteers between 20 and 50 years of age. Clin. Biomech. 10(7), 352–361.

Janda, V., 1978. Muscles, central nervous motor regulation and back problems. In: Korr, I. (Ed.), The neurobiological mechanisms in manipulative therapy. Plenum Press, London, p. 27.

Janda, V., 1986. Muscle weakness and inhibition (pseudoparesis) in back pain syndromes. In: Grieve, G.P. (Ed.), Modern manual therapy of the vertebral column. Churchill Livingstone, Edinburgh, pp. 197–201.

Järvinen, M., Jozsa, L., Kannus, P., et al., 1997. Histological findings in chronic tendon disorders. Scand J Med Sci Sports 7, 86–95.

Jensen, G., 1989. Musculoskeletal analysis. Thoracic spine. In: Scully, R.M., Barnes, R.M. (Eds.), Physical Therapy. JB Lippincott, Philadelphia, PA, pp. 429–437.

Jensen, M.C., Brant-Zawadski, M.N., Obuchowski, N., et al., 1994. Magnetic resonance imaging of the lumbar spine in people without back pain. N. Engl. J. Med. 331, 69–73.

Jiang, H.X., Russell, G., Raso, V.J., et al., 1995. The nature and distribution of the innervation of human supraspinal and interspinal ligaments. Spine 20, 869–876.

Johnson, T.B., Whillis, J. (Eds.), 1944. Gray's anatomy. Descriptive and applied. Longmans & Green, London.

Jones, L.H., 1981. Strain and counterstrain. American Academy of Osteopathy, Colorado Springs, CO.

Jull, G.A., Richardson, C.A., Toppenberg, R., et al., 1993. Towards a measurement of active muscle control for lumbar stabilization. Aust. J. Physiother. 39, 187–193.

Jull, G.A., Richardson, C.A., 2000. Motor control problems in patients with spinal pain: a new direction for therapeutic exercise. J. Manipulative Physiol. Ther. 23, 115–117.

Jurriaans, E., Friedman, L., 1997. CT and MRI of the sacroiliac joints. In: Vleeming, A., Mooney, V., Dorman, T. et al. (Eds.), Movement, stability & low back pain. The essential role of the pelvis. Churchill Livingstone, Edinburgh, p. 347.

Kaigle, A.M., Wessberg, P., Hansson, T. H., 1998. Muscular and kinematic behavior of the lumbar spine during flexion-extension. J. Spinal Disord. 11(2), 163–174.

Kapandji, I.A., 1974. The physiology of the joints. III. The trunk and vertebral column, second ed. Churchill Livingstone, Edinburgh.

Kassarjian, A., Brisson, M., Palmer, W.E., 2007. Femeroacetabular impingement. Eur. J. Radiol. 63, 29.

Keating, J.C., Bergman, T.F., Jacobs, G.E., et al., 1997a. Fluoroscopically guided therapeutic sacroiliac joint injections. J. Clin. Exp. Neuropsychol. 19, 838–839.

Keating, J.G., Avillar, M.D., Price, M., 1997b. Sacroiliac joint arthrodesis in selected patients with low back pain. In: Vleeming, A., Mooney, V., Dorman, T. et al. (Eds.), Movement, stability & low back pain. The essential role of the pelvis. Churchill Livingstone, New York, pp. 573–594.

Kegel, A.H., 1948. Progressive resistance exercise in the functional restoration of the perineal muscles. Am. J. Obstet. Gynecol. 56, 238–248.

Kerman, I.A., 2008. Organization of brain somatosensory-sympathetic circuits. Exp. Brain Res. 187, 1–16.

Kesson, M., Atkins, E., 1999. The thoracic spine and sport. J. Orthop. Med. 21, 80–86.

Kieffer, S.A., Cacayorin, E., Sherry, R.G., 1984. The radiological diagnosis of herniated lumbar intervertebral disc. A current controversy. J. Am. Med. Assoc. 251, 1192.

Kirkaldy-Willis, W.H., Cassidy, J.D., 1985. Spinal manipulation in the treatment of low back pain. Can. Fam. Phys. 31, 535–540.

Kirkaldy-Willis, W.H., Hill, R.J., 1979. A more precise diagnosis for low back pain. Spine 4, 102–109.

Kirschner, J.S., Foye, P.M., Cole, J.L., 2009. Piriformis syndrome, diagnosis and treatment. Muscle & Nerve 40, 10–18.

Kissling, R.O., Jacob, H.A.C., 1997. The mobility of sacroiliac joints in healthy subjects. In: Vleeming, A., Mooney, V., Dorman, T. et al. (Eds.), Movement, stability & low back pain. The essential role of the pelvis. Churchill Livingstone, Edinburgh, pp. 177–185.

Klauser, A., Halpern, E.J., Frauscher, F., et al., 2005. Inflammatory low back pain: high negative predictive value of contrast-enhanced color Doppler ultrasound in the detection of inflamed sacroiliac joints. Arthritis Rheum. 53, 440–444.

Klein, K.K., 1973. Progression of pelvic tilt in adolescent boys from elementary through high school. Arch. Phys. Med. Rehabil. 54, 57–59.

Klein, K.K., Buckley, J.C., 1968. Asymmetries of growth in the pelvis and legs of growing children. Am. Correct. Ther. J. 22, 53–55.

Klein, R.G., Dorman, T.A., Johnson, C.E., 1989. Proliferant injections for low back pain: histologic changes of injected ligaments and objective measurements of lumbar spine mobility before and after treatment. J. Neurolog. Orthop. Med. Surg. 10, 123–126.

Klein, R.G., Eek, B.C., DeLong, W.B., et al., 1993. A randomized double-blind trial of dextrose-glycerine-phenol injections for chronic, low back pain. J. Spinal Disord. 6, 23–33.

Korr, I.M., 1978. Neurobiological mechanisms of manipulative therapy. Plenum Press, New York.

Korr, I.M., 1986. Somatic dysfunction, osteopathic manipulative treatment and the nervous system: a few facts, some theories, many questions. J. Am. Osteopath. Assoc. 86, 109–114.

Kostopoulos, D.C., Keramidas, G., 1992. Changes of elongation of falx cerebri during craniosacral therapy techniques applied to the skull of an embalmed cadaver. Cranio 10(1), 9–12.

Kravitz, S.R., 1987. The mechanics of dance and dance-related injuries. Bull. Hosp. Jt. Dis. Orthop. Inst. 47, 203–210.

Kumar, S., 1990. Cumulative load as a risk factor for back pain. Spine 15, 1311–1316.

Kurica, K.B., 1995. A prospective study of sacroiliac joint arthrodesis with one to six year patient follow-up. In: Vleeming, A., Mooney, V., Dorman, T. et al. (Eds.), The integrated function of the lumbar spine and sacroiliac joint. European Conference Organizers, Rotterdam, pp. 367–368.

Kvist, M., Jozsa, L., Järvinen, M., 1992. Vascular changes in the ruptured Achilles tendonand its paratenon. Int Orthop 16, 377–382.

Lamoth, C.J., Meijer, O.G., Wuisman, P. I., et al., 2002. Pelvis-thorax coordination in the transverse plane during walking in persons with non-specific low back pain. Spine 27, E92–E99.

Langevin, H.M., Storch, K.N., White, S. L., et al., 2006. Fibroblast spreading induced by connective tissue stretch involves intracellular redistribution of alpha- and beta-actin. Histochem. Cell Biol. 125, 487–495.

Langevin, I.L.M., Churchill, D.L., Wu, J., et al., 2002. Evidence of connective tissue involvement in acupuncture. FASEB J. 16, 872–874.

Langnes, D., 2009. Personal communication

LaTouche, R., Escalante, K., Linares, M. T., 2008. Treating non-specific chronic low back pain through the Pilates method. J. Body Move. Ther. 12(4), 364–370.

Laws, K., 1984. The physics of dance. Oxford University Press, Oxford.

Lee, A.S., Cholewicki, J., Reeves, N.P., et al., 2010. Comparison of trunk proprioception between patients with low back pain and healthy controls. Arch. Phys. Med. Rehabil. 91(9), 1327–1331.

Lee, D.G., 1992a. Intra-articular versus extra-articular dysfunction of the sacroiliac joint – a method of differentiation, IFOMT Proceedings, 5th International Conference, p. 69. Vail, CO.

Lee, D.G., 1992b. The relationship between the lumbar spine, pelvic girdle and hip. In: Vleeming, A., Mooney, V., Snijders, C. et al. (Eds.), Low back pain and its relation to the sacroiliac joint. European Conference Organizers, Rotterdam, pp. 464–478.

Lee, D.G., 1993a. Biomechanics of the thorax: a clinical model of in vivo function. J. Man. Manipulative Ther. 1, 13–21.

Lee, D.G., 1994a. Biomechanics of the thorax. In: Grant, R. (Ed.), Physical therapy of the cervical and thoracic spine. Churchill Livingstone, New York, Ch 3.

Lee, D.G., 1994b. Manual therapy for the thorax: a biomechanical approach. Delta Orthopedic Physiotherapy Clinic, Delta, BC.

Lee, D.G., 1997. Instability of the sacroiliac joint and the consequences for gait. In: Vleeming, A., Mooney, V., Dorman, T. et al. (Eds.), Movement, stability & low back pain. The essential role of the pelvis. Churchill Livingstone, Edinburgh, pp. 231–233.

Lee, D.G., 1998. Video teaching tapes. 1: Assessment – articular function of the sacroiliac joint. 2: Manual therapy techniques for the sacroiliac joint. 3: Exercises for the unstable pelvis. Available at: www.dianelee.ca or www.discoverphysio.ca.

Lee, D.G., 1999. The pelvic girdle: an approach to the examination and treatment of the lumbo–pelvic–hip region. Churchill Livingstone, Edinburgh.

Lee, D.G., 2002. The Com-Pressor. Available online at: www.dianelee.ca or www.optp.com.

Lee, D.G., 2003. The thorax – an integrated approach. Diane G Lee Physiotherapist Corporation, Surrey, Canada. Available: www.dianelee.ca or www.optp.com.

Lee, D.G., 2004a. The pelvic girdle: An approach to the examination and treatment of the lumbopelvic-hip region, third ed. Churchill Livingstone, Edinburgh.

Lee, D.G., 2007a. The evolution of myths and facts regarding function and dysfunction of the pelvic girdle. In: Vleeming, A., Mooney, V., Stoeckart, R. (Eds.), Movement, stability & lumbopelvic pain: integration of research and therapy, second ed. Churchill Livingstone, Edinburgh, pp. 191–200.

Lee, D.G., 2007b. An integrated approach for the management of low back and pelvic girdle pain: a case report. In: Vleeming, A., Mooney, V., Stoeckart, R. (Eds.), Movement, stability & lumbopelvic pain: integration of research and therapy, second ed. Churchill Livingstone, Edinburgh, pp. 593–620.

Lee, D.G., 2007c. Clinical expertise: show me the patient. Presented at the Sixth World Congress on low back and pelvic pain, Barcelona.

Lee, D.G., 2011. The pelvic girdle, fourth ed. An integration of clinical expertise and research. Churchill Livingstone, Edinburgh.

Lee, D.G., Vleeming, A., 1998. Impaired load transfer through the pelvic girdle – a new model of altered neutral zone function. In: Proceedings from the Third Interdisciplinary World Congress on low back and pelvic pain, Vienna, Austria.

Lee, D.G., Vleeming, A., 2003. The management of pelvic joint pain and dysfunction. In: Boyling, J.D., Jull, G. (Eds.), Grieve's modern manual therapy of the vertebral column, third ed. Elsevier Science, Edinburgh.

Lee, D.G., Vleeming, A., 2007. An integrated therapeutic approach to the treatment of pelvic girdle pain. In: Vleeming, A., Mooney, V., Stoeckart, R. (Eds.), Movement, stability & lumbopelvic pain. Integration of research and therapy, second ed. Churchill Livingstone, Edinburgh, pp. 621–638.

Lee, D.G., Walsh, M.C., 1996. Workbook of manual therapy techniques for the vertebral column and pelvic girdle, second ed. Friesen Printers, Altona, MB.

Lee, L.-J., 2004b. An integrated approach to the assessment and treatment of the lumbopelvic-hip region. DVD available at: www.dianelee.ca.

Lee, L.J., Coppieters, M.W., Hodges, P.W., 2009. Anticipatory adjustments to arm movement reveal complex control of paraspinal muscles in the thorax. J. Electromyogr. Kinesiol. 19(1), 46.

Lehmann, R.C., 1988. Thoracoabdominal musculoskeletal injuries in racquet sports. Clin. Sports Med. 7, 267–276.

Lenehan, K.I., Fryer, G., McLaughlin, P., 2003. The effect of muscle energy technique on gross trunk range of motion. J. Osteo. Med. 6(1), 13–18.

Lentell, G.L., Katzman, L.L., Walters, M.R., 1992. The relationship between muscle function and ankle stability. J. Orthop. Med. 14, 85–90.

Letson, A.K., Dahners, L.E., 1994. The effect of combinations of growth factors on ligament healing. Clin. Orthop. Relat. Res. 308, 207–212.

Li, J., He, W., Yao, J., et al., 1996. Possibility of observing the changes of cerebrospinal fluid pulse waves as a substitute for volume pressure test. Clin. Med. J. (England) 109(5), 411–413.

Liboff, A.R., 1997. Bioelectromagnetic fields and acupunture. J Altern Complement Med 3(Suppl 1), S77–S87.

Lieberman, D.E., 2008. Running barefoot. Br. J. Sports Med. 27, 51–59.

Lieberman, D.E., Venkadesan, M., Werbel, W.A., et al., 2010. Foot strike patterns and collision forces in habitually barefoot versus shod runners. Nature 463, 531–535.

Lippitt, A.B., 1995a. Recurrent subluxation of the sacroiliac joint: diagnosis and treatment. Bulletin Hospital for Joint Diseases 54(2), 94–102.

Lippitt, A.B., 1995b. Percutaneous fixation of the sacroiliac joint. In: Vleeming, A., Mooney, V., Dorman, T. et al. (Eds.), The integrated function of the lumbar spine and sacroiliac joint. European Conference Organizers, Rotterdam, pp. 369–390.

Little, P., Lewith, G., Webley, F., et al., 2008. Randomised controlled trial of Alexander technique lessons, exercise, and massage (ATEAM) for chronic and recurrent back pain. BMJ 337, a884.

Loken, N.C., Willoughby, R.J., 1977. The complete book of gymnastics, third ed. Prentice Hall, Englewood Cliffs, NJ.

Lovett, R.W., 1903. A contribution to the study of the mechanics of the spine. Am. J. Anat. 2, 457–462.

Lundborg, G., 1988. Nerve injury and repair. Churchill Livingstone, Edinburgh.

Luttgens, K., Deutsch, H., Hamilton, N., 1992. Kinesiology: scientific basis of human locomotion, eighth ed. Brown & Benchmark, Dubuque, IA.

Maffetone, P., 1999. Complementary sports medicine. Human Kinetics, Champaign, IL.

Magora, A., Schwartz, A., 1976. Relation between the low back pain syndrome and X-ray findings. 1. Degenerative osteoarthritis. Scand. J. Rehabil. Med. 8, 115–125.

Magoun, H.I., 1951. Osteopathy in the cranial field. Compiled by the Osteopathic Cranial Association, p. 17.

Maigne, J.-Y., 1997. Lateral dynamic X-rays in the sitting position and coccygeal discography in common coccydynia. In: Vleeming, A., Mooney, V., Dorman, T. et al. (Eds.), Movement, stability & low back pain. The essential role of the pelvis. Churchill Livingstone, Edinburgh, pp. 385–391.

Maigne, J-Y, 2002. Management or common coccygodynia. www.coccyx.org>medical papers.

Maigne, J.-Y., Chatellier, G., 2001. Comparison of three manual coccydynia treatments: a pilot study. Spine 26, E479–E484.

Maigne, J.-Y., Straus, G.S., 1994. Idiopathic coccygodynia: lateral roentgenograms in the sitting position and coccygeal discography. Spine 19, 930–934.

Maigne, J.-Y., Lazareth, J.P., Guerin-Surville, H., et al., 1986. The lateral cutaneous branches of the dorsal rami of the thoracolumbar junction: an anatomical study of 37 dissections. J. Surg. Radiol. Anat. 8, 251–256.

Maigne, J.-Y., Aivaliklis, A., Pfefer, S., 1996. Results of sacroiliac joint double block and value of sacroiliac pain provocation tests in 54 patients with low back pain. Spine 21, 1889–1892.

Maigne, R., 1972. Orthopedic medicine. Charles C. Thomas, Springfield, IL.

Maigne, R., 1980. Low back pain of thoracolumbar origin. Arch. Phys. Med. Rehabil. 61, 389–395.

Maigne, R., 1995. Thoraco-lumbar junction syndrome: a source of diagnostic error. J. Orthop. Med. 17, 84–89.

Maitland, G.D., 1977. Vertebral manipulation. Butterworth, London.

Malyak, M., 1997. Fibromyalgia. In: West, S.G. (Ed.), Rheumatology secrets. Hanley & Belfus, Philadelphia, PA, pp. 354–363.

Maniol, L., 1938. Histologic effects of various sclerosing solutions used in the injection treatment of hernia. Arch. Surg. 36, 171–189.

Mann, R., 1982. Biomechanics of running. In: Mack, R.P. (Ed.), American Academy of Orthopedic Surgeons symposium on the foot and leg in running sports. CV Mosby, St Louis, pp. 1–29.

Marnach, M.L., Ramin, K.D., Ramsey, P.S., et al., 2003. Characterization of the relationship between joint laxity and maternal hormones in pregnancy. Obstet. Gynecol. 101(2), 331–335.

Marks, M.R., Haas, S.S., Wiesel, S.W., 1988. Low back pain in the competitive tennis player. Clin Sports Med 7(2), 277–287.

Marr, M., 2007. Effects of the Bowen technique on flexibility levels: implications for fascial plasticity. Presentation at the First Scientific Exploration of Fascia from an Interdisciplinary Perspective, Harvard University.

Masi, A.T., Benjamin, M., Vleeming, A., 2007. Anatomical, biomechanical, and clinical perspectives on sacroiliac joints: an integrative synthesis of biodynamic mechanisms related to ankylosing spondylitis. In: Vleeming, A., Mooney, V., Stoeckart, R. (Eds.), Movement, stability & lumbopelvic pain. Integration of research and therapy. second ed. Churchill Livingstone, Edinburgh, pp. 205–227.

Matheny, F., 1989. Bicycling Magazine's complete guide to riding and racing techniques. Rodale Press, Emmaus, PA.

Mayer, D., Liebeskind, J., 1974. Pain reduction by focal electrical stimulation of the brain: an anatomical and behavioral analysis. Brain Res. 68, 73–93.

McArdle, W.D., Katch, F.I., Katch, V.L., 1986. Exercise physiology: energy, nutrition and human performance. Lea & Febiger, Philadelphia, PA.

McCall, I.W., Park, W.M., O'Brien, J.P., 1979. Induced pain referral from posterior lumbar elements in normal subjects. Spine 4, 441–446.

McCallum, D.J. 1999. Unpublished data.

McGill, S., 2002. Low back disorders – evidence based prevention and rehabilitation. Human Kinetics, Canada.

McGill, S.M., Grenier, S., Kavcic, N., et al., 2003. Coordination of muscle activity to assure stability of the lumbar spine. J. Electromyogr. Kinesiol. 13, 353.

McGivney, J.Q., Cleveland, B.R., 1965. The levator syndrome and its treatment. South. Med. J. 58, 505–509.

McGuckin, N., 1986. The T4 syndrome. In: Grieve, G.P. (Ed.), Modern manual therapy of the vertebral column. Churchill Livingstone, Edinburgh, pp. 370–376.

McLain, R.F., 1994. Mechanoreceptor endings in human cervical facet joints. Spine 19, 495–501.

McLain, R.F., Pickar, J.G., 1998. Mechanoreceptor endings in human thoracic and lumbar facet joints. Spine 23(2), 168.

Mehling, W., Hamel, K., 2005. Randomized, controlled trial of breath therapy for patients with low back pain. Altern. Ther. Health Med. 11(4), 44–52.

Melzack, R., 1981. Myofascial trigger points: relation to acupuncture and mechanisms of pain. Arch. Phys. Med. Rehabil. 62, 114–117.

Melzack, R., 1999. Pain – an overview. Acta Anesth. Scand. 43, 880–884.

Melzak, R., 2005. Evolution of the neuromatrix theory of pain. Pain Pract. 5(2), 85.

Melzack, R., Wall, P., 1965. Pain mechanisms: a new theory. Science 150, 971–979.

Menezes, A., 2000. The complete guide to Joseph H. Pilates techniques of physical conditioning. Hunter House, CA.

Mens, J.M.A., Stam, H.J., Stoeckart, R., et al., 1992. Peripartum pelvic pain: a report of the analysis of an inquiry among patients of a Dutch patients' society. In: Vleeming, A., Mooney, V., Snijders, C. et al. (Eds.), Low back pain and its relation to the sacroiliac joint. European Conference Organizers, Rotterdam, pp. 519–533.

Mens, J.M.A., Vleeming, A., Snidjers, C., et al., 1997. Active straight leg raising test: a clinical approach to the load transfer function of the pelvic girdle. In: Vleeming, A., Mooney, V., Dorman, T. et al. (Eds.), Movement, stability & low back pain. The essential role of the pelvis. Churchill Livingstone, Edinburgh, pp. 425–431.

Mens, J.M.A., Vleeming, A., Snijders, C.J., et al., 1999. The active straight leg raising test and mobility of the pelvic girdle. Eur. Spine J. 8, 468–473.

Mens, J.M.A., Vleeming, A., Snijders, C. J., et al., 2001. Reliability and validity of the active straight leg raise test in posterior pelvic pain since pregnancy. Spine 26(10), 1167.

Mens, J.M.A., Vleeming, A., Snijders, C. J., et al., 2002. Validity of the active straight leg raising test for measuring disease severity in patients with posterior pelvic pain after pregnancy. Spine 27(2), 196–200.

Mens, J.M.A., Damen, L., Snijders, C.J., et al., 2006. The mechanical effect of a pelvic belt in patients with pregnancy-related pelvic pain. Clin. Biomech. 21, 122–127.

Mens, J.M.A., Vleeman, A., Snijders, C. J., 2007. Active straight leg raising: a clinical approach to the load transfer functions of the pelvic girdle. J. Man Manipulative Ther. 15, 133–141.

Meyer, G.H., 1878. Der mechanismus der symphysis sacroiliaca. Archiv für Anatomie und Physiologie 1, 1.

Meyers, H.L., 2006. Clinical application of counterstrain. Osteopathic Press, Tucson, AZ.

Micheli, L.J., 1979. Low back pain in the adolescent: differential diagnosis. Am. J. Sports Med. 7, 362–364.

Micheli, L.J., 1983. Back injuries in dancers. Clin. Sports Med. 2, 473–484.

Micheli, L.J., 1985. Back injuries in gymnastics. Clin. Sports Med. 4, 85–93.

Midttun, A., Bojsen-Moller, F., 1986. The sacrotuberous ligament pain syndrome. In: Grieve, G.P. (Ed.), Modern manual therapy of the vertebral column. Churchill Livingstone, Edinburgh, pp. 815–818.

Millar, W.J., 1996. Chronic pain. Health Rep. 7, 47–53.

Miller, J.A.A., Schultz, A.B., Andersson, G.B.J., 1987. Load-displacement behaviour of sacroiliac joints. J. Orthop. Res. 5, 92–101.

Mirman, M.J., 1989. Sclerotherapy, fourth ed. E. Springfield, Springfield, PA.

Mitchell, Jr., F.L., Mitchell, P.K.G., 2005. The muscle energy manual, Vol I: Concepts and mechanisms, the musculoskeletal screen, cervical region evaluation and treatment. MET Press, East Lansing, MI.

Mitchell, Sr., F.L., Mitchell, Jr., F.L., 1979. An evaluation and treatment manual of osteopathic muscle energy procedures. Moran and Pruzzo Associates, Valley Park, MO.

Mitchell, P.K.G., 2009a. Muscle energy technique: history, model, research. Edition VOD. Verband der Osteopathen, Germany.

Mitchell, P.K.G., 2009b. Personal communication.

Mixter, W.J., Barr, J.S., 1934. Rupture of the intervertebral disc with involvement of the spinal canal. N. Engl. J. Med. 211, 210–215.

Mok, N., Brauer, S.G., Hodges, P.W., 2004a. Different range and temporal pattern of lumbopelvic motion accompanies rapid upper limb flexion in people with low back pain. In: Vleeming, A., Mooney, V., Tischler, H. et al. (Eds.), Fifth Interdisciplinary World Congress on low back and pelvic pain. Melbourne, Australia, p. 295.

Mok, N.W., Brauer, S.G., Hodges, P.W., 2004b. Hip strategy for balance control in quiet standing is reduced in people with low back pain. Spine 29, E107–E112.

Mok, N.W., Brauer, S.G., Hodges, P.W., 2007. Failure to use movement in postural strategies leads to increased spinal displacement in low back pain. Spine 32(19), E537.

Mooney, V., Robertson, J., 1976. The facet syndrome. Clin. Orthop. Relat. Res. 115, 149–156.

Mooney, V., Pozos, R., Vleeming, A., et al., 1997. In: Vleeming, A., Mooney, V., Dorman, T. et al. (Eds.), Movement, stability & low back pain. The essential role of the pelvis. Churchill Livingstone, Edinburgh, pp. 115–122.

Morris, R., McKay, W., Mushlin, P., 1987. Comparison of pain associated with intradermal and subcutaneous infiltration with various local anaesthetic solutions. Anesth. Analg. 66, 1180–1182.

Moseley, G.L., 2007. Motor control in chronic pain: new idea for effective intervention. In: Vleeming, A., Mooney, V., Stoeckart, R. (Eds.), Movement, stability & lumbopelvic pain: Integration of research and therapy. second ed. Churchill Livingstone, Edinburgh, pp. 513–525.

Moseley, G.L., Hodges, P.W., 2005. Are the changes in postural control associated with low back pain caused by pain interference? Clin. J. Pain 21(4), 323–329.

Moseley, G.L., Hodges, P.W., Gandevia, S.C., 2002. Deep and superficial fibres of the lumbar multifidus muscle are differentially active during voluntary arm movements. Spine 27(2), E29.

Moseley, G.L., Hodges, P.W., Gandevia, S.C., 2003. External perturbation of the trunk in standing humans differentially activates components of the medial back muscles. J. Physiol. 547(2), 581.

Mueller, M.J., Minor, S.D., Schaaf, J.A., et al., 1995. Relationship of plantar-flexor peak torque and dorsiflexion range of motion to kinetic variables during walking. Phys. Ther. 75, 684–693.

Murphy, B.A., Dawson, N.J., Slack, J.R., 1995. Sacroiliac joint manipulation decreases the H-reflex. Electromyogr. Clin. Neurophysiol. 35, 87–94.

Murphy, M., 1992. The future of the body: explorations into the further evolution of human nature. Tarcher Putnam, New York.

Naeim, F., Froetscher, L., Hirschberg, G.G., 1982. Treatment of the chronic iliolumbar syndrome by infiltration of the iliolumbar ligament. West. J. Med. 136, 372–374.

Nilsson, N., Christensen, H., Hartvigsen, J., 1996. Lasting changes in passive range motion after spinal manipulation: a randomized, blind, controlled trial. J. Manipulative Physiol. Ther. 19, 165–168.

Nixon, J.E., 1983. Injuries to the neck and upper extremities of dancers. Clin. Sports Med. 2, 459–472.

Norman, G.F., 1968. Sacroiliac disease and its relationship to lower abdominal pain. Am. J. Surg. 116, 54–56.

O'Brien, C.P., 1992a. Case history: footballer's ankle (anterior impingement of the ankle). J. Orthop. Med. 14, 91.

O'Brien, R.F., 1992b. Ron O'Brien's diving for gold. Leisure Press, Champaign, IL.

O'Neill, J.M.D., Jurriaans, E., 2007. CT and MRI of the sacroiliac joints.

In: Vleeming, A., Mooney, V., Stoeckart, R. (Eds.), Movement, stability & lumbopelvic pain: integration of research and therapy. second ed. Churchill Livingstone, Edinburgh, pp. 311–326.

O'Sullivan, P.B., 2000. Lumbar segmental 'instability': clinical presentation and specific stabilizing exercise management. Man. Ther. 5(1), 2–12.

O'Sullivan, P.B., 2005. Diagnosis and classification of chronic low back pain disorders: maladaptive movement and motor control impairment as underlying mechanisms. Man. Ther. 10(4), 242.

O'Sullivan, P.B., Beales, D., 2007. Diagnosis and classification of pelvic girdle pain disorders – Part 1: a mechanism based approach within a biopsychosocial framework. Man. Ther. 12, 86.

O'Sullivan, P.B., Beales, D., Beetham, J., et al., 2002. Altered motor control strategies in subjects with sacroiliac joint pain during the active straight-leg-raise test. Spine 27(1), E1–E8.

O'Sullivan, P.B., Burnett, A., Floyd, A.N., et al., 2003. Lumbar repositioning deficit in a specific low back pain population. Spine 28, 1074–1079.

Ogata, K., Naito, M., 1986. Blood flow of peripheral nerve: Effects of dissection, stretching and compression. J. Hand Surg. 11B, 10–14.

Ongley, M.J., Klein, R.G., Dorman, T.A., et al., 1987. A new approach to the treatment of chronic low back pain. Lancet 2, 143–146.

Ongley, M.J., Dorman, T.A., Eek, B.C., et al., 1988. Ligament instability of knees. A new approach to treatment. Man Med. 3, 152–154.

Östgaard, H.C., 1998. Assessment and treatment of low back pain in working pregnant women. In: Vleeming, A., Mooney, V., Tischler, H. et al. (Eds.), Third Interdisciplinary World Congress on low back and pelvic pain. European Conference Organizers, Rotterdam, pp. 161–171.

Östgaard, H.C., 2007. What is pelvic girdle pain? In: Vleeming, A., Mooney, V., Stoeckart, R. (Eds.), Movement, stability & lumbopelvic pain: integration of research and therapy. second ed. Churchill Livingstone, Edinburgh, pp. 353–360.

Östgaard, H.C., Anderson, G.B.J., 1992. Low back pain post partum. Spine 17(1), 53–55.

Östgaard, H.C., Zetherstroem, G., Roos-Hanson, E., 1996. Regression of back and posterior pelvic pain after pregnancy. Spine 21, 2777–2780.

Pace, J.B., Nagle, D., 1976. Piriformis syndrome. West. J. Med. 124, 435–439.

Paish, W., 1976. Track and field athletics. Lupus Books, London.

Panjabi, M.M., 1992a. The stabilizing system of the spine. I. Function, dysfunction, adaptation, and enhancement. J. Spinal Disord. 5(4), 383–389.

Panjabi, M.M., 1992b. The stabilization system of the spine. II. Neutral zone and instability hypothesis. J. Spinal Disord. 5(4), 390.

Panjabi, M.M., 2006. A hypothesis of chronic back pain: ligament subfailure injuries lead to muscle control dysfunction. Eur. Spine J. 15(5), 668–676.

Pansky, B., House, E.L., 1975. Review of gross anatomy. Macmillan, New York.

Papadopoulos, E.C., Khan, S.N., 2004. Piriformis syndrome and low back pain: a new classification and review of the literature. Orthop. Clin. North Am. 35, 65–71.

Paris, S.V., 1990. Foundations of clinical orthopaedics. Institute Press, St Augustine, FL.

Paris, S.V., Viti, J., 2007. Differential diagnosis of low back pain. In: Vleeming, A., Mooney, V., Stoeckart, R. (Eds.), Movement, stability & lumbopelvic pain: integration of research and therapy. second ed. Churchill Livingstone, Edinburgh, pp. 381–390.

Parker, P., 1988. Free heel skiing: the secrets of telemark and parallel techniques – in all conditions. Chelsea Green Publishing, Chelsea, VT.

Pearcy, M., Tibrewal, S.B., 1984. Axial rotation and lateral bending in the normal lumbar spine measured by three-dimensional radiography. Spine 9, 582.

Pearson, W.M., 1951. A progressive structural study of school children. J. Am. Osteopath. Assoc. 51, 155–167.

Pearson, W.M., 1954. Early and high incidence of mechanical faults. J. Osteopath. 61, 18–23.

Pećina, M., 1979. Contribution to the etiological explanation of the piriformis syndrome. Acta Anat. 105, 181–187.

Perry, J.D., 1997. How effective is EMG biofeedback in treating incontinence? www.incontinet.com/effective.htm.

Perry, J.D., Hullett, L.T., 1990. The role of home trainers in Kegel's home exercise program for treatment of incontinence. Ost. Wound Manage 30, 46–57.

Perry, J.D., Hullett, L.T., Bollinger, J.R., Biofeedback treatment of incontinence: California Biofeedback 1988. 79, 18–19.1.

Petersen, C., 2009. Fit 2 ski: A complete guide to fitness, second ed. BK Media c/o Fit to Play Int. Inc., Vancouver, Canada.

Petersen, C., Nittinger, N., 2006. Fit to play tennis: High performance playing tips, second ed. Racquet Tech Publishing, Vista, CA.

Pitkin, H.C., Pheasant, H.C., 1936. Sacrathrogenetic telalgia. A study of sacral mobility. J. Bone Joint Surg. 18A, 365–374.

Pitman, B., 1988. Fencing: techniques of foil, epée and saber. Crowood Press, Swindon.

Pohl, H., 2007. Changes in the structure of collagen distribution in the skin, caused by manual technique. Unpublished work from the First

Scientific Exploration of Fascia from an Interdisciplinary Perspective, Harvard University.

Pomeranz, B., 1975. Brain's opiates at work in acupuncture. New Sci. 73, 12–13.

Pomeranz, B.H., Chiu, D., 1976. Naloxone blocks acupuncture analgesia and causes hyperalgesia: Endorphin is implicated. Life Sci. 19, 1757–1762.

Pool-Goudzwaard, A., Hoek van Dijke, G., Mulder, P., et al., 2003. The iliolumbar ligament: its influence on stability of the sacroiliac joint. Clin. Biomech. (Bristol, Avon) 18(2), 99–105.

Pool-Goudzwaard, A., van Dijke, G.H., van Gurp, M., et al., 2004. Contribution of pelvic floor muscles to stiffness of the pelvic ring. Clin. Biomech. (Bristol, Avon) 19, 564–571.

Pool-Goudzwaard, A., Slieker ten Hove, M.C., Vierhout, M.E., et al., 2005. Relations between pregnancy-related low back pain, pelvic floor activity and pelvic floor dysfunction. Int. Urogynecol. J. Pelvic Floor Dysfunct. 16(6), 468–474.

Porterfield, J.A., DeRosa, C., 1998. Mechanical low back pain. Perspectives in functional anatomy. WB Saunders, Philadelphia, PA.

Porterfield, J.A., DeRosa, C., 2004. Mechanical low back pain. WB Saunders, Philadelphia, PA.

Porterfield, J.A., DeRosa, C., 2007. Conditions of weight bearing: asymmetrical overload syndrome (AOS). In: Vleeming, A., Mooney, V., Stoeckart, R. (Eds.), Movement, stability & lumbopelvic pain. Integration of research and therapy. second ed. Churchill Livingstone, Edinburgh, pp. 391–403.

Prechtl, J.C., Powley, T.L., 1990. B-afferents: a fundamental division of the nervous system mediating homeostasis? Behav. Brain Sci. 13, 289–331.

Proulx, W.R., 1990. Comparison of efficacy of prolotherapy versus steroid injection in the treatment of low back pain. Presented at the annual meeting of the American Association of Orthopedic Medicine, Denver, CO.

Queen, J.A., 1993. Karate basics. Sterling Publishing Co Inc, New York.

Radebold, A., Cholewicki, J., Panjabi, M.M., et al., 2000. Muscle response pattern to sudden trunk loading in healthy individuals and patients with chronic low back pain. Spine 25(8), 947.

Radebold, A., Cholewicki, J., Polzhofer, G.K., et al., 2001. Impaired postural control of the lumbar spine is associated with delayed muscle response times in patients with chronic idiopathic low back pain. Spine 26(7), 724–730.

Ravin, T., 2007. Visualization of pelvic biomechanical dysfunction. In: Vleeming, A., Mooney, V., Stoeckart, R. (Eds.), Movement, stability & lumbopelvic pain. Integration of research and therapy. second ed. Churchill Livingstone/ Elsevier, Edinburgh, pp. 327–339.

Reeves, K.D., 1994. Treatment of consecutive severe fibromyalgia patients with prolotherapy. J. Orthop. Med. 16, 84–85.

Reeves, K.D., Hassanein, K.M., 2000. Randomized, prospective, placebo-controlled double-blind study of dextrose prolotherapy for osteoarthritic thumb and finger (DIP, PIP and trapeziometacarpal) joints: evidence of clinical efficacy. J. Altern. Complement. Med. 6, 311–320.

Reeves, K.D., Hassanein, K.M., 2003. Long term effects of dextrose prolotherapy for anterior cruciate ligament laxity: A prospective and consecutive patient study. Altern. Ther. Health Med. (US) 9, 58–62.

Resnick, D., 2002. AS. In: Resnik, D. (Ed.), Diagnosis of bone and joint disorders. fourth ed. WB Saunders, Philadelphia, PA, pp. 1023–1081.

ResnicK, D., Niwayama, G, 1988. Plain film radiology: Sources of diagnostic error. In: Diagnosis of bone and joint disease, second ed. WB Saunders, Philadelphia, PA.

Resnick, D., Niwayama, G., Georgen, T. G., 1975. Degenerative disease of the sacroiliac joint. Invest. Radiol. 10(6), 608–621.

Rice, C.O., 1937. Injection treatment of hernia. FA Davis, Philadelphia, PA.

Rice, C.O., Mattson, H., 1936. Histologic changes in the tissues of man and animals following the injection of irritating solutions intended for the cure of hernia. Ill. Med. J. 70, 271–278.

Richard, R., 1986. Osteopathic lesions of the sacrum. Physio-pathology and corrective techniques. (D. Louch, Trans.). Thorsons Publishing, Wellingborough (original work published in 1978).

Richardson, A.R., 1986. The biomechanics of swimming: the shoulder and knee. Clin. Sports Med. 5, 103–113.

Richardson, C.A., Jull, J.A., Hodges, P.W., et al., 1999. Therapeutic exercise for stabilization in low back pain: scientific basis and clinical approach. Churchill Livingstone, Edinburgh.

Richardson, C.A., 2004. Impairment in muscles controlling pelvic orientation and weightbearing. In: Richardson, C.A., Hodges, P.W., Hides, J.A. (Eds.), Therapeutic exercise for lumbopelvic stabilization. Churchill Livingstone, Edinburgh, pp. 3–7.

Richardson, C.A., Jull, G.A., 1995. Muscle control – pain control. What exercises would you prescribe? Man. Ther. 1, 2–10.

Richardson, C.A., Snijders, C.J., Hides, J.A., et al., 2002. The relationship between the transversus abdominis muscles, sacroiliac joint mechanics and low back pain. Spine 27, 399–405.

Richardson, C.A., Hides, J.A., Hodges, P.W., 2004. Principles of the therapeutic 'segmental stabilization' exercise model. In: Richardson, C.A., Hodges, P.W., Hides, J.A. (Eds.), Therapeutic exercise for lumbopelvic stabilization. A motor control approach for treatment and prevention of low back pain. second ed. Churchill Livingstone, Edinburgh, pp. 175–183.

Robinson, D., 1947. Piriformis syndrome in relation to sciatic pain. Am. J. Surg. 73, 356–358.

Robinson, H.S., Brox, J.I., Robinson, R., et al., 2007. The reliability of motion- and pain provocation tests for the sacroiliac joint. Man. Ther. 12(1), 72.

Rydevik, B., Lundborg, G., Bagge, U., 1981. Effects of graded compression on intraneural blood flow: An in-vivo study on rabbit tibial nerve. J. Hand Surg. 6, 3–12.

Sahrmann, S.A., 2002. Diagnosis and treatment of movement impairment syndromes. Mosby, St. Louis, MI.

Sahrmann, S.A., 2010. Movement system impairment syndromes of the extremities, cervical and thoracic spines. Elsevier Mosby, St. Louis, MI.

Sammarco, G.J., 1983. The dancer's hip. Clin. Sports Med. 2, 485–498.

Samorodin, F.T., 2002. Treatment: manual therapy modes. In: Schamberger, W. (Ed.), The malalignment syndrome: implications for medicine and sport. first ed. Churchill Livingstone, Edinburgh, pp. 387–400.

Sanford, A.H., Granata, K.P., Orishimo, K.F., 1997. Co-contraction of core muscles detected on fine-wire electromyography. J. Electromyogr. Kinesiol .

Sapolsky, R.M., Spencer, E.M., 1997. Insulin growth factor 1 is suppressed in socially subordinate male baboons. Am. J. Physiol. 273(4 Pt 2), 1346.

Sapolsky, R.M., Alberts, R.C., Altmann, J., 1997. Hypercortisolism associated with social subordinance isolation among wild baboons. Arch. Gen. Psychiatry 54, 1137–1143.

Sapsford, R.R., Hodges, P.W., Richardson, C.A., et al., 1997. Activation of pubococcygeus during a variety of isometric abdominal exercises. Abstract. International Continence Society Conference Japan.

Sapsford, R.R., Hodges, P.W., Richardson, C.A., et al., 2001. Co-activation of the abdominal and pelvic floor muscles during voluntary exercises. Neurourol. Urodyn. 20, 31–42.

Sapsford, R.R., Richardson, C.A., Maher, C.F., et al., 2008. Pelvic floor muscle activity in different sitting postures in continent and incontinent women. Arch. Phys. Med. Rehabil. 89(9), 1741–1747.

Sashin, D., 1930. A critical analysis of the anatomy and the pathologic changes of the sacro-iliac joints. J. Bone Joint Surg. 12A, 891–910.

Saunders, S., Coppieters, M., Hodges, P.W., 2004. Reduced tonic activity of the deep trunk muscles during locomotion in people with low back pain. In: Proceedings of the World Congress of low back and pelvic pain, Melbourne, Australia.

Saunders, S.W., Schache, A., Rath, D., et al., 2005. Changes in three-dimensional lumbo-pelvic kinematics and trunk muscle activity with speed and mode of locomotion. Clin. Biomech. 20, 784–793.

Savage, J., 1996. Wresting basics – an introduction to the history and basic techniques of wrestling. Capstone Press, Mankato, MN.

Schamberger, W., 1983. Orthotics for athletes: attacking the biomechanical roots of injury. Can. Fam. Phys. 29, 1670–1680.

Schamberger, W., 1987. Nerve injuries around the foot and ankle. Med. Sport Sci. 23, 105–120.

Schamberger, W., 2002. The malalignment syndrome: implications for medicine and sport. Churchill Livingstone, Edinburgh, pp. 127–128.

Schamberger, W., 2003. The malalignment syndrome: treating a common cause of pelvic, back and leg pain. Vancouver, BC. DVD available at: www.backhealthworks.ca or www.plazaphysio.ca.

Schleifer, L.M., Ley, R., Spalding, T.W., 2002. A hyperventilation theory of job stress and musculoskeletal disorders. Am. J. Ind. Med. 41, 420–432.

Schleip, R., 2008. The nature of fascia: latest news from connective tissue research. DVD available at: www.info@fasciaresearch.com.

Schleip, R., Klingler, W., Lehmann-Horn, F., 2007. Fascia is able to contract in a smooth muscle-like manner and thereby influence musculoskeletal mechanics. In: Sixth Interdisciplinary World Congress on low back and pelvic pain. Barcelona, pp. 62–64.

Schunke, G.B., 1938. The anatomy and development of the sacroiliac joint in man. Anat. Rec. 72, 313.

Schwartz, B.C., Dazet, C.A., 1998. Competitive tennis. Human Kinetics, Champaign IL.

Schwarzer, A.C., Aprill, C.N., Bogduk, N., 1995. The sacroiliac joint in chronic low back pain. Spine 20, 31–37.

Selby, P., 1992. Dysfunction of the pelvic floor. Presentation to Northwest Association of Rehabilitation Medicine, San Diego, CA.

Shaw, J.L., 1992. The role of the sacroiliac joint as a cause of low back pain and dysfunction. In: Vleeming, A., Mooney, V., Snijders, C. et al. (Eds.), Low back pain and its relation to the sacroiliac joint. European Conference Organizers, Rotterdam, pp. 67–80.

Shibata, Y., Shirai, Y., Miyamoto, M., 2002. The aging process in the sacroiliac joint: helical computed tomography analysis. J. Orthop. Sci. 7(1), 12.

Simons, D.G., Travell, J.G., Simons, L.S., 1999. Travell and Simons' Myofascial pain and dysfunction: Trigger point manual, vol.1, second ed. Lippincott Williams & Wilkins, Baltimore, MD.

Sjolund, B., Terenius, L., Eriksson, M., 1977. Increased cerebrospinal fluid levels of endorphins after electro acupuncture. Acta Physiol. Scand. 100, 382–384.

Smidt, G.L., McQuade, K., Wei, S.H., et al., 1995. Sacroiliac kinematics for reciprocal straddle positions. Spine 20(9), 1047–1054.

Smith, M.D., Russell, A., Hodges, P.W., 2006. Disorders of breathing and continence have a stronger association with back pain than obesity and physical activity. Aust. J. Physio. 52, 11–15.

Smith, M.D., Coppieters, M.W., Hodges, P.W., 2007. Postural response of the pelvic floor and abdominal muscles in women with and without incontinence. Neurourol. Urodyn. 26(3), 377.

Snijders, C.J., Vleeming, A., Stoeckart, R., 1993a. Transfer of lumbosacral load to iliac bones and legs. I. Biomechanics of self-bracing of the sacroiliac joints and its significance for treatment and exercise.. Clin. Biomech. (Bristol, Avon) 8(6), 285–295.

Snijders, C.J., Vleeming, A., Stoeckart, R., 1993b. Transfer of lumbosacral load to iliac bones and legs. II. The loading of the sacroiliac joints when lifting in a stooped posture. Clin Biomech (Bristol, Avon) 8(6), 295–301.

Snijders, C.J., Vleeming, A., Stoeckart, R., et al., 1995a. Biomechanics of sacroiliac joint stability: validation experiments on the concept of self-locking. In: Vleeming, A., Mooney, V., Snijders, C. et al. (Eds.), The integrated function of the lumbar spine and the sacroiliac joint. European Conference Organizers, Rotterdam, pp. 75–91.

Snijders, C.J., Vleeming, A., Stoeckert, R., et al., 1995b. Biomechanical modelling of sacroiliac stability in different postures. Spine: State of the Art Reviews. Hanley & Belfus, Philadelphia, PA, p. 23.

Solonen, K.A., 1957. The sacroiliac joint in the light of anatomical, roentgenological and clinical studies. Acta Orthop. Scand. Suppl. 26, 1–127.

Standring, S., 2008. Gray's anatomy, fortieth ed. The anatomical basis of clinical practice. Churchill Livingstone/Elsevier.

Stashak, T.S. (Ed.), 2002. Adam's lameness in horses. fifth ed. Lippincott Williams & Wilkins, Philadelphia, PA.

Steege, J.F., Metzger, D.A., Levy, B.S. (Eds.), 1998. Chronic pelvic pain: an integrated approach. WB Saunders, Philadelphia.

Sterling, M., Jull, G.A., Wright, A., 2001. Cervical mobilization: concurrent effects on pain, sympathetic nervous system activity and motor activity. Man. Ther. 6, 72–81.

Stevens, A., 1992. Side-bending and axial rotation of the sacrum inside the pelvic girdle. In: Vleeming, A., Mooney, V., Snijders, C. et al. (Eds.), Low back pain and its relation to the sacroiliac joint. First Interdisciplinary World Congress on Low Back Pain and its Relation to the Sacroiliac Joint. San Diego. European Conference Organizers, Rotterdam, pp. 209–230.

Stevens, A., Vyncke, G., 1986. Sacrum rotation in the horizontal plane on lateral bending. In: Eighth Congress of the International Federation for Manual Medicine, Madrid.

Stewart, J.D., 2003. The piriformis syndrome is overdiagnosed. Muscle Nerve 28, 644–646.

Still, A.T., 1902. The philosophy and mechanical principles of osteopathy. Hudson-Kimberly, Kansas MO.

Stinson, J.T., 1993. Spondylolysis and spondylolisthesis in the athlete. Clin. Sports Med. 12, 517–528.

Stokes, M., Hides, J., Elliott, J., et al., 2007. Rehabilitative ultrasound imaging of the posterior paraspinal muscles. J. Orthop. Sports Phys. Ther. 37, 581–595.

Strachan, W.F., 1939. Applied anatomy of the pelvis and perineum. J. Am. Osteopath. Assoc. 38, 359–360.

Strasser, H., Kells, S., 1998. A lifetime of soundness: the keys to optimal horse health, lameness rehabilitation, and the high-performance barefoot horse, third ed. (Revised). Self-published, Sabine Kells, PO Box 44, Qualicum Beach, BC, Canada V9K 1S7.

Sturesson, B., Selvik, G., Uden, A., 1989. Movements of the sacroiliac joints. A roentgen stereophotogrammetric analysis. Spine 14(2), 162–165.

Sturesson, B., Uden, A., Onsten, I., 1999. Can an external frame fixation reduce the movements in the sacroiliac joint? A radiostereometric analysis of 10 patients. Acta Orthop. Scand. 70, 42–46.

Sturesson, B., Uden, A., Vleeming, A., 2000a. A radiostereometric analysis of the movements of the sacroiliac joints in the reciprocal straddle position. Spine 25(2), 214–217.

Sturesson, B., Uden, A., Vleeming, A., 2000b. A radiostereometric analysis of movements of the sacroiliac joints during the standing hip flexion test. Spine 25(3), 364–368.

Sunderland, S., 1978a. Traumatized nerves, roots and ganglia: musculo-skeletal factors and neuropathological consequences. In: Korr, I.M. (Ed.), The neurobiologic mechanisms in manipulative therapy. Plenum Press, London, p. 137.

Sunderland, S., 1978b. Nerves and nerve injuries, third ed. Churchill Livingstone, Melbourne.

Sweeting, R.C., Fowler, C., Crocker, B., 1989a. Anterior knee pain and spinal dysfunction in adolescents. J. Man Med. 4, 65–68.

Sweeting, R., et al., 1989b. Unpublished; personal communications: Dynamometer detection of unilateral weakness in those with malalignment and seemingly strong muscles on manual testing. Obvious asymmetric weakness with malalignment; response to realignment.

Swift, S., 1985. Centered riding. St Martin's Press, New York.

Taylor, H., Murphy, B., 2006. Altered sensorimotor integration with cervical spine manipulation. J. Manipulative Physiol. Ther. 31, 115–126.

Thabe, H., 1986. Electromyography as tool to document diagnostic findings and therapeutic results associated with somatic dysfunctions in the upper cervical spinal joints and sacroiliac joints. Man. Med. 2, 53–58.

Thiele, G.H., 1936. Tonic spasm of the levator ani, coccygeus and piriformis muscle. Trans. Am. Proctol. Soc. 37, 145–155.

Thiele, G.H., 1937. Coccydynia and pain of the superior gluteal muscle. JAMA 109, 1271–1275.

Thiele, G.H., 1963. Coccygdynia: cause and treatment. Diseases of the colon and rectum 6(6), 422–436.

Thompson, J.A., O'Sullivan, P.B., Briffa, N.K., et al., 2006. Altered muscle activation patterns in symptomatic women during pelvic floor muscle contraction and Valsalva manoeuvre. Neurourol. Urodyn. 25, 268–276.

Travell, J.G., Simons, D.G., 1983. Myofascial pain and dysfunction. The trigger point manual. Williams & Wilkins, Baltimore.

Travell, J.G., Simons, D.G., 1992. Myofascial pain and dysfunction: the trigger point manual. The lower extremities, vol. 1. Williams & Wilkins, Baltimore, MD.

Tsai, L., Wredmark, T., 1993. Spinal posture, sagittal mobility, and subjective rating of back problems in former female elite gymnasts. Spine 18, 872–875.

Tsao, H., Galea, M.P., Hodges, P.W., 2008. Reorganization of the motor cortex is associated with postural control deficits in recurrent low back pain. Brain 131(8), 2161–2171.

Upledger, J.E., 1987. Craniosacral therapy II: beyond the dura. Eastland Press, Seattle, WA.

Upledger, J.E., Larni, Z., 1990. Somato-emotional release and beyond. U1 Publishing, Palm Beach Gardens, FL.

Upledger, J., Vredevoogd, J.D., 1983. Craniosacral therapy. Eastland Press, Chicago, IL.

Urquhart, D.M., Hodges, P.W., 2005. Postural activity of the abdominal muscle varies between body regions and between body positions. Gait Posture 22, 295–301.

Valojerdy, M.R., Salsabili, N., Hogg, D. A., 1989. Age changes in the human sacroiliac joint: joint fusion. Clin. Anat. 2, 253–261.

van der Wurff, P., Buijs, E.J., Groen, G.J., 2006. A multitest regimen of pain provocative tests as an aid to reduce unnecessary minimally invasive sacroiliac joint procedures. Arch. Phys. Med. Rehabil. 87, 10–14.

van Dieën, J.H., 2007. Low back pain and motor behaviour: contingent adaptations, a common goal. In: Proceedings from the Sixth Interdisciplinary World Congress on Low Back and Pelvic Pain. Barcelona, November, 7–10 p. 3.

van Dieën, J.H., de Looze, M.P., 1999. Directionality of anticipatory activation of trunk muscles in a lifting task depends on load knowledge. Exp. Brain Res. 128(3), 397–404.

van Dieën, J.H., Cholewicki, J., Radebold, A., 2003. Trunk muscle recruitment patterns in patients with low back pain enhance the stability of the lumbar spine. Spine 28(8), 834–841.

van Ingen Schenau, G.J., 1982. The influence of air friction in speed skating. J. Biomech. 15, 449–458.

van Ingen Schenau, G.J., De Boer, R.W., De Groot, G., 1989. Biomechanics of speed skating. In: Vaughan, C.L. (Ed.), Biomechanics of sport. CRC Press, Boca Raton, FL, pp. 121–167.

van Wingerden, J.P., Vleeming, A., Snijders, C.J., et al., 1993. A functional anatomical approach to the spine–pelvis mechanism interaction between the biceps femoris muscle and the sacrotuberous ligament. Eur. Spine J. 2, 140–144.

van Wingerden, J.P., Vleeming, A., Buyruk, H.M., et al., 2001. Muscular contribution to force closure; sacroiliac joint closure in vivo. In: Proceedings from the Fourth Interdisciplinary World Congress on Low Back and Pelvic Pain. Montreal, Canada, pp. 153–159.

van Wingerden, J.P., Vleeming, A., Buyruk, H.M., et al., 2004. Stabilization of the sacroiliac joint in vivo: verification of muscular contribution to force closure of the pelvis. Eur. Spine J. 13(3), 199.

Vlaeyen, J.W.S., Linton, S.J., 2000. Fear-avoidance and its consequences in chronic musculoskeletal pain: a state of the art. Pain 85, 317–332.

Vlaeyen, J.W.S., Vancleef, L.M.G., 2007. Behavioral analysis, fear of movement/(re)injury, and cognitive- behavioral management of chronic low back pain. In: Vleeming, A., Mooney, V., Stoeckart, R. (Eds.), Movement, stability & lumbopelvic pain. Integration of research and therapy. second ed. Churchill Livingstone, Edinburgh, pp. 475–485.

Vleeming, A., Mooney, V., Stoeckart, R. (Eds.), 2007. Movement, stability & lumbo-pelvic pain: Integration of research and therapy, second ed. Churchill Livingstone, Edinburgh.

Vleeming, A., Stoeckart, R., 2007. The role of the pelvic girdle in coupling the spine and the legs: a clinical-anatomical perspective on pelvic stability. In: Vleeming, A., Mooney, V., Stoeckart, R. (Eds.),

Movement, stability & lumbopelvic pain: integration of research and therapy. second ed. Churchill Livingstone, Edinburgh, pp. 113–137.

Vleeming, A., Stoeckart, R., Snijders, D. J., 1989a. The sacrotuberous ligament: a conceptual approach to its dynamic role in stabilizing the sacro-iliac joint. Clin. Biomech. 4, 201–203.

Vleeming, A., Van Wingerden, J.P., Snijders, C.J., et al., 1989b. Load application to the sacrotuberous ligament; influences on sacro-iliac joint mechanics. Clin. Biomech. 4, 204–209.

Vleeming, A., Stoeckart, R., Volkers, A. C.W., et al., 1990a. Relation between form and function in the sacroiliac joint. 1. Clinical anatomical aspects. Spine 15(2), 130–132.

Vleeming, A., Volkers, A.C.W., Snijders, C.J., et al., 1990b. Relation between form and function in the sacroiliac joint. II. Biomechanical aspects. Spine 15(2), 133–136.

Vleeming, A., Van Wingerden, J.P., Dijkstra, P.F., et al., 1992a. Mobility in the sacroiliac joints in the elderly: a kinematic and radiological study. Clin. Biomech. 7, 170–176.

Vleeming, A., Stoeckart, R., Snijders, C. J., 1992b. A short history of sacroiliac research. Developmental biology of the sacroiliac joint. Regional anatomy of the sacroiliac joint. Investigating sacroiliac mobility. In: Vleeming, A., Mooney, V., Snijders, C. et al. (Eds.), Course proceedings of the First Interdisciplinary World Congress on low back pain and its relation to the sacroiliac joint, San Diego, 5–6 November. European Conference Organizers, Rotterdam, pp. 1–64.

Vleeming, A., Snijders, C.J., Stoeckart, R., et al., 1995a. A new light on low back pain. In: Proceedings from the Second Interdisciplinary World Congress on low back pain, San Diego, CA.

Vleeming, A., Pool-Goudzwaard, A.I., Stoeckart, R., et al., 1995b. The posterior layer of the thoracolumbar fascia; its function in load transfer from spine to legs. Spine 20(7), 753–758.

Vleeming, A., Pool-Goudzwaard, A.L., Hammudoghlu, D., et al., 1996. The function of the long dorsal sacroiliac ligament: its implication for understanding low back pain. Spine 21(5), 556.

Vleeming, A., Snijders, C.J., Stoeckart, R., et al., 1997. The role of the sacroiliac joint in coupling between spine, pelvis, legs and arms. In: Vleeming, A., Mooney, V., Dorman, T. et al. (Eds.), Movement, stability & low back pain. The essential role of the pelvis. Churchill Livingstone, Edinburgh, pp. 53–71.

Vleeming, A., de Vries, H., Mens, J.M., et al., 2002. Possible role of the long dorsal sacroiliac ligament in women with peripartum pelvic pain. Acta Obstet. Gynecol. Scand. 81, 430.

Wagner-Chazalon, A., 2000. Back in the saddle. Chiropractor and vet find link between horses, riders and backs. Canadian Horseman, Mar/Apr. 18–21.

Walheim, G.G., 1984. Stabilization of the pelvis with the Hoffman frame. Acta Orthop. Scand. 55, 319–324.

Walheim, G.G., Selvic, G., 1984. Mobility of the pubic symphysis. Clin. Orthop. Relat. Res. 191, 129–135.

Walker, J.M., 1986. Age-related differences in the human sacroiliac joint. a histological study; implications for therapy. J. Orthop. Sports Phys. Ther. 7, 325.

Walker, J.M., 1992. The sacroiliac joint: a critical review. Phys. Ther. 72, 903–916.

Wallace, K.A., 1994. Pelvic floor muscle dysfunction and its behavioral treatment. In: Agostini, R. (Ed.), Medical and orthopedic issues of active and athletic women. Hanley & Belfus, Philadelphia, PA, pp. 200–212.

Wanless, M., 1995. Ride with your mind: a right brain approach to riding. Hamlyn, London.

Watanabe, K., 1989. Ski-jumping, alpine-, cross-country- and Nordic-combination skiing. In: Vaughan, C.L. (Ed.), Biomechanics of sport. CRC Press, Boca Raton, FL, pp. 239–261.

Weinberg, S.K., 1986. Medical aspects of synchronized swimming. Clin. Sports Med. 5, 159–167.

Weishaupt, D., Zanetti, M., Hadler, J., et al., 1998. MRI imaging of the lumbar spine: prevalence of intervertebral disk extrusion and sequestration, nerve root compression, end plate abnormalities, and osteoarthritis of the facet joints in asymptomatic volunteers. Radiology 209, 661–666.

Weisl, H., 1955. Movements of the sacro-iliac joint. Acta Anat. 23, 80–91.

Wells, J., 2009. Pelvic floor dysfunction: diagnosis and treatment. Personal communications.

Wells, P.E., 1986. Movement of the pelvic joints. In: Grieve, G.P. (Ed.), Modern manual therapy of the vertebral column. Churchill Livingstone, Edinburgh, pp. 176–181.

West, J., 1989. Water skiing: skills of the game. Crowood Press Ltd, Marlborough.

Whatmore, G.B., Kohli, D.R., 1974. The physiopathology and treatment of functional disorders. Grune & Stratton, New York.

White, A.A., Panjabi, M.M., 1978. The basic kinematics of the human spine. Spine 3, 12.

Whittaker, J.L., 2004. Abdominal ultrasound imaging of pelvic floor muscle function in individuals with low back pain. J. Man Manip. Ther. 12, 44.

Whittaker, J.L., 2007. Ultrasound imaging for rehabilitation of the lumbo-pelvic region – a clinical approach. Churchill Livingstone/Elsevier, Edinburgh.

Whittaker, J.L., 2010. Assessment of pelvic floor muscle function in women with and without low back pain using transabdominal ultrasound. J. Man Manip. Ther. 15, 235–239.

Willard, F.H., 1995. The lumbosacral connection: the ligamentous structure of the low back and its relation to pain. In: Vleeming, A., Mooney, V., Dorman, T. et al. (Eds.), The integrated function of the lumbar spine and sacroiliac joint. European Conference Organizers, Rotterdam, pp. 29–58.

Willard, F.H., 1997. The muscular, ligamentous and neural structure of the low back and its relation to back pain. In: Vleeming, A., Mooney, V., Dorman, T. et al. (Eds.), Movement, stability & low back pain. The essential role of the pelvis. Churchill Livingstone, Edinburgh, pp. 3–35.

Willard, F.H., 2007. The muscular, ligamentous and neural structure of the lumbosacrum and its relationship to low back pain. In: Vleeming, A., Mooney, V., Stoeckart, R. (Eds.), Movement, stability & lumbopelvic pain. Integration of research and therapy. second ed. Churchill Livingstone, Edinburgh, pp. 5–45.

Williams, P.L., Warwick, R. (Eds.), 1980. Gray's anatomy. thirtysixth ed. The joints of the lower limb: the sacro-iliac joint Churchill Livingstone, Edinburgh, pp. 473–477.

Woo, C.C., 1997. World class female windsurfing championships: a pilot study of physical characteristics and injuries. Sports Chiropract. Rehab. 11, 11–17.

Worth, D.R., 1986. Movements of the cervical spine. In: Grieve, G.P. (Ed.), Modern manual therapy of the vertebral column. Churchill Livingstone, Edinburgh, pp. 77–85.

Worth, S. (Ed.), 1990. The rules of the game. St. Martin's Press, New York.

Wyke, B.D., 1985. Articular neurology and manipulative therapy. In: Glasgow, E.F., Twomey, L.T., Scull, E.R. et al. (Eds.), Aspects of manipulative therapy. second ed. Churchill Livingstone, New York, pp. 72–77.

Yamashita, T., Cavanaugh, J.M., El-Bohy, A.A., et al., 1990. Mechanosensitive afferent units in the lumbar facet joint. J. Bone Joint Surg. (Am.) 72(A), 865–870.

Yeomans, W., 1928. The relation of arthritis of the sacro-iliac joint to sciatica. Lancet 2, 1119–1122.

Index

Note: Page number followed by *b* indicate boxes and *f* indicate figures.

A

B

C

D

E

F

G

J

M

N

O

P

Q

R

S

T

U

V

W

X

Y

Z